Comprehensive MEDICINE
for Dental Students

Comprehensive MEDICINE for Dental Students

Archith Boloor MBBS MD (Internal Medicine)
Additional Professor
Department of Medicine
Kasturba Medical College, Mangalore
Manipal Academy of Higher Education
Karnatake, India
archithb@gmail.com

Mohammed Shaheen MBBS
Kasturba Medical College, Mangalore
Manipal Academy of Higher Education
Karnatake, India

Forewords
V Surendra Shetty
Dilip G Naik

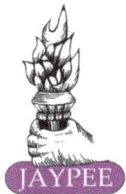

JAYPEE BROTHERS MEDICAL PUBLISHERS
The Health Sciences Publisher
New Delhi | London

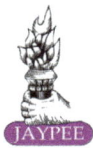 **Jaypee Brothers Medical Publishers (P) Ltd**

Headquarters
EMCA House
23/23-B, Ansari Road, Daryaganj
New Delhi 110 002, India
Landline: +91-11-23272143, +91-11-23272703
+91-11-23282021, +91-11-23245672
E-mail: jaypee@jaypeebrothers.com

Corporate Office
Jaypee Brothers Medical Publishers (P) Ltd.
4838/24, Ansari Road, Daryaganj
New Delhi 110 002, India
Phone: +91-11-43574357
Fax: +91-11-43574314
E-mail: jaypee@jaypeebrothers.com

Overseas Office
JP Medical Ltd.
83, Victoria Street, London
SW1H 0HW (UK)
Phone: +44-20 3170 8910
Fax: +44(0)20 3008 6180
E-mail: info@jpmedpub.com

Website: www.jaypeebrothers.com
Website: www.jaypeedigital.com

© 2022, Jaypee Brothers Medical Publishers

The views and opinions expressed in this book are solely those of the original contributor(s)/author(s) and do not necessarily represent those of editor(s) of the book.

All rights reserved. No part of this publication may be reproduced, stored or transmitted in any form or by any means, electronic, mechanical, photocopying, recording or otherwise, without the prior permission in writing of the publishers.

All brand names and product names used in this book are trade names, service marks, trademarks or registered trademarks of their respective owners. The publisher is not associated with any product or vendor mentioned in this book.

Medical knowledge and practice change constantly. This book is designed to provide accurate, authoritative information about the subject matter in question. However, readers are advised to check the most current information available on procedures included and check information from the manufacturer of each product to be administered, to verify the recommended dose, formula, method and duration of administration, adverse effects and contraindications. It is the responsibility of the practitioner to take all appropriate safety precautions. Neither the publisher nor the author(s)/editor(s) assume any liability for any injury and/or damage to persons or property arising from or related to use of material in this book.

This book is sold on the understanding that the publisher is not engaged in providing professional medical services. If such advice or services are required, the services of a competent medical professional should be sought.

Every effort has been made where necessary to contact holders of copyright to obtain permission to reproduce copyright material. If any have been inadvertently overlooked, the publisher will be pleased to make the necessary arrangements at the first opportunity.

Inquiries for bulk sales may be solicited at: jaypee@jaypeebrothers.com

Comprehensive Medicine for Dental Students

First Edition: **2022**

ISBN 978-93-5465-491-6

Dedication

To all the students of dentistry;
who work to put a smile on people's face.
You are appreciated and loved.
May your kind grow.

Foreword

The current academic scenario in our country is witnessing the mushrooming of textbooks. This is a sign of enterprise and effort on the part of our teachers. Having over 300 dental colleges in our country admitting 25,000 students every year, there is a need for a quality textbook of general medicine for dental students.

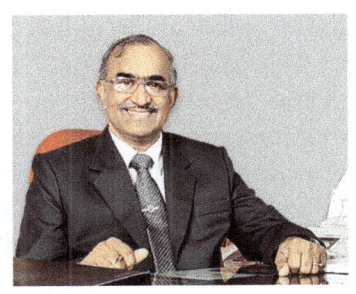

One needs to separate the wheat from the chaff and direct one's interest towards textbooks with quality content such as this one authored by Dr Archith Boloor. It is a matter of great pride to me personally, since the author of the book is a faculty member and gifted teacher at Kasturba Medical College, Mangaluru, Karnataka, India of which Manipal College of Dental Sciences is a sister institute.

A brief overview of the book reveals the amount of effort put by the authors. This book comprehensively covers the latest Dental Council of India (DCI) prescribed syllabus. The authors have innovated and added aspects of clinical medicine, medical emergencies and highlighting the relevance of certain topics to dentists.

This book will be useful not just for BDS students but also to general dental practitioners as a ready reference. I would like to congratulate the authors for their brilliant effort in bringing out this book and wish them all the success in their future endeavors.

V Surendra Shetty
Former Pro-Vice-Chancellor
Manipal Academy of Higher Education
Karnataka, India
surendra.shetty@manipal.edu

Foreword

It is my pleasure to write a foreword for the textbook on general medicine written by Dr Archith Boloor. The dental graduates need a thorough understanding of the systemic signs and symptoms of various ailments accompanying oral manifestations. An in-depth knowledge of the etiopathogenesis, clinical examination methods, investigations, and differential diagnosis must be known for dental graduates. Dr Boloor is a good teacher who has won "Good Teacher Award" from Kasturba Medical College, Mangalore, Karnataka, India, who has the knack of making challenging concepts clear in simple words. He has authored many textbooks for MBBS students, and this is his first venture for dental graduates.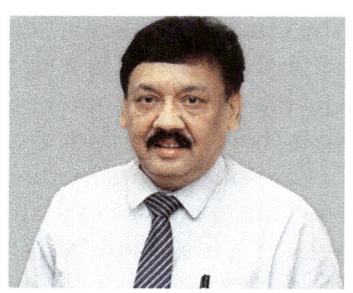

The textbook has incorporated procedures involved in general medicine, including history taking, clinical procedures of various systemic ailments related to dentistry, including medical emergencies, and crisis management in the era of pandemics.

I wish all the best to both the authors for compiling a concise textbook of general medicine for dental graduates and dentists.

Dilip G Naik
Pro-Vice-Chancellor – Mangalore Campus
Manipal Academy of Higher Education
Karnataka, India
dilip.naik@manipal.edu

Preface

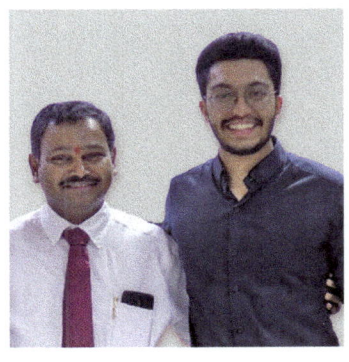

As healthcare workers learning, graduating and working through our latest occupational hazard, our job has become rather demanding. You wake up. You have to power through all of your patients for the day—some glad to see you, some not so much, some who would not even see you tomorrow. Donning, doffing through the PPEs (Punishing Perspiratory Equipment, do not let anyone tell you otherwise). You come back home, tired from explaining to the concerned Ola driver that the vaccine does not make you infertile, or worse, impotent. You watch the news. A couple of calls from your relatives later, each conversation undulating between a spectrum of "No, I have not found a cure for corona yet" and "Yes, please wear your mask for your son's wedding, you have invited hundreds of people" – You finally go to bed. With no foreseeable end in sight, the pandemic is seeming to be more of an unfortunate living condition at this point. One does not complain about the malaria in Mangaluru anymore, or the state of the petrol prices: just little factoids that we have reluctantly chosen to live with. Every day, we think about ways in which we can make this "new normal" easier. Less monotonous. More rewarding.

When we set out to write this book, there were several challenges in front of us: how deep do we dive into medicine? How relevant will this book be to a dentist? Why are we doing this during a pandemic? To answer each of these separately; after carefully coursing through the nationally approved syllabus for dentistry students, getting in touch with several students around the country, the book is an attempt to patch up all the gaps that we thought existed. A lot of the material in this book fits into the "Must Know" category, but we have taken good care to include the juicy "Nice-to-Know" bits as well. This book has all the necessary contents to become a book-shelf staple for any dentist, tailored for the new curriculum.

Why are we doing this during a pandemic? Because never before in the history of modern medicine have we faced such an acute shortage of healthcare workers. The lines that once divided interdisciplinary care have become the tally marks counting the number of patients who do not have access to any doctor. Now, more than ever—health needs to be united under its original purpose.

So, when we thought about ways in which we can make this "new normal" more rewarding. We came up with a short-term solution and a long-term investment. The short-term solution is this book, which we hope you will accept whole heartedly. Though we know that this book will not magically fill the gaping cavities smiling back at us; we do hope that it will help set in motion many of the changes that we need to see.

Our long-term investment is you. You, the reader of this book, who will wake up tomorrow, power through all your patients in your PPE, answer a truckload of questions from a lot of well-informed and equally ill-informed people, and you will go to bed knowing fully well that a clone of the previous day awaits you when you wake up.

But through it all, you will remember to smile. A gentle touch, a kind ear, a tiny nod, and most importantly, a smile. Things which you can do, that undeniably have the power to change a person's day.

The original purpose of health is not to treat illness. It is to provide healing.

Archith Boloor
Mohammed Shaheen

Acknowledgments

It is both an equally fun and daunting task to write a book. This was a very new experience for us, and the people who helped us at every step of the way have our eternal gratitude.

We thank Dr Anudeep Padakanti, Dr Nikhil Kenny Thomas, Dr Vivek K Koushik, Dr Abu Thajudeen, Dr Madhav Hande, Dr Aditya Ramanathan, Dr Aditya Narayan, Dr Nandan Padmanabha and Dr Srinath Rajashekar, for their presence in our lives: a source of constant inspiration, encouragement and joy.

We thank our family and our friends, both in and out of the medical fraternity, who have played their irreplaceable role in bringing us to where we are today.

We thank all the healthcare workers who have worked through this pandemic. Your sacrifice and your perseverance is the kind of magic that the world needs to see today.

We convey our sincere thanks to Shri Jitendar P Vij (Group Chairman) of M/s Jaypee Brothers Medical Publishers (P) Ltd, New Delhi, India, for having been the guiding force behind all our works.

We also thank Dr Sneha Kashyap (Development Editor) and Ms Sunita Katla (Executive Assistant to Group Chairman and Publishing Manager) of M/s Jaypee Brothers Medical Publishers (P) Ltd, New Delhi, India, for their help in the formatting and their well-received technical assistance and unwavering support during the process of developing this project.

We thank Dr V Surendra Shetty and Dr Dilip G Naik, our teachers, and guides for having written the forewords for the book.

Lastly, we thank the student community who have loved, accepted and used all our previous works. We welcome any and every feedback, and we assure you that we will strive to improve our book and keep it up to date for the further editions.

Archith Boloor
Mohammed Shaheen

Contents

1. History Taking — 1
- Importance of History Taking 1
- Detailed Assessments versus Problem-Focused Assessments 1
- Writing a Case Sheet 1
- Etiquette During History Taking 2
- Components of History Taking 2
- Examination of the Patient 4
- Protecting Yourself: Hygiene for the Healthcare Worker 4
- Patient–Doctor Privilege 4
- Model Case Sheet–I 6
- Outcome-based Education 8

2. Vital Signs and General Physical Examination — 9

Vitals Examination 9
- Pulse 9
- Respiration 16
- Blood Pressure 17
- Jugular Venous System 19
- Body Temperature 23
- Pain: The Fifth Vital Sign 27
- Pallor 28
- Icterus 29
- Cyanosis 31
- Clubbing 32
- Edema 35
- Lymphadenopathy 36
- Anthropometry 43

3. Gastrointestinal Tract Examination — 49
- Case Sheet Format 49
- Diagnosis Format 51
- Discussion on Cardinal Symptoms 51
- Discssion on Examination 59

4. Respiratory System Examination — 82
- Case Sheet Format 82
- Diagnosis Format 85
- Discussion on Cardinal Symptoms 86
- Discussion on Examination 93

5. Cardiovascular System Examination — 114
- Case Sheet Format 114
- Diagnosis Format 116
- Discussion of Symptoms 117
- Discussion on Examination 122

6. Gastroenterology   144

- Symptomatology 144
- Dyspepsia 147
- Gastrointestinal Bleeding 148
- Diarrhea 151
- Diseases of the Esophagus 154
- Gastroesophageal Reflux Disease 155
- Barrett's Esophagus 158
- Hiatus Hernia 158
- Achalasia of the Esophagus 158
- Diseases of the Stomach and Duodenum 159
- Peptic Ulcer Disease 159
- Diseases of the Intestine 164
- Inflammatory Bowel Disease 166

7. Hepatobiliary Disorders   170

- Functions of Liver 170
- Liver Function Tests 170
- Jaundice 174
- Chronic Parenchymal Liver Disease 181
- Chronic Hepatitis B 182
- Chronic Hepatitis C 184
- Fulminant Hepatitis Failure 185
- Reye's Syndrome 186
- Fatty Liver/Steatosis 187
- Alcoholic Liver Disease 187
- Nonalcoholic Fatty Liver Disease, Nonalcoholic Steatosis, Nonalcoholic Steatohepatitis 187
- Cirrhosis 188
- Portal Hypertension 190
- Variceal Bleeding 191
- Hepatic (Portosystemic) Encephalopathy 193
- Hepatorenal Syndrome 195
- Ascites 196
- Spontaneous Bacterial Peritonitis 199
- Drug and Liver 200
- Budd–Chiari Syndrome 200
- Hepatocellular Carcinoma 201
- Pyogenic Liver Abscess (Bacterial Liver Abscess) 202
- Amebic Liver Abscess 202
- Hereditary Hemochromatosis 202
- Wilson's Disease 203

8. Respiratory System   206

- Bronchial Asthma 206
- Chronic Obstructive Pulmonary Disease 215
- Pulmonary Tuberculosis 224
- Suppurative Lung Disease 236
- Atelectasis 239
- Lung Abscess 240
- Pleural Effusion 242
- Empyema Thoracis 245

- Pneumothorax 246
- Pneumonia 249
- Occupational Lung Diseases 257
- Respiratory Failure 257
- Acute Lung Injury and the Acute Respiratory Distress Syndrome 258
- Bronchopulmonary Aspergillosis 260
- Pulmonary Eosinophilic Syndromes 261

9. Cardiology 266

- Ischemic Heart Disease 266
- Acute Coronary Syndrome 271
- Hypertension 280
- Acute Rheumatic Fever 288
- Valvular Heart Disease 293
- Infective Endocarditis 302
- Heart Failure 309
- Pulmonary Edema 313
- Cardiac Arrhythmias 315
- Cardiomyopathy 318
- Congenital Heart Diseases 320
- Cardiac Arrest 321
- Syncope 324
- Investigations 324
- Cor Pulmonale 324
- Circulatory Failure: Shock 325
- Deep Venous Thrombosis 328
- Pulmonary Embolism 329
- Hyperlipidemia 329

10. Renal System 333

- Functions of Kidney 333
- Terminologies 333
- Glomerulonephritis 335
- Post-streptococcal (Postinfectious) Glomerulonephritis 336
- Nephrotic Syndrome 337
- Acute Kidney Injury (Acute Renal Failure) 340
- Chronic Kidney Disease 344
- Urinary Tract Infections 349

11. Neurology 354

- Symptomatology 354
- Dysarthrias 355
- Headache 355
- Migraine 356
- Cluster Headache 359
- Tension-type Headache 360
- Stroke and Cerebrovascular Disease 360
- Subarachnoid Hemorrhage 363
- Seizures and Epilepsy 364
- Status Epilepticus 368
- Meningitis 369
- Neurosyphilis 372

- Encephalitis 373
- Diseases of Cranial Nerves 373
- Bell's Palsy 374
- Intracranial Pressure 376
- Coma 376
- Brain Death 378

12. Hematology 380

- Disorders of Red Blood Cell 380
- Anemia 380
- Platelet Disorders 401
- Clotting Disorders 403
- Thrombosis 405
- Leukemia 409
- Myeloproliferative Diseases 417
- Plasma Cell Dyscrasias 421
- Lymphoma 422
- Blood Transfusion 428
- Stem-Cell Therapy 430
- Bone Marrow Transplantation 430

13. Nutrition 432

- Nutritional Assessment 432
- Vitamin A 434
- Vitamin B Complex 436
- Vitamin C 440
- Scurvy 440
- Vitamin D 441
- Vitamin E (Tocopherol) 445
- Vitamin K 445
- Calcium Homeostasis 446
- Hyperparathyroidism 446
- Hypercalcemia 449
- Hypoparathyroidism 450
- Tetany 451
- Trace Elements 452
- Protein-Energy Malnutrition 452
- Obesity 454

14. Endocrinology 460

- Disorders of Pituitary and Hypothalamus 460
- Acromegaly 462
- Prolactinoma 464
- Diabetes Insipidus 465
- Thyroid Disorders 467
- Thyrotoxicosis 468
- Hypothyroidism 474
- Thyroiditis 477
- Adrenal Gland Disorders 479
- Cushing's Syndrome 479
- Addison's Disease 483
- Acute Adrenal Crisis 485

- Steroid Therapy 486
- Pheochromocytoma 486
- Diabetes Mellitus 489
- Chronic Complications of Diabetes 505
- Metabolic Syndrome 508

15. Infectious Diseases 511

- Measles 511
- Rubella 513
- Mumps 513
- Infectious Mononucleosis 514
- Herpesviruses Infecting Humans 515
- Chickenpox (Varicella) 515
- Shingles 517
- Arboviral Diseases 518
- Dengue Fever 518
- COVID-19 520
- Diphtheria 523
- Plague 523
- Botulism 524
- Pertussis (Whooping Cough) 524
- Typhoid (Enteric Fever) 524
- Food Poisoning 526
- Dysentery 527
- Amebiasis 528
- Cholera 530
- Leptospirosis 530
- Rickettsial Diseases 531
- Candidiasis (Moniliasis) 532
- Mucormycosis 532
- Malaria 533
- Kala-azar or Visceral Leishmaniasis 536
- Sepsis 537
- HIV/AIDS 538
- Sexually Transmitted Infections 544
- Syphilis 545
- Pyrexia of Unknown Origin 548

16. Emergencies in Medicine 551

- List of Common Emergencies in Medical Practice 551

Hypersensitivity Reactions 551
- Urticaria ("Hives") 551
- Angioedema 552
- Systemic Anaphylaxis 553

17. Viva Voce: Instruments, Procedures, and X-rays 557

Instruments and Procedures 557
- Gastric Lavage Tube 557
- Laryngoscope 558
- Metal Tracheostomy Tube 558
- Endotracheal Tube 558

- Ambu Bag 559
- Ryles Tube—Nasogastric Tube 559
- Suction Catheter 560
- Foley Catheter 560
- Sahli's Hemoglobinometer 561
- Neubauer Chamber/Hemocytometer 561
- Insulin Syringe 561
- Tuberculin Syringe 561
- Vim Silverman Liver Biopsy Needle 562
- Trucut Biopsy Gun 562
- Bone Marrow Aspiration Needle (Klima Needle) 562
- Bone Marrow Biopsy Needle (Jamshidi Needle) 562
- Lumbar Puncture Needle 563
- Intravenous Drip Set 563
- Intravenous Cannula 564
- Oxygen Mask 564
- Inhaler Devices 564
- Urinometer 566
- Westergren Tube 566
- Discussion of Common X-rays 567

18. Normal Laboratory Values   571

- Laboratory Values of Clinical Importance 571
- Commonly Used Formulas in Medicine 575

Index   577

CHAPTER 1

History Taking

CHAPTER OUTLINE

- Importance of History Taking
- Detailed Assessments versus Problem-Focused Assessments
- Writing a Case Sheet
- Etiquette During History Taking
- Components of History Taking
- Examination of the Patient
- Protecting Yourself: Hygiene for the Healthcare Worker
- Patient–Doctor Privilege
- Model Case Sheet–I
- Outcome-based Education

IMPORTANCE OF HISTORY TAKING

A good history and detailed examination forms the foundation of medical practice. Whether you are a physician, a dentist, an emergency medical technician, or a first responder, an extensive, precise, and accurate initial assessment sets the pace for further care, evaluation, and testing. From a clinical standpoint, the decision making of the patient's treatment depends solely on the information gathered during your history and examination. These are also the skills that a medical professional carries with themselves, their till the end of their practice. As one garners more experience, you will become faster, more concise, and will be able to derive more information out of less questions.

With more and more emphasis being placed on the integration of health care across specialties, the basics of medical knowledge have become irreplaceable. Each of your patients is going to be a different and unique individual—spanning various ages, gender identities, sexualities, socioeconomic backgrounds, and ethnicities. The essentials of health care—empathy, listening, clinical reasoning, and deduction—are skills that will help you to understand the psyche and the mindset of every patient. History taking and examination is thus, the vital first step in developing a meaningful therapeutic relationship with your patient.

DETAILED ASSESSMENTS VERSUS PROBLEM-FOCUSED ASSESSMENTS (TABLE 1.1)

While encountering a patient for the first time, one should make the decision of doing a detailed assessment or a problem-focused assessment. It is also always prudent to make adjustments into your history as you go along; if a patient presents with a fresh wound, you may start with a problem-based approach. But as you take history, you may find out that the patient is diabetic, in which case you may need to go into further detail.

Table 1.1: Detailed and problem-focused assessments.

Detailed	Problem-focused
Essential for forming the initial framework of a patient's symptoms	Essential for returning patients, emergent patients, or follow-up cases
Provides a baseline for future reference	Saves time in dire situations for quick intervention
Holistic approach to the patient as an individual	Assessment of only a particular system with respect to the chief symptom

As students of medicine, it is encouraged to do a detailed history. This helps you to develop pace and flow, two very important qualities when interviewing a patient. However, the ground reality is very different. As you become interns and residents, you may have to allocate time and resources to your patient based on the urgency of their problem. This equity of health care is what we refer to as triaging—the patient that needs attention the most gets it first. In such situations, a short, focused history is preferred.

WRITING A CASE SHEET

In the era of evidence-based medicine, documentation has become a skill that doctors need to master. A good, crisp case sheet can make the difference in pattern of care; especially in larger hospitals where a patient is treated upon by a team of healthcare professionals. Even in smaller clinics, it is impractical to expect a doctor or a nurse to remember every detail about every patient. Hence, good documentation paves the way for good clinical outcomes.

Unfortunately for the students, like most things in medicine, a universally accepted format for case sheets does not exist. Keep in mind that it is more important to include everything than to nitpick about the order of the information presented. Students are always encouraged to find a format that is comfortable to them and stick to that while taking history, so that they do not miss out on any vital information. The final case sheet can then be tailored to the hospital, clinic, or institutions requirement.

Around the world, different countries practice different ways of case sheet writing. However, the one thing that is always common is the S-O-A-P approach.

The subjective: The first part of the case sheet always consists of the subjective history provided by the patient. This includes all the information that is given by the patient verbally. More often than not, this cannot be verified by the clinician. A patient might tell you that he feels a rat gnawing away in his stomach. This is his subjective way of expressing his discomfort to you. As a clinician, you have no way of confirming this. The subjective part includes the chief complaints, history of presenting illness, past, personal, and family histories.

The objective: The objective part of the case sheet includes all the information that is elicited by the doctor, which he can verify. This usually includes the examination findings and their interpretations. A patient may tell you that his legs have been feeling weak since a month, this is subjective. However, once you test the power in his lower limbs and verify that he cannot move his leg against resistance, it is an objective finding. The objective part usually includes the general physical examination and the systemic examination.

The assessment: The assessment is the part of the case sheet, which consists of the summarization of the subjective and the objective findings. A concise summary with all the positive findings, a preliminary diagnosis and any recent investigations or reports may be included in the assessment portion.

The plan: The plan is the part of the case sheet, which outlines the diagnostic and therapeutic interventions that the patient must receive under your care. This includes all the investigations, interventions, procedures, and the drug charting that needs to be done. If the patient is admitted in your facility, then it is of utmost importance to include a daily follow-up note. The follow-up note consists of the patient's general condition, relevant examination findings, and any changes to his/her initial plan that may be recommended as per the patient's prognosis.

Note: Though it is rare that doctors will encounter this terminology in India, in several countries, the case sheet itself is known as the SOAP note. As members of a quickly growing global health network, this was added here in an attempt to sensitize the Indian healthcare community toward this format. It is also good to notice that it is not very different from what we follow in India.

ETIQUETTE DURING HISTORY TAKING

More often than not, medical professionals are accused of taking their position of respect for granted. This is definitely not an appreciable quality. As doctors, we must hold ourselves to an extremely high standard especially when we deal with patients and their families. It is imperative that we follow all the general rules of social etiquette—dress well, talk empathetically, and use respectful language. It is always recommended to introduce yourself to the patient before the interview, state the purpose of the interview, and approximately how long it will take. This is also a good time to ask if the patient has any pressing concern, which needs immediate attention. Reassure the patient that all the information provided during this interview is completely confidential.

COMPONENTS OF HISTORY TAKING

- **Initial information:** The initial information during history taking entails the date and time of evaluation. In situations where several clinicians are handling multiple cases, it may also be prudent to add the name of the evaluating physician. This is exceptionally important in situations of emergency where the physician performing the initial assessment needs to be readily available for assistance.
- **Personal details:** This includes all the details that help us in identifying the patient. A good rule of thumb to follow is name, age, gender identity, occupation, and marital status. In a multicultural society such as India, the patient's native village or town is also a good point of identification. If the patient is referred from a different center, that can also be entered here.
- **Source of history and reliability:** The source of history or reliability is usually a must-have in pediatric cases. Though not always necessary, it is a good practice to mention this in adult history taking as well. This is exceptionally useful when the patient himself is poorly oriented or unable to give clear history. It reflects the accuracy of the information in the case sheet.
- **Chief complaints:** The chief complaint is the immediate and emergent complaint, which brings the patient to you. Try to use the patient's own words when writing the chief complaint. Arranging the chief complaints chronologically can also help to streamline your thought process while interpreting your case sheet at a later time.

Note: A point to keep in mind is that more often than not, it is the history-taker's duty to arrange and make sense out of the information. Do not be afraid to ask leading questions to clarify the time and intensity of each symptom. For example, a patient may present with a fluid-filled abdomen, as his chief complaint since 1 month. It may strike as odd to you that the patient noticed his abdomen enlarging for an entire month and decided to come to the hospital on this particular day. However, upon further probing, it will be clear that the patient's family brought him to the hospital because he was somnolent since 2 days.

- **History of presenting illnesses:** This column provides the descriptive aspect of the chief complaints. It is a comprehensive, clear, and chronological account of the patient's problems. This includes all the details that come with the famous mnemonic OLD-CHART:
  - *Onset:* Sudden, insidious, immediate, or emergent.
  - *Location:* Site of the symptom.

- *Duration:* How long has the symptom been bothering the patient?
- *Character:* Any descriptive words that the patient may use to help narrow down the cause of his symptom. A common example is seen in pain, where patients can describe it as stabbing, crushing, burning, dull-aching, etc.
- *Aggravating factors:* Are there any actions that increase the symptom?
- *Relieving factors:* Are there any actions that reduce the symptom?
- *Temporal pattern:* Does the intensity of the symptom change throughout the day? This can also be extrapolated to seasonal variations also.

As illnesses affect different parts of the body, and many illnesses may be multisystem, it is important to ask about connected symptoms. You need to cover the following areas:

- **Respiratory system:** Dyspnea, wheeze, cough, sputum, hemoptysis, and chest pain
- **Cardiovascular system:** Chest pain, orthopnea, paroxysmal nocturnal dyspnea, ankle swelling, palpitations, and intermittent claudication
- **Gastrointestinal system:** Abdominal pain, nausea, vomiting, hematemesis, bowel habit, bleeding per rectum, and melaena
- **Urogenital system:** Frequency, nocturia, polydypsia, loin pain, and hematuria
- Menarche, menopause, cycle, intermenstrual bleeding, and postcoital bleeding
- **Central nervous system:** Headaches, visual disturbances, sleep, hearing, tinnitus, light headedness, blackouts, fits, unsteady gait, weakness, and paresthesias
- **Musculoskeletal:** Myalgia, arthralgia, back pain, and joint swelling
- **Psychiatric:** The mental state examination will be taught more formally in your psychiatric attachment. Remember, depression is common and may often coexist with physical ill health.

The best way to round out a good history of presenting illness note is to include relevant positive history and relevant negative history. There are several commonly encountered cases which are diagnoses of exclusions. Noting down these points of exclusion (often called negative history) can help you to arrive at a provisional diagnosis easily.

- **Past (medical or surgical) history:** Broadly, the past medical or surgical history can be divided into three categories—childhood illnesses, adult illnesses, and screening tests. Childhood illnesses are usually not mentioned in the past history, unless there is a significant residual morbidity or chronicity of the condition.

In order to give a complete picture of the patient's health status, adult past history can be divided into medical, surgical, obstetric/gynecological, and psychiatric. In each of these categories, always focus on the past illnesses, which might give a clue to the patient's current ailment. A great rule of thumb to follow is disease-duration-drug, i.e., name of the ailment, followed by duration, and then the therapeutic intervention that was used.

In elderly patients, screening tests are done to rule out certain predictable age-dependent conditions. The results of these screening tests can be mentioned in the past history. This saves both time and resources for the treating clinician as these tests need not be repeated again.

- **Personal history:** In personal history, we comment on the person's temperament. An additional note on the patient's appetite, sleep, bowel, and bladder habits is encouraged, especially if there is any variation from his normal patterns. If the patient is sexually active, the clinician should elicit history about his sexual practices and evaluate whether the patient engages in high-risk sexual behavior.

Lastly, it is always prudent to ask the patient about his addictions and allergies. Tobacco usage, drug addictions, and alcohol consumption are all commonly encountered addictions, which can alter or change the course of both the patient's condition and your treatment. When eliciting such history, it is always important to be open-minded and to make the patient feels safe enough to share that information with you.

> **Note:** A common situation that can be encountered is family members and patient bystanders asking prying questions about the patient's addictions, sexuality, or gender identity. Similarly, an employer or manager may contact you in order to gain information about the patient's condition. Handling these situations tactfully is of paramount importance. Trust is the foundation of a good doctor–patient relationship. It is, therefore, extremely necessary to keep the information furnished in the personal history between the treating doctor and his patient. Learning to intersperse questions about personal details within regular history taking is very helpful to establish the rapport with the patient.

- **Family history:** Under family history, outline the present or past health conditions of any immediate family members. These include but are not limited to hypertension, cardiovascular disease, diabetes, cancer, autoimmune conditions, and untimely deaths. If the patient has a known genetically transmitted disease, a pedigree chart may also be added.
- **Review of systems:** Review of systems is an additional column that can be added when a clinician is evaluating a patient for a routine health checkup. It is very similar to the "head-to-toe" examination part except that questions are asked pertaining to the patient's general health status. Go from the head to the toe of the patient, asking questions that may be significant to his quality of life such as "How is your vision?" and "How is your hearing?" and "Do you have any skin rashes?"

Do keep in mind that when a patient presents with a chief complaint, the history and your line of questions will be streamlined to include all the details that contribute to his current ailment. As such, a review of systems is not necessary in those situations since all those points would have been covered previously.

EXAMINATION OF THE PATIENT

Setting up the Examination

Before you examine the patient, take your time and prepare yourself for the sequence in which you wish to go about. Approach the patient with calmness and be as professional as one can be. Introduce yourself as a student, ask if he/she has any urgent discomfort, which needs attending and then request the patient to let you examine them.

Once the patient has agreed to the examination, it is both your responsibility and in your best interest to make the patient as comfortable as possible. It is very common for patients to feel vulnerable and uneasy during examination. This may be in anticipation of pain or the uncertainty of what the doctor may find. But an uncomfortable patient begets an uncomfortable doctor. Adjust the height of the bed, the lighting, and your stance based on the patient's requirement. Take extra steps to protect the patient's modesty. The extra work done in preparation tells a patient that you are genuinely concerned about his/her health and the patient will show his/her appreciation in the form of cooperation.

"A doctor is one of the only jobs where you can ask someone to take off his/her clothes and he/she will do it without question". This trust is a unique aspect of the doctor–patient relationship which is your responsibility to safeguard. Close the doors, place blinds or partitions, and ask the patient, if he/she wants anyone in the room to leave and comply with his/her requests. Wash and warm your hands before you touch the patient.

During the Examination

A seasoned clinician completes the physical examination in a quick, thorough, and gentle manner. He notices the body language and the mannerisms of the patient, empathizes with his condition, and provides reassurance in the best way possible. It is very normal to forget a particular part of the examination during the process. Go back to the patient and request his permission to do the parts that you missed out.

During examination, it might take time for you, as a student, to appreciate certain findings. No clinician expects a 2nd or 3rd year student to properly diagnose a heart murmur. As such, if you find yourself spending some extra time trying to learn the nature of a finding, it is always a good practice to inform the patient that you are doing so because of your desire to learn and not because there is something wrong with them.

Another common happening in the wards is the patient or his/her bystanders asking you to interpret your findings to them. In the eyes of the patient, you are another doctor and he/she can use your knowledge as a "secondary opinion". As an inexperienced doctor, who is not the patient's primary clinician, you may find yourself in a situation trying to give information that you yourself are unsure of. Be respectful and mindful of the patient bystanders concerns, but also be gracious enough to accept what you know and do not know. As a student, it is more fruitful to share findings with your peers and your professors. Discuss the diagnosis and plan with them so that you can be an active part of the treating team.

After the Examination

Write down your findings in a streamlined and systemic manner. Go through your pre-examination list and fill in any gaps in your case sheet. It is also a good practice to thank the patient for his cooperation and to offer them some positive reassurance.

PROTECTING YOURSELF: HYGIENE FOR THE HEALTHCARE WORKER

> **CDC Recommendations for Hand Hygiene**
> - **Key situations where hand hygiene should be performed include:**
>   - Before touching a patient, even if gloves are worn
>   - Before exiting the patient's care area after touching the patient or the patient's immediate environment
>   - After contact with blood, body fluids, or excretions, or wound dressings
>   - Prior to performing an aseptic task (e.g., placing an intravenous drip, preparing an injection)
>   - If hands are moving from a contaminated-body site to a clean-body site during patient care
>   - After glove removal
> - Use soap and water when hands are visibly soiled (e.g., blood and body fluids), or after caring for patients with known or suspected infectious diarrhea (e.g., *Clostridium difficile* and *norovirus*). Otherwise, the preferred method of hand decontamination is with an alcohol-based hand rub.

In a hospital, your chances of being cured of a disease and your chances of contracting a disease are both extremely high. Healthcare workers are constantly at the risk of life-threatening illnesses because of the close proximity with which they work with sick patients. Even after countless years of research, effort, and studies, hospital infections are an occupational hazard that we may never be able to completely eliminate due to the nature of our jobs. Hence, it is always important for a doctor to adopt certain practices to put his/her health and safety first.

Universal precautions are a set of guidelines by the CDC that have been recommended in an effort to reduce the risk of parenteral, mucous membrane, and non-contact exposure of healthcare workers to harmful blood-borne pathogens. The following body fluids are considered potentially harmful—blood, blood products, semen, vaginal secretions, synovial fluid, pleural fluid, peritoneal fluid, pericardial fluid, and amniotic fluid. All healthcare workers must be cautious to prevent injury through needlestick and exposure to these hazards. Further, with the rise of severe acute respiratory syndrome coronavirus 2 (SARS-Cov-2) or the coronavirus, it is now more important than ever to maintain a strict level of hand and hospital hygiene.

PATIENT–DOCTOR PRIVILEGE

As a doctor, it is a very natural and expected part of your profession to ask extremely embarrassing, secretive, and personal information. Your clinical reasoning relies entirely upon your ability to convince a patient that he/she can trust you with the most intimate parts of his/her lives; information, which he/she has perhaps not shared with anyone else. It is very important for you, as a doctor, to be receptive to such information and to accept it with an open mind. These may include sensitive information pertaining to his/her daily habits, drug addictions, sexual activity, sexuality, gender identity, criminal activity, or prior illnesses. The conversation between a doctor and a patient is not the place for prejudice or judgment, especially if it is against your cultural and religious beliefs. If you feel like you cannot get past your inhibition when dealing with a patient, be respectful and ask a peer or colleague to take over.

Furthermore, if a patient provides you with such information, it is your duty to keep that information a secret. This is exceptionally important when a patient bystander, distant relative, or employer asks you for details pertaining to the patient's condition. In the western countries, it is illegal for you to provide confidential details even to the next of kin without the patient's consent. However, in the Indian scenarios, due to the close-knit nature of families and communities, privacy is often taken for granted. As a doctor, it is your responsibility to uphold the patient's dignity.

Always ask for the patient's consent before sharing sensitive information to his/her family, friends, or employers. When the patients are teenagers or under-aged, ask the patient, if he/she needs some time to speak alone away from his/her parents. It is always a good practice to ask the patient bystanders to leave during the examination process. This is the ideal time to elicit sensitive history from the patient.

MODEL CASE SHEET-I

Outpatient department, 8:32 AM, 26th July 2021

—Dr XYZ

ABC, a 45-year-old businessperson identifying as male, hailing from Someshwar presented to the outpatient department (OPD) with chief complaints of:
- Abdominal distension since 6 months
- Abdominal discomfort and heaviness since 6 months
- Scanty micturition since 2 months
- Weakness, loss of appetite, and malaise since 1.5 months

History of Presenting Illness

The patient states that he was in reasonably good health until 6 months ago when he developed abdominal distension. It was insidious in onset and gradually progressive over the last few months. It is not associated with abdominal pain; however, it is associated with discomfort and heaviness.

The patient has also been experiencing reduce micturition since 2 months. This has also been associated with loss of appetite and malaise. The patient has noticed that he passes dark-colored stools, especially after 1–2 days of constipation.

There are no aggravating or relieving factors. The patients cannot appreciate any temporal or seasonal variations in his symptoms.

The patient does not give any history of fever, shortness of breath, cough, facial puffiness, joint pain, skin rash, hematemesis, or loss of consciousness.

Past History

- **Medical:** The patient was hospitalized 3 years ago for jaundice. The symptoms lasted for around 4–5 months and gradually subsided. Hospital records are unavailable. Patient does not give any history of blood transfusion.
- **Surgical:** No significant history
- **Pediatric:** No significant history

Personal History

The patient is calm and oriented. His appetite has reduced since 1.5 months. Bowel and bladder habits have become infrequent. The patient claims that he has been feeling sleepy during the day since the last 2 days. Patient is sexually active with his wife. They use condoms inconsistently. The patient claims that his libido has reduced since 2 months.

The patient smokes about 10 cigarettes a day for the last 20 years (10 pack years). He drinks alcohol amounting to 180–240 mL of whiskey per week. He is allergic to peanuts. He does not give any history of drug allergies.

Family History

The patient's father passed away 6 years ago. He was in good health. The patient's mother is alive and in good health. His wife and his two children do not have any similar complaints and are in good health.

General Physical Examination

The patient is well oriented to time, place, and person. He is in a good mood and not irritable. He is seated upright on the examination table. He appears ill and emaciated.
- **Vitals:** Pulse—88 bpm; blood pressure (BP)—110/76 mm Hg, temperature—99°F; and respiratory rate—18 breaths/min
- **Pallor:** Present
- **Icterus:** Present
- **Cyanosis:** Absent
- **Clubbing:** Absent
- **Lymphadenopathy:** Absent
- **Edema:** Present

Head to Toe Examination
- Eyes are icteric. Hollowed temporal fossa can be appreciated. Patient is pale.
- Multiple spider nevi can be seen on the upper torso and back.
- Generalized ecchymotic spots can also be seen
- Gynecomastia is seen.
- There are leukonychia and palmar erythema.
- Lower limbs show pitting pedal edema.

Systemic Examination

Gastrointestinal System

Lips, gums, teeth, and buccal cavity: Cheilitis and stomatitis are present. Gingiva appears normal. Gums do not bleed. There is no fetor hepaticus.

Per abdominal examination:

Inspection:
- Abdomen is distended and flanks are full.
- Umbilicus is everted.
- Visible superficial veins with flow away from the umbilicus.
- No visible peristalsis or scar marks.

Palpation:
- No tenderness
- Liver is not palpable.
- Spleen is palpable—4 cm from the left costal margin in the anterior axillary line toward the right iliac fossa. The surface is smooth, consistency is firm, and the spleen is nontender.
- **Testes:** Both testes are atrophied.
- Fluid thrill is present.

Percussion: Shifting dullness is appreciated.

Auscultation: There is no significant finding on auscultation.

Brief Examination of Other Systems

- **Central nervous system:** Patient is right handed. Constructional apraxia is present. No flapping tremors. Normal deep tendon reflexes
- **Respiratory system:** Normal vesicular breath sounds on all lung fields.
- **Cardiovascular system:** S1 and S2 heard clearly on all cardiac areas. No added sounds or murmurs

Summary

A 45-year-old male presented with abdominal distention, discomfort, and heaviness since 6 months and scanty micturition and loss of appetite since 1.5 months. He has a prior history of hospitalization due to jaundice, consumes 6 units of alcohol per week, and has 10 pack-year smoking history.

On examination, the abdomen is distended with fluid. Fluid thrill and shifting dullness are appreciated. Several signs of liver cell failure can be seen. Constructional apraxia is also present.

Provisional Diagnosis

Chronic liver disease is probably due to alcoholic etiology with ascites, portal hypertension, and early hepatic encephalopathy.

Investigations

- Complete blood count
- Prothrombin time/international normalized ratio (PT/INR)
- Fasting blood sugar (FBS)/postprandial blood sugar (PPBS)
- Serum electrolytes
- Liver function test (LFT)
- Renal function test (RFT)
- HIV
- Hepatitis B surface antigen (HBsAg)
- Chest X-ray

Drug Charting

- Tablet furosemide 40 mg 1-1-0
- Tablet spironolactone 25 mg 1-1-0
- Tablet pantoprazole 40 mg 1-0-0
- Tablet propranolol 20 mg 0-0-1
- Injection thiamine 100 mg IV once daily
- Syrup lactulose 20 mL 1-0-1

Note: This is a model case sheet. It is not a one-size-fits-all template that you can use throughout every set up. Please keep in mind that ultimately, a case sheet is just a tool for effective patient care; to facilitate easy communication between healthcare professionals, nitpicking on individual details while disregarding the safety, privacy, and health of the patient must be avoided at all costs. As a new resident or intern, it is a good practice to ask the consultant doctors and staff nurses how they prefer the health documents to be written, charted, and maintained. Some seniors may be used to a different format, which enables them to take better decisions. If it is in the patient's best interest to adopt certain variations in case sheet writing, then it should be done without question.

OUTCOME-BASED EDUCATION

Deciding outcomes for academic achievements and its attainment for assessment and formulation is based on a learning theory called outcome-based education (OBE). OBE is an educational theory that bases each part of an educational system around goals (outcomes). By the end of the educational experience, each student should have achieved the goal.

Course outcomes (COs): POs are attained through program specific core courses, which has their own previously set outcomes to attain. These course-specific outcomes are called course outcomes. Outcomes are stated in such a way that they can be actually measured. COs are set by the institution, by consulting with the department heads, faculty, students and other stakeholders.

The central theme of OBE are the learning outcomes, and the curriculum is woven around to make the learner achieve the 'higher order thinking skills'. These skills enable the learner to perform under various settings and circumstances with precision. Such adaptive quality practice is what is needed for our healthcare providing environment.

The following are the course outcomes for general medicine:
- Demonstrate understanding of the pathophysiologic basis, epidemiological profile, signs and symptoms of disease and their investigation and management
- Competently interview and examine an adult patient and make a clinical diagnosis
- Appropriately order and interpret laboratory tests
- Initiate appropriate cost-effective treatment based on an understanding of the rational drug prescriptions, medical interventions required and preventive measures
- Follow up of patients with medical problems and refer whenever required
- Communicate effectively, educate and counsel the patient and family
- Manage common medical emergencies and refer when required
- Independently perform common medical procedures safely and understand patient safety issues.

In our book we have covered the medical topics under specific learning outcomes. The assessment questions at the end of each chapter also integrate the specific outcomes for assessment.

Vital Signs and General Physical Examination

CHAPTER 2

CHAPTER OUTLINE

- **Vitals Examination**
  - Pulse
  - Respiration
  - Blood Pressure
  - Jugular Venous System
- Body Temperature
- Pain: The Fifth Vital Sign
- **Physical Examination**
  - Pallor
  - Icterus
- Cyanosis
- Clubbing
- Edema
- Lymphadenopathy
- Anthropometry

VITALS EXAMINATION

PULSE

Definition

Pulse is pressure distension wave produced by contraction of left ventricle against a partially filled aorta, which is transmitted to peripheries and is felt on a peripheral artery against a bony prominence.

Assessment of arterial pulse	
Characteristics	**Best assessed by palpating**
Rate	Radial artery
Rhythm	
Volume	Carotid artery
Character or quality	Carotid artery Exceptions: • Collapsing pulse, which is appreciated better at radial artery • Pulsus bisferiens best appreciated in brachial artery
Radioradial and radiofemoral delay:	
Whether all peripheral vessels are felt	
Condition of vessel wall	
Example: 72 beats/min regular rhythm, normal volume and character, all peripheral pulses are well felt, no radioradial or radiofemoral delay, and no vessel wall thickening	

Method of Palpation of Radial Artery (Fig. 2.1)

Radial artery is felt using three fingers. The distal finger is to block the backflow, proximal finger is to stabilize artery on the bone, and middle finger is used to feel and count the pulse (3-finger method).

This method can be used for all the peripheral pulses, except carotid.

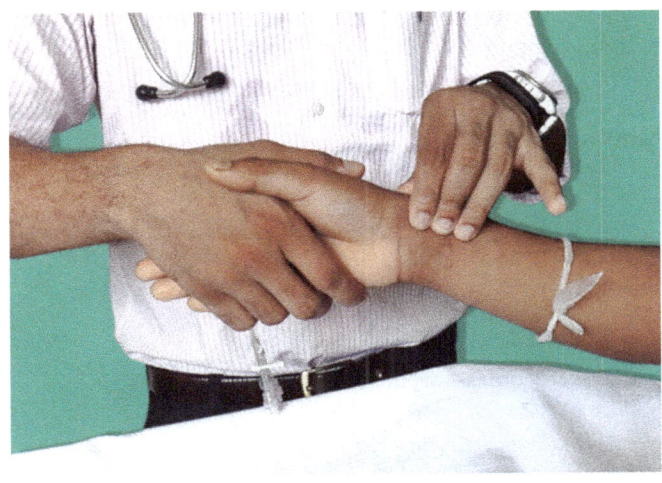

Fig. 2.1: Method of palpation of radial artery.

Pulse Rate

Calculate the rate by counting the radial pulse for one full minute.

Normal rate = 60–100	
<60 (Bradycardia)	**>100 (Tachycardia)**
Physiological: Athletes and sleep **Pathological:** • Severe hypoxia • Hypothyroidism/myxedema • Obstructive jaundice • Hypothermia • Sick sinus syndrome • Vasovagal syncope • Drugs—β-blockers, verapamil, and digoxin • Heart block • Raised intracranial tension (Cushing's phenomenon)	**Physiological:** Infants, children, emotion, exertion, and pregnancy **Pathological:** • Tachyarrhythmias • High-output states: Anemia, pyrexia, anxiety, beriberi, and thyrotoxicosis • Cardiac failure • Cardiogenic shock • Drugs (e.g., atropine, nifedipine, salbutamol, terbutaline, nicotine, and caffeine)

Relationship between pulse and temperature	
1°F temperature rise = Increase in pulse rate by 10 beats/min	
Relative tachycardia	Relative bradycardia

• Acute rheumatic carditis
• Diphtheric myocarditis
• Tuberculosis
	• Any viral fever (dengue, yellow fever: *Faget's sign*)
	• Enteric fever 1st week
	• Pyogenic meningitis/intracerebral abscess
	• *Brucellosis*
	• *Legionella*
	• Psittacosis
	• Typhus
	• Q fever
	• Leptospirosis
	• Noninfectious causes:
	  ▪ Patients on β-blockers
	  ▪ CNS lesions
	  ▪ Lymphomas
	  ▪ Factitious fever
	  ▪ Drug fever

Rhythm

Rhythm is assessed by palpating the radial pulse. The normal rhythm is **regular**.

Causes of irregular rhythm
Regularly irregular: • Atrial tachyarrhythmias, sinus arrhythmia, partial/2nd-degree AV blocks • Ventricular bigeminy and trigemini
Irregularly irregular: • Ventricular ectopics/VPCs • Atrial fibrillation • Atrial tachyarrhythmia with varying AV blocks
Regular with occasional irregularity: • Extra systoles

(AV: atrioventricular; VPC: ventricular premature complex)

Pulse Deficit (Apex–Pulse Deficit) (Fig. 2.2)

It is the difference between the heart rate (counted by auscultation) and pulse rate when counted simultaneously for one full minute.

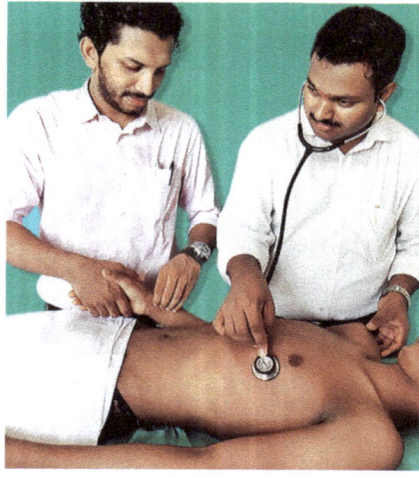

Fig. 2.2: Demonstration of apex pulse deficit.

Causes

Pulse deficit of >10 beats/min occurs in atrial fibrillation and <10 beats/min may be found with ventricular premature beats or slow/controlled atrial fibrillation (AF).

Differences Between Atrial Fibrillation and Ventricular Premature Complexes (VPCs)

	Atrial fibrillation	VPCs
Apex pulse deficit	Usually >10	Usually <10
JVP "a" wave	Absent	Normal
S1	Variable intensity	Normal
Effect of exercise/hand grip	Irregularity perisists	Pulse becomes regular

Volume of the Pulse

It is measure of pulse pressure (pulse pressure is difference between systolic and diastolic blood pressure).

Normal pulse pressure = 30–60	
<30 mm Hg (low volume): Hypokinetic pulse	**>60 mm Hg (high volume): Hyperkinetic pulse**
• Congestive cardiac failure • Hypovolemia • Shock • Mitral stenosis • Aortic stenosis (*pulsus parvus*) • Constrictive pericarditis	**Physiological:** Fever, pregnancy, alcoholism, and exercise **Pathological:** *High-output states*: Anemia, beriberi, cor pulmonale, cirrhosis liver (hypoproteinemia), thyrotoxicosis, AV fistula, and Paget's disease *Cardiac causes (pulsus magnus)*: Aortic regurgitation, bradycardia, complete heart block, PDA, systolic HTN, rupture of sinus Valsalva into heart chamber, aortopulmonary window

Varying volume: It is seen in atrial fibrillation.
Anisosphygmia: This is defined as varying volume of pulses in bilateral brachial/radial vessels. It is seen in Takayasu's arteritis.
Coanda effect: In supravalvular aortic stenosis, pulse volume is better in the right upper limb compared to left due to the selective jet of the blood directed to the right subclavian vessel.
Note: Pulsus alternans, pulsus bigeminus, and pulsus paradoxus are also abnormalities in volume. (described under the section of character of pulse)

(HTN: hypertension; PDA: patent ductus arteriosus)

Grading of Pulse

The examination of the arterial pulses is tabulated using a scale as follows:

Grade	Description
0	Complete absence of pulsation
1	Small or feeble/reduced pulsation
2	Palpable but diminished as compared to other side
3	Normal pulsation
4	Large or high volume/bounding pulsation

Chapter 2: Vital Signs and General Physical Examination

Character of Pulse
- Best assessed in the carotids
- **Exceptions:**
  - Collapsing pulse, which is appreciated better at radial artery
  - Pulsus bisferiens is best appreciated in brachial artery.

Trisection Method
Varying degrees of pressure is applied with the finger pads of the thumb or first two fingers to assess upstroke, systolic peak, and diastolic slope of the *pulse*.

Components of Pulse Wave (Figs. 2.3A and B)

Individual components of pulse waveform	
Wave	**Description**
Percussion wave	It is due to arrival of the impulse generated by LV ejection
Tidal wave	It is due to reflection of the upper part of the body
Dicrotic wave	It is due to reflection from the lower part of the body
Dicrotic notch or incisura	This corresponds to S_2

Speed of Pulse Wave and Time Taken to Reach the Peripheral Arteries

Speed of pulse wave	5 m/s
Speed of blood flow	0.5 m/s
Time taken for transmission of pulse to:	
Carotid	30 ms
Brachial	60 ms
Femoral	75 ms
Radial	80 ms

- Normally, radial pulse is felt 5–10 ms later that femoral pulse

Types of characters of pulse (Fig. 2.4):		
Catacrotic pulse	It is the normal character of the pulse	
Pulsus parvus et tardus	A low amplitude (parvus) with a slow rising and late peak (tardus)	Severe aortic stenosis (AS)
Pulsus anacroticus	Single peak low volume	Severe aortic stenosis (AS)
Water hammer pulse or collapsing pulse or Watson's pulse or pulsus celer	High (large) volume pulse, sharp rise (systolic pressure is high), ill-sustained, sharp fall (diastolic pressure is low), and pulse pressure is at least 60 mm Hg	Aortic regurgitation, patent ductus arteriosus (PDA), AP window, rupture of sinus Valsalva, arteriovenous fistula, and hyperdynamic circulation states
Twin beating pulse		
Pulsus bisferiens	Rapid rising, twice beating, and both waves felt in systole	Severe aortic regurgitation (AR), moderate AR +AS, hypertrophic obstructive cardiomyopathy (HOCM)
Pulsus dicroticus/ dicrotic pulse	Twice beating First wave in systole, second wave in diastole Seen when pulse rate and diastolic pressure are low	Typhoid fever, severe left ventricular failure (LVF), dehydration, dilated cardiomyopathy, and endotoxic shock
Alternating volume pulses		
Pulsus alternans	Alternating weaker and stronger volume pulses in regular rhythm, doubling rate of Korotkoff sound on lowering cuff pressures	Left ventricular failure
Pulsus bigeminus	Pulse wave with normal beat followed by a premature beat and a compensatory pause, occurring in rapid succession, resulting in alteration of the strength of pulse	Digoxin toxicity

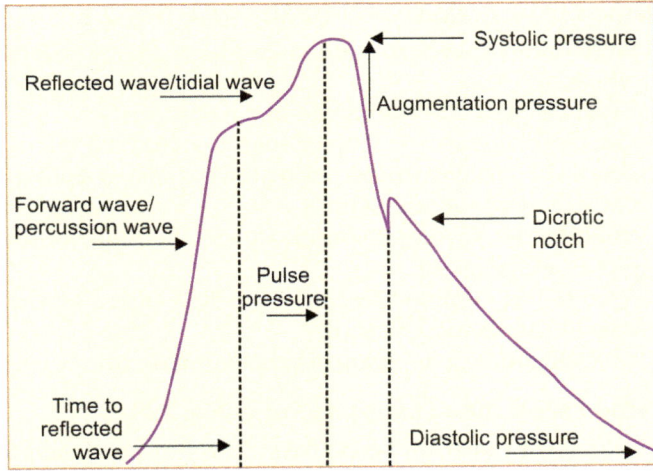

Fig. 2.3A: Image of jugular venous pressure (JVP) and different waveforms.

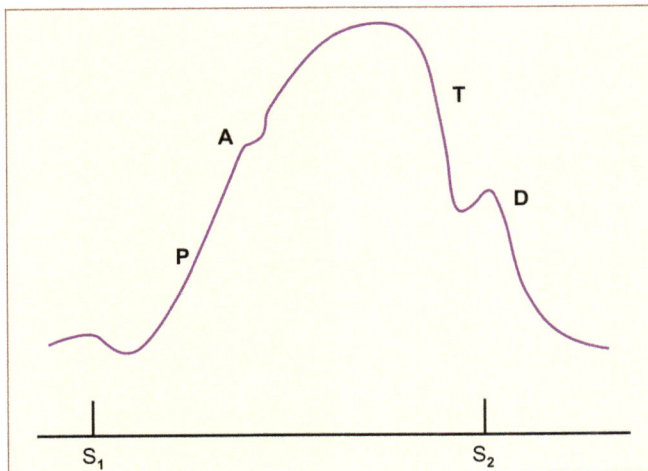

Fig. 2.3B: Waveform showing different components of pulse wave.

Contd...

Contd...

Pulsus paradoxus		
Pulsus paradoxus	Systolic blood pressure falls more than 10 mm Hg during inspiration (exaggeration of normal phenomenon)	Constrictive pericarditis, acute severe asthma/COPD, cardiac tamponade, tension pneumothorax, massive pulmonary embolism Others are anaphylactic shock and obesity

Reverse pulsus paradoxus (inspiratory rise in pulse volume and pressure): It is seen in positive pressure ventilation, HOCM (hypertrophic obstructive cardiomyopathy), and isorhythmic AV dissociation.

Absent pulsus paradoxus in constrictive pericarditis: If associated with large ASD/VSD/ AR/pericardial adhesions

(ASD: atrial septal defect; COPD: chronic obstructive pulmonary disease; VSD: ventricular septal defect)

Method of Eliciting Pulsus Paradoxus (Fig. 2.5)

- Pulsus paradoxus refers to an exaggerated fall in a patient's blood pressure during inspiration by greater than 10 mm Hg.
- Patient is placed in a semirecumbent position; respirations should be normal. *Do not instruct them to change their breathing pattern, as the depth of respiration influences the magnitude of pulsus paradoxus and will be amplified in patients with pulmonary disease.*
- The blood pressure cuff is inflated to at least 20 mm Hg above the systolic pressure and slowly deflated until the first Korotkoff sounds heard.
- Initially sounds will be heard only during expiration. Note the level.
- As the cuff is further deflated, the point at which the first Korotkoff sound is audible during both inspiration and expiration is recorded. Note the level.
- If difference between the two is more than 10 mm Hg, then it is pulsus paradoxus.
- This is not a true paradox, as it is an exaggeration of normal phenomenon of fall of BP during inspiration.

Then, What is the Paradox?

The paradox is that in patients with constrictive pericarditis, during inspiration, the blood pressure might drop significantly that the peripheral pulses will be absent; however, the heart sounds will still be heard.

Other paradoxus in medicine:
- **French paradox:** The observation that the French suffers a relatively low incidence of coronary heart disease, despite having a diet relatively rich in saturated fats
- "Thrombotic paradox" of hypertension (or "**Birmingham paradox**")
- **Venous paradox:** *Kussmaul sign* is a *paradoxical* rise in jugular *venous* pressure (JVP) on inspiration, or a failure in the appropriate fall of the JVP with inspiration
- **Ulnar paradox:** Higher the lesion minimal is the deficit
- **Paradoxical respiration:** It causes the chest to contract during inhaling and to expand during exhaling, the opposite of how it should move. The most common causes of paradoxical breathing include—chest trauma, including injuries from a fall, a sports injury, or a car accident. Neurological problems that can paralyze the diaphragm
- **Kinesia paradox:** It is seen in Parkinsonism and patients who generally cannot move but under certain circumstances exhibit a sudden and brief period of mobility (walking or even running).

Method of Elicitation of Pulsus Alternans (Fig. 2.6)

- Pulsus alternans refers to alternating high and low volume pulses
- Patient is placed in a semirecumbent position
- The blood pressure cuff is inflated to at least 20 mm Hg above the systolic pressure and slowly deflated until the first Korotkoff sounds heard
- Initially, the Korotkoff sounds due to the high volume pulses will be heard.
- As you lower the blood pressure, both high volume and low volume pulses will be heard.
- This will produce doubling of Korotkoff sounds

Method of Eliciting Collapsing Pulse (Fig. 2.7)

- Palpate the radial artery and trace the artery proximally to a point where it is just felt.

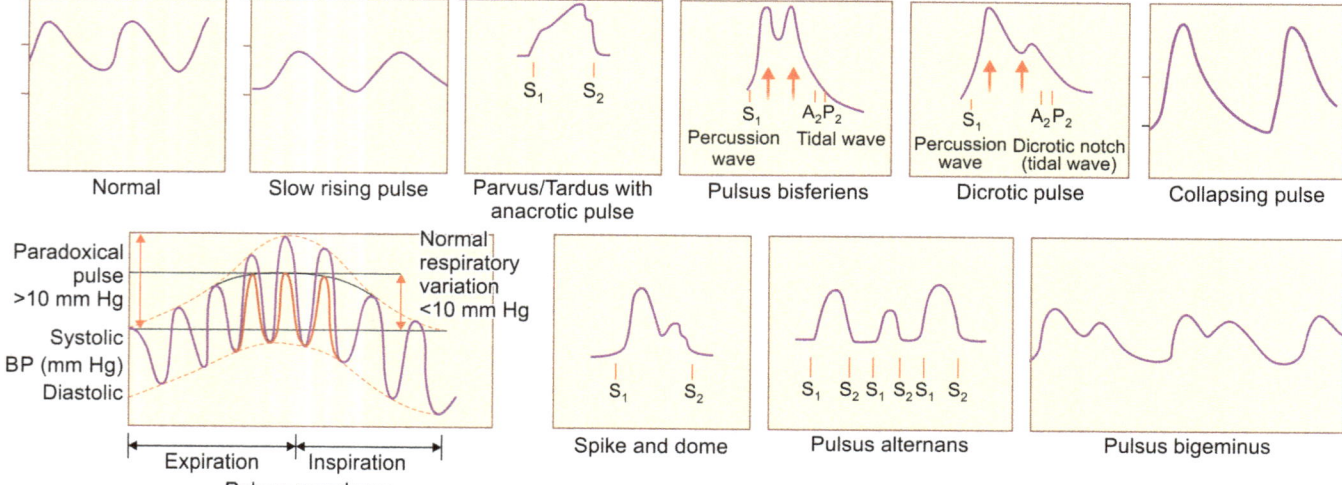

Fig. 2.4: Image showing different pulse waveforms.

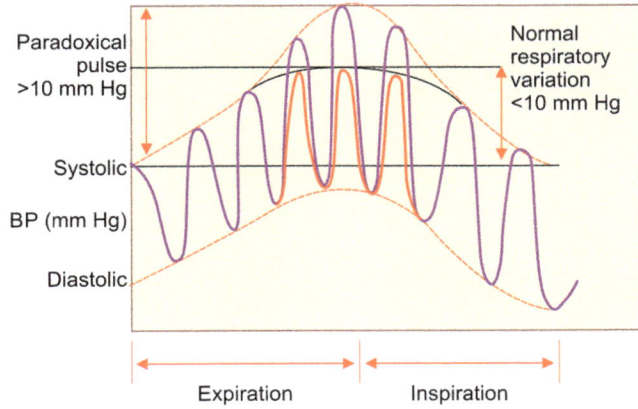

Fig. 2.5: Pulsus paradoxus.

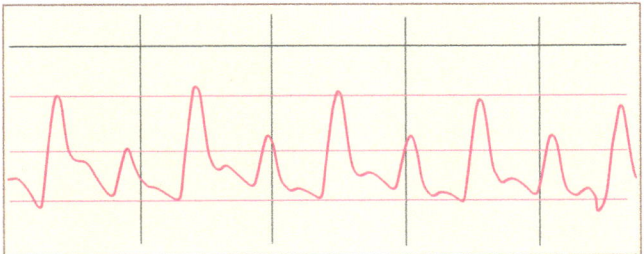

Fig. 2.6: Pulsus alternans.

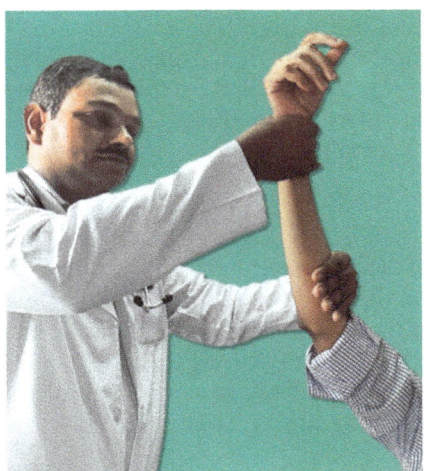

Fig. 2.7: Demonstration of collapsing pulse.

- At this point, wrap around your wrist so as place the metacarpal heads of your palm on the artery.
- Simultaneously, palpate the radial and ulnar arteries by encircling the wrist with other hand.
- Now, abruptly raise the patients hand above the shoulder (artery becomes in line with the central aorta, allowing direct systolic ejection and diastolic backflow).
- In collapsing pulse, both radial and ulnar arteries are felt distinctly and, there is an abrupt thrust/knock and collapse under the metacarpal heads on elevation.
- Thrust produced is similar to the one produced by tilting of water hammer toy. It is due to diastolic runoff in aortic regurgitation.

Collapsing pulse is characterized by rapid upstroke (percussion wave) followed by rapid descent (collapse) of the pulse wave without dicrotic notch, which reflects low systemic vascular resistance.
- Rapid upstroke is due to the rapid ejection of greatly increased stroke volume.
- The rapid descent or collapsing character is due to:
  - Diastolic "run-off" (backflow) into the left ventricle
  - Reflex vasodilation mediated by carotid baroreceptors secondary to large stroke volume
  - The rapid run-off to the periphery due to decreased systemic vascular resistance

Corrigan's pulse/sign is largely used to describe the abrupt distension and quick collapse of carotid pulse in aortic regurgitation whereas the term Watson's water hammer pulse' is used for the characteristic pulse seen in peripheral arteries such as the radial artery

- Make sure the patient does not have any shoulder pain before doing this.

Method of Eliciting Pulsus Bisferiens
- Best felt in brachial and carotid arteries
- Felt by applying graded pressure
- With fingers press and occlude the brachial artery
- On slowly releasing the pressure, the double peaking of the pulse is appreciated

Condition of Vessel Wall
Vessel wall thickening is assessed by using Osler's sign (described under the pseudohypertension).

Peripheral Pulses (Fig. 2.8)

Palpation of Carotid Pulse (Figs. 2.9 and 2.10):
- Ask the patient to relax neck.
- Palpate the right carotid artery by placing examiner's left thumb near the upper neck between the sternomastoid and trachea roughly at the level of cricoid cartilage.
- Note the character of the pulse.

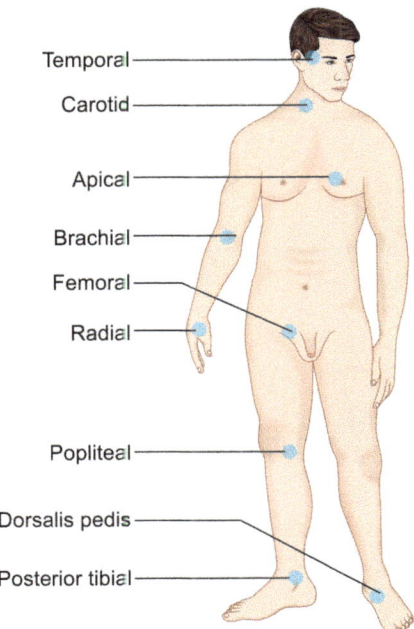

Fig. 2.8: Image showing site of different peripheral pulses.

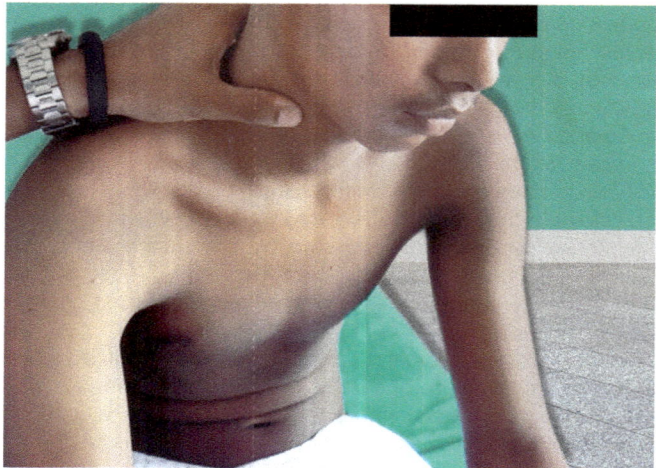

Fig. 2.9: Demonstration of palpation of right carotid pulse.

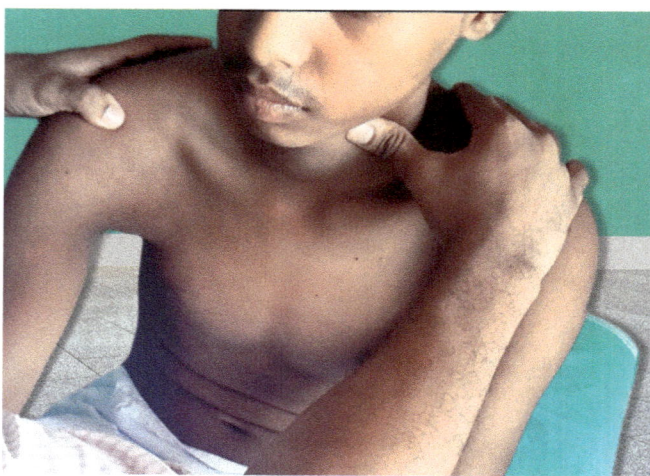

Fig. 2.10: Demonstration of palpation of left carotid pulse.

- Now, repeat the procedure on other side by placing the examiners right thumb over the patient's left carotid.

  Note: Make sure not to compress the carotid sinus and also it is advisable to auscultate for carotid bruit prior to palpation, to prevent possible dislodgment of the atherosclerotic plaque (if present).

Palpation of Branchial Pulse (Fig. 2.11)
- To examine the *brachial artery* in the right arm, the examiner supports the patient's forearm in his left hand.
- Patient's upper arm is abducted, the elbow is slightly flexed, and the forearm is externally rotated.
- The examiner's right hand is then curled over the anterior aspect of the elbow to palpate along the course of the artery just medial to the biceps tendon and lateral to the medial epicondyle of the humerus.
- The position of the hands should be switched when examining the opposite limb.

Palpation of Abdominal Aorta
- The *abdominal aorta* is best palpated by applying firm pressure with the flattened fingers of both hands to indent the epigastrium toward the vertebral column.
- For this examination, it is essential that the subject's abdominal muscles be completely relaxed; such relaxation can be encouraged by having the subject flex the hips and by providing a pillow to support the head.
- In extremely obese individuals or in those with massive abdominal musculature, it may be impossible to detect aortic pulsation.

Palpation of Common Femoral Artery (Fig. 2.12)
- The *common femoral artery* emerges into the upper thigh from beneath the inguinal ligament one-third of the distance from the pubis to the anterior superior iliac spine.
- It is best palpated with the examiner standing on the ipsilateral side of the patient and the fingertips of the examining hand pressed firmly into the groin.

Palpation of Popliteal Artery (Fig. 2.13)
- *The popliteal artery* passes vertically through the deep portion of the popliteal space just lateral to the midplane.
- Generally, this pulse is felt most conveniently with the patient in the supine position and the examiner's hands are encircling and supporting the knee from each side.
- The pulse is detected by pressing deeply into the popliteal space with the supporting fingertips.

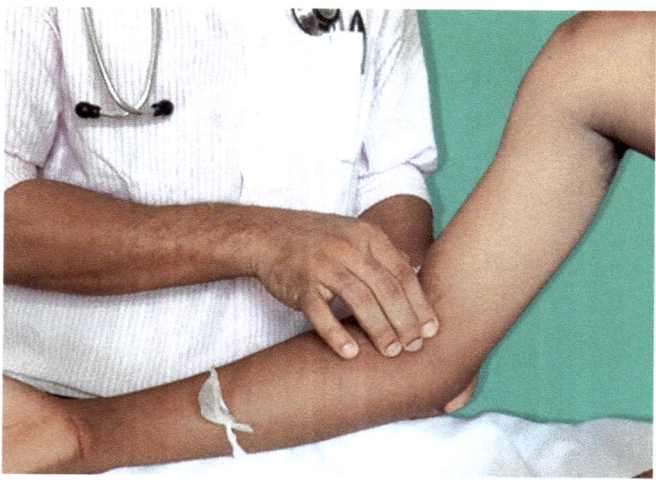

Fig. 2.11: Demonstration of palpation of brachial pulse.

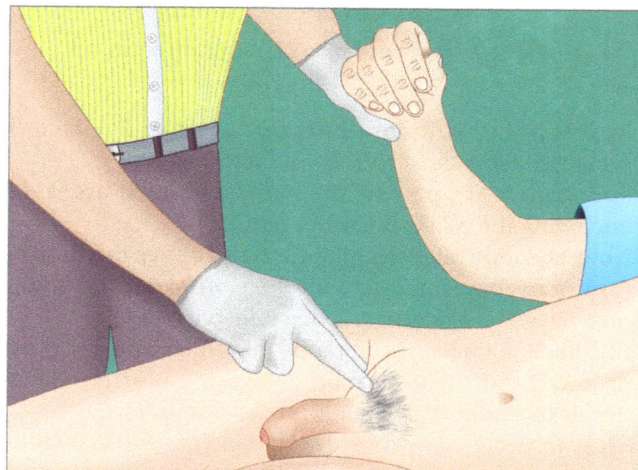

Fig. 2.12: Site of examination of femoral pulse.

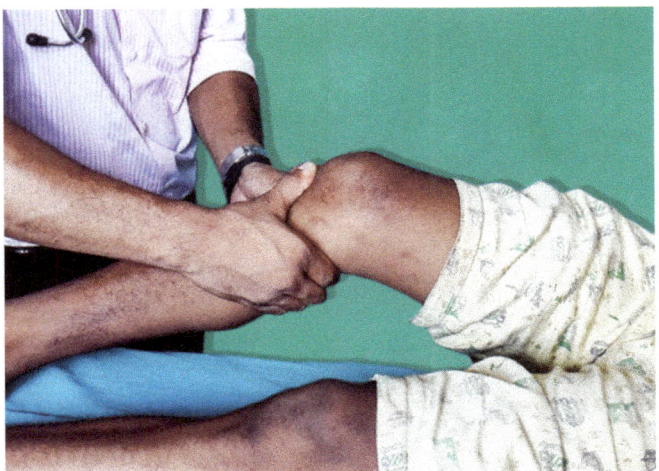

Fig. 2.13: Demonstration of palpation of popliteal artery.

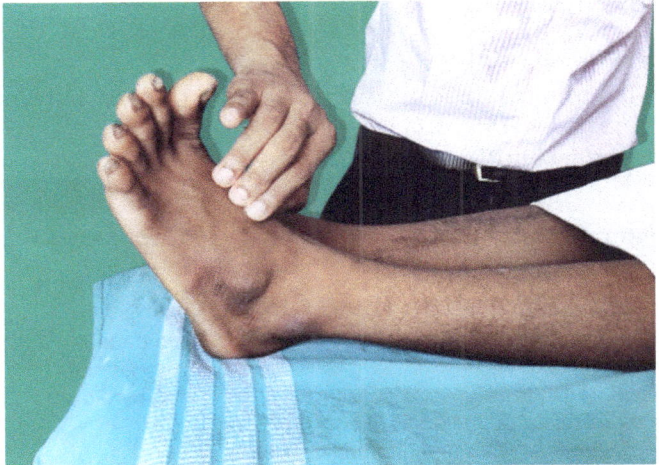

Fig. 2.15: Demonstration of palpation of dorsalis pedis artery.

- Since complete relaxation of the muscles is essential to this examination, the patient should be instructed to let the leg "go limp" and to allow the examiner to provide all the support needed.

Palpation of Posterior Tibial Artery (Fig. 2.14)
- The *posterior tibial artery* lies just posterior to the medial malleolus.
- It can be felt most readily by curling the fingers of the examining hand anteriorly around the ankle, indenting the soft tissues in the space between the medial malleolus and the Achilles tendon, above the calcaneus.
- The thumb is applied to the opposite side of the ankle in a grasping fashion to provide stability.

Palpation of Dorsalis Pedis Artery (Fig. 2.15)
- The *dorsalis pedis artery* is examined with the patient in the recumbent position and the ankle relaxed.
- The examiner stands at the foot of the examining table and places the fingertips transversely across the dorsum of the forefoot near the ankle.
- The artery usually lies near the center of the long axis of the foot, lateral to the extensor hallucis tendon, but it may be aberrant in location and often requires some searching.
- This pulse is congenitally absent in approximately 10% of individuals.

Radioradial Delay
Proceed to palpate both radial pulses simultaneously to detect any inequality in timing. This is known as radioradial delay. Causes include:
- Presubclavian coarctation
- Thoracic inlet syndrome—cervical rib
- Takayasu's disease
- Aortic arch aneurysm

Check for inequality in the strength of the radial pulses. Strength inequality of arm pulses has been shown to be a highly sensitive sign in diagnosing aortic dissection.

Radiofemoral Delay (Fig. 2.16)
Radiofemoral delay is the sign that is present, if the femoral pulse comes after the radial pulse. Delay of the femoral compared with the right radial pulse is found in coarctation of the aorta. Rarely, it can be seen in aortoarteritis.

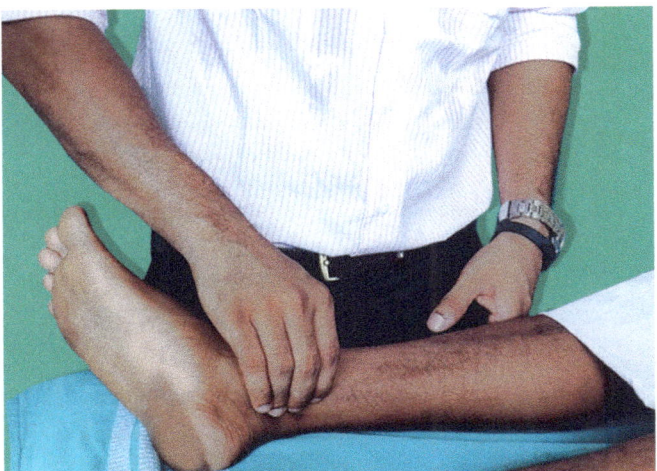

Fig. 2.14: Demonstration of palpation of posterior tibial pulse.

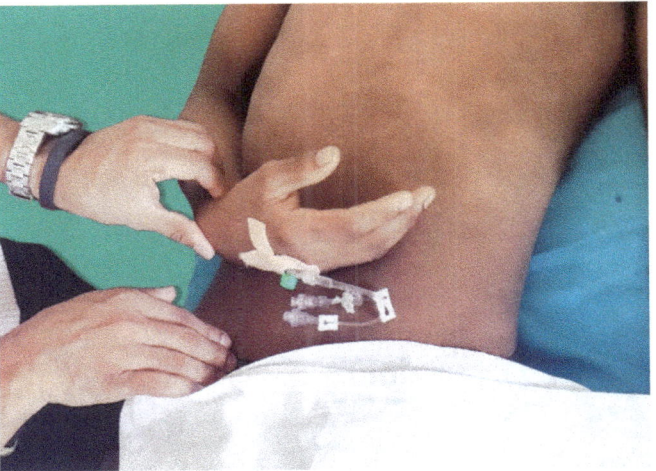

Fig. 2.16: Demonstration of radiofemoral delay.

RESPIRATION

Respiratory Rate
- It is counted while measuring the pulse rate and diverting the patient **(Fig. 2.17)**.
- Normal PR:RR = 4:1

Normal (16–20 breaths/min)	
Tachypnea	**Bradypnea**
>20 breaths/min	<10 breaths/min
Physiological: • Anxiety • Exertion **Pathological:** • Local diseases of chest wall and lung • Systemic hypoxia and metabolic acidosis	Narcotics Head trauma Hypothermia Hypothyroidism

Muscles of Respiration

Inspiration	Expiration
Main: • External IC • Diaphragm	Predominantly passive process
Accessory muscles: • SCM • Scalenus anterior • Pectoralis • Trapezius	**Accessory muscles (used in forceful expiration):** • Internal intercostals • Abdominals • Quadratus lumborum • Latissimus dorsi

(SCM: sternocleidomastoid muscle)

Types of Respiration

Keep two hands flat, one on the chest and other on the abdomen and watch for movements of hand **(Fig. 2.18)**.
In abdominothoracic—movements of hand over the abdomen are more prominent.
In thoracoabdominal—movements of hand over the thorax are more prominent.

Abdominothoracic	Thoracoabdominal
Due to well-developed abdominal muscles	Well-formed internal intercostal muscles
Seen in males	Seen in females

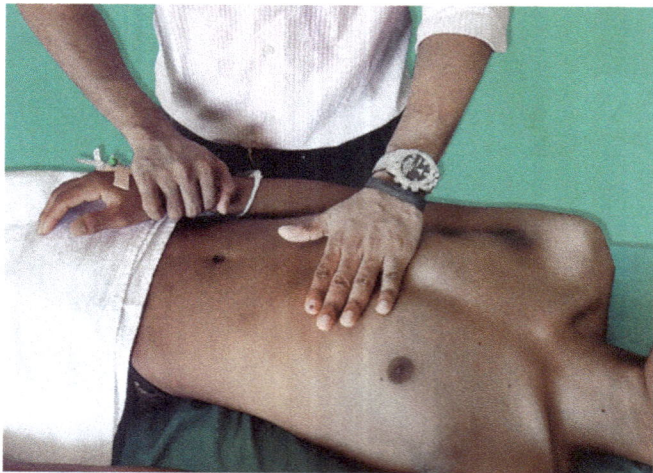

Fig. 2.17: Method of calculating respiratory rate.

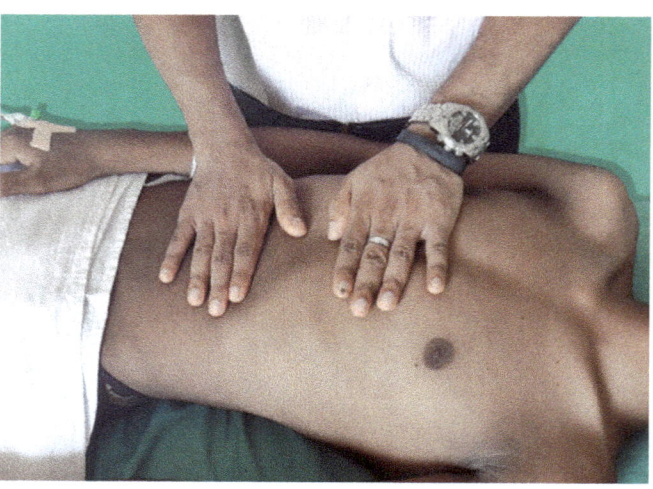

Fig. 2.18: Method of assessing type of respiration.

Variants

Purely thoracic	Purely abdominal
Abdominal movement during respirations is absent	Thoracic movement during respiration is absent
Peritonitis Pregnancy Ascites/ovarian cyst	Pleuritic chest pain Defective chest wall Respiratory muscle paralysis (neurogenic, NMJ, and muscular)

Abnormal Patterns of Breathing (Fig. 2.19)

Regular	Irregular
Cheyne–Stokes (periods of apnea alternating with hyperapnea): Cardiac failure (LVF)—most common cause Raised ICP Brainstem lesions	*Biot's:* Meningitis
Kussmaul's (rapid deep breathing): Metabolic acidosis (DKA and renal failure) Pontine lesions	*Ataxic:* Brainstem disorders
	Apneustic: Pontine lesions

(DKA: diabetic ketoacidosis; ICP: intracranial pressure; LVF: left ventricular failure)

Condition	Description
Eupnea	Normal breathing rate and pattern
Tachypnea	Increased respiratory rate
Bradypnea	Decreased respiratory rate
Apnea	Absence of breathing
Hyperpnea	Normal rate, but deep respirations
Cheyne-Stokes	Gradual increases and decreases in respirations with periods of apnea
Biot's	Rapid, deep respirations (gasps) with short pauses between sets
Kussmaul's	Tachypnea and hyperpnea
Apneustic	Prolonged inspiratory phase with shortened expiratory phase

Fig. 2.19: Different type of breathing patterns.

Pursed Lip Breathing

- It is seen with chronic obstructive pulmonary disease (COPD)
- Mechanism of auto-positive end-expiratory pressure (PEEP)
- The purpose of this breathing is to slow down the airflow during the exhalation to build up back pressure in the airway to avoid a sudden drop in intrapulmonary pressure resulting in alveolar and airway collapse.

Airway Obstruction

- Upper airway obstruction—prolonged inspiration
- Lower airway obstruction—prolonged expiration

BLOOD PRESSURE

Definition

Arterial blood pressure can be defined as the lateral pressure exerted by the moving column of blood on the walls of the arteries.

$$BP = Cardiac\ output \times Peripheral\ resistance$$

Systolic BP (SBP)	Diastolic BP (DBP)
It is defined as the maximum BP in the arteries attainable during systole. Normal range is 120 + 20 mm Hg	It is defined as the minimum pressure that is obtained at the end of the ventricular diastole. Normal range is 60–90 mm Hg
Pulse Pressure (PP)	**Mean Arterial Pressure (MAP)**
It denotes the difference between systolic and diastolic pressure. PP = SBP − DBP = 40 mm Hg	DBP + 1/3 pulse pressure Normal = 95 mm Hg

Korotkoff Sounds

Korotkoff sounds	SBP	120 mm Hg	Tapping sound 1
		110 mm Hg	Murmurish 2
		95 mm Hg	Banging sound 3
		85 mm Hg	Muffing sound 4
	DBP	80 mm Hg	No sound 5

Types and Character of Korotkoff Sounds

American Heart Association (AHA), 2017 classification:

BP category	Systolic BP		Diastolic BP
Normal	<120 mm Hg	and	<80 mm Hg
Elevated	120–129 mm Hg	and	<80 mm Hg
Stage 1 hypertension	130–139 mm Hg	Or	80–89 mm Hg
Stage 2 Hypertension	≥140 mm Hg	Or	≥90 mm Hg

Steps of Examination of Blood Pressure

Key steps	Specific instructions
Step 1: Properly prepare the patient	- Have the patient relax, sitting in a chair (feet on floor, back supported) for >5 min **(Fig. 2.20)**. - The patient should avoid caffeine, exercise, and smoking for at least 30 min before measurement. - Ensure patient has emptied his/her bladder.

Contd...

Key steps	Specific instructions
	- Neither the patient nor the observer should talk during the rest period or during the measurement. - Remove all clothing covering the location of cuff placement. - Measurements made while the patient is sitting or lying on an examining table do not fulfill these criteria.
Step 2: Use proper technique for BP measurements	- Use a BP measurement device that has been validated, and ensure that the device is calibrated periodically. - Support the patient's arm (e.g., resting on a desk). - Position the middle of the cuff on the patient's upper arm at the level of the right atrium (the midpoint of the sternum) **(Fig. 2.21)**. - Use the correct cuff size, such that the bladder encircles 80% of the arm, and note if a larger- or smaller-than-normal cuff size is used. - Either the stethoscope diaphragm or bell may be used for auscultatory readings.
Step 3: Take the proper measurements needed for diagnosis and treatment of elevated BP/hypertension	- At the first visit, record BP in both arms. Use the arm that gives the higher reading for subsequent readings. - Separate repeated measurements by 1–2 minute - For auscultatory determinations, use a palpated estimate of radial pulse obliteration pressure to estimate SBP. Inflate the cuff 20–30 mm Hg above this level for an auscultatory determination of the BP level. - For auscultatory readings, deflate the cuff pressure 2 mm Hg per second, and listen for Korotkoff sounds.
Step 4: Properly document accurate BP readings	- Record SBP and DBP. If using the auscultatory technique, record SBP and DBP as onset of the first Korotkoff sound and disappearance of all Korotkoff sounds, respectively, using the nearest even number. - Note the time of most recent BP medication taken before measurements.
Step 5: Average the readings	- Use an average of ≥2 readings obtained on ≥2 occasions to estimate the individual's level of BP. - In presence of atrial fibrillation, minimum of 3 BP readings have to be estimated.
Step 6: Provide BP readings to patient	- Provide patients the SBP/DBP readings both verbally and in writing.

(SBP: systolic blood pressure; DBP: diastolic blood pressure)

Selection Criteria for BP Cuff Size for Measurement of BP in Adults

Arm circumference	Usual cuff size
22–26 cm	Small adult
27–34 cm	Adult
35–44 cm	Large adult
45–52 cm	Adult thigh

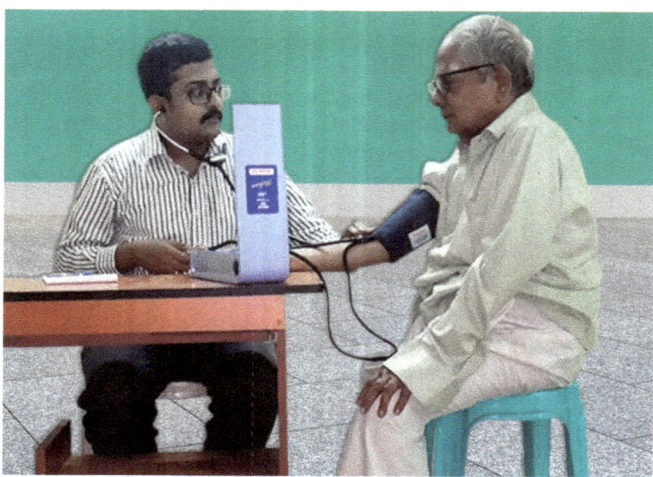

Fig. 2.20: Demonstration of blood pressure (BP) measurement.

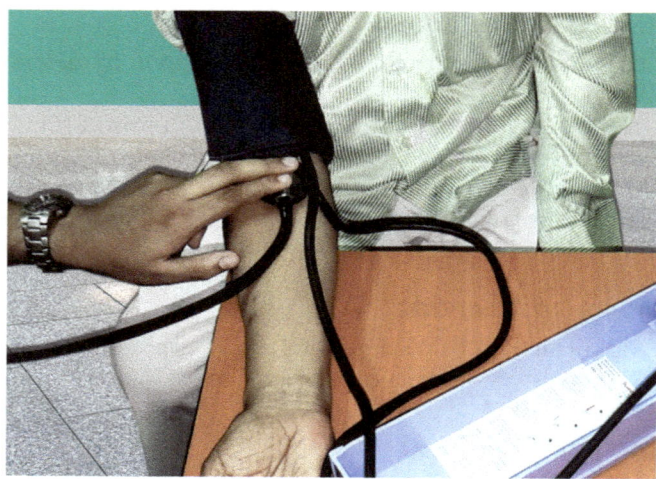

Fig. 2.21: Demonstration of placement of blood pressure (BP) cuff.

White Coat Hypertension
Higher office BPs than out-of-office BPs

Masked Uncontrolled Hypertension
Controlled office BPs but uncontrolled BPs in out-of-office settings

Paroxysmal Hypertension—Episodic Elevated BP

- Pheochromocytoma
- Pseudopheochromocytoma—panic disorders and labile hypertension
- Carcinoid
- Clonidine withdrawal
- Renovascular hypertension
- Hypoglycemia
- Cheese reaction

Pseudohypertension
It is a condition in which indirect blood pressure (BP) measured by the cuff method overestimates the true intra-arterial BP. A palpable although pulseless, radial artery, while the BP cuff is inflated above systolic pressure, is a positive *Osler sign*. Osler sign occurs due to Monckeberg's sclerosis of arteries.

Paradoxical Hypertension
On starting treatment with antihypertensives, the BP rises instead of falling in the following conditions:
- Angiotensin-converting enzyme (ACE) inhibitors or angiotensin-receptor blockers (ARBs) for a patient with renal artery stenosis
- Beta-blockers given to a patient with pheochromocytoma
- Beta-blockers in a patient with diabetic autonomic neuropathy

Hypotension
It is defined as blood pressure below 90/60 mm Hg.

Causes
Cause of hypotension according to age group shown in **Figure 2.22**.

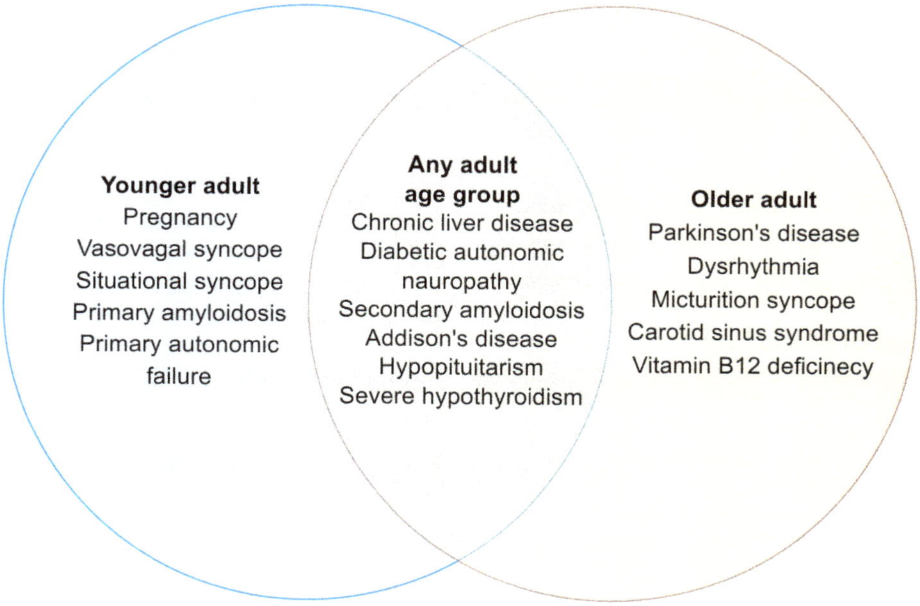

Younger adult
Pregnancy
Vasovagal syncope
Situational syncope
Primary amyloidosis
Primary autonomic failure

Any adult age group
Chronic liver disease
Diabetic autonomic nauropathy
Secondary amyloidosis
Addison's disease
Hypopituitarism
Severe hypothyroidism

Older adult
Parkinson's disease
Dysrhythmia
Micturition syncope
Carotid sinus syndrome
Vitamin B12 deficinecy

Fig. 2.22: Cause of hypotension according to age group.

Postural Hypotension/Orthostatic Hypotension

- A drop in blood pressure (hypotension) due to a change in body position (posture) when a person moves to a more vertical position (i.e.) from sitting to standing or from lying down to sitting or standing.
- Postural (orthostatic) hypotension is diagnosed when, within 2–5 minutes of quiet standing (after a 5-minute period of supine rest), one or both of the following is present:
  - At least, a 20 mm Hg fall in systolic pressure
  - At least, a 10 mm Hg fall in diastolic pressure
- Many disorders can cause orthostatic hypotension, with the two major mechanisms being autonomic failure, which can be caused by multiple disorders, and severe volume depletion.

Autonomic failure	Volume depletion
Diabetic neuropathy Parkinson disease Dementia with Lewy bodies MSA (Shy–Drager syndrome) Spinal cord transaction Chronic kidney disease Amyloidosis Guillain–Barré syndrome Paraneoplastic autonomic neuropathy Familial dysautonomia (Riley–Day syndrome) Primary autonomic failure (Bradbury–Eggleston syndrome)	Acute or subacute volume depletion (due to diuretics, hyperglycemia, hemorrhage, or vomiting) Chronic hypovolemia, a frequent feature of autonomic failure, exacerbates orthostatic symptoms

JUGULAR VENOUS SYSTEM

Jugular Venous Pulse

It is defined as undulating top of oscillating column of blood in right internal jugular vein (IJV) that faithfully represents the pressure and volumetric changes in the right side of heart, which changes with various stages of cardiac cycle and respiration.

Why Right Side IJV is Preferred?

- Right side IJV is in direct connection and in straight line (Fig. 2.23).
- Also, left innominate may be compressed or kinked by dilated aorta/aneurysm

Why internal jugular vein is preferred over external jugular vein for JVP assessment?	
Internal jugular	**External jugular**
Straight communication with right atrium	Not in straight communication with right atrium
Less valves	More valves
Less influenced by fascial planes	More kinked by fascial planes
Less effected by sympathetic system	More effected by sympathetic system
	Vasoconstriction secondary to hypotension (in CCF) can make EJV small and barely visible

Differences between carotid and JVP:	
Carotid pulse	**Jugular venous pulse**
Better felt	Better seen
Cannot be obliterated	Can be obliterated (by pressure on root of neck)
One positive wave	2 positive and 2 negative
Medially seen	Laterally seen
Seen in lower part	Seen in upper part
Definite upper level absent	Definite upper level in present
Expansile impulse (outward)	Retractile impulse (inward)
Does not change with position	Changes with position
Does not change with respiration	Changes with respiration
Does not change with abdominal compression	Changes with abdominal compression

Steps of Examination of JVP (Figs. 2.24 and 2.25)

- Patient comfortably lying in semi-reclined position (45° position).
- Patient neck slightly turned on the left side.
- Shine torch form left side tangentially.

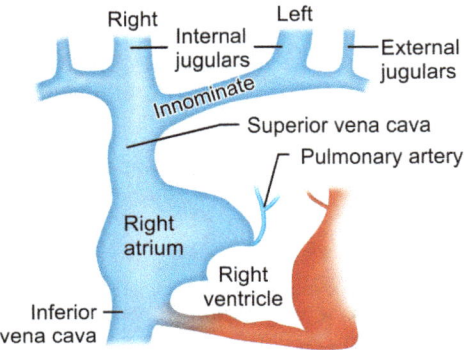

Fig. 2.23: Right jugular vein is in the straight continuity with right atrium.

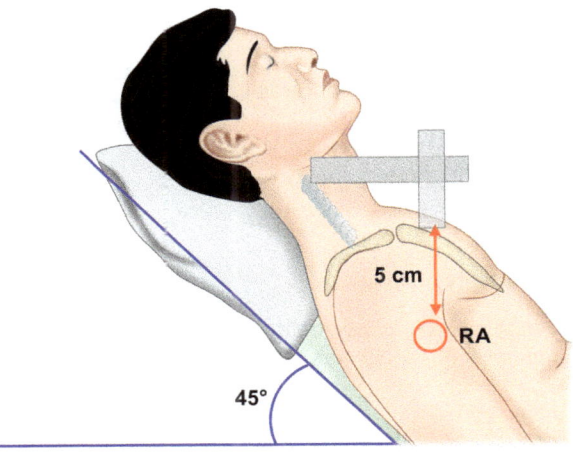

Fig. 2.24: Pictorial image showing method of examination of jugular venous pressure (JVP).

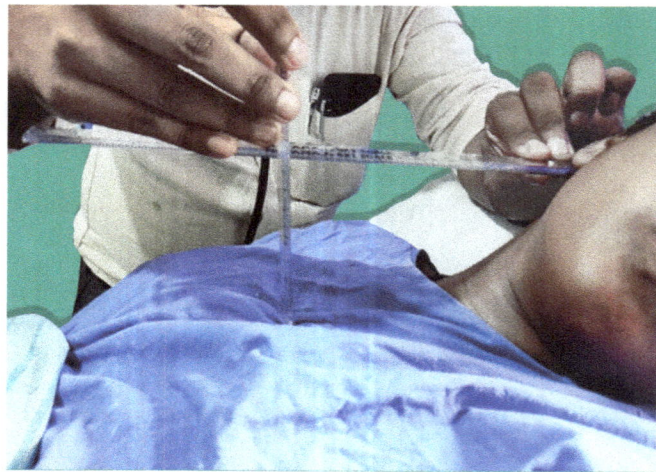

Fig. 2.25: Examination of height of jugular venous pressure (JVP).

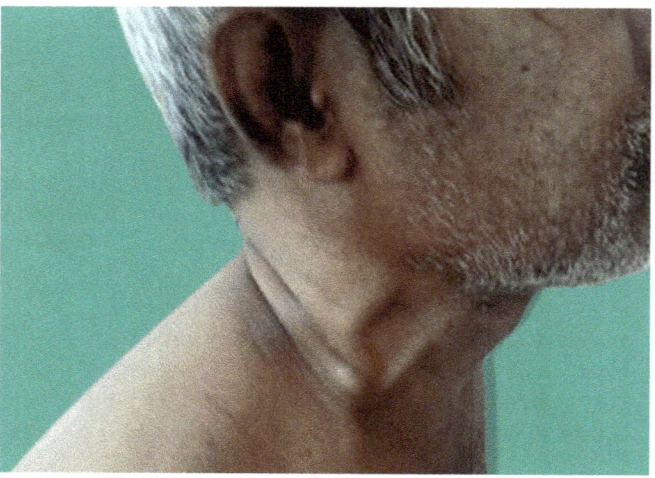

Fig. 2.26: Image showing engorged neck veins.

- Observe for pulsation between two heads of sternocleidomastoid.
- Trace the pulsation and locate the upper level.
- Take two scales.
- Place first scale at the upper level of JVP and the scale has to be parallel to the ground.
- Now, place the second scale at the level of sternal angle and scale has to be perpendicular to the first scale.
- The vertical distance has to be measured on the second scale.
- Express as ___ cm of water above sternal angle (for total JVP/central venous pressure (CVP) from right atrium, add 5 cm to this value)
- *Conversion*: 1.36 cm of H_2O or blood = 1 mm Hg
- Normal is less than 4 cm or just visible above clavicle in 45° position.
- Normal CVP is <7 mm of Hg or 9 cm H_2O

Causes of Raised JVP

Engorged (Fig. 2.26) and pulsatile neck vein	Engorged and nonpulsatile neck vein
Cardiac causes: • Right heart failure • Congestive cardiac failure • Chronic constrictive pericarditis • Cardiac tamponade • Complete heart block • Restrictive cardiomyopathy • SVC obstruction • Tricuspid stenosis	• Superior mediastinal syndrome • Valsalva maneuver • Chronic constrictive pericarditis (advance stage)
Noncardiac causes: • Pulmonary thromboembolism • Pulmonary hypertension • Acute nephritis • Pregnancy • Fluid overload status	

JVP Components and Waveforms (Figs. 2.27 and 2.28)

Component	Cardiac event responsible
A wave	Atrial contraction/systole
X wave (initial x descent)	Atrial relaxation
C wave	Cusp bulge (some consider c wave is due to the impact of carotid pulsation)
"X" wave (x descent following "c" wave)	Descent in floor of RA with downward pull of TV with continued ventricular contraction
V wave	Atrial filling during ventricular systole
Y wave	RA emptying during ventricular diastole
H wave (Hirschfelder wave)	Seen in diastasis

(RA: right atrium)

"a" wave (most prominent of JVP):			
Absent	Atrial fibrillation		
Large/giant "a" wave	• TS • TA • RA myxomas	• RV infarct • RV cardiomyopathy	PH PS PE
	AS* HCM* (Bernheim effect*)		
Canon "a" waves	Regular	Junctional rhythm VT (1:1 retrograde conduction)	
	Irregular	CHB AV dissociation Ventricular ectopics VT V pacing	

(RV: right ventricular; PH: pulmonary hypertension; PS: pulmonary stenosis; PE: pulmonary embolism; AV: atrioventricular; CHB: complete heart block)

Bernheim effect: Left-sided diseases causing prominent a wave, i.e., severe LVH with septal thickening interfere with RV filling resulting in prominent a wave.

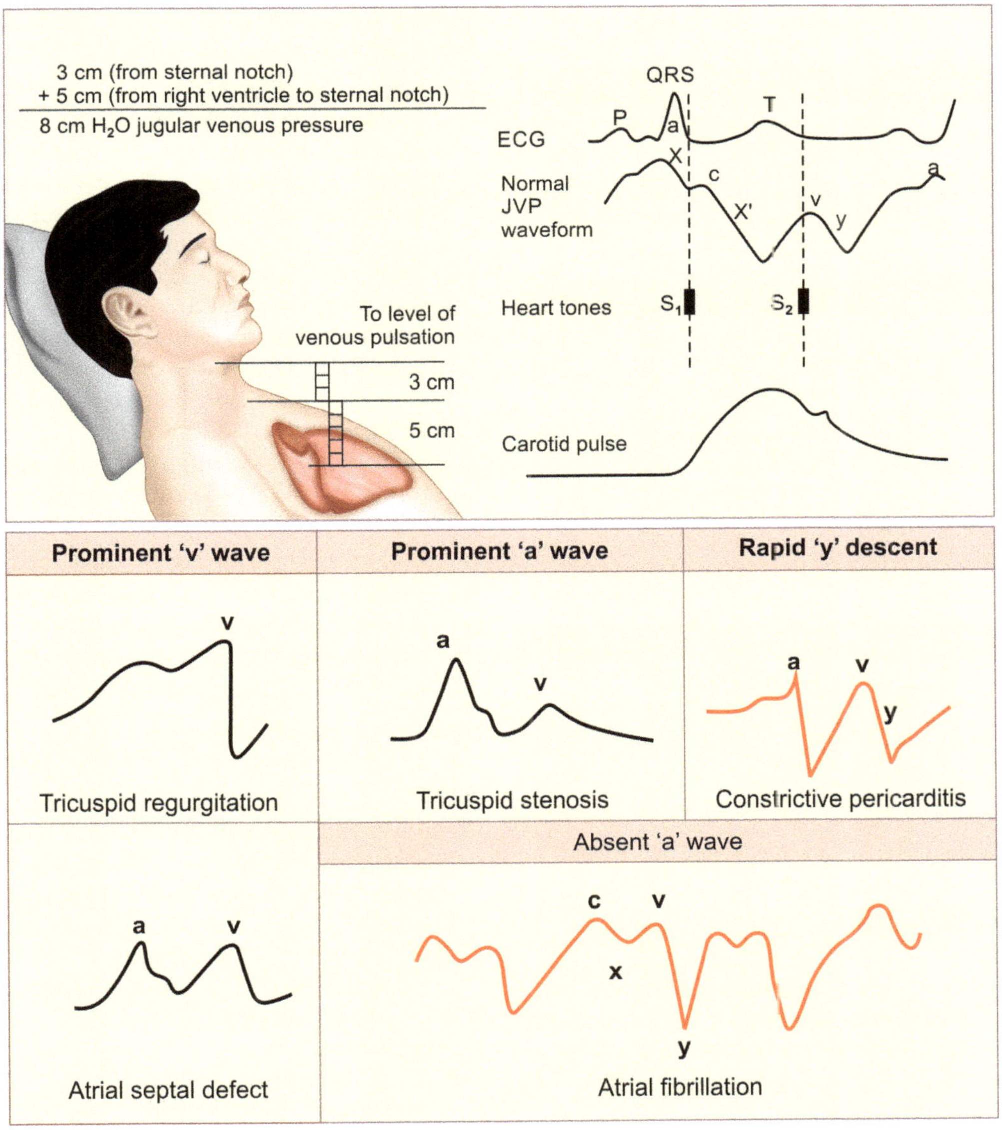

Fig. 2.27: Jugular venous pressure (JVP) demonstration.

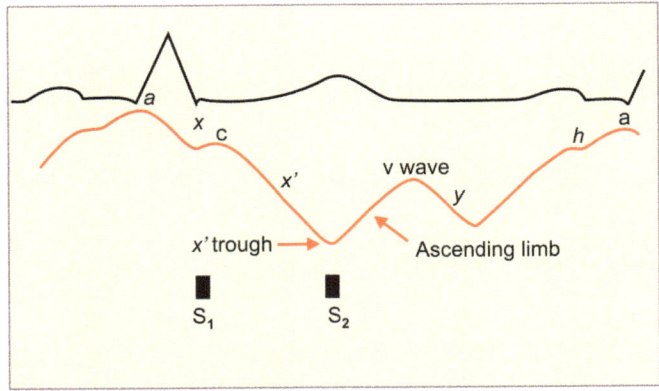

Fig. 2.28: Jugular venous pressure wave pattern.

"v" wave:	
Diminished	Hypovolemia
Prominent	TR* ASD VSD (Gerbode defect—LV → RA defect) CHF Atrial fibrillation Cor pulmonale

(ASD: atrial septal defect; CHF: congestive heart failure; LV: left ventricular; RA: right atrium; VSD: ventricular septal defect)

*In TR, due to absent x and prominent v wave merging with c wave, it results in large positive systolic and regurgitant waves (CV wave) followed by a rapid deep Y descent.

Lancisi's sign—may cause subtle motion of ear lobe with each heartbeat.

"X" descent (systolic collapse):	
Absent	Tricuspid regurgitation
Prominent	Tamponade
	ASD
	Pericarditis—constrictive

(ASD: atrial septal defect)

"Y" descent (diastolic collapse):	
Slow descent	Tamponade
	TS
	RA myxoma
Rapid descent	Constrictive pericarditis
	Severe TR
	Severe RV failure

(RA: right atrium; RV: right ventricular)

Differences between constrictive pericarditis and cardiac tamponade (Fig. 2.29):

	X wave	Y wave
Pericarditis – constrictive	+	++ (prominent Y)
Tamponade	++ (prominent X)	—
TR	—	++

(Mnemonic: Prominent y and x waves can be remembered with mnemonic PaY TaX)

Other Sites of JVP Estimation

Gaertner's method:
Normally, the superficial veins of dorsum of hand collapse when raised above the sternal angle. Persistent prominence is suggestive of raised central venous pressure (*Anthem sign*—when the same is tested by asking the patient to make fist, raised arm like an anthem pledge).

May's sign:
- Visible engorged vein on the undersurface of tongue in sitting posture.

Abdominojugular (AJR) reflux of Rundott (previously known as hepatojugular reflux):
Demonstration (Fig. 2.30):
- Examine patient at 45° semirecumbent position and firm consistent abdominal pressure of around 40 mm Hg is applied (an inflated BP cuff may be used)
- Site of compression is not mandatorily on liver and can be anywhere in the abdomen preferably on the right side.
- Historically, pressure was applied for 15 seconds; however, recent studies suggest 10 seconds is adequate
- **Normal response:** Transient rise of around 4 cm for about 4–5 cardiac cycles (approximately 5 seconds)
- **Sustained response/positive response:** Earliest sign of RHF, also seen in TR
- **Absent response/negative response:** Obstruction/thrombosis of IVC or hepatic veins as seen in Budd-Chiari syndrome

Friedreich's sign of constrictive pericarditis:
Friedreich's sign describes a rapid fall and rise in the JVP. It occurs when stiff ventricles are unable to accommodate the rapid ventricular filling that should follow opening of the tricuspid valve in the presence of elevated atrial pressure.

Square root sign of JVP:
Dip and plateau pattern of JVP is seen in constrictive pericarditis.

Kussmaul's sign of JVP:
- Normally, when the patient inspires there is fall in the height of JVP due to increased negative intrathoracic pressure.
- However in certain conditions, there is an inspiratory rise in upper level of JVP and this is known as Kussmaul sign.
- It is true venous paradox.
- It is seen in:
  - Constrictive pericarditis
  - Right heart failure (RHF)
  - Right ventricular (RV) infarction
  - Restrictive cardiomyopathy

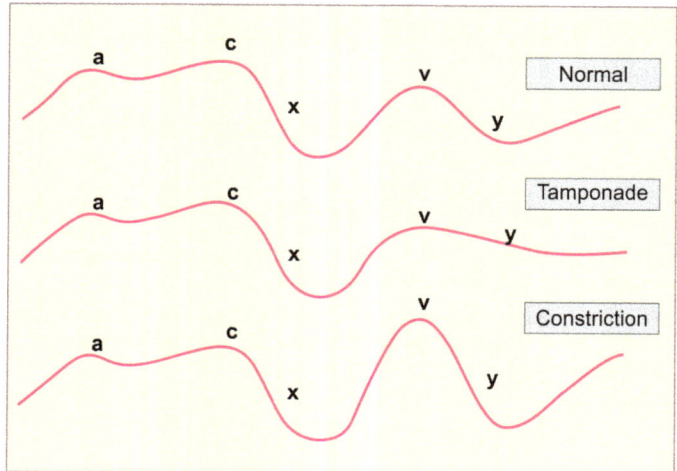

Fig. 2.29: Waveforms of jugular venous pressure (JVP) in tamponade versus constrictive pericarditis.

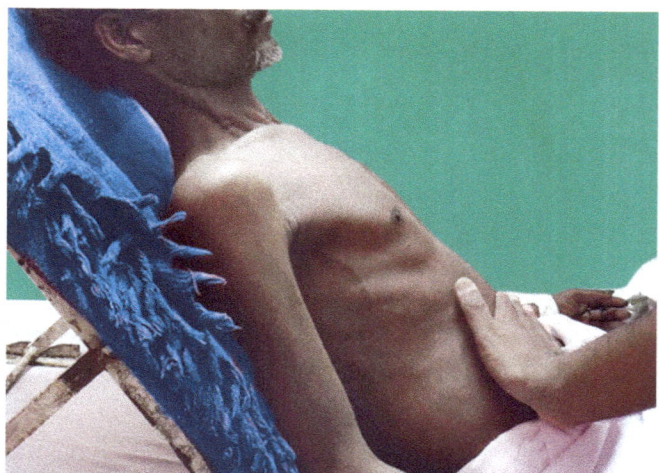

Fig. 2.30: Demonstration of abdominojugular reflux.

M pattern in JVP:		
Constrictive pericarditis	Due to prominent x and y waves	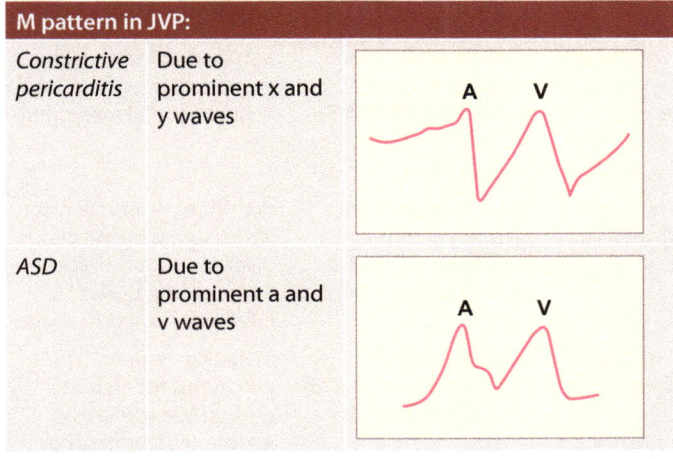
ASD	Due to prominent a and v waves	

Raised jugular venous pressure with shock:
- Congestive heart failure
- Cardiac tamponade
- Right ventricular infarction
- Tension pneumothorax
- Massive pulmonary embolism

BODY TEMPERATURE

Temperature

It is a measure of heat content.

Body Core Temperature

It usually refers to the temperature of the internal body core, measured under the tongue, in the ear canal or in the rectum.

Normal range (oral): 36.8 ± 0.4°C (98.2 ± 0.7°F)

Regulation of temperature: Under the control of neurons of preoptic anterior hypothalamus and posterior hypothalamus

Site of Examination of Temperature

Oral temperature	• Probe placed under the tongue into the sublingual pockets and the lips closed around the instrument • The patient should not have recently smoked or ingested cold or hot food or drink • Usually tested for about 3 minutes (It follows changes in core body temperature, as branch of external carotid artery perfuses the area of posterior sublingual pockets.)
Rectal temperature	• Measured with a lubricated blunt-tipped glass thermometer inserted 4–5 cm (2.5 cm in children) into the anal canal at an angle 20° from the horizontal with the patient lying prone • Usually tested for about 3 minutes • Lags behind changes at other core sites, as it is located for from the central nervous system as well as from the pulmonary artery (Indication of deep visceral temperature, modified by the temperature of the skin of the buttocks, the iliac artery, and iliac vein)
Tympanic temperature	• The scanning tip should be gently placed in the ear canal and then slowly inserted against the tympanic membrane snugly • Measures the infrared heat waves from the tympanic membrane • Close to hypothalamus and rapid measurement of core body temperature
Axillary temperature	• Thermometer placed in the axilla and shoulder adducted • Convenient for patient • Core temperature cannot be assessed directly • Lags behind the changes in core body temperature
Temporal artery skin thermometer	• Placed on the skin of the forehead over the temporal artery • An electronic thermometer that is fast and accurate • Less invasive than the tympanic thermometer and more reliable when used correctly

Thermometers (Fig. 2.31)

Glass Thermometer and Electric Digital Thermometer

☐ Glass thermometers bulb contains an alloy of elements called Galinstan.

☐ Electric digital thermometers are more convenient than glass instruments because the probe cover is disposable, response time is quicker (allowing accurate measurements within 10–20 seconds), and there is a signal when the rate of change in temperature becomes insignificant.

The most common methods of temperature assessment that carry the least amount of risk for patient injury are the use of glass or electronic digital thermometers to measure oral, rectal, axillary, or vaginal temperatures; basal thermometers; temporal artery thermometers; tympanic thermometers; and liquid crystal forehead temperature strips. These methods can be utilized in healthcare settings and also within the patient's home.

Although the more invasive methods are more accurate, they carry a higher risk of potential complications, so they are not routinely utilized in areas outside of a critical care or surgical setting. Examples of invasive methods of temperature assessment are esophageal and rectal temperature probes, temperature-sensing indwelling urinary catheters, temperature-sensing pulmonary artery (PA) catheters, a cardiopulmonary bypass (CPB) machine, and extracorporeal membrane oxygenation (ECMO).

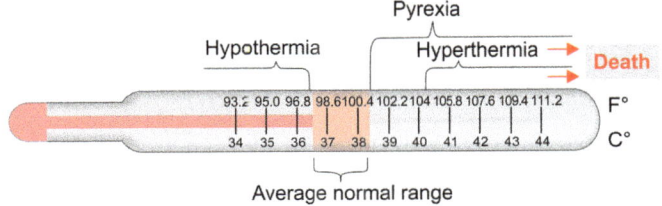

Fig. 2.31: Thermometer showing marking in both Celsius and Fahrenheit.

Circadian Variation of Temperature

- Circadian rhythm is governed by suprachiasmatic nuclei in anterior hypothalamus.
- Normal variation is 0.5–1.0°C variation over the day
- Lowest temperature is noted at 6:00 AM
- Peaks at 4:00–6:00 PM

Variation of Temperature during Menstrual Cycles

An abrupt increase of 0.3–0.5°C accompanies ovulation and may be useful as a fertility guide.

Fever

Fever is an elevation of body temperature that exceeds the normal daily variation and occurs in conjunction with an *increase in the hypothalamic set point.*

It can be defined as temperature of >37.2°C (98.9°F) at 6 AM or >37.7°C (99.9°F) at 4–6 PM.

When the hypothalamic set point is raised, the body is perceived to be cooler than the new set point. Shivering is initiated to generate heat. Blood is shunted from the periphery to the core to conserve heat and sweating is diminished. The generated heat will raise the body temperature to match the elevated set point. When the hypothalamic set point is lowered, either as part of the normal diurnal fluctuations that occur during an infection or in response to antipyretic agents, heat is lost by evaporation (sweating) and radiation (cutaneous vasodilation).

Types of fever based on duration:		
Acute fevers	<7 days	Infectious diseases, such as malaria and viral-related upper respiratory tract infections
Subacute fevers	Usually not more than 2 weeks in duration	Typhoid fever and intra-abdominal abscess
Chronic or persistent fevers	>2-week duration	Chronic bacterial infections, such as tuberculosis, viral infections, such as HIV, cancers, and connective tissue diseases

Grading of Fever Based on Body Temperature

Body temperature	°C	°F
Normal	37–38	98.6–100.4
Mild-/low-grade fever	38.1–39	100.5–102.2
Moderate-grade fever	39.1–40	102.2–104.0
High-grade fever	40.1–41.1	104.1–106.0
Hyperpyrexia	>41.1	>106.0

The conversion formula is:
1. $T°F = 9/5 (T°C) + 32$
2. $T°C = 5/9 (T°F) - 32$

For axillary, oral, and rectal temperature, there is an approximately 0.8°F or 0.4°C difference between each site and the next higher one. For convenience, it is rounded up to 1°F or 0.5°C.

Patterns of fever (Fig. 2.32)		
Continuous or sustained fever	Defined as fever that does not fluctuate more than about 1°C (1.5°F) during 24 h, but at no time touches normal	Lobar and gram-negative pneumonia, typhoid, and acute bacterial meningitis
Remittent fever	Defined as fever with daily fluctuations exceeding 2°C, but at no time touches normal	Remittent fevers are often associated with infectious diseases, such as infective endocarditis, rickettsia infections, and brucellosis
Intermittent fever	Defined as fever present only for several hours during the day	Malaria, pyogenic infections, tuberculosis (TB), schistosomiasis, lymphomas, *Leptospira, Borrelia,* kala-azar, or septicemia
	Double quotidian fever (12-hour periodicity)	Kala-azar, gonococcal endocarditis. Adult onset stills disease
	Quotidian fever (periodicity of 24 hours)	Mixed falciparum and vivax
	Tertian fever (periodicity of 48 hours)	*Plasmodium falciparum, ovale,* and *vivax*
	Quartan fever (periodicity of 72 hour)	*Plasmodium malariae*
	Pel-Ebstein's fever (intermittent low-grade fever characterized by 3–10 days of fever with subsequent afebrile periods of 3–10 days)	It is thought to be atypical, but rare manifestation of Hodgkin's lymphoma
Relapsing fevers	Refer to those that are recurring and separated by periods with low-grade fever or no fever	Seen in malaria, lymphoma, *Borrelia,* cyclic neutropenia, and rat-bite fever

Fever with Night Sweats

It has been described in infectious diseases, such as TB, *Nocardia,* brucellosis, liver or lung abscess, and subacute infective endocarditis, as well as in noninfectious diseases, such as polyarteritis nodosa and cancers, such as lymphomas.

Fever with Bradycardia

It is a feature of untreated typhoid, leishmaniasis, brucellosis, Legionnaire's disease and psittacosis, and yellow fever.

Fever with Unknown Origin

In 1961, pyrexia of unknown origin (PUO) was originally defined by Petersdorf and Beeson as an illness of more than 3-week duration, fever higher than 38.3°C (101°F) on several occasions and diagnosis uncertain after 1 week of study in hospital.

This definition has been modified, removing the requirement that the evaluation must take place in the hospital and refined to include four different sub-groups, each requiring different investigative strategies—classical, nosocomial, neutropenic, and human immunodeficiency virus (HIV)-related.

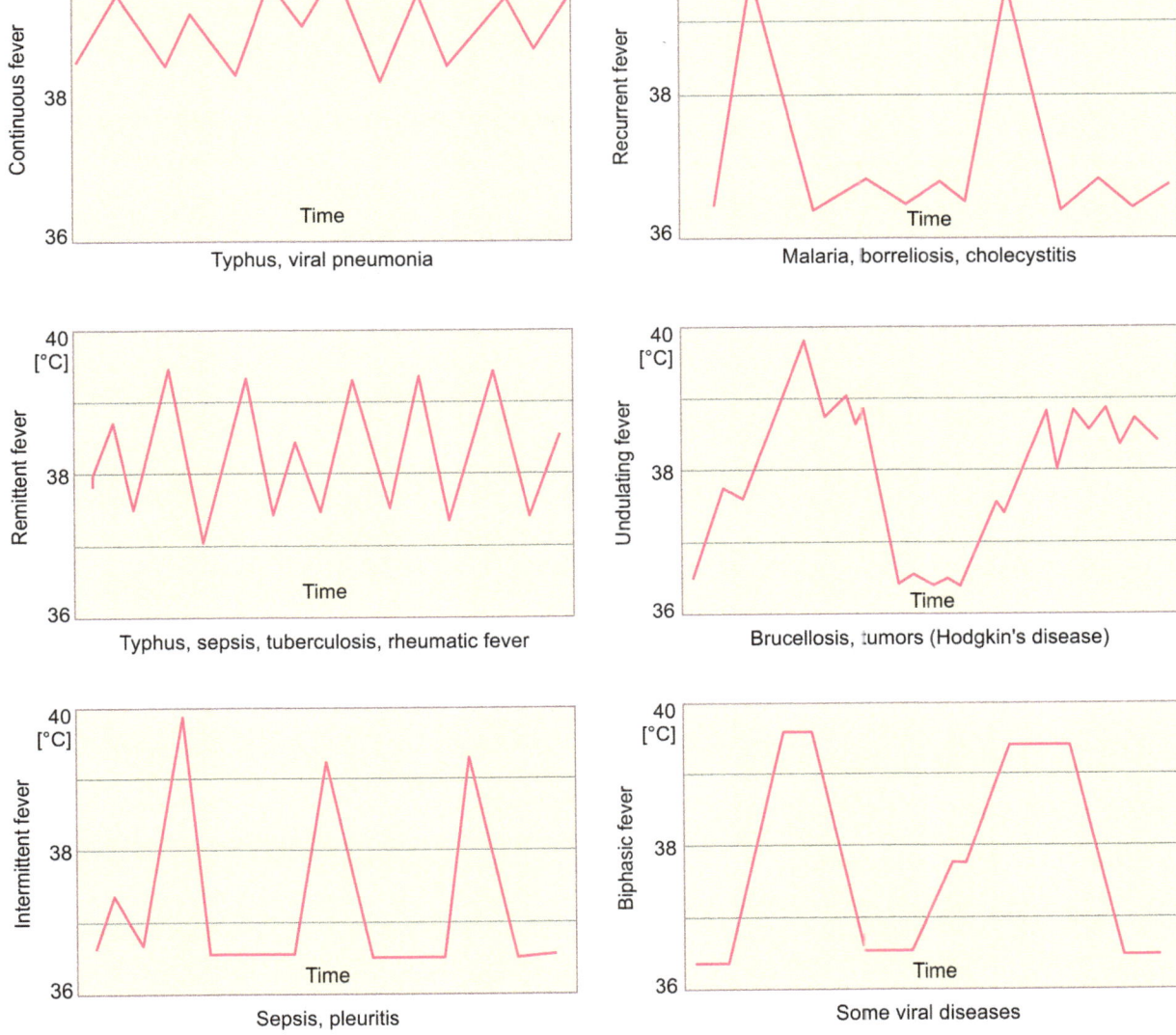

Fig. 2.32: Clinical pattern of fevers.

Hyperpyrexia:
(Body temperature >105°F)

Causes include:
- Pontine hemorrhage
- Rheumatic fever
- Meningococcal meningitis
- Cerebral malaria
- Septicemia
- Encephalitis
- Serotonin syndrome
- Thyroid storm
- Neuroleptic malignant syndrome

Aseptic fever:
- Malignancies
- Acute myocardial infarction
- Sarcoidosis
- Chronic renal failure
- Collagen vascular diseases
- Drug fever
- Radiation sickness
- Postsurgical patients

Drug fever:
It is a prolonged fever with relative bradycardia and hypotension. It persists 2–3 days even after drug is withdrawn and is associated with rash and eosinophilia, e.g., penicillin, procainamide, propylthiouracil, sulfonamides, anticonvulsant, etc.

Note: All drugs except digitalis can cause drug-induced fever.

Nature of defervescence:
The *nature of fever defervescence* may also provide some diagnostic clues.

Defervescence by crisis (Fig. 2.33)	Defervescence by lysis (Fig. 2.34)
Within hours	Gradually over days
Example: Effective antimalarial therapy leads to fever defervescence by crisis	*Example*: Typhoid fevers resolution occurs by lysis following effective antibiotics

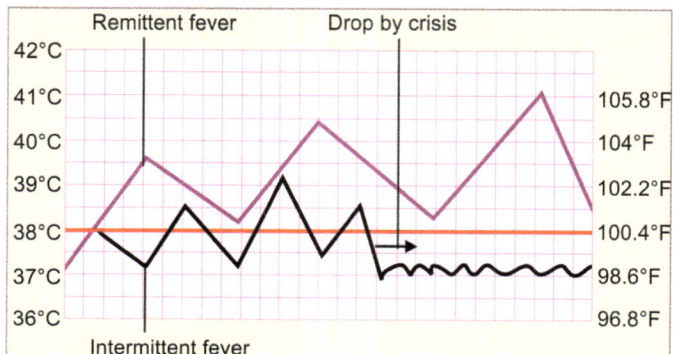

Fig. 2.33: Defervescence by crisis.

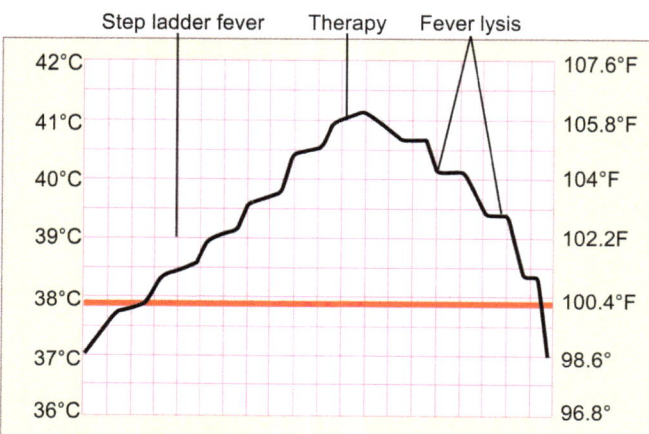

Fig. 2.34: Defervescence by lysis in typhoid fever.

Disorders of Increased Body Temperature

Hyperpyrexia	The body's temperature regulation mechanism sets the body temperature above the normal temperature then generates heat to achieve this temperature.
Hyperthermia	Unchanged (normothermic) setting of the thermoregulatory center in conjunction with an uncontrolled increase in body temperature that exceeds the body's ability to lose heat
Heat stroke	Acute condition of hyperthermia that is caused by prolonged exposure to excessive heat /± humidity. The heat-regulating mechanisms of the body eventually become overwhelmed and unable to effectively deal with the heat, causing the body temperature to climb uncontrollably.
Malignant hyperthermia	It occurs in individuals with an inherited abnormality of skeletal–muscle sarcoplasmic reticulum that causes a rapid increase in intracellular calcium levels in response to halothane and other inhalational anesthetics or to succinylcholine.
Neuroleptic malignant syndrome (NMS)	It is seen with neuroleptic use (antipsychotic phenothiazines, haloperidol, prochlorperazine, and metoclopramide) or the withdrawal of dopaminergic drugs characterized by "lead-pipe" muscle rigidity, extrapyramidal side effects, autonomic dysregulation, and hyperthermia.

Hypothermia

Hypothermia is defined as a core temperature below 35°C (95°F)	
Mild hypothermia	Core temperature 32–35°C (90–95°F)
Moderate hypothermia	Core temperature 28–32°C (82–90°F)
Severe hypothermia	Core temperature below 28°C (82°F)
Profound hypothermia	Core temperature <24°C (75°F) or <20°C (68°F)

Causes of hypothermia:

Decreased heat production:
- Hypopituitarism
- Hypoadrenalism
- Hypothyroidism

Increased heat loss:
- Burns
- Cold immersion injuries
- Vasodilatation from pharmacologic or toxicologic agents
- Cold infusions
- Overenthusiastic treatment of heat stroke

Impaired thermoregulation:
- Central nervous system (CNS) trauma
- Strokes
- Toxicologic and metabolic derangements
- Intracranial bleeding
- Parkinson disease
- CNS tumors
- Wernicke disease
- Multiple sclerosis

Miscellaneous causes:
- Sepsis
- Multiple trauma
- Pancreatitis
- Prolonged cardiac arrest
- Uremia

Named fevers	Disease/organism
Glandular fever	Infectious mononucleosis (EBV)
Pappataci, 3 day, sandfly fever	Phlebotomus fever
Goal fever	Rickettsia prowazekii
Malta, undulating fever	Brucellosis
Relapsing fever	Borrelia recurrentis (louse) B. duttoni (tick)
Rat bite fever	Spirillum minus Streptobacillus moniliformis
Trench or 5-day fever	Bartonella quintana
Oroya fever	Bartonella bacilliformis
Q fever	Coxiella burnetii
7-day fever	Leptospira hepdomadis
Pretibial fever	L. autumnale
Haverhill fever	Streptobacillus moniliformis
Pontiac fever	Legionella
Monkey fever	Kyasanur forest disease
Biphasic fever	• Dengue • Kala-azar • Chikungunya • Polio
Valley fever	Coccidioidomycosis
Dumdum/Burdwan fever	Kala-azar
Brazilian purpuric fever	H. aegypticus

PAIN: THE FIFTH VITAL SIGN

Pain is recognized as the fifth vital sign.

Assessment should include:
- Location
- Intensity
- Character/quality
- Frequency
- Duration
- Pattern

Standardized pain scale is used for assessment.

Location: Determine as precisely as possible where the pain is felt. Indicate, if the pain radiates or moves.

Intensity: A grade of how severe the pain is documented using a pain assessment tool, the resident finds easy to use, e.g., a numerical, verbal descriptor, faces, or behavioral.

Frequency:
- The occurrence of the pain
- How often the pain occurs?
- Is it breakthrough pain?

Quality: The qualities are aching, annoying, cramping, exhausting, nauseating, pounding, sharp, throbbing, stabbing, agonizing, blowing, dull, fearful, nagging, penetrating, quivering, shooting, suffocating, numbness, tingling, weakness, spasm, burning, gnawing, pressure, squeezing, radiating, tingling, touch sensitive, etc.
- *Pain behaviors:* Facial (wrinkled forehead, tightly closed eyes, grimacing, and frowning), nonverbal behavior (bracing, rubbing, and guarding), and vocalizations (crying, yelling, groaning, and moaning).

Nonverbal indicators of discomfort: These are aggressiveness, crying, fearful, noisy respirations, pacing, repetitive, restless, rocking, confusion, irritability, increased activity, withdrawal, tense, calling out, grunting, knees pulled up, other change in usual activities, or behavior patterns/routine.

Duration:
- How long the pain lasts (minutes or hours)?
- Sudden or gradual onset
- Is it consistent or persistent?
- Does it change over time or come and go (intermittent)? If intermittent—frequency, duration, and circumstances in which it occurs.

Pattern: How the pain starts, what was being done when it started, what makes it better, and what makes it worse.

Types of Pain

- **Somatic pain (bone and muscle) is:**
  - Relatively well localized
  - Worse on movement
  - Tender to pressure over the area
  - Often accompanied by a dull background aching pain
- **Visceral pain is:**
  - Often poorly localized, deep, and aching
  - Usually constant
  - Often referred (e.g., diaphragmatic irritation may be referred to the right shoulder; pelvic visceral pain is often referred to the sacral or perineal area)
- **Neuropathic pain is:**
  - A constant, superficial burning sensation or a deeply aching quality that may be accompanied by some sudden, sharp, shooting, and lancinating (stabbing) pain.
  - In a relatively constant area of the body surface (dermatome), if caused by actual damage to a specific peripheral nerve, plexus, root, or spinal cord.

Pain assessment model		
S	Site	Where exactly is the pain?
O	Onset	What were they doing when the pain started?
C	Character	What does the pain feel like?
R	Radiates	Does the pain go anywhere else?
A	Associated symptoms	For example, nausea vomiting
T	Time/duration	How long have they had the pain?
E	Exacerbating/relieving factors	Does anything make the pain better or worse?
S	Severity	Obtain an initial pain score

Pain assessment scales:
- Wong-Baker Faces scale
- Numerical rating scale (NRS)
- Visual analog scale (VAS)

PHYSICAL EXAMINATION

PALLOR

Definition
It is defined as paleness of skin and mucous membranes.

Sites of Examination
- Conjunctiva (**Fig. 2.35**)
- Tongue
- Oral mucosa
- Palmar crease (**Fig. 2.36**)
- Nail bed (Hb <8 g/dL)

Grading of Pallor

Mild	Moderate	Severe
Cannot be detected clinically	Clinically visible	Clinically visible plus one of the following features: 1. Palmar crease disappearance 2. Cervical venous hum (suggestive of chronic compensation)

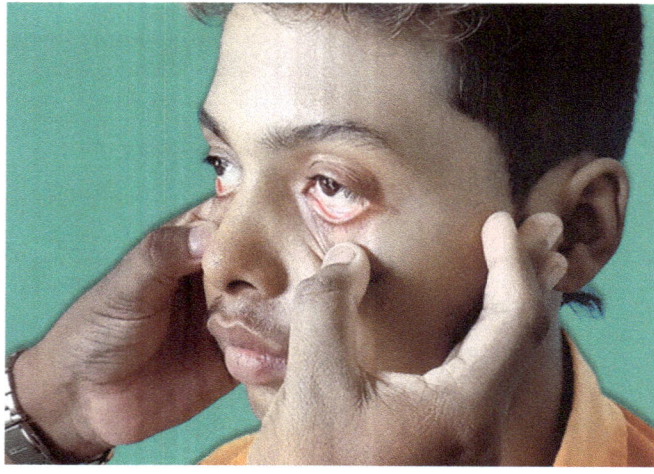

Fig. 2.35: Method of demonstration of pallor over conjunctiva.

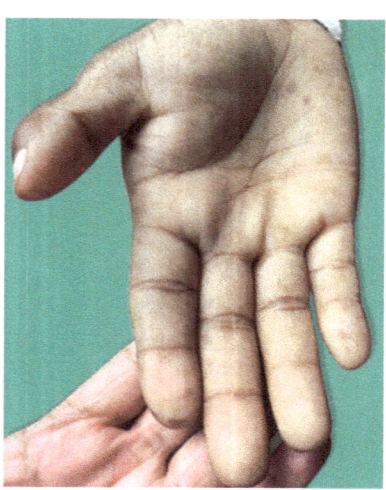

Fig. 2.36: Demonstration of pallor in hands.

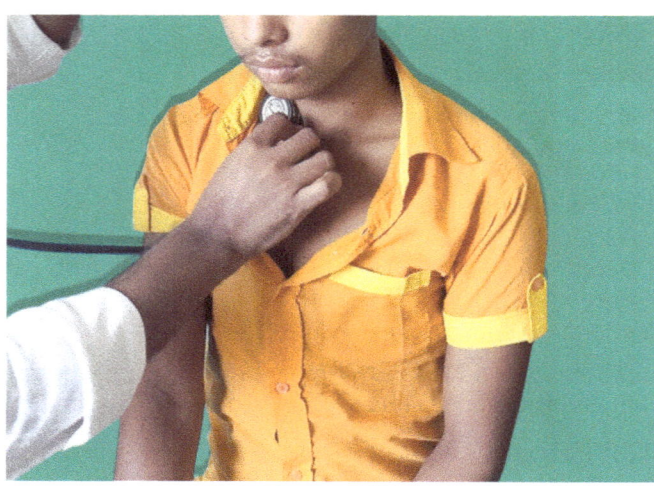

Fig. 2.37: Demonstration of cervical venous hum.

Method of Elicitation of Cervical Venous Hum (Fig. 2.37)
- Auscultate the root of the neck on the right side with bell of stethoscope, with patient in standing or sitting position.
- A continuous murmur will be heard.
- The cervical venous hum was first described by Pontain and hence called *Pontain's murmur.*
- The presence indicates chronic compensated severe anemia.

Conditions Causing Pallor without Anemia
- Hypopituitarism
- Hypothyroidism
- Hypogonadism
- Shock
- Left heart failure

Definition of Anemia
Anemia is defined as decrease in circulating red blood cell mass. It is characterized by decrease of hemoglobin concentration (Hb)/RBC count/hematocrit (PCV) below normal for the patient's age, sex, and altitude of residence.

Normal adult hemoglobin level is in the range of 13–17 g/dL in males and 12–15 g/dL in females.

Clues for Etiology of Anemia

Iron deficiency anemia:	
Specific symptoms	Pica, dysphagia, restless leg syndrome, and Malena
Specific sign	Bald tongue (**Fig. 2.38**) Koilonychia (**Fig. 2.39**) Blue sclera (**Fig. 2.40**)
Peripheral smear	Microcytic hypochromic red cells
Other specific investigation	Iron studies, BM staining for iron, stool/urine for occult blood, and endoscopy
Megaloblastic anemia:	
Specific symptoms	Tingling and numbness Sensory ataxia

Contd...

Contd...

Specific sign	Glossitis, knuckle pigmentation **(Fig. 2.41)**, absent DTRs, sensory loss, positive Romberg's test
Peripheral smear	Macrocytic RBCs, hypersegmented neutrophils, and pancytopenia
Other specific investigation	Serum vitamin B12 levels, red cell folate levels, bone marrow examination, and schilling's test
Anemia of chronic disease:	
Specific symptoms	Symptoms of chronic kidney, liver disease, and connective tissue disorders
Specific sign	Hypertension, AV fistula—CKD Signs of liver cell failure—CLD Signs of rheumatoid arthritis, SLE, etc.
Peripheral smear	Normocytic normochromic anemia ± pancytopenia
Other specific investigation	Renal function test, liver function tests, autoantibodies, and raised serum ferritin
Hemolytic anemia:	
Specific symptoms	History of associated jaundice, developmental delay, family history positivity, recurrent blood transfusions, and gallstones
Specific sign	Triad of anemia + jaundice + splenomegaly Hemolytic (Chipmunk) facies **(Fig. 2.42)** Hyperpigmentation **(Fig. 2.43)**, short stature, and leg ulcers
Peripheral smear	Microcytic hypochromic (thalassemia) Microspherocytes (hereditary spherocytosis) Sickle cells Reticulocytosis
Other specific investigation	Hemoglobin electrophoresis, Coombs test, sickling test, and osmotic fragility
Aplastic anemia:	
Specific symptoms	Recurrent infections Bleeding manifestations
Specific sign	Signs of pancytopenia No organomegaly
Peripheral smear	Pancytopenia
Other specific investigation	Bone marrow examination Cytogenetics

(BM: bone marrow; CKD: chronic kidney disease; CLD: chronic liver disease; DTR: deep tendon reflex; SLE: systemic lupus erythematosus)

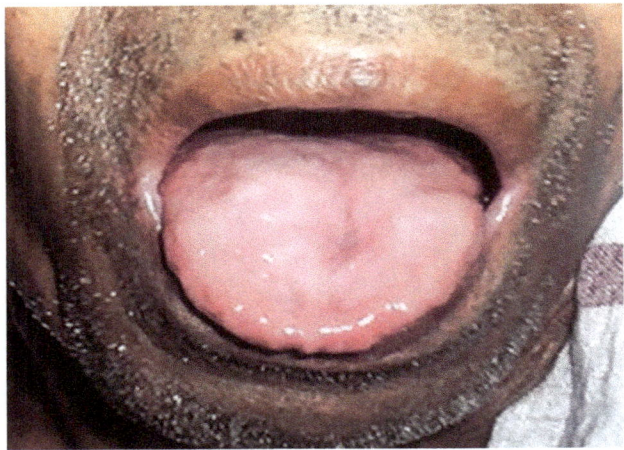

Fig. 2.38: Bald tongue.

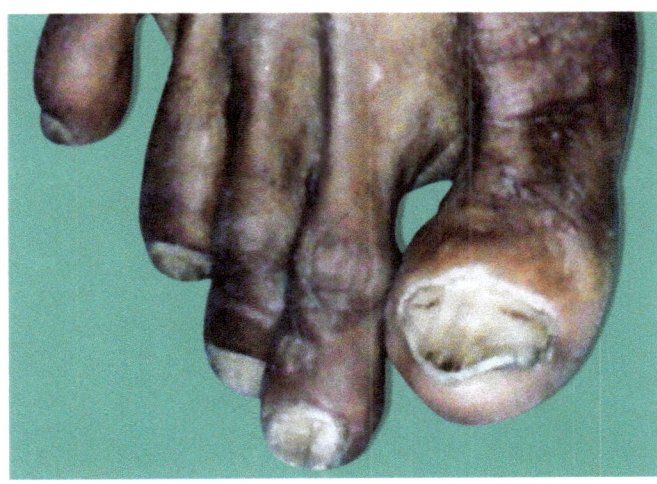

Fig. 2.39: Koilonychia.

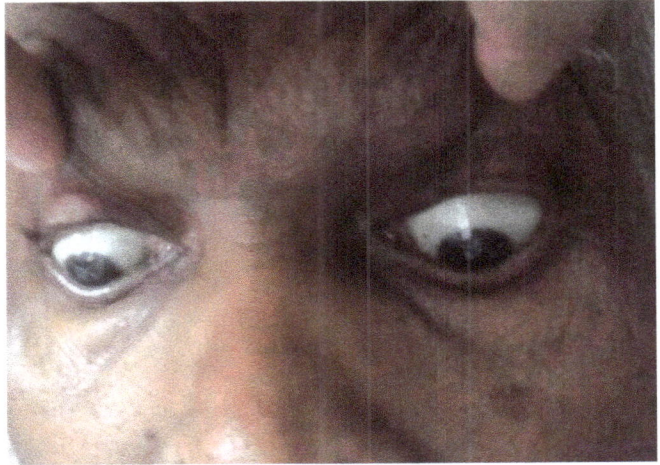

Fig. 2.40: Blue sclera.

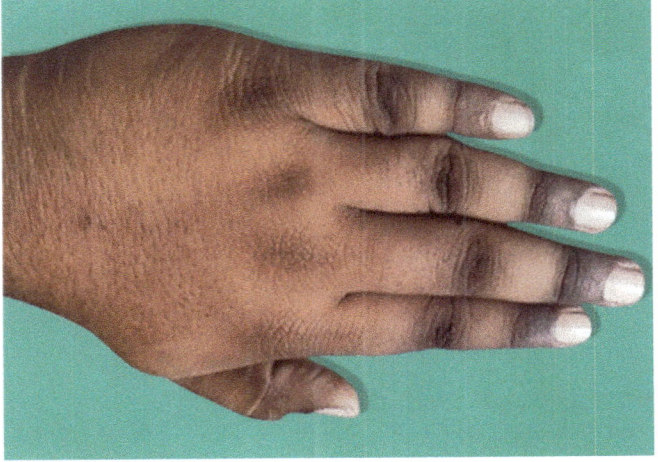

Fig. 2.41: Knuckle pigmentation.

ICTERUS

Definition

It is defined as yellowish discoloration of skin, mucous membranes, sclera, and blood vessels secondary to increased bilirubin (bile pigments have affinity to elastin tissue).

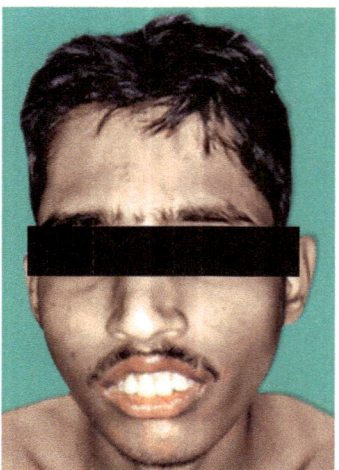

Fig. 2.42: Chipmunk facies.

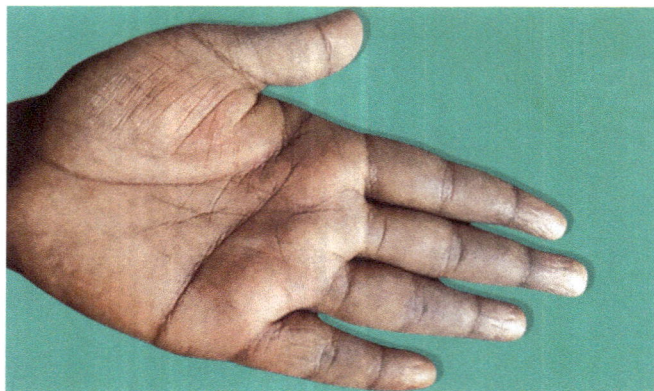

Fig. 2.43: Hyperpigmentation of palm.

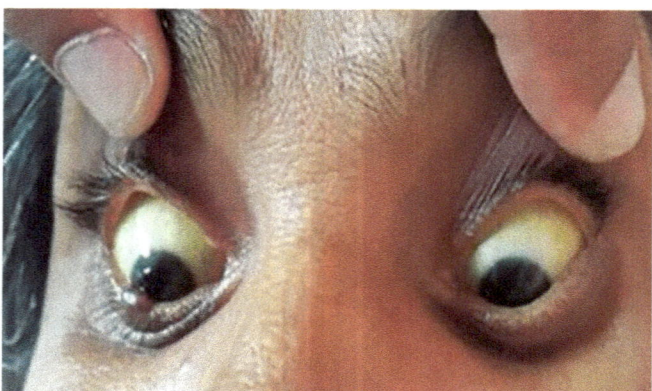

Fig. 2.44: Demonstration of icterus.

Sites to Look for Jaundice
- Sclera (**Fig. 2.44**)
- Sublingual mucosa
- Oral cavity
- Palms and soles
- Skin

Scleral icterus is a term commonly used, but from a histopathologic perspective, it is a misnomer. Bilirubin has a high affinity for elastin, which is an abundant protein in the conjunctivae as well as the superficial, fibrovascular episclerae, but not the sclerae proper. One actually is observing icterus of the bulbar conjunctiva against the white background provided by sclera. Conjunctival icterus is often the first sign of hyperbilirubinemia. Hence, we recommend for the use of term "conjunctival icterus" instead of "scleral icterus".

Why unexposed sclera/conjunctiva seen?
- Since the exposed part of sclera/conjunctiva is exposed to sunlight, bilirubin gets converted to soluble form and hence exposed part of conjunctiva may not reveal mild jaundice.
- Yellowish discoloration is seen some times in the exposed sclera/conjunctiva normally also and it is called as muddy conjunctiva.

Serum Bilirubin Levels and Jaundice

0.3–1.2 mg/dL	Normal
1.2–2.5 mg/dL	Latent jaundice (generally not appreciated on clinical examination)
>2.5 mg/dL	Clinically appreciated

Yellowish Discoloration without Jaundice
- Hypercarotenemia (here sclera is not affected)
- Hypothyroidism (due to decrease metabolism of carotene)
- Excessive exposure to phenols/nitric acid
- Quinacrine intake

Differentiating Type of Jaundice Based on Scleral Color

Lemon yellow	Most likely hemolytic jaundice
Dark yellow (**Fig. 2.45**)	Obstructive jaundice
Greenish dark yellow	Long-standing obstructive jaundice due to oxidation of bilirubin to biliverdin

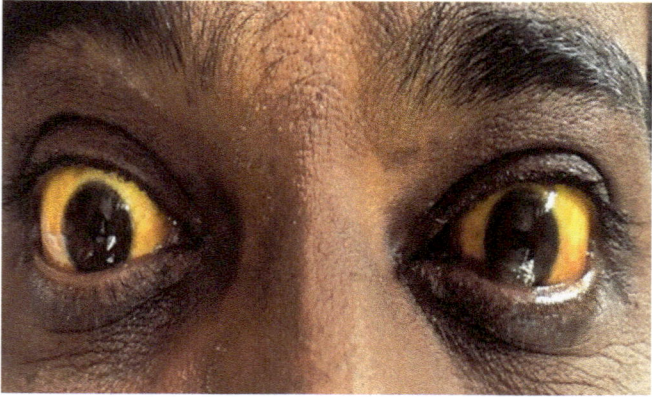

Fig. 2.45: Dark yellow icterus.

Differentiating Jaundice based on Clinical and Laboratory Findings

	Prehepatic (hemolytic)	Hepatic	Posthepatic (obstructive/surgical)
History:			
Urine	Normal	Yellow	Yellow
Stools	Normal	Normal	Pale Clay like
Pruritus	-	±	++
Examination:			
Bradycardia	-	-	+
Pallor	Present	Absent	Absent
Jaundice	Mild	Moderate	Severe
Splenomegaly	Present	Variable	Absent
Palpable gall bladder	±	-	++
Features of liver cell failure	Absent	+ (Early feature)	± (Late feature)
Laboratory data:			
Serum bilirubin	UCB↑	UCB↑ + CB↑	CB↑
Serum enzymes	LDH↑	AST↑ ALT↑	ALP↑
Urine bilirubin	-	+	+
Urine urobilinogen	+	+	-
Examples:			
Examples	Thalassemia Sickle cell anemia Spherocytosis Malaria Immune hemolytic anemias	Hepatitis (viral/alcoholic/drug induced) Infiltrative disorders Ischemic hepatitis	CBD stones Helminths in the CBD Carcinoma—head of pancreas Primary biliary cirrhosis Primary sclerosing cholangitis

(ALT: alanine transaminase; ALP: alkaline phosphatase; AST: aspartate aminotransferase; UCB: unconjugated bilirubin; CB: conjugated bilirubin; LDH: lactate dehydrogenase)

CYANOSIS

Definition
It is defined as bluish color of skin and mucous membranes resulting from an increased quantity of reduced hemoglobin (deoxygenated) or hemoglobin derivatives (methemoglobin or sulfhemoglobin) in the small vessels of those tissues.

Criteria
Deoxyhemoglobin >5 g% or abnormal Hb (methemoglobin or sulfhemoglobin) ± oxygen saturation (SaO_2) <85%

Classification
- **True cyanosis:**
  - Central cyanosis
  - Peripheral cyanosis
  - Mixed cyanosis
- **Pseudocyanosis**

Etiology of Cyanosis

True cyanosis	
Central cyanosis:	
Cardiac:	**Cyanotic heart diseases:**
T	• Truncus arteriosus
T	• Transposition of great arteries
T	• TAPVC
T	• Tetralogy of Fallot
T	• Tricuspid atresia
E	• Ebstein's anamoly
E	• Eisenmengerization (*tardive cyanosis*)
Pulmonary	• Asthma • COPD • Cor pulmonale • Respiratory failure of any cause, such as pneumonia, tension pneumothorax, massive pleural effusion, and acute pulmonary edema

Others	• High altitude
	• Polycythemia
	• *Enterogenous or pigment cyanosis (replacement cyanosis):*
	  ▪ Methemoglobinemia (>1.5 g/dL)
	  ▪ Sulfhemoglobinemia (>0.5 g/dL)
	• Carboxyhemoglobin (produces cherry red discoloration)

Peripheral cyanosis:	
• Low cardiac output • Local vasoconstriction (cold, frostbite, and Raynaud's phenomenon) • Arterial obstruction • Venous obstruction • Hyperviscosity conditions (multiple myeloma and polycythemia) • Cryoglobulinemia	
Mixed cyanosis:	
• Left ventricular failure (has both central and peripheral cyanosis)	
Pseudocyanosis:	

• **Metals:**
  ▪ Gold
  ▪ Silver
  ▪ Mercury
  ▪ Arsenic
• **Drugs:**
  ▪ Minocycline
  ▪ Chloroquine
  ▪ Amiodarone	

(COPD: chronic obstructive pulmonary disease; TAPVC: total anomalous pulmonary venous connection)

Chapter 2: Vital Signs and General Physical Examination

Atypical presentation of cyanosis		
	Description	Example
Differential cyanosis	Cyanosis is seen in only lower limbs	PDA with eisenmengerization
Reverse differential cyanosis	Cyanosis is seen in only upper limbs	PDA with eisenmengerization and transposition of great arteries
Cyanosis absent despite of sufficient reduced hemoglobin		In severe anemia, carbon monoxide poisoning

Differences between Central and Peripheral Cyanosis

Central cyanosis	Peripheral cyanosis
It is due to inadequate oxygenation of systemic circulation	It is due to sluggish peripheral circulation
It is an hypoxic hypoxia	It is a stagnant hypoxia
Site of examination: • Tongue (Fig. 2.46) • Oral mucosa (Fig. 2.47)	Site of examination: • Tip of nose • Ear lobule • Outer lips • Finger tips • Nail bed • Extremities
Extremities are warm	Extremities are cold
Does not improve on rewarming	Improves on rewarming
SpO_2: <85%	SpO_2: >85%
Improves on oxygenation	Does not improve with oxygenation
Dyspnea and high volume pulse seen	Usually absent
Exercise may worsen	Exercise may improve
May be associated with clubbing and polycythemia	

(PaO_2: partial pressure of oxygen)

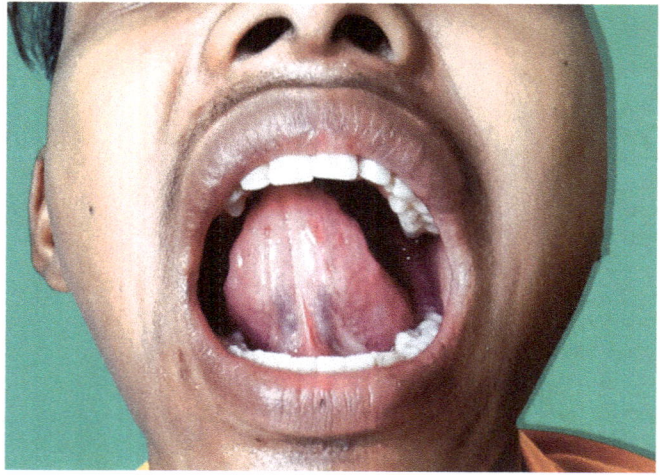

Fig. 2.46: Demonstration of central cyanosis.
(In this patient, mucosa is pink and lingual veins are clearly demarkable—which is normal.)

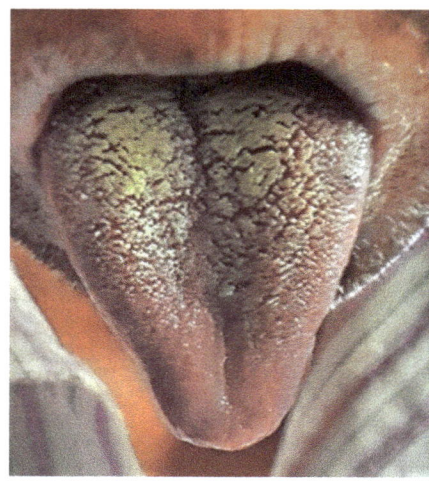

Fig. 2.47: Bluish discoloration of tongue and oral mucosa suggestive of central cyanosis.

Note: Cyanosis is best appreciated in areas of the body where the overlying epidermis is thin and the blood vessel supply abundant, such as the lips, malar prominences (nose and cheeks), ears, and oral mucous membranes (buccal and sublingual); it is better appreciated in fluorescent lighting.

Hyperoxia Test (Cardiac versus Pulmonary Cyanosis)

After giving 100% oxygen for 10 minutes, a repeat arterial blood gas (ABG) is done and if partial pressure of oxygen (PaO_2) is <150 mm Hg then the cause is cardiac and if the PaO_2 improves to >200 mm Hg, the cause is respiratory.

CLUBBING (HIPPOCRATES FINGERS)

Definition

It is defined as selective bulbous enlargement of distal segment of digits with subsequent loss of normal angle between the nail and nail bed.

Theories of Clubbing

PDGF (role of platelet)	The megakaryocytes preferably lodge in the tips of the digits and locally release platelet-derived growth factor (PDGF) and vascular endothelial growth factor (VEGF). These growth factors along with other mediators increase endothelial permeability and activate and cause proliferation of connective tissue cells (e.g., fibroblasts).
Neurogenic	Persistent vagal stimulation causes vasodilation and clubbing (e.g., lung carcinoma)
Hypoxic	Causes opening of deep arteriovenous fistula in fingers (e.g., tetralogy of Fallot)
Ferritin Prostaglandins Bradykinin Adenine nucleotides 5-hydroxytryptamine	Circulating vasodilators, which are usually inactivated as blood passes through the lungs, bypass the inactivation process in the patients with right to left shunts

Grading

Grades of clubbing (Figs. 2.48 to 2.53):	
Grade 1	Increased fluctuation of nail bed
Grade 2	Loss of Lovibond angle/onychonychial angle (normal is <180°) Profile sign Schamroth sign
Grade 3	Parrot beaking Drumstick fingers (seen in severe cyanotic heart disease, bronchiectasis, and empyema)
Grade 4	Pain along the distal ends of long bone due to subperiosteal new bone formation Condition seen generally seen with bronchogenic carcinoma

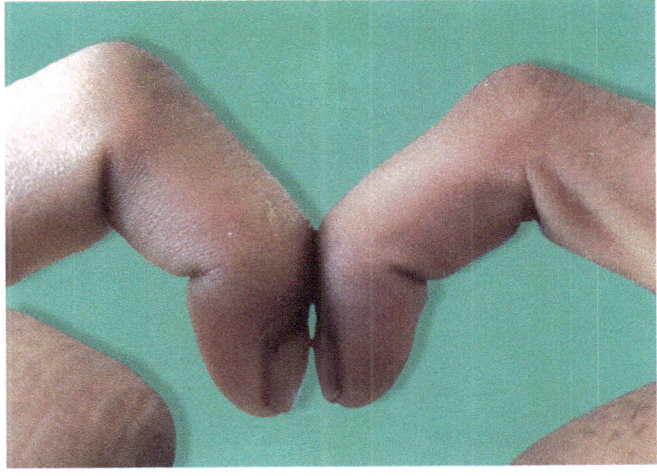

Fig. 2.50: Demonstration of Schamroth's sign.

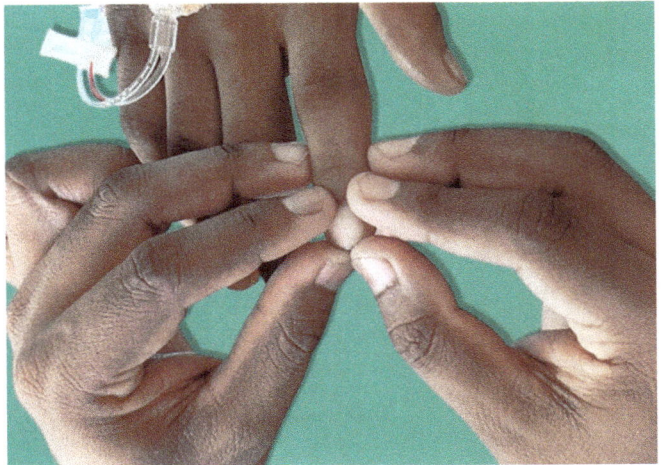

Fig. 2.48: Demonstration of Grade 1 clubbing.

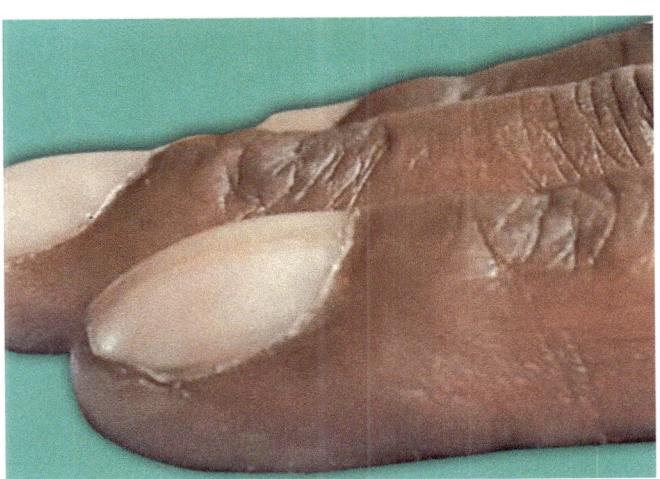

Fig. 2.51: Demonstration of Grade 3 clubbing.

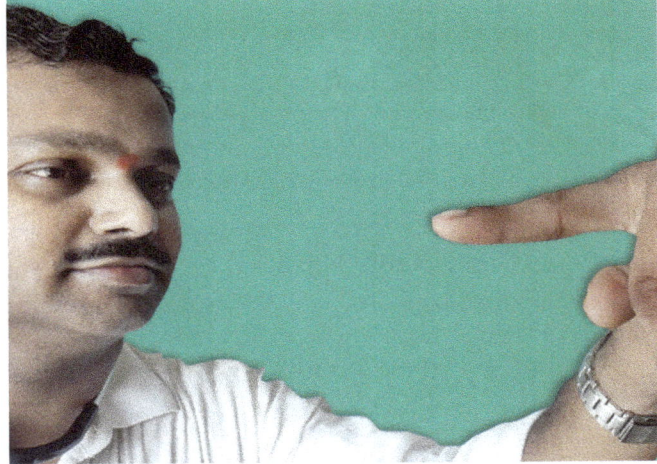

Fig. 2.49: Demonstration of profile sign.

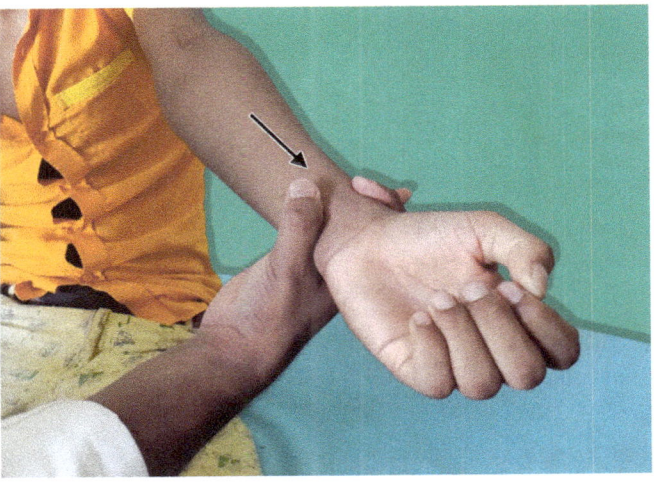

Fig. 2.52: Demonstration of Grade 4 clubbing.

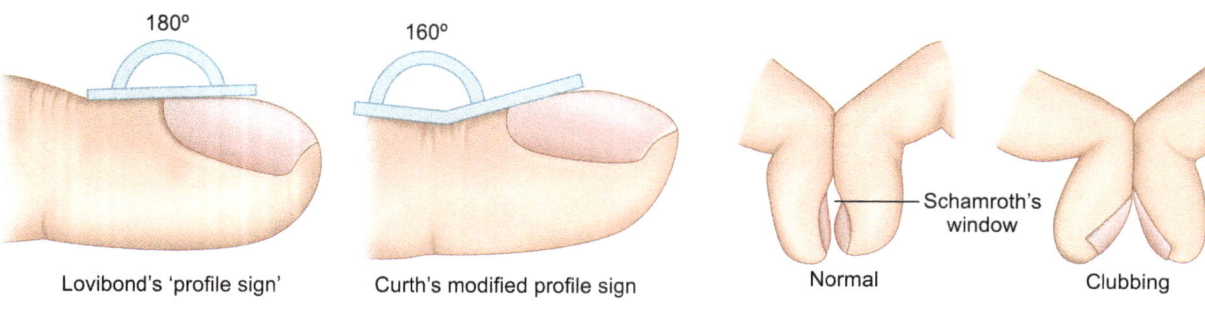

Fig. 2.53: Image depicting profile sign and Schamroth's sign.

Causes of Clubbing

Respiratory causes	
Malignancies	Bronchogenic carcinoma Mesothelioma
Suppurative diseases	Bronchiectasis Lung abscess Empyema
Interstitial lung diseases	
Tuberculosis	Seen in 30% cases as a sequela to complications
Sarcoidosis	Can be seen
COPD	Never

Cardiac causes
Subacute bacterial endocarditis Atrial myxoma Cyanotic heart disease Acyanotic heart disease with eisenmengerization

Gastrointestinal causes
Inflammatory bowel disease: • Ulcerative colitis • Crohn's disease Primary biliary cirrhosis Hepatocellular carcinoma

Neurological causes
• Syringomyelia • Median nerve injury • Hemiplegia

Miscellaneous
• Pachydermoperiostosis (pan digital hereditary clubbing) • Touraine–Solente–Gole syndrome

Atypical presentation of clubbing	
Acute clubbing	• Subacute bacterial endocarditis • Lung abscess • Empyema

Atypical presentation of clubbing	
Unilateral clubbing	• Hemiplegia • Aneurysm of subclavian artery • Pancoast tumor
Pseudoclubbing	• Leprosy • Leukemia infiltration • Hyperparathyroidism • Thyroid acropachy • Sclerodactyly • Exposure to vinyl chloride • Subungual tumor or cyst
Painful clubbing	• Bronchogenic carcinoma • Subacute bacterial endocarditis • Lung abscess
Reversible clubbing	• Lung abscess • Empyema
Unidigital clubbing	• Median nerve injury • Trauma
Clubbing with cyanosis	• Cyanotic congenital heart diseases • ILD
Differential clubbing: • Upper limb (N) • Lower limb (clubbing)	• PDA with reversal of shunt
Reverse differential clubbing: • Upper limb (clubbing) • Lower limb (N)	• PDA + TGA + reversal of shunt

(ILD: interstitial lung disease; PDA: patent ductus arteriosus; TGA: transposition of the great arteries)

Phalangeal Depth Ratio (Fig. 2.54)

☐ Ratio of distal phalangeal depth (DPD) with interphalangeal depth (IPD)
☐ <1 is normal and >1 is suggestive of clubbing.

Digital Index

☐ It is sum of phalangeal depth ratio of 10 fingers.
☐ A digital index of 10.2 or higher is indicative of clubbing. Although a phalangeal depth ratio of 1.0 or greater in any finger is suggestive of clubbing, digital index is more specific for clubbing.

Chapter 2: Vital Signs and General Physical Examination

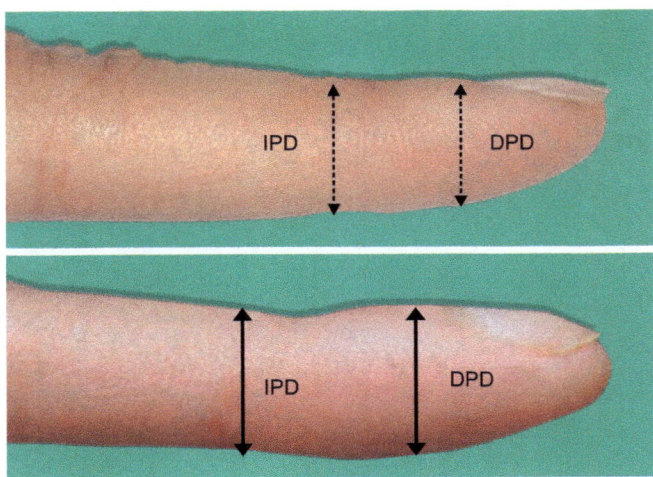

Fig. 2.54: Picture depicting the phalangeal depth at proximal and distal interphalangeal joints.

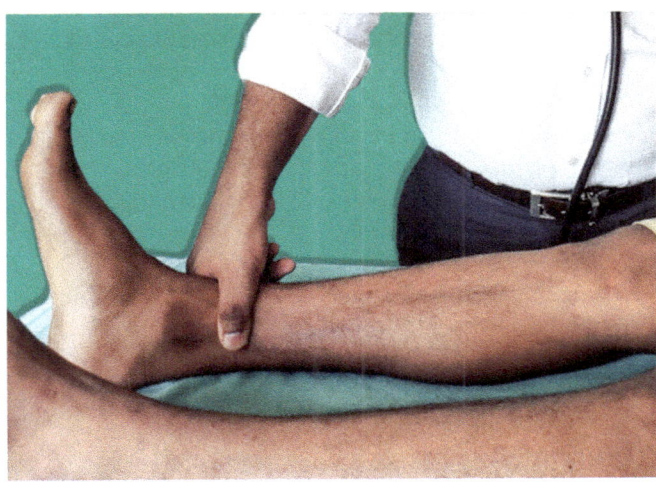

Fig. 2.55: Method of eliciting pedal edema.

Other Nail Changes

Nail changes	Causes
Koilonychia	• IDA • Hemochromatosis
Beaus lines	• Measles • Pneumonia • Pulmonary infarction
Plummer nails	Rat bitten nail
Red nails	CCF
Blue nails	Copper or silver deposit
Black nails	• Peutz–Jeghers syndrome • Cushing's disease • Addison's disease
White nails	• Anemia • Hypoalbuminemia • DM • CCF • Rheumatoid arthritis

(IDA: iron deficiency anemia; CCF: congestive cardiac failure)

EDEMA

Definition
It is defined as abnormal accumulation of fluid in interstitium.

Sites of Examination of Edema

In mobile patient	• Legs 2–3 cm above the medial malleolus
In bed-ridden supine patient	• Sacrum • Back over the scapula
To check for abdominal wall edema	• Pinch the skin over the abdomen

Technique (Fig. 2.55)
Press the skin and subcutaneous tissue for at least 15–20 seconds against bony prominence except for checking abdominal wall edema (where we pinch the skin and subcutaneous tissue).

Grading of Pitting Edema (Fig. 2.56)

1+	2-mm depression, immediate rebound
2+	4-mm deep pit, a few seconds to rebound
3+	6-mm deep pit, 10–12 seconds to rebound
4+	8-mm deep pit, >20 seconds to rebound

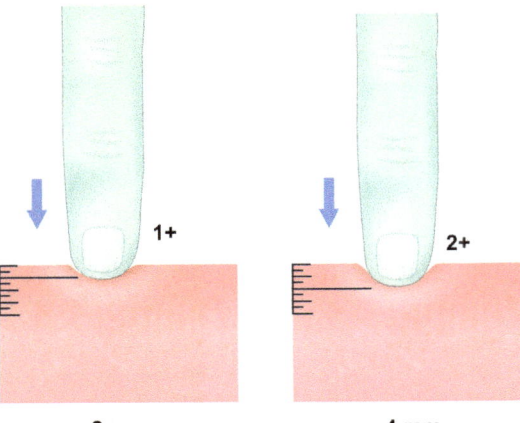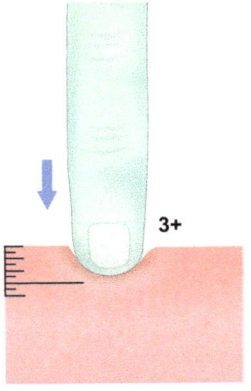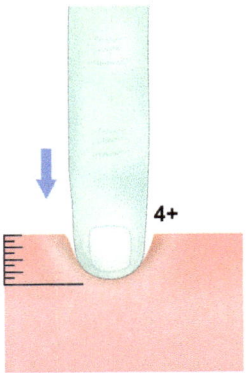

Fig. 2.56: Grading of pitting edema.

Edema:		
Pitting		**Nonpitting (Brawny edema)**
Rapid recovery	*Slow recovery*	Does not pit or recover in few seconds
Recovers in <40 seconds	Recovery takes >40 seconds	Nontender Skin shows hyperkeratosis
Mechanism: ↓Oncotic pressure	Mechanism: ↑Hydrostatic pressure	Mechanism: Lymphedema
Low serum protein	(N) Serum protein	Lymphatic obstruction
Causes: Increased protein loss: • Burns • Nephrotic • Bowel disease *Decreased intake or synthesis:* • Kwashiorkor • Malabsorption • Liver disease	*Causes: Systemic venous HTN:* • CHF **(Fig. 2.57)** • Pericarditis • Tricuspid valve diseases *Local venous HTN:* • DVT • Inferior venacaval syndrome	*Causes:* Myxedema **(Fig. 2.58)**—hypothyroidism *Pretibial myxedema*—Graves's disease *Upper limb:* • Breast cancer • Radiation induced *Lower limb:* • Aplasia cutis • Congenital (praecox, tarda, Milroy's disease, and Meigs' disease) • Filariasis **(Fig. 2.59)** • Recurred streptococcal infection • Malignancies

Facial edema: Trichinosis, hypothyroidism, allergies, nephrotic syndrome, and angioedema (Quincke's edema)
Pretibial myxedema: Grave's thyrotoxicosis
Neurogenic edema: Secondary to autonomic dysfunction
Drug-induced edema: Nifedipine, corticosteroids, estrogen, NSAIDs, and insulin
- *May–Thurner syndrome*: Chronic, unilateral, and pitting edema due to left iliac vein is compressed by the right iliac artery
- *Idiopathic edema*: Chronic, bilateral, and pitting
  - In females <50 years of age, more during menstrual cycles

(HTN: hypertension; DVT: deep vein thrombosis; NSAID: nonsteroidal anti-inflammatory drugs)

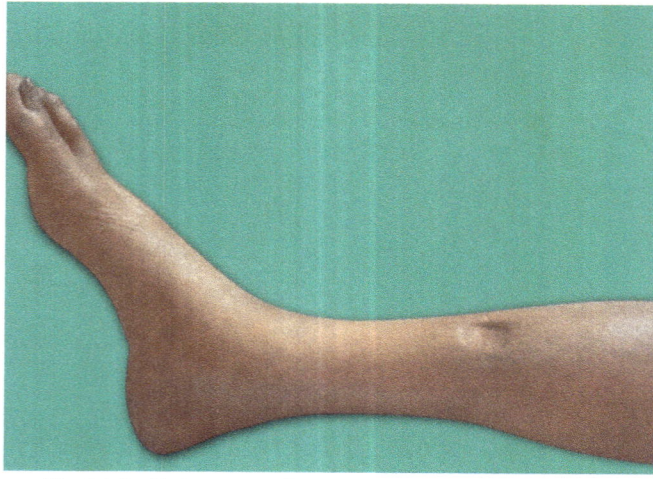

Fig. 2.57: Pitting type of pedal edema seen in congestive cardiac failure.

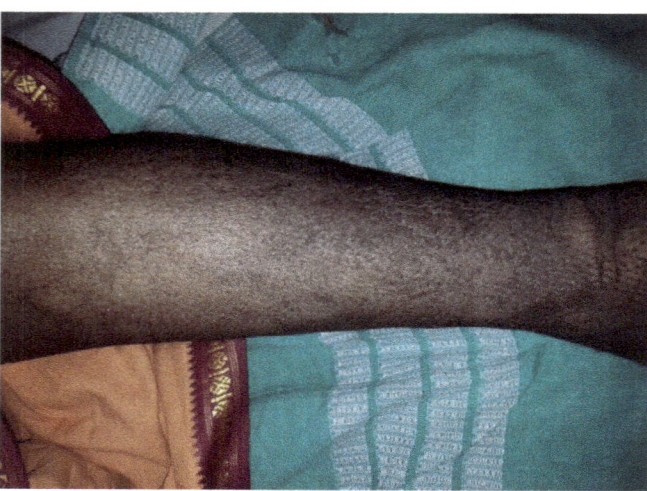

Fig. 2.58: Nonpitting type of pedal edema seen in myxedema.

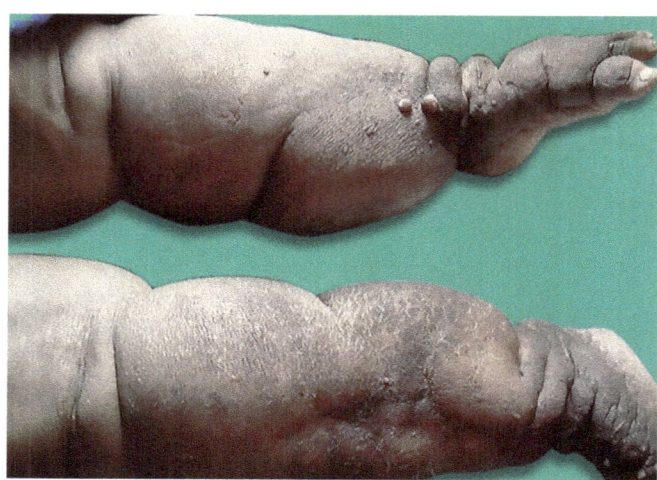

Fig. 2.59: Nonpitting type of pedal edema seen in filariasis.

LYMPHADENOPATHY

Definitions

Generalized Lymphadenopathy

Two or more noncontinuous groups of significant lymph node involvement. (Examples of significant lymphadenopathy are given in the below table.)

Significant Lymphadenopathy

Size >2 cm in	Inguinal region
Size >1 cm in	Extrainguinal region
Any size	• Supraclavicular • Epitrochlear • Popliteal • Any lymph node in draining area
Based on fixity	• Fixed to each other (matting) • Fixed to underlying tissues • Fixed to skin
Based on consistency	• Hard/firm lymph nodes

Persistent Generalized Lymphadenopathy

It is defined as lymph nodes of more than 1 cm in size, in 2 or more areas persisting for 3 or more months (mnemonic **1-2-3**). It is commonly seen in HIV/AIDS.

Causes of Generalized Lymphadenopathy

Infections	Bacterial	• Disseminated TB • Secondary syphilis
	Viral	• HIV • Infectious mononucleosis
	Parasitic	• Toxoplasmosis
	Fungal	• Histoplasmosis • Coccidioidomycosis • Paracoccidioidomycosis
Malignancy		• Lymphomas • Acute leukemias • CLL • CML (in blast crisis)
Immunological		• SLE • Adult onset still disease • JRA • Sjogren's disease • Kawasaki disease • Serum sickness (postzone phenomenon—excess of antibody)
Granulomatous		• Sarcoid • Amyloidosis • Histiocytosis X
Endocrine		• Hyperthyroidism
Drugs		• Phenytoin (pseudolymphoma) • Primidone • Carbamazepine • Allopurinol • Captopril • Bactrim DS • Sulindac (NSAIDS) • Hydralazine • Beta-blockers
Syndromic lymphadenopathy		• Kikuchi–Fujimoto disease • Castleman disease • Kimura disease • Rosai–Dorfman syndrome • Familial Mediterranean fever
Miscellaneous		• Niemann–Pick disease

(TB: tuberculosis; CLL: chronic lymphocytic leukemia; CML: chronic myeloid leukemia; SLE: systemic lupus erythematosus; JRA: juvenile rheumatoid arthritis)

Describing a Lymph Node

- Size (significant or not)
- Site
- Number
- Consistency
- Overlying skin
- Mobility
- Tenderness
- Draining area

Consistency:

Soft	Normal consistency
Hard	Malignancy
Indian rubber	Hodgkin's lymphoma
Shotty lymph node (discrete shots of gun)	Syphilis
Bubo (large LN with central necrosis)	Lymphogranuloma venereum
Matted	Tuberculosis due to periadenitis
Hard LN in tuberculosis	Hyperplastic tuberculosis lymphadenopathy

(LN: lymph node)

Different Group of Lymph Nodes (Fig. 2.60)

Cervical Lymph Node

This is divided into:
- Superficial or deep (based on whether above or below deep cervical fascia)
- Vertical or horizontal

Superficial Cervical Lymph Nodes

- They are superficial to deep cervical fascia
- These include:
  - External Waldeyer's ring:
    - Submental
    - Submandibular (B/L)
    - Preauricular (B/L)
    - Postauricular (B/L)
    - Occipital lymph nodes
  - Pretracheal
  - Paratracheal
  - Post-triangle lymph nodes

Deep Cervical Lymph Nodes

- **Horizontal:** Supraclavicular lymph nodes
- **Vertical:** Jugulodigastric and jugulo-omohyoid lymph nodes

Examination of Cervical Lymph Nodes

- *Examination of anterior group* of lymph nodes is done by standing behind the patient → flex the neck to relax the fascia → first feel for the submental group (using a single finger) **(Fig. 2.61)** and then → bilateral submandibular **(Fig. 2.62)** → bilateral preauricular **(Fig. 2.63)** → jugulodigastric **(Fig. 2.64)** → jugulo-omohyoid **(Fig. 2.65)** → supraclavicular groups **(Fig. 2.66)** (± pre- and paratracheal)
- **Examination of posterior group** of lymph nodes is done by standing in front of the patient → feel for the postauricular **(Fig. 2.67)** → occipital **(Fig. 2.68)** → posterior triangle group of lymph nodes **(Fig. 2.69)**

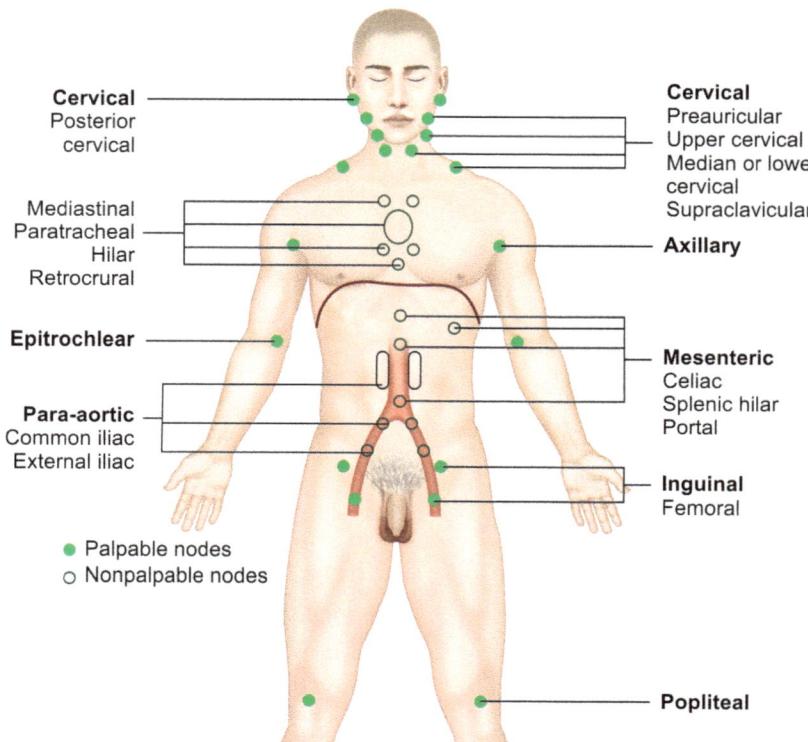

Fig. 2.60: Image showing different groups of lymph nodes.

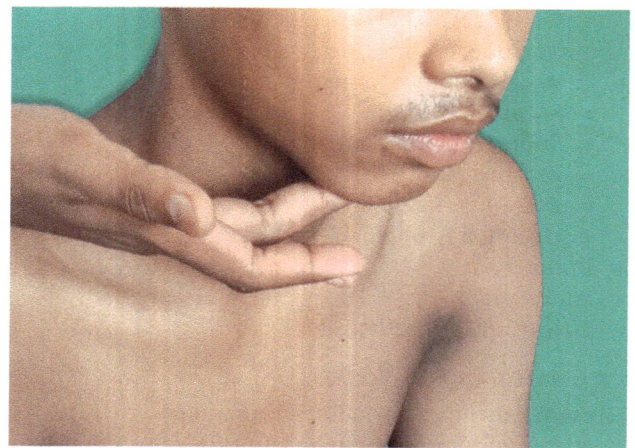

Fig. 2.61: Method of examining submental group of lymph node.

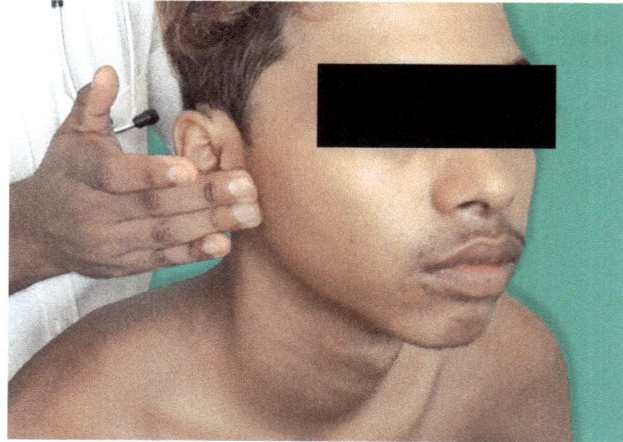

Fig. 2.63: Method of examining preauricular lymph nodes.

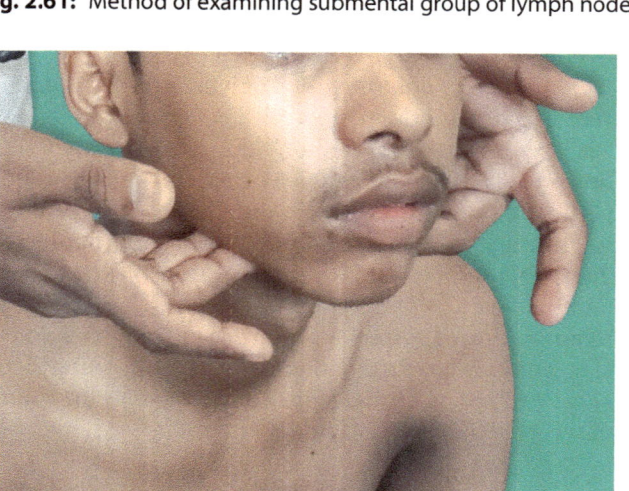

Fig. 2.62: Method of examining submandibular lymph nodes.

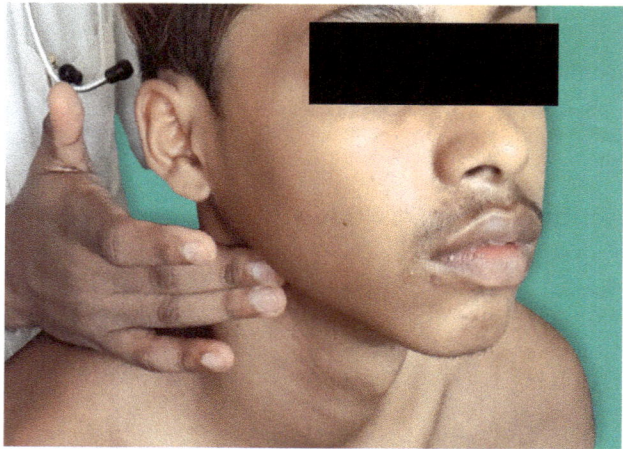

Fig. 2.64: Method of examining jugulodigastric lymph nodes.

Chapter 2: Vital Signs and General Physical Examination

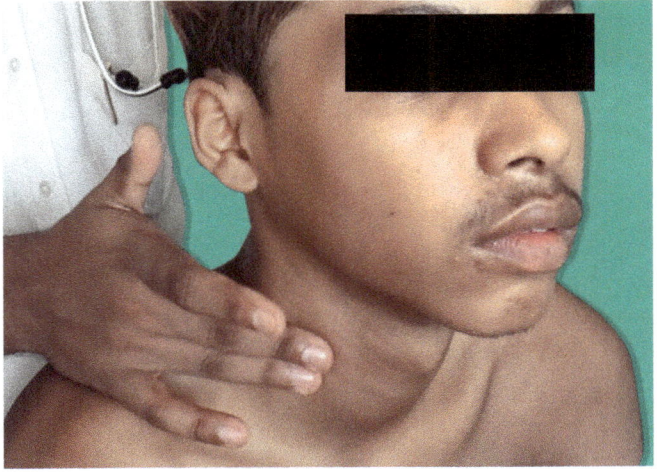

Fig. 2.65: Method of examining jugulo-omohyoid lymph nodes.

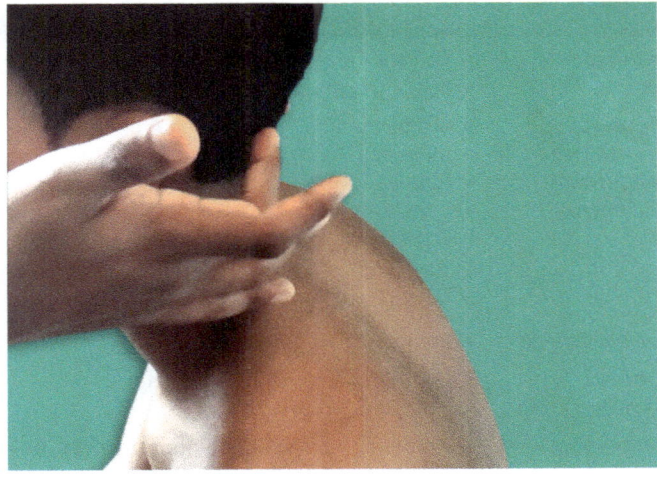

Fig. 2.68: Method of examining occipital lymph nodes.

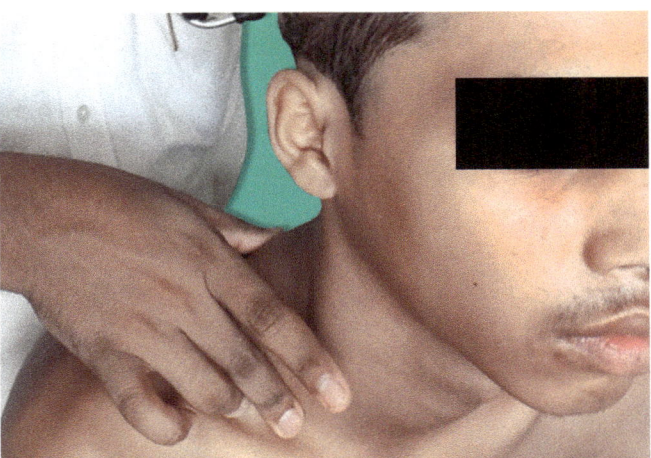

Fig. 2.66: Method of examining supraclavicular lymph nodes.

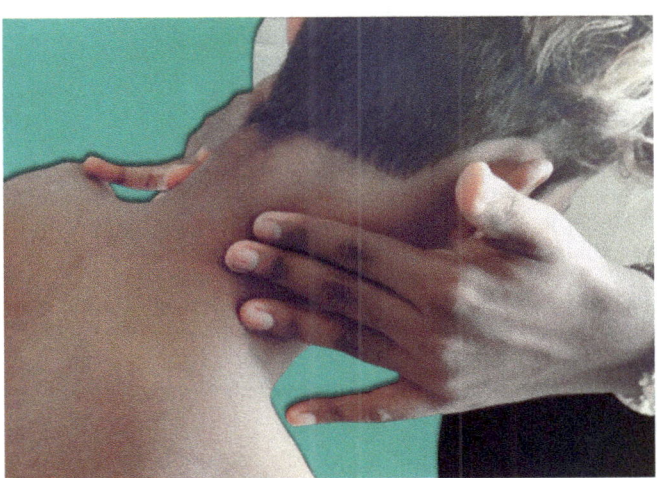

Fig. 2.69: Method of examining posterior triangle lymph nodes.

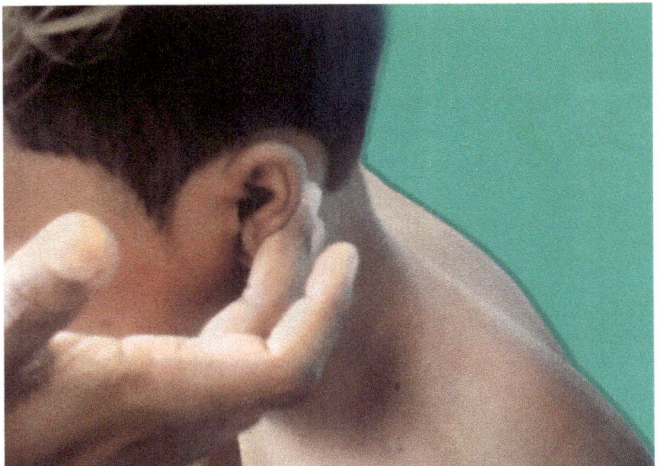

Fig. 2.67: Method of examining postauricular lymph nodes.

Supraclavicular Lymph Nodes and Drainage

Right supraclavicular	Left supraclavicular
Right lung (all three lobes) Left lung lower lobe	Left lung upper lobe
	1. Breast 2. Bronchus 3. Bowel 4. Bladder 5. Gonads (testis/ovaries)

Other named lymph nodes	
Virchow node	*Left supraclavicular node*
Scalene node (Fig. 2.70)	• Sentinel node of bronchogenic carcinoma • Relax neck • Palpate (deep) between the two heads of SCM

Other named lymph nodes	
Winterbottom sign	• Posterior triangle lymph node enlargement • Seen in early phase of African trypanosomiasis
Causes of posterior triangle lymph node enlargement	• Scalp infection • Measles • Rubella • Infectious mononucleosis • Trypanosomiasis
Node of woods	• Jugulodigastric lymph node enlargement seen in TB when spread via tonsils
Delphian node	• Pretracheal node
External Waldeyer's ring	• Commonly seen to be enlarged in non-Hodgkin's lymphoma
Berry's node	• Jugulo-omohyoid lymph nodes seen in thyroid malignancy

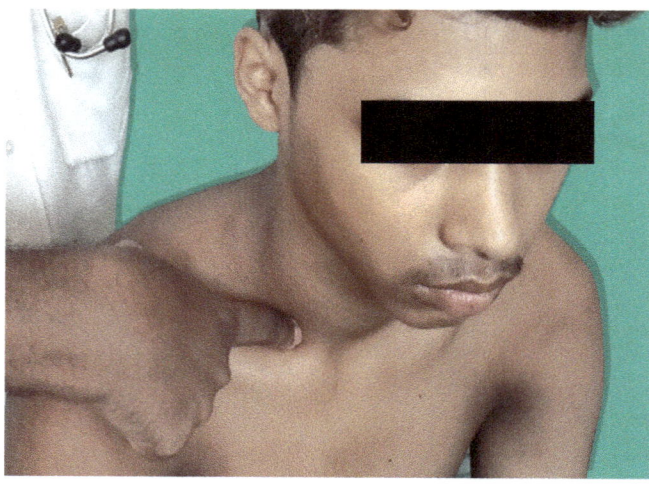

Fig. 2.70: Method of examining scalene lymph nodes.

Axillary Group of Lymph Nodes
- There are five axillary lymph node groups
- Lymph nodes include:
    1. Lateral (humeral)
    2. Anterior (pectoral)
    3. Posterior (subscapular)
    4. Central
    5. Apical nodes

The apical nodes are the final common pathway for all of the axillary lymph nodes.

Note: Examine the right axillary lymph nodes with the left hand except for humeral group (which is examined with right hand).

Examination of Right Axillary Lymph Nodes (Figs. 2.71 to 2.80)

Hyperabduct the right arm of patient
↓
Insinuate your left hand finger tips deep in axilla of patient
↓
Place the right forearm of patient on your left forearm
↓
With right hand palm, compress or give pressure over the patients right shoulder joint and feel for the apical group of lymph nodes
↓
Central group can be felt just below the apical group
↓
Anterior group can be felt on the anterior axillary fold
↓
Posterior group can be felt on the posterior axillary fold
↓
Lateral group is felt with examiner's right hand by palpating over the patient's humerus

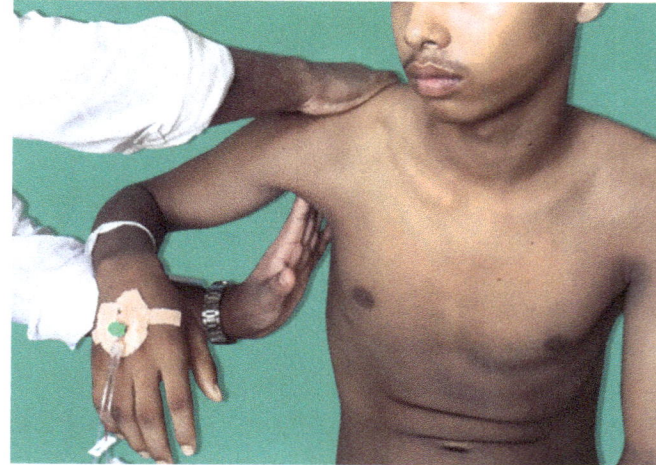

Fig. 2.71: Method of examining right apical group (axillary) lymph nodes.

Drainage Areas of Axillary Lymph Nodes
☐ Chest wall with breast
☐ Parietal pleura
☐ Hand

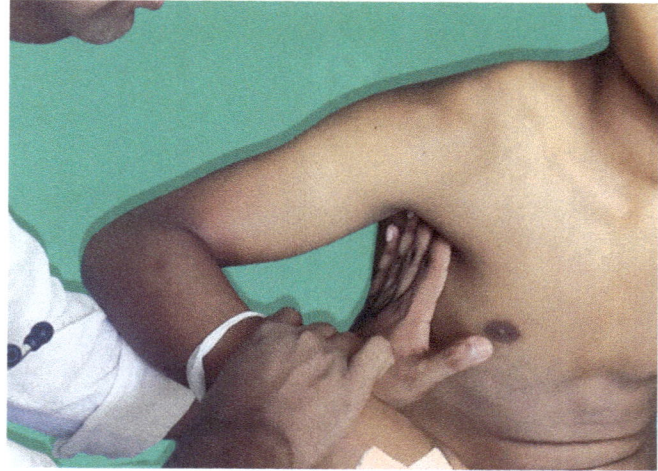

Fig. 2.72: Method of examining right central group (axillary) lymph nodes.

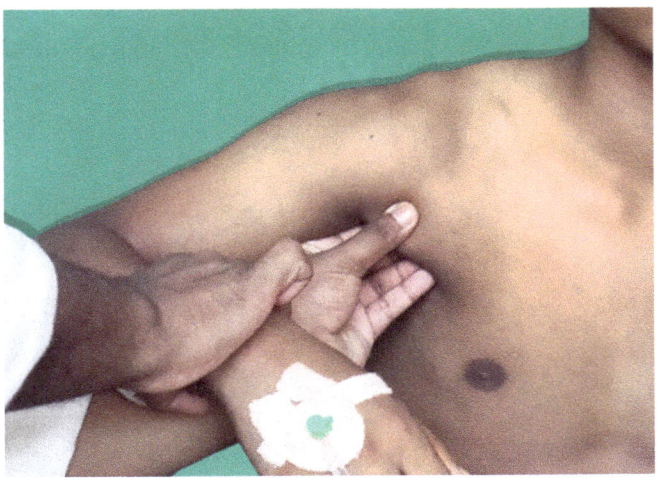

Fig. 2.73: Method of examining right anterior group (axillary) lymph nodes.

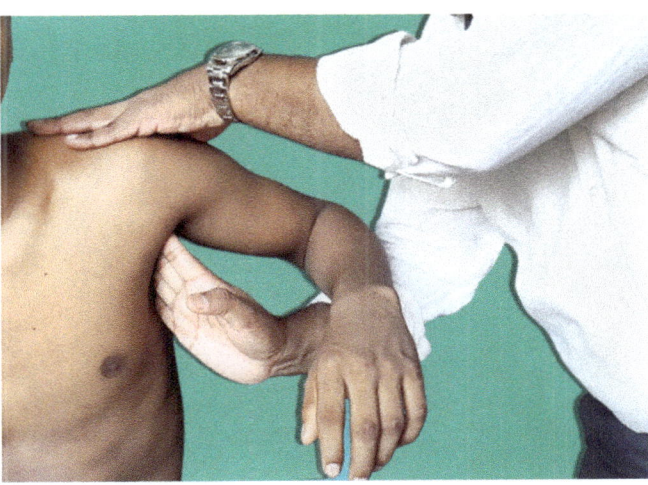

Fig. 2.76: Method of examining left apical group (axillary) lymph nodes.

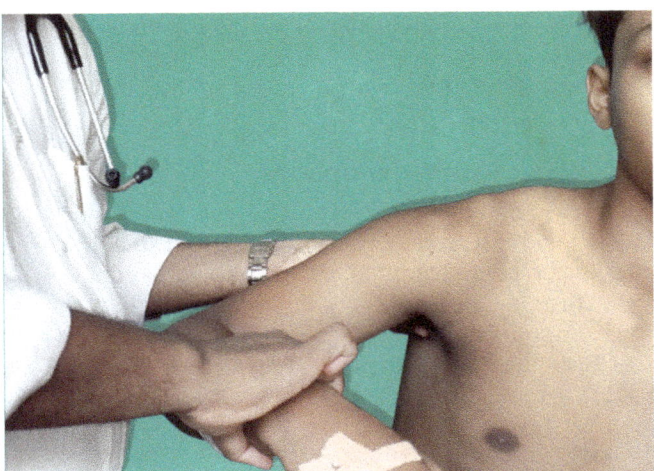

Fig. 2.74: Method of examining right posterior group (axillary) lymph nodes.

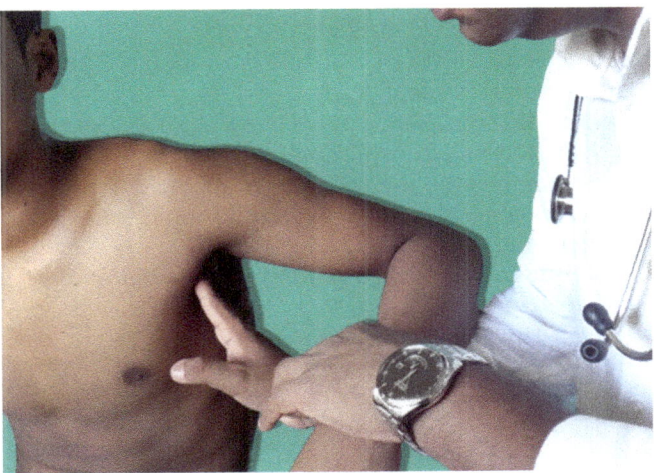

Fig. 2.77: Method of examining left central group (axillary) lymph nodes.

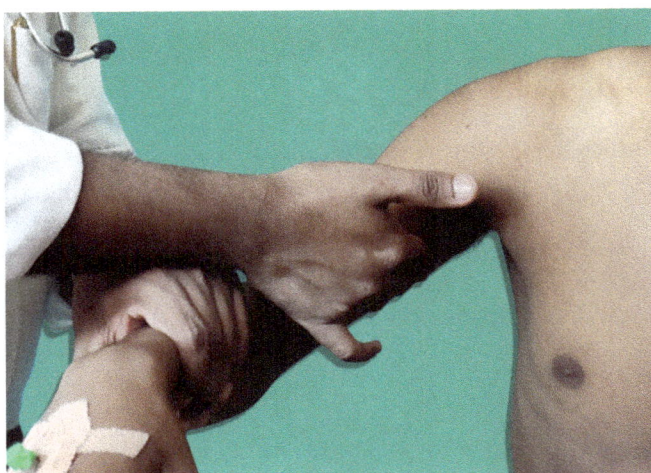

Fig. 2.75: Method of examining right lateral group (axillary) lymph nodes.

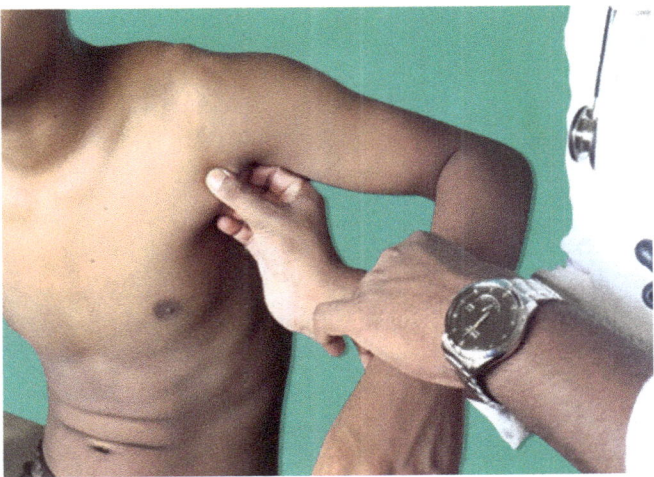

Fig. 2.78: Method of examining left anterior group (axillary) lymph nodes.

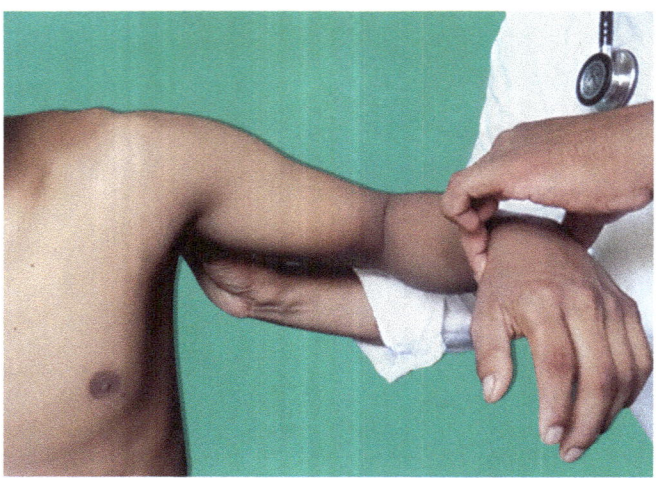

Fig. 2.79: Method of examining left posterior group (axillary) lymph nodes.

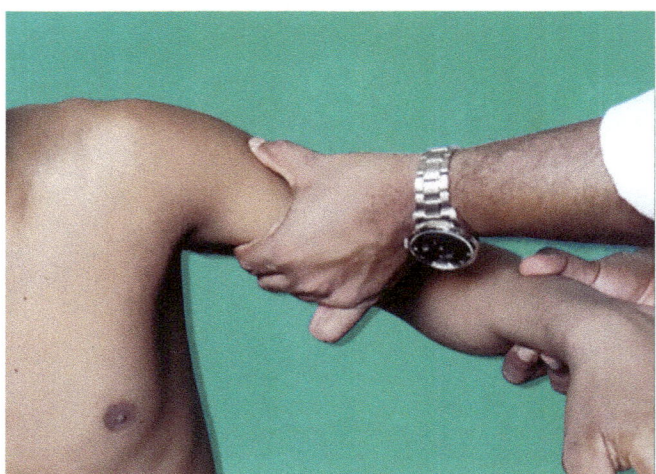

Fig. 2.80: Method of examining left lateral group (axillary) lymph nodes.

Epitrochlear Group of Lymph Nodes

- Situated on medial aspect of the elbow, about 4–5 cm above the humeral epitrochlea
- Epitrochlear station drains the lymph from the last two or three fingers and from the medial aspect of the hand itself.
- For examining the right elbow, rest the right elbow of the patient on the right hand palm of the examiner and feel the lymph node with thumb.
- **Systemic causes of epitrochlear lymphadenopathy:**
  - Secondary syphilis
  - Non-Hodgkin lymphoma (NHL)
  - HIV
  - Disseminated tuberculosis
  - Sporothrix
  - Cat scratch disease

Inguinal Lymph Nodes

Horizontal group	Vertical group
Palpated along the inguinal ligament	Palpated vertically downwards from the midpoint of inguinal ligament
Drains: • External genitalia • Scrotum • Perineum • Anal canal below dentate line	*Drains:* • Lower limb

Popliteal Lymphadenopathy

- Palpate the popliteal fossa with the knee in semiflexed position

- Systemic diseases associated with enlargement include:
  - NHL
  - Disseminated TB
  - HIV

Para-aortic Lymphadenopathy

- Relax abdomen
- With two hand placed over the epigastrium, one should feel for the enlarged lymph nodes by deep palpation.
- Enlarged in:
  - Lymphomas
  - Testicular malignancies
  - Tuberculosis

Mesenteric Lymph Nodes

- These are examined along the line of attachment of the mesentery, from the right iliac fossa medially toward the umbilicus.
- Enlarged in:
  - HIV
  - Lymphomas
  - Ulcerative colitis

Mediastinal Lymph Nodes

- *D'Espine sign* is a bronchophony/whispering pectoriloquy heard over the vertebral spines (on the back) below the level of tracheal bifurcation; below the fourth thoracic spine (T_4) in adults.
- It indicates tracheobronchial (mediastinal) lymphadenopathy.

ANTHROPOMETRY

Height

Method of Measurement of Length/Height

- Recumbent length **(Fig. 2.81)** is measured using an infantometer with a fixed head piece and horizontal backboard, and an adjustable foot piece. The *recorder supports the child's head* while the *examiner positions the feet* and ensures that the head lies in the Frankfort horizontal plane.
- Standing height **(Fig. 2.82)** is an assessment of maximum vertical size. This stature measurement is collected on all SPs aged 2 years and older who are able to stand unassisted. Standing height is measured using a stadiometer with a fixed vertical backboard and an adjustable headpiece. Instruct the SP to stand with the *heels together and toes apart*. The toes should point slightly outward at approximately a 60° angle. Check that the back of the *head, shoulder blades, buttocks, and heels makes contact with the backboard*.

Short Stature

Short stature is defined as a height that is below the 2.5th percentile or two or more standard deviations below the mean for age and gender for a given population. A growth velocity that is below the 5th percentile for age and gender is called growth deceleration (e.g., <5 cm/year after the age of 5 years). Dwarfism is defined as short stature for the age of the patient. Most common causes of dwarfism are familial short stature and constitutional delay of growth and puberty.

Cause of short stature	
Constitutional (hereditary)	Gurkhas and African pygmies
Endocrine	• Cretinism • Pituitary dwarf • Frohlich's syndrome • Cushing syndrome
Genetic	• Turner syndrome • Noonan syndrome • Hurler's syndrome • Morquio's syndrome • Multiple lentigines syndrome
Skeletal	• Ellis-van Creveld syndrome • Achondroplasia • Osteogenesis imperfecta
Acquired (in children)	• Rickets • Pott's spine

Note: For detail list and differential diagnosis of short stature, refer to page no 74–75 in Exam Preparatory Manual for Undergraduates by Archith Boloor.

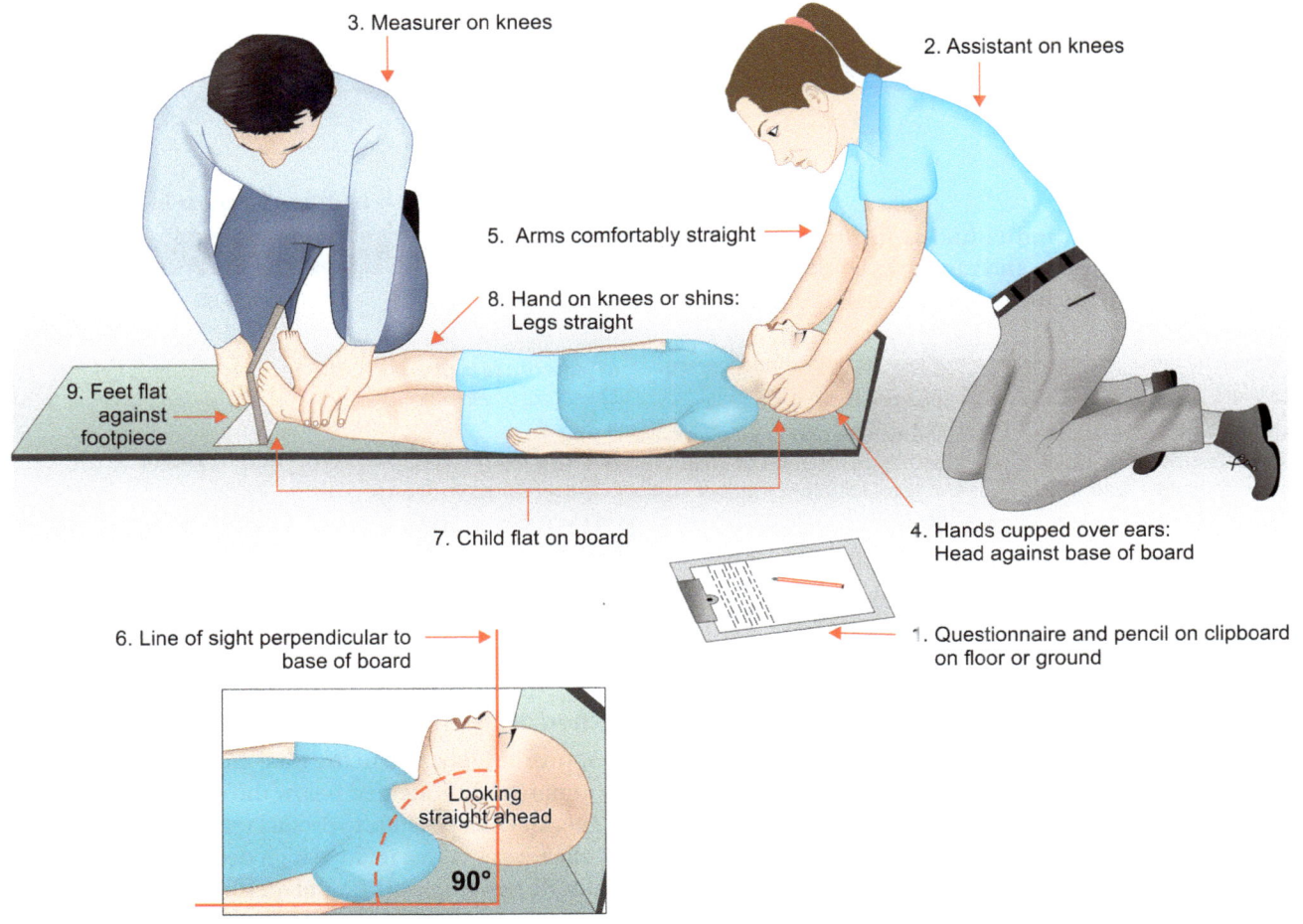

Fig. 2.81: Measurement of recumbent length.

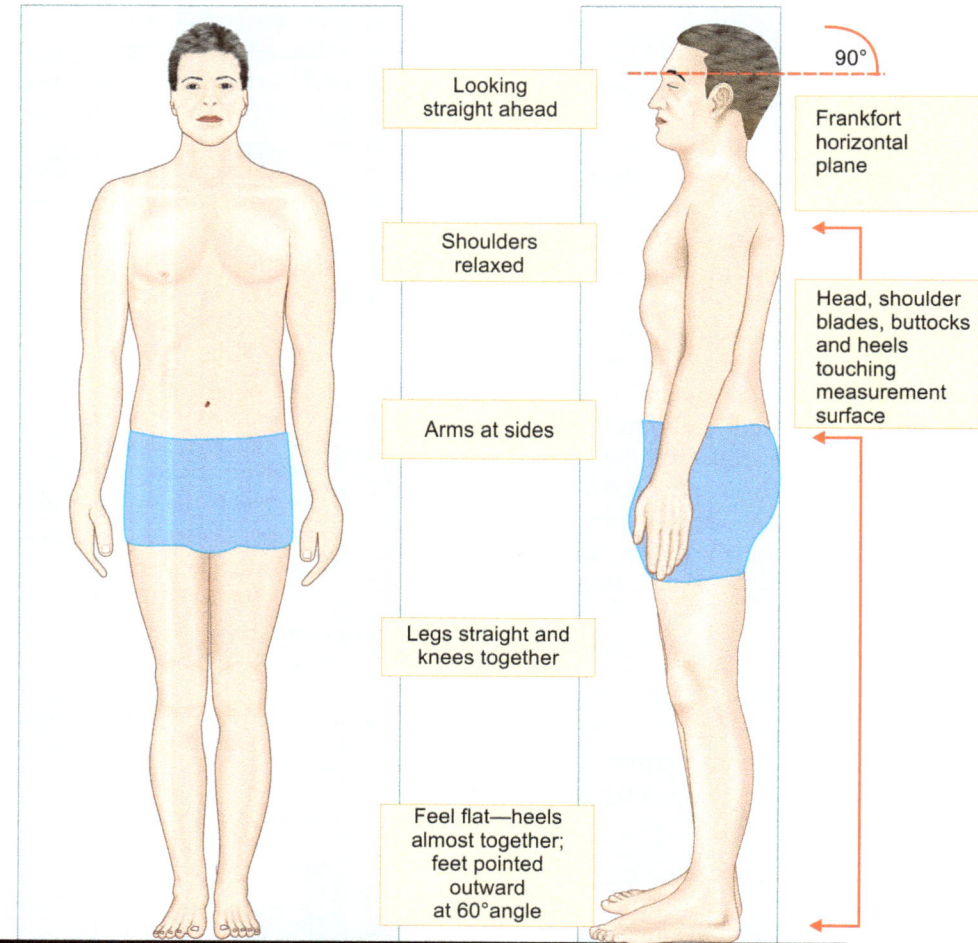

Fig. 2.82: Measurement of vertical height.

Tall Stature

When the height of an individual is far in excess of the average normal for the age and race (≥2 standard deviation of the mean height), the individual is considered to be tall in stature.

Causes of tall stature:	
Tall stature with equal upper and lower segments or equal arm span to height ratio	Tall stature with unequal upper to lower segment (ratio of ≤0.8) or arm span to height (ratio of ≥1.05)
Constitutional tall stature Pituitary giants Sexual precocity Thyrotoxicosis	Marfan syndrome Homocystinuria Klinefelter syndrome

Arm Span

Method of Measurement of Arm Span

It is the distance between the tips of the middle fingers of one hand to the other with arms abducted in horizontal plane. The arm span to height ratio is normally equal or ≤1.05.

Clinical implication—arm span versus height ratio:

Age	Ratio
At birth	The arm span is typically less than length (by at least 2.5 cm)
10 years of age in boys and 12 years of age in girls	The arm span exceeds height

Cause of increased arm span–height ratio:
- Klinefelter syndrome
- Homocystinuria
- Marfan's syndrome
- Sotos syndrome
- Hypogonadism

Skinfold Thickness

Method of Measurement

- Approximately, half of the total amount of fat tissue in the human body is located below the surface of the skin.
- This makes it possible to predict total body fat from skinfold thicknesses with a relative high degree of accuracy using a simple two-compartmental method.

Chapter 2: Vital Signs and General Physical Examination

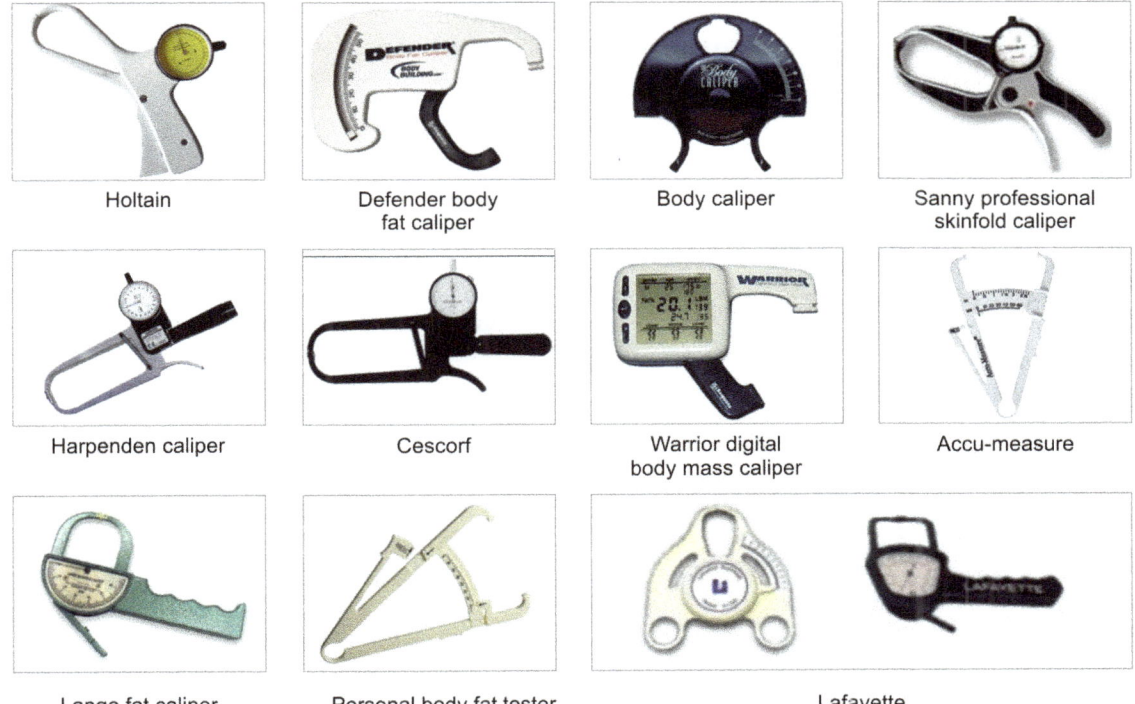

Fig. 2.83: Different types of skinfold calipers.

- This accuracy is confirmed by CT scan as well as ultrasonic and radiographic techniques used to measure subcutaneous fat.
- In general, when measuring skinfold thickness:
  - The assessor, using the forefinger and the thumb, grasps and lifts the subcutaneous tissue and skin from the underlying muscle.
  - Places the pincers of the skinfold caliper (Fig. 2.83), applying a constant pressure, 2 cm below the fingers at a depth of 1 cm
  - Holds this position for 3–4 seconds
  - Takes three measurements for accuracy
  - Provides the actual skinfold thickness in mm

Triceps skinfold (TSF) (Fig. 2.84):
- A measure of subcutaneous fat stores taken at the midpoint of the posterior aspect of the humerus
- Correlates closely with percentage of body fat and with total body fat
- Triceps skinfold thickness varies between 6 and 12 mm in lean individuals and between 40 and 50 mm in obese individuals.
- Subject should be *standing* with *arms hanging loosely at the sides.*
- Assessor to be positioned behind the subject
- To locate the triceps skinfold site, *locate the site previously marked for the mid-arm circumference measurement (MAC).*
- The triceps skinfold site is on the posterior surface of the arm, midway between the shoulder and the elbow.

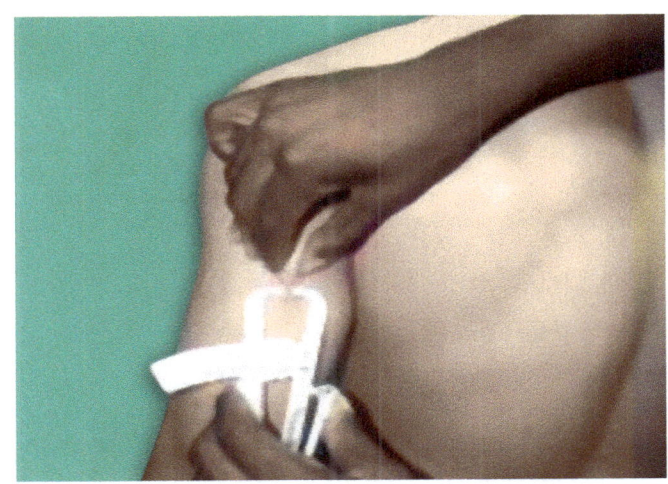

Fig. 2.84: Image showing *triceps skinfold (TSF).*

- *Using the forefinger and the thumb,* the assessor *grasps and lifts the subcutaneous tissue and skin 2 cm above TSF site.*
- Place the *pincers of the skinfold caliper* at the *TSF point at a depth of 1 cm.*
- Hold this position for 3–4 seconds.
- Take three measurements for accuracy.
- Provide the actual skinfold thickness in mm.

Body Mass Index

Calculation

Formula is weight (kg)/height^2 (meters).

Body Mass Index

	WHO	SEAC
Underweight	<18.5	<18.5
Normal	18.5–24.9	18.5–22.9
Overweight	25–29.9	23–24.9
Preobese	—	25–29.9
Obese	≥30	≥30
Obese 1	30–40	30–40
Obese 2 (morbid)	40.1–50	40.1–50
Obese 3	>50	>50

(SEAC: South East Asian Countries)

Metabolic syndrome	
NCEP ATP-III, 2005*	WHO, 1999
Essential criteria:	
—	Insulin resistance
Additional criteria (≥3 of following)	*Additional criteria* (≥2 of following)
Waist circumference: • >90 cm (males) • >80 cm (females)	WHR: • >0.9 (males) • >0.85 (females) • BMI ≥30
Glucose ≥100 mg/dL or on Rx	
TG ≥150 mg/dL or on Rx	TG ≥150 mg/dL
HDL: <40 (males) <50 (females) or on Rx	HDL: <35 (males) <40 (females)
HTN ≥130/85 or on Rx	HTN ≥140/90

(ATP: Adult Treatment Panel; NCEP: National Cholesterol Education Program; HDL: high-density lipoprotein; HTN: hypertension; TG: triglyceride: WHR: waist hip ratio)
*Most commonly followed.

Waist Hip Ratio

Method of Measurement

Waist circumference:
- Locate the narrowest point between ribs and iliac crests.
- Ensure that the tape measure is at the same height around the waist.
- Measure and state the measurement correctly to the nearest centimeter.
- ≥90 cm (adult male) and ≥80 cm (adult female) considered having abdominal obesity for south Asians.
- Differences in cut points abdominal obesity for south Asians and Europids:

Abdominal obesity	South Asians	Europids
Men	WC ≥ 90 cm	WC ≥ 102 cm
Women	WC ≥ 80 cm	WC ≥ 88 cm

(WC: waist circumference)

Hip circumference:
- Hip measurement is taken at the widest lateral extension of the hips.
- Ensure that the tape measure is horizontal.
- Measure and state the measurement correctly to the nearest centimeter.
- Calculate waist/hip ratio to 2 decimal places **(Fig. 2.85)**.

Clinical Implication

0.9 (males) or >0.85 (females) is criterion for metabolic syndrome.

Mid-arm Circumference (Figs. 2.86 and 2.87)

- Locate the midpoint of the arm.
- Nondominant arm elbow flexed at 90° with palm facing upward
- Measurer stands behind the subject and locates the lateral tip of the acromion and the most distal point on the olecranon process
- Place a tape measure so that it passes between these 2 landmarks and mark the midpoint. Measure the mid-arm circumference.
- The subject stands erect with arms hanging freely at the sides and the palms facing the thighs.
- Place the tape measure perpendicular to the long axis of the arm at the marked midpoint and measure the circumference to the nearest mm (e.g., 18.1 cm)
- Provide the actual MAC in cm.

Neck Circumference

- Neck circumference (NC) measurement as a simple and time-saving screening measure could be used to identify overweight and obese population.
- Measured on a plane as horizontal as possible, at a point just below the larynx (thyroid cartilage) and perpendicular to the long axis of the neck (the tape line in front of the neck at the same height as the tape line in the back of the neck).
- It varies based on population. Among south Asians, an NC of >34.9 cm for men and >31.25 cm for women were the best predictors for identifying metabolic syndrome.

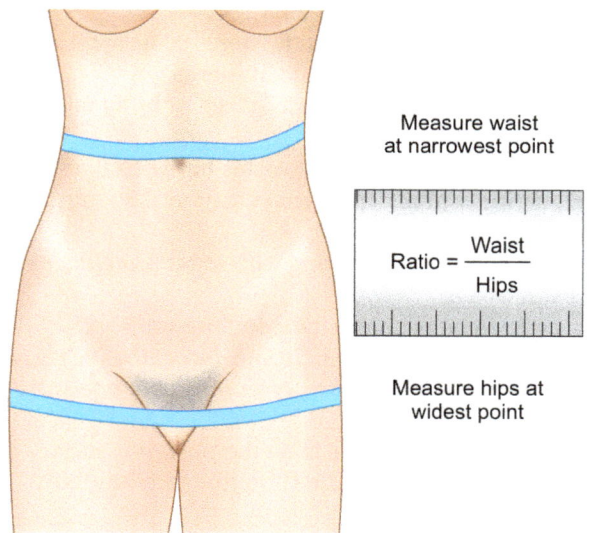

Fig. 2.85: Image showing examination of waist–hip ratio.

Chapter 2: Vital Signs and General Physical Examination

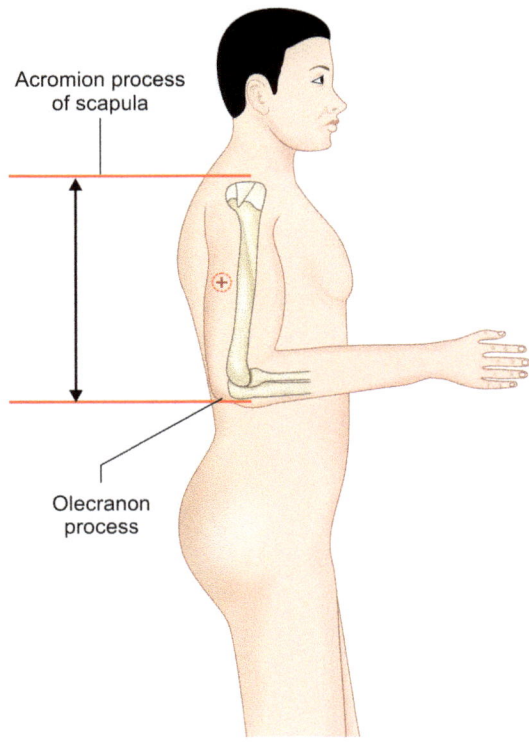

Fig. 2.86: Image showing method of marking midpoint for measuring mid-arm circumference.

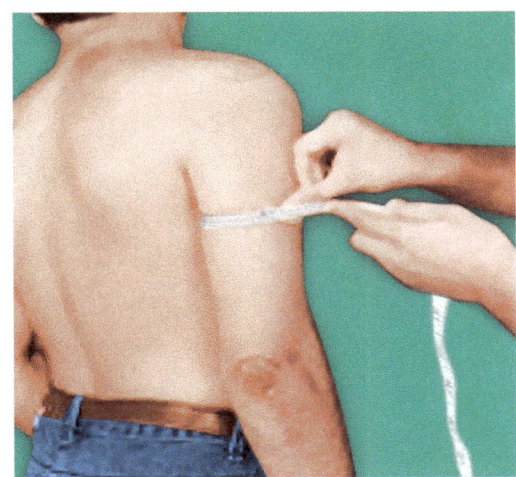

Fig. 2.87: Image showing method of measuring mid-arm circumference.

Miscellaneous Topics

Significant Weight Loss
- \>10% of body weight × 6 month
- 5 kg or more × 1 month

Cachexia
Complex metabolic syndrome is associated with underlying illness, and is characterized by the loss of muscle with/without loss of fat mass.

Emaciation
Emaciation is extreme weight loss and unnatural thinness due to a of subcutaneous fat (the fatty, adipose tissue beneath the skin) muscle throughout body.

OBJECTIVE-BASED SELF-EVALUATION

SHORT ANSWER QUESTIONS

1. List the clinical differences between central and peripheral cyanosis.
2. What are the precautions to be taken while measuring the blood pressure?
3. Mention the types of jaundice. Tabulate the differences between each type.
4. Define generalized lymphadenopathy. List the common causes.
5. Discuss the clinical relevance of body mass index.
6. List two causes each for pitting and nonpitting edema.
7. List the differences between jugular and carotid pulsations.

MULTIPLE CHOICE QUESTIONS

1. **A 22-year-old female with mitral stenosis with atrial fibrillation comes to your OPD. The radial pulse examination will reveal:**
   a. High volume pulse
   b. Pulsus paradoxus
   c. Irregularly irregular pulse
   d. Pulsus bisferiens
2. **Matted cervical lymph nodes are seen in:**
   a. Toxoplasmosis   b. Brucellosis
   c. Lymphoma   d. Tuberculosis
3. **Nonpitting edema is classically seen with:**
   a. Filariasis
   b. Nephrotic syndrome
   c. Heart failure
   d. Hypoalbuminemia
4. **A young male on examination has differential cyanosis and clubbing. Most possible diagnosis is:**
   a. Bronchiectasis
   b. Patent ductus arteriosus with reversal of shunt
   c. Infective endocarditis
   d. Heart failure
5. **Persistent generalized lymphadenopathy is characteristic of:**
   a. Lymphoma   b. HIV/AIDS
   c. Tuberculosis   d. Syphilis
6. **Absent 'a' wave in jugular venous pulse is characteristic of:**
   a. Tricuspid stenosis
   b. Complete heart block
   c. Atrial fibrillation
   d. Constrictive pericarditis

7. A patient is admitted with history of intermittent fever with a periodicity of 48 hours. He is diagnosed to have vivax malaria. This pattern of fever is called:
   a. Tertian fever
   b. Quatran fever
   c. Quotidian fever
   d. Remittent fever
8. All of the following are associated with hypothermia, *except*:
   a. Hypopituitarism
   b. Hyperthyroidism
   c. Burns
   d. Hypoadrenalism
9. Phalangeal depth ratio and digital index is used to measure:
   a. Body surface area
   b. Edema
   c. Clubbing
   d. Temperature
10. Short stature is seen in all of the following syndromes, *except*:
    a. Turner syndrome
    b. Noonan syndrome
    c. Hurler's syndrome
    d. Marfan's syndrome

ANSWERS

| 1. c | 2. d | 3. a | 4. b | 5. b |
| 6. c | 7. a | 8. b | 9. c | 10. d |

CHAPTER 3

Gastrointestinal Tract Examination

CHAPTER OUTLINE

- Gastrointestinal Tract: Case Sheet Format
- Gastrointestinal Tract: Diagnosis Format
- Discussion on Cardinal Symptoms
- Discussion of Examination
- Oral Cavity Examination
- Examination of Individual Organs

GASTROINTESTINAL TRACT: CASE SHEET FORMAT

History Taking
- Name:
- Age:
- Sex:
- Residence:
- Occupation:

Chief Complaints
1. _____ × days
2. _____ × days
3. _____ × days

History of Presenting Illness

Abdominal distention:
- Duration
- Onset
- Progression
- Aggravating factors
- Relieving factors
- Associated symptoms
- Is it preceded by pedal edema or followed by it?

Pedal edema
- Duration
- Onset
- Progression
- Aggravating factors
- Relieving factors
- Is it preceded by facial puffiness or followed by it?

Abdominal pain
- Onset
- Site
- Type of pain
- Radiation
- Aggravating factors
- Relieving factors
- Associated symptoms

Nausea and vomiting:
- Episodes
- Contents
- Blood tinged or not
- How many hours after consumption of food?
- Associated with pain abdomen?
- Conditions with nausea and vomiting but not associated with pain abdomen

Other symptoms
- Heart burn, flatulence, and water brash
- Hematemesis and melena
- Dysphagia
- Constipation and diarrhea

Altered bowel habit
- Stool color
- Stool odor
- Stool frequency
- Blood tinged or melena

Other symptoms
- Fever
- Weight loss
- Pain in oral cavity
- Halitosis
- Hiccups
- Other relevant history

Past History
- Asthma
- Chronic obstructive airway disease
- Tuberculosis
- History of contact with tuberculosis
- Diabetes mellitus (DM)

- ❏ Hypertension (HTN)
- ❏ Ischemic heart disease (IHD)
- ❏ Seizure disorder

Family History

Draw a three generation pedigree chart

Personal History
- ❏ Bowel habits
- ❏ Bladder habits
- ❏ Appetite
- ❏ Loss of weight
- ❏ Occupational exposure
- ❏ Sleep
- ❏ Dietary habits and taboo
- ❏ Food allergies
- ❏ Smoking Index or Pack years
- ❏ Alcohol history

Menstrual and Obstetric History
- ❏ G__P__ L__A__
- ❏ Age of menarche __
- ❏ Menopause at __
- ❏ Flow—ameno/oligo/menorrhagia

Summarize

(*Write brief summary of the history*)

Differential Diagnosis
1.
2.
3.

General Examination

Patient
- ❏ Conscious
- ❏ Coherent
- ❏ Cooperative
- ❏ Obeying commands

Body Mass Index (BMI)

Weight (kg)/ Height^2 (meters)

Vitals
- ❏ **Pulse**
  - Rate:
  - Rhythm:
  - Volume:
  - Character:
  - Vessel wall thickening:
  - Radio-radial delay and radio-femoral delay:
  - Peripheral pulses:
- ❏ **Blood pressure**
  - Right arm:
  - Left arm:
  - Leg:
- ❏ **Respiratory rate**
  - Regular/irregular
  - Abdominothoracic (male)/thoracoabdominal (female)
  - Usage of accessory muscles:
- ❏ **Jugular venous pressure**
  - __ cm of blood above sternal angle (+ 5 cm water from right atrium)
- ❏ **Jugular venous pulse**
  - Waveform (describe waves)
- ❏ **Pulse oximetry**

On Physical Examination
- ❏ Pallor:
- ❏ Icterus:
- ❏ Cyanosis:
- ❏ Clubbing:
- ❏ Lymphadenopathy:
- ❏ Edema:

Other Head-to-Toe Signs of Chronic Liver Cell Failure
- ❏ Alopecia
- ❏ Fetor hepaticus
- ❏ Jaundice
- ❏ Parotid swelling
- ❏ Gynecomastia
- ❏ Testicular atrophy
- ❏ Loss of secondary sexual characters
- ❏ Spider nevi
- ❏ Palmar erythema
- ❏ Duputryen's contracture
- ❏ Asterixis
- ❏ Xanthelasma
- ❏ Signs of chronic cholestasis (scratch marks due to pruritus)

Systemic Examination

The order of examination of abdomen is preferably done—Inspection → Auscultation → Palpation and percussion (as the auscultatory findings might change post-palpation and percussion).

Inspection
- ❏ Spine
- ❏ Shape/distention (localized/generalized), flanks (free/full)
- ❏ Skin over the abdomen
- ❏ Symmetry
- ❏ Umbilicus
- ❏ Movement of corresponding quadrants with respiration
- ❏ Dilated veins
- ❏ Visible mass
- ❏ Visible pulsations
- ❏ Visible peristalsis
- ❏ Scars or sinuses
- ❏ Divarication of recti

Palpation
- ❏ Superficial palpation
  - Warmth
  - Tenderness
  - Guarding
  - Rigidity
- ❏ Deep palpation
  - Liver
    - Size
    - Shape
    - Border or edge
    - Surface
    - Tenderness
    - Consistency
    - Movement with respiration
    - Pulsation
  - Spleen
    - Location
    - Size
    - Shape
    - Consistency
    - Surface
    - Edge
    - Tenderness
    - Movement with respiration
  - Gallbladder
  - Other palpable mass
- ❏ Bimanual palpation
  - *Kidneys*
    - Location
    - Size
    - Shape
    - Consistency
    - Surface
    - Edge
    - Tenderness
    - Movement with respiration
- ❏ Dipping method (in case of large ascites)
- ❏ Hernia orifices

Percussion
- ❏ Liver
- ❏ Spleen
- ❏ Traube's space
- ❏ Fluid
  - Shifting dullness
  - Fluid thrill
  - Puddle sign

Auscultation
- ❏ Bowel sounds
- ❏ Succussion splash
- ❏ Bruit
- ❏ Venous hum
- ❏ Friction rub

Examination of
- ❏ Scrotum
- ❏ Spine
- ❏ Supraclavicular fossa

Per Rectal Examination

Per Vaginal Examination

GASTROINTESTINAL TRACT: DIAGNOSIS FORMAT

For Cirrhosis
- ❏ Compensated or decompensated
- ❏ Possible etiology—alcohol/postviral/toxin/nonalcoholic steatohepatitis (NASH)
- ❏ With complications—portal HTN with or without gastrointestinal (GI) bleed/hepatic encephalopathy (preferable to mention stage)/spontaneous bacterial peritonitis/hepatocellular carcinoma (HCC)/hepatorenal syndrome/others.

Example
Decompensated chronic liver disease—cirrhosis secondary to alcohol, with portal HTN, with upper GI (UGI) bleed, patient in stage 2 hepatic encephalopathy with no evidence of spontaneous bacterial peritonitis or other complications.

DISCUSSION ON CARDINAL SYMPTOMS

Abdominal Swelling
Abdominal swelling is a manifestation of numerous diseases. Patients may complain of bloating or abdominal fullness. Patients with abdominal distention from *ascites* may report the new onset of an inguinal or umbilical hernia. Dyspnea may result from pressure against the diaphragm.

Causes
The causes of abdominal swelling can be remembered conveniently as the *seven F's*: flatus, fat, fluid, fetus, feces, full bladder, or a "fatal growth"/neoplasm **(Table 3.1)**.

Jaundice
Discussed in detail in Chapter 2c: Physical Examination.

Gastrointestinal Bleeding
Gastrointestinal bleeding (GIB) presents as either overt or occult bleeding **(Table 3.2)**.
Gastrointestinal bleeding is also categorized by the site of bleeding as:
1. **Upper gastrointestinal bleeding (UGIB):** Esophagus, stomach, duodenum
2. **Lower gastrointestinal bleeding (LGIB):** (colonic), small intestinal, or obscure GIB (if the source is unclear).

Table 3.1: Causes of abdominal swelling.

Causes	Description
Flatus	• The normal small intestine contains ~200 mL of gas made up of nitrogen, oxygen, carbon dioxide, hydrogen, and methane • *Aerophagia*, the swallowing of air, can result in increased amounts of oxygen and nitrogen in the small intestine and lead to abdominal swelling • Increased intestinal gas is the consequence of bacterial metabolism of excess fermentable substances such as lactose and other oligosaccharides, which can lead to production of hydrogen, carbon dioxide, or methane
Fat	• Weight gain with an increase in abdominal fat can result in an increase in abdominal girth. • Visceral obesity is associated with metabolic syndrome, insulin resistance, and cardiovascular disease. • It also can be a manifestation of certain diseases, such as Cushing's syndrome.
Fluid	• The accumulation of fluid within the abdominal cavity (ascites) often results in abdominal distention
Fetus	• Pregnancy results in increased abdominal girth. Typically, an increase in abdominal size is first noted at 12–14 weeks of gestation, when the uterus moves from the pelvis into the abdomen.
Feces	• In the setting of severe constipation or intestinal obstruction, increased stool in the colon leads to increased abdominal girth. These conditions are often accompanied by abdominal discomfort or pain, nausea, and vomiting and can be diagnosed by imaging studies.
Fatal growth/ neoplasm	• An abdominal mass can result in abdominal swelling. Neoplasms, abscesses, or cysts can grow to sizes that lead to increased abdominal girth. Enlargement of the intra-abdominal organs, specifically the liver (hepatomegaly) or spleen (splenomegaly), or an abdominal aortic aneurysm can result in abdominal distention.
Full bladder	• Bladder distention also may result in lower abdominal swelling. It will be associated with anuria

Table 3.2: Types of gastrointestinal bleeding.

Overt gastrointestinal bleeding	Occult gastrointestinal bleeding
Overt GIB is manifested by *hematemesis*, vomitus of red blood or "coffee-grounds" material; *melena*, black, tarry stool; and/or *hematochezia*, passage of red or maroon blood from the rectum.	**Occult GIB** may present with *symptoms of blood loss or anemia* such as lightheadedness, syncope, angina, or dyspnea; or with iron-deficiency anemia or a positive fecal occult blood test on routine testing.

Hematemesis is the vomiting of blood, which may be obviously red or have an appearance similar to coffee grounds.

Melena is the passage of black, tarry stools due to altered blood (usually blood should remain in the gut for 14 hours approximately). It usually means bleeding episodes from sites above the ligament of Treitz. However, even up to middle of transverse colon can produce melena. It takes 60 mL or more of blood in the stomach to turn stools black. One episode of bleed can produce 5–7 episodes of melena.

Hematochezia is the passage of fresh blood per anus, usually in or with stools.

Upper Gastrointestinal Sources of Bleeding

The upper gastrointestinal sources of bleeding have been shown in **Table 3.3**.

Lower Gastrointestinal Bleeding

The causes of LGIB have been shown in **Table 3.4** and **Figure 3.1**.

Nausea and Vomiting

Definitions

Nausea is the subjective feeling of need to vomit. **Vomiting** (emesis) is the oral expulsion of gastrointestinal contents due to gut and thoracoabdominal wall contractions.

Table 3.3: Causes of upper gastrointestinal bleeding.

Causes		
Esophageal causes	**Gastric causes**	**Duodenal causes**
• Esophageal varices • Esophagitis • Esophageal cancer • Esophageal ulcers • Mallory-Weiss tear	• Gastric ulcer • Gastric cancer • Gastritis • Gastric varices • Dieulafoy's lesions • Gastric antral vascular ectasia • Portal hypertensive gastropathy	• Duodenal ulcer • Vascular malformation including aortoenteric fistulae • Hematobilia, or bleeding from the biliary tree • Hemosuccus pancreaticus, or bleeding from the pancreatic duct • Severe superior mesenteric artery syndrome

Table 3.4: Causes of lower gastrointestinal bleeding.

Colonic bleeding (95%)	Small intestinal bleeding (5%)
• Diverticular disease	• Angiodysplasia
• Anorectal disease (hemorrhoid, anal fissure, fistula in ano, solitary rectal ulcer, etc.)	• Crohn's disease and infectious disease
• Neoplasia (polyp, ulcerated lesions)	• Neoplasia (polyp, ulcerated lesions)
• Inflammatory bowel diseases	• Radiation
• Infectious colitis	• Meckel's diverticulum
• Angiodysplasia	• Aortoenteric fistula
• Radiation colitis/proctitis	• Mesenteric ischemia
• Other	

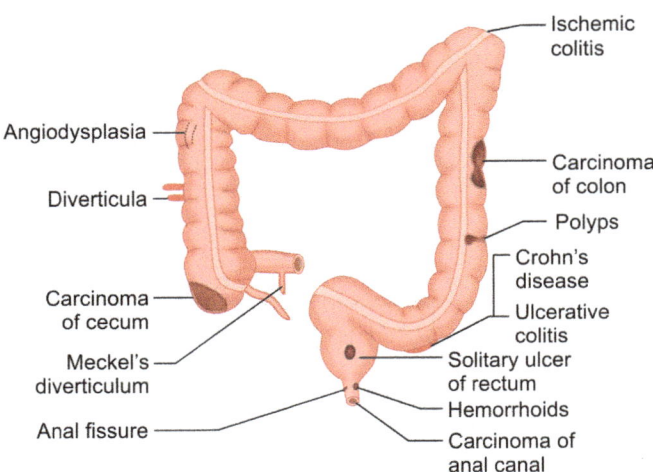

Fig. 3.1: Causes of lower gastrointestinal bleeding.

Mechanism of Initiation of Emesis

Brainstem nuclei—including the nucleus tractus solitarius; dorsal vagal, and phrenic nuclei; medullary nuclei regulating respiration; and nuclei that control pharyngeal, facial, and tongue movements—coordinate initiation of emesis involving neurokinin NK1, serotonin 5-HT3, and vasopressin pathways. The causes of nausea and vomiting are described in **Table 3.5**.

Clinical Clues for Diagnosis

1. Gastroparesis and pyloric obstruction elicit vomiting within an hour of eating.
2. Emesis from intestinal blockage occurs later.
3. Vomiting occurring minutes after meal consumption prompts consideration of rumination syndrome.
4. With severe gastric emptying delays, the vomitus may contain food residue ingested days before.
5. Feculent emesis is noted with distal intestinal or colonic obstruction.
6. Bilious vomiting excludes gastric obstruction, whereas emesis of undigested food is consistent with a Zenker's diverticulum or achalasia.
7. Vomiting can relieve abdominal pain from a bowel obstruction, but has no effect in pancreatitis or cholecystitis.
8. Profound weight loss raises concern about malignancy or obstruction.
9. An intracranial source is considered if there are headaches or visual field changes.
10. Vertigo or tinnitus indicates labyrinthine disease.

Projectile vomiting is a type of severe **vomiting** in which stomach contents are forcefully propelled several feet away from the patient and is usually not associated with nausea. It is a classical feature of raised intracranial tension.

Diarrhea

Definitions

Diarrhea is defined as passage of abnormally liquid or unformed stools at an increased frequency. For adults on a typical Western diet, stool weight >200 g/day can generally be considered diarrhea.

Diarrhea may be further defined as *acute* if <2 weeks, *persistent* if 2–4 weeks, and *chronic* if >4 weeks in duration **(Tables 3.6 and 3.7)**.

Types of Diarrhea

- **Inflammatory diarrhea** is characterized by frequent, small-volume, bloody stools, and may be accompanied by tenesmus, fever, or severe abdominal pain. Inflammatory diarrhea is suspected with the demonstration of leukocytes

Table 3.5: Causes of nausea and vomiting.

Intraperitoneal	Extraperitoneal	Medications/metabolic disorders

• Obstructing disorders
  ▪ Pyloric obstruction
  ▪ Small-bowel obstruction
  ▪ Colonic obstruction
  ▪ Superior mesenteric artery syndrome
• Enteric infections
  ▪ Viral
  ▪ Bacterial
• Inflammatory diseases
  ▪ Cholecystitis
  ▪ Pancreatitis
  ▪ Appendicitis
  ▪ Hepatitis
• Altered sensorimotor function
  ▪ Gastroparesis
  ▪ Intestinal pseudo-obstruction
  ▪ Gastroesophageal reflux
  ▪ Chronic nausea vomiting syndrome
  ▪ Cyclic vomiting syndrome
  ▪ Cannabinoid hyperemesis syndrome
  ▪ Rumination syndrome
• Biliary colic
• Abdominal irradiation
	• Cardiopulmonary disease
	  ▪ Cardiomyopathy
	  ▪ Myocardial infarction
	• Labyrinthine disease
	  ▪ Motion sickness
	  ▪ Labyrinthitis
	  ▪ Malignancy
	• Intracerebral disorders
	  ▪ Malignancy
	  ▪ Hemorrhage
	  ▪ Abscess
	  ▪ Hydrocephalus
	• Psychiatric illness
	  ▪ Anorexia and bulimia nervosa
	  ▪ Depression
	• Postoperative vomiting
		• Drugs
		  ▪ Cancer chemotherapy
		  ▪ Antibiotics
		  ▪ Cardiac antiarrhythmic
		  ▪ Digoxin
		  ▪ Oral hypoglycemics
		  ▪ Oral contraceptives
		  ▪ Antidepressants
		  ▪ Restless legs/Parkinson's therapies
		  ▪ Smoking cessation agents
		• Endocrine/metabolic disease
		  ▪ Pregnancy
		  ▪ Uremia
		  ▪ Ketoacidosis
		  ▪ Thyroid and parathyroid disease
		  ▪ Adrenal insufficiency
		• Toxins
		  ▪ Liver failure
		  ▪ Ethanol

Table 3.6: Large-volume versus small-volume diarrhea.

Large volume diarrhea	Small volume diarrhea
Right colonic or small bowel disorders	Left colonic disorders
The rectosigmoid reservoir is intact	Compromises this rectosigmoid reservoir capacity
Individual bowel movements are less frequent and larger.	Frequent small-volume bowel movements.

Note: Normal rectosigmoid colon functions as a storage reservoir.

Table 3.7: Acute and chronic diarrhea.

Acute diarrhea	Chronic diarrhea
More than 90% of cases of acute diarrhea are caused by infectious agents; these cases are often accompanied by vomiting, fever, and abdominal pain. The remaining 10% or so are caused by medications, toxic ingestions, ischemia, food indiscretions, and other conditions.	Diarrhea lasting >4 weeks warrants evaluation to exclude serious underlying pathology. In contrast to acute diarrhea, most of the causes of chronic diarrhea are noninfectious.

Table 3.8: Causes of acute diarrhea.

Cause	Description
Viral infection	Viral gastroenteritis: Norovirus or rotavirus
Bacterial infection	**Cause:** *Compylobacter, Escherichia coli, Salmonella,* or *Shigella*
Parasitic infection	*Cryptosporidium, Entamoeba histolytica,* or *Giardia*
Travelers' diarrhea	**Cause:** Consuming food or drinks contaminated with bacteria, parasites, or viruses
Medication	Antibiotics and long-term use of proton pump inhibitors: Increased risk of *Clostridium difficile* infection
Food allergy or intolerance	Cow's milk, egg, seafood, soy, or fructose or lactose intolerance
Digestive disorder	Celiac disease, Crohn disease, irritable bowel syndrome, or ulcerative colitis
Artificial sweetener	Mannitol, sorbitol, or xylitol found in sugar-free candies and gum

or leukocyte proteins (e.g., calprotectin or lactoferrin) on stool examination.

- **Fatty stools** are suggested by a history of weight loss, greasy, or bulky stools that are difficult to flush, and oil in the toilet bowl that requires a brush to remove **floating stools** indicate gas production by colonic bacteria, not steatorrhea.
- **Watery diarrhea** can be further classified as osmotic or secretory in origin. Osmotic diarrhea is due to the ingestion of poorly absorbed ions or sugars. Secretory diarrhea is due to disruption of epithelial electrolyte transport.

Causes of Acute Diarrhea
The causes of acute diarrhea are described in **Table 3.8**.

Causes of Chronic Diarrhea
The causes of chronic diarrhea are described in **Table 3.9**.

Mimics of Diarrhea
Pseudodiarrhea, or the frequent passage of small volumes of stool, is often associated with rectal urgency, tenesmus, or a feeling of incomplete evacuation, and accompanies irritable bowel syndrome (IBS) or proctitis.

Fecal incontinence is the involuntary discharge of rectal contents and is most often caused by neuromuscular disorders or structural anorectal problems.

Overflow diarrhea may occur in nursing home patients due to fecal impaction that is readily detectable by rectal examination.

Table 3.9: Causes of chronic diarrhea.

Fatty diarrhea	Watery diarrhea

1. **Malabsorption syndromes**
    • Mucosal diseases (e.g., celiac disease and Whipple's disease)
    • Mesenteric ischemia
    • Short bowel syndrome
    • Small intestinal bacterial overgrowth
2. **Maldigestion**
    • Inadequate luminal bile acid concentration
    • Pancreatic exocrine insufficiency
Inflammatory diarrhea
• Diverticulitis
• Infectious diseases
    • Invasive bacterial infections (e.g., tuberculosis and yersiniosis)
    • Invasive parasitic infections (e.g., amebiasis and strongyloidiasis)
    • Pseudomembranous colitis (*Clostridium difficile* infection)
    • Ulcerating viral infections (e.g., cytomegalovirus, herpes simplex virus)
• Inflammatory bowel diseases: Crohn's disease, ulcerative colitis
• Ischemic colitis
• Neoplasia: Carcinoma of colon, lymphoma
• Radiation colitis
	• Osmotic diarrhea
	    • Carbohydrate malabsorption
	    • Osmotic laxatives
	• Secretory diarrhea
	• Bacterial toxins
	• Congenital syndromes (e.g., congenital chloridorrhea)
	• Disordered motility, regulation
	    • Diabetic autonomic neuropathy
	    • Irritable bowel syndrome
	    • Postsympathectomy diarrhea
	    • Postvagotomy diarrhea
	• Diverticulitis
	• Endocrinopathies: Addison's disease, carcinoid syndrome, gastrinoma, hyperthyroidism, mastocytosis, medullary carcinoma of thyroid, pheochromocytoma, somatostatinoma, and VIPoma
	• Laxative abuse (stimulant laxatives)
	• Medications and toxins

Constipation

Definition

- ***Constipation*** refers to bowel movements that are infrequent or hard to pass.
- ***Obstipation*** is intractable constipation that has become refractory to cure or control. There is inability to pass any feces or flatus.
- ***Tenesmus*** is stated by patients as the unpleasant symptom that there remains something to evacuate from the rectum despite passing a stool. It is often painful. Indicate rectal inflammation.

Etiology of Constipation

The etiology of constipation is described in **Table 3.10**.

Dyspepsia

Definition

Rome III criteria for dyspepsia
More than or equal to one of the following:
- Postprandial fullness
- Early satiation (inability to finish a normal sized meal)
- Epigastric pain or burning

Causes of Dyspepsia

The causes of dyspepsia have been described in **Box 3.1**.

Dysphagia

Definition

Dysphagia, from the Greek *dys* (difficulty, disordered) and *phagia* (to eat), refers to the sensation that food is hindered in its passage from the mouth to the stomach **(Tables 3.11 and 3.12)**.

Table 3.10: Etiology of constipation.

Etiology	Features
Functional (nonorganic) or retentive	Includes constipation due to fecal withholding behaviors and when all organic causes have been ruled out.
Anatomic causes	Include anal stenosis or atresia, anteriorly displaced anus, imperforate anus, intestinal stricture, anal stricture
Abnormal musculature	Related causes include Prune-Belly syndrome, gastroschisis, Down syndrome, muscular dystrophy.
Intestinal nerve abnormality	Related causes include Hirschsprung disease, pseudo-obstruction, intestinal neuronal dysplasia, spinal cord defects, tethered cord, spina bifida
Drugs	Anticholinergics, narcotics, antidepressants, lead, vitamin D intoxication
Metabolic and endocrine causes	Hypokalemia, hypercalcemia, hypothyroidism, diabetes mellitus (DM), or diabetes insipidus.
Other causes	Celiac disease, cystic fibrosis, cow milk protein allergy, inflammatory bowel disease, scleroderma, among others

Box 3.1: Causes of dyspepsia.

Luminal gastrointestinal tract
- Chronic gastric or intestinal ischemia
- Food intolerance
- Functional dyspepsia
- Gastroesophageal reflux disease
- Gastric or esophageal neoplasms
- Gastric infections (e.g., cytomegalovirus, fungus, tuberculosis, syphilis)
- Gastroparesis (e.g., diabetes mellitus, post-vagotomy, scleroderma, chronic intestinal pseudo-obstruction, postviral, idiopathic)
- Irritable bowel syndrome
- Peptic ulcer disease
- Parasites (e.g., *Giardia lamblia*, *Strongyloides stercoralis*)

Medications
Acarbose, aspirin, other nonsteroidal anti-inflammatory drugs (including cyclooxygenase-2 selective agents), colchicine, digitalis preparations, estrogens, ethanol, glucocorticoids, iron, levodopa, niacin, narcotics, nitrates, orlistat, potassium chloride, quinidine, sildenafil, theophylline

Pancreaticobiliary disorders
- Biliary pain: Cholelithiasis, choledocholithiasis, sphincter of Oddi dysfunction
- Chronic pancreatitis
- Pancreatic neoplasms

Systemic conditions
Adrenal insufficiency, congestive heart failure, diabetes mellitus, hyperparathyroidism, myocardial ischemia, pregnancy, renal insufficiency, thyroid disease

Table 3.11: Causes of oropharyngeal dysphagia.

Neuromuscular causes	Structural causes
• Amyotrophic lateral sclerosis (ALS) • Multiple sclerosis • Muscular dystrophy • Myasthenia gravis • Parkinson's disease • Polymyositis or dermatomyositis • Stroke • Thyroid dysfunction	• Carcinoma • Infections of pharynx or neck • Osteophytes and other spinal disorders • Prior surgery or radiation therapy • Proximal esophageal web • Plummer–Vinson syndrome • Thyromegaly • Zenker's diverticulum

Odynophagia

Definition

Odynophagia, or painful swallowing, is specific feature for esophageal involvement. It usually reflects an inflammatory process in the esophageal mucosa.

Causes of Odynophagia

The causes of odynophagia are described in **Box 3.2**.

Pain Abdomen

The history of a patient with abdominal pain includes determining whether the pain is acute or chronic and a detailed description of the pain and associated symptoms, which should be interpreted with other aspects of the medical history.

Table 3.12: Causes of esophageal dysphagia.

Motility (neuromusclar) disorders	Structural (mechanical) disorders
Primary disorders • Achalasia • Diffuse esophageal spasm • Hypertensive LES • Ineffective esophageal motility • Nutcracker (high-pressure) esophagus	**Intrinsic** • Carcinoma and benign tumors • Diverticula • Eosinophilic esophagitis • Esophageal rings and webs (other than Schatzki ring) • Foreign body • Lower esophageal (Schatzki) ring • Medication-induced stricture • Peptic stricture
Secondary disorders • Chagas' disease • Reflux-related dysmotility • Scleroderma and other rheumatologic disorders	**Extrinsic** • Mediastinal mass • Spinal osteophytes • Vascular compression

---

Box 3.2: Causes of odynophagia.

Caustic ingestion: Acid, alkali
Pill-induced Injury
❖ Alendronate and other bisphosphonates
❖ Aspirin and other NSAIDs
❖ Iron preparations
❖ Potassium chloride (especially slow-release form)
❖ Tetracycline and its derivatives
❖ Quinidine
❖ Zidovudine
Infectious esophagitis
❖ *Viral*: Cytomegalovirus, Epstein-Barr virus, herpes simplex virus, human immunodeficiency virus
❖ *Bacteria*: Mycobacteria (tuberculosis or *Mycobacterium avium* complex)
❖ *Fungal: Candida albicans,* histoplasmosis
❖ *Protozoan: Cryptosporidium, Pneumocystis*
Severe reflux esophagitis
Esophageal carcinoma

Acute versus Chronic Pain

There is no strict time period that will classify the differential diagnosis unfailingly. A clinical judgment must be made that considers whether this is an accelerating process, one that has reached a plateau, or one that is longstanding but intermittent. Patients with chronic abdominal pain may present with an acute exacerbation of a chronic problem or a new and unrelated problem. Pain of less than a few days' duration that has worsened progressively until the time of presentation is clearly "acute". Pain that has remained unchanged for months or years can be safely classified as chronic. Pain that does not clearly fit either category might be called subacute and requires consideration of a broader differential than acute and chronic pain.

Description of Pain

Pain is discussed under following headings:
- **Location and radiation:** The location of abdominal pain helps narrow the differential diagnosis as different pain syndromes typically have characteristic locations. For example, pain involving the liver or biliary tree is generally located in the right upper quadrant, but it may radiate to the back or epigastrium. Because hepatic pain only results when the capsule of the liver is "stretched", most pain in the right upper quadrant is related to the biliary tree. Pain radiation is also important: the pain of pancreatitis classically bores to the back, while renal colic radiates to the groin.
- **Temporal elements:** The onset, frequency, and duration of the pain are helpful features. The pain of pancreatitis may be gradual and steady, while perforation and resultant peritonitis begins suddenly and is maximal from the onset.
- **Quality:** The quality of the pain includes determining whether the pain is burning or gnawing, as is typical of gastroesophageal reflux and peptic ulcer disease, or colicky, as in the cramping pain of gastroenteritis or intestinal obstruction.
- **Severity:** The severity of the pain generally is related to the severity of the disorder, especially if acute in onset. For example, the pain of biliary or renal colic or acute mesenteric ischemia is of high intensity, while the pain of gastroenteritis is less marked. Age and general health may affect the patient's clinical presentation. A patient taking corticosteroids may have significant masking of pain, and older adult patients often present with less intense pain.
- **Precipitants or palliation:** Determining what precipitates or palliates the pain can help narrow the differential. The pain of chronic mesenteric ischemia usually starts within 1 hour of eating, while the pain of duodenal ulcers may be relieved by eating and recur several hours after a meal.
- **Position/posture:** The pain of pancreatitis is classically relieved by sitting up and leaning forward. Peritonitis often causes patients to lie motionless on their backs because any motion causes pain. Obtaining a history of pain occurring in relationship to eating lactose- or gluten-containing foods may be helpful in identifying sensitivities to these food constituents. Patients with foodborne illness may become ill after eating certain foods.

Associated Symptoms

- **Other gastrointestinal symptoms:** We ask about associated nausea, vomiting, diarrhea, constipation, hematochezia, melena, and changes in stool (e.g., change in caliber). For patients with right upper quadrant pain or concern for liver disease, we also ask about jaundice and changes in the color of urine and stool. The bowel habit is an important part of the history for chronic abdominal pain. While many organic lesions can result in chronic diarrhea, IBS often presents with swings between diarrhea and constipation, a pattern that is much less likely with organic disease.
- **Genitourinary symptoms:** Patients with symptoms such as dysuria, frequency, and hematuria are more likely to have a genitourinary cause for their abdominal pain.
- **Constitutional symptoms:** Symptoms such as fevers, chills, fatigue, weight loss, and anorexia would be concerning for infection, malignancy, or systemic illnesses [e.g., inflammatory bowel disease (IBD)].

- **Cardiopulmonary symptoms:** Symptoms such as cough, shortness of breath, orthopnea, and exertional dyspnea suggest a pulmonary or cardiac etiology. Orthostatic hypotension may indicate early shock or be associated with adrenal insufficiency.
- **Other:** Patients with diabetic ketoacidosis will have symptoms of polyuria and thirst. Patients with suspected IBD should be asked about extraintestinal manifestations.

Other Medical History

- **Specific questions for women:** Women should be screened for sexually transmitted diseases and risks for pelvic inflammatory disease (e.g., new or multiple partners). Premenopausal women should be asked about their menstrual history (last menstrual period, last normal menstrual period, previous menstrual period, and cycle length) and use of contraception. They should also be asked about vaginal discharge or bleeding, dyspareunia or dysmenorrhea, as these symptoms suggest a pelvic pathology.
- **Past medical history:** A history of surgeries and procedures should be obtained to assess risk for differing etiologies (e.g., a history of abdominal surgery is a risk factor for obstruction). A history of cardiovascular disease (CVD) or multiple risk factors for CVD in a patient with epigastric pain raises concern for a myocardial ischemia.
- **Medications:** A comprehensive medication list should be elicited as this can inform the differential. For example, patients taking high doses of nonsteroidal anti-inflammatory drugs (NSAIDs) are at risk for gastropathy and peptic ulcer disease. Patients with recent antibiotics use or hospitalization are at risk for *Clostridioides* (formerly *Clostridium*) *difficile*. Patients on chronic steroids are at risk for adrenal insufficiency and may be immunosuppressed with atypical presentations of abdominal pain.
- **Other history**
  - Alcohol: It is important to ask about alcohol intake to assess for the possibility of liver disease and pancreatitis.
- **Family history:** Family history should be asked as appropriate based on other history. For example, patients with history concerning for IBD or cancer should also be asked about family history.
- **Travel history:** A travel history is important to elicit in patients with symptoms consistent with gastroenteritis or colitis (e.g., nausea, vomiting, and diarrhea) to consider infectious etiologies.
- **Sick contacts:** Often patients are in contact with someone with gastroenteritis before having similar symptoms. Patients with foodborne illness may also have close contacts with similar illness.

Site of Pain and Possible Etiology

Right upper quadrant
The causes of right upper quadrant abdominal pain are described in **Table 3.13**.

Epigastric pain
The causes of epigastric abdominal pain are described in **Table 3.14**.

Left upper quadrant
The causes of left upper quadrant abdominal pain are described in **Table 3.15**.

Table 3.13: Causes of right upper quadrant (RUQ) abdominal pain.

RUQ	Clinical features
Biliary colic	Intense, dull discomfort located in the RUQ or epigastrium. Associated with nausea, vomiting and diaphoresis. Generally lasts at least 30 minutes, plateauing within one hour. Benign abdominal examination
Acute cholecystitis	Prolonged (>4–6 hours) RUQ or epigastric pain, fever. Patients will have abdominal guarding and Murphy's sign.
Acute cholangitis	Fever, jaundice, RUQ pain
Sphincter of Oddi dysfunction	RUQ pain similar to other biliary pain
Hepatic	
Acute hepatitis	RUQ pain with fatigue, malaise, nausea, vomiting and anorexia. Patients may also have jaundice, dark urine, and light-colored stools
Perihepatitis (Fitz-Hugh-Curtis syndrome)	RUQ pain with a pleuritic component, pain is sometimes referred to the right shoulder
Liver abscess	Fever and abdominal pain are the most common symptoms
Budd-Chiari syndrome	Symptoms include fever; abdominal pain, abdominal distention (from ascites), lower extremity edema, jaundice, gastrointestinal bleeding, and/or hepatic encephalopathy
Portal vein thrombosis	Symptoms include abdominal pain, dyspepsia, or gastrointestinal bleeding

Table 3.14: Causes of epigastric abdominal pain.

Epigastric	Clinical features
Acute myocardial infarction	May be associated with shortness of breath and exertional symptoms
Acute pancreatitis	Acute-onset, persistent upper abdominal pain radiating to the back
Chronic pancreatitis	Epigastric pain radiating to the back
Peptic ulcer disease	Epigastric pain or discomfort is the most prominent symptom
Gastroesophageal reflux disease	Associated with heartburn, regurgitation, and dysphagia
Gastritis/gastropathy	Abdominal discomfort/pain, heartburn, nausea, vomiting, and hematemesis
Functional dyspepsia	The presence of one or more of the following: Postprandial fullness, early satiation, epigastric pain, or burning
Gastroparesis	Nausea, vomiting, abdominal pain, early satiety, postprandial fullness, and bloating

Table 3.15: The causes of left upper quadrant (LUQ) abdominal pain.

LUQ	Clinical features
Splenomegaly	Pain or discomfort in LUQ, left shoulder pain and/or early satiety
Splenic infarct	Severe LUQ pain
Splenic abscess	Associated with fever and LUQ tenderness
Splenic rupture	May complain of LUQ, left chest wall, or left shoulder pain that is worse with inspiration

Table 3.16: Causes of lower abdominal pain.

Lower abdomen	Localization	Clinical features
Appendicitis	Generally right lower quadrant	Periumbilical pain initially that radiates to the right lower quadrant. Associated with, anorexia, nausea and vomiting
Diverticulitis	Generally left lower quadrant; right lower quadrant more common in Asian patients	Pain usually constant and present for several days prior to presentation. May have associated nausea and vomiting
Nephrolithiasis	Either	Pain most common symptom, varies from mild to severe. Generally flank pain, but may have back or abdominal pain
Pyelonephritis	Either	Associated with dysuria, frequency, urgency, hematuria, fever, chills, flank pain, and costovertebral angle tenderness
Acute urinary retention	Suprapubic	Present with lower abdominal pain and discomfort; inability to urinate
Cystitis	Suprapubic	Associated with dysuria, frequency, urgency and hematuria
Infectious colitis	Either	Diarrhea as the predominant symptom, but may also have associated abdominal pain, which may be severe.

Lower abdominal pain
The causes of lower abdominal pain are described in **Table 3.16**.

Diffuse abdominal pain
The causes of diffuse abdominal pain are described in **Table 3.17**.

Table 3.17: Causes of diffuse abdominal pain.

Diffuse/poorly characterized	Clinical features
Bowel obstruction	• Most common symptoms are nausea, vomiting, crampy abdominal pain, and obstipation • Distended, tympanic abdomen with high-pitched or absent bowel sounds
Perforation of the gastrointestinal tract	Severe abdominal pain, particularly following procedures
Acute mesenteric ischemia	Acute and severe onset of diffuse and persistent abdominal pain, often described as pain out of proportion to examination.
Chronic mesenteric ischemia	Abdominal pain after eating ("intestinal angina"), weight loss, nausea, vomiting, and diarrhea
Inflammatory bowel disease (ulcerative colitis/Crohn disease)	Associated with bloody diarrhea, urgency, tenesmus, bowel incontinence, weight loss, and fevers
Viral gastroenteritis	Diarrhea accompanied by nausea, vomiting and abdominal pain
Spontaneous bacterial peritonitis	Fever, abdominal pain, and/or altered mental status
Dialysis-related peritonitis	Abdominal pain and cloudy peritoneal effluent. Other symptoms and signs include fever nausea, diarrhea, abdominal tenderness, and rebound tenderness
Colorectal cancer	Variable presentation, including obstruction and perforation
Other malignancy	Vary depending on malignancy
Celiac disease	Abdominal pain in addition to including diarrhea with bulky, foul-smelling, floating stools due to steatorrhea and flatulence
Ketoacidosis	Diffuse abdominal pain and nausea and vomiting
Adrenal insufficiency	Diffuse abdominal pain and nausea and vomiting
Foodborne Illness	Mixture of nausea, vomiting, fever, abdominal pain and diarrhea
Irritable bowel syndrome	Chronic abdominal pain with altered bowel habits
Constipation	
Diverticulosis	May have symptoms of abdominal pain and constipation
Lactose intolerance	Associated with abdominal pain, bloating, flatulence and diarrhea. Abdominal pain may be cramping in nature

GASTROINTESTINAL TRACT: DISCUSSION

General Examination

Peripheral signs of chronic liver disease

Skin, nail, and hands

- Spider nevi (telangiectatic superficial blood vessels with central feeding vessel)
- Clubbing of hands (especially biliary cirrhosis and hepatocellular carcinoma)
- Leukonychia
- Palmar erythema (blotchy appearance over the thenar and hypothenar eminence)
- Bruising
- Duputryen's contracture (sign of alcoholism)
- Scratch marks (cholestatic jaundice)

Endocrine—due to estrogen excess

- Gynecomastia
- Atrophy of testis
- Loss of axillary and pubic hair

Others

- Parotid and lacrimal gland swelling (alcoholic liver disease)
- Fetor hepaticus (characteristic sweet smelling breath)
- Asterixis

Signs of Cirrhosis of Liver

Jaundice

- Jaundice is not a common feature of cirrhosis; it is more common with acute diseases.
- Mechanisms of jaundice in cirrhosis:
  - Failure to excrete bilirubin (mainly)
  - Intrahepatic cholestasis (superadded hepatitis/tumor)
  - Hemolysis due to hypersplenism (not a major contributor).

Hepatomegaly

- **Early stages:** Liver is enlarged, firm to hard, irregular, and nontender. Hepatomegaly is not common in cirrhosis but common when the cirrhosis is due to alcoholic liver disease, NASH, and hemochromatosis. Hepatomegaly may indicate transformation into HCC.
- **Late stages:** Liver decreases in size and nonpalpable due to progressive destruction of liver cells and accompanying fibrosis.

Ascites

- Ascites due to liver failure and portal HTN.
- It signifies advanced disease.

(discussed in detail later)

Spider Nevi

Spider nevi **(Fig. 3.2)**, also known as spider telangiectasia; vascular spiders; spider angiomas; arterial spiders, and nevus araneus.

Spider nevi (spider telangiectasia; vascular spiders; spider angiomas; arterial spiders, nevus araneus)	
Description	Consists of a central arteriole from which numerous small vessels radiate peripherally-resembling spider's legs. Whole spider disappears when central arteriole is compressed with a pinhead. When compression is released filling occurs from center to periphery.
Pathophysiology	Due to arteriolar changes induced by hyperestrogenism.
Location	Usually found only in the necklace area, i.e., above the nipples, territory drained by the superior vena cava, such as head and neck, upper limbs, front and back of upper chest.
Size	Vary from pin head to 0.5 mm in diameter.
Clinical demonstration	Applying pressure over the body of spiders with a glass slide (diascopy) **(Fig. 3.3)**, or pin head **(Fig. 3.4)** leading to pallor with refilling following the release of pressure
Significance	They are a strong indicator of liver disease but can be found in other conditions
Causes	**Liver disorders** • Viral hepatitis • Alcoholic hepatitis • Hepatocellular carcinoma • Treatment with sorafenib	**Others** • Third trimester of pregnancy • Rheumatoid arthritis • Thyrotoxicosis • Also normally seen in 2% of healthy population
Differential diagnosis	Venous star, Campbell de Morgan spots, petechiae and hereditary hemorrhagic telangiectasias

Note:
- Florid spider telangiectasia, gynecomastia and parotid enlargement are most common in alcoholic hepatitis.
- Florid spiders and new onset clubbing in a patient with cirrhosis indicates hepatopulmonary syndrome.

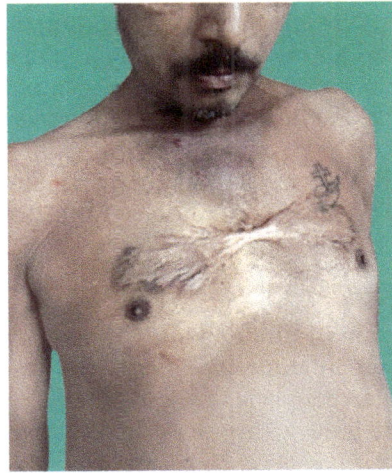

Fig. 3.2: Cirrhosis of liver with ascites and spider nevi. Patient in addition has tattoo and keloid, which may suggest viral hepatitis as the cause of cirrhosis.

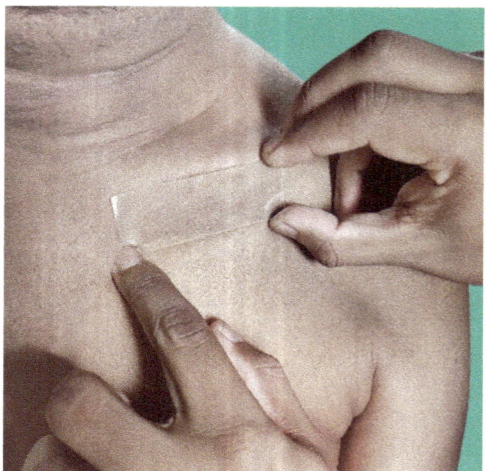

Fig. 3.3: Demonstration of spider nevi (glass-slide method).

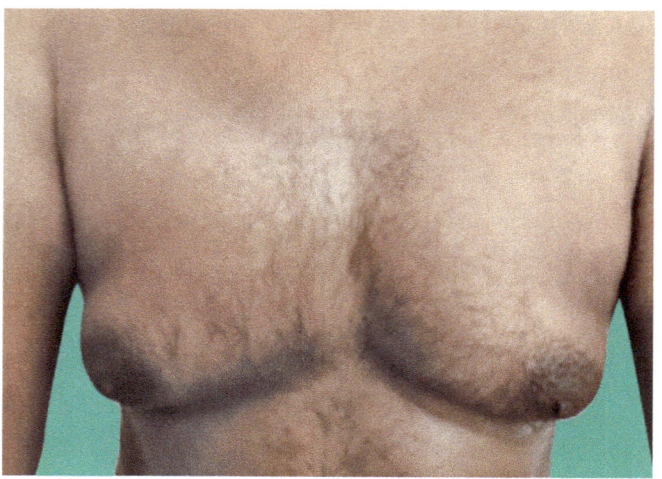

Fig. 3.5: Gynecomastia.

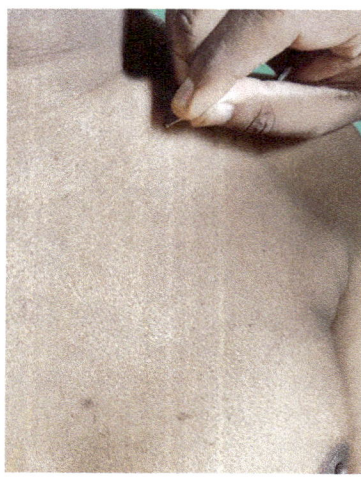

Fig. 3.4: Demonstration of spider nevi (pin-head method).

Palmar Erythema (Liver Palm)

- Palmar erythema can be seen early but is of limited diagnostic value, as it occurs in many conditions associated with a hyperdynamic circulation (e.g., normal pregnancy).
- **Cause:** Develops due to increased peripheral blood flow. In cirrhosis, circulatory changes results in increased peripheral blood flow and decreased visceral blood flow (especially to the kidneys).
- **Sites involved:** Prominent in the thenar and hypothenar eminences of palm. Spares the central portion of the palm. May be seen on the sole.

Endocrine Changes

- **Diminished body hair and loss of hair**
  - This is seen mainly in males with loss of male hair distribution. Alopecia affects usually the face, axilla, and chest and is due to hyperestrogenism.
  - *Causes of hyperestrogenism*: Due to increased peripheral formation of estrogen resulting from diminished hepatic clearance of the precursor, androstenedione.
  - *Effects of hyperestrogenism*: Alopecia, gynecomastia, and testicular atrophy.

- **Hyperglycemia:**
  - In hyperglycemia, 80% of cirrhotics have impaired glucose tolerance, 20% develop diabetes.
- **Gynecomastia (Fig. 3.5)**
  - Found in males (atrophy of breasts in females).
  - *Cause:* Due to increased estradiol/free testosterone ratio **(Box 3.3)**.
  - *Examination (Fig. 3.6):* Appear as palpable nodule (4 cm, subareolar).
  - **Microscopy**: Proliferation of glandular tissue of breast.
  - *Pseudogynecomastia* is accumulation of subareolar fat tissue without palpable nodule.

Testicular Atrophy

- Due to hyperestrogenic state, it is characterized by a small size compared with Prader's orchidometer **(Fig. 3.7)**, soft testes with loss of testicular sensation (sickening sensation in epigastrium on squeezing the testes). The dimensions of the average adult testicle are 4.5 × 3.5 × 2.5 cm and the volume is 15–25 mL.
- **Female:** Irregular menses, amenorrhea, and atrophy of breast.

Duputryen'ss Contracture (It is a Sign of Alcoholism)

- **Pathophysiology:** Fibrosis of palmar aponeurosis probably caused by local microvessel ischemia. Platelet and fibroblast-derived growth factors promote fibrosis.

Box 3.3: Causes of gynecomastia.

- Cirrhosis of liver
- Drugs:
  - Spironolactone
  - Cimetidine
  - Digoxin
  - Ketoconazole
  - Estrogens
  - Isoniazid
- Physiological (puberty/aging)
- Klinefelter's syndrome
- Hypogonadism
- Tumor:
  - Testes
  - Lung

- **Sites involved:** Flexion contracture of the fingers **(Fig. 3.8)** (especially ring and little fingers).
- **Other causes of Duputryen's contracture:** DM, rheumatoid arthritis, and manual labor (workers exposed to repetitive handling tasks or vibration).

Clubbing and Central Cyanosis
- Due to development of pulmonary arteriovenous shunts that leading to hypoxemia.

Nail Changes
- **White (Terry's)** chalky and brittle nails **(Fig. 3.9)**. And it can be easily demonstrated on comparison with normal person nails when placed side by side **(Fig. 3.10)**.
- **Muehrcke's nails:** Characterized by transverse white lines that disappear on applying pressure and these lines do not move with growth of nail.
- **Clubbing** is present in primary biliary cholangitis or hepatoma.

Parotid and Lacrimal Gland Enlargement (Fig. 3.11)
Observed commonly in alcoholic cirrhosis due to associated autonomic dysfunction.

Anemia
It can be due to various causes:
- Acute and chronic blood loss from varices
- Nutritional deficiency of vitamin B12 and folate
- Hypersplenism

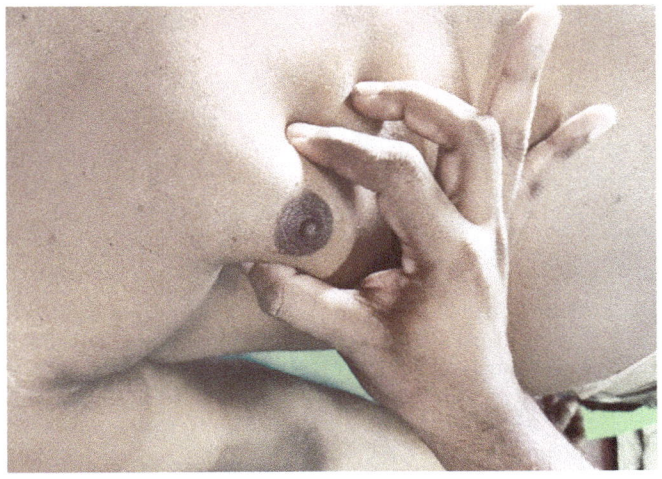

Fig. 3.6: Palpation breast bud in gynecomatia.

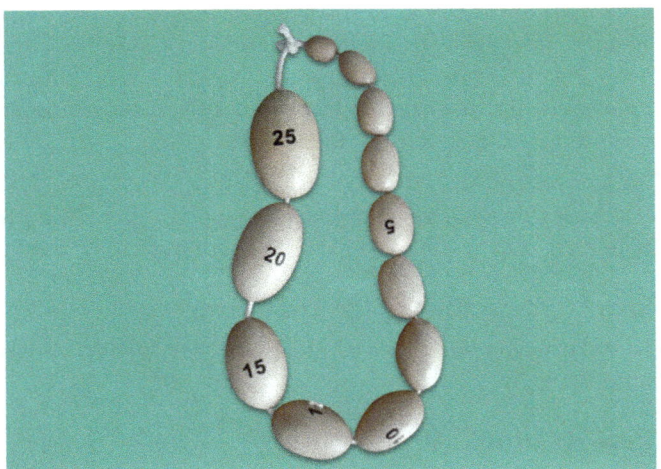

Fig. 3.7: Prader's orchidometer.

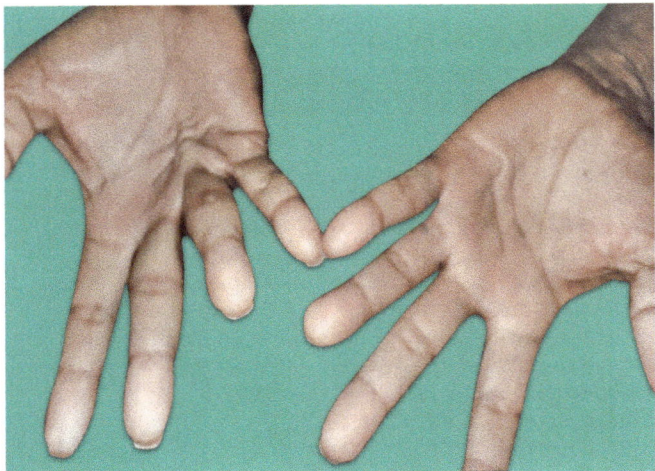

Fig. 3.8: Duputryen's contracture.

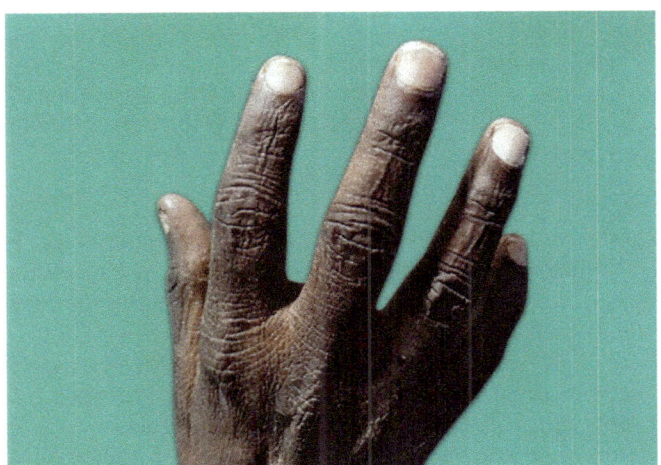

Fig. 3.9: White nails.

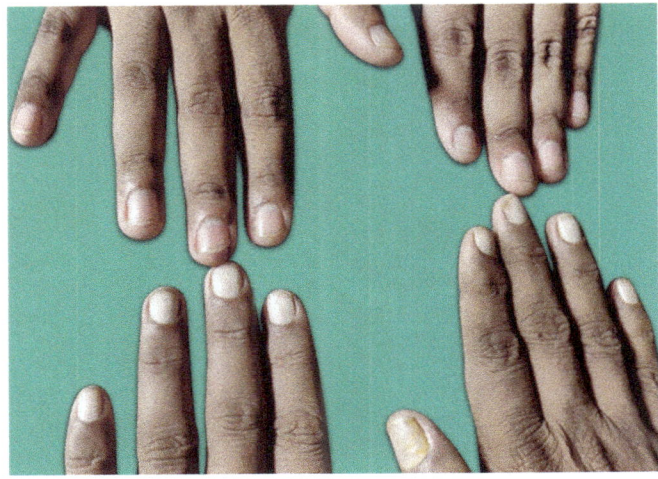

Fig. 3.10: Leukonychia—compare with nails of normal person (preferably hands to be placed side by side).

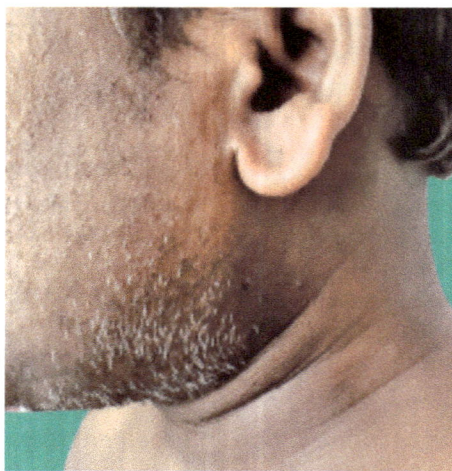

Fig. 3.11: Diminished facial hair with parotid enlargement.

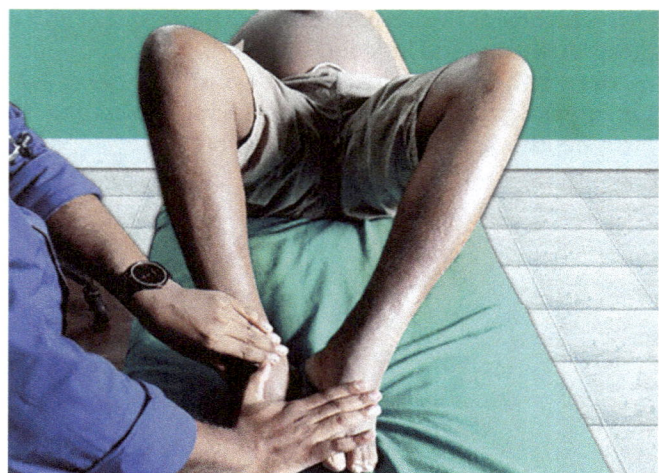

Fig. 3.13: Demonstration of flapping tremors in legs—on leaving the legs to fall apart a negative myoclonus can be noticed by observing the knee.

- Bone marrow suppression by alcohol
- Hemolysis.
- **Zieves syndrome:** Alcohol-induced hemolytic anemia with hypercholesterolemia

Fetor Hepaticus
- Sweet, pungent smelling odor
- It is due to volatile **dimethyl sulfide**, especially in portosystemic shunting and liver failure and hepatic encephalopathy

Asterixis
- Asterixis is a disorder of motor control characterized by an inability to actively maintain a position and consequent irregular myoclonic lapses of posture affecting various parts of the body independently.
- It is a type of negative myoclonus characterized by a brief loss of muscle tone in agonist muscles followed by a compensatory jerk of the antagonistic muscles.
- **Demonstration of asterixis of hand (Fig. 3.12):**
  - Asterixis is tested by extending the arms, dorsiflexing the wrists, and spreading the fingers to observe for the "flap" at the wrist. The flap is due to irregular myoclonic lapses of posture caused by involuntary 50–200 m silent periods appearing in tonically active muscles.
- **Demonstration of asterixis of leg (Fig. 3.13):** Testing asterixis at the hip joint involves keeping the patient in a supine position with knees bent and feet flat on the table, leaving the legs to fall to the sides. Negative myoclonus of the lower limbs at the hip joints repetitively occurs and is appreciated by looking at the knees.

Causes of asterixis
The causes of asterixis (flapping tremor) are described in **Table 3.18**.

Signs Pointing the Etiology of Cirrhosis
The etiology and signs of cirrhosis are described in **Table 3.19**.

Signs of Chronic Alcoholism
- *Parotid swelling*
- *Duputryen's contracture*

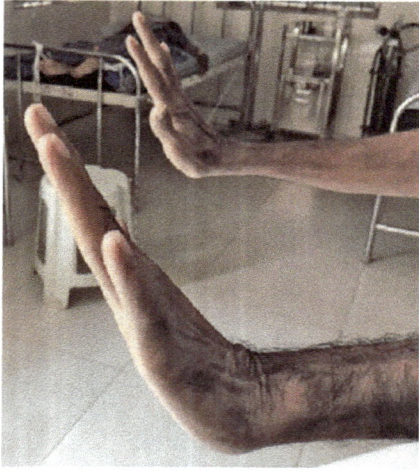

Fig. 3.12: Demonstration of asterixis in hands.

Table 3.18: Causes of asterixis.

Bilateral	Unilateral
Metabolic: Liver failure, azotemia, respiratory failure **Sedatives:** Benzodiazepines, barbiturates **Anticonvulsants:** Phenytoin (phenytoin flap), carbamazepine, valproic acid, gabapentin **Antipsychotics:** Lithium **Antibiotics:** Ceftazidime **Others:** Metoclopramide **Dyselectrolytemia:** Hypomagnesemia, hypokalemia **Bilateral structural brain lesions**	**Focal brain lesions at:** • Thalamus • Corona radiata • Anterior cerebral artery territory • Primary motor cortex • Parietal lobe • Cerebellum • Midbrain • Pons

Table 3.19: Signs and etiology of cirrhosis.

Signs	Etiology of Cirrhosis
Parotid enlargement, Duputryen's contracture	Alcohol
Tattoo marks, Jaundice	Hepatitis B/C
Metabolic syndrome	NASH
Xanthoma, xanthelasma, obstructive jaundice	Primary biliary cirrhosis
Skin hyperpigmentation, organomegaly, diabetes	Hemochromatosis
Emphysema and cirrhosis	Alpha-1 antitrypsin deficiency
Long-standing heart failure	Cardiac cirrhosis
Tender liver with absent abdominojugular reflux	Budd–Chiari syndrome
Arthritis, skin changes, nephritis	Autoimmune
Deforming arthritis on treatment	Methotrexate induced
KF ring on cornea	Wilsons disease

ORAL CAVITY EXAMINATION

A torch, tongue depressor, and gloves (for palpation) needed

Lips
- Angular stomatitis, cheilitis—iron deficiency, riboflavin deficiency
- Herpes labialis
- Circumoral pigmentation

Teeth
- Caries
- Color/staining: Tobacco, tetracycline (yellow), fluorosis (chalk white), red/erythrodontia (porphyria)
- Shape of teeth: Peg-shaped incisors and moon molars in congenital syphilis, widely spaced teeth in acromegaly.

Gums
- Gingivitis
- **Gum bleeding:** Scurvy, vitamin K deficiency, acute leukemia, thrombocytopenia, coagulopathies, gingivitis
- **Gum hypertrophy**
  - Drugs: Phenytoin, nifedipine, cyclosporine
  - Pregnancy
  - AML—M4, M5
  - Chronic gingivitis
  - Tumors: Epulis
- Ulcers, pyorrhea

Tongue
- **Macroglossia:** Acromegaly, myxedema, amyloidosis, Downs' syndrome
- **Coated tongue:** Typhoid, candidiasis
- **Color of tongue:**
  - *Pale:* Anemia
  - *Red beefy:* B12 deficiency
  - *Magenta:* B2 deficiency
  - *Bluish:* Cyanosis
  - *Yellowish:* Jaundice
  - *Strawberry:* Scarlet fever
- **Dry tongue:** Dehydration, anticholinergics, diabetes
- Leukoplakia, hairy leukoplakia
- Fissuring
- **Geographic tongue:** Desquamated epithelium
- Median rhomboid glossitis

Buccal Mucosa
- Ulcers
- Pigmentation
- Candidiasis
- Koplik spots

Palate/Pharynx
- Ulcers
- Postnasal drip
- **White patch of tonsil:**
  - Candidiasis
  - Diphtheria
  - Agranulocytosis
  - Infectious mononucleosis
  - Follicular tonsillitis
  - Vincent's angina
  - Malignancy
  - Tonsillolith

Causes of Oral Ulcers
The causes of oral ulcers have been described in **Table 3.20**.

Pigmentation of Oral Mucosa
- Addison's disease
- Peutz-Jegher syndrome
- Hemochromatosis
- Heavy metal: Lead (Burtonian line)

Table 3.20: Causes of oral ulcers.

Aphthous ulcer	
Infections	**Gastrointestinal disease**
• Herpetic stomatitis	• Celiac disease
• Chickenpox	• Crohn's disease
• Hand, foot, and mouth disease	• Ulcerative colitis
• Herpangina	**Connective tissue disorders**
• Infectious mononucleosis	• Lupus erythematosus
• HIV	• Behçet's syndrome
• Acute necrotizing gingivitis	• Reiter's disease
• Tuberculosis	
• Syphilis	
Candida	
Dermatological disorders	**Malignancy**
• Lichen planus	**Drugs:** Cytotoxic agents, antibiotics
• Pemphigus	**Radiation**
• Pemphigoid	**Trauma**
• Erythema multiforme	
• Dermatitis herpetiformis	
• Linear IgA disease	
• Epidermolysis bullosa	

- Acanthosis
- Drugs like, hormones, oral contraceptives, cyclophosphamide, busulfan, bleomycin clofazimine, chloroquine
- Pregnancy
- Laugier-Hunziker Syndrome
- Nevi
- Malignant melanoma

Systemic Examination

The order of examination of abdomen is preferably done: Inspection → Auscultation → Palpation and Percussion. (*As the auscultatory findings might change post palpation and percussion*)

Inspection

Position of Patient

- Most of the GIT examination (inspection) is done in supine position (standing position is adapted for examination of dilated veins).
- Expose from chest to mid-thigh preferably.
- Relax abdominal wall muscles by flexing the thigh with arms by the side of the patient.

Shape of Abdomen

Shape	Condition seen
Scaphoid	Normal
Generalized abdominal distention (The 7Fs)	1. Fluid 2. Fat 3. Flatus 4. Feces 5. Fetus 6. Full bladder 7. Fatal neoplasm
Localized abdominal distention	Indicate a organomegaly or mass
Fullness of flanks indicates	Free fluid

Skin over the Abdomen

Findings	Seen in
Discoloration	**Pancreatitis** • *Cullen's sign:* Discoloration around umbilicus • *Grey Turner's sign:* Discoloration over the flanks
Ecchymosis or purpura	Coagulopathy
Striae atrophica or gravidarum (white or pink wrinkled linear marks)	• Recent change in size of the abdomen • Pregnancy • Ascites • Wasting diseases and • Severe dieting
Wide purple striae	Cushing's syndrome (pigmented)
Linea nigra	Pigmentation of the abdominal wall in the midline below the umbilicus, seen in pregnancy

Contd...

Contd...

Findings	Seen in
Erythema ab igne	• Brown mottled pigmentation produced by constant application of heat, usually a hot water bottle or heat pad, on the skin of the abdominal wall. • It is a **sign of chronic pain** as in chronic pancreatitis.
Paracentesis marks	Indicate diagnostic/therapeutic ascitic tapping
Sinuses	• Tuberculosis • Crohn's disease
Stretched shiny skin	Indicate tense ascites

Scars

Few commonly employed incisions over the abdomen as shown in **Figure 3.14**:

Quadrants of Abdomen

Abdomen can be grossly divided into four quadrants as shown in **Figure 3.15** with the help of transumbilical plane and median plane.

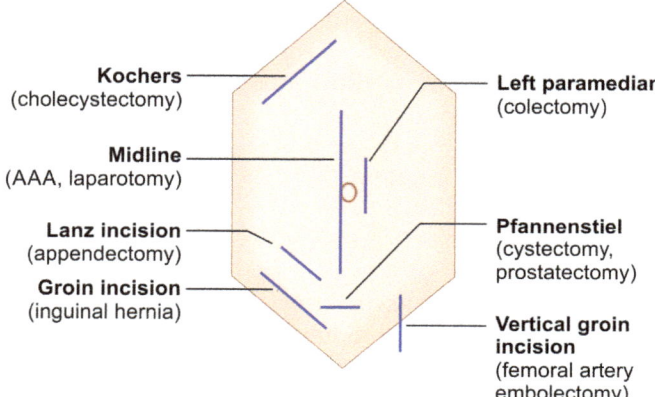

Fig. 3.14: Surgical scar commonly employed.

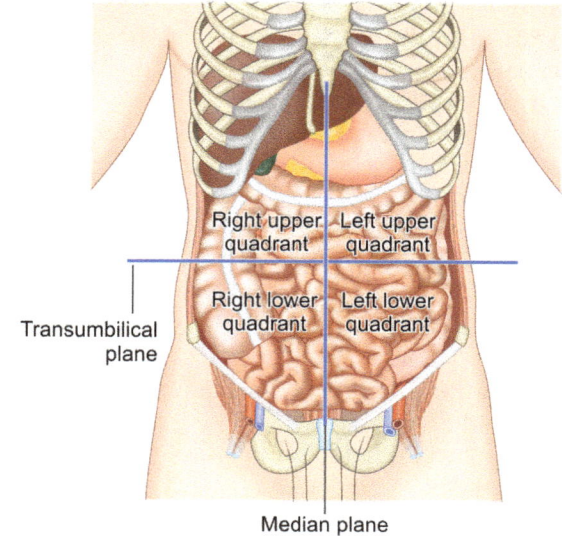

Fig. 3.15: Four quadrants of the abdomen.

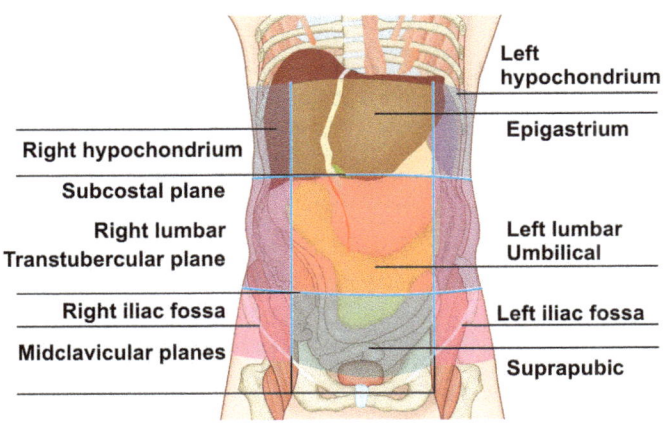

Fig. 3.16: Planes and nine areas of the abdomen.

Regions of Abdomen

Abdomen can also divided into nine regions with the help of right and left mid clavicular line, transtubercular plane, and subcostal plane as shown in the **Figure 3.16**.

Umbilicus

Finding	Seen in
Slightly retracted and inverted	Normal
Everted	Suggestive of tense ascites
Umbilical hernia	Indicate lax abdominal wall with gross ascites
Umbilical node	Sister Mary Joseph node seen in metastasis from GIT cancers
Normally, $\frac{\text{(distance between xisphisternum and umbilicus)}}{\text{(distance between umbilicus and pubis symphysis)}} = 1.6$	
Ratio decreased-umbilicus is displaced up (smiling umbilicus)	• Pelvic mass • Ovarian tumors
Ratio increased-umbilicus displaced down (weeping umbilicus)	• Upper abdominal mass • Ascites
Spinoumbilical distance (distance between ASIS to umbilicus)	• Normally—equidistant • Shift of umbilicus to one side indicates tumors/mass originating from other side

Movement with Respiration

Method of examination: Shine a light, across the patient's abdomen, and watch for the abdominal wall movements.

Finding	Seen in
Normal	• Gentle rise in the abdominal wall during inspiration and a fall during expiration • Corresponding areas move equally on both sides
Diminished or absent movements	Generalized peritonitis (**the still, silent abdomen**)

Visible Peristalsis

The direction of peristalsis and site of obstruction is seen in **Table 3.21**.

Visible Mass

The **Figure 3.17** demonstrates the underlying intra-abdominal structures with respect to the regions.

Divarication of Recti (Diastasis of Recti)

It is a gap between the rectus abdominis muscle, which becomes prominent on straining (**Fig. 3.18**). Make the patient

Table 3.21: Site of obstruction and direction of peristalsis.

Site of obstruction	Direction of peristalsis
Obstruction at the pylorus	Peristalsis from left costal margin to right
Obstruction in the distal small bowel	Right to left (or) Irregular pattern

Note: visible peristalsis may be a normal finding in very thin elderly patients with lax abdominal muscles.

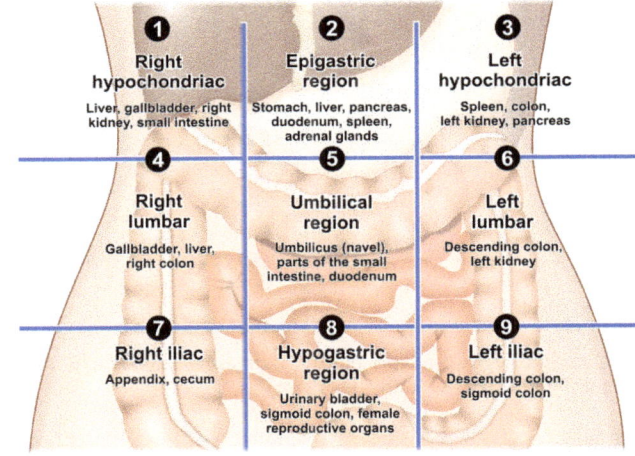

Fig. 3.17: Pictorial representation of corresponding areas and underlying structures.

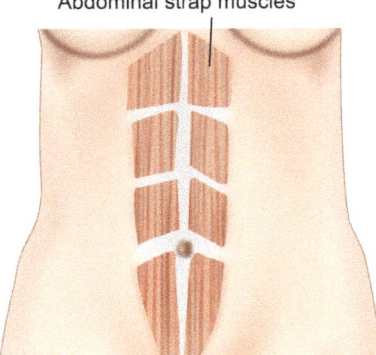
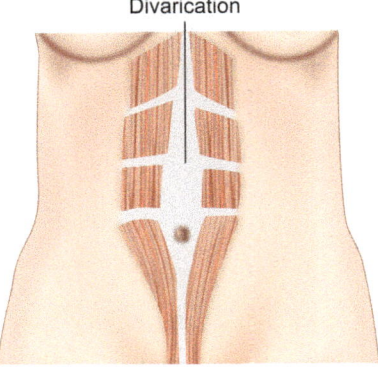

Fig. 3.18: Image showing divarication of recti.

Chapter 3: Gastrointestinal Tract Examination

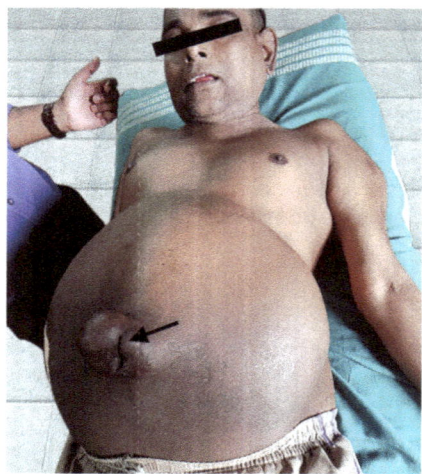

Fig. 3.19: Midline defect suggestive of divarication of recti and umblical hernia (arrow) on asking the patient to raise the head off the bed.

lie supine and tense the abdominal muscles by lifting the head **(Fig. 3.19)**, a midline defect can be seen and felt. It is common after postpartum, and also can be seen with tense ascites.

Auscultation

Note that the abdomen should be auscultated prior to palpation. Auscultate in all four quadrants of the abdomen.
1. Bowel sounds
2. Bruits
3. Venous hum
4. Rubs
5. Succussion splash

Bowel Sounds* (Fig. 3.20)

Normal	7–35 per minute
Increased (borborygmus)	• Intestinal obstruction • Diarrhea • Laxative use • Carcinoid syndrome • Massive GI bleed
Decreased	Paralytic ileus and peritonitis

*When bowel sounds are not present, one must auscultate for full 3 minutes before saying that bowel sounds are absent.

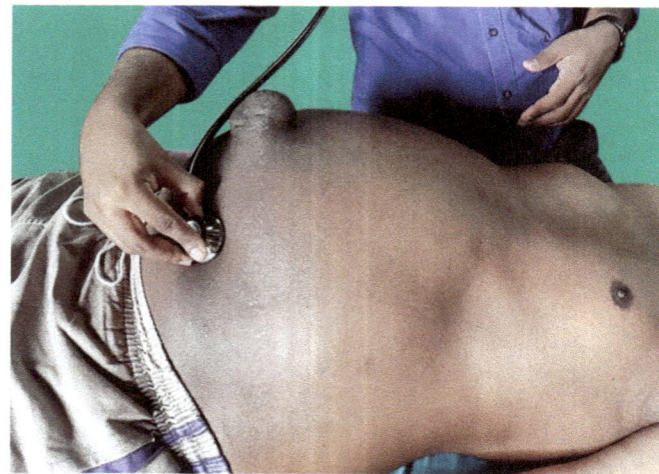

Fig. 3.20: Auscultation of bowel sounds.

Bruits

Renal artery bruit (Fig. 3.21)	• 2.5 cm above and lateral to the umbilicus in transpyloric plane • Indicates partial renal artery stenosis
Abdominal aorta (Fig. 3.22)	• Epigastrium in aortic aneurysm or aortoarteritis
Hepatic bruit (Fig. 3.23)	• HCC • Acute alcoholic hepatitis • Hemangioma
Iliac bruit (Fig. 3.24)	• 2.5 cm below and lateral to the umbilicus

Venous Hum

Cruveilhier baumgarten murmur (Fig. 3.25)
❒ It is a continuous murmur, produced due to the opening of the paraumbilical vein in the falciform ligament.
❒ It is heard midway between the xiphisternum and umbilicus on to the right side of the epigastrium.
❒ A patent umbilical vein excludes an extrahepatic cause of portal hypertension because the umbilical vein arises from the intrahepatic portion of the left portal vein.

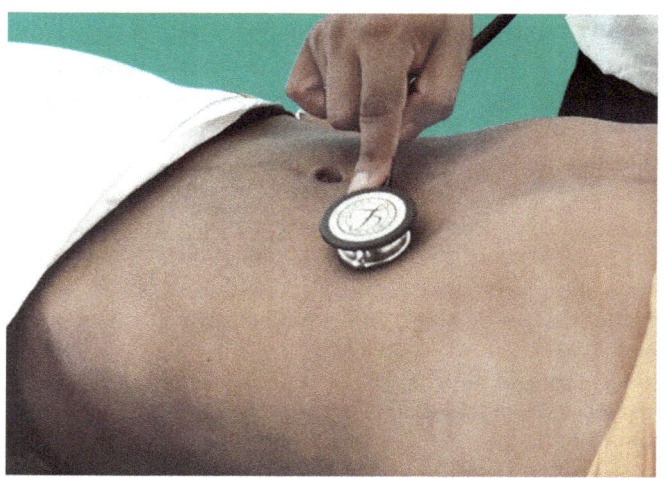

Fig. 3.21: Renal artery bruit—2.5 cm above and later to umbilicus in transpyloric plane.

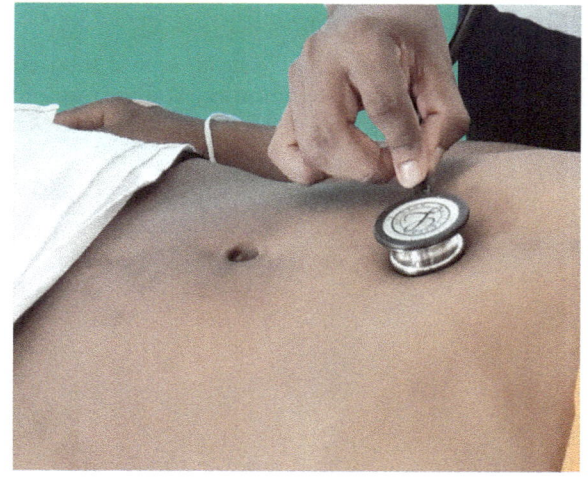

Fig. 3.22: Abdominal aorta bruit—in epigastrium in midline.

Chapter 3: Gastrointestinal Tract Examination

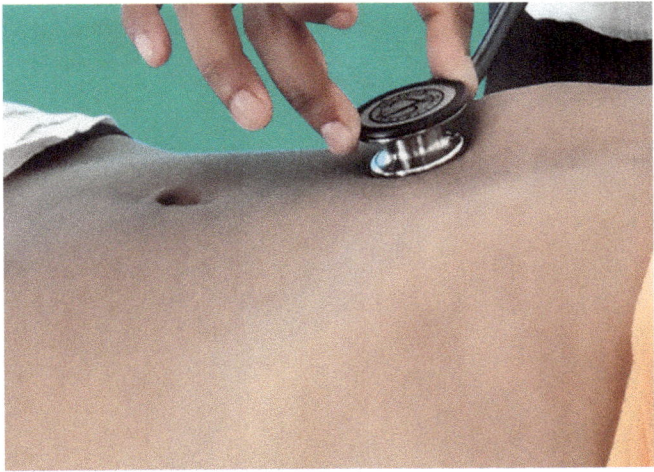

Fig. 3.23: Hepatic bruit.

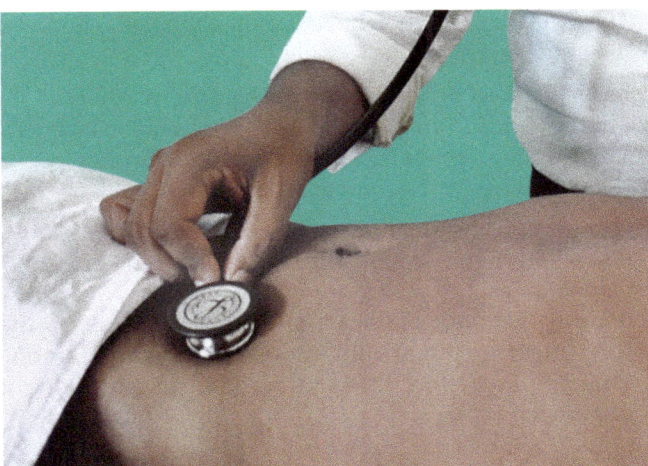

Fig. 3.24: Iliac bruit—2.5 cm below and lateral to umbilicus.

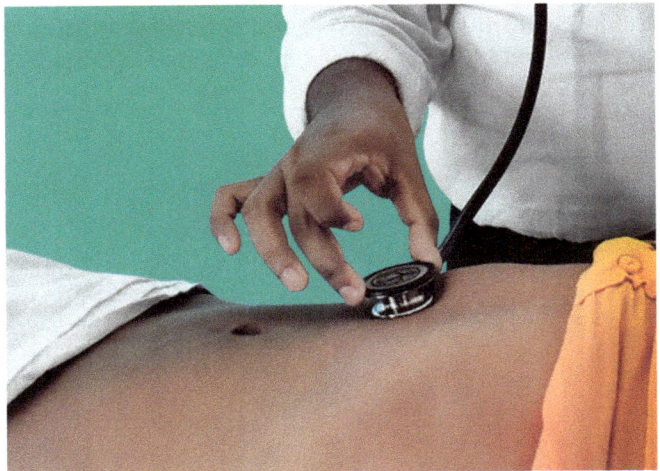

Fig. 3.25: Cruveilhier Baumgarten murmur heard midway between the xiphisternum and umbilicus on to the right side of the epigastrium.

Rubs
- Hepatic friction rub is superficial, scratchy sound heard on the liver.

Commonly seen with:
- HCC,
- Postliver biopsy,
- Hepatic infarcts, and
- Gonococcal peritonitis (Fitz–Hugh–Curtis syndrome).
- Splenic rub is a coarse, scratching sound coinciding with inspiration over the left upper quadrant due to splenic infarct.

Commonly seen with:
- Subacute bacterial endocarditis
- Chronic myeloid leukemia.
- Sickle cell anemia.
- After splenic puncture (e.g., in diagnosis of chronic kala-azar).

Succussion Splash
- When you auscultate the patient's epigastric/left upper quadrant and then shake the patient a "splash-like" noise is heard
- If heard after several hours after eating, it suggests delayed gastric emptying, which may be due to gastric outlet obstruction.
- Thoracic succussion splash has been described in achalasia cardia, hydropneumothorax, and large hiatal hernia.

Palpation and Percussion of the Abdomen
The following scheme is suggested for palpating abdomen:
- Start in lower left quadrant of abdomen and repeat all quadrants as described below.
- Palpate lightly initially, followed by deep palpation.
- Feel for left kidney → spleen → right kidney → liver → aorta and para-aortic glands → common femoral vessels → urinary bladder → both groins → external genitalia.

EXAMINATION OF INDIVIDUAL ORGANS
Examination of Liver
Location
- Right hypochondriac region
- Epigastric region
- Left hypochondriac region

Extent
- Upper border—6th rib anteriorly
- Inferior border—crosses midline at the level of transpyloric plane (at the level of L1 vertebrae)

Inspection
- Watch for the fullness in the right hypochondrium and epigastrium (epigastrium usually represents left lobe).
- Direction of enlargement is toward the right iliac fossa.

Palpation
Following methods of palpation have been discussed:
- Traditional method/conventional method
- Preferred method
- Alternate method
- Hooking method
- Dipping method

Traditional method/conventional method (Fig. 3.26)
- Place right hand on the right iliac fossa, parallel to the costal margin
- Keep the hand steady during inspiration and feel for the liver edge as it descends with each inspiration
- If edge is not felt, move the hand upward toward costal margin by 1 cm during expiration.
- Repeat the procedure till the liver border is felt.

Preferred method (Fig. 3.27)
- Sit on the right side the patient facing the head end of the patient.
- Now place both hands side-by-side flat on the abdomen in the right subcostal region lateral to the rectus with the fingers pointing toward the ribs.
- If resistance is felt, move the hands further down until resistance disappears.
- Exert gentle pressure and ask the patient to inspire deeply.
- The border of the liver can be felt on the tips of the fingers.
- This procedure can be repeated from lateral to medial to trace the entire edge of the liver.

Alternate method (Fig. 3.28)
- Place the right hand below and parallel to the right subcostal margin.

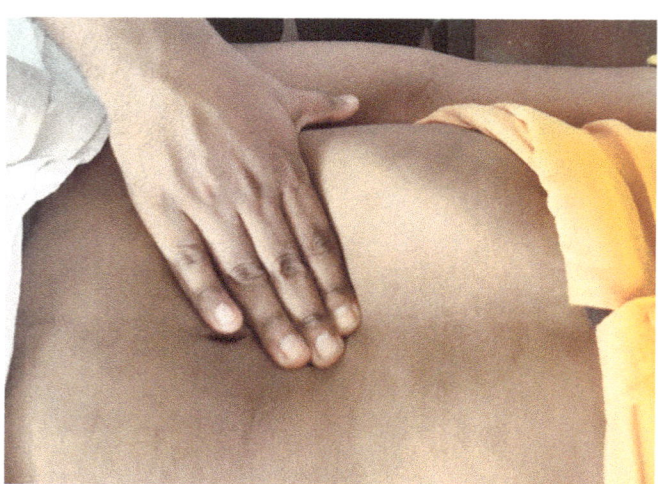

Fig. 3.28: Alternate method of palpation of liver.

- The liver edge will then be felt against the radial border of the index finger.

Hooking method of liver examination (Fig. 3.29)
Examiner stands from the patient's right shoulder, facing the foot end, and examines the lower edge of the liver by curling the fingertips under the right costal margin.

Dipping method of liver palpation in ascites (Fig. 3.30)
- Place both hand one over the other, over the area to be palpated.
- Rapidly flex your metacarpophalangeal joints, so that your fingers suddenly dip into the patient's abdomen.
- This displaces the fluid, enhancing the palpation of underlying organ.

Liver Span
- The liver span is the distance in centimeters between the upper border of the liver in the right midclavicular line, as determined by percussion (i.e., where lung resonance changes to liver dullness), and the lower border, as determined by either percussion or palpation (**Figs. 3.31 to 3.33**).

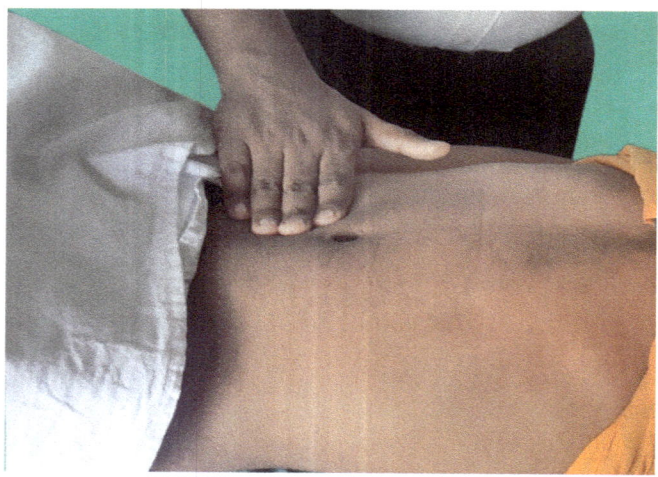

Fig. 3.26: Traditional method of palpation of liver.

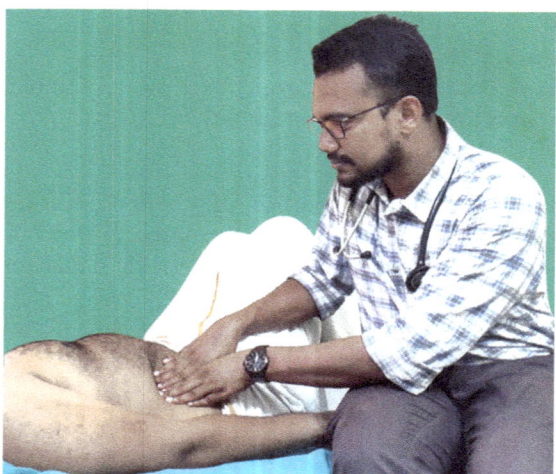

Fig. 3.27: Preferred method of palpation of liver.

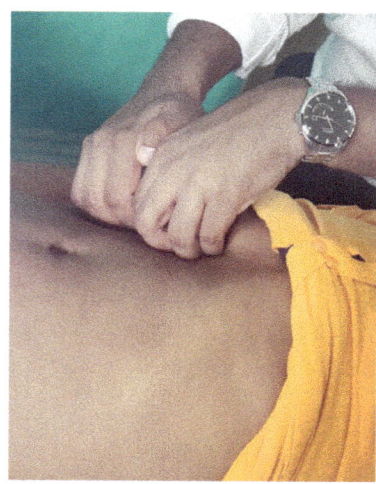

Fig. 3.29: Hooking method of palpation of liver.

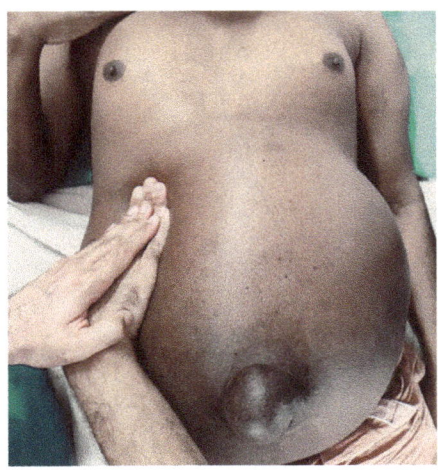

Fig. 3.30: Dipping method of palpation of liver.

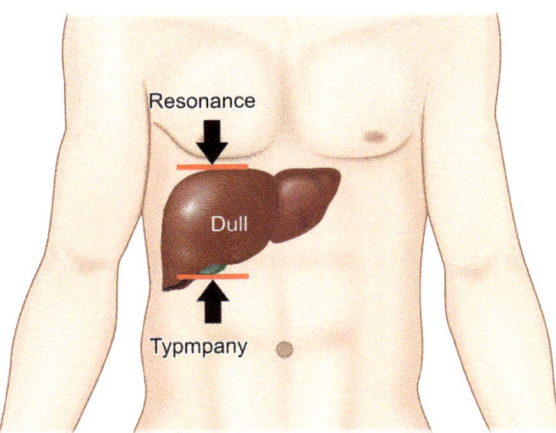

Fig. 3.31: Illustration showing liver span.

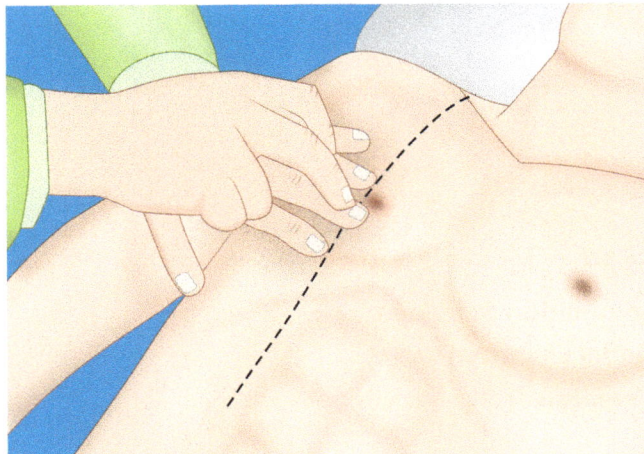

Fig. 3.32: Percuss along the midclavicular line.

- The upper border of the liver is assessed using a heavy percussion technique. Light percussion is used to locate the lower edge of the liver. Light percussion is required because heavy percussion may underestimate the lower extent of the liver border.

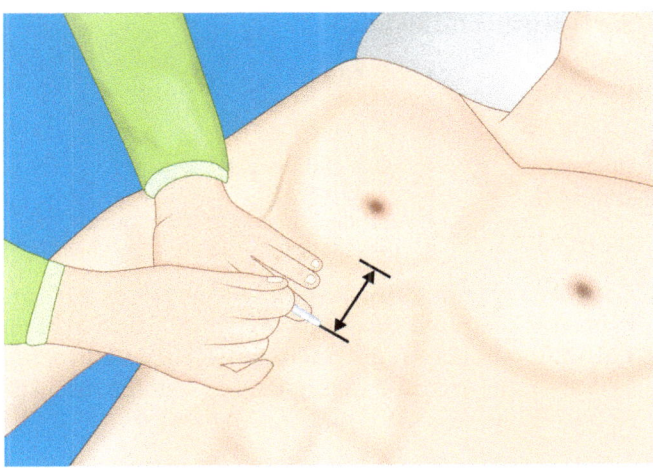

Fig. 3.33: Mark the upper and lower border of dullness.

- The normal liver span is less than 13 cm.
  - In midclavicular line: normally 6–12 cm.
  - In midsternal line (left lobe): Normally 4–8 cm.
- The clinical estimate of the liver span is usually an under-estimation of the actual liver size by about 2–5 cm **(Table 3.22)**.

If the liver is enlarged and palpable, assess the following:
- **Location** of the edge in cm below the costal margin in the midclavicular or anterior axillary line.
- **Span** (in cm)
- **Tenderness** (tender/nontender) **(Table 3.23)**
- **Margins** (regular, irregular; rounded or sharp). In cancer, the liver edge may be irregular.

Rounded	Infiltrative disorders
Sharp	• Secondary metastases • Biliary obstruction • Hepatitis

Table 3.22: Liver span and its condition.

Liver span	Condition seen
Increased	Hepatomegaly
Decreased	Shrunken liver as in cirrhosis
False positive for enlarged liver	• Right-sided pleural effusion • Right lower lobe consolidation

Note: In conditions like emphysema of the lung, the liver may be pushed down. The edge may be palpable, leading the examiner to believe that the patient has hepatomegaly when the real problem is a hyperdistended lung. Percussion will reveal that the upper border is lower than expected.

Table 3.23: Tender and painless hepatomegaly.

Tender hepatomegaly	Painless hepatomegaly
• Right heart failure • Acute hepatitis (viral/alcoholic/drug induced) • Liver abscess (amebic/pyogenic) • Hepatoma • Infarcts • Actinomycosis • Acute Budd-Chiari syndrome	• Fatty liver • Infiltrative and storage disorders • Malaria • Leukemia • Lymphoma

- **Surface** (smooth, nodular)

Smooth	• Malaria • Acute hepatitis • Infiltrative disorders, etc.
Nodular	• Metastatic cancers • Hepatoma • Alcoholic cirrhosis (micronodular) • Posthepatic cirrhosis (macronodular)

- **Consistency (soft/firm/hard):** In metastatic cancers and in obstructive jaundice, the liver is typically firm to hard.
- **Pulsatility (pulsatile/not pulsatile):** A pulsatile liver may be present in tricuspid regurgitation (systolic), tricuspid stenosis (diastolic), HCC and hemangiomas.

Ausculto Percussion Method (The Scratch Test)
- The diaphragm of the stethoscope is placed either over the xiphoid process or just superior to the costal margin along the midclavicular line.
- The examiner then gently scratches the skin along the right midclavicular line, starting in the lower abdomen, and advancing toward the head **(Fig. 3.34)**.
- The sound produced by the scratching changes in quality and intensity when over the liver, as sounds are much more easily transmitted through the solid organ.

Causes of Hepatomegaly
Causes of hepatomegaly can be grossly grouped under the headings of infections, malignancies, infiltrative disorders, hematological disorders, and vascular disorders as shown in **Figure 3.35**.

Caudate Lobe (Fig. 3.36)
- Arises from the right lobe of the liver, on the posteriosuperior surface.
- Hypertrophy of caudate lobe is characteristic hepatic outflow obstruction (Budd-Chiari syndrome).

Riedels Lobe (Fig. 3.37)
- Congenital variant projecting from the right lobe of the liver
- May be mistaken for gallbladder or right kidney.

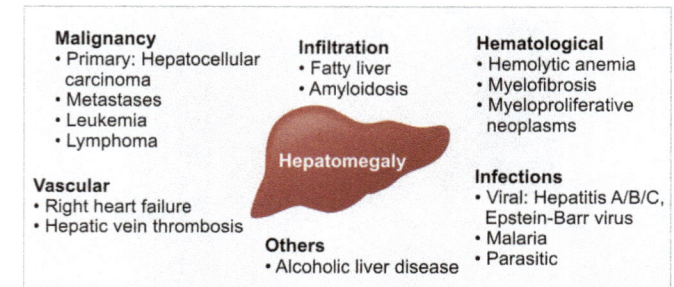

Fig. 3.35: Causes of hepatomegaly.

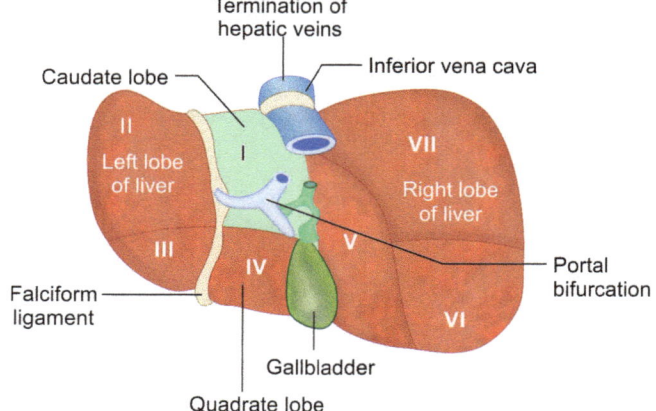

Fig. 3.36: Caudate lobe location and boundaries.

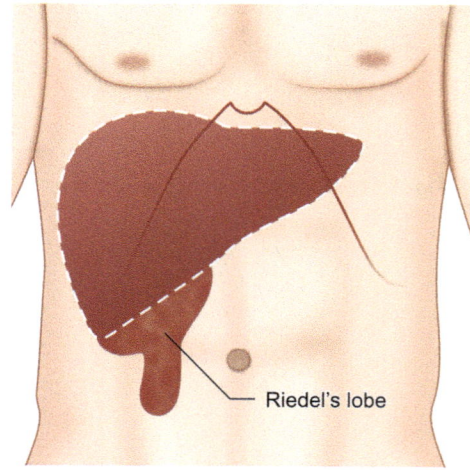

Fig. 3.37: Anomalous lobe of the liver projecting from right lobe.

Examination of Spleen
Normal Characteristics

Dimensions	• 12 cm length, 7 cm width • 13 cm craniocaudal diameter
Weight	• <250 g
Location (Fig. 3.38)	• Along - 9th, 10th, 11th ribs mid-axillary line • Long axis along line of 10th rib.
Extent	• **Anteriorly (lower pole):** Up to mid-axillary line. • **Posteriorly:** The superior angle of spleen is 4 cm lateral to D10 spine.
Margin	• There is a **notch** on the inferolateral border, and this may be palpated when the spleen is enlarged

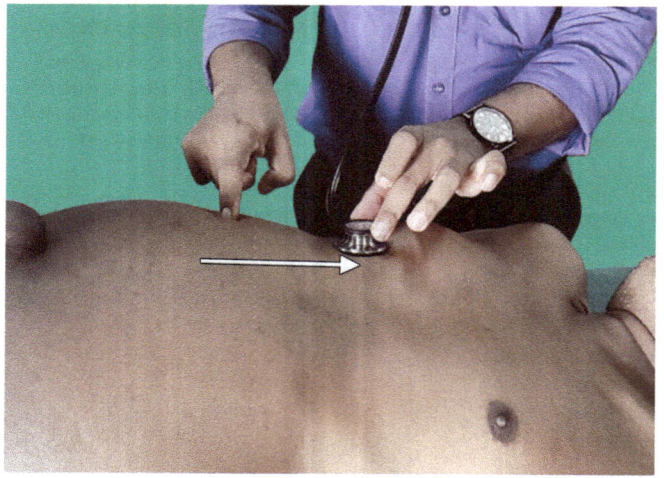

Fig. 3.34: Demonstration of ausculto-percussion method.

Chapter 3: Gastrointestinal Tract Examination

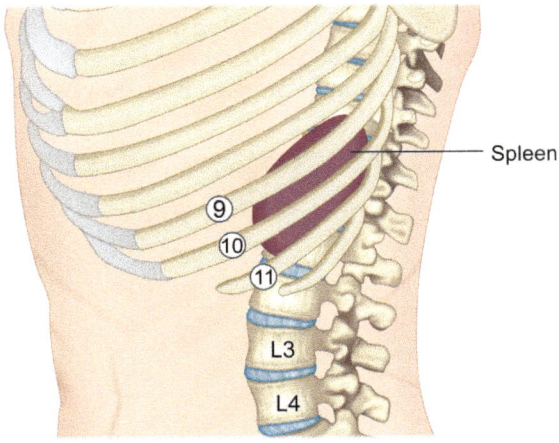

Fig. 3.38: Surface marking of spleen.

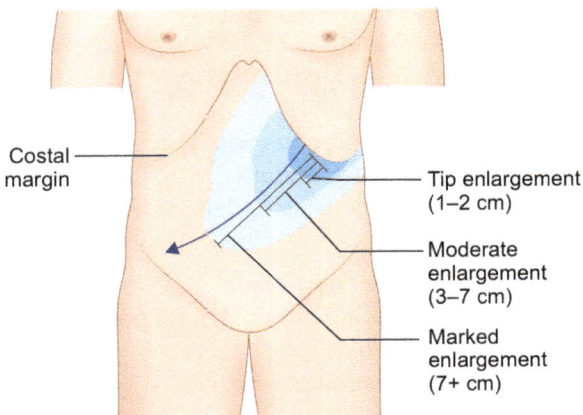

Fig. 3.39: Grading of splenomegaly.

Normal spleen is NOT palpable clinically except in following scenarios:
- Only occasionally palpable in 1–3% of New Guinea population.
- Tip may be palpable in newborn up to 3 months of age.

Splenic Enlargement
- Before clinically palpable—spleen enlarges in superior and posterior direction.
- It has to enlarge 2–3 times to normal to become palpable.
- Once palpable, it appears (felt) below tip of 10th rib (beneath/under the left costal margin) and further enlarges downward, medially (inward), and forward toward umbilicus (LHC to RIF).

Grading of Enlargement/Splenomegaly

Based on largest dimension	
Moderate splenomegaly	Severe splenomegaly
11–20 cm	>20 cm

Based on distance from costal margin (Fig. 3.39)		
Mild (Tip) enlargement	Moderate enlargement	Severe (Marked) enlargement
1–2 cm (<3 cm)	3–7 cm (3–8 cm) Between costal margin and umbilicus	7+ cm (>8 cm / >1,000 g) Beyond umbilicus crossing midline

Note: Size of the spleen is measured from the left coastal margin to the tip along the long axis of spleen.

Hackett's grading system for palpable splenomegaly (Fig. 3.40)

Grade	Description
Grade 0	Normal impalpable spleen
Grade 1	Spleen palpable only in deep inspiration
Grade 2	Spleen palpable on midclavicular line half way between umbilicus and costal margin
Grade 3	Spleen expands toward the umbilicus
Grade 4	Spleen goes past the umbilicus
Grade 5	Spleen expands toward pubic symphysis

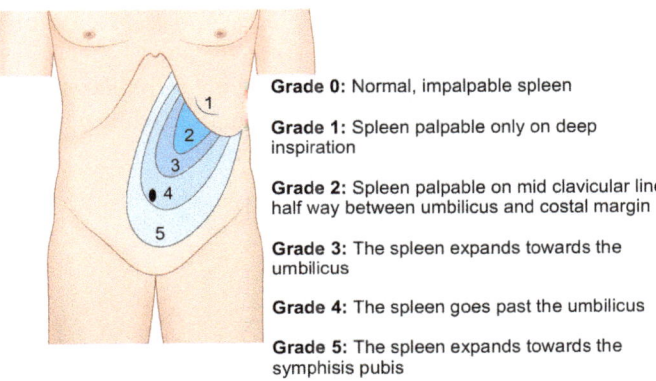

Fig. 3.40: Hackett's grading system for palpable splenomegaly.

Inspection
Fullness may be seen emerging from left upper quadrant extending diagonally toward the right lower quadrant (RLQ).

Palpation
Following methods of palpation have been discussed
- Classical method
- Bimanual method
  - In supine position
  - In right lateral position
- Hooking method
  - In supine position
  - In right lateral position
- Dipping method

Classical method (Fig. 3.41)
- Patient in supine position, examine with single hand (right).
- Place the hand in the RLQ in RIF and move diagonally toward left upper quadrant
- Hand should be firmly placed one the abdominal wall.
- Keep the hand steady during inspiration and feel for the splenic edge as it descends with each inspiration.
- If edge is not felt move the hand diagonally toward LUQ by 1 cm during expiration.
- Repeat the procedure.
- Tip of the finger are used to feel the splenic tip.

Bimanual (supine position) (Fig. 3.42)
- Place palm of left hand over the left lowermost ribcage posterolaterally, restricting the expansion of left lower ribs on inspiration.
- While applying firm pressure with the left hand, ask the patient to take deep inspiration.
- Insinuate right hand beneath the left costal margin and feel for the splenic edge.

Bimanual (right lateral position):
- Done with patient lying in right lateral position with the left hip and knee flexed.
- Rest of maneuver is similar to above

Hooking method (supine position) (Fig. 3.43)
- The physician hooks his fingers beneath the left costal margin as the patient inspires.
- For better appreciability, patient asked to lie down on his left fist just inferior to his left scapula **(Middleton's maneuver) (Figs. 3.44A and B)**.
- From above, spleen may be continently palpable with two hands arching below the left costal margin while patient is asked to take deep breath in/out slowly.

Hooking maneuver (right lateral position)
- Examiner stands on left side facing toward foot end.
- With one hand hook the left lower costal margin and with other hand, give a counter-pressure from the posterolateral aspect.

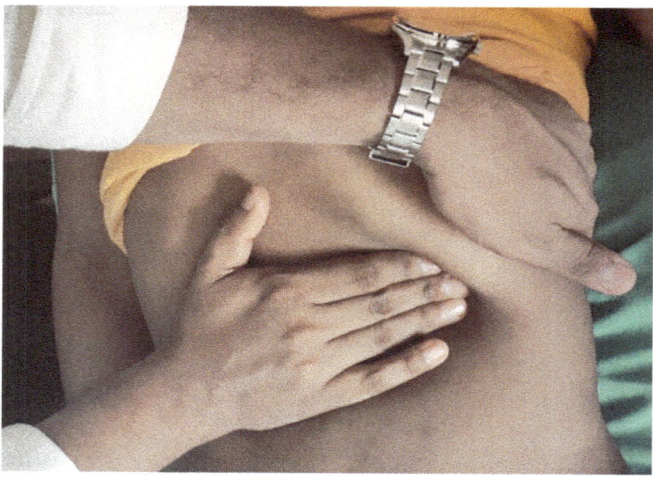

Fig. 3.42: Demonstration of bimanual method (supine position) of spleen palpation.

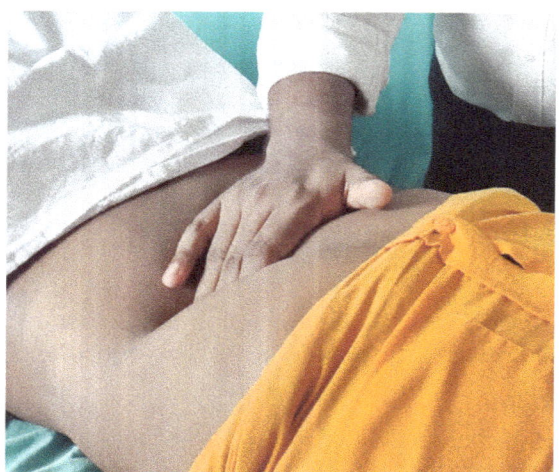

Fig. 3.41: Demonstration of classical method of spleen palpation.

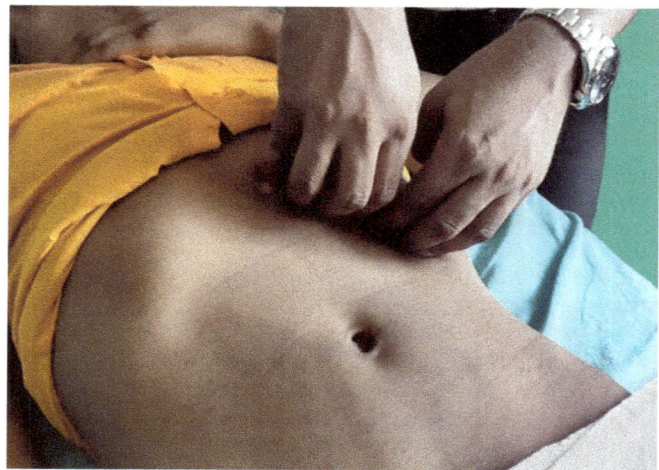

Fig. 3.43: Demonstration of hooking method (supine position) of spleen palpation.

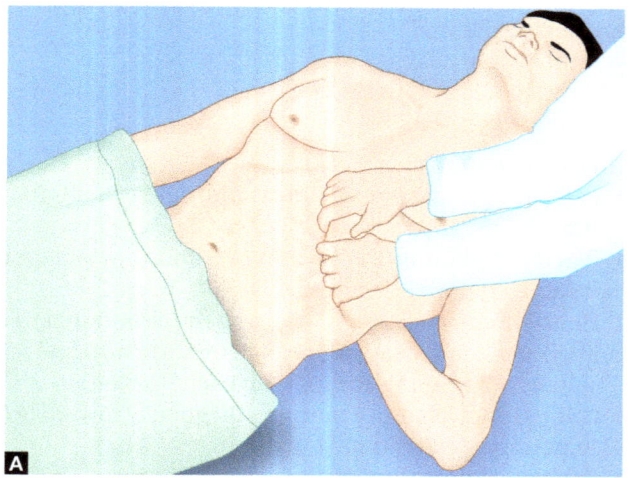
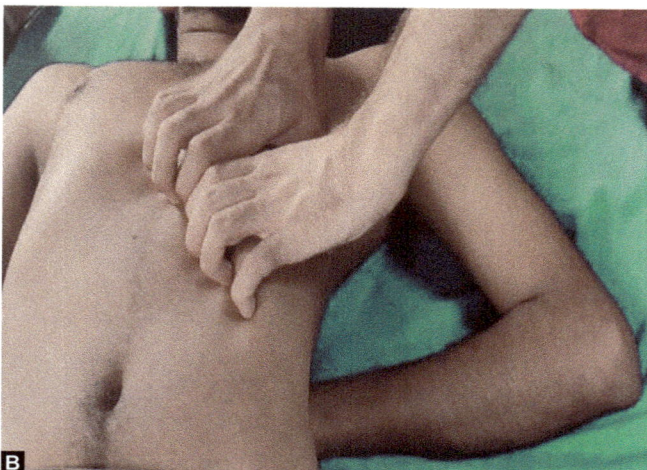

Figs. 3.44A and B: Demonstration of hooking method with Middleton's maneuver.

- Now ask the patient to take deep inspiration and feel for the tip of the spleen, by the hooking fingers.

Dipping method
- It is done in marked ascites
- Similar to dipping method of liver (as described later, under the palpation of liver).

Percussion
Following methods of percussion have been discussed:
- Castell's method
- Traube's space percussion
- Nixon's method of percussion

Percussion by Castell's method (spleen percussion sign)
- With patient in supine position, percuss in the lowest left intercostal space in the anterior axillary line **(Figs. 3.45 and 3.46)** (usually the 8th or 9th IC space–Castell's point)
- This space should remain resonant during full inspiration.
- Dullness on full inspiration indicates possible splenic enlargement (a positive Castell's sign).
- Most sensitive of all clinical signs with sensitivity 82% and specificity 83%.

	Full inspiration	Full expiration
Normal	Resonant	Resonant
Mild splenomegaly*	Dull	Resonant
Moderate/severe splenomegaly	Dull	Dull

*Percussion sign is considered positive, when a change in percussion note is observed between full expiration and full inspiration

Percussion of Traube's (semilunar) space
- It is a semilunar space in the left anterior chest bounded by:
  - Above by 6th rib
  - Below by left costal margin
  - Laterally by mid axillary line
- With patient supine, percuss inferior to lung resonance from medial to lateral **(Figs. 3.46 and 3.47)**, as described by **Barkun**. Normally, a tympanic note heard due to gastric air bubble.

Obliteration of Traube's space	• Massive splenomegaly • Left-sided pleural effusion • Pericardial effusion • Enlarged left lobe of the liver • Full stomach or fundic mass
Upward shift of Traube's space	• Left diaphragmatic paralysis • Left lower lobe collapse or fibrosis

Percussion by Nixon's method:
- Patient is first placed in the right lateral decubitus position.
- Percussion starts at the midpoint of the left costal margin and is continued upward perpendicular to the left costal margin **(Figs. 3.48 and 3.49)**.
- Normally, the level of dullness does not extend more than 8 cm above the costal margin and splenomegaly is diagnosed if the dullness extends beyond 8 cm.

Causes of Splenomegaly
The causes of splenomegaly are shown in **Table 3.24.**

Causes of Hepatosplenomegaly
Common causes of hepatosplenomegaly and associated features have been illustrated in the **Figure 3.50.**

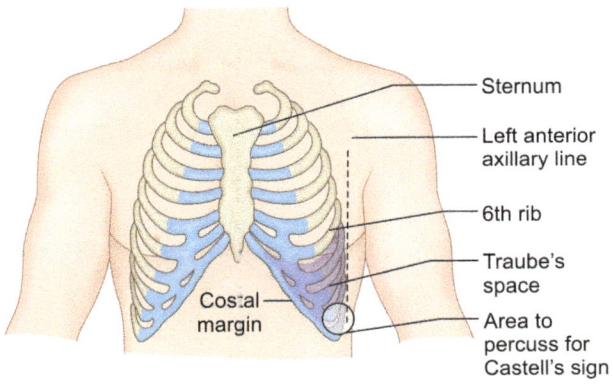

Fig. 3.46: Landmarks of Traube's space and castell sign.

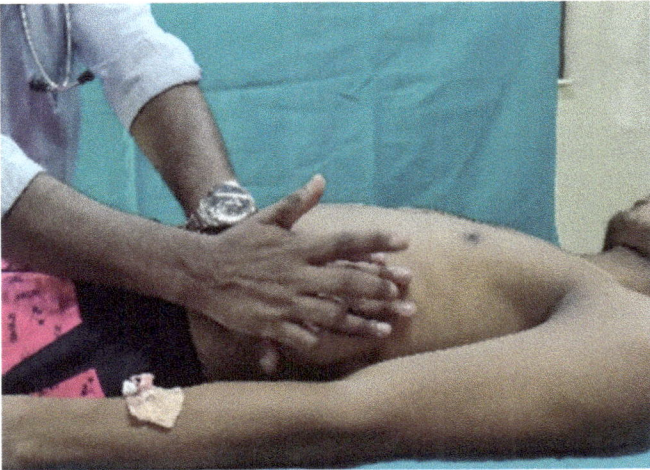

Fig. 3.45: Percussing the lowest left intercostal space in anterior axillary line—castells method of splenic percussion.

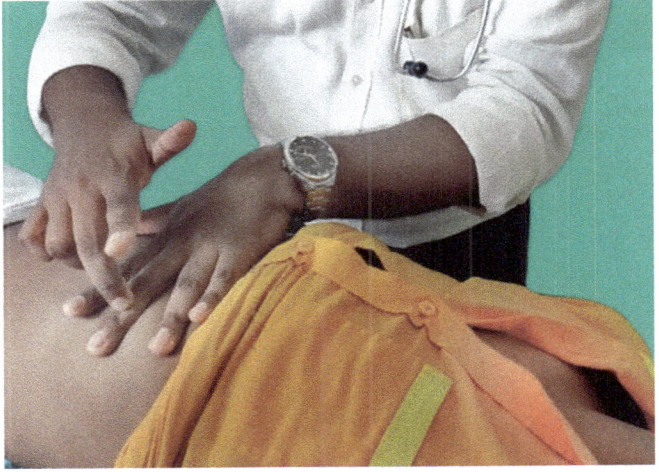

Fig. 3.47: Percussion of Traube's space.

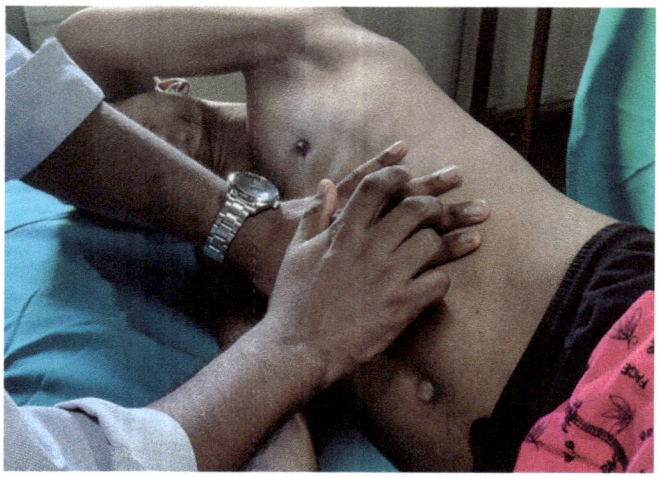

Fig. 3.48: Percussing the posterior axillary line in right lateral position (Nixon's method).

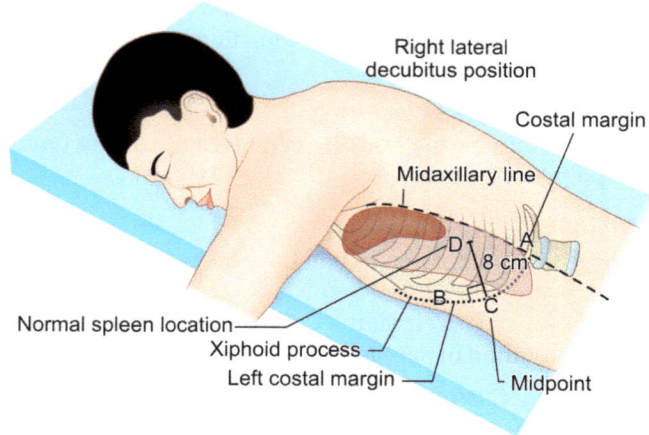

Fig. 3.49: Landmarks for Nixon's method.

Table 3.24: Causes of splenomegaly.

Mild splenomegaly	
Acute infections	Septic shock, infective endocarditis, enteric fever, infectious hepatitis, infectious mononucleosis, brucellosis, cytomegalovirus, toxoplasmosis
Chronic infections	Tuberculosis, syphilis, brucellosis, chronic bacteremia, HIV
Parasitic infestations	Malaria, kala-azar, and schistosomiasis
Inflammation	Rheumatoid arthritis, sarcoidosis, SLE
Others	Congestive cardiac failure, thalassemia minor
Moderate splenomegaly	
Neoplastic	Lymphomas, acute leukemia, chronic lymphocytic leukemia, chronic myeloid leukemia
Non-neoplastic	Cirrhosis of liver (with portal hypertension), chronic hemolytic anemia, malaria, kala-azar, sarcoidosis, infectious mononucleosis, splenic abscess, amyloidosis, hemochromatosis, polycythemia vera
Severe (massive) splenomegaly	
Common causes	Chronic myeloid leukemia, myelofibrosis, kala-azar, hairy cell leukemia, tropical splenomegaly, portal hypertension (extrahepatic portal vein thrombosis), hyper-reactive malarial splenomegaly
Uncommon causes	Lymphomas, Gaucher's disease, Niemann-Pick disease, thalassemia major, splenic cysts and tumors of spleen, myeloid metaplasia, hairy-cell leukemia, sarcoidosis, MAC infection in HIV patients

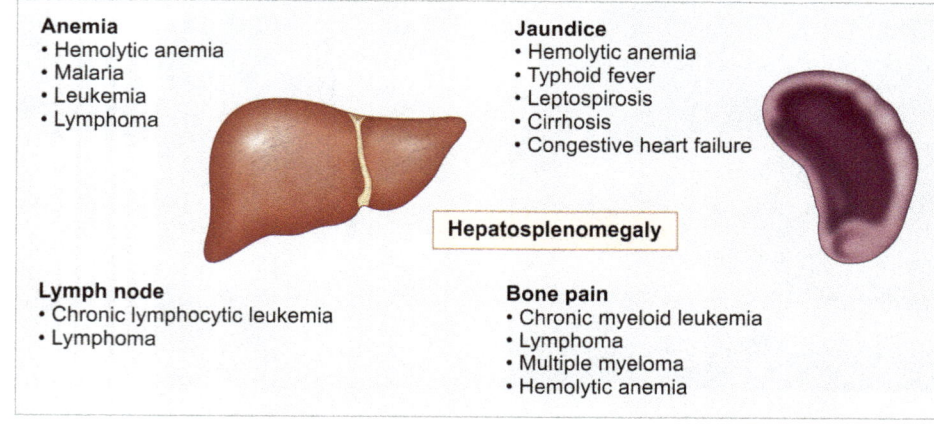

Fig. 3.50: Causes of hepatosplenomegaly.

Examination of Gallbladder

- Location—lateral edge of rectus abdominis near the tip of right 9th costal margin
- Moves with respiration
- Upper border continues with liver
- Causes of enlarged gallbladder
  - Carcinoma head of pancreas
  - CBD obstruction
  - Mucocele of gallbladder
  - Carcinoma of gallbladder
- **Murphy's sign:** In acute cholecystitis, at the high of inspiration, patient stops breathing with gasp as mass in felt.
- **Courvoisier's law:** In a jaundiced patient, if the gallbladder is palpable, it is unlikely due to CBD gallstone obstruction.

Examination of Kidney

Examination of Left Kidney

- The right hand is placed anteriorly in the left lumbar region while the left hand is placed posteriorly in the left loin (**Fig. 3.51**).
- Ask the patient to take a deep breath in, press the left hand forward and the right hand backward, upward, and inward.
- Left kidney is usually not palpable (except whey low lying or enlarged)
- If palpable, it is described as bimanually palpable and ballotable.
- **Bimanually palpable:** As it can be felt as a swelling between both right and left hands
- **Ballotable:** It can be pushed from one hand to the other. It is due to perinephric fat which allows the free movement of the kidney in the retroperitoneum.

Palpation of Right Kidney

- Place the right hand horizontally in the right lumbar region anteriorly with the left hand placed posteriorly in the right loin (**Fig. 3.52**).
- Push forward with the left hand, press the right hand inward and upward and ask the patient to take a deep breath in.

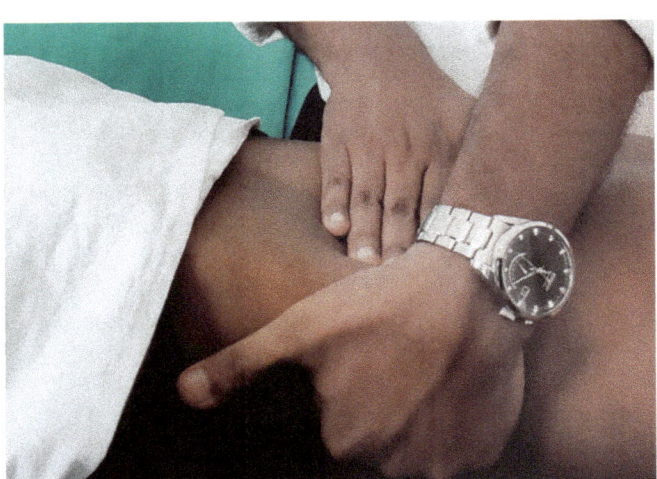

Fig. 3.51: Palpation of left kidney.

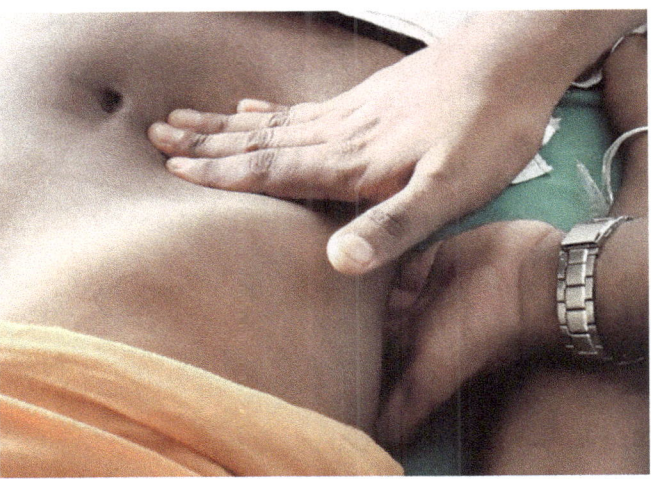

Fig. 3.52: Palpation of right kidney.

- The lower pole of the right kidney, unlike the left, is commonly palpable in thin patients and is felt as a smooth, rounded swelling which descends on inspiration
- It is also bimanually palpable and ballotable.

Causes of Unilateral and Bilateral Kidney Enlargement

Causes of unilateral and bilateral kidney enlargement are shown in **Table 3.25**.

Spleen and Left Kidney

Difference between spleen and left kidney is shown in **Table 3.26**.

The differences between liver, spleen and kidney are shown in **Table 3.27**.

Table 3.25: Causes of unilateral and bilateral kidney enlargement.

Unilateral kidney enlargement	Bilateral kidney enlargement
• Renal cell carcinoma	• Polycystic kidneys
• Hydronephrosis	• Bilateral hydronephrosis

Table 3.26: Difference between spleen and left kidney.

Characteristics	Spleen	Left kidney
Location	Left hypochondrium	Left lumbar
Direction of enlargement	Toward RIF	Toward left hypochondrium and LIF
Movement with respiration	+	–
Insinuation between left costal margin and organ	Not possible	Possible
Bimanual palpation	–	+
Ballotability	–	+
Crossing midline	Can cross midline	Never cross midline
Notch	+	–
Band of colonic resonance	–	+

Table 3.27: Difference points between liver versus spleen versus kidney.

Features	Liver	Spleen	Kidney
Location	Right hypochondrium	Left hypochondrium	Lumbar
Direction of enlargement	Toward RIF	Toward RIF	Toward hypochondrium and iliac fossa
Movement with respiration	+	+	–
Insinuation of fingers between the costal margin and organ	Not possible	Not possible	Possible
Bimanually palpable	–	–	+
Ballotablity	–	–	+
Anterior percussion	Dull	Dull	Tympanic

Examination of Free Fluid in Abdomen

Ascites

Definition
Ascites is defined as the accumulation of free fluid in the peritoneal cavity. The peritoneal cavity can accumulate as much as 60 L fluid.

Massive ascites and tense ascites are the clinical terms and are described at the end.

The etiology of ascites is described in **Table 3.28.**

Ascites Praecox
Defined as appearance of **ascites** before the generalized edema. It is usually associated with chronic constrictive pericarditis.

Causes of ascites without significant edema:
- Chronic constrictive pericarditis
- Tuberculous peritonitis
- Malignant peritonitis
- Pancreatic ascites
- Acute Budd-Chiari syndrome

Following methods have been discussed of demonstration of ascites
- Fullness of flanks/horse-shoe dullness
- Shifting dullness
- Fluid wave/fluid thrill
- Puddle sign
- Ausculto-percussion sign of Guarino

Bulging flanks/fullness of flanks/horse-shoe dullness:
- Occurs when the weight of abdominal free fluid is sufficient to push the flanks outward **(Fig. 3.53).**
- On inspection, it can be seen as fullness of flanks or bulging of flanks.
- Bulging flanks can be caused by ascites or by obesity.

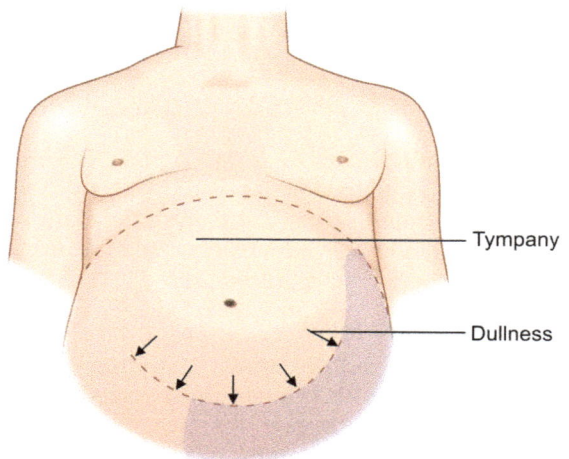

Fig. 3.53: Illustration showing horse-shoe dullness.

Table 3.28: Etiology of ascites.

Nonperitoneal causes		Peritoneal causes	
Intrahepatic portal hypertension	• Cirrhosis • Fulminant hepatic failure • Veno-occlusive disease	Granulomatous peritonitis	• Tuberculous peritonitis • Fungal and parasitic infections • Sarcoidosis • Foreign bodies (cotton, starch, barium)
Extrahepatic portal hypertension	• Hepatic vein obstruction (i.e., Budd-Chiari syndrome) • Congestive heart failure	Malignant ascites	• Primary peritoneal mesothelioma • Secondary peritoneal • Carcinomatosis
Hypoalbuminemia	• Nephrotic syndrome • Protein-losing enteropathy • Malnutrition	Vasculitis	• Systemic lupus erythematosus • Henoch-Schönlein purpura
Miscellaneous disorders	• Myxedema • Ovarian tumors • Pancreatic and biliary ascites	Miscellaneous disorders	• Eosinophilic gastroenteritis • Whipple disease • Endometriosis
Chylous	Secondary to malignancy, trauma		

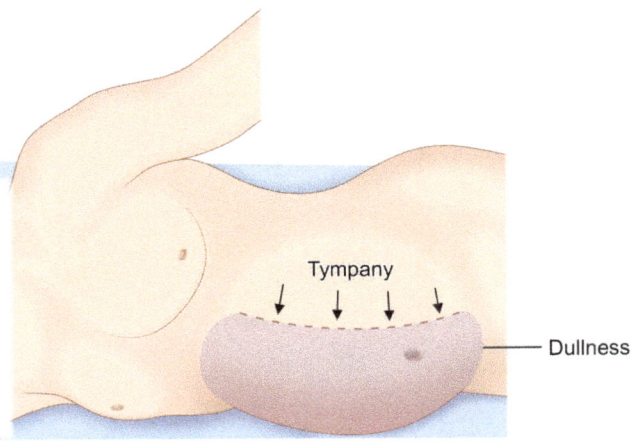

Fig. 3.54: Illustrations showing shift of dullness on lying lateral decubitus position.

- One method for discriminating between the two is to test for flank dullness.
- With the patient recumbent, gas-filled loops of bowel will characteristically float on top of ascites, making the percussion note tympanic at the umbilicus and dull beyond the fluid meniscus into the flanks —*Horse-shoe dullness*

Shifting dullness (Fig. 3.54):
Presence of shifting dullness indicates at least 1.5 L of free fluid in the peritoneal space.

Examination (Figs. 3.55A to K)
- Patient in supine position, start percussion from above downward in the midline till below the umbilicus till you get dullness.
- This dullness could be due to distended urinary bladder, hence repeat this after making the patient empty the bladder.
- Now, begin by percussing at the umbilicus and moving toward the flanks.
- The transition from air to fluid can be identified when the percussion note changes from tympanic to dull.
- Mark the dullness—tympany transition point.
- Turn the patient to opposite lateral side and wait for 30–60 seconds.
- Now percuss area again.
- The area of tympany will shift toward the top and the area of dullness shifts toward the bottom.
- Repeat the same maneuver on the opposite side.

Causes of ascites without shifting dullness
- Massive ascites
- Loculated ascites

Fluid thrill (fluid wave) assessment for ascites:
- In supine position, ask the patient or an assistant to place the ulnar surface of one hand above the umbilicus, pressing firmly (so the subcutaneous tissue and fat does not jiggle) with the hand pointing toward the patient's toes **(Fig. 3.56)**
- Use one hand to palpate and one hand to percuss.
- Place a hand on the lateral aspect of the patient's abdomen between the costal margin and the ilium in the anterior axillary line.
- Tap one side of the patients flank sharply with your fingertips.
- Feel on the opposite flank for an impulse transmitted through the fluid.
- Repeat procedure by flicking on the other side.
- **Results:**
  - *Positive:* An easily palpable impulse is felt on opposite of tapping suggests ascites of around more than 2 L.
  - *Negative:* No impulse is felt
  - *False positive:* Can be felt over large ovarian cyst or large hydatid cyst or large hydronephrosis.

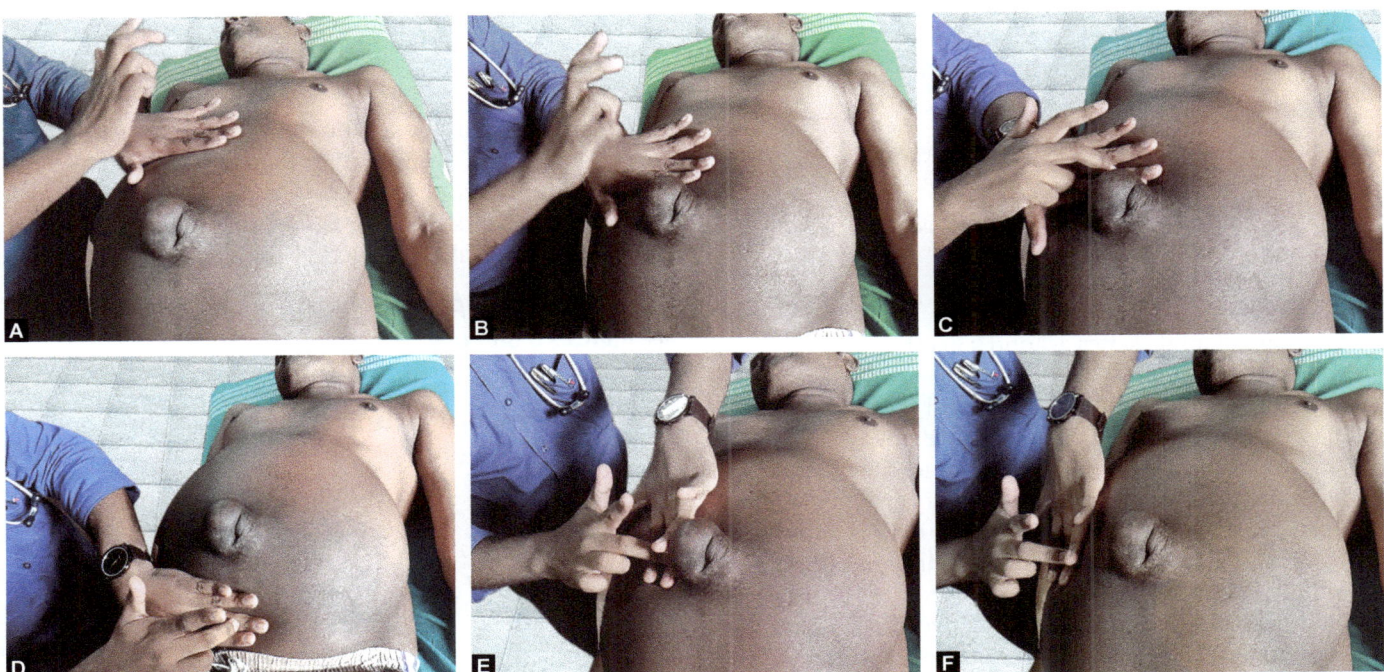

Figs. 3.55A to F

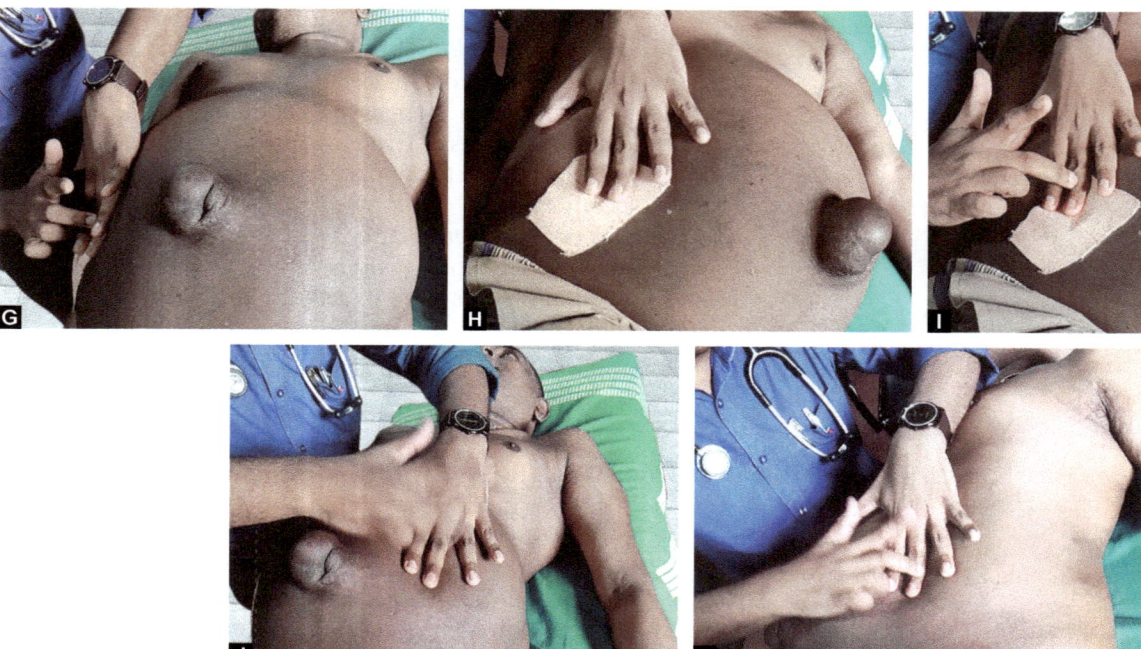

Figs. 3.55G to K

Figs. 3.55A to K: Demonstration of shifting dullness.

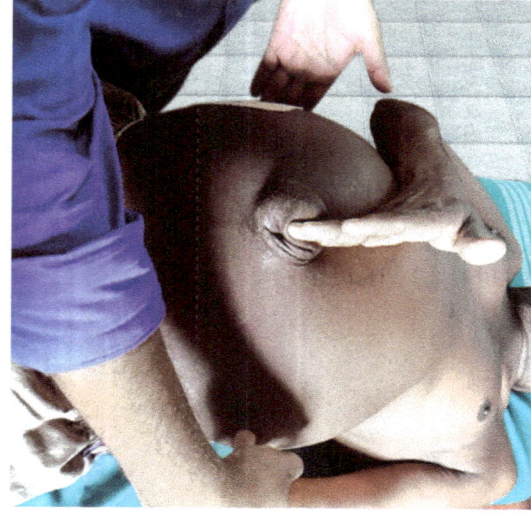

Fig. 3.56: Demonstration of fluid thrill.

Puddle sign:
- It is a sign of mild ascites around 250 mL.
- No frequently done
- Patient is prone for 3–5 minutes and then examined in knee-elbow position as shown in the **Figure 58E.**
- Diaphragm of the stethoscope is placed over the most dependent area of the abdomen.
- Place diaphragm of the stethoscope over the umbilical region and scratch the abdominal wall from periphery to umbilicus.
- Sudden change in the note is a positive sign.
- Sign can be false positive in case of massive splenomegaly or distended urinary bladder.

Different Methods of Examination of Ascites

The sensitivity, specificity, and likelihood ratio of different methods of examination of ascites is shown in **Table 3.29**.

What is tense ascites and massive ascites?
- The earliest clinical sign of ascites is puddle sign, which is positive with as low as 250 mL of ascitic fluid.
- Shifting dullness is specific sign of ascites, which occurs due to the floating of the bowel loops in ascitic fluid. This appears when the fluid accumulation is around 1.2 L.
- As the fluids accumulate further, fluid thrill appears (at around 2 L). Appearance of fluid thrill makes the ascites tense.

As the ascitic fluid fills, the mesentery is stretched and bowel loops float in the ascitic fluid. As the mesentery can only stretch up to a limit, further fluid accumulation results in the submersion of bowel loops. At this stage, shifting dullness disappears however fluid thrill persists **(Fig. 3.57)**. This condition is called as massive ascites.

Diagrammatic Representation of Signs of Ascites
See **Figures 3.58A to E**.

Table 3.29: Different methods of examination of ascites.

Method	Amount of fluid	LR+	LR−	Sn	Sp
Fullness of flanks		2.0	0.3	0.81	0.59
Horse-shoe dullness		2.0	0.3	0.84	0.59
Shifting dullness	1.5 L	2.7	0.3	0.77	0.72
Fluid thrill	>2 L	6.0	0.4	0.62	0.9
Puddle sign	250 mL	1.6	0.8	0.45	0.73

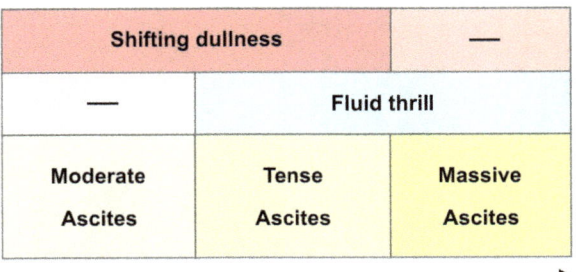

Fig. 3.57: Schematic representation showing relationship between shifting dullness and fluid thrill with respect to increasing ascites.

Examination of Dilated Veins

Position of Patient

Make the patient stand and examine the anterior abdominal wall, the flanks, and back for dilated veins. Dilated tortuous veins are significant.

Steps of Examination (Harvey's Sign) (Fig. 3.59)

- The direction of blood flow in the veins is examined by placing the tips of the index fingers together and compressing the vein.
- Then, the finger tips are slid apart producing an empty segment of the vein between the fingers **(Fig. 3.60A)**.
- Then, one finger is removed and filling of the vein is observed **(Fig. 3.60B)**.
- The procedure is repeated but, now the opposite finger is removed and filling is observed **(Fig. 3.60C)**.
- The direction of flow of the veins is the direction in which the filling was rapid and more **(Table 3.30)**.

Per Rectal Examination

Rectal examination consists of:
- Visual inspection of the perianal skin,
- Digital palpation of the rectum, and
- Assessment of neuromuscular function of the perineum.

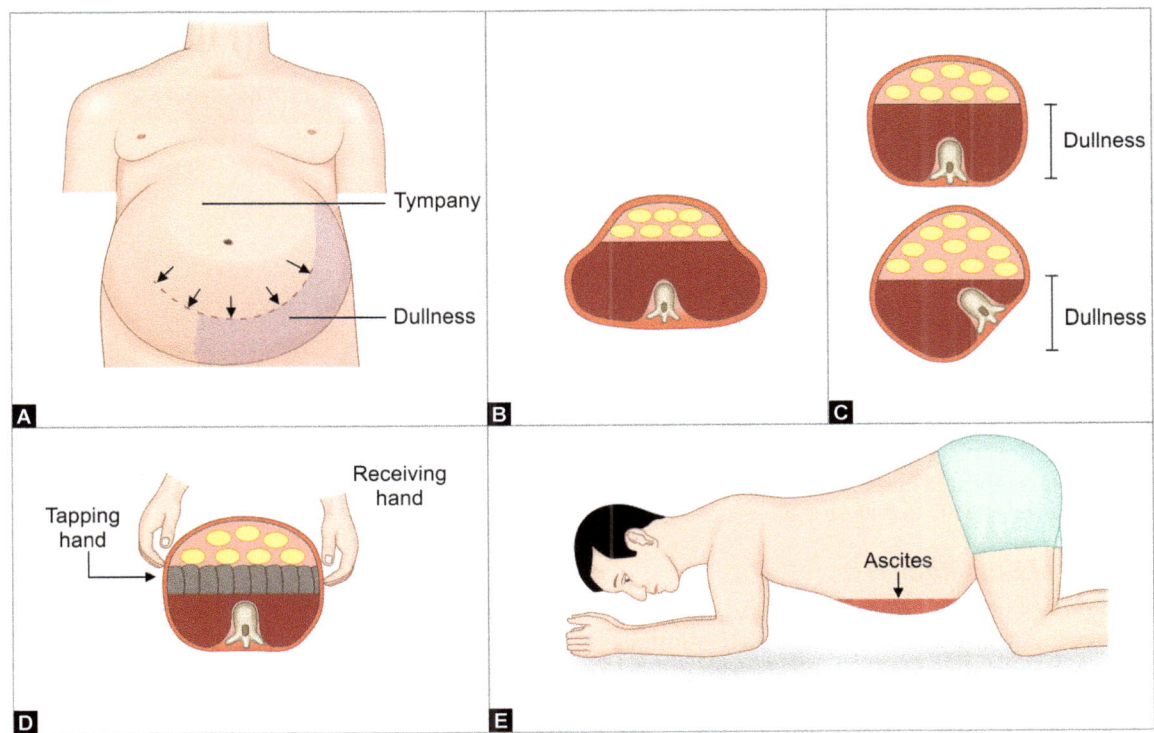

Figs. 3.58A to E: Signs of ascites: (A) Horse-shoe dullness; (B) Fullness (bulging) of flanks; (C) Shifting dullness; (D) Fluid thrill/fluid wave; (E) Puddle sign.

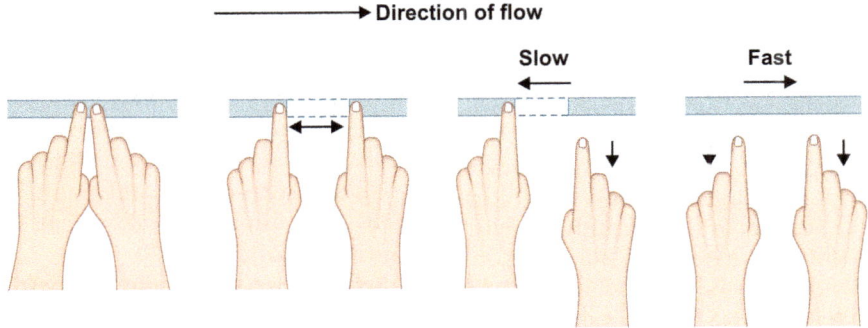

Fig. 3.59: Illustration of Harvey's sign.

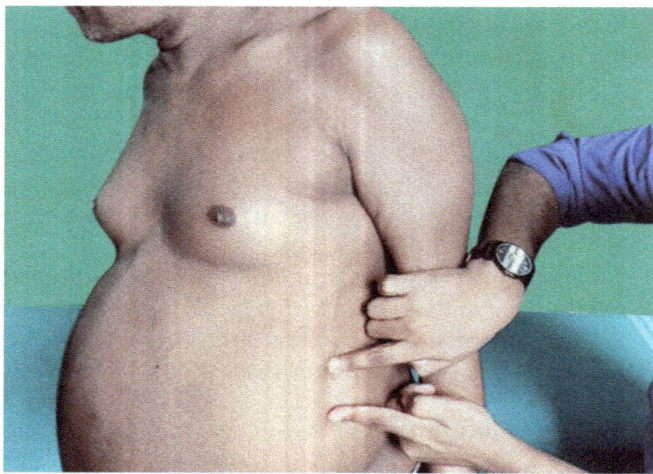

Fig. 3.60A: The finger tips are slid apart producing an empty segment of the vein between the fingers.

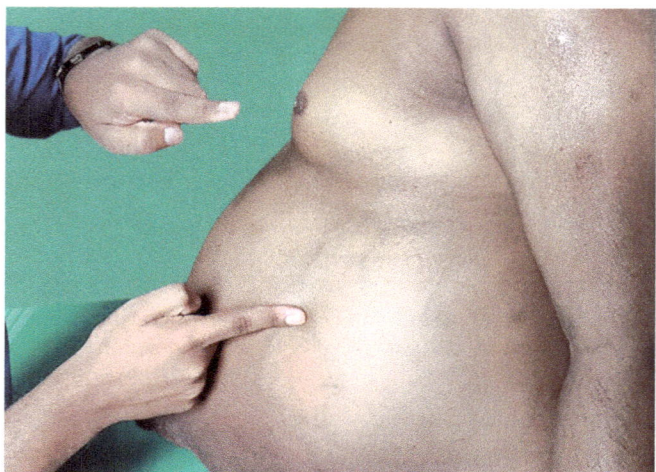

Fig. 3.60B: One finger is removed and filling of the vein is observed.

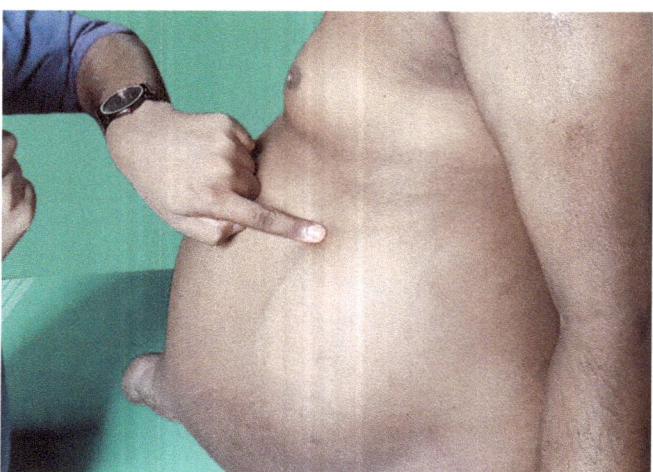

Fig. 3.60C: Procedure is repeated but, now the opposite finger is removed and filling is observed.

Preferred Position of Examination

The *lateral decubitus*, or *Sim's position*, provides optimal examination. The patient lies on the left side with the buttocks near the edge of the examining table or bedside with the right knee and hip in slight flexion.

The rectal examination involves both inspection and palpation. First, using a gloved hand, the examiner inspects the buttocks for fistulous tracts, the skin tags, excoriations, blood, fissures in patients with IBD, rectal prolapse, and superficial ulcers.

Palpation of the rectum can reveal ulcers, masses.

Tenderness may be felt with prostatitis, pelvic inflammatory disease, tubo-ovarian abscesses, ovarian cysts, ectopic pregnancy, and IBD.

Also note the consistency, color, and presence of frank or occult blood in the stool (melena). Black stools result from degraded blood (melena), iron, licorice, bismuth, rhubarb, or overindulgence in chocolate cookies. Red-colored stools may be due to brisk bleeding known as hematochezia (usually distal to the ligament of Treitz).

Hemorrhoids are usually not felt unless thrombosed. Proctoscopy is the best way to look for hemorrhoids.

Table 3.30: Direction of flow in veins above and below umbilicus.

Condition (Fig. 3.61)	Direction of flow in veins above umbilicus	Direction of flow in veins below umbilicus
normal (veins not visible)	Upward	Downward
Portal hypertension (veins are visible and tortuous)	Upward	Downward
Portal vein thrombosis	Downward	Upward
SVC obstruction	Downward	Downward
IVC obstruction	Upward	Upward

Caput medusa: Dilated tortuous veins around the umbilicus resembling a head of medusa.

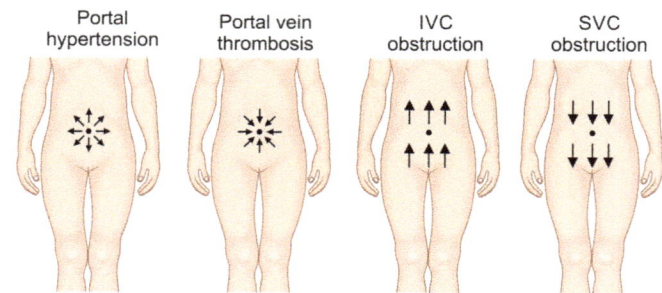

Fig. 3.61: Illustration showing direction of flow of veins.

Others

Per Vaginal/Per Speculum Examination

In female patients with ascites, ovarian neoplasms, pelvic tumor, per vaginal mass/bleeding can be detected.

Gastrointestinal tract examination is incomplete without examination of the **three S—Scrotum, Spine, and Supraclavicular fossa.**

- **Scrotum:** Hydrocele, hernia, testicular atrophy, testicular tumors
- **Spine:** Metastasis, Pott's spine
- **Supraclavicular fossa:** Metastasis to left scalene node.

OBJECTIVE-BASED SELF-EVALUATION

SHORT ANSWER QUESTIONS

1. List the differences between spleen and left kidney on clinical examination.
2. List the causes of abdominal distension.
3. What are the clinical signs to detect ascites?
4. List the causes of massive splenomegaly.
5. List the causes of tender hepatomegaly.
6. List the clinical signs of chronic liver disease.
7. Spider nevi.
8. List causes of gum hyperplasia.
9. What is asterixis? List the causes.
10. List the causes of oral ulcers.
11. Enumerate the methods of palpation of liver.
12. List the percussion methods for splenic examination.
13. List causes of hepatosplenomegaly.
14. Traube's space.
15. List the features in examination that would be present if kidneys were enlarged.

MULTIPLE CHOICE QUESTIONS

1. Direction of flow away from the umbilicus in dilated veins is seen in:
   a. Portal hypertension
   b. SVC obstruction
   c. IVC obstruction
   d. Portal vein thrombosis
2. Puddle sign in the abdomen is used to detect:
   a. Spleen
   b. Liver
   c. Ascites
   d. Kidney
3. Ascites praecox is seen in:
   a. Chronic constrictive pericarditis
   b. Tuberculous peritonitis
   c. Malignant peritonitis
   d. All of the above
4. Bimanually palpable and ballotable organ is:
   a. Spleen
   b. Liver
   c. Kidney
   d. Gallbladder
5. Massive splenomegaly is seen in:
   a. Chronic myeloid leukemia
   b. Myelofibrosis
   c. Kala-azar
   d. All of the above
6. Obliteration of Traube's space is seen with:
   a. Hepatomegaly
   b. Splenomegaly
   c. Right sided pleural effusion
   d. Pneumothorax
7. Tender hepatomegaly is seen in:
   a. Fatty liver
   b. Infiltrative and storage disorders
   c. Right heart failure
   d. Malaria
8. Cullen's sign and Grey Turner's sign is seen in:
   a. Aortic regurgitation
   b. Pancreatitis
   c. Infective endocarditis
   d. Splenic rupture
9. Macroglossia is a feature of:
   a. Acromegaly
   b. Myxedema
   c. Amyloidosis
   d. All the above
10. Parotid enlargement and Duputryens contracture are seen in:
    a. Alcoholic cirrhosis
    b. Posthepatitic cirrhosis
    c. Primary biliary cirrhosis
    d. Budd–Chiari syndrome

ANSWERS

| 1. a | 2. c | 3. d | 4. c | 5. d |
| 6. b | 7. c | 8. b | 9. d | 10. a |

Respiratory System Examination

CHAPTER 4

CHAPTER OUTLINE

- Case Sheet Format
- Diagnosis Format
- Discussion on Cardinal Symptoms
- Discussion on Examination

RESPIRATORY SYSTEM: CASE SHEET FORMAT

History Taking
- Name:
- Age:
- Sex:
- Residence:
- Occupation:

Chief Complaints
1. _____ × days
2. _____ × days

History of Presenting Illness

Cough:
- Duration
- Onset
- Progression
- **Variation:**
  - Diurnal variation
  - Seasonal variation
  - Postural variation
- Aggravating factors
- Relieving factors

Expectoration:
- Duration
- Onset
- Progression
- **Variation:**
  - Diurnal variation
  - Seasonal variation
  - Positional variation
- Aggravating and relieving factors
- Quantity of sputum
- Color
- Smell

- **Blood tinged:**
  - How often
  - Quantity
  - Fresh or altered
  - Associated epistaxis

Dyspnea:
- Duration
- Onset
- Grade
- Progression
- Aggravating factors
- Relieving factors
- Orthopnea
- Trepopnea
- Platypnea
- Paroxysmal nocturnal dyspnea (PND)

Any respiratory system complaints:
- Wheeze
- Cough with expectoration

Chest pain:
- Duration
- Onset
- Site
- Type of pain
- Radiation
- Diurnal variation (nocturnal angina)
- Variation with respiration
- Aggravating factors
- Relieving factors
- **Associated symptoms:** Nausea, vomiting, and sweating
- Dyspepsia
- Local tenderness

Wheeze:
- Duration
- Onset

- ❑ Progression
- ❑ Episodic or continuous
- ❑ Variation
- ❑ Allergy
- ❑ Skin rashes
- ❑ Aggravating and relieving factors

Fever:
- ❑ Episodic or continuous
- ❑ Grade
- ❑ Chill and rigors
- ❑ Aggravating factors
- ❑ Relieving factors
- ❑ **Variation:** Diurnal variation

History of
- ❑ Nasal discharge
- ❑ Recurrent cold
- ❑ Recurrent headaches
- ❑ Weight loss
- ❑ Anorexia
- ❑ Evening rise of temperature
- ❑ Smoking
- ❑ Belching
- ❑ Regurgitation of food
- ❑ Hoarseness of voice

Past History
- ❑ Asthma
- ❑ Chronic obstructive airway disease
- ❑ Tuberculosis
- ❑ History of contact with tuberculosis
- ❑ Diabetes mellitus (DM)
- ❑ Hypertension (HTN)
- ❑ Ischemic heart disease (IHD)
- ❑ Seizure disorder

Family History
Draw pedigree chart representing three generations.

Personal History
- ❑ Bowel habits
- ❑ Bladder habits
- ❑ Appetite
- ❑ Loss of weight
- ❑ Occupational exposure
- ❑ Sleep
- ❑ Dietary habits and taboo
- ❑ Food allergies
- ❑ Smoking (in smoking Index or Pack years)
- ❑ Alcohol history (_____ g of alcohol/day or _____ units of alcohol/week)

Menstrual and Obstetric History
- ❑ G___P___L___A___
- ❑ Age of menarche __
- ❑ Menopause at __
- ❑ Flow–ameno/oligo/menorrhagia

Summarize
Write a brief summary

Differential Diagnosis
1.
2.
3.

General Examination
Patient
- ❑ Conscious
- ❑ Coherent
- ❑ Cooperative
- ❑ Obeying commands

Body Mass Index (BMI)
- ❑ Weight (kg)/Height^2 (meters)
- ❑ Grading according to WHO for south east Asian countries

Vitals
- ❑ Pulse
  - Rate
  - Rhythm
  - Volume
  - Character
  - Vessel wall thickening
  - Radio-radial delay and radiofemoral delay
  - Peripheral pulses
- ❑ **Blood pressure:**
  - Right arm
  - Left arm
  - Leg
- ❑ **Respiratory rate:**
  - Regular
  - Abdominothoracic (male) or thoracoabdominal (female)
  - Usage of accessory muscles
- ❑ **Jugular venous pulse:** Waveform
- ❑ **Jugular venous pressure:**
  - _____ cm of blood above sternal angle (+ 5 cm water)
  - Pulse oximetry
  - Pain

On Physical Examination
- ❑ Pallor:
- ❑ Icterus:
- ❑ Cyanosis:
- ❑ Clubbing:
- ❑ Lymphadenopathy:
- ❑ Edema:

Others Head to Toe
- ❑ Oral cavity examination
- ❑ Use of accessory muscles of respiration
- ❑ External markers of tuberculosis
- ❑ External markers of malignancy
- ❑ Features suggesting type of respiratory failure

Systemic Examination

Upper Respiratory Tract Examination
- Nostrils:
- Nasal septum:
- Nasal polyps:
- Sinus tenderness:
- Tonsils:
- Postpharyngeal wall:

Lower Respiratory Tract

Inspection:
- Shape and symmetry:
- Spine:
- Subcostal angle:
- Trachea:
- Apex beat:
- Respiratory movements:

Area	Right	Left
Supraclavicular		
Infraclavicular		
Mammary		
Suprascapular		
Infrascapular		

- Visible pulsations/sinus/scars:
- Diaphragm movements:

Palpation:
(Warm the palms by rubbing against each other before palpation)
- Spine–position and tenderness:
- Trachea:
- Apex:
- Respiratory movements:

Area	Right	Left
Supraclavicular		
Infraclavicular		
Mammary		
Suprascapular		
Infrascapular		

Dimensions:

T diameter		
AP diameter		
T : AP diameter		
Chest circumference	Expiration	
	Inspiration	
Right hemithorax	Expiration	
	Inspiration	
Left hemithorax	Expiration	
	Inspiration	
Chest expansion	Right hemithorax	
	Left hemithorax	
	Total	
Spinoscapular distance	(right side) and (left side)	
Spinoacromial distance	(right side) and (left side)	

Vocal fremitus

Areas	Right	Left
Supraclavicular		
Infraclavicular		
Mammary		
Axillary		
Infra-axillary		
Suprascapular		
Interscapular		
Infrascapular		

- Tactile fremitus:
- Friction fremitus:
- Tenderness:
- Subcutaneous emphysema:
- Rib crowding:
- Bony tenderness:

Percussion:

Areas	Right	Left
Supraclavicular		
Clavicular		
Infraclavicular		
Mammary		
Axillary		
Infra-axillary		
Suprascapular		
Interscapular		
Infrascapular		

- Shifting dullness:
- Tidal percussion:
- Traube's space:
- Kronig's isthmus:
- Liver dullness:
- Liver span:

Heart border on
- Right side:
- Left side:

Auscultation:
Breath sounds:
(Vesicular/bronchial/amphoric/cavernous)

Areas	Right	Left
Supraclavicular		
Infraclavicular		
Mammary		
Axillary		
Infra-axillary		
Suprascapular		
Interscapular		
Infrascapular		

Vocal resonance:

Areas	Right	Left
Supraclavicular		
Infraclavicular		
Mammary		
Axillary		
Infra-axillary		
Suprascapular		
Interscapular		
Infrascapular		

Adventitious sounds:
- Crepitations
- Rhonchi (Inspiratory or expiratory/Polymorphic or monomorphic)
- Rubs

Additional tests:
- Coin test:
- Bronchophony:
- Egophony:
- Succussion splash:
- Post-tussive creps:

Other Systems

Cardiovascular system:
- Inspection:
- Palpation:
- Percussion:
- Auscultation:

Gastrointestinal system:
- Inspection:
- Palpation:
- Percussion:
- Auscultation:

Nervous system:
- Higher mental functions:
- Cranial nerves:
- Sensory system:
- Motor system:
- Reflexes:
- Cerebellar system:
- Meningeal signs:

RESPIRATORY SYSTEM: DIAGNOSIS FORMAT

Anatomical Diagnosis
- Lung—(Right/Left/Bilateral) disease with (upper/middle/lower) lobe
- Pleural—

Pathological Diagnosis
- Consolidation/fibrosis/collapse/obstructive lung disease/restrictive lung disease/effusion/pneumothorax.

Etiological Diagnosis
Tuberculosis bronchogenic carcinoma/smoking/occupation/trauma

Complications
Respiratory failure (type I or type II)/cor pulmonale

Examples

Example 1
Right upper lobe fibrosis post-tubercular etiology, no evidence of respiratory failure or cor-pulmonale.

Example 2
Bilateral obstructive lung disease—emphysema secondary to smoking with evidence of type 2 respiratory failure and cor-pulmonale.

Example 3
Left-sided pleural effusion secondary to malignancy with no evidence of respiratory failure or cor-pulmonale.

RESPIRATORY SYSTEM: DISCUSSION ON CARDINAL SYMPTOMS

Symptoms discussed include:
- Cough
- Expectoration
- Hemoptysis
- Dyspnea
- Chest pain (wrt Respiratory system)
- Others

Cough

Definition
A sudden and variable expiratory thrust of air from the lungs through the air passages associated with phonation, which momentarily interrupts the physiological pattern of breathing.

Mechanism of Cough Production
Cough reflex initiated by chemical/mechanical stimuli. This is carried by the afferents which are type C and type 1 fibers and innervate pharynx, larynx, large airways, terminal bronchiole, and lung parenchyma. Afferents travel via vagus and superior laryngeal nerve. Nucleus tractus solitarius (NTS) in brain stem is the cough center. Efferents travel via vagus, phrenic, spinal motor nerves to the larynx, trachea, bronchi, and diaphragm-producing cough (**Flowchart 4.1**).

Mechanical events during cough production: The mechanical events involved in a typical cough are rapid successions of:
- A fairly deep initial inspiration;
- The tight closure of the glottis, reinforced by the supraglottic structures;
- The quick and forceful contraction of the expiratory muscles; and
- The sudden opening of the glottis while the contraction of the expiratory muscles continues.

Classification can be based on following heading (Table 4.1)
- *Based on etiology:* The etiology can be classified into respiratory causes and nonrespiratory causes.
- *Based on duration of cough:* Cough has been classified into acute (less than 3 weeks), subacute (3-8 weeks), and chronic (more than 8 weeks).

Table 4.1: Classification of cough.

Cough	Duration	Respiratory causes	Nonrespiratory causes
Acute cough	Less than 3 weeks	• Tracheobronchitis • Bronchopneumonia • Viral pneumonia • Acute-on-chronic bronchitis • Pulmonary embolism **Sudden onset:** • Bronchial asthma • Asthmatic bronchitis • Whooping cough • Foreign body	LVF GERD
Sub-acute cough	3–8 weeks	• Tuberculosis, pneumonia (bacterial, viral, fungal) • B. pertussis • Bronchiectasis • Post-viral tussive syndrome	• GERD • Tourette's syndrome • Intentional cough
Chronic cough	Lasting for more than 8 weeks	• COPD, asthma • ILD • Tuberculosis • Lung cancer • Pneumoconiosis (asbestosis, silicosis, anthracosis, etc.), • Mesothelioma of lung • Upper airway cough syndrome	• Drug-induced (ACE inhibitors, beta blockers, NSAIDs) • Habit cough syndrome

Note: Chronic cigarette smoking is the most common cause of chronic cough.
(COPD: chronic obstructive pulmonary disease; GERD: gastroesophageal reflux disease; NSAIDs: nonsteroidal anti-inflammatory drugs; ACE: angiotensin-converting enzyme)

- *Based on expectoration:* It is also classified into productive or dry cough depending on the presence or absence of expectoration, respectively.

Types of Cough
Different types of cough are shown in **Table 4.2**.

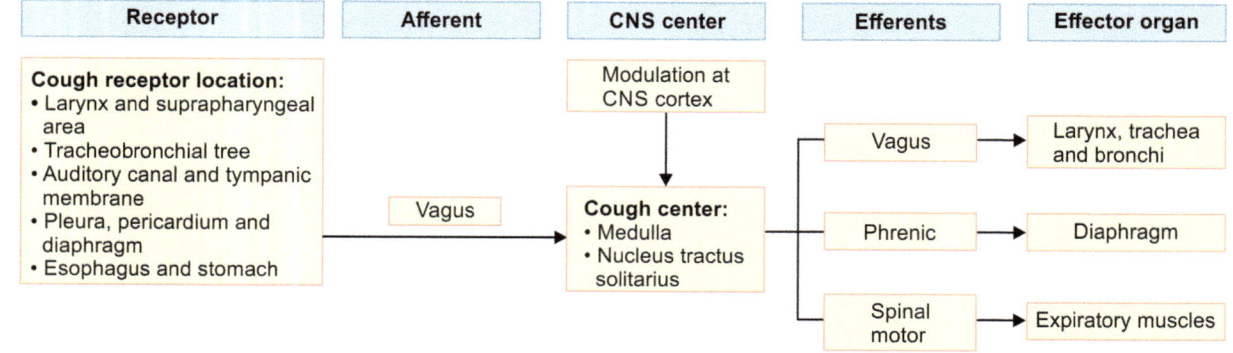

Flowchart 4.1: Cough reflex.

Table 4.2: Different types of cough.

Types	Features
Dry cough	Pleural disorders, diseases of interstitium, mediastinal lesions
Productive cough	Suppurative lung disease, airway diseases
Brassy/Gander cough	Metallic sound due to compression of trachea by intrathoracic space occupying lesions or aortic aneurysms also known as leopards grow
Bovine cough	Loss of expulsive nature as in a tumor pressing on the recurrent laryngeal nerve
Paroxysmal cough	Whooping cough, chronic bronchitis, foreign body, bronchial asthma
Barking cough	Involvement of epiglottis, croup (laryngo-tracheobronchitis), hysteria
Spluttering cough	T-E fistula, cough while swallowing
Hacking cough	Heavy smokers, chronic pharyngitis or laryngitis
Otogenic cough	Due to stimulation of Arnold's nerve in the external auditory meatus (impacted wax/foreign body)

Chronic cough with normal chest X-ray
❖ Cough variant asthma
❖ Tropical eosinophilia
❖ Upper airway cough syndrome
❖ Aspiration
❖ Habitual cough
❖ Foreign body
❖ Drugs angiotensin-converting enzyme inhibitors
❖ Chronic bronchitis
❖ Chronic idiopathic cough

Expectoration/Sputum

Sputum can be described under the following headings
- Quantity
- Quality
- Odor

Quantity	
Normal	10–15 mL/24 hours
Bronchorrhea	• Production of more than 100 mL/day • Bronchiectasis • Lung abscess • Bronchoalveolar carcinoma • Organophosphorus poisoning
Quality	
Mucoid	Chronic bronchitis, bronchial asthma
Mucopurulent	Infections
Purulent	Lung abscess, bronchiectasis
Rust-colored purulent sputum	Pneumococcal pneumonia
Currant jelly and sticky sputum	*Klebsiella pneumoniae*
Blood-tinged foamy sputum	Pulmonary edema (pink frothy)
Greenish	*Pseudomonas*
Granules—yellow/black	Actinomycosis
Anchovy sauce (brown)	Amebic abscess rupturing into lung
Black (melanoptysis)	Carbon particles discolor the sputum gray (as in cigarette smokers) or black (as in coal miners or with smoke inhalation)
Odor	
Foul smelling sputum	Anaerobic infection seen in lung abscess, bronchiectasis

Special Points
- Chronic expectoration of large amounts of purulent and foul-smelling sputum is strongly suggestive of bronchiectasis.
- Sudden production of such sputum in a febrile patient indicates a lung abscess.
- **Three-layer sputum** consisting of a foamy upper layer, mucous middle layer, and viscous purulent bottom layer is pathognomonic of bronchiectasis
- **Postural variation in sputum:** Bronchiectasis, lung abscess.

Hemoptysis

Definition
Hemoptysis is defined as coughing of blood originating from below the vocal cords. Hemoptysis can range from blood-streaking of sputum to the presence of gross blood in the absence of any accompanying sputum.

Massive Hemoptysis
Life threatening (or) massive hemoptysis is defined as coughing of blood >150 mL/time (or) >600 mL/24 hours. Only 5% of hemoptysis is massive, but mortality is 80%. Clinical definition of massive hemoptysis is any bleeding that result in a threat to life because of airway or hemodynamic compromise due to bleeding.

Causes of Hemoptysis
Causes of hemoptysis are described in **Table 4.3**.

Causes of Massive Hemoptysis
Causes of massive hemoptysis are described in **Table 4.4**.

Clinical Clues of Hemoptysis
Clinical clues for the diagnosis of hemoptysis are described in **Table 4.5**.

True and False Hemoptysis
Differences between true and false hemoptysis is shown in **Table 4.6**.

Table 4.3: Causes of hemoptysis.

Structure involved	Common causes	Uncommon causes
Bronchial disease	Bronchial carcinoma, bronchiectasis, acute and chronic bronchitis	Bronchial adenoma, foreign body
Parenchymal disease of lung	Pulmonary tuberculosis (Rasmussen's aneurysm-dilation of a pulmonary artery in a tuberculous cavity), lung abscess, pneumonia (particularly *Klebsiella*), fungal infections (aspergilloma and invasive aspergillosis, pulmonary contusion/laceration (traumatic)	Parasites (e.g., hydatid disease, flukes), trauma, actinomycosis, mycetoma
Vascular diseases of lung	Pulmonary infarction	Goodpasture's syndrome, polyarteritis nodosa, idiopathic, pulmonary hemosiderosis, primary pulmonary hypertension
Cardiovascular disease	Acute left ventricular failure	Mitral stenosis, aortic aneurysm, pulmonary thromboembolism
Hematological disorders		Leukemia, hemophilia, anticoagulants, hemorrhagic diathesis

Table 4.4: Causes of massive hemoptysis.

- Pulmonary tuberculosis
- Pulmonary infarction
- Bronchiectasis
- Bronchogenic carcinoma
- Cystic fibrosis
- Lung abscess
- Necrotizing pneumonia
- Mitral stenosis
- Pulmonary arteriovenous malformation

Table 4.5: Clinical clues for the diagnosis of hemoptysis.

Clinical clues	Suggested diagnosis
Anticoagulant use	Medication effect, coagulation disorder
Tobacco use	Acute bronchitis, chronic bronchitis, pneumonia, lung cancer
Dyspnea on exertion, fatigue, orthopnea, paroxysmal nocturnal dyspnea, frothy pink sputum	Congestive heart failure, left ventricular failure, mitral stenosis
Fever, productive cough	Upper respiratory tract infection, acute bronchitis, pneumonia, lung abscess
History of cancer (e.g., breast, colon, or kidney)	Endobronchial metastasis from carcinoma
History of chronic lung disease, recurrent lower respiratory tract infection, cough with copious purulent sputum	Bronchiectasis, lung abscess
Pleuritic chest pain, calf tenderness	Pulmonary embolism or infarction
Toxic symptoms	Tuberculosis
Weight loss	Emphysema, lung cancer, tuberculosis, bronchiectasis, lung abscess
Melena, alcoholism, chronic use of NSAIDs	Gastritis, gastric or peptic ulcer, esophageal varices
Association with menses	Catamenial hemoptysis
Cachexia, clubbing, hoarseness	Lung cancer, small cell carcinoma
Clubbing	Lung cancer, bronchiectasis, lung abscess
Dullness to percussion, fever, crepitations	Pneumonia

(NSAIDs: non-steroidal anti-inflammatory drugs)

Table 4.6: Differences between true and false hemoptysis.

True hemoptysis	False hemoptysis (Spurious)
Below vocal cords	Above vocal cords
Persists as blood tinged sputum	Does not persist
May be mixed with sputum	Not mixed with sputum
History of cardiopulmonary disease	Obvious by ENT examination
Chest X-ray may be abnormal	Normal chest X-ray

Hemoptysis and Hematemesis

Differences between hemoptysis and hematemesis is shown in **Table 4.7**.

Dyspnea

Definition

"Dyspnea" is a term used to characterize a subjective experience of breathing discomfort that is comprised of qualitatively distinct sensations that vary in intensity. (Undue awareness of unpleasant breathing)

Table 4.7: Differences between hemoptysis and hematemesis.

Hemoptysis	Hematemesis
Coughing of blood. Cough precedes hemoptysis	Vomiting of blood. Nausea and vomiting precedes hematemesis
History of cardiopulmonary disease	History of gastrointestinal disease
Bright red in color	Dark brown in color
Sputum remains blood stained after the attack for few days	Usually followed by melena
Mixed with sputum	Mixed with gastric contents
Blood is frothy due to admixture of air	Airless and not frothy
Alkaline	Acidic
Sputum contains hemosiderin laden macrophages	No
Melena absent	Melena present

Mechanism of Dyspnea

Chemoreceptors
- **Peripheral:** Carotid and aortic bodies (sensitive to changes pO_2, pCO_2 and H^+)
- **Central:** Medulla (sensitive only to changes pCO_2, not pO_2, change in pH of CSF).

Increased work of breathing:
- **Airflow obstruction:** Bronchial asthma, COPD, tracheal obstruction
- **Decreased pulmonary compliance:** Pulmonary edema, fibrosis, allergic alveolitis
- **Restricted chest expansion:** Ankylosing spondylitis, respiratory paralysis, and kyphoscoliosis.

Increased ventilatory drive
- **Increased physiological dead space (V/Q mismatch):** Consolidation, collapse, pulmonary embolism (PE), pulmonary edema

Hyperventilation due to receptor stimulation
- **Chemoreceptors:** Acidosis, hypoxia (shock, pneumonia), hypercapnia
- **J receptors at alveolo-capillary junction:** Pulmonary edema, pulmonary embolism, pulmonary congestion (activates Hering-Breuer reflex, which terminates inspiratory effort before full inspiration is achieved—rapid and shallow)
- **Muscle spindles in intercostal muscles:** Tension-length disparity
- **Central:** Exertion, anxiety, thyrotoxicosis, pheochromocytoma

Impaired respiratory muscle function
- **Diseases with impaired muscle function:** Poliomyelitis, Guillain-Barre syndrome (GBS), myasthenia gravis.

Orthopnea
Dyspnea develops in recumbent position and is relieved by sitting up or by elevation of the head with pillows.

The severity can be graded by the number of pillow used at night, e.g., three pillow orthopnea

Mechanism:
- Pulmonary congestion during recumbency (cannot be pumped out of LV) seen in congestive heart failure (CHF), chronic obstructive pulmonary disease (COPD), and bronchial asthma.
- Increased venous return.
- Diaphragm elevation leading to decreased vital capacity.

Seen in:
Orthopnea is classically seen in left heart failure but can also occur in constrictive pericarditis, COPD, bilateral diaphragmatic palsy, asthma triggered by gastric reflux, and gross ascites.

Paroxysmal Nocturnal Dyspnea (PND)
Attacks of dyspnea occur at night and awaken the patient from sleep.

Mechanism
- It is due to decreased responsiveness of respiratory center in brain during sleep and pulmonary congestion (due to increased sympathetic activity during REM sleep) 2-3 hours after onset of sleep.
- Absorption of edema fluid with increase in right ventricular output causing over filling the lungs
- Takes 10–30 minutes for recovery after upright posture (Fig. 4.1).

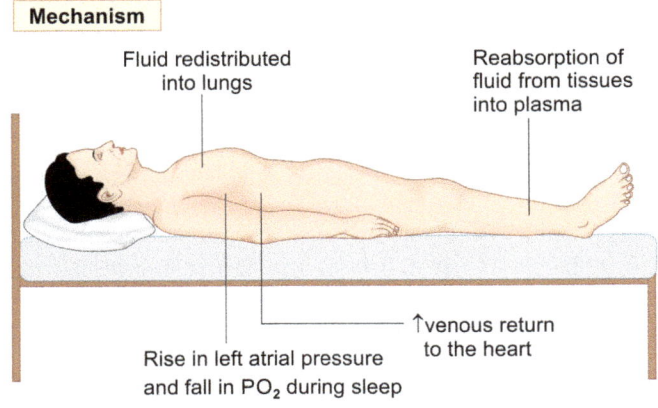
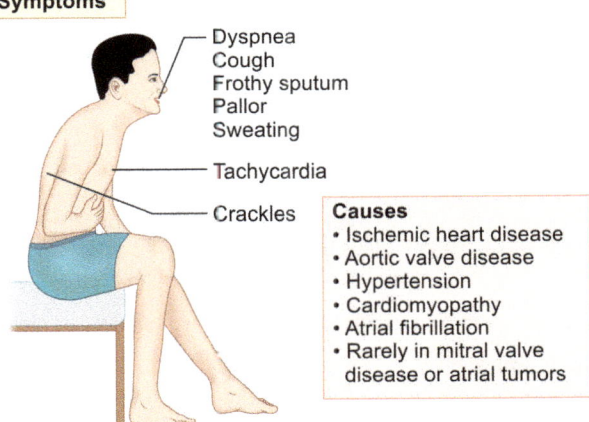

Fig. 4.1: Mechanism of paroxysmal nocturnal dyspnea.

Causes:
- Specific sign of LV dysfunction and includes IHD, aortic valve disease, hypertension, and cardiomyopathy.
- It has low sensitivity (<30%) but 75% specificity to diagnose heart disease.

Differences Between Orthopnea and PND
Differences between orthopnea and PND is shown in **Table 4.8.**

Differential Diagnosis for Paroxysmal Nocturnal Dyspnea
- Left heart failure
- Nocturnal episodes of asthma
- Postnasal discharge with attendant severe cough
- Sleep apnea with arousal
- Nightmares
- Nocturnal angina with dyspnea (angina equivalent)
- Nocturnal aspiration in gastroesophageal reflux disease
- Nocturnal episodes of recurrent minute pulmonary emboli
- Nocturnal hypoglycemia

Trepopnea
Aggravation of dyspnea when lying on one side and relieved by lying on opposite side.

Causes
- Unilateral lung disease: Uninvolved normal lung receives more blood supply due to gravity.
- Congestive heart failure: Lying on right side enhances venous return and sympathetic activity.
- Lung tumor: Gravity induced compression of blood vessels or lung.

Platypnea
Dyspnea on sitting or standing and relieved by supine position.

Causes
- Venous to arterial shunting (lung bases)
- Intracardiac shunts (ASD, pneumonectomy)
- Intrapulmonary right to left shunt [hepatopulmonary syndrome, pulmonary embolism (PE), COPD]
- Acute respiratory distress syndrome (ARDS).

Bendopnea
A newly described symptom in patients with heart failure is mediated via a further increase in ventricular filling pressures during bending in subjects whose sitting ventricular filling pressures are already high, particularly in patients with low cardiac index **(Fig. 4.2)**.

Approach to Dyspnea

Onset and duration	
Minutes to hours (rapid onset)	Pneumothorax, acute asthma, PE, pulmonary edema, foreign body
Hours to days (gradual onset)	Pneumonia, pleural effusion, anemia, Guillain–Barre syndrome (GBS)
Months to years (slow onset)	Pulmonary tuberculosis (PTB), COPD, carcinoma, fibrosing alveolitis
Severity (grading systems)*	
MRC	
mMRC	Discussed later
NYHA	
Aggravating and relieving factors	
Improves on weekend/holidays	Occupational asthma, extrinsic allergic alveolitis
Recumbency/sleep	Orthopnea/paroxysmal nocturnal dyspnea (PND)
Associated symptoms	
Pleuritic chest pain	Pneumonia, pulmonary infarction, rib fracture, pneumothorax
Central non-pleuritic chest pain	Myocardial infarction, massive pulmonary embolism
Cough or wheeze	Asthma, pulmonary embolism, pneumothorax.

Table 4.8: Differences between orthopnea and PND.

	Paroxysmal nocturnal dyspnea	Orthopnea
Definition	Episode of sudden onset of dyspnea 2–2.5 hours after sleep	Dyspnea in recumbent posture
Timing	Patient wakes up from rapid eye movement (REM) sleep	Occurs soon after lying down
Method of relief	Sits up with legs hanging down, stands up, air hunger, self ventilates to comfort	Gets up, uses more pillows, sleeps in erect posture
Mechanism	Depressed respiratory center. Sympathetic over activity during REM → catecholamine surge resulting in tachycardia → interstitial pulmonary congestion → respiratory center lags behind → perceived as acute dyspnea. There is sudden transient increase in PCWP	Shifting of venous blood (>400 Ml) into pulmonary circulation, V/Q mismatch, compression of diaphragm, postural diastolic dysfunction. There is a slow sustained rise in pulmonary capillary wedge pressure (PCWP)
Associated symptoms	Angina, perspiration, palpitation, rarely hemoptysis	All the symptoms of congestive cardiac failure (CCF)
Oxygen saturation	Transient hypoxia	Normal
Differential diagnosis	Night mares/panic attacks/nocturnal hypoglycemia/obstructive sleep apnea (OSA)	COPD/gross obesity/acute asthma/gross ascites

Chapter 4: Respiratory System Examination

New York Heart Association (NYHA) Classification
Classification by New York Heart Association is described in **Table 4.10**.

Causes of Acute and Chronic Dyspnea
Causes of acute and chronic dyspnea are shown in **Table 4.11**.

Acute Severe Breathlessness
- Pulmonary edema
- Massive pulmonary embolism
- Acute severe asthma

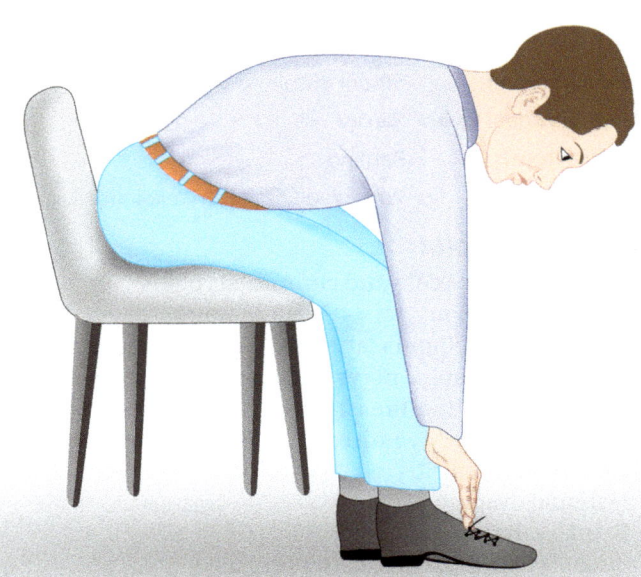

Fig. 4.2: A patient sits in a chair, bends at the waist, and touches his/her feet. Bendopnea is considered present, if dyspnea occurs within 30 seconds of bending.

Grading Systems
Grading system are explained in **Box 4.1** and **Table 4.9**.

Pitfalls of mMRC Grading
- The mMRC dyspnea scale quantifies disability attributable to breathlessness, and is useful for characterizing baseline dyspnea in patients with respiratory diseases.
- Describes baseline dyspnea, but does not accurately quantify response to treatment of COPD.

Box 4.1: MRC grading of breathlessness.

Medical Research Council (MRC) grading of severity of dyspnea
1. Not troubled by breathlessness except on strenuous exertion
2. Short of breath when hurrying on level ground or walking up slight hill
3. Walks slower than people of same age or stops after 15 minutes when walking at own pace on level
4. Stops after 100 yards (90 m) or after few minutes in level ground
5. Too breathless to leave house, dress or undress

Table 4.9: mMRC grading of breathlessness.

Grade	Description of breathlessness
Grade 0	I only get breathless with strenuous exercise
Grade 1	I get short of breath when hurrying on level ground or walking up a slight hill
Grade 2	On level ground, I walk slower than people of the same age because of breathlessness, or I have to stop for breath when walking at my own pace on the level
Grade 3	I stop for breath after walking about 100 yards or after a few minutes on level ground
Grade 4	I am too breathless to leave the house or I am breathless when dressing

Table 4.10: NYHA classification.

NYHA Class	Patients with cardiac disease (Description of HF related symptoms)
Class I (Mild)	Patients with cardiac disease but without resulting in limitation of physical activity. Ordinary physical activity does not cause undue fatigue, palpitation, dyspnea, or angina pain
Class II (Mild)	Patients with cardiac disease resulting in slight limitation of physical activity. They are comfortable at rest. Ordinary physical activity results in fatigue, palpitation, dyspnea, or angina pain
Class III (Moderate)	Patients with cardiac disease resulting in marked limitation of physical activity. They are comfortable at rest. Less than ordinary activity causes fatigue, palpitation, dyspnea, or angina pain
Class IV (Severe)	Patients with cardiac disease resulting in the inability to carry on any physical activity without discomfort. Symptoms of heart failure or the anginal syndrome may be present even at rest. If any physical activity is undertaken, discomfort is increased

Table 4.11: Causes of acute and chronic dyspnea.

Acute dyspnea	Chronic dyspnea
Cardiovascular system	
Cardiogenic acute pulmonary edema	Chronic heart failure, myocardial ischemia
Respiratory system	
• Acute severe bronchial asthma • Acute exacerbation of COPD • Spontaneous pneumothorax • Pneumonia • Acute pulmonary embolism • ARDS • Inhaled foreign body (especially in children) • Lobar collapse • Laryngeal edema (e.g., anaphylaxis) or obstruction • Metabolic acidosis (e.g., diabetic ketoacidosis, lactic acidosis, uremia, overdose of salicylates, ethylene glycol poisoning) • Psychogenic hyperventilation (anxiety or panic-related)	• COPD • Chronic bronchial asthma • Bronchial carcinoma • Interstitial lung disease (e.g., sarcoidosis, fibrosing alveolitis, extrinsic allergic alveolitis, pneumoconiosis) • Chronic pulmonary thromboembolism • Lymphatic carcinomatosis • Large pleural effusion(s) • Severe anemia • Obesity • Deconditioning

- Acute exacerbation of COPD
- Severe pneumonia
- Tension pneumothorax
- Foreign body/mucous plug
- Epiglottitis (children)
- Metabolic acidosis
- Psychogenic

Chest Pain

(Discussed in cardiovascular system)

Respiratory Causes of Chest Pain

- Raw upper sternal: Tracheitis
- Pleuritic: associated with breathing
- Neurologic: invasion of nerves

Pleuritic chest pain is characterized by sudden and intense sharp, stabbing, or burning pain in the chest when inhaling and exhaling. It is exacerbated by deep breathing, coughing, sneezing, or laughing. When pleuritic inflammation occurs near the diaphragm, pain can be referred to the neck or shoulder. Pleuritic chest pain is caused by inflammation of the parietal pleura and can be triggered by a variety of causes.

- Pulmonary embolism, myocardial infarction, pericarditis, aortic dissection, pneumonia, and pneumothorax are the six serious conditions that cause pleuritic pain.

Other Symptoms

Noisy Breathing (Partial Obstruction of Airway)

Laryngeal level	Stridor (Inspiratory sound)
Oropharyngeal level	Stertor
Tracheal level	Rattling
Bronchial level	Wheezing (inspiratory/expiratory)

Hoarseness of Voice

- Inflammatory: Acute and chronic laryngitis
- Smoke inhalation
- Neoplastic carcinoma laryngeal papillomatosis
- Recurrent laryngeal nerve damage: Post-thyroidectomy
- Carcinoma of lung/breast
- Neurological: Myasthenia gravis, hypothyroidism, rheumatoid arthritis
- Habitual dysphonias
- Reinke's dysphonia
- Singer's nodules/vocal cord polyps,
- GERD reflux

Hiccoughs

Respiratory causes include basal pneumonia and pleurisy

Snoring

Feature of obstructive sleep apnea

RESPIRATORY SYSTEM: DISCUSSION ON EXAMINATION

General Examination

Built and Nourishment
Body mass index and anthropometry have been discussed in detail in General Examination.

Respiratory diseases associated with emaciation
- Respiratory diseases associated with HIV
- Pulmonary tuberculosis
- Malignancy

Pickwickian syndrome (obesity hypoventilation syndrome)
- Obesity
- Hypoxia
- Pulmonary HTN

Vital Examination (with respect to RS)

Pulse:
- **Rate:** Tachycardia (any pneumonia, febrile illness, hypoxia)
- Irregular pulse seen in multifocal atrial tachycardia, atrial fibrillation
- Character
- Bounding pulse—CO_2 retention
- Pulsus paradoxus—acute exacerbation of COPD/Asthma

Respiratory rate:
(Discussed in Chapter 2)

Blood pressure:
- **Wide pulse pressure:** In hypercapnia
- **Low blood pressure:** Seen with hypoxia, acute respiratory distress
- **Postural hypotension:** Addison's disease, paraneoplastic.

JVP:
- **Elevated:** In corpulmonale, tricuspid regurgitation
- **Nonpulsatile JVP:** SVC obstruction

Temperature:
- Evening rise of temperature: Tuberculosis
- High spiking fevers: Lung abscess, empyema, pneumonias.
- Temperature fall by crisis: Pneumonias

Pallor:
- Tuberculosis
- Malignancy
- Any cause of massive hemoptysis

Polycythemia:
Chronic respiratory diseases usually associated with polycythemia so if patient with COPD, if he has anemia look for other causes, such as GI bleed, CKD, or coexistent malignancy.

Icterus:
- Hepatitis secondary to ATT drugs
- Atypical pneumonias (hemolytic jaundice)
- As a part of MODS
- Rarely metastasis to liver

Edema:
- Cor-pulmonale
- Bronchiectasis leading to hypoproteinemia (due to loss of protein in the sputum and nephrotic syndrome secondary to amyloidosis)—100 mL of sputum can cause 3–4 g of protein loss.
- Hypercapnia-induced dilation of the precapillary sphincters.
- Reduced renal blood flow with relatively preserved glomerular filtration rate and elevated levels of renin, aldosterone, arginine vasopressin, and atrial natriuretic peptide

Cyanosis, clubbing, and lymphadenopathy described in detail in the chapter General examination.

Lymphatic drainage of lung	
Most of the lung (Right upper lobe Right middle lobe Right lower lobe Left lower lobe)	Right tracheobronchial → right bronchomediastinal right supraclavicular lymph node
Left upper lobe	Left tracheobronchial → left bronchomediastinal → left supraclavicular lymph node

Lymphatic drainage of pleura (Fig. 4.3)	
Cervical pleura	Axillary lymph nodes
Parietal pleura	Anterior: internal mammary nodes Posterior: extrapleural nodes
Diaphragmatic pleura	Internal mammary nodes cardiophrenic nodes Para-aortic, intercostal and posterior mediastinal nodes
Mediastinal pleura	Internal mammary nodes

ORAL CAVITY EXAMINATION
- Halitosis seen in suppurative lung diseases
- Tobacco staining of the teeth
- Poor oral hygiene
- Cyanosis or polycythemia

Skin

External Markers of Tuberculosis
- Matted lymph nodes
- Erythema nodosum
- Phlyctenular conjunctivitis
- Choroid tubercle
- Discharging sinuses
- Scrofuloderma
- Lupus vulgaris
- Beaded vas deferens
- Positive Mantoux test
- Generalized tinea versicolor
- Uveitis

External Markers of Malignancy
- Cachexia
- Grade IV clubbing (HPOA)

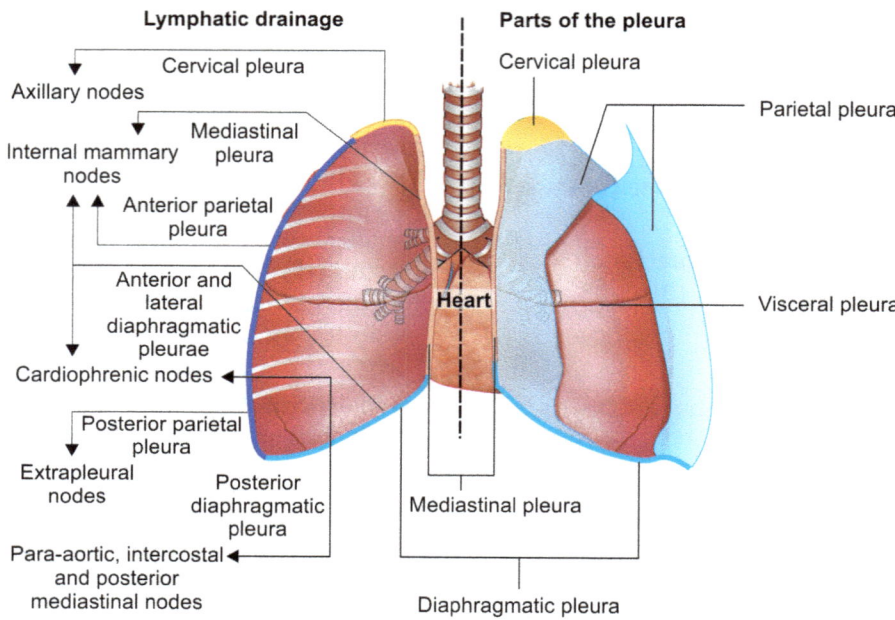

Lymph fluid from the visceral pleura drains into the subpleural lymphatic plexus and into the bronchopulmonary nodes at the hilum of the lung

Fig. 4.3: Parts of pleura with corresponding lymphatic drainage.

- Hard lymph nodes
- Acanthosis nigricans
- Horner's syndrome
- SVC obstruction features

Features of Respiratory Failure

Features of respiratory failure are shown in **Table 4.12**.

Features of Cor-pulmonale

- Right ventricular dilatation
  - Parasternal heave
  - Epigastric pulsation
- Right ventricular failure
  - Raised JVP
  - Pedal edema
  - Tender hepatomegaly
  - Ascites
  - Positive hepatojugular reflex is first sign of RVF

EXAMINATION OF RESPIRATORY SYSTEM

Examination of Upper Respiratory Tract System

Demarcation of URTI and LRTI

- Externally: demarcated by cricoid cartilage
- Internally: demarcated by glottis

LRTI Diseases Associated with URTI

- Nasal turbinate hypertrophy or polyps causing airway obstruction
- Sinus tenderness suggestive of sinusitis
- Kartageners syndrome:
  - Recurrent sinusitis with ciliary dyskinesia
  - Bronchiectasis

Table 4.12: Features of respiratory failure.

	Type 1	Type 2
Definition	Hypoxemic respiratory failure (type I) is characterized by an arterial oxygen tension (PaO_2) lower than 60 mm Hg with a normal or low arterial carbon dioxide tension ($PaCO_2$)	Hypercapnic respiratory failure (type II) is characterized by a $PaCO_2$ higher than 50 mm Hg
Sensorium	Anxious agitated	Drowsy to comatose
Peripheries	Cold	Warm
Pulse	Feeble	Bounding
Blood pressure	Low	Wide pulse pressure
Cyanosis	+	-
Asterixis	-	+
Respiratory rate	Tachypneic	Normal to low
Papilledema	-	+
Cause	ARDS Pneumonia Acute severe asthma Tension pneumothorax	COPD Obesity Respiratory paralysis

Type 3 (Perioperative):
Functional residual capacity falls below closing volume as a result of atelectasis in post-operative patients. This is generally a subset of type 1 failure but is sometimes considered separately because it is common.
Type 4 (Shock):
Secondary to cardiovascular instability.

(ARDS: acute respiratory distress syndrome; COPD: chronic obstructive pulmonary disease)

- Situs inversus
- Male infertility
- ❏ **Wegeners granulomatosis:** Necrotizing granuloma
- ❏ **Samter's triad:**
  - Aspirin sensitivity
  - Bronchial asthma
  - Ethmoidal polyps
- ❏ **Young's syndrome:**
  - Sinopulmonary disease
  - Azoospermia
- ❏ **Churg-Strauss syndrome:**
  - Asthma
  - Eosinophilia
  - Vasculitis
  - Granuloma

Inspection (Lower Respiratory Tract)

Surface Marking of Lung

Right side three lobes	Left side two lobes
• Right upper lobe (RUL) • Right middle lobe (RML) • Right lower lobe (RLL)	• Left upper lobe (LUL) • Left lower lobe (LLL)

Demarcating Lower Lobe of Either Side (Figs. 4.4 to 4.7)

Lower lobe of either lung can be demarcated from other lobes by drawing a curvilinear line (major interlobar fissure/oblique fissure) joining three bony points:

1. Starting from T2/T3 spinous process, curvilinear line along the medial border of scapula
2. Crossing the 5th rib in the mid-axillary line
3. Reaching the 6th rib in mid-clavicular line

Part of lung below this line is lower lobe

Marking right middle lobe

Draw a straight line (Minor IL fissure/horizontal fissure) from the 4th rib at right sternal border toward the MAL cutting the major inter lobar fissure at 5th rib. The triangular area represents RML.

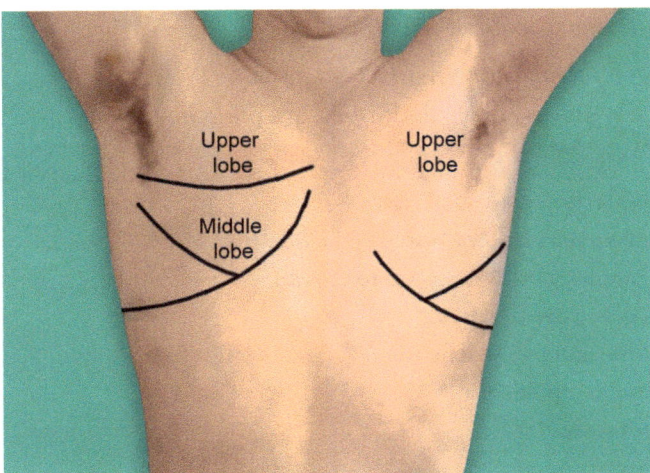

Fig. 4.4: Anterior view of chest showing surface marking of lung lobes.

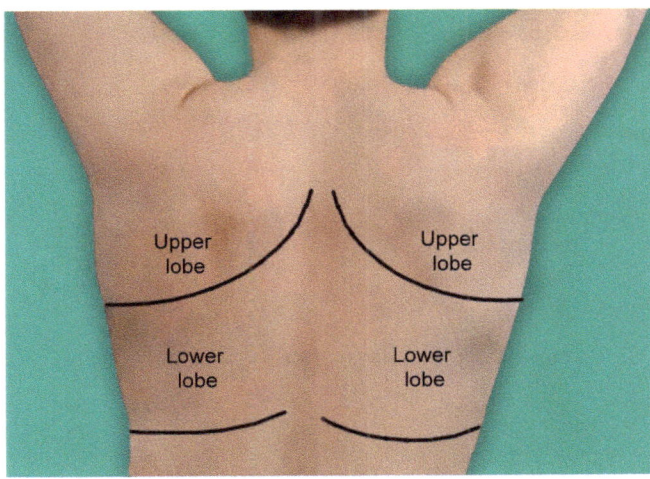

Fig. 4.5: Posterior view of chest showing surface marking of lung lobes.

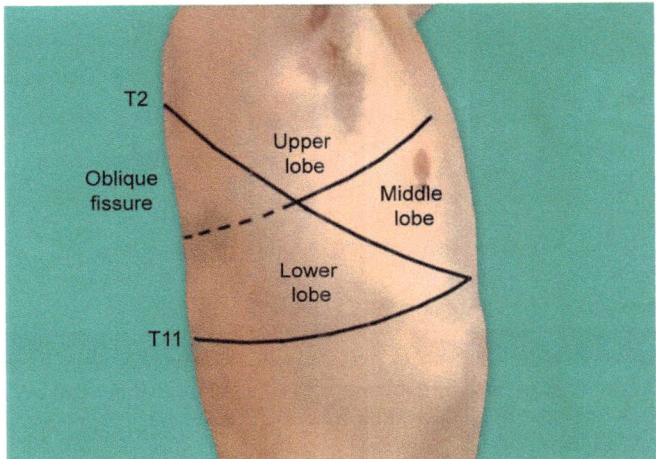

Fig. 4.6: Right lateral view of chest showing right major interlobar fissure and right minor interlobar fissure.

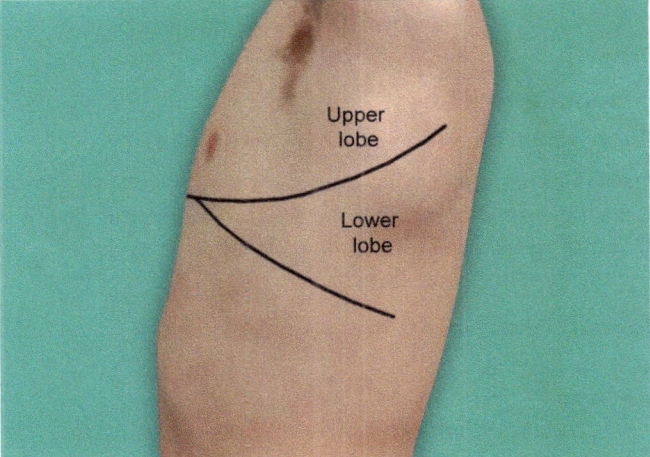

Fig. 4.7: Left lateral view of chest showing left major interlobar fissure.

Level of lower border	MCL	MAL	Scapular
Lung (Figs. 4.8 and 4.9)	6th rib	8th rib	10th rib
Pleura	8th rib	10th rib	12th rib

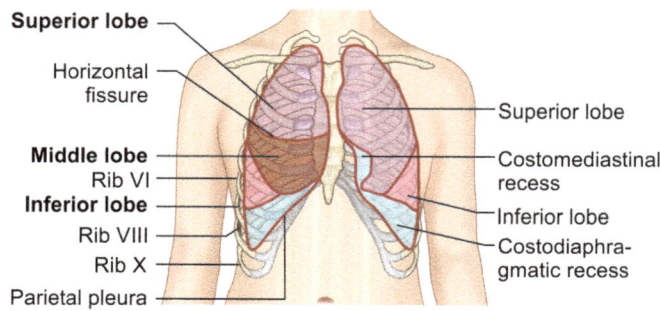

Fig. 4.8: Lower margin of lung in MCL and MAL.

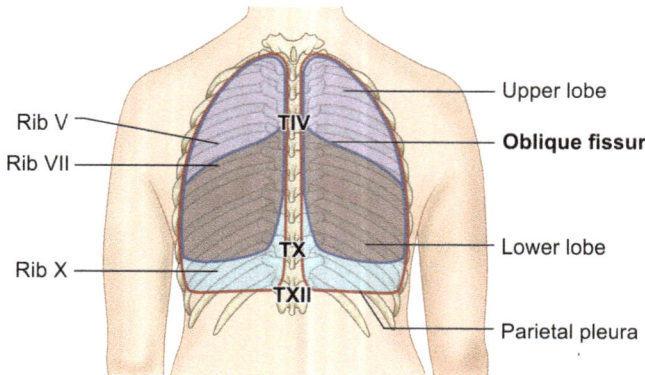

Fig. 4.9: Lower margin of lung in scapular line.

Table 4.13: Chest examination.

Front examination	Back examination	Axillary examination
Predominantly to look for upper and middle lobe	Predominantly to look for lower lobe pathology	All three lobes can be assessed
Examined in Sitting upright with hand by the side	Examined in Sitting upright with hands placed on the opposite shoulder and neck flexed	Examined in the sitting position with hands raised opposite the shoulder and placed on the occiput

Examination of Chest

Chest examination is described in **Table 4.13**.

Position of patient during examination can be
- Sitting—most of the examination is done in this position
- Standing—spine and shoulder droop
- Supine—shifting dullness

Normal Chest (Fig. 4.10)
- Spine central
- Shape
  - Circular: infants and early childhood
  - Elliptical: adults
  - Circular: old age
- Vertical >transverse >AP
- Transverse: AP = 7:5 (called as **Hutchinson's index**)
- Subcostal angle ≤ 90 (more acute in males)

Deformities of Chest

Chest deformities are described in **Table 4.14**.

Asymmetry of Chest

Asymmetry of chest is shown in **Table 4.15**.

Trachea

Normally central or slightly deviated to right

Trails Sign (Fig. 4.12)

In the presence of tracheal deviation, there is prominence of the clavicular head of sternocleidomastoid of same side.

The investing layer of cervical fascia splits to enclose the sternocleidomastoid and then falls back and continues as the pretracheal fascia. When there is tracheal shift to one side, the fascia covering the ipsilateral sternocleidomastoid relaxes. The sternocleidomastoid goes into a state of contraction making the clavicular head prominent.
- Clinical implication of tracheal shift: It suggests upper mediastinal shift.
- Indicates upper lobe fibrosis or collapse

Apical Impulse
- Normally 10 cm from sternal margin.
- Clinical implication—suggests lower mediastinal shift

Examination of Drooping of Shoulder (Fig. 4.13)

Examine the standing patient from behind to look for position of shoulder. Drooping of shoulder indicates volume loss on that side (collapse/fibrosis/fibrothorax/pneumonectomy). It can be seen rarely with paralysis of trapezius.

Associated features include:
- Prominent medial border of scapula on the affected side
- Space between medial border of scapula and spine is decreased
- Inferior angle of scapula is at the lower lever (normally it is at level of T_7 vertebra)

Examination of Spine
- Look for position of spine
- Look for scoliosis/kyphosis/lordosis/gibbus **(Fig. 4.14)**
- In emphysema, there is exaggerated thoracic kyphosis

Causes of Scoliosis

Causes of scoliosis are shown in **Table 4.16**.

Differentiation of congenital versus acquired scoliosis

On bending forward acquired scoliosis disappears but congenital scoliosis persists.

Respiratory Movements

(Describe as equal/diminished in a particular area)

Area	Right	Left
Supraclavicular		
Infraclavicular (Arbitrarily up to 3rd rib)		
Mammary (Arbitrarily 3rd to 6th rib)		
Axillary (Up to 6th rib)		
Infra-axillary (Beyond 6th rib)		
Suprascapular		
Infrascapular		
Interscapular		
Scapular (Mentioned in some books)		

Note: That there is no inframammary area.

Chapter 4: Respiratory System Examination

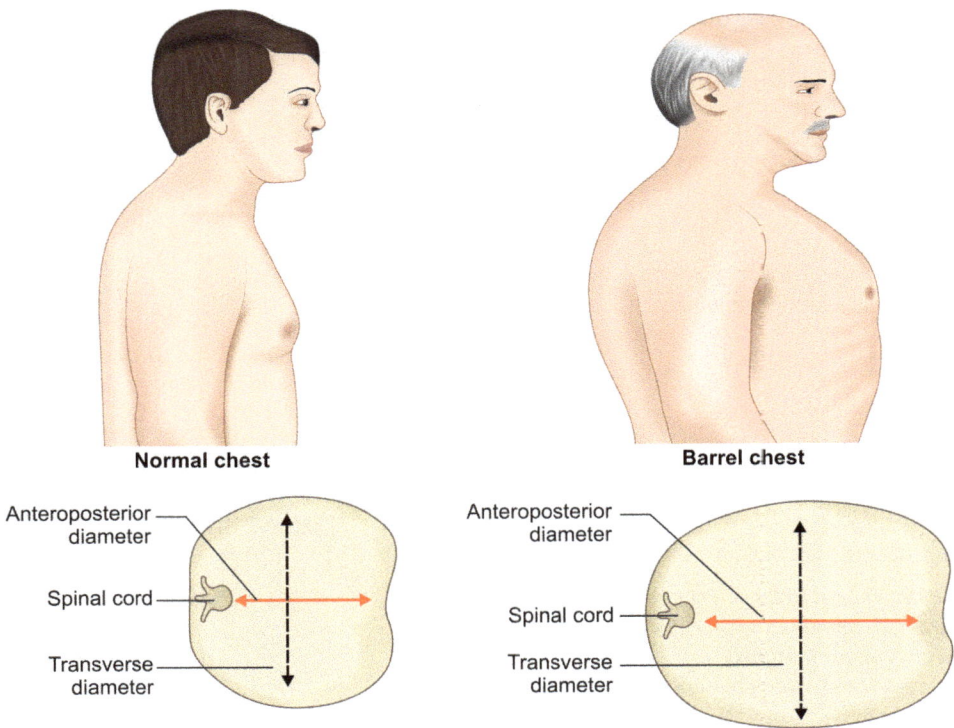

Fig. 4.10: Normal and barrel-shaped chest.

Table 4.14: Chest deformities.

Deformities of chest	
1. Flat chest (alar chest)	Anteroposterior ratio is 2:1
2. Pectus carinatum (Figs. 4.11A and B) (Pigeon chest/keel chest)	Forward protrusion of sternum seen in rickets and childhood respiratory disease, such as asthma. Can also be seen in Marfan's syndrome
3. Pectus excavatum (Figs. 4.11A and B) (Funnel chest, cobbler's chest)	Funnel-like depression. At the lower end of the chest, seen in Marfan's syndrome. Displaces the heart to the left. Ventilation capacity of the lung is restricted
4. Rachitic chest	Funnel-shaped Keel breast Harrison sulci (horizontal groove where the diaphragm attaches to the ribs—seen in rickets, chronic asthma, and COPD) Vertical grooves on either side of sternum Rachitic rosary (bead-like enlargement of costochondral enlargement especially 4/5/6 ribs)—painless and seen in vitamin D deficiency
5. Scorbutic rosary	Sharp angulation of the ribs arising due to backward displacement of sternum Painful and seen in vitamin C deficiency
6. Barrel-shaped chest (Fig. 4.10)	COPD—emphysema • Anteroposterior: Transverse diameter is 1:1 • Exaggerated thoracic kyphosis • Wide subcostal angle
7. Phthinoid chest	Combination of alar and flat chest
8. Flail chest	Paradoxical movement of the chest in fracture of three or more consecutive ribs
9. Shield-like chest	Turners and Noonan syndrome

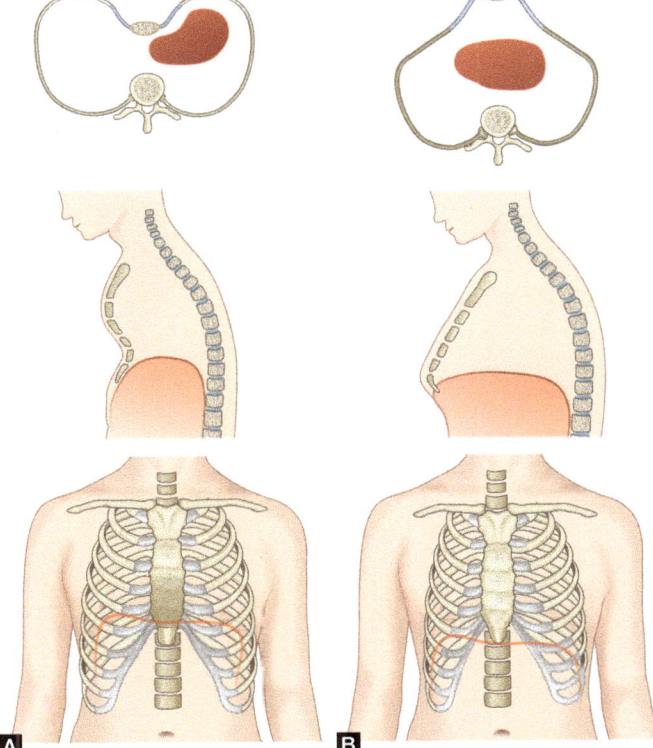

Figs. 4.11A and B: (A) Pectus excavatum; (B) Pectus carinatum.

Abnormal signs in respiratory system
Abnormal signs in respiratory system are shown in **Table 4.17**.

Inspiratory Intercostal Retraction (Fig. 4.16)
☐ Mild degree of intercostal retraction in the lower chest is normal

Chapter 4: Respiratory System Examination

Table 4.15: Asymmetry of chest.

Asymmetry	Features
Deformity of spine	• Scoliosis • Kyphoscoliosis • Gibbus
U/L bulge	• Pleural effusion • Pneumothorax • Compensatory hypertrophy • Malignancy of lung or pleura
U/L flattening	• Fibrosis • Collapse • Fibrothorax • Pneumonectomy • Agenesis of one lung (McLeod's syndrome/Swyer-James syndrome) • Mastectomy • Absent pectoralis (Poland's syndrome)
Local bulging (fullness)	• Supraclavicular fullness (Pancoast tumor/lymphadenopathy/massive pleural effusion/tension pneumothorax) • Empyema necessitans (cough impulse present) • Aortic aneurysm • Malignant infiltration • Pericardial effusion • Surgical emphysema
Local retraction	• Apical TB (Mohrenheim's fossa/infraclavicular fossa) • Lung fibrosis

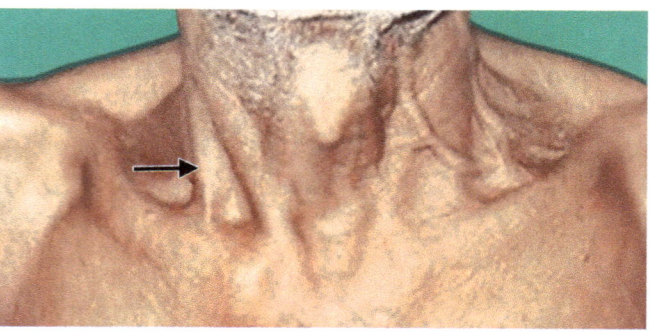

Fig. 4.12: Trail's sign showing undue prominence of sternocleidomastoid on the right side due to tracheal shift to right.

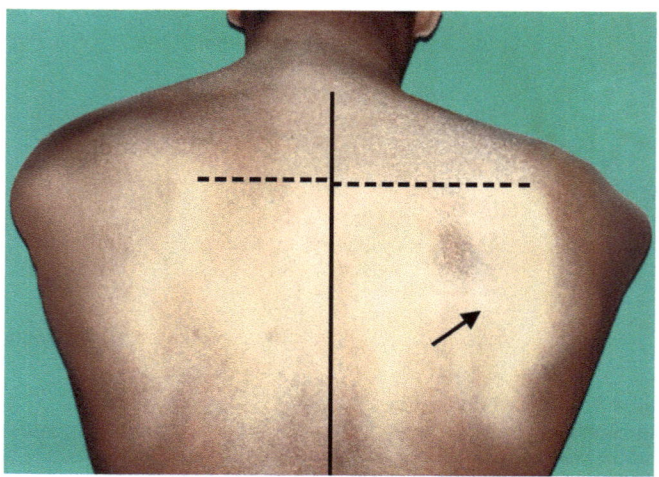

Fig. 4.13: Shoulder drooping on right side.

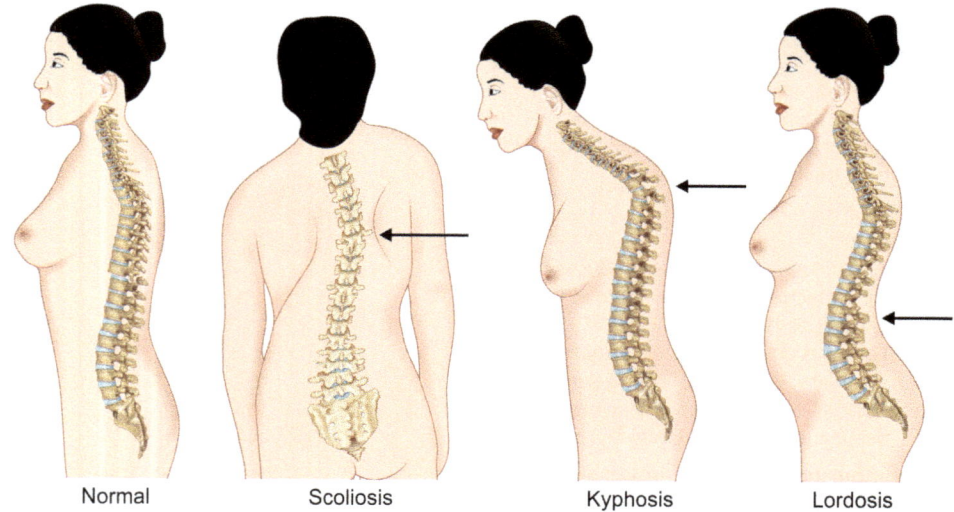

Fig. 4.14: Spine deformities.

▫ Differences between unilateral and bilateral intercostal retraction is shown in **Table 4.18**.

Visible Pulsations/Scars/Sinuses

Visible pulsation or vessels:
▫ **Collaterals around scapula:** Coarctation of Aorta (Suzman's sign)
▫ **Engorged veins over the anterior part of chest**
  • **SVC obstruction**
    ▪ Bronchogenic carcinoma
    ▪ Mediastinal growth
    ▪ Mediastinal lymphnodes
    ▪ Aortic aneurysm
    ▪ Chronic mediastinal fibrosis

- **Pulsatile swelling in anterior chest wall:** Aortic aneurysm.

Visible scars:
- Previous surgery (lobectomy)
- Pleural fluid aspiration site
- Lymphnode biopsy site

Sinuses:
- Abscess draining points
- Empyema thoracis (usually in tuberculosis/actinomycosis))

Palpation (Lower Respiratory Tract)

Trachea
- Normal length: 4–5 cm above suprasternal notch

Table 4.16: Causes of scoliosis.

Scoliosis	Causes
Neuromuscular causes	• Spina bifida • Marfan's syndrome • Cerebral palsy • Federick's ataxia • Spinocerebellar degenerations • Charcot marie tooth disease • Syringomyelia • Poliomyelitis • Muscular dystrophy (Duchene's, Fascioscapulo humeral, Myotonic dystrophy)
Degenerative	Osteoporosis Postspine surgery
Osteopathic	Klippel feil syndrome
Congenital scoliosis	Down's syndrome Prader-Willi syndrome
Respiratory diseases	Fibrosis Fibrothorax
Idiopathic	-

- Normal cricoid to suprasternal notch distance is 3–4 finger breadth (decreased in COPD due to hyperinflation)

Method of Palpation

> Keep the index and ring finger of the right hand on medial ends of the clavicle
> ↓
> With middle finger trace the trachea from above downward **(Fig. 4.17)**
> ↓
> Then, insinuate the middle finger between the trachea and sternal head of sternocleidomastoid, and feel for resistance **(Fig. 4.18)**

Implication of tracheal shift: Upper mediastinal shift

Oliver's Sign (Tracheal Tug Sign) (Fig. 4.19)
- Stand behind patient and hold cricoid cartilage give a slight upward thrust.

Positive test	Downward pull with each heart beat suggestive of aortic aneurysm
Negative test	Normal
False positive	Mediastinal tumor attached to abdominal aorta
False negative	Thrombosed aortic aneurysm

- **Tracheal descent on inspiration (Campbell sign):** Due to downward pull of the depressed diaphragm in long-standing hyperinflation of lung.
- **Laryngeal fixation:** Increased pressure on cricoid cartilage due to inflammatory or neoplastic lesion in mediastinum.

Apical Impulse
- Confirm the position of apex
- Comment on character
- Watch for thrills and other palpable heart sounds
- Implication of apical shift: it suggests lower mediastinal shift

Table 4.17: Abnormal signs of respiratory system.

Abnormal signs	Description
Sitting up and catching the edge	Described in COPD where the patient sits up and fixes shoulders to use latissimus dorsi for expiration
Tripod position (Fig. 4.15A)	Patient is sitting in leading forward posture with their outstretched hands on their knees. This position fixes and lifts the shoulder girdle and improves the function of pectoralis major and minor
Hoover sign	It paradoxical inspiratory indrawing of lateral rib cage (costal margin). It is a sign of chronic airflow obstruction. Pulmonary hyperinflation leads to loss of apposition of the diaphragmatic fibers resulting in horizontal orientation of fires. When these horizontally oriented fibers contract, the costal margins gets pulled inwards
Pursed lip breathing (Fig. 4.15B)	Seen in COPD to increase the intra-alveolar pressure to maintain a positive intraluminal pressure, which reduces the airway collapse, air way resistance, and residual volume and hence improves ventilation
Dahl's sign	Patches of hyperpigmentation/bruising above the knees due to constant tenting position of the hands and elbows
Littens sign	To look for the diaphragmatic movement Sit to one side of the patient lying in supine position and look at the diaphragmatic movements
Excessive usage of SCM and scalene	COPD or asthma
Paradoxical respiration	Indrawing of abdominal wall when the rib case moves outwards. Best felt by bimanual palpation with one hand over the patient's chest and other on the abdomen. Indicates respiratory muscle weakness

(COPD: chronic obstructive pulmonary disease)

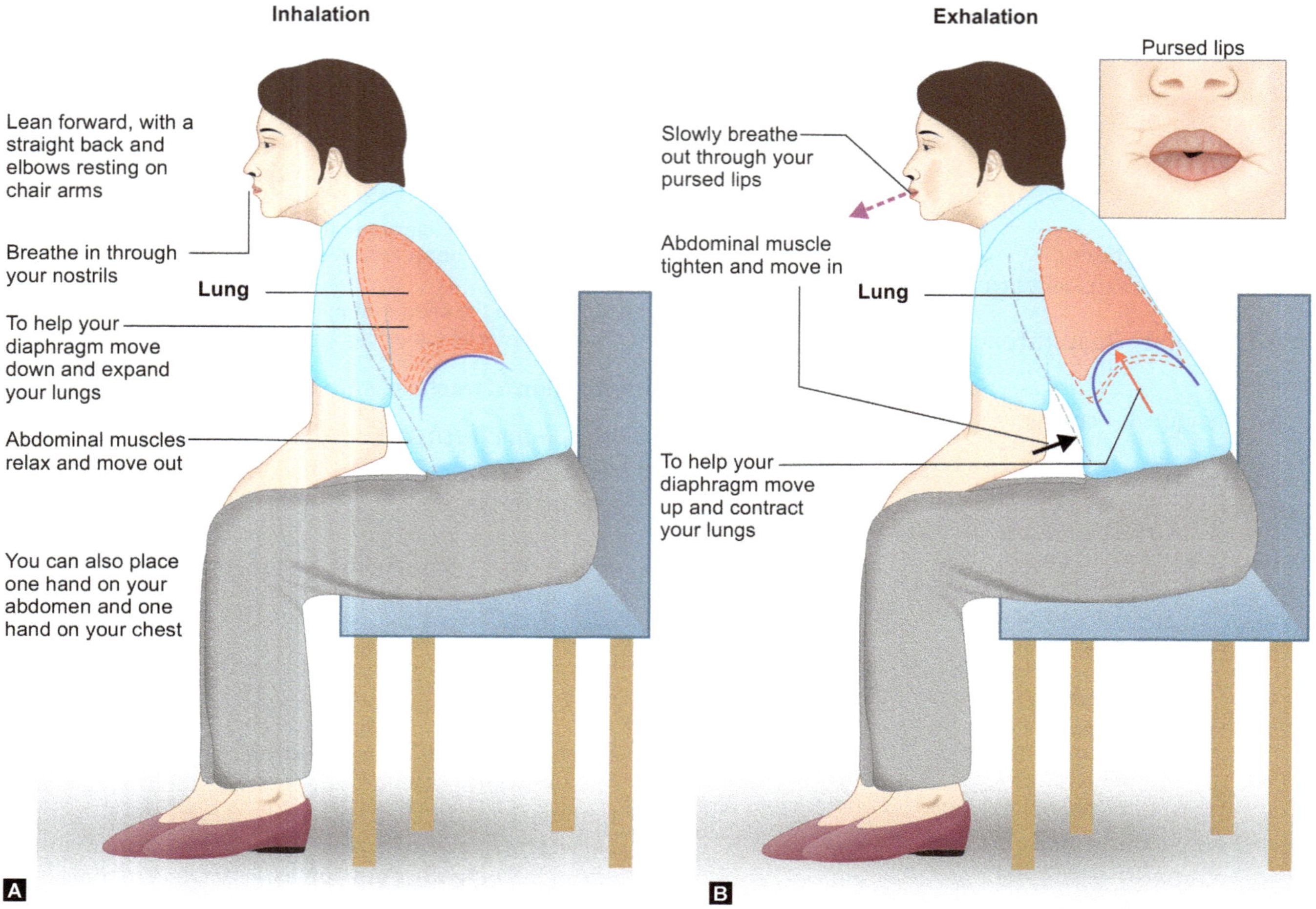

Figs. 4.15A and B: Tripod position with pursed lip breathing.

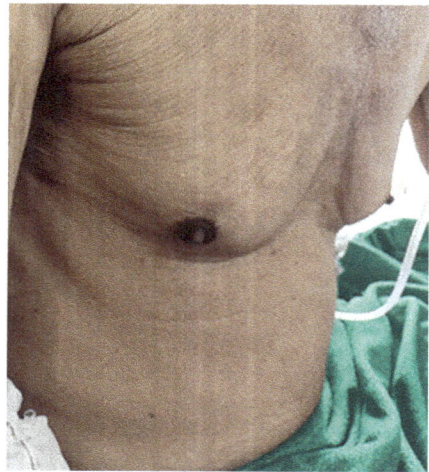

Fig. 4.16: Intercostal retractions.

Table 4.18: Differences between unilateral and bilateral intercostal retraction.

Unilateral intercostal retraction	Bilateral intercostal retraction
• Collapse • Fibrosis • Adherent pericarditis (Broadbent's sign–indrawing of lower anterior chest wall with each ventricular systole)	• Indicates upper air way obstruction (adenoids/foreign body) • Hyperinflation of chest

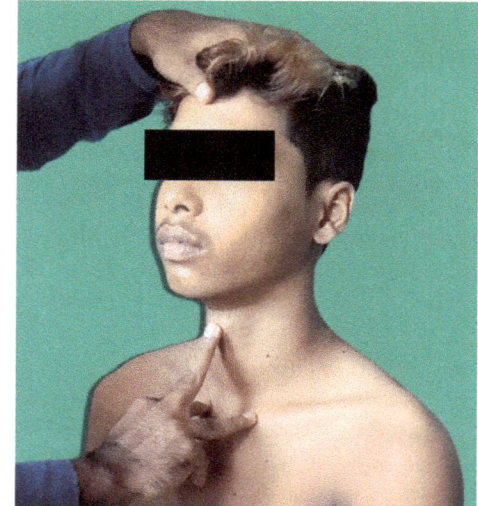

Fig. 4.17: Tracing the trachea down with the middle finger.

Apex not felt/seen in respiratory diseases:
- Emphysema
- Left-sided pleural effusion
- Left-sided pneumothorax

Mediastinal shift with respect to respiratory disease

Mediastinal shift with respect to respiratory disease is shown in **Table 4.19**.

Chapter 4: Respiratory System Examination

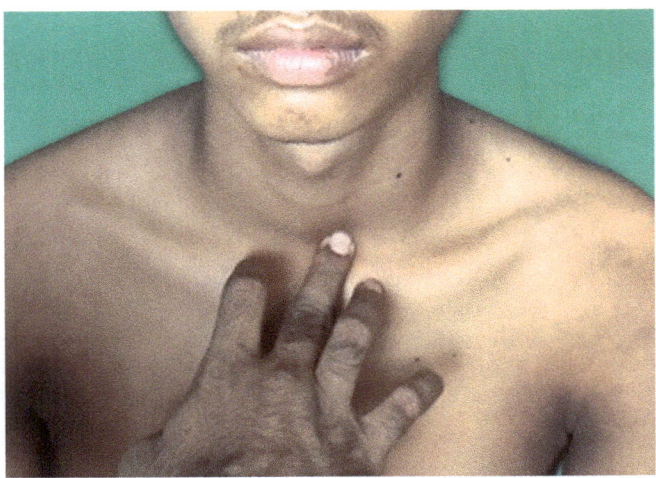

Fig. 4.18: Insinuate the middle finger between the trachea and sternal head of sternocleidomastoid, and feel for resistance.

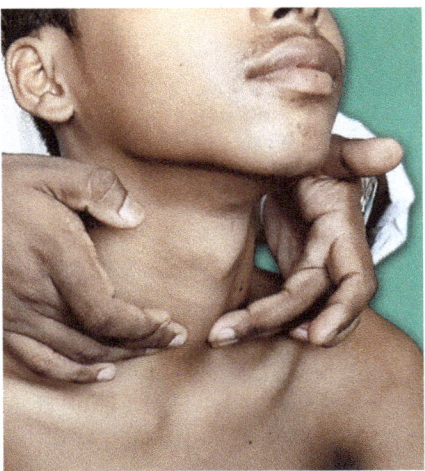

Fig. 4.19: Demonstration of Oliver's sign.

Table 4.19: Mediastinal shift with respect to respiratory diseases.

Mediastinal shift	Disease
Shift to same side	Fibrosis Collapse
Shift to opposite side	Pleural effusion Pneumothorax Tumor or mass
No shift of mediastinum	Unilateral disease • Pneumonia disease • Bilateral disease • COPD • Asthma • Bronchiectasis • Interstitial lung disease

Examination of respiratory movements	
Upper anterior chest (Fig. 4.20)	• Examined by placing the palms in the infraclavicular areas • Look for superio-anterior movement of the palms • This examines the pump handle movement of the upper lobes.

Contd...

Contd...

Examination of respiratory movements	
Lower anterior chest (Fig. 4.21)	• Grasp the sides of the chest and approximate the tips of the thumbs in the mammary area with loose fold of skin in between • Watch for separation of the thumbs and compare the movements with each respiration • It demonstrates the buckle handle movements of the lower chest
Upper posterior chest (Fig. 4.22)	• Examine from the back by placing hand in the supraclavicular fossa and watch for movements superiorly • This demonstrates the movement of the apical segment
Lower posterior chest (Fig. 4.23)	• Grasp the sides of the chest and approximate the tips of the thumbs in the infrascapular area with loose fold of skin in between • Watch for separation of the thumbs and compare the movements with each respiration • This demonstrate the lower lobe movements

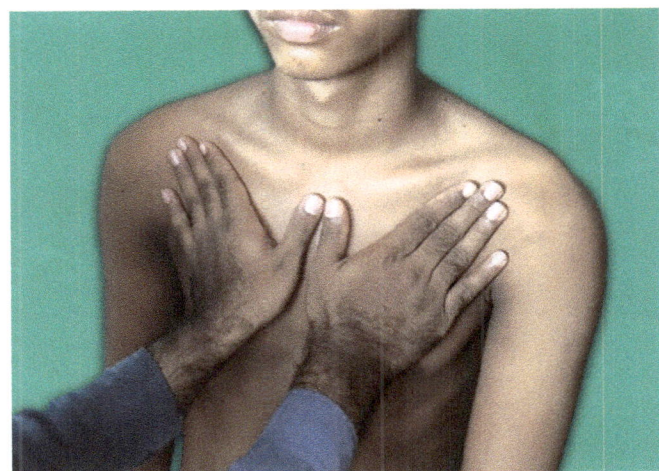

Fig. 4.20: Examination of respiratory movements of upper anterior chest.

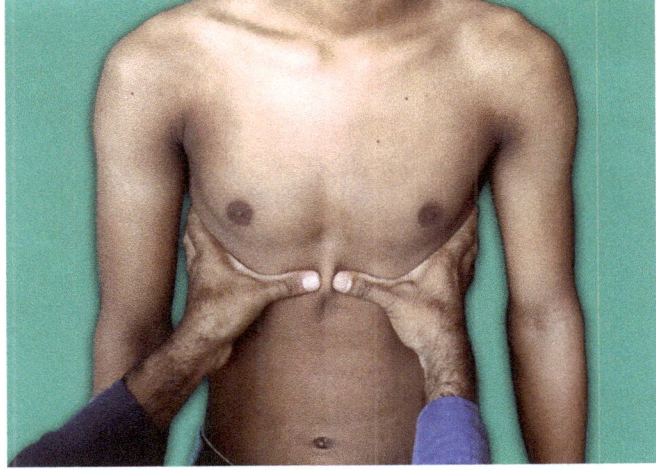

Fig. 4.21: Examination of respiratory movements of lower anterior chest.

Chapter 4: Respiratory System Examination

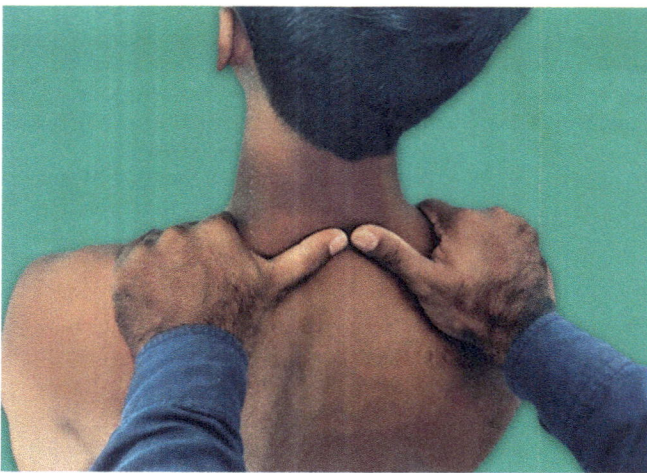

Fig. 4.22: Examination of respiratory movements of upper posterior chest.

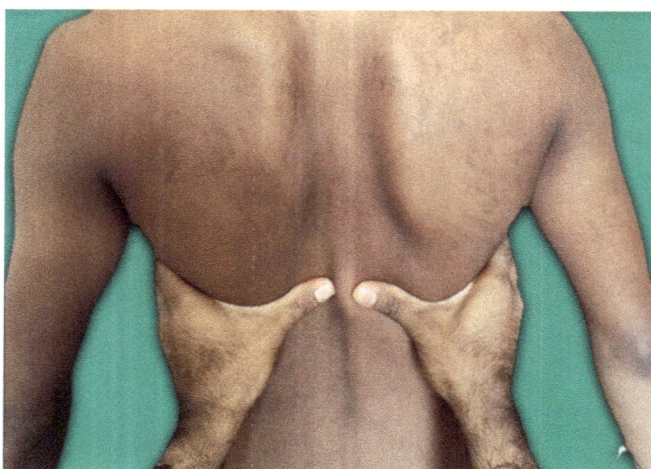

Fig. 4.23: Examination of respiratory movements of lower posterior chest.

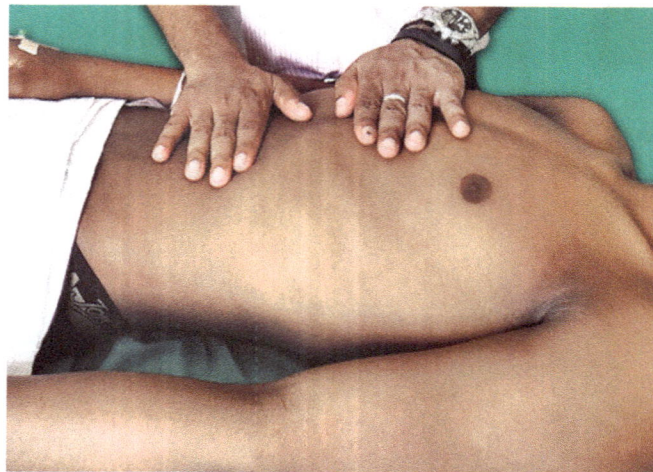

Fig. 4.24: Examination of diaphragmatic movements.

Diaphragmatic movements:
- Place one hand on chest and other hand on the abdomen (**Fig. 4.24**)

Table 4.20: Causes of decreased chest movements.

Unilateral	Bilateral
• Pleural effusion • Empyema • Pneumothorax • Fibrosis • Collapse	• COPD • Asthma • ILD • Ankylosing spondylosis • Systemic sclerosis

Table 4.21: Measurement of chest movement.

Measurements	Description
AP diameter (Fig. 4.25)	Use two cardboards and place as shown in the Figure 4.25
Transverse diameter (Fig. 4.26)	Normal ratio of AP to T = 5:7
Chest expansion (Fig. 4.27)	Normal = 5–8 cm (adult), decreases with age (e.g., 60 year ≥ 3 cm is considered normal) COPD/ILD expansion is <1.5 cm
Hemithorax expansion (Figs. 4.28A and B)	Stand on one side and place the tape from spine to mid sternal as shown in **Figures 4.28A and B**

Note: Chest expansion should be assessed as the difference of measurement between deep inspiration and deep expiration.

"The most important examination finding is to check for hemithorax expansion and hemithorax measurement".

- Normally both hands are lifted during inspiration
- If chest (rise) but abdomen (static)—suggests and abdominal pathology, which is fixing the abdomen
- If chest (rises) but abdomen (retracts)—suggests diaphragmatic palsy

Causes of chest movements
The causes of decreased chest movements are shown in **Table 4.20**.

Measurements of chest dynamics
Table 4.21 shows measurement of chest movements.

Remember: *"The side that moves less is the site of disease".*

Increased hemithorax size with decreased hemithorax movement	Decreased hemithorax size with decreased hemithorax movement	Normal hemithorax size with decreased hemithorax movement
Pleural effusion Pneumothorax	Fibrosis Collapse	Consolidation

Examination of Spinoscapular Distance (Fig. 4.29)

It is the distance between the spine and the scapular line (scapular line is the vertical line passing through the inferior angle of scapula).

Examination of Spino-acromion Distance (Fig. 4.30)

It is the distance measured between the spine and the tip of acromion process.

Chapter 4: Respiratory System Examination

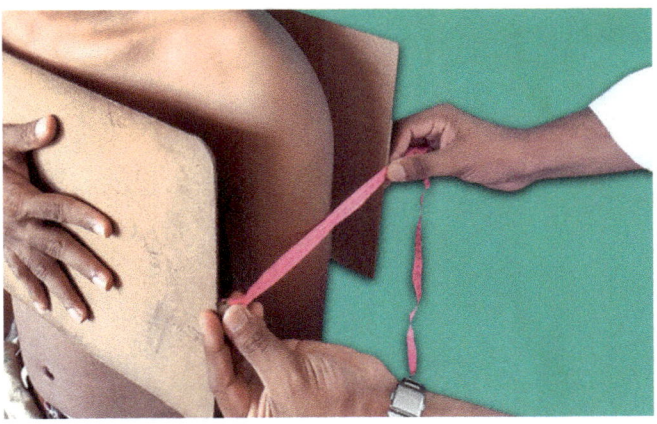
Fig. 4.25: Examination of anteroposterior diameter.

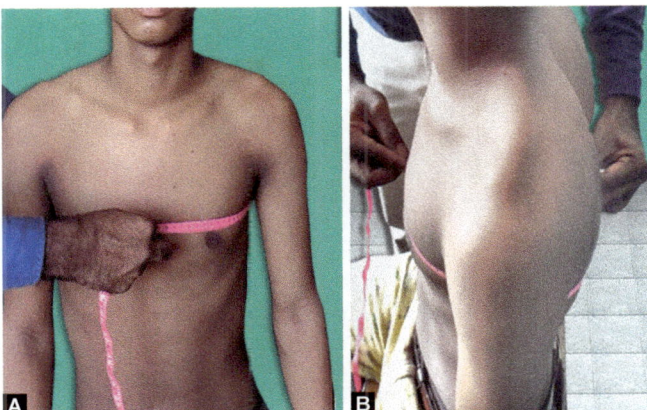
Figs. 4.28A and B: Examination of hemithorax circumference.

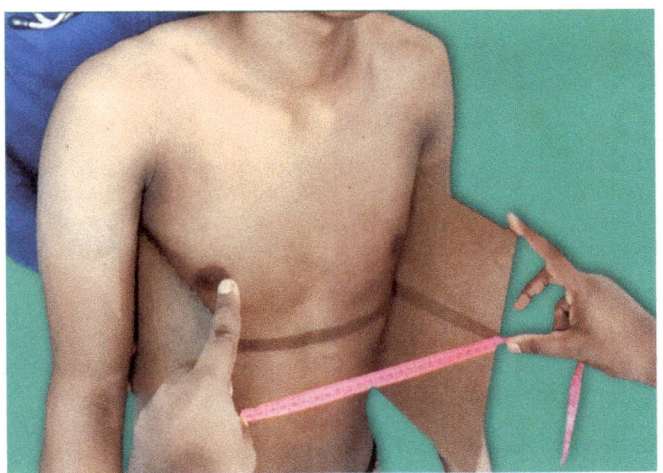
Fig. 4.26: Examination of transverse diameter.

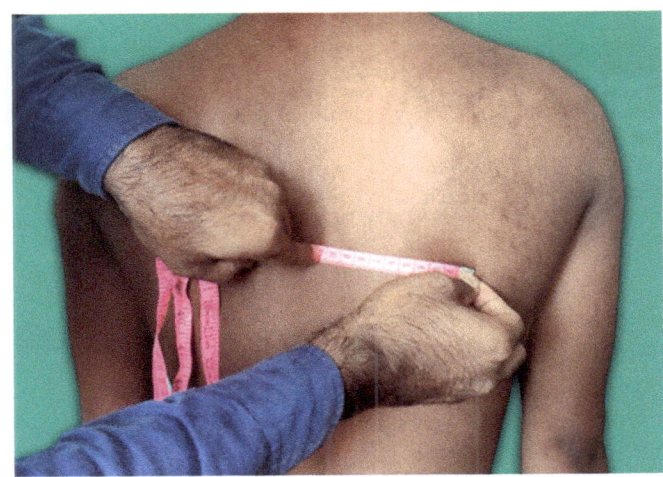
Fig. 4.29: Examination of spino-scapular distance.

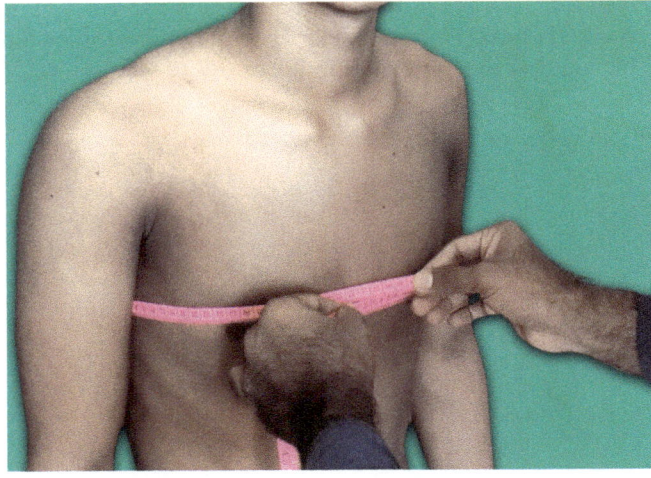
Fig. 4.27: Examination of chest expansion (crossed tape).

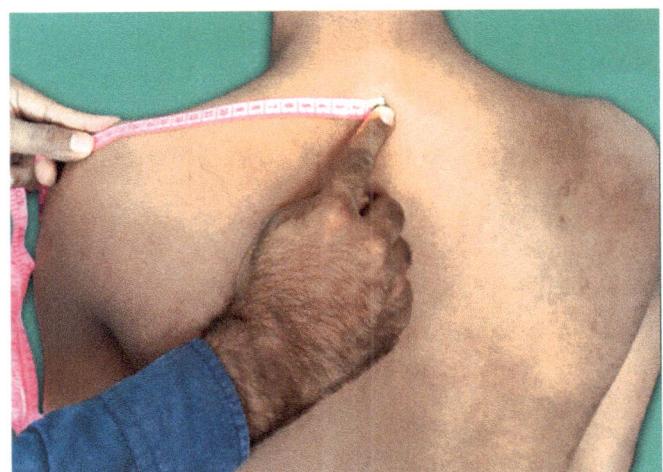
Fig. 4.30: Examination of spino-acromion distance.

Vocal Fremitus

- The sounds produced by vocal cords are transmitted along the tracheobronchial tree and heard/felt over the chest wall.
- Place the ulnar border of the hands on identical areas on both sides of the chest (**Fig. 4.31**)
- Ask the patient to repeat "one – one – one - "

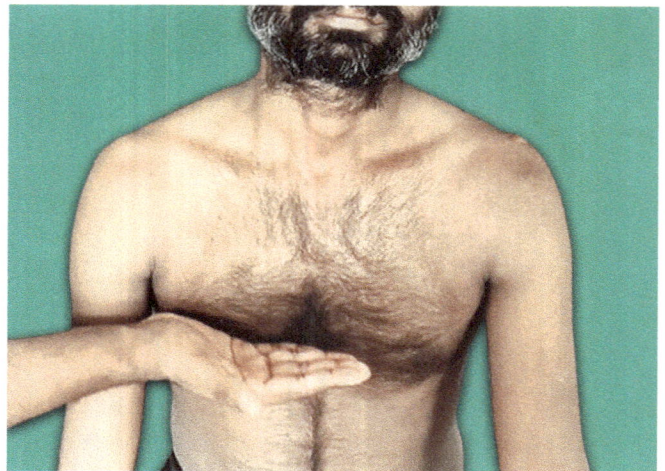

Fig. 4.31: Demonstration of vocal fremitus.

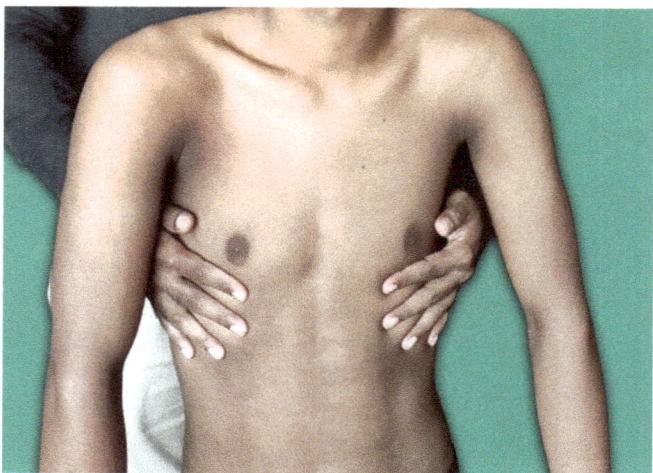

Fig. 4.32: Examination of rib crowding.

Vocal fremitus	
Increased	Decreased
• Consolidation • Large cavity • Bronchopleural fistula	• Pleural effusion • Pneumothorax • Fibrosis • Collapse • Asthma • Emphysema • Thick pleura

Rib crowding		Intercostal widening	
u/L	B/L	U/L	B/L
Atelectasis Collapse Fibrosis Pneumonectomy	ILD Fibrosis (bilateral)	Pneumothorax Pleural effusion	Emphysema

Tactile Fremitus
☐ These are palpable adventitious sounds
☐ It could be coarse crepitations or rhonchi

Friction Fremitus
These include palpable pericardial rub or pleural rub (e.g., dry pleurisy)

Tenderness
Seen in
☐ Empyema (intercostal tenderness)
☐ Local inflammation of soft tissue
☐ Osteomyelitis/rib fractures/costeochondritis (Tietz syndrome)
☐ Tumor infiltration
☐ Amebic liver abscess
☐ Subphernic abscess

Detection of Subcutaneous Emphysema
Spongy crepitant feeling on palpation:
☐ Injury to chest wall
☐ Pneumothorax
☐ Rupture of esophagus

Rib Crowding/Intercostal Widening
☐ Stand behind the patient and place the fingers in the intercostal spaces simultaneously on both sides as shown in **Figure 4.32**.
☐ Observe for the separation of the fingers

Percussion (Lower Respiratory Tract)
Preferably done in sitting position, supine position is needed for demonstrating shifting dullness.

Position of Patient for Percussion
☐ **Anterior chest (Fig. 4.33):** Sits up straight with hands by his side
☐ **Axilla (Fig. 4.34):** Raise the arm over the head and place over the back of head
☐ **Back of chest (Fig. 4.35):** Sits up with hands crossed and placed over the opposite shoulders.

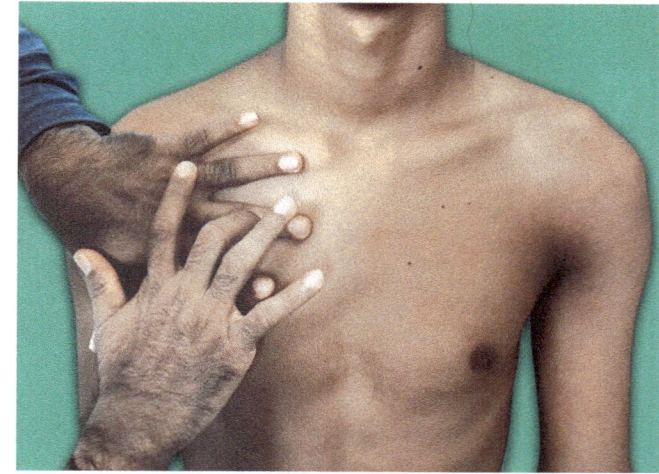

Fig. 4.33: Demonstration of percussion of anterior chest.

Chapter 4: Respiratory System Examination

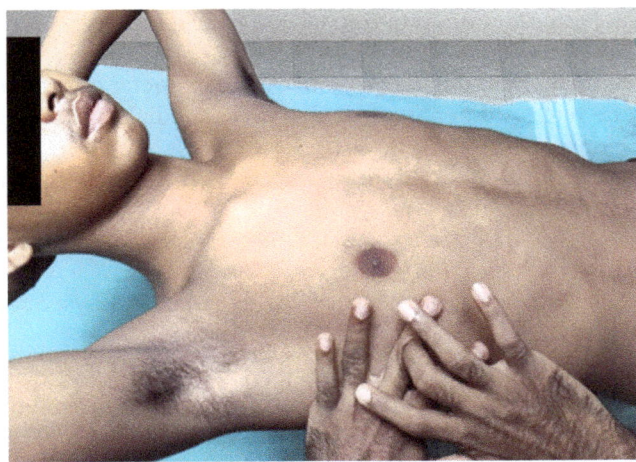

Fig. 4.34: Demonstration of percussion of axillary area.

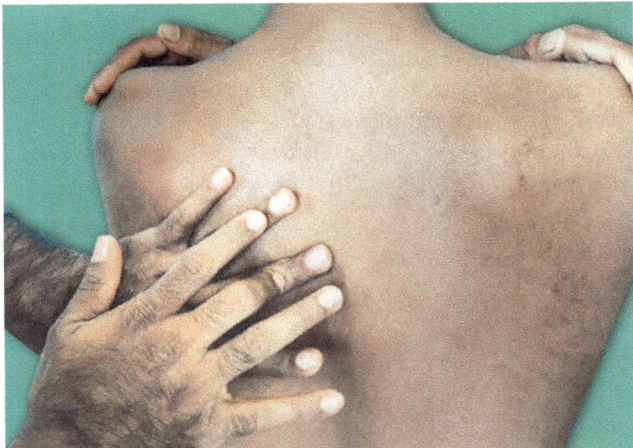

Fig. 4.35: Demonstration of percussion over the posterior chest.

Rules of Percussion
- **Direction of percussion:** Always percuss from resonant to nonresonant area.
- **Pleximeter** is usually the middle phalynx of middle finger of left/non dominant hand) is firmly placed on the surface while rest of fingers are slightly lifted off.
- **Plexor/plessor** (percussing finger) is middle finger of the right/dominant hand.
- The movement of the plexor hand should be sudden and originating from the wrist.
- The pleximeter must be kept parallel to the border to be percussed.
- Percuss around 2–3 time over each area.
- Percussion has to be heard as well as felt.
- Always percuss the identical areas of chest for comparison.
- The distance between the pleximeter finger and the ear should preferably maintained.

Types of Percussion
Types of percussion are described in **Table 4.22**.

Table 4.22: Types of percussion.

Heavy percussion	Light percussion
Posterior part of chest	Anterior part of chest and abdomen

Direct percussion	Indirect percussion	Auscultatory percussion
Directly over the bony structures like clavicle	By percussing the pleximeter finger with the plexor/plessor	Was first described by Laennec and used to delineate the size of organs by placing the stethoscope directly above the structure to be outlined, followed by percussion from the periphery toward the organ of interest

Direct percussion (Fig. 4.36)
- Percuss the middle third of the clavicle with plexor finger.
- Stretch the skin over the clavicle using the left hand as shown in **Figure 4.36**.
- Normally middle third of the clavicle is resonant whereas the medial and lateral thirds are dull (because of muscles attached).

Impaired note	Heard in apical fibrosis
Dull note	Mass lesion-like Pancoast tumor
Widening of zone of resonance	Heard in seen in pneumothorax or emphysema

Lung resonance:
Normal:
- Vesicular resonance
- Front of chest more resonant
- Lesion >5 cm from chest wall or <2–3 cm in size will not alter the percussion note

Abnormal Types of Percussion Note
Abnormal types of percussion note are described in **Table 4.23**.

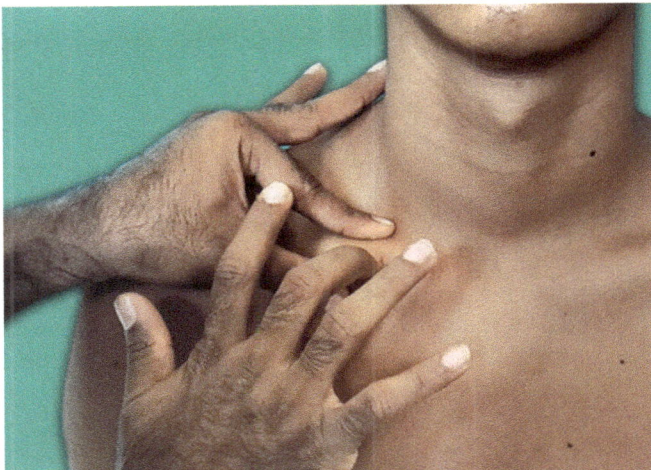

Fig. 4.36: Demonstration of direct clavicular percussion.

Table 4.23: Abnormal types of percussion note.

Quantitative	Qualitative
1. Tympanic note	1. Crackpot
2. Subtympanic note	2. Amphoric
3. Hyperresonant note	3. Bell tympany
4. Impaired note	
5. Dull/woody dull note	
6. Stony dull note	

Quantitative types:
- **Tympanic:**
  - It is a drum-like note
  - Normally seen over the stomach, intestine—Traube's space.
  - In chest—superficial cavity, subcutaneous emphysema (metallic tympanic note)
- **Sub-tympanic (skodiac):**
  - It is Boxy quality
  - Seen just above pleural effusion
- **Hyper-resonant:**
  - Intermediate between normal and tympanic note
  - B/L—emphysema
  - U/L—pneumothorax, compensatory emphysema
  - Large bullae
- **Impaired note:** Airless areas (fibrosis, collapse)
- **Dull note:**
  - Consolidation
  - Thick pleura
- **Flat dull:**
  - Elicted by percussing the thigh
  - Seen in pleural effusion
- **Stony dullness:**
  - Pain over the pleximeter finger with resistance felt by plexor
  - Large pleural effusion
  - Large solid tumor

Qualitative types
- **Cracked pot resonance:**
  - Normally seen in chest of infants or child during the act of crying
  - Pathological slung cavity with communication with bronchus due to sudden expulsion of air form the cavity to bronchus
  - Artificially imitated by beating clasped hands over the knee
- **Amphoric:**
  - Low-pitched hollow note
  - Normal seen in trachea and cheek distended with air
  - Pathologically seen in pneumothorax and large cavity
- **Bell tympany:**
  - High pitched metallic or tympanic note
  - Seen in massive pneumothorax
  - Place coin on effected side of chest and percuss with another coin while simultaneously auscultating the back.
- **Dullness in presence of fluid in lung:**
  - Straight line dullness: Hydropneumothorax
  - S-shaped curve of ellis: Pleural effusion

5-7-9 rule
The upper border of liver dullness is at 5th ICS in mid clavicular line, 7th ICS in the midaxiallary line, and 9th ICS in the scapular line.

Topographical Percussion of Lung
Apical percussion:
- **Kronigs isthmus:** It is band of resonance in the supraclavicular area bounded anteriorly by the posterior border of the clavicle, medially by the neck muscles, posteriorly by the anterior border of trapezius, extended laterally till the acromioclavicular joint.
- Stand behind the patient, place the pleximeter finger over the neck and percuss from lateral to medial as shown in **Figure 4.37**.
- On percussion there is dull zone medially and laterally, and only middle part is resonant.
- Dullness in this area suggests apical tuberculosis, Pancoast tumor or apical fibrosis.
- The zone of resonance may be widened in emphysema or apical pneumothorax.

Tidal percussion
- Tidal percussion is measure of diaphragmatic excursion
- It is used to differentiate whether the causes of dullness are above the diaphragm (subpulmonic effusion) or below (sub phrenic collections).
- Patient in sitting position, percuss the right side of the chest from above downward till you get the liver dullness. Normally, it is in 5th Intercostal space.
- Ask the patient to take deep inspiration and hold his breath.
- Now percuss the same area
- Normally, dullness moves down by 1–2 intercostal spaces as shown in **Figures 4.38A and B**.

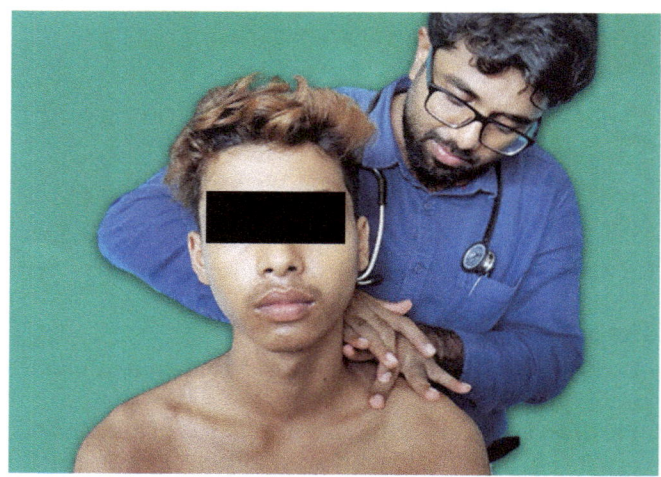

Fig. 4.37: Percussion of apical area (Kronig's isthmus).

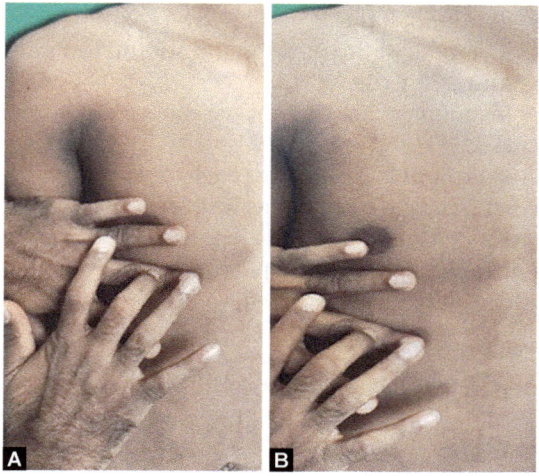

Figs. 4.38A and B: Demonstration of tidal percussion: (A) Expiration; (B) Inspiration.

Chapter 4: Respiratory System Examination

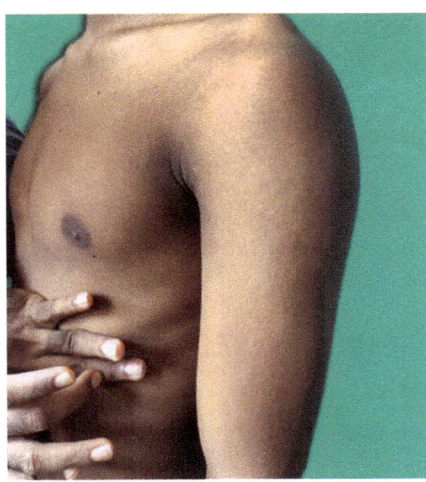

Fig. 4.39: Percussion of Traube's space.

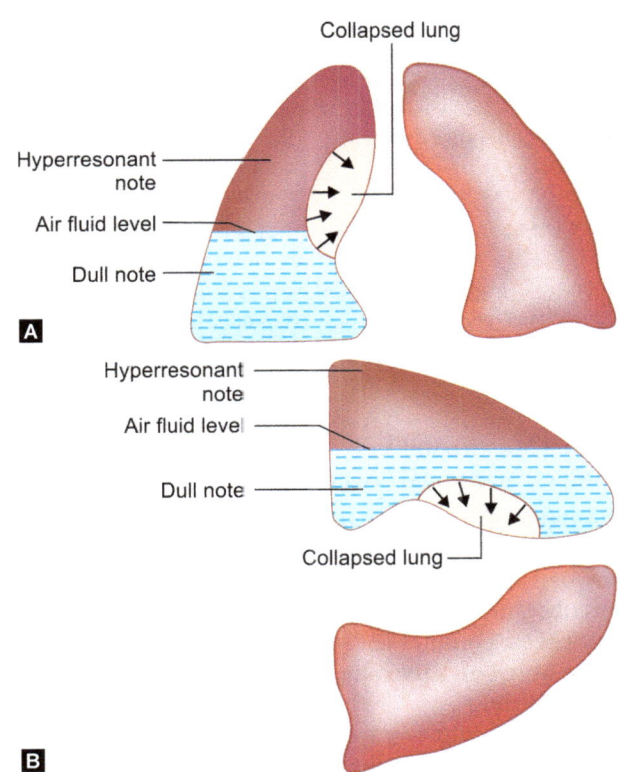

Figs. 4.40A and B: (A) Sitting position; (B) Left lateral position.

- Tidal percussion is negative in subpulmonic effusion, diaphragmatic paralysis.
- In emphysema, since the lung is already fully expanded tidal percussion will be negative

Percussion of Traube's Space (Fig. 4.39)
- It is a semilunar space in the left anterior chest bounded by
  - Above by 6th rib
  - Below by left-costal margin
  - Laterally by midaxillary line

Normal traube's space percussion	Tympanic note
Obliteration of Traube's space	• Left-sided pleural effusion • Pericardial effusion • Massive splenomegaly • Enlarged left lobe of the liver • Full stomach or fundic mass
Upward shift of Traube's space	• Left diaphragmatic paralysis • Left lower lobe collapse or fibrosis

Shifting dullness
Classically described for hydropneumothorax. It can also be demonstrated in pleural effusion.

Steps:
- Percuss the anterior chest in sitting position, from above downwards to get upper border of dullness. You will get a level of straight line dullness perpendicular to long axis of body as shown in **Figure 4.40A**. Mark this level.
- Now, make the patient lie down in opposite lateral position for approximately 5–10 minutes (may take around 30–40 minutes in case of pleural effusion). Now, note the change in the straight line dullness which will now be parallel to long axis of body as shown in **Figure 4.40B**.

Special findings in percussion
Special findings with clinical condition in percussion are shown in **Table 4.24**.

Table 4.24: Special findings in percussion.

Special finding	Clinical condition
Shifting dullness	Hydropneumothorax
S-shaped curve of Ellis (Damoiseau curve)	Pleural effusion (moderate)
Obliteration of Traube's space	Pleural effusion (left sided)

Auscultation
Position of Patient

In upright position	Front	Sitting or standing
	Back	Preferably sitting and leaning forward with neck flexed and arms crossed in front
In recumbent position	Back	Turn the patient sideways or slip the steth underneath the patient

Breathing Advice
Ask the patient to breathe through the mouth. If not cooperating, ask the patient to count numbers or cough successively and then observe during the deep inspiration.

Normal Physiology of Breath Sounds
Table 4.25 shows the mechanism of sound production.

Grading of breath sound intensity
0: Absent breath sounds
1: Barely audible breath sound
2: Faint but definitely audible breath sound

Table 4.25: Mechanism of sound production.

In larger airways (Pharynx, large airways of trachea and lung)	In smaller airways
Sounds are generated due to turbulence	Higher frequencies are lost due to dampening when they travel from higher to smaller airways
They are the source of sound	They are just filter sounds and not source of sound
Sound frequencies are of range 200–2,000 Hz	Sound frequencies are of range 200–400 Hz
Heard over the upper sternum	Heard over the most other areas of lung

3: Normal breath sound
4: Louder than normal breath sound

Graphical representation of breath sounds:
- **Upstroke:** Inspiratory element
- **Downstroke:** Expiratory element
- **Length:** Duration or timing
- **Thickness:** Loudness or intensity
- **Angle between upstroke and downstroke made with a vertical line:**
  - Pitch of respiratory sound
  - Lower the angle higher is the pitch

Types of normal breathing
- **Vesicular breathing:** Most areas of chest
- **Tracheal/bronchial breathing:**
  - Larynx
  - Trachea
  - Between C7 and T3
- **Bronchovesicular**
  - Anteriorly 1st and 2nd ICS
  - Posteriorly between the scapula

VESICULAR BREATH SOUNDS

Characteristics
- Rustling or breezy quality
- Longer duration of inspiratory phase (which includes both tubular and alveolar phase)
- Higher pitch of inspiratory sound
- I:E = 3:1
- Absence of pause between I and E

Distribution
Most areas of the chest

Intensity
- Louder : IC, axillary and ISC areas
- Diminished : lower margins of lung and over the scapular areas.

Mode of Production
Distension and separation of alveolar walls by the in rushing current of air.

Graphical Representation

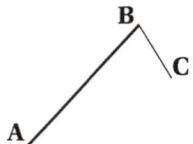

A—Tubular phase of inspiration
B—Alveolar phase of inspiration
C—Expiration

TRACHEAL (BRONCHIAL) BREATH SOUNDS

Characteristics
- Character is aspirate or guttural
- Expiration in longer
- Expiration is louder
- Expiration has high pitch
- I:E = 1:1
- There pause between inspiration and expiration (due to absence of alveolar phase)

Distribution
- Larynx
- Trachea

Mode of Production
Due to in and out movement of air through narrow aperture of glottis

Graphical Representation

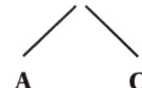

Type of Bronchial Breathing
- **Tubular:**
  - High pitched sounds at the bronchioles are conducted to the chest wall without modification.
  - For example,
    - Consolidation
    - Above the level of pleural effusion
    - Massive pericardial effusion (Ewart's sign)
- **Amphoric:**
  - Low pitched bronchial breathing with high pitched overtones producing a metallic quality.
  - For example,
    - Open pneumothorax due to bronchopleural fistula
    - Large communicating cavity
- **Cavernous:** Low pitched sound with peculiar hollow quality, e.g., cavity

BRONCHOVESICULAR BREATH SOUNDS
It is also known as vesicular breath sounds with prolonged expiration.

Table 4.26: Diminished intensity of breath sounds.

Defect in production	Defect in transmission
Bronchial obstruction	Pleural effusion
Emphysema	Pneumothorax
Respiratory muscle paralysis	Thickened pleura
	Thick chest wall
	Fibrosis

Characteristics

- Intermediate in character between vesicular and bronchial breath sounds
- Expiratory phase is louder, longer, and higher pitch than inspiratory, or hollow character.

Distribution

- Upper part of sternum
- Up to 3rd/4th dorsal spines between scapula
- At times over the lung apices particularly on right side

Mode of Production

Usually seen when air containing lung tissue is interposed between a large bronchus and the chest wall—thus combining the characteristics of both vesicular and bronchial breath sounds.

Graphical Representation

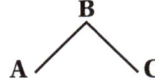

It is the hallmark auscultatory finding of obstructive lung disease like COPD and asthma.

Diminished Intensity of Breath Sounds

Diminished intensity of breath sounds is described in **Table 4.26.**

ADVENTITIOUS SOUNDS (FLOWCHART 4.2)

See **Flowchart 4.2**.

Flowchart 4.2: Adventitious sounds.

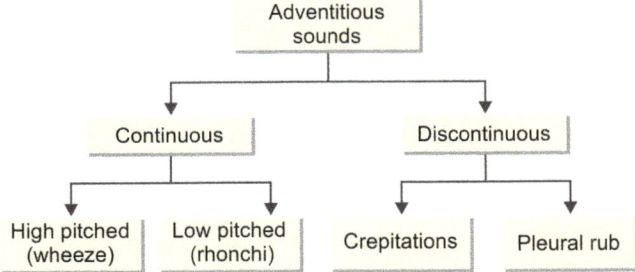

Continuous Adventitious Sounds

- Lasts for more than 250 ms
- Musical in quality
- **Mechanism of production of sound:** Important prerequisite for the production of wheeze is airflow limitation. Narrowing of airways along with increased intrathoracic pressure results in airflow limitation producing sinusoidal oscillations, e.g., wheeze and rhonchi **(Table 4.27).**

Table 4.27: Differences between wheeze and rhonchi.

Wheeze	Rhonchi
High-pitched sounds	Low-pitched sounds
400 Hz	200 Hz
Hissing quality (sibilant)	Snoring quality (sonorous)
Predominantly arise from small airways obstruction	Usually produced when air moves through tracheal-bronchial passages in the presence of mucous or respiratory secretions

Classification of Wheezes/Rhonchi (Table 4.28)

1. Monophonic or polyphonic
2. Inspiratory or Expiratory

Discontinuous Adventitious Sounds (Rales/Crepitations/Crackles)

- These are discontinuous, explosive, nonmusical, and harsh in quality
- Mainly inspiratory (can be in expiratory or both)

Mechanism of Crepitation

1. Bubbling sounds produced by passage of air through accumulated secretions.
2. Sudden snapping opening of successive small airways when airflow is through it.

Fine and Coarse Crepitations

Differences between fine and coarse crepts is shown in **Table 4.29**.

Inspiratory and Expiratory Crepitations

Differences between inspiratory and expiratory crepitation is shown in **Table 4.30.**

Few Named Crepitations

- **Coarse leathery:** Bronchiectasis
- **Velcro crepitations:** ILD
- **Posture-induced crackles:** Appearance of fine crackles while changing of posture (sitting to supine or supine with passive leg elevation). Auscultate in the posterior axillary line in the 8th 9th 10th intercostal spaces after 3 minute of supine position. It indicates ischemic heart disease with heart failure.
- **Post-tussive crepitations:** Crepitations, which are not present normally but appear after a bout of cough. Seen in early pneumonia, early tuberculosis and lung abscess.

Table 4.28: Classification of wheeze/rhonchi.

Monophonic	Polyphonic
Single tones	Diffuse, multiple tones, both phases
Due to local pathology producing bronchial obstruction	Due to dynamic compression
1. Tumor 2. FB aspiration 3. Bronchostenosis 4. Mucous plug 5. Lymph node compression	1. COPD 2. Bronchial asthma 3. Tropical pulmonary eosinophilia 4. Hypersensitive pneumonitis 5. Eosinophilic pneumonia 6. Churg-Strauss syndrome

Table 4.29: Differences between fine and coarse crepitations.

Fine crepitations	Coarse crepitations
Due to snapping opening of successive small airways	Due to bubbling sounds produced by passage of air through accumulated secretions
High-pitched (Soft)	Low-pitched (Loud)
Smaller airways	Larger airways
Heard during inspiration	Heard during inspiration and expiration
Not modified by coughing	Modified by coughing
Not palpable	Palpable
For example, 1. Indux crepitations (Initial stages of pneumonia) 2. Pulmonary edema (early phase) 3. Interstitial lung disease 4. Asbestosis 5. Hypersensitivity pneumonitis 6. Sarcoidosis	For example, 1. Redux crepitations (Resolution phase of pneumonia) 2. Pulmonary edema (Late phase) 3. Bronchiectasis 4. Lung abscess 5. Bronchitis

Table 4.30: Differences between Inspiratory and expiratory crepitations.

Inspiratory crepitations		Expiratory crepitations
Early	Acute bronchitis Chronic bronchitis	Redux crepitations (Resolution phase of pneumonia) • Pulmonary edema (Late phase) • Bronchiectasis • Lung abscess • Bronchitis
Mid	Bronchiectasis resolving phase of pneumonia	
Late	ILD Asbestosis Early pneumonia Pulmonary edema	

Stridor
- High-pitched whistling or grating sound which is produced by upper airway obstruction.
- It is louder over the neck than the chest wall.
- Indicates extrathoracic upper airway obstruction (such as vocal cord paralysis, supraglottic growths, etc.)
- It usually seen during inspiration however can be seen in expiration in intrathoracic tracheobronchial obstruction.

Pleural Rub
- It is harsh discontinuous, localized, nonmusical, and superficial grating sound due to rubbing of the inflamed pleural surface against each other.
- It is heard in both phases of respiration and disappear on holding the breath

Causes
- Dry pleurisy
- Consolidation
- Infarction

Pleural Rub and Crepitations
Differences between pleural rub and crepitations are described in **Table 4.31**.

Table 4.31: Differences between pleural rub and crepitations.

Pleural rub	Crepitations
Both inspiratory and expiratory phases	Inspiratory/expiratory or both
Localized to small area	Wide spread
No change after coughing	May clear after coughing
Pressure on stethoscope increases the sound	No effect
Associated with pleuritic chest pain and local tenderness	No pain or tenderness

Vocal Resonance
- Make the patient sit
- Place the stethoscope firmly on the chest wall
- Ask the patient to speak "one–one–one" or "ninety nine" repeatedly
- Compare corresponding areas anteriorly, in axilla and in back.
- Increased vocal resonance **(Table 4.32)**

Variations of vocal resonance
Bronchophony
- Increase in loudness as well as clarity of the sound.
- Seen in:
  - Consolidation
  - Just above level of pleural effusion
  - On spine up to T4

Egophony
- Selected amplification of high frequency sounds. "E" is hear as "A".
- **Seen in:** Consolidation (It is the aucultatory sign of consolidation)

Whispering pectoriloquy
- When the whispered sound in the chest wall is heard clearly and distinguishably as if uttered directly into the external ear.
- Seen in:
  - Consolidation
  - Cavity with communication with bronchus

Other Auscultatory Features
Post-tussive suction
It is a sign of superficial collapsible cavity seen in active tuberculosis. When you auscultate a cavernous bronchial breathing (which indicates a cavity), ask the patient to cough. A suction sound will be heard, if the cavity collapses.

Table 4.32: Vocal resonance.

Increased	Decreased
• Consolidation • Large cavity • Bronchopleural fistula	• Pleural effusion • Pneumothorax • Fibrosis • Collapse • Asthma • Emphysema • Thick pleura

Note: In upper lobe fibrosis, VR is increased due to the pulled trachea.

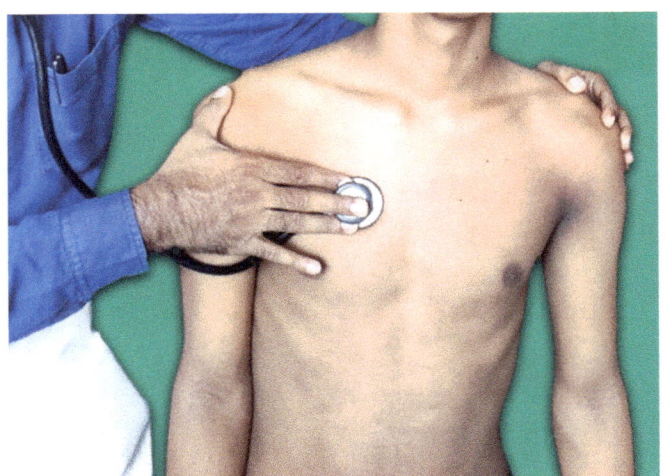

Fig. 4.41: Demonstration of succussion splash.

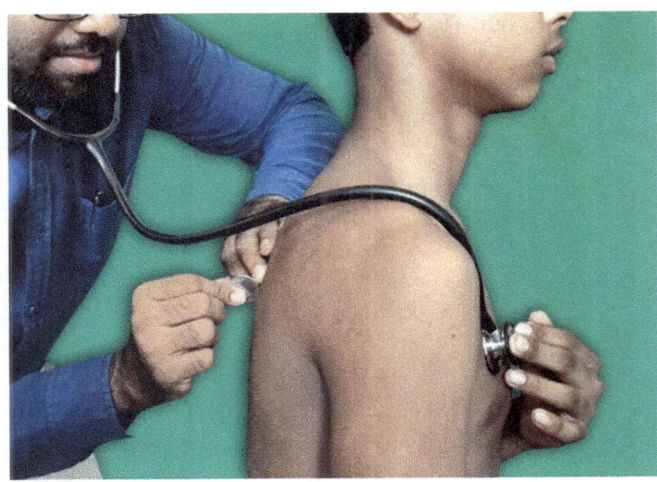

Fig. 4.42: Demonstration of coin test.

Prerequisites for post-tussive suction:
- Superficial cavity
- Thin-walled cavity
- Has to be communicating with bronchus
- Surrounding lung should be normal

Succussion splash (Hippocrates succussion)
- It is seen in hydropneumothorax.
- First percuss and get the air fluid level in hydropneumothorax.
- Keep the diaphragm at the air-fluid level
- Hold the opposite shoulder of the patient and shake vigorously as shown in **Figure 4.41**.
- Tinkling or splashing sound will be heard.
- Other conditions, such as large cavity with fluid, diaphragmatic hernia can also produce succussion splash.

Coin test
- High-pitched metallic or tympanic note
- Place one coin flat on affected side of chest (posteriorly/anteriorly) and percuss with another coin perpendicularly on it, while simultaneously auscultating from the opposite direction of the same affected side as shown in **Figure 4.42**.
- Seen in massive pneumothorax/hydropneumothorax.

Hamman's mediastinal crunch
- Loud cracking or clicking sound heard in the 3rd–5th intercostal spaces near the left sternal border synchronous with the heart beat.
- Its sign of mediastinal emphysema (pneumomediastinum) or can also be seen in left sided pneumothorax.

Forced expiratory time (FET)
- It is a simple inexpensive and sensitive bedside test to detect airflow obstruction.
- Instruct the patient to inhale up tot the total lung capacity and then blow it as fast and complete as possible.
- Place the bell of stethoscope in suprasternal notch and time the audible expiration
- A value less than 5 seconds indicates FEV1/FEC more than 60%, where as FET >6 seconds **indicates** FEV1/FEC less than 50%.

Clinical examination findings in common diseases are shown in **Table 4.33**.

Chapter 4: Respiratory System Examination

Table 4.33: Clinical examination findings in common diseases.

	Findings	Fibrosis	Collapse	Pleural effusion	Pneumothorax	Hydropneumothorax	Consolidation	Cavity	Emphysema	ILD
Inspection	Trachea/Mediastinum	Pulled to same side	Pulled to same side	Pushed to opposite side	Pushed to opposite side	Pushed to opposite side	Central	Central	Central	Central
	Retraction/bulge	Retraction on the affected side	Retraction on the affected side	Bulging/fullness on the affected side	Bulging/fullness on the affected side	Bulging/fullness on the affected side	-	-	Barrel shaped chest	B/L diminished movements
	Chest expansion	Reduced on the effected side	Reduced on the effected side	Reduced on the effected side	Reduced on the effected side	Reduced on the effected side	Reduced on the effected side	Reduced on the effected side	Reduced bilaterally	Reduced bilaterally
Palpation	Hemithorax dimension	Reduced on the effected side	Reduced on the effected side	Increased on the effected side	Increased on the effected side	Increased on the effected side	Normal dimensions	Normal dimensions	Bilaterally inflated lungs with AP:T diameter = 1:1	Decreased or normal chest dimensions
	Vocal fremitus	Reduced	Reduced	Reduced	Reduced	Reduced	Increased	Increased in the presence of communication with bronchus	Bilaterally equal	Bilaterally equal
Percussion	Percussion note	Impaired note over fibrosed lung	Dull note over the collapse lung	Stony dull note over the pleural effusion and skodiac dullness at the level of pleural effusion	Hyperresonant note over the pneumothorax	Hyperresonant note above the air fluid level and dull note below the air fluid level	Woody Dull note over the cnsolidation	Large cavity gives resonant note	Hyperresonant note over bilateral lung fields	Resonant note heard over bilateral lung fields
	Special findings	William's tracheal resonance		Ellis Curve pattern of upper level of effusion Grocco's triangle Obliteration of Traube's space Garland's triangle	Bell tympany can be appreciated. (Coin test positive)	Shifting dullness, Straight line dullness, Succussion splash, Bell tympany can be appreciated (Coin test positive)		Wintrich's sign (cavity communicating with bronchus) Friedrich's sign Gerhardt's sign	Liver dullness is pushed down. Negative for tidal percussion	
Auscultation	Breath sounds	Diminished breath sounds	Absent breath sounds	Absent breath sounds	Absent breath sounds	Absent breath sounds	Tubular breath sounds	Cavernous breath sounds	Vesicular breath sounds with prolonged expiration	Vesicular breath sounds
	Adventitious sounds/special findings	Fine crepitations	-	-	Bell tympany can be appreciated (Coin test positive)	Bell tympany can be appreciated (Coin test positive)	Crepitations heard	Post-tussive suction (in superficial cavity)	Rhonchi heard over the bilateral lung fields	Fine Velcro crepitations
	Vocal resonance	Reduced	Reduced	Reduced	Reduced	Reduced	Increased (Bronchophony Egophony Whispering petroloquey)	Increased in the presence of communication with bronchus	Bilaterally equal	Bilaterally equal

OBJECTIVE-BASED SELF-EVALUATION

SHORT ANSWER QUESTIONS

1. List the common causes of chronic cough.
2. List the differences between hemoptysis and hematemesis.
3. Mention the common causes for hemoptysis.
4. List the causes of acute severe dyspnea.
5. Paroxysmal nocturnal dyspnea (PND).
6. Differences between orthopnea and PND.
7. mMRC grading of breathlessness.
8. NYHA classification.
9. Describe the respiratory signs of a patient with right upper lobe pneumonia.
10. Describe the respiratory signs of a patient with left pleural effusion.
11. Describe the respiratory signs of a patient with right sided hydropneumothorax.
12. Describe the respiratory signs of a patient with left upper lobe fibrosis.
13. Describe the respiratory signs of a patient with emphysema.
14. Describe the respiratory signs of a patient with bilateral bronchiectasis.
15. Describe the respiratory signs of a patient with bronchial asthma.

MULTIPLE CHOICE QUESTIONS

1. Succussion splash in respiratory examination is seen in:
   a. Hydropneumothorax
   b. Pneumothorax
   c. Pneumonia
   d. Pleural effusion
2. Egophony is the auscultatory sign of:
   a. Hydropneumothorax
   b. Pneumothorax
   c. Pneumonia
   d. Fibrosis
3. Vocal resonance is decreased in all conditions, *except*:
   a. Consolidation
   b. Pleural effusion
   c. Pneumothorax
   d. Fibrosis
4. Coarse leathery crepitations are classical of:
   a. Bronchiectasis
   b. Pneumothorax
   c. Pneumonia
   d. Fibrosis
5. Cavernous bronchial breathing is classical of:
   a. Consolidation
   b. Cavity
   c. Pleural effusion
   d. Fibrosis
6. All are characteristics of vesicular breath sounds, *except*:
   a. Rustling or breezy quality
   b. Longer duration of inspiratory phase (which includes both tubular and alveolar phase)
   c. Higher pitch of inspiratory sound
   d. Pause between inspiration and expiration
7. Percussion note of Traube's space is normally:
   a. Resonant
   b. Dull
   c. Tympanic
   d. Hyper-resonant
8. Intercostal tenderness is classical of:
   a. Rib fracture
   b. Empyema
   c. Fibrosis
   d. Pneumonia
9. Patient in tripod position with pursed lip breathing is suggestive of:
   a. Heart failure
   b. Renal failure with metabolic acidosis
   c. Emphysema
   d. Severe anemia
10. Right supraclavicular lymph node drains all the following parts of lung, *except*:
    a. Right upper lobe
    b. Right lower lobe
    c. Left upper lobe
    d. Left lower lobe

ANSWERS

1. a
2. c
3. a
4. a
5. b
6. d
7. c
8. b
9. c
10. c

Cardiovascular System Examination

CHAPTER OUTLINE

- Case Sheet Format
- Diagnosis Format
- Discussion on Symptoms
- Discussion on Examination

CARDIOVASCULAR SYSTEM: CASE SHEET FORMAT

History Taking

Name:
Age:
Sex:
Residence:
Occupation:
Chief complaints (describe in chronological order):
1. _____ × days
2. _____ × days

Dyspnea:
- Duration
- Onset
- Grade
- Progression
- Aggravating factors
- Relieving factors
- Orthopnea
- Trepopnea
- Platypnea
- Bendopnea
- Paroxysmal nocturnal dyspnea
- Any respiratory system complaints:
  - Wheeze
  - Cough with expectoration

Chest pain:
- Duration
- Onset
- Site
- Type of pain
- Radiation
- Diurnal variation (nocturnal angina)
- Aggravating factors
- Relieving factors
- Associated symptoms:
  - Nausea, vomiting, and sweating
- Dyspepsia
- Local tenderness
- Angina equivalents:
  - Dyspnea
  - Diaphoresis
  - Discomfort in lower jaw
  - Dyspeptic symptoms
  - Fatigue

Palpitations:
- Duration
- Onset
- Fast or slow
- Regular or irregular
- Precipitating factors
- Associated symptoms:
  - Stoke–Adams
- Post-palpitation diuresis

Syncope:
- Duration
- Onset
- Number of attacks
- Awareness
- Precipitating factors
- Associated symptoms

Pedal edema:
- Duration
- Onset
- Progression
- Aggravating factors
- Relieving factors
- Is it preceded by facial puffiness or followed by facial puffiness?

Other symptoms:
- Hemoptysis
- Cyanosis
- Decreased urine output
- Gastrointestinal symptoms
- Right hypochondrial pain

- Fatigability
- Fever
- Rheumatic fever history
- Infective endocarditis
- Cyanotic spells
- Squatting after exertion

Past history:
- Asthma
- Chronic obstructive airway disease
- Tuberculosis
- History of contact with tuberculosis
- Diabetes mellitus
- Hypertension
- Ischemic heart disease (IHD)
- Seizure disorder

Family history:
- 3-generation pedigree chart to be drawn

Personal history:
- Bowel habits
- Bladder habits
- Appetite
- Loss of weight
- Occupational exposure
- Sleep
- Dietary habits and taboo
- Food allergies
- Smoking Index or Pack years
- Alcohol history (if yes mention in grams of alcohol)

Treatment history:
- Drugs using
- Frequency of drug (example—drug taken 5 times a week most likely to be digoxin)
- Duration of usage
- Any blood test to be monitored [example—international normalized ratio (INR) for warfarin]
- Any intramuscular injections (once in 3 weeks IM injection most likely to be benzathine penicillin for rheumatic heart disease prophylaxis)

Menstrual and obstetric history:
- G__P__L__A__
- Age of menarche __
- Menopause at __
- Flow—amenorrhea/oligomenorrhea/menorrhagia

Summarize:
Differential diagnosis:
1.
2.
3.

General Examination

Patient:
- Conscious
- Coherent
- Cooperative
- Obeying commands

Body mass index (BMI):
- W (kg)/h² (meters)
- Grading according to World Health Organization (WHO) for south east Asian countries

Vitals examination:
- Pulse:
  - Rate
  - Rhythm
  - Volume
  - Character
  - Vessel wall thickening
  - Radio-radial delay and radio femoral delay
  - Peripheral pulses
- Blood pressure:
  - Right arm
  - Left arm
  - Leg
  - Postural drop in BP
- Respiratory rate:
  - Regular/irregular
  - Abdominothoracic (male) or thoracoabdominal (female)
  - Usage of accessory muscles
- Jugular venous pressure:
  - __ cm of water (blood) above sternal angle (+5 cm from the right atria)
- Jugular venous pulse:
  - Waveform
- Pulse oximetry

Physical examination:
- Pallor:
- Icterus:
- Cyanosis:
- Clubbing:
- Lymphadenopathy:
- Edema:

Others:
- Signs of infective endocarditis
- Signs of rheumatic fever

Systemic Examination

Inspection:
- Chest shape and symmetry
- Breast abnormalities
- Spine deformity
- Precordial prominence
- Pulsations:
  - Apical pulse
  - Pulsation in aortic and pulmonary area
  - Sternoclavicular pulsations
  - Left parasternal pulsations
  - Epigastric pulsations
  - Ectopic pulsations
- Distended veins

Palpation:
- Confirmation of shape and symmetry
- Palpation of precordium

- Palpation of cardiovascular pulsation for sounds, thrills, and rubs
- Tracheal tug

Percussion:
- Right heart border
- Left heart border
- 2nd intercostal (IC) space
- Sternal percussion

Auscultation:
- *Apex (mitral area)*:
  - S1
  - S2
  - S3 and S4
  - *Murmur*:
    1. Timing
    2. Grade
    3. Quality
    4. Pitch
    5. Configuration
    6. Radiation
    7. Best heard with diaphragm or bell
    8. Patient position
    9. With breath held in inspiration or expiration
    10. Variation with other maneuvers
- *Tricuspid area*:
  - S1
  - S2
  - S3 and S4
  - *Murmur*:
    1. Timing
    2. Grade
    3. Quality
    4. Pitch
    5. Configuration
    6. Radiation
    7. Best heard with diaphragm or bell
    8. Patient position
    9. With breath held in inspiration or expiration
    10. Variation with other maneuvers
- *Erb's neoaortic area:*
  - S1
  - S2
  - S3 and S4
  - *Murmur*:
    1. Timing
    2. Grade
    3. Quality
    4. Pitch
    5. Configuration
    6. Radiation
    7. Best heard with diaphragm or bell
    8. Patient position
    9. With breath held in inspiration or expiration
    10. Variation with other maneuvers
- *(R) 2nd IC space (aortic area)*:
  - S1
  - S2
  - S3 and S4
  - *Murmur*:
    1. Timing
    2. Grade
    3. Quality
    4. Pitch
    5. Configuration
    6. Radiation
    7. Best heard with diaphragm or bell
    8. Patient position
    9. With breath held in inspiration or expiration
    10. Variation with other maneuvers
- *(L) 2nd IC space (pulmonary area)*:
  - S1
  - S2
  - S3 and S4
  - *Murmur*:
    1. Timing
    2. Grade
    3. Quality
    4. Pitch
    5. Configuration
    6. Radiation
    7. Best heard with diaphragm or bell
    8. Patient position
    9. With breath held in inspiration or expiration
    10. Variation with other maneuvers
- *Other areas*:
  - Axilla
  - Epigastrium
  - Clavicle
  - Carotid

Other System Examination

(Relevant findings in other systems to be noted)

CARDIOVASCULAR SYSTEM: DIAGNOSIS FORMAT

For Acquired Heart Disease
- Acquired heart disease possible etiology (rheumatic/ischemic/cardiomyopathy/degenerative)
- Valvular involvement [mitral stenosis (MS)/mitral regurgitation (MR)/aortic stenosis (AS)/ aortic regurgitation (AR)/others] with severity grading
- With/without evidence of pulmonary artery hypertension (grading)
- Patient in or not in atrial fibrillation (if AF present, look for signs of thromboembolism)
- With or without evidence of heart failure (right/left/congestive)
- With or without signs of infective endocarditis
- With or without signs of active rheumatic carditis
- Patient is in New York Heart Association (NYHA) Class (I/II/III/IV)

Examples: Acquired valvular heart disease possibly rheumatic etiology, with severe mitral stenosis and moderate mitral regurgitation, with severe pulmonary artery hypertension, patient in atrial fibrillation and congestive cardiac failure, with no signs of infective endocarditis, thromboembolism, or active rheumatic carditis. Patient is in NYHA class III.

CARDIOVASCULAR SYSTEM: DISCUSSION OF SYMPTOMS

Chest Pain

Chest pain is a common symptom of cardiac disease. It can be due to noncardiac causes such as anxiety or diseases involving the respiratory, musculoskeletal, or gastrointestinal systems.

Causes of Chest Pain

See **Figure 5.1**.

Differential Diagnosis of Chest Pain

Potentially life-threatening causes	Common non-life-threatening causes

• Acute coronary syndromes: Acute myocardial infarction (MI), ST-segment elevation MI, non-ST-segment elevation MI
• Unstable angina
• Pulmonary embolism
• Aortic dissection
• Myocarditis
• Tension pneumothorax
• Acute chest syndrome/crisis in sickle cell anemia
• Pericarditis
• Boerhaave's syndrome (perforated esophagus)
• Gastrointestinal: Perforated peptic ulcer, acute pancreatitis, acute cholecystitis
	• Gastrointestinal:
	  ■ Biliary colic
	  ■ Gastroesophageal reflux disease
	  ■ Peptic ulcer disease
	• Pulmonary:
	  ■ Pneumonia
	  ■ Pleuritis
	• Musculoskeletal pain: Costochondritis (Tietze's syndrome), intercostal myalgia/neuralgia, fracture of the ribs (cough, trauma), secondaries in the ribs, Bornholm disease
	• Thoracic radiculopathy: Texidor's twinge (precordial catch syndrome)
	• Emotional: Anxiety
	• Neural: Shingles/herpes zoster

Differential Features of Ischemic Cardiac and Noncardiac Pain

Features	Ischemic cardiac pain	Noncardiac pain
Site	Central, diffuse	Peripheral, localized
Character of pain	Tight, squeezing, dull, constricting, choking or 'heavy'	Sharp, stabbing, catching
Precipitation/provocation	Exertion, emotion	Spontaneous, not related to exertion
Radiation	Jaw/neck/shoulder	Usually no radiation
Relieving factors	Rest (in less than 5 minutes), nitrates	Not relieved by rest or by nitrates
Associated features	Breathlessness, diaphoresis	Depends on the cause

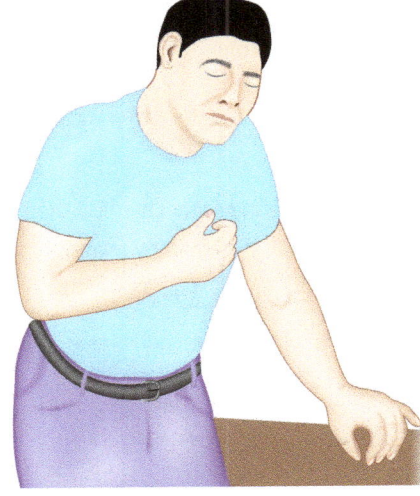

Fig. 5.1: Causes of chest pain.

Differentiating Features of the Common Causes of Chest Pain

Disease	Description	Location	Radiation	Associations
Acute coronary syndromes	Crushing, tightening, squeezing, or pressure like	Retrosternal, left anterior chest or epigastric	Right (R) or left (L) shoulder, R or L arm/hand/jaw	Dyspnea, diaphoresis, nausea
Pulmonary embolism	Heaviness, tightness	Whole chest (massive) or focal chest (segmental)	None	Dyspnea, unstable vital signs, feeling of impending doom if massive or just tachycardia, tachypnea if segmental
Aortic dissection	Ripping, tearing	Midline, substernal	Interscapular area of back	Secondary arterial branch occlusion (paraplegia)
Pericarditis/cardiac tamponade	Sharp, constant or pleuritic	Substernal	None	Fever, dyspnea, pericardial friction rub
Pneumothorax	Sudden, sharp, lancinating, pleuritic	One side of chest	Shoulder, back	Dyspnea
Perforated esophagus	Sudden, sharp, after forceful vomiting	Substernal	Back	Dyspnea, diaphoresis, signs of sepsis

Types of Angina

Angina	Angina is a symptom of myocardial ischemia that is recognized clinically by its character, its location, and its relation to provocative stimuli.
Stable angina	Angina is stable when it is not a new symptom and when there is no deterioration in frequency, severity, or duration of episodes.
Unstable angina	This is a form of acute coronary syndrome. It has at least one of these three features: 1. It occurs at rest (or with minimal exertion), usually lasting more than 10 minutes 2. It is severe and of new onset (i.e., within the prior 4–6 weeks) 3. It occurs with a crescendo pattern (i.e., distinctly more severe, prolonged, or frequent than before).
Variant angina/ prinzmetal angina	It is caused due to coronary vasospasm.
Microvascular angina/ cardiac syndrome X	Angina-like chest pain, in the context of normal epicardial coronary arteries on angiography
Episodic angina	This syndrome is one in which pains having the characters of angina of effort occur at longer or shorter intervals.
Nocturnal angina	Seen in severe aortic regurgitation *Proposed mechanisms are:* • Prolonged diastole at night: Regurgitation time is prolonged. • Dilated LV, increased LV mass, and increased demand • Diastolic coronary stealing and Venturi effect of AR jet
Angina decubitus	It is angina that occurs when a person is lying down (not necessarily only at night) without any apparent cause. It occurs because gravity redistributes fluids in the body.
Second wind, or warm up, angina	Describes patients with ischemic heart disease and exertional angina that forces them to stop; after the first bout of angina, they are able to continue with minor, or even without any further symptoms, ischemic preconditioning and collateral recruitment are proposed mechanisms.
Linked angina	It is associated with: • Gastroesophageal and duodenal disorders and diseases • Gallbladder disease • Cervical spondylitis
Refractory angina	Angina that cannot be controlled with optimal medical therapy and where revascularization is unfeasible
Status anginosus	It is a clinical term denoting periods of frequently recurring anginal pain at rest, indistinguishable from the pain of cardiac infarction or from its prodromal manifestation, but without the electrocardiographic and laboratory evidences of classical cardiac infarction.
Vincent's angina	Fusospirochetal infection of the pharynx and palatine tonsils, causing "ulceromembranous pharyngitis and tonsillitis"
Ludwig's angina	Severe diffuse cellulitis that presents an acute onset and spreads rapidly, bilaterally affecting the submandibular, sublingual, and submental spaces
Abdominal angina	Postprandial pain that occurs in the mesenteric vascular occlusive disease
Angina sine dolore	It is a painless episode of coronary insufficiency. It is associated with diabetes mellitus also called silent ischemia

(LV: left ventricle; AR: aortic regurgitation)

Canadian Cardiovascular Society (CSS) Functional Classification of Angina

Class I	Ordinary activity (e.g., walking, climbing stairs at own pace) does not bring on angina. Angina occurs only with strenuous, rapid, or prolonged exertion at work or during recreation.
Class II	Slight limitation of ordinary activity. Symptoms occur when walking or climbing stairs rapidly, walking up a hill, walking upstairs after a meal, in cold weather, in wind, or when under emotional stress, or only a few hours after waking, and climbing more than one flight of ordinary stairs at a normal pace and in normal conditions.
Class III	Marked limitation of ordinary activity. Symptoms occur after walking 50–100 yards on the level, or climbing more than one flight of ordinary stairs in normal conditions.
Class IV	Inability to carry on any physical activity without discomfort. Angina may be present at rest.

Angina equivalents:
These are commonly seen in elderly and diabetics (with autonomic neuropathy) where ischemic angina is absent and they present with:
- Shortness of breath
- Perspiration/diaphoresis
- Syncope
- Gastrointestinal (GI) symptoms—upper abdominal pain, nausea, and vomiting
- Fatigue
- Confusion

Palpitations

Definition

Palpitation is the term used to describe an uncomfortable increased awareness of one's own heartbeat or the sensation of slow, rapid, or irregular heart rhythms.
- Palpitations do not always indicate the presence of arrhythmia and conversely, an arrhythmia can occur without palpitations.
- Palpitations are usually noted when the patient is quietly resting.
- Palpitation can be either intermittent or sustained and either regular or irregular.
- A change in the rate, rhythm, or force of contraction can produce palpitations.

Causes of Palpitations

Cardiac causes	Drug-induced

• **Cardiac arrhythmias:**
  ■ Premature atrial and ventricular contractions
  ■ Supraventricular and ventricular arrhythmias
• **Structural heart diseases:**
  ■ Atrial myxoma, valvular heart disease
	• Alcohol (use or withdrawal)
	• Atropine
	• Amphetamines
	• Caffeine, nicotine
	• Cocaine
	• Beta agonists, theophylline

• Congenital heart disease, cardiomyopathy • Mitral valve prolapse, pacemaker	
Psychosomatic disorders: Generalized anxiety, major depression, and panic disorder	**Endocrine:** Hyperthyroidism, hypoglycemia, and pheochromocytoma
High output states: Anemia, beriberi, fever, pregnancy, and thyrotoxicosis	**Miscellaneous and idiopathic:** Emotional stress, hyperventilation, premenstrual syndrome, and strenuous physical activity

Duration and frequency of palpitations:
- Duration may be either short lasting or persistent.
- Note onset and offset of palpitations.
- *Frequency*: It may occur daily, weekly, monthly, or yearly.

Types of Palpitations

Extrasystolic palpitations	Due to ectopic beats, these usually produce feelings of "missing/skipping a beat" and/or a "sinking of the heart" interspersed with periods during which the heartbeats are normal. Patients report that the heart seems to stop and then start again. It can often be seen even in young individuals, usually without any disease of the heart, and generally benign.
Tachycardiac palpitations	These are the rapid fluctuation such as "beating wings" in the chest. It may be regular (e.g., in atrioventricular tachycardia, atrial flutter, or ventricular tachycardia) or irregular or arrhythmic (e.g., in atrial fibrillation).
Anxiety-related palpitations	These are perceived as a form of anxiety. They begin and end gradually.

Associated symptoms and circumstances:
- Palpitations developing after sudden changes in posture are usually due to intolerance to orthostatic or to episodes of atrioventricular nodal reentrant tachycardia.
- Occurrence of syncope or other symptoms, such as severe fatigue, dyspnea, or angina, in addition to palpitations, is more common with structural heart disease.
- Hypersecretion of natriuretic hormone results in polyuria/post-palpitation diuresis in atrial fibrillation.
- Palpitations associated with anxiety or during panic attacks are usually due to sinus tachycardia secondary to the mental disturbance.
- Palpitations may be produced by an increase in the sympathetic drive during physical exercise.

Typical Descriptions of Palpitations

Flip-flopping in the chest	Palpitations are sensed as the heart seeming to stop and then start again, producing a pounding or flip-flopping sensation. This type of palpitation is generally caused by supraventricular or ventricular premature contractions.
Rapid fluttering in the chest	It is due to a sustained ventricular or supraventricular arrhythmia, including sinus tachycardia.

Contd...

Contd...

Pounding in the neck	An irregular pounding feeling in the neck is caused by atrioventricular dissociation, with independent contraction of the atria and ventricles, resulting in occasional atrial contraction against a closed tricuspid and mitral valve. This produces cannon A waves, which are intermittent increase in the "A" wave of the jugular venous pulse. *Cannon A* waves may be seen with ventricular premature contractions, third degree or complete heart block, or ventricular tachycardia (VT).

Dyspnea

Dyspnea is discussed in detail in respiratory examination section.

Syncope

Definition

Syncope is defined as a transient loss of consciousness due to inadequate cerebral blood flow with loss of postural tone. It is associated with loss of postural tone, with spontaneous return to baseline neurologic function without any resuscitative efforts.

- *Presyncope* is the term used for lightheadedness in which the individual thinks he/she may black out.
- *Classical vasovagal syncope:* Syncope triggered by emotional or orthostatic stress such as venipuncture (experienced or witnessed), painful or noxious stimuli, fear of bodily injury, prolonged standing, heat exposure, or exertion.

Mechanism

- Global hypoperfusion of cerebral cortices or focal hypoperfusion of the reticular activating system
- About one-third of individuals may develop a syncopal episode during their lifetime.
- Its incidence increases with age (sharp rise at age of 70 years).
- Cardiac syncope has a high incidence (about 24%) of subsequent cardiac arrest.

Causes of True Syncope

Cardiac causes	Noncardiac causes
• **Cardiac arrhythmias:** Ventricular tachycardia, paroxysmal supraventricular tachycardia, long QT syndrome, Brugada syndrome, bradycardia (Mobitz type II or 3rd degree heart block) • **Structural cardiac or cardiopulmonary disease:** Cardiac valvular disease (AS, MS, PS), obstructive cardiomyopathy, atrial myxoma, acute aortic dissection, pericardial disease/tamponade, pulmonary embolus/pulmonary hypertension, acute myocardial infarction/ischemia	• **Neurocardiogenic syncope 'vasovagal or vasodepressor syncope':** Classical vasovagal syncope, situational syncope, carotid sinus syncope, glossopharyngeal neuralgia, micturation syncope • **Orthostatic hypotension:** Autonomic failure which may be primary (e.g., pure autonomic failure, multiple system atrophy, Parkinson's disease with autonomic failure) or secondary (e.g., diabetic neuropathy) • **Neurovascular syncope:** Vascular steal syndromes

Causes of pseudosyncope
- ❖ Seizures
- ❖ **Metabolic or toxic abnormalities:** Hypoglycemia and encephalitis rarely syncope.
- ❖ **Neurologic syncope:** Subarachnoid hemorrhage, transient ischemic attack, complex migraine headache.
- ❖ **Psychiatric syncope**
- ❖ **Drug induced loss of consciousness:** Drugs of abuse and alcohol

Pedal Edema

Definition

Edema is defined as the abnormal fluid accumulation in the interstitial space that exceeds the capacity of physiological lymphatic drainage. Pedal edema is a common presentation of various systemic and nonsystemic diseases.

Approach to Pedal Edema

Site and distribution	*Whether the pedal edema is unilateral or bilateral*: • Unilateral edema results mainly due to local causes such as deep vein thrombosis (DVT), cellulitis, compartment syndrome, and filarial lymphatic obstruction • Bilateral pedal edema is mainly due to systemic causes such as congestive cardiac failure, anemia, chronic kidney disease, and chronic liver disease.
Duration of illness	• Short duration of the illness indicates an acute cause, such as cellulitis, DVT, and compartment syndrome, which usually occurs in 72 hours.
Association with pain	**Painless:** Edema due to heart failure, hypoproteinemia, and lymphedema **Painful:** Deep vein thrombosis and cellulitis. *A dull aching type of pain is seen in chronic venous insufficiency.*
Variability of edema	Venous edema due to congestive cardiac failure and venous insufficiency is aggravated by standing and improves with overnight limb elevation during sleep. *Idiopathic edema,* which is seen in females, increases throughout the day during upright posture.
History of systemic illness	• Symptoms of systemic diseases such as exertional dyspnea, orthopnea, paroxysmal nocturnal dyspnea, and chest pain point to cardiac failure • History of oliguria and puffiness of face suggests renal etiology • Long-term alcohol consumption, yellowish discoloration of eyes and urine, and abdominal distension point to cirrhosis of liver • Symptoms of endocrine disorders such as hypothyroidism are often missed. • Similar history about all other systemic causes of pedal edema should be elicited in detail. • Patients who are bed-ridden for a prolonged period of time have dependent edema over the sacral area.

Contd...

Contd...

History of drug intake	Drugs such as calcium channel blockers, NSAIDs, and steroids can cause pedal edema.
History of trauma and radiation	Trauma and radiation can cause cellulitis and compartment syndrome leading to pedal edema. Long-term radiation can also cause lymphedema in some patients.
Miscellaneous causes	Obstructive sleep apnea can also cause pedal edema due to right ventricular failure.

(DVT: deep vein thrombosis; NSAID: nonsteroidal anti-inflammatory drug)

Other Symptoms

- *Symptoms of low-cardiac output:* Fatigue, dizziness, and syncope
- *Symptoms of pulmonary hypertension:* Exertional fatigue, exertional chest pain, exertional dyspnea
- *Fever:* Rheumatic and infective endocarditis
- *Symptoms of heart failure:* Fatigue, anorexia, weight gain, leg swelling, exertional fatigue, decreased urine output, perspiration, confusion, cough, hemoptysis, and wheezing

Chapter 5: Cardiovascular System Examination

CARDIOVASCULAR SYSTEM: DISCUSSION ON EXAMINATION

General Examination

Vitals
Pulse, blood pressure, and jugular venous pressure (JVP)

Anthropometry
It is discussed in detail in chapter on General Examination.

Physical Examination
Signs of infective endocarditis (Figs. 5.2A to F):
- Fever
- Pallor
- Clubbing
- Splinter hemorrhages
- Mucosal petechiae
- Janeway lesions
- Osler's nodes
- Roth spots on fundus

Signs of rheumatic fever:
- Fever
- Arthritis
- Erythema marginatum
- Subcutaneous nodules
- Tachycardia

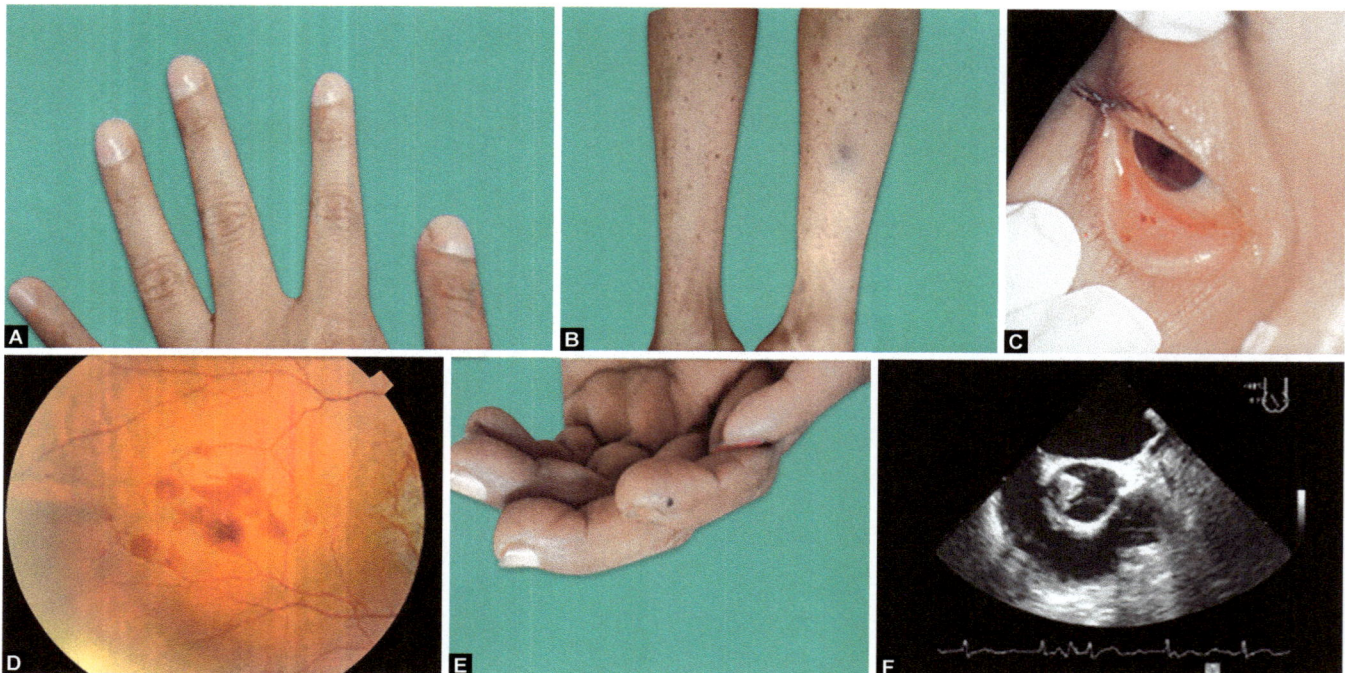

Figs. 5.2A to F: Signs of infective endocarditis: (A) Clubbing; (B) Petechiae; (C) Subconjunctival hemorrhage; (D) Roth spots; (E) Osler's nodes; (F) Echocardiography showing vegetation.

Stigmata of Congenital Heart Disease

Syndrome	Cardiac defects	Other features	
Down syndrome (trisomy 21) (child has many problem)	ECD and VSD	• Cataract • Hypotonia • Hypothyroidism • Increased gap between 1st and 2nd toe (sandal toe) • Leukemia • Duodenal atresia • Hirschsprung's disease • Alzheimer's disease • Simian crease • Mental retardation • Micrognathia • Atlantoaxial instability • Nystagmus	• Protruding tongue • Poor hearing • Round face • Respiratory infections • Occiput is flat • Oblique palpebral fissure • Brushfield spots • Brachycephaly • Low nasal bridge • Language problem • Epicanthic fold • Ear folded • Mongolian slant • Myoclonus

Contd...

Contd...

Syndrome	Cardiac defects	Other features
Marfan syndrome	Aortic aneurysm, aortic and/or mitral regurgitation	Arachnodactyly with hyperextensibility, subluxation of lens, and other joint deformities
William's syndrome	Supravalvular AS, and PA stenosis	Varying degrees of mental retardation, so-called elfin facies (consisting of some of the following: upturned nose, flat nasal bridge, long philtrum, flat malar area, wide mouth, full lips, widely spaced teeth, periorbital fullness), and hypercalcemia of infancy
Rubella syndrome	PDA and PA stenosis	*Triad of the syndrome is* deafness, cataract, and CHDs. Others include intrauterine growth retardation, microcephaly, microphthalmia, hepatitis, and neonatal thrombocytopenic purpura
Noonan's syndrome (Turner-like syndrome)	PS (dystrophic pulmonary valve), LVH (or anterior septal hypertrophy)	Similar to Turner's syndrome but may occur in phenotypic male and without chromosomal abnormality
LEOPARD syndrome (multiple lentigines syndrome)	PS, HOCM, and long PR interval	Lentiginous skin lesion, ocular hypertelorism, pulmonary stenosis, abnormal genitalia, retarded growth, and deafness
Holt-Oram syndrome (cardiac limb syndrome)	ASD and VSD	Defects or absence of thumb or radius
Ellis–van Creveld syndrome (chondroectodermal dysplasia)	ASD and single atrium	Short stature of prenatal onset, short distal extremities, narrow thorax with short ribs, polydactyly, nail hypoplasia, and neonatal teeth
DiGeorge syndrome	Interrupted aortic arch, truncus arteriosus, VSD, PDA, and TOF	Hypertelorism, short philtrum, downslanting eyes, hypoplasia or absence of thymus and parathyroid, hypocalcemia, deficient cell-mediated immunity
Cornelia de Lange's (de Lange's) syndrome	VSD	Hirsutism, prenatal growth retardation, microcephaly, anteverted nares, downturned mouth, and mental retardation
CHARGE syndrome	TOF, truncus arteriosus, aortic arch anomalies (e.g., vascular ring, interrupted aortic arch)	Coloboma, choanal atresia, growth or mental retardation, genitourinary anomalies, ear anomalies, and genital hypoplasia

(AS: aortic stenosis; ECD: endocardial cushion defect; VSD: ventricular septal defect; PA: pulmonary artery; PDA: patent ductus arteriosus; PS: pulmonary stenosis; LVH: left ventricular hypertrophy; HOCM: hypertrophic obstructive cardiomyopathy; ASD: atrial septal defect; TOF: tetralogy of Fallot)

Systemic Examination

All examinations of cardiovascular examination have to be simultaneously timed with carotid pulse. Findings synchronous with carotid upstroke is systolic and if it asynchronous, it is diastolic.

Inspection and Palpation of Heart
Chest deformity and associated clinical diseases

Chest deformity	Associated diseases
Barrel shaped	COPD and cor pulmonale
Broad shield-like chest	• Turner syndrome • Noonan syndrome
Pectus carinatum	• Marfan's syndrome • Noonan syndrome
Pectus excavatum	• Marfan's syndrome • Homocystinuria
Straight back syndrome	• Loss of normal kyphosis • Expiratory splitting of S2 • Mid-systolic murmur • Prominent pulmonary artery
Male gynecomastia	Digitalis or spironolactone
Female hypomastia	MVP

(COPD: chronic obstructive pulmonary disease; MVP: mitral valve prolapse)

Topographical areas of the heart:
See **Figure 5.3**.

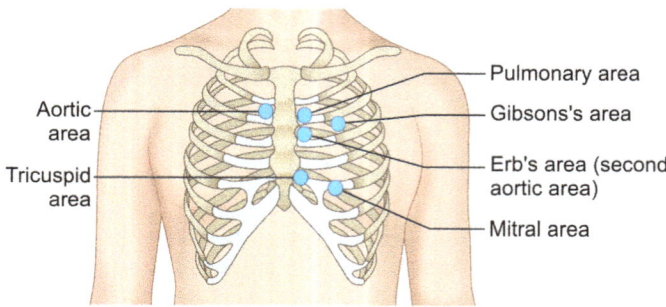

Fig. 5.3: Illustration showing areas of heart.

Precordial bulge:
- Patient in supine position, stand at the foot end of the bed, and look for precordial bulge
- If present, it indicates right ventricular dilatation in childhood.
- Classically seen only with congenital heart diseases such as atrial septal defect (ASD).
- Costal cartilage fuses by 16 years of age, so cardiac diseases, which are acquired beyond 16 years, may not have a precordial bulge.
- Acquired heart disease that can produce precordial bulge is juvenile mitral stenosis.

Causes of precordial bulge

Cardiovascular causes:	
Ribs involved, e.g., cardiac enlargement of long duration	Ribs not involved, e.g., pericardial effusion
Noncardiovascular causes:	
• Skeletal deformity • Bronchogenic carcinoma • Mediastinal growth	

Apical impulse:
Definition:
It is the outermost and lowermost point of maximum impulse (PMI) in early systole, which imparts a perpendicular gentle thrust to a palpating finger, followed by a slight medial retraction in the late systole.

Method of examination of apical impulse: First observe the *position* of apical impulse, then comment on the *character*.
- Patient should be in supine position
- First palpate the apex with the palm (**Fig. 5.4**), then localize it with fingertip (**Fig. 5.5**).
- Observe the amplitude and duration of the lift of the palpating finger.
- If apical impulse is not palpable in supine position, the patient can be put in left lateral position and examination done.

Features of normal cardiac impulse

Location	Left 5th ICS, 1–2 cm medial to MCL (or) ≤10 cm from the midsternal line (**Fig. 5.6**)
Extent	<3 cm diameter or one ICS
Duration	<50% of diastole

(ICS: intercostal space; MCL: midclavicular line)

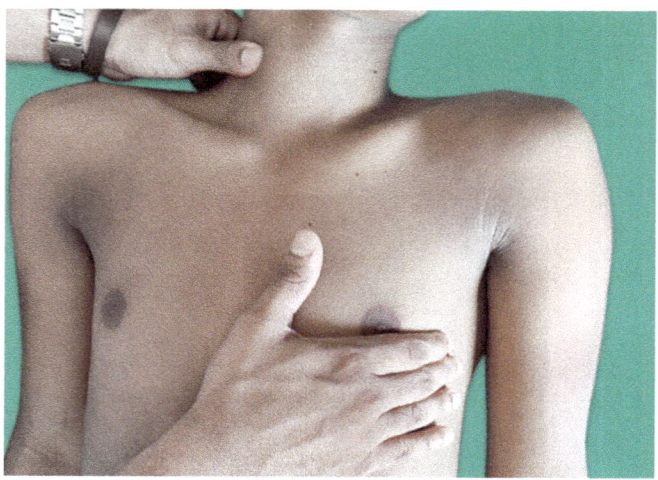

Fig. 5.4: Palpating the apex with palm flat on the chest.

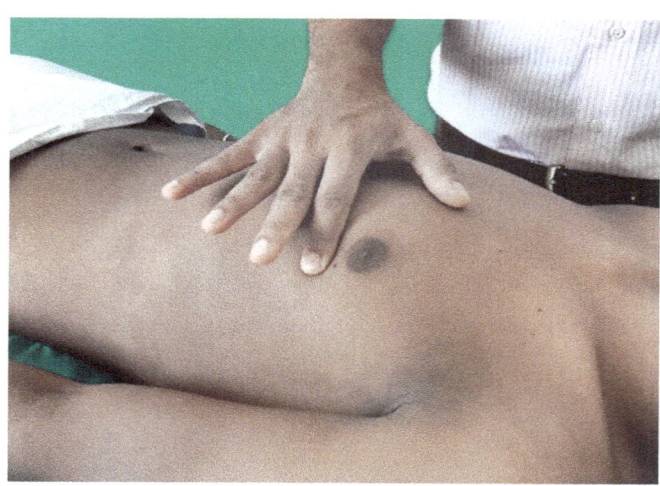

Fig. 5.5: Localizing the apex with the finger tip.

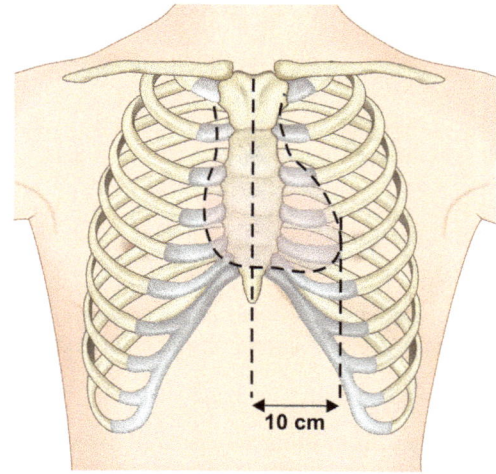

Fig. 5.6: Location of cardiac impulse.

Mechanism of normal apical impulse:
- Anterior and counter clock-wise rotation of LV due to isovolumetric contraction during early systole and medical retraction due to clock-wise rotation of the LV during late systole.

Abnormalities of apex (Fig. 5.7)

Absent	*Cardiovascular causes:* • Pericardial effusion • Dextrocardia *Noncardiac causes:* • Behind rib • Obesity or thick chest wall • COPD/emphysema • Left-sided pleural effusion • Left-sided pneumothorax
Tapping	Mitral stenosis (palpable S1—closing snap)
Hyperdynamic	Increased in amplitude Duration is >1/3 to <2/3 of systole Occupies more than one intercostal space (hence called *diffuse apex*) Occurs in LV *volume overload* conditions *Physiological:* • Thin chest • Pectus excavatum • High output states *Pathological:* • AR • MR • VSD • PDA • AV fistula
Heaving	• Increase in amplitude • Duration is >2/3 of systole • Confined to one intercostal space. • Occurs in LV *pressure overload* • AS • Systemic hypertension • HCM • Coarctation of aorta
Double apical impulse	• HOCM • LV aneurysm • LV dyssynergy
Triple or quadruple or wavy impulse	HOCM
Retractile	Severe TR
Seesaw apex	LV aneurysm

(AR: aortic regurgitation; MR: mitral regurgitation; VSD: ventricular septal defect; PDA: patent ductus arteriosus; AV: atrioventricular; LV: left ventricle; COPD: chronic obstructive pulmonary disease; HCM: hypertrophic cardiomyopathy; HOCM: hypertrophic obstructive cardiomyopathy)

Which ventricle is causing the apical impulse?
☐ The heart during systole, becoming smaller, generally withdraws from the chest wall except for the apex. The effect of this withdrawal on the chest wall can be observed as an inward movement of the chest wall during systole called "RETRACTION".
☐ The presence of lateral retraction identifies the apical impulse to be formed by the right ventricle, which is an abnormal state.
☐ A wide area apex beat with medial retraction implies left ventricular enlargement.

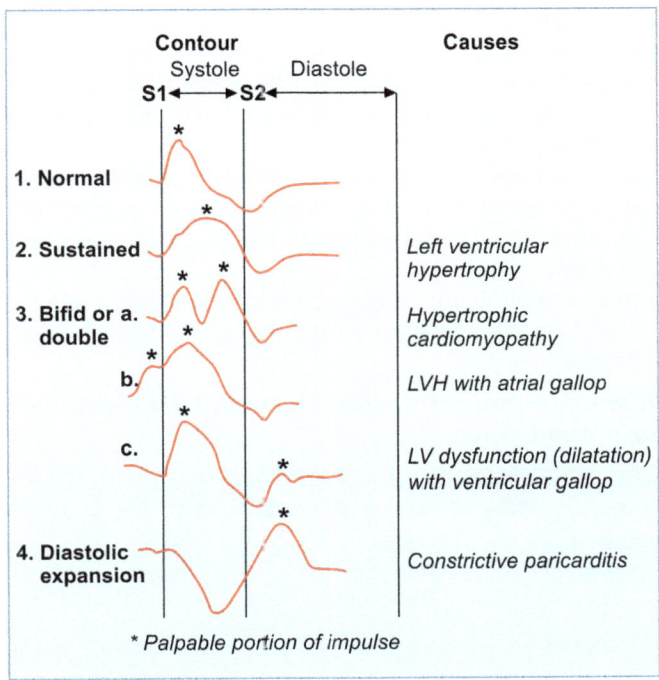

Fig. 5.7: Apicogram showing different types of cardiac apex.

Right ventricle (RV) apex versus left ventricle (LV) apex

RV apex	LV apex
Apex rotated and shifted laterally but does not cross midline	Apex may be shifted down and out
Lateral retraction	Medial retraction

Note: In adhesive pericarditis, systolic retraction of the apex followed by diastolic expansion is described in constrictive pericarditis—**Skoda's sign**.

Displacement of apex:

Upward displacement	• Children • Ascites • Abdominal tumor • Pericardial effusion
Downward displacement	• Mediastinal growth • Aortic aneurysm
Lateral displacement	If trachea is also shifted along with the displacement of apex beat, then it is due to mediastinal shift as a result of conditions such as lung fibrosis, collapse, pneumothorax, or skeletal abnormalities. If the trachea is central but the apex is displaced, the causes may be: • *Left ventricular enlargement:* The apex will be displaced *downward and laterally* • *Right ventricular enlargement:* The apex will be displaced *laterally*

Left parasternal (LPS) pulsation/heave:
☐ It is produced by either by right ventricle (RV) or left atrium (LA).
☐ Normally, RV activity is neither visible nor palpable.

Examination of LPS area:

- Heal of hand with wrist is cocked up **(Fig. 5.8)** (or) ulnar border of hand **(Fig. 5.9)** is applied over 3/4/5 intercostal space (ICS) in left sternal margin, and feel for the pulsations.
- In children or thin patients, parasternal heave can be demonstrated by placing a pen over the parasternal area parallel to the sternal margin and watch for the movement of the tip of the pen.
- In case of difficulty in appreciating the parasternal heave from breathing, ask the patient to momentarily hold the breath.

All India Institute of Medical Sciences (AIIMS) grading of parasternal heave.

Grade I	Grade II	Grade III
Visible Not palpable	Visible Palpable Obliterable	Visible Palpable Not obliterable
Ill sustained	>50% of systole	Full systole

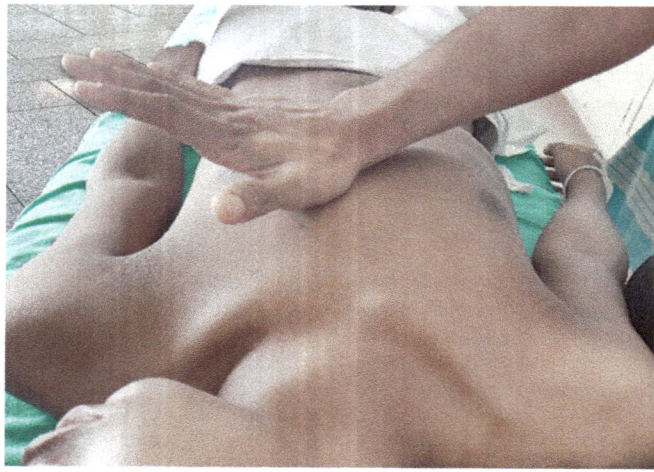

Fig. 5.8: Examination of parasternal heave.

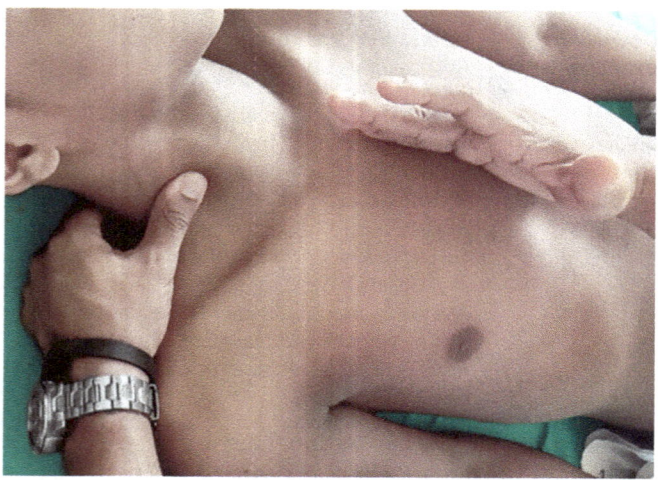

Fig. 5.9: Examination of parasternal heave.

How to differentiate RV and LA parasternal heave?

RV parasternal heave	LA parasternal heave
• Synchronous with apex • Systolic	• Not synchronous with apex • Diastolic

(RV: right ventricle; LA: left atrium)

Conditions where LPS pulsations seen

Physiological	• Children • Reduced AP diameter
Right ventricular hypertrophy associated	*Pressure overload:* • Pulmonary HTN • Pulmonary stenosis *Volume overload:* • TR • ASD • VSD
Normal RV	• *Moderate-to-severe MR* (jet or squid effect)—regurgitant jet of blood into LA pushes the RV anteriorly • *RWMA of LV*—dyskinetic motion of LV septum pushes RV forwards during the systole

Note:
1. There is no parasternal heave in TOF
2. In MS with MR, there are both LAE and RVH hence very prominent parasternal heave seen

(ASD: atrial septal defect; VSD: ventricular septal defect; HTN: hypertension; LV: left ventricle; RV: right ventricle; LA: left atrium; TOF: tetralogy of Fallot; MS: mitral stenosis; MR: mitral regurgitation; LAE: left atrial enlargement; RVH: right ventricular hypertrophy)

Aortic and pulmonary pulsations (base of the heart):

These are examined in sitting and leaning forward position with breath held in expiration (*Erb's maneuver*—described in auscultation section).

Aortic area	Pulmonary area
Right 2nd ICS area	Left 2nd ICS area
Visible pulsations:	
For example: • Aneurysm of aorta • Chronic AR	For example: • Pulmonary HTN • Pulmonary artery dilatation • Pulmonary artery aneurysm • Hyperdynamic pulmonary artery circulation
Palpable heart sounds:	
• A2 (sHTN) • Ejection click (bicuspid aortic valve)	• P2 (pHTN)—*diastolic shock* • Ejection click (pulmonary stenosis)
Palpable murmurs:	
• AS • AR (dilated root—AR)	• PS • PDA (Gibson's area left 1st ICS) • Graham steel murmur

(AR: aortic regurgitation; AS: aortic stenosis; HTN: hypertension; PDA: patent ductus arteriosus; PS: pulmonary stenosis)

Sternoclavicular pulsations:

Suprasternal pulsations	• Aneurysm of arch of aorta • Thyroid ima artery
Right sternoclavicular joint	• Aortic dissection • Aneurysm of aorta • Aortic regurgitation • Right aortic arch • Blalock–Taussig shunt

Epigastric pulsations:
- The subxiphoid region should be palpated by placing the thumb/index finger/palm of the hand over the epigastrium with the fingertips pointing up toward the patient's head (**Fig. 5.10**).
- Gentle pressure is applied downward (posteriorly) and upward toward the head.
- The patient should be asked to take a deep inspiration in order to move the diaphragm down. This facilitates the palpation of the right ventricle.
- If the impulse was palpable pushing the tip of the thumb/fingertips downward (toward the feet), it would indicate a palpable right ventricular impulse.
- Transmitted abdominal aortic pulsations will cause the impulse to strike the palmar aspect of the thumb/hand.
- Transmitted hepatic pulsations are felt from the right side onto lateral surface of the examining finger.

Causes of epigastric pulsations:

Cardiac causes	RVH (d/t any cause)
Aortic causes	• Thin build • Aneurysm of descending aorta • Aortic regurgitation
Hepatic causes	• *Presystolic/diastolic*: TS • *Systolic*: TR

(TR: tricuspid regurgitation; TS: tricuspid stenosis)

Other pulsations:

At back	• *Suzman's sign* in coarctation of aorta • Pulmonary AV fistula
At neck	• Aortic regurgitation • Carotid aneurysm • Subclavian artery aneurysm

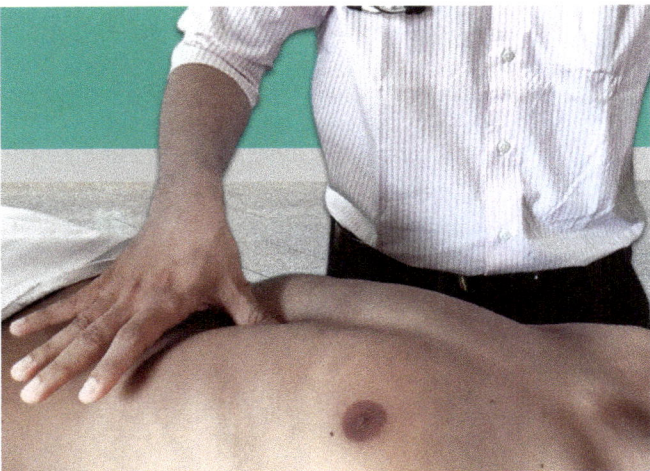

Fig. 5.10: Demonstration of epigastric pulsations.

Thrills:
- Thrills are palpable murmurs (grade IV or more intensity).
- It is described as purring of the cat.
- It is best felt with head of the metacarpal bones.
- It can be systolic, diastolic, or continuous.

Area	Timing	Cause
Mitral (apex)	Systolic	Severe MR
	Diastolic	MS
Left sternal border	Systolic	VSD
Pulmonary area	Systolic	PS
Aortic area	Systolic	AS
	Diastolic	Acute severe AR
Left 1st ICS	Continuous	PDA Or Rupture of sinus of Valsalva

Note: As a rule, thrills in the apex of heart are diastolic and thrills in the base of the heart are systolic (exceptions systolic thrill of acute severe MR and diastolic thrill of acute severe AR)

(AS: aortic stenosis; AR: aortic regurgitation; MS: mitral stenosis; PDA: patent ductus arteriosus; VSD: ventricular septal defect)

Others sounds palpable at apex:

Low-frequency sounds:	
LV S3	• Non-CVS: A, T, and P • CVS: LVF and MR
LV S4 (LVEDP >15–18 mm Hg)	• AS • HCM • MR/AR • CAD
Pericardial knock	Constrictive pericarditis—systolic retraction of whole pericardium)
High-frequency sounds:	
S1	Tapping apex of MS
OS	Early diastolic sound in MS
Ejection systolic click	AS (congenital—bicuspid aortic valve)
Tumor flap	LA/RA myxomas
Murmurs (thrills):	
Systolic	MR AS VSD
Diastolic	MS

(AS: aortic stenosis; AR: aortic regurgitation; CVS: cardiovascular system; HCM: hypertrophic cardiomyopathy; LVF: left ventricular failure; MR: mitral regurgitation; MS: mitral stenosis; VSD: ventricular septal defect; LA: left atrium; RA: right atrium)

Other palpable sounds in parasternal area:

Low-frequency sounds:	
RV S3 (increased flow to ventricles)	• RV failure • Chronic TR • ASD
RV S4 (against increased pressures of ventricle)	• PS • Decreased RV compliance

Contd...

Contd...

High-frequency sounds:	
OS of TS	
Murmurs (thrills):	
Systolic	TR
Diastolic	TS

(ASD: atrial septal defect; PS: pulmonary stenosis; RV: right ventricle; TR: tricuspid regurgitation; TS: tricuspid stenosis)

> **Note:**
>
> | | |
> |---|---|
> | *Palpable S1* | Tapping apex |
> | *Palpable S2* | Diastolic shock (palpable P2) |
> | *Constrictive pericarditis* | Diastolic knock or pericardial knock |

Dilated vessels:
1. *Dilated veins*: Caudal flow (SVC obstruction); cranial flow (IVC obstruction)
2. Collaterals are seen with coarctation of aorta (COA)

For example, *Suzman's sign*—seen in COA where collaterals are seen in interscapular and infrascapular region.

Scars (Fig. 5.11):

Median sternotomy (generally done when there is need for connecting a heart lung machine)	CABG
Lateral thoracotomy	All valve replacement surgeries PDA surgery scar

(CABG: coronary artery bypass graft; PDA: patent ductus arteriosus)

Tracheal tug (Oliver's sign):
- Raise the chin of patient and apply the upward pressure on two sides of cricoid cartilage **(Fig. 5.12)**.

Positive	Downward pull with each heart beat	Aortic aneurysm
False positive		Due to mediastinal mass
False negative	Does not move with heart beat	Thrombosed aortic aneurysm

Percussion

Determination of Heart Border

Right heart border
- Percuss from above downward in midclavicular line up to the liver dullness **(Fig. 5.13)**.
- Start percussing one space above the liver dullness **(Fig. 5.14)**, from the right midclavicular line to the sternum keeping the pleximeter finger parallel to the sternal edge **(Figs. 5.15A and B)**.
- Repeat this in two more consecutive spaces above.

Dullness corresponding to right sternal margin	Normal
Dullness outside the R-sternal margin laterally	• Pericardial effusion • Dextrocardia • Cardiac enlargement • Right atrial enlargement • Mediastinal mass • Lung pathology

Left heart border:
- Palpate the apex
- In same intercostal space (ICS), go to the midaxillary line and start percussing medially.
- Direction of percussion should be parallel to the apparent left heart border **(Figs. 5.16A and B)**

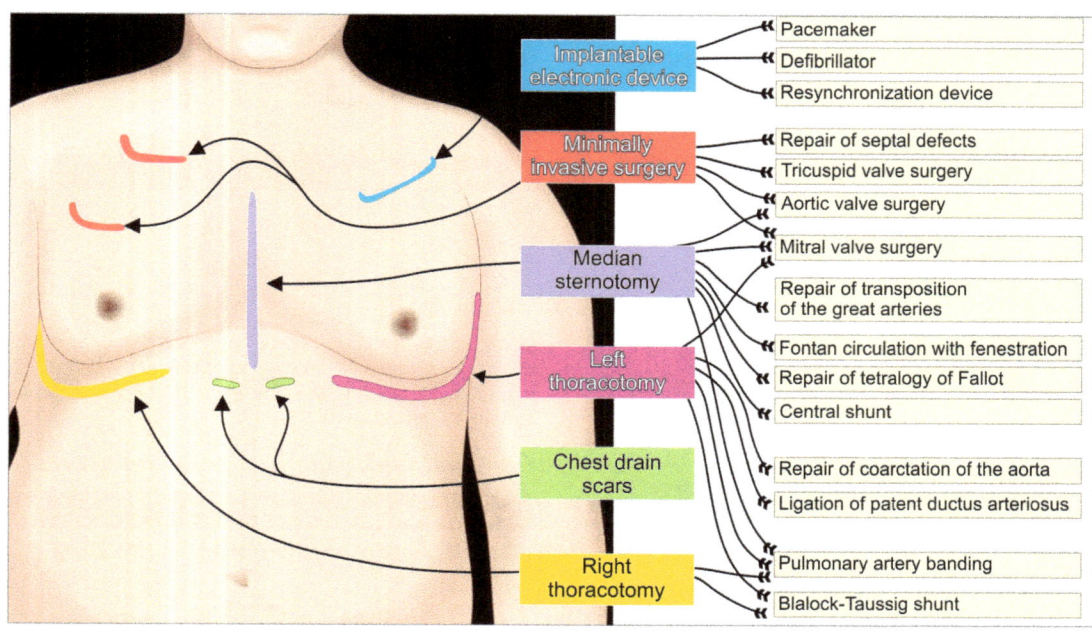

Fig. 5.11: Different surgical scars for cardiac disease.

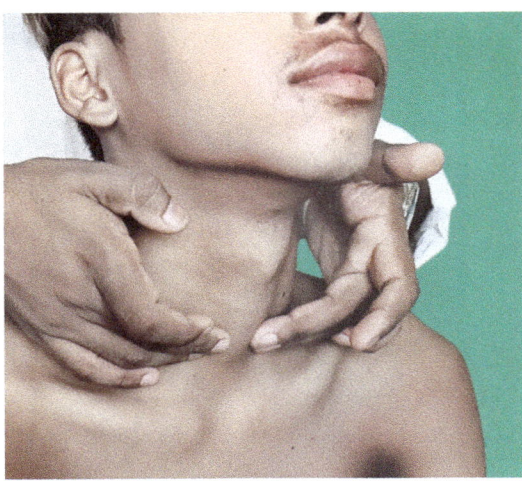

Fig. 5.12: Demonstration of Oliver's sign.

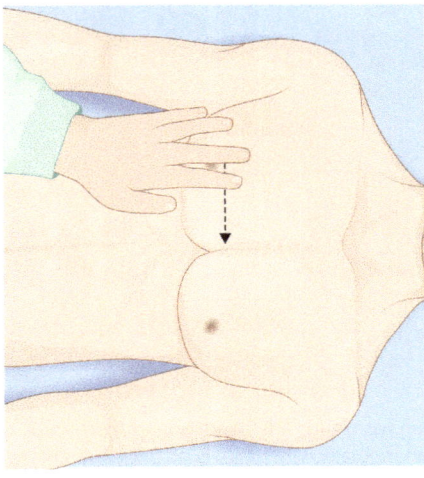

Fig. 5.15A: Illustration showing direction of percussion of right heart border.

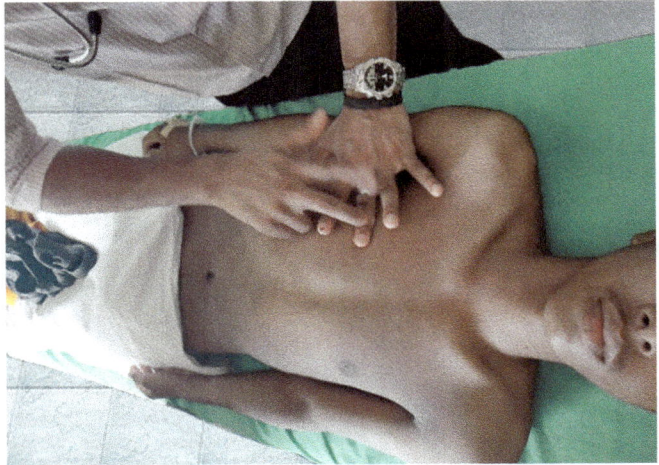

Fig. 5.13: Percuss from above downward in midclavicular line up to the liver dullness.

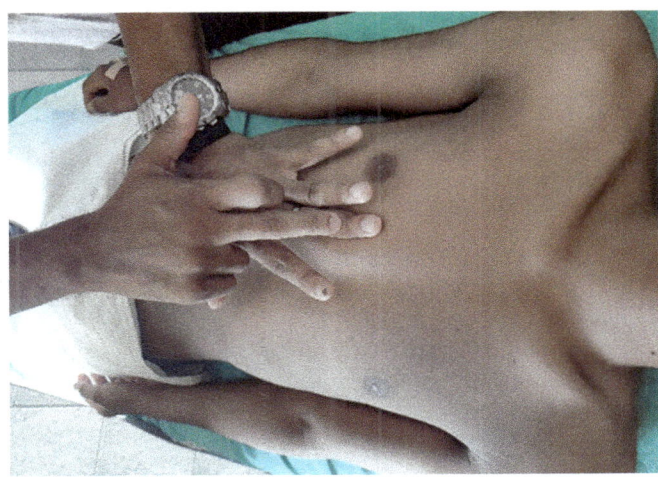

Fig. 5.15B: Change the direction of percussing finger parallel to heart border and move medially till you get dullness (due to right heart border).

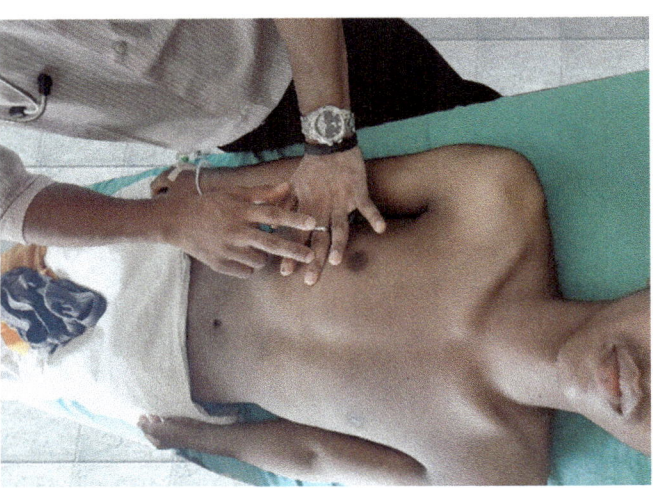

Fig. 5.14: Now, go one space above the liver dullness.

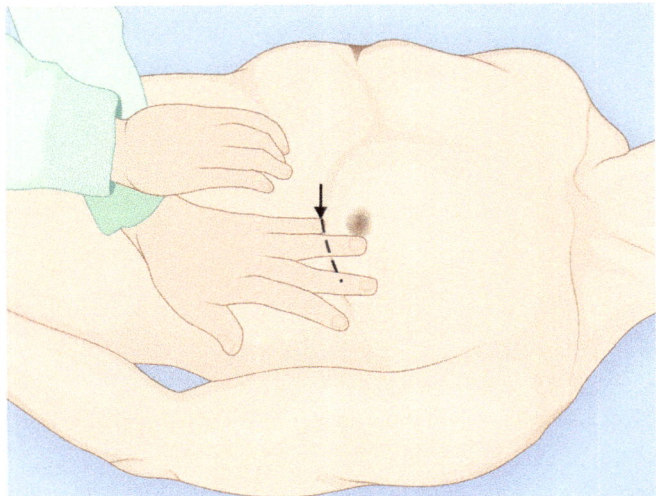

Fig. 5.16A: Illustration showing direction of percussion of left heart border.

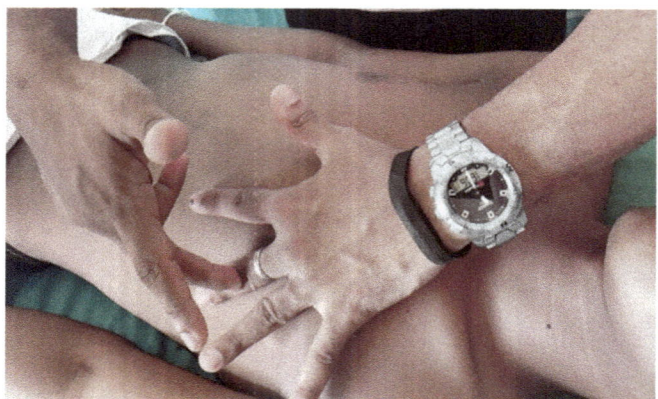

Fig. 5.16B: Percussion for left heart border from midaxillary line and start percussing medially with percussing finger parallel to heard border.

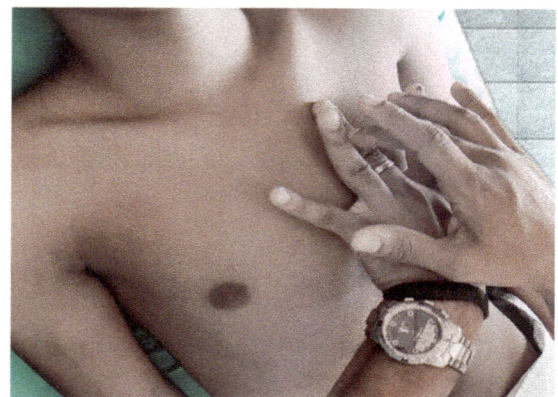

Fig. 5.18: Percussion of left 2nd intercostal space.

Normally	Corresponds to the apex
Dullness outside apex seen in:	• Large pericardial effusion • LV aneurysm

(LV: left ventricle)

Note: Position of pleximeter while percussing the heart border showing be always parallel to presumed borders of heart as showed in the **Figure 5.17**.

Percussion of aortic and pulmonary areas:
☐ *For aortic area*: Start percussing parallel to the right sternal edge and percuss laterally.
☐ *For pulmonary area*: Start percussing parallel to the left sternal edge and percuss laterally.
☐ Normally, it is resonant.

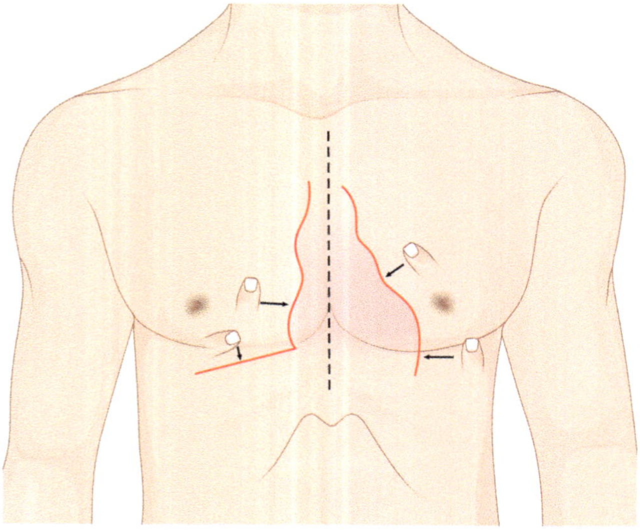

Aortic area	Pulmonary area (Fig. 5.18)
Resonant (normal)	Resonant (normal)
Dullness: • Dilated aorta • Aortic aneurysm • Superior mediastinal mass	*Dullness:* • Dilated PA • PAH • PDA

(PA: pulmonary artery; PAH: pulmonary arterial hypertension; PDA: patent ductus arteriosus)

Auscultation
Hearing of human beings:
☐ Capability is 20–20,000 Hz
☐ Sensitivity is 1,000–5,000 Hz
Minimum time gap to differentiate two sounds by human ear is 20 ms.

Characters of cardiac sounds:
☐ *Loudness*—implies amplitude or intensity
☐ *Pitch*—implies frequency

Difference between low and high frequency heart sounds:

Low frequency	High frequency
<125 Hz	>300 Hz
Low pitch	High pitch
Rough Rumbling	Soft blowing
For example: • S3, S4, and pericardial knock • MDM (TS/MS)	For example: • S1, S2, ESC, OS • Systolic murmur of (MR and AR)
Better appreciated with *bell* of stethoscope by applying low pressure over the chest piece.	Better appreciated with *diaphragm* of stethoscope by applying firm pressure over the chest piece.

Fig. 5.17: Illustration showing placement of pleximeter finger during percussion of heart borders.

(AR: aortic regurgitation; MR: mitral regurgitation; MS: mitral stenosis; TS: tricuspid stenosis)

Topographical areas of heart (Fig. 5.19):

Mitral area	Corresponds to apex (normally in left 5th ICS 1–2 cm medial to midclavicular line
Tricuspid area	Lower left sternal edge corresponding to 5th ICS
Aortic area	Right 2nd ICS
Neoaortic area (Erb's neoaortic area)	Left 3rd ICS
Pulmonary area	Left 2nd ICS
Other areas:	
Axilla	PSM of MR
Epigastrium area	PSM of TR
Carotid artery	Conduction of AS murmur Carotid bruit
Gibson's area	Left 1st ICS (PDA)
Roger's area	Left 4th ICS (VSD)
Interscapular area	Coarctation of aorta Aneurysm of descending aorta
Subclavian artery (supraclavicular area)	Bruit over this area heard in aortoarteritis
Femoral artery	Duroziez's murmur of AR

(ICS: intercostal space; MR: mitral regurgitation; TR: tricuspid regurgitation; PDA: patent ductus arteriosus; VSD: ventricular septal defect)

Sequence of auscultation:

Levine and Harvey inching method of auscultation
↓
Apex
↓
Left axilla
↓
Tricuspid area
↓
Epigastrium
↓
Neoaortic area
↓
Base of heart (aortic and pulmonary area)
↓
Clavicle, above and below
↓
Carotids

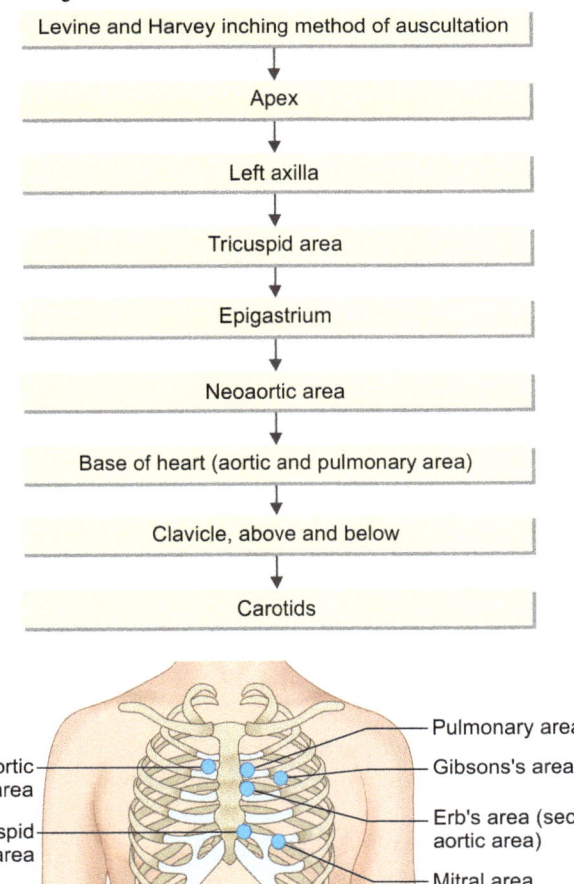

Fig. 5.19: Illustration of areas of auscultation.

Position of patient during auscultation:

Left lateral decubitus	Mitral area
Supine	Tricuspid area
Sitting and leaning forward (Erb's maneuver)	Aortic or pulmonary area

Heart Sounds

First Heart Sound (S1)

- Two audible components (M1 and T1)
- Two inaudible components (muscular in origin coinciding with beginning of LV contraction and opening with semilunar valves, respectively)
- M1-T1 interval = 20 ms
- It is loudest at apex.
- It coincides with carotid upstroke.
- *Determinants of S1:*
  - Structural integrity of valve
  - Position of the valve at the onset of ventricular systole
  - PR interval (inversely proportional)
  - Increased ionotropic activity of heart (directly proportional)
  - Loss of isovolumetric contraction leads to soft S1 (MR, AR, and VSD)
  - Thoracic cavity and chest wall (high-frequency murmurs are more attenuated with soft tissues)

Variations of S1:

Loud	Soft	Variable
• MS (mild to moderate) and TS • ASD (loud T1)	• Muffled in pansystolic murmurs—MR, TR (here valves are wide and do not coaptate)	• Atrial fibrillation • Ventricular tachycardia (AV dissociation)
• Tachycardia • Short PR interval • Hyperdynamic circulation • Thin people	• MS (severe calcification) • AR (increased LV filling and premature closure of mitral valve) • Bradycardia • Long PR and heart blocks • Obesity, emphysema, and effusion	• Complete heart blocks (cannon sound)

When do you say loud S1?
- When S1 is heard with the same intensity as of mitral area in the base of heart (aortic and pulmonary areas)

Splitting of S1:

Wide splitting	Reverse splitting (T1 before M1)
• Ebstein's anomaly • ASD • Complete RBBB • LV pacing	• Ectopics • Severe MS • Complete LBBB • RV pacing

Note: Ebstein's anomaly on can hear S1 split, S2 split, OS, S4 and pulmonary ejection click.

(MS: mitral stenosis; TS: tricuspid stenosis; ASD: atrial septal defect; RBBB: right bundle branch block; LBBB: left bundle branch block; RV: right ventricle; LV: left ventricle; MR: mitral regurgitation; TR: tricuspid regurgitation)

Second Heart Sound (S2)

- Two components (A2 and P2)
- A2-P2 time interval is <30 ms (expiration) and 40-50 ms (inspiration)
- Heard best in base of the heart (pulmonary and aortic areas)
- The loudest component of S2 in pulmonary area is A2
- The loudest component of S2 in aortic area is A2
- *Hangout interval*: The time interval from the crossover of pressures between ventricles and the arteries to the actual closure of valves is called hangout interval.
- Mechanism of normal split of S2:
  - During inspiration, there is an increase in the capacitance of pulmonary vascular bed, this results in the delay of rise of pulmonary arterial pressure resulting in prolonged pulmonary hangout interval.
  - Early A2 (contributes around 27%)
  - Delayed P2 (contributes for 73%)
- Physiological split is inspiratory and disappears on standing, due to decreased venous return (while pathological split persists on standing).

Variations of S2 (Fig. 5.20):

A2	
Loud	**Soft**
• Hyperdynamic state • sHTN • Aneurysm of aorta • Aortic root dilatation (e.g., syphilis and ankylosing spondylosis) • TGA • Pulmonary atresia	• AS • AR • Aortic sclerosis (elderly) • Thick chest wall, obesity, and emphysema

When do you say loud A2?
Normally, A2 is loudest at the base (aortic and pulmonary area). A2 is considered to be loud, if the intensity in the mitral area is same as the base of the heart.

P2:	
Loud	**Soft**
• Hyperkinetic states • pHTN • Dilation of pulmonary trunk • Aneurysm of pulmonary artery • Thin chest wall • Condition with left to right shunt	• PS • Dysplastic pulmonary valve • Thick chest wall, obesity, and emphysema

When do you say loud P2?
Normally, A2 is louder than P2 even in pulmonary area but if P2 is as loud as A2 then P2 is considered as loud P2.

Single S2:
• Severe AS and aortic atresia • Severe PS and pulmonary atresia • Fallot's tetralogy (A2 becomes loud and P2 disappears)

(AR: aortic regurgitation; AS: aortic stenosis; HTN: hypertension; PS: pulmonary stenosis; TGA: transposition of the great artery)

Splitting of 2nd heart sound:

Narrow split	Wide split	
	Variable	**Fixed**
Severe pHTN	• *Chest deformity*— funnel chest and straight back syndrome • *Due to early A2*—MR and VSD • *Due to late P2*—RBBB, LV pacing, and ectopics from LV	• ASD • Severe RV failure • Acute pulmonary embolism

Note:
Why do you get wide fixed split in ASD?

Wide split is due to:	Fixed split is due to:
• Increased RV ejection time • Prolonged pulmonary hangout interval • RBBB	• Free communication between two atria equalizes the pressure during inspiration and expiration • Already prolonged pulmonary hangout interval cannot be further prolonged

Paradoxical split (reverse split):	
• P2 comes before A2 • Split is prominent and wider during expiration, while it narrows during inspiration • Causes due to either early P2 or late A2	
Early P2	**Late A2**
• Complete LBBB • RV pacing • PVCs of RV	• Severe AS • Severe sHTN • HCM

(AS: aortic stenosis; ASD: atrial septal defect; HTN: hypertension; HCM: hypertrophic cardiomyopathy; LBBB: left bundle branch block; RBBB: right bundle branch block; PVC: premature ventricular contraction; RV: right ventricle; LV: left ventricle)

Diastolic Heart Sounds

(S3, Pericardial knock, and S4)

Third Heart Sound (S3)

- Third heart sound (S3) is a low-pitched early diastolic sound best heard with the bell.
- It coincides with rapid ventricular filling immediately after opening of the atrioventricular valves and is therefore heard after the second as "lub-dub-dum"
- It is almost never heard at the base of heart (aortic and pulmonary area).
- It is less palpable than S4.
- It is sign of ventricular systolic dysfunction.
- *Prerequisite*:
  - Nonobstructed AV valve
- *Best heard with bell*:
  - LVS3—left lateral position at apex during expiration
  - RVS3—left sternal edge in supine during inspiration

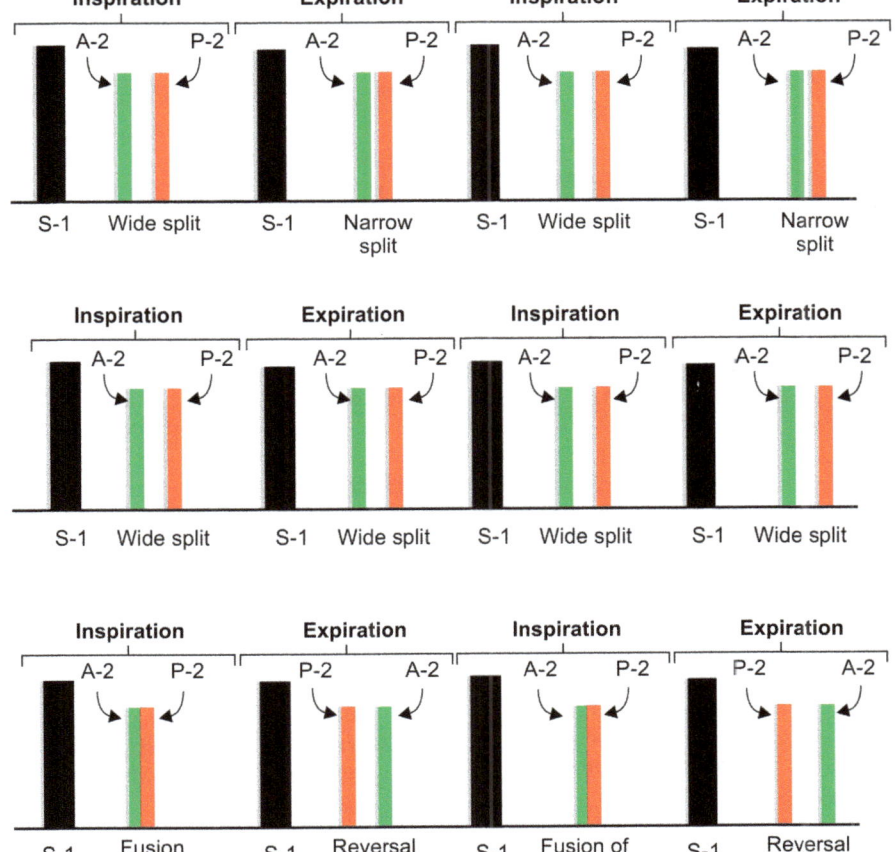

Fig. 5.20: Variations of 2nd heart sound.

Causes of S3:

Physiological and hyperdynamic states	Pathological LV S3	Pathological RV S3
• Children • Under 40 years • Athletes • Pregnancy • and • Other hyperdynamic states	• Left ventricular failure • Aortic regurgitation • Mitral regurgitation • Ischemic heart disease • Cardiomyopathy	• Right ventricular failure • Endomyocardial fibrosis

Pericardial knock:

☐ *Cause*—sudden cessation of ventricular filling
☐ Seen in—constrictive pericarditis
☐ Timing—comes earlier than S3
☐ Frequency—higher than S3
☐ *Diastolic knock* is palpable pericardial knock in constrictive pericarditis
☐ Correlates with other clinical findings such as:
  • Rapidly descent
  • Kussmaul's sign
  • Systolic retraction of apex (Broadbent's sign)
  • Congestive hepatomegaly with ascites

Fourth Heart Sound (S4)

☐ It is a low frequency late diastolic or presystolic sound heard during atrial contraction.
☐ It is also called as a presystolic or an atrial diastolic gallop (even though its ventricular in origin).
☐ Prerequisites
☐ Healthy contracting atrium
☐ Nonobstructive AV valve
☐ Noncomplaint (stiff) ventricle
☐ Theories of production of S4
☐ Ventricular theory (rapid deceleration of incoming blood)
☐ Impact theory (dynamic impact of the heart with chest wall)
☐ Best head with bell
☐ LVS4—left lateral position at apex during expiration
☐ RVS4—left sternal edge in supine position during inspiration
☐ S4 may be confused with spilt S1. Firm pressure by the diaphragm of stethoscope eliminates S4 but not split S1.

Causes of S4:

☐ Physiological: >60 years
☐ Pathological:

Pathological S4:

RV S4	LV S4
Right ventricular hypertrophy due to: • Pulmonary hypertension • Pulmonary stenosis	• Systemic hypertension • Hypertrophic cardiomyopathy • Ischemic heart disease (especially acute myocardial infarction) • Acute mitral regurgitation • Anemia, thyrotoxicosis, and AV fistula

(AV: atrioventricular; LV: left ventricle; RV: right ventricle)

> **Note:**
> - **Triple gallop rhythm:** S1, S2, and S3 (or S4) with HR >100
> - **Summation rhythm:** S1, S2, S3, and S4 with HR >100

Clicks and Snaps

Clicks	Snaps
High-pitched systolic sounds	High-pitched diastolic sounds
Produced by aortic and pulmonary valve opening	Produced by mitral and tricuspid valve opening

Clicks

Clicks	Ejection clicks		Nonejection clicks
Timing	Early systolic		Mid-to-late systolic
Pathology	Vascular (dilated vessel)	Valvular (diseased valve)	Valve prolapse
Left-sided causes	• Systemic hypertension • Aneurysm of aortic root	Bicuspid aortic valve	Mitral valve prolapse
Right-sided causes	Dilated pulmonary artery (idiopathic or secondary to PAH)	Congenital pulmonary stenosis	Tricuspid valve prolapse

(PAH: pulmonary arterial hypertension)

> **Note:** Pulmonary valvular ejection click seen in congenital pulmonary stenosis is the only event occurring in the right side of the heart, which is better heard on expiration.

Opening snap:
- It is high-pitched diastolic sound occurring 0.04–0.12 seconds after A2 (S3 occurs 0.12 second after A2) due to opening of mitral or tricuspid valves.
- It occurs after S2 and before S3
- *Mechanism of opening snap (OS):*
  - Stenotic anterior mitral/tricuspid valve leaflet suddenly bulging downward into the ventricular cavity such as a dome, with a snapping sound when the valve is rapidly opened during diastole. So, OS is heard only if leaflets are mobile.
  - OS occurs when movement of valve suddenly stops, at point when ventricular pressure drops below that of atrial pressure.

In mitral stenosis:
- It is the most important auscultatory sign of valvular involvement in MS (pathognomonic sign)
- Absent OS indicates the calcification of body of the mitral leaflets.
- The time interval between A2 and OS is inversely proportional to the severity of the MS.
- *Best heard:* During expiration, just medial to the cardiac apex with the diaphragm of the stethoscope.

Other conditions with OS:
- Mitral regurgitation (10%)
- Tricuspid stenosis
- Atrial septal defect

Differences between OS, split S2, and S3:

	Opening snap (OS)	S2 split	S3
Area	Medial to apex	Base of heart	At the apex
On standing	A2-OS increases	A2-P2 decreases	Disappears
Pitch	High	High	Low
Best heard	Diaphragm	Diaphragm	Bell

Other sounds:

Tumor plop	Seen in myxomas
Prosthetic valve sounds	• Metallic S1 heard with mechanical mitral valve • Metallic S2 heard with mechanical aortic valve • Bioprosthetic valves heart sounds are normal

Pericardial Rub

It is the sound produced due to sliding (apposition) of the two inflamed layers (visceral and parietal pericardium) of the pericardium.
- **Phases:** It is triphasic
  1. Mid-systolic
  2. Mid-diastolic
  3. Presystolic
- **Character:** It is scratchy, grating, leathery, or creaking in character. Its intensity varies over time, and with the position of the patient.
- **Best heard:** With diaphragm of stethoscope on the left sternal border (3rd and 4th intercostal space) leaning over at the end of expiration. It may be audible over any part of the precordium but is often localized. It can be better appreciated with patient in knee elbow position.
- A pleuropericardial rub is a similar sound that occurs in time with the cardiac cycle but is also influenced by respiration and is pleural in origin.

Murmurs

Sudden deceleration of blood produces heart sounds while heart murmurs are produced by turbulent flow (Reynolds number >2,000) across an abnormal valve, septal defect or outflow obstruction, or by increased volume or velocity of flow through a normal valve.

Mechanism
- Increased blood velocity
- Decreased blood viscosity
- *Valve*: Narrowed or incompetent; organic or relative
- Abnormal connection
- Vibration of loose structure
- Diameter of vessel increased or decreased

Murmurs are described under the following headings:
- Timing
- Grade
- Quality
- Pitch
- Configuration
- Radiation
- Best heard with diaphragm or bell

- Patient position
- With breath held in inspiration or expiration
- Variation with other maneuvers
- Location of maximum intensity

1. *Timing (Fig. 5.21):*

Timing refers to the portion of the cardiac cycle that the murmur occupies. Murmurs may be systolic, diastolic, or continuous.

Systolic murmurs may be:
- Early systolic murmurs
- Mid-systolic murmurs
- Late systolic murmurs
- Pansystolic murmurs

Systolic murmurs:

Murmur and description	Example
Early systolic murmurs (begin with the first heart sound and extend to middle or late systole)	• VSD (small muscular VSD/large VSD with pulmonary hypertension) • Acute severe MR • Acute severe TR
Mid-systolic/ejection systolic murmurs [begin following a murmur-free interval in early systole and end with a murmur-free interval (of variable duration) in late systole]	• Aortic stenosis • Pulmonary stenosis • HOCM
Late systolic murmurs (begin during the last half of systole and may or may not extend to the second heart sound)	• Mitral valve prolapse • Tricuspid valve prolapse • Papillary muscle dysfunction
Pansystolic murmurs (begin with the first heart sound and extend to or through the second heart sound)	• Mitral regurgitation • Tricuspid regurgitation • Ventricular septal defect • Rare—early PDA/PDA with Eisenmenger

(HOCM: hypertrophic obstructive cardiomyopathy; PDA: patent ductus arteriosus; VSD: ventricular septal defect)

Diastolic murmurs may be:
- Early diastolic
- Mid-diastolic
- Late diastolic/presystolic

Diastolic murmur:

Murmur	Example
Early diastolic murmur	• Aortic regurgitation • Pulmonary regurgitation

Mid-diastolic murmur	• Mitral stenosis
	• Tricuspid stenosis
	• Carrey Coombs murmur of acute rheumatic fever
	• Austin Flint murmur of chronic aortic regurgitation
	• Flow MDM:
	  ▪ Across mitral valve
	    – MR, AR, VSD, and PDA
	  ▪ Across tricuspid valve
	    – ASD, TR, and TAPVC
	• Atrial myxoma
	• Ball valve thrombus
	• Cor triatriatum
	• Rytand's murmur of complete heart block

Late diastolic murmurs/presystolic murmur	• Mitral stenosis • Tricuspid stenosis • Myxoma

(AR: aortic regurgitation; ASD: atrial septal defect; MR: mitral regurgitation; PDA: patent ductus arteriosus; VSD: ventricular septal defect; TAPVC: total anomalous pulmonary venous connection)

Continuous murmurs:

The continuous murmur is the murmur that begins in systole and continues without interruption, *encompassing the second sound,* throughout diastole or part of diastole.

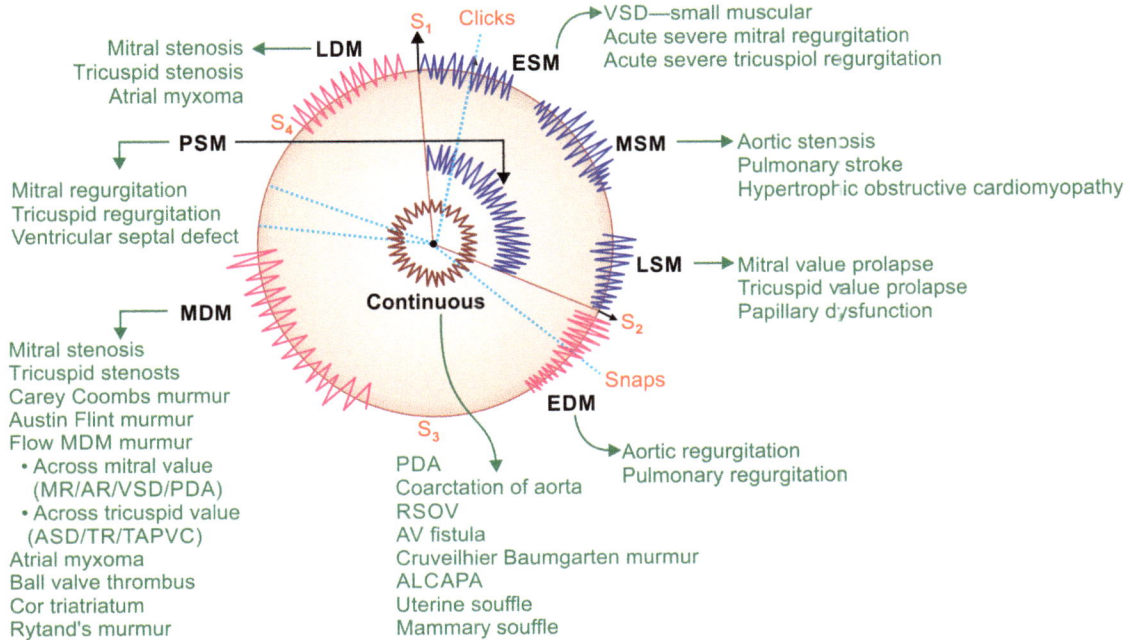

Fig. 5.21: Timing of murmurs and examples.

Classification of continuous murmurs:

Systemic to pulmonary communication:
- Patent ductus arteriosus
- Aortopulmonary window
- Anomalous origin of left coronary artery from pulmonary artery (ALCAPA)
- Tricuspid atresia
- Truncus arteriosus
- Shunts for TOF surgery—Waterson, Potts, or Blalock–Taussig shunt

Systemic to right heart connection:
- Coronary AV fistula
- Rupture sinus of Valsalva

Left atrium to right atrium connection:
- Lutembacher syndrome

Arteriovenous fistula:
- Systemic
- Pulmonary

Normal flow through constricted arteries:
- Coarctation of aorta
- Peripheral pulmonary stenosis
- Renal artery stenosis

Increased flow through normal vessels:
- Venous:
  - Cervical venous hum
  - Cruveilhier–Baumgarten murmur
- Arterial:
  - Mammary soufflé
  - Uterine soufflé
  - Thyrotoxicosis
  - Tumors—hepatoma and hypernephroma

Differential diagnosis of continuous murmur:

Systolic–diastolic murmurs	To and fro murmurs
Murmur in systolic and murmur in diastolic but S2 is heard distinctly. The two murmurs are separated by small silence differentiating them from continuous murmurs.	
Occurs through different orifices:	*Occurs through same orifice:*
• VSD with AR • MR with MS	• AS with AR • Pulmonary hypertension with Pulmonary regurgitation

(AR: aortic regurgitation; AS: aortic stenosis; MR: mitral regurgitation; MS: mitral stenosis; VSD: ventricular septal defect)

2. Grading of murmurs:
Systolic murmurs:
Levine and Freeman grading of systolic murmurs:

Grade	Description	Thrill
Grade 1	Murmur so faint that it can be heard only with special effort.	Absent
Grade 2	Murmur is faint, but is immediately audible	
Grade 3	Murmur that is moderately loud	
Grade 4	Murmur that is very loud	Present
Grade 5	A murmur is extremely loud and is audible with one edge of the stethoscope touching the chest wall	
Grade 6	A murmur is so loud that it is audible with the stethoscope just removed from contact with the chest wall	

Diastolic murmurs (by AIIMS):

Grade	Description	Thrill
Grade 1	Very soft	
Grade 2	Soft	Absent
Grade 3	Loud	
Grade 4	Very loud	Present

3. Character/quality:
Quality refers to the tonal effect of the murmurs. Frequently used descriptors are *blowing, musical, squeaking, whooping, honking, harsh, rasping, grunting, and rumbling.*

4. Frequency or pitch:
- It relates to the velocity of blood at the site of origin of the murmur and is designated as high, medium, or low. In general, the higher the velocity, the higher the pitch of the murmur.
- Murmurs that emanate from areas of stenosis where velocity is lower are typically low-to-medium pitched.

5. Configuration (Figs. 5.22 to 5.24):
Configuration of a murmur refers to its shape.
- To a large degree, it is a function of intensity and duration.
- Crescendo murmurs progressively increase in intensity.

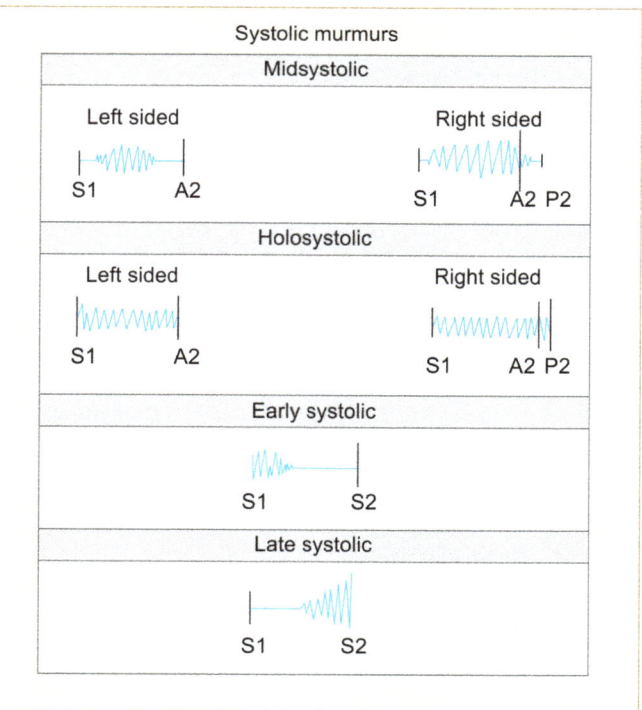

Fig. 5.22: Configuration of systolic murmurs.

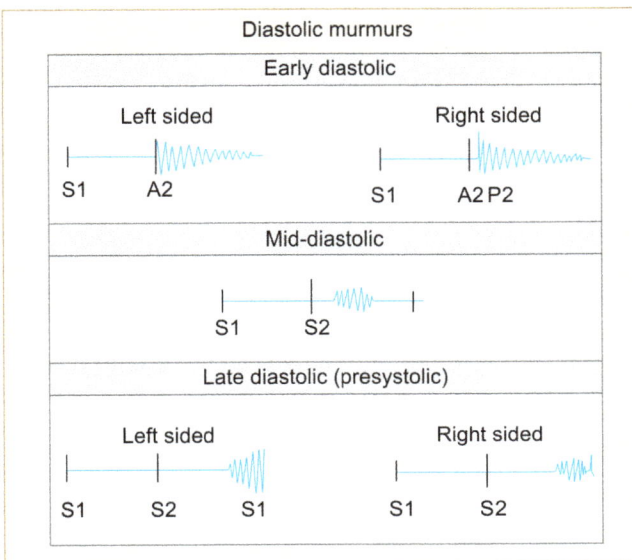

Fig. 5.23: Configuration of diastolic murmurs.

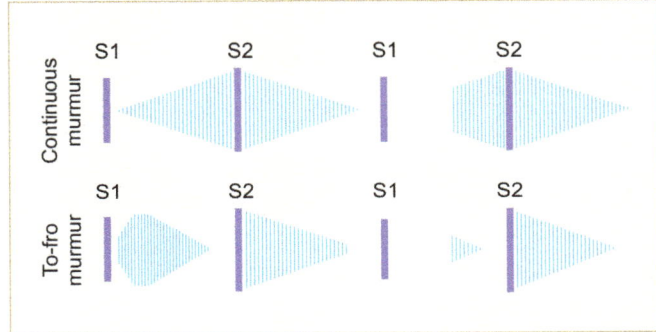

Fig. 5.24: Configuration of continuous and to-and-fro murmurs.

- Decrescendo murmurs progressively decrease in intensity.
- With crescendo–decrescendo murmurs (diamond or kite-shaped murmurs), a progressive increase in intensity is followed by a progressive decrease in intensity.
- Plateau murmurs maintain a relatively constant intensity.

6. Radiation/conduction (Fig. 5.25):
It reflects the intensity of the murmur and the direction of blood flow.

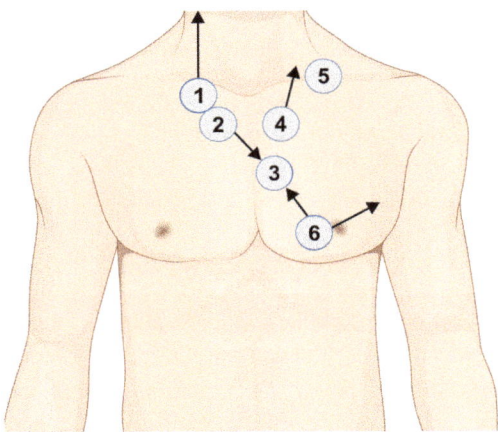

Fig. 5.25: Figure showing radiation of murmurs.

Radiation	Conduction
It is through noncardiac structures	It is through anatomical continuity
Intensity decreases with distance	Intensity remains same or decreases with distance
• Mitral regurgitation murmur (PSM) radiates to axilla. • Tricuspid regurgitation radiates to epigastrium.	Aortic stenosis murmur (ESM) conducts to the carotid.

(PSM: pansystolic murmur; ESM: early systolic murmur)

- Early systolic murmur (ESM) of AS conducting to carotids
- Early diastolic murmur (EDM) of AR in right 2nd ICS radiating to left 3rd ICS
- Pansystolic murmur (PSM) of TR radiating to upper left sternal border
- ESM of PS conducting toward clavicle
- Murmur of PDA at infraclavicular area radiates to back
- PSM of MR radiating to axilla or base of heart

7. Best heard with bell or diaphragm:

Best heard with bell	Best heard with diaphragm
MDM of MS and TS (other sounds: S3, S4, and pericardial knock)	Systolic murmur of MR, TR, AS, and diastolic murmur of AR (other sounds: S1, S2, ESC, and OS)

(AR: aortic regurgitation; AS: aortic stenosis; MS: mitral stenosis; TS: tricuspid stenosis; MR: mitral regurgitation; TR: tricuspid regurgitation)

8. Variation with position:

Left lateral recumbent position	Sitting and leaning forward	Lying flat or passive leg raising in supine position
Accentuates: Sounds: • S1 • LVS3 and LVS4 • OS of MS Murmurs: • MS • MR • Click and murmur of MVP • Austin Flint murmur	Accentuates: Murmurs: • AR • PR	Accentuates: Sounds: • S3 and S4 Murmurs: • Valvular AS/PS • TR Attenuates: • EDM of AR • Murmur of HOCM • MVP murmur and click are delayed

(AR: aortic regurgitation; AS: aortic stenosis; HOCM: hypertrophic obstructive cardiomyopathy; LV: left ventricle; PR: pulmonary regurgitation; PS: pulmonary stenosis; MS: mitral stenosis; MR: mitral regurgitation; EDM: early diastolic murmur; TR: tricuspid regurgitation)

9. Variation with respiration:
Breathing produces a greater effect on the right side of the heart than the left side.

Right-sided murmurs increase on inspiration	Left-sided murmurs increase on expiration
Inspiration increases venous return to the right side of the heart by increasing flow in the vena cava, but decreases venous return to the left side of the heart due to pooling of blood in pulmonary venous capacitance vessels	Expiration decreases venous return to the right side of the heart by reducing vena cava flow, but increases venous return to the left side of the heart due to collapse of pulmonary venous capacitance vessels

Contd...

Contd...

Right-sided murmurs increase on inspiration	Left-sided murmurs increase on expiration
• TS • TR (Carvallo's sign*) • PR • Mild or moderate PS • Severe PS	• MS • MR • AS • AR • VSD • Pericardial rub

(AR: aortic regurgitation; AS: aortic stenosis; MR: mitral regurgitation; MS: mitral stenosis; PR: pulmonary regurgitation; PS: pulmonary stenosis; TR: tricuspid regurgitation; TS: tricuspid stenosis; VSD: ventricular septal defect)

- *Carvallo's sign**—when the murmur of tricuspid valve regurgitation gets louder with deep inspiration.
- The effects of inspiration on systolic murmurs can be accentuated by employing Mueller's maneuver (forced inspiration on a closed glottis).

10. Variation with other maneuvers:
- The physiologic maneuvers are breathing, standing, sudden squatting, isometric hand grip exercise, Valsalva maneuver (described at the end), passive leg raising, and attention to the beat following a post-extrasystolic pause.
- The pharmacologic interventions used most commonly in clinical practice are amyl nitrite administration and intravenous infusion of alpha-adrenergic agonists (phenylephrine or methoxamine).

Valvular disease	Accentuated by	Attenuated by
MS	Expiration Exercise, squatting, amyl nitrate, and isometric handgrip	Inspiration, sudden standing
MR	• Expiration • Squatting • Isometric exercise	• Sudden standing • Valsalva • Amyl nitrate
AS	Expiration Post-PVC beat • Squatting • Lying flat from standing	• Valsalva • Standing • Handgrip
AR	• Expiration • Sitting up and leaning forward • Squatting • Isometric exercise • Vasopressors	• Amyl Nitrate • Valsalva
MVP	Murmur and click later If LV volume increases: • Squatting • Postectopic • Isometric exercise (intensity increases)	Murmur and click Earlier: If LV volume decreases: • Standing • Valsalva
HOCM	• Expiration • Valsalva strain • Standing • Postectopic • Amyl nitrate	• Inspiration • Sustained handgrip • Squatting • Methoxamine

(AR: aortic regurgitation; AS: aortic stenosis; HOCM: hypertrophic obstructive cardiomyopathy; MR: mitral regurgitation; MS: mitral stenosis; LV: left ventricle)

11. Location of maximum intensity of murmur:
- Location refers to the point on the precordium where the murmur is heard with maximum intensity.
- Many systolic murmurs are audible over multiple areas of the precordium. Localizing their point of maximum intensity may aid greatly in determining their site of evolution.

For example:
In aortic stenosis/aortic sclerosis, Gallavardin phenomenon is seen. Two distinct systolic murmurs are heard one high-pitched murmur in the aortic area and the other musical systolic murmur in the mitral area. This is due to periodic wake phenomena.

Examples for how to describe a murmur:

The murmur of mitral stenosis is a mid-diastolic low-pitched rough rumbling murmur with presystolic accentuation is best audible at the apex (mitral area), in the left lateral position with the bell of the stethoscope, patients breath held in expiration. The murmur increases on isometric hand grip.
The murmur of aortic regurgitation is a soft, high-pitched, early diastolic, decrescendo murmur usually heard best at the third intercostal space on the left (Erb's point) with the diaphragm of the stethoscope at end expiration with the patient sitting up and leaning forward.

Innocent murmurs:
Innocent murmurs are those not due to recognizable lesions of the heart or blood vessels. They are most common in children and adolescents.

The Seven S's of innocent murmurs:

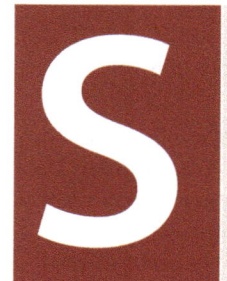

1. Sensitive (changes with child's position or with respiration)
2. Short duration (not holosystolic)
3. Single (no associated clicks or gallops)
4. Small (murmur limited to a small area and nonradiating)
5. Soft (low amplitude)
6. Sweet (not harsh sounding)
7. Systolic (occurs during and is limited to systole)

Examples of innocent murmurs:

Systolic	• Vibratory systolic murmur (Still's murmur) • Pulmonic systolic murmur (pulmonary trunk) • Mammary soufflé • Peripheral pulmonic systolic murmur (pulmonary branches) • Supraclavicular or brachiocephalic systolic murmur • Aortic systolic murmur • Still's murmur
Diastolic	*All diastolic murmurs are pathological* (not innocent)
Continuous	• Venous hum • Continuous mammary soufflé

Named murmurs	
Carey Coombs murmur	Mid-diastolic murmur, in rheumatic fever
Austin Flint murmur	Mid-late diastolic murmur, in aortic regurgitation

Contd...

Contd...

Named murmurs	
Graham–Steel murmur	High-pitched, diastolic, in pulmonary regurgitation
Rytand's murmur	Mid-diastolic atypical murmur, in complete heart block
Dock's murmur	Diastolic murmur, left anterior descending (LAD) artery stenosis
Mill–Wheel murmur	Due to air in RV cavity following cardiac catheterization
Still's murmur	Inferior aspect of lower left sternal border, systolic ejection sound, vibratory/musical quality, in subaortic stenosis, and small VSD
Gibson's murmur	Continuous machinery murmur of PDA
Key–Hodgkin murmur	Diastolic murmur of aortic regurgitation. Hodgkin correlated this diastolic murmur with retroversion of the aortic valve leaflets, seen in syphilitic aortic regurgitation.
Cabot–Locke murmur	Diastolic murmur is heard best at the left sternal border, heard in anemic patients. The murmur resolves with treatment of anemia.
Roger's murmur	It is the loud pansystolic murmur, which is heard maximally at the left sternal border in small VSD.
Pontains murmur	Cervical venous hum in severe anemia
Cole-Cecil murmur	AR murmur in left axilla due to higher position of apex
Cruveilhier–Baumgarten venous hum	It is diagnostic of portal hypertension

(AR: aortic regurgitation; PDA: patent ductus arteriosus; RV: right ventricle; VSD: ventricular septal defect)

Auscultation for mitral stenosis (Fig. 5.26):
☐ Patient in left lateral position

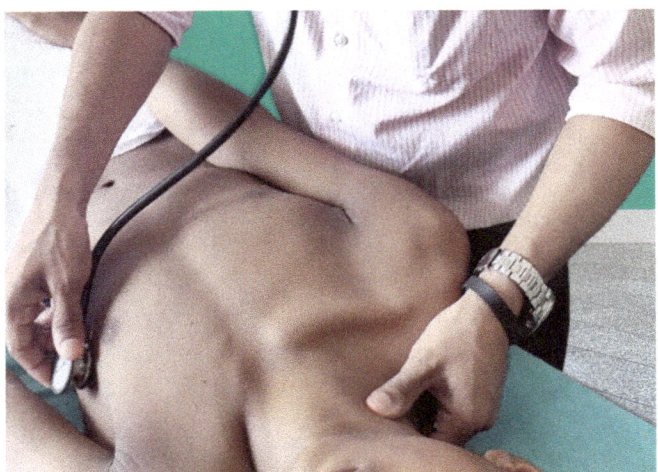

Fig. 5.26: Auscultation of mitral area MDM of mitral stenosis.

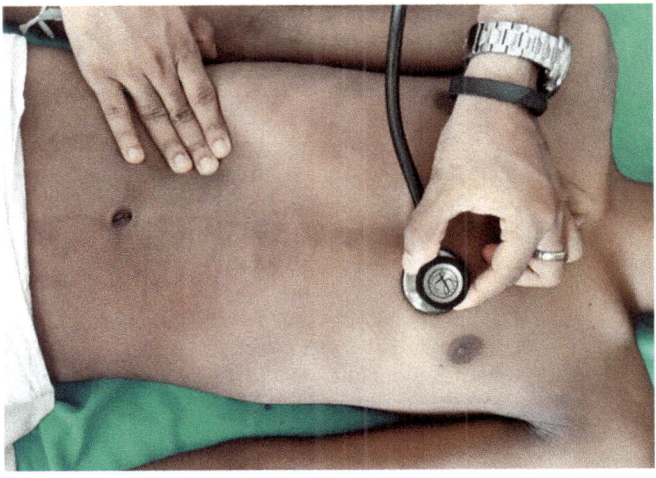

Fig. 5.27: Auscultation of tricuspid regurgitation.

☐ Breath held in expiration
☐ Using bell of stethoscope
☐ Time the murmur with carotid

Auscultation of tricuspid area (Fig. 5.27):
☐ Patient in supine position
☐ Breath held in inspiration
☐ Using diaphragm of stethoscope
☐ Murmur increased on hepatic compression

Auscultation of aortic area (Fig. 5.28):
☐ Patient in sitting up and leaning forward position
☐ Breath held in expiration
☐ Using diaphragm of stethoscope
☐ Time the murmur with carotid

Changing murmurs:
Murmurs, which change in character or intensity from moment to moment:
- Carey-Coombs' murmur
- Infective endocarditis
- Atrial thrombus
- Atrial myxomas

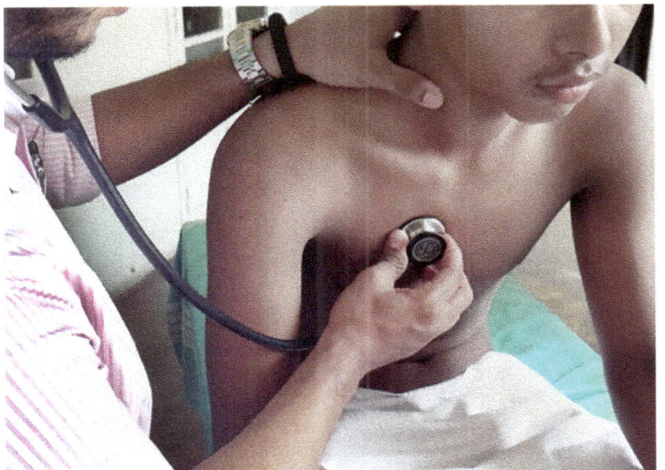

Fig. 5.28: Auscultation of aortic area (Erb's maneuver).

Other system examination:

Respiratory system	• Hoarseness of voice (enlarged left atrium—Ortner's syndrome) • Hemoptysis • Left lower lobe collapse or consolidation (pericardial effusion) • Basal crepitations (LVF) • Pleural effusion (LVF) • Rhonchi (pulmonary edema)
GIT	• Tender hepatomegaly (right heart failure) • Splenomegaly (infective endocarditis) • Ascites (right heart failure) • Dysphagia (due to large left atrium)
Nervous system	• Stroke (hemiplegia/Horner's syndrome and cranial nerve palsies)

(GIT: gastrointestinal tract; LVF: left ventricular failure)

Pulsatile liver:
Examination of pulsatile liver:
☐ Patient in 45° recumbent position
☐ Two methods are described
1. *Bimanual palpation* **(Fig. 5.29)**: Place one palm over the anterior surface of the right lower chest and other palm on the posterolateral surface of the right lower chest. Pulsations of the liver are felt between the two palms.
2. *Make fist of the* right hand **(Fig. 5.30)** and place the knuckles and fingers in the right lower intercostal spaces and feel for the pulsatile liver as shown in **Figure 5.30**.

Systolic pulsation	Diastolic pulsations (presystolic)
• TR • AR	TS

(AR: aortic regurgitation; TR: tricuspid regurgitation; TS: tricuspid stenosis)

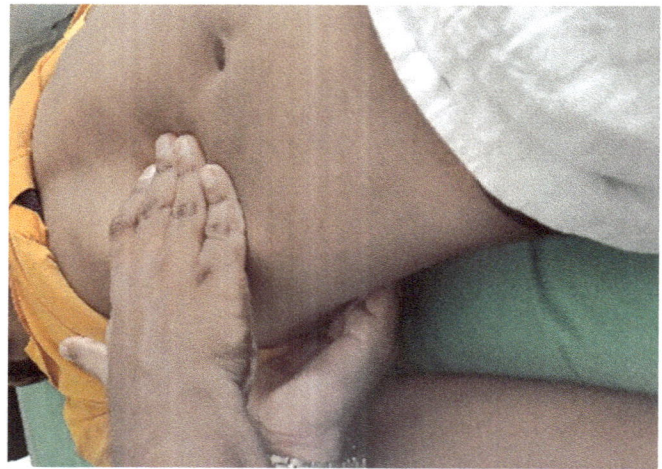

Fig. 5.29: Bimanual method of palpation of pulsatile liver.

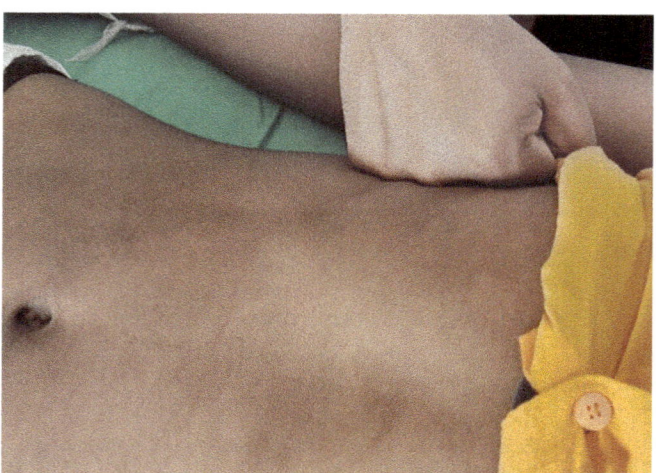

Fig. 5.30: Examining the pulsatile liver by making fist and placing the knuckles and fingers in the intercostal spaces.

Findings	MS	MR	AS	AR	TR	ASD	VSD	PDA
Pulse	Low volume Irregularly irregular (if associated with AF)	High volume Irregularly irregular (if associated with AF)	Low volume Pulsus parvus et tardus Anacrotic pulse Apicocarotid delay—severe AS	High volume Collapsing pulse Water hammer pulse Pulsus bisferiens	Normal	Normal Irregularly irregular (if associated with AF)	High volume	High volume, collapsing
Blood pressure	Low BP Mean of 3 readings to be taken, if atrial fibrillation is present	Wide pulse pressure Mean of 3 readings to be taken, if atrial fibrillation is present	Low BP Systolic decapitation Coanda effect: Right upper limb BP > left upper limb BP (supravalvular AS)	Wide pulse pressure Hill's sign—lower limb BP >20 mm of upper limb BP	Normal	Normal	Wide pulse pressure	Wide pulse pressure
JVP	Raised in heart failure Prominent a waves—pulmonary hypertension without atrial fibrillation Absence of a wave—atrial fibrillation Prominent v waves (c-v waves) and rapid y descent—tricuspid regurgitation	Raised in heart failure Prominent a waves—pulmonary hypertension without atrial fibrillation Absence of a wave—atrial fibrillation Prominent v waves (c-v waves) and rapid y descent—tricuspid regurgitation	Usually normal Raised in heart failure Rarely prominent a wave—Bernheim effect	Usually normal Raised in heart failure	Raised with most prominent "giant" v wave in the jugular venous pulse (a cv wave replaces the normal x descent) Earlobe pulsations (Lancisi's sign)	"M" pattern—a and v waves have equal height a wave becomes taller when pulmonary hypertension develops or associated mitral stenosis (MS)	Raised in heart failure	Raised in heart failure
Apex	Tapping apex	Hyperdynamic Down and out apex	Heaving	Hyperdynamic Down and out apex	Normal	Normal	Mild displaced down and out	Hyperdynamic Down and out apex
Parasternal heave	Present (RVH or left atrial enlargement)	Present (RVH or left atrial enlargement)	No	No		Present	Present	±
Thrills	Diastolic thrill at apex	Systolic thrill at apex in acute or severe MR	Systolic thrill over the aortic and carotid area	Diastolic thrill in aortic/neoaortic area	Systolic thrill in left lower sternal edge	Nil	Left 4–5 ICS parasternal area	Continuous thrill at the upper-left sternal edge

Contd...

Contd...

Findings		MS	MR	AS	AR	TR	ASD	VSD	PDA
Heart sounds	S1	Loud	Soft	Normal	Soft	Soft	Loud	Soft	Loud
	S2	Loud P2 (pulmonary hypertension) Narrow split (pulmonary hypertension)	Loud P2 (pulmonary hypertension) Narrow split (pulmonary hypertension)	Soft A2 (valvular AS) Loud A2 (bicuspid aortic valve) Paradoxical split (severe AS)	Normal Tambour A2 in syphilitic AR	Loud P2 with narrow split (pulmonary hypertension)	P2 loud Wide fixed split	P2 loud	P2 loud Paradoxical split
	S3	RV S3 (present in failure)	RV/LV S3 (present in failure)	LVS3 in failure	LVS3 in severe AR	RVS3	RVS3	±	±
	S4	Never	Present in acute MR	Present Indicates severe AS	±	—	RVS4 (Eisenmenger's)	RVS4 (Eisenmenger's)	RVS4 (Eisenmenger's)
	Others	Opening snap	OS in 10%	AEC in bicuspid aortic valve	—	—	PEC (Eisenmenger's)	PEC (Eisenmenger's)	PEC (Eisenmenger's)
Murmurs		MDM at mitral area PSM at tricuspid area ESM at pulmonary area EDM (Graham Steel) at pulmonary area	PSM in mitral area radiation to axilla/base Flow MDM at mitral area PSM at tricuspid area ESM at pulmonary area EDM (Graham Steel) at pulmonary area	ESM in aortic area conducting to carotid Systolic murmur at mitral area (Gallavardin phenomenon)	EDM in aortic/neoaortic area Flow ESM in aortic area MDM at mitral area (Austin Flint) Diastolic murmur in left axilla (Cole–Cecil murmur)	Blowing PSM At the lower-left sternal border that is increased during inspiration and reduced during expiration (de-Carvallo's sign)	ESM in pulmonary area and MDM in tricuspid area Once Eisenmenger's—EDM in pulmonary area and PSM in tricuspid area	PSM heard best at the left sternal edge (3rd, 4th and 5th intercostal space)	Continuous harsh "machinery-like/Gibson's murmur heard with late systolic accentuation in the first left intercostal space below the clavicle
Other features		Palpable P2 (diastolic shock)	Palpable P2 (diastolic shock)	—	Peripheral signs	Pulsatile liver	Precordial bulge	Aortic insufficiency in approximately 5%	Differential cyanosis and clubbing when Eisenmenger's develops

(AF: atrial fibrillation; MS: mitral stenosis; MR: mitral regurgitation; AS: aortic stenosis; AR: aortic regurgitation; TR: tricuspid regurgitation; ASD: atrial septal defect; VSD: ventricular septal defect; PDA: patent ductus arteriosus; JVP: jugular venous pressure; EDM: early diastolic murmur; ESM: early systolic murmur; PSM: pansystolic murmur; ICS: intercostal space)

OBJECTIVE-BASED SELF-EVALUATION

SHORT ANSWER QUESTIONS

1. Differenting features of ischemic cardiac and noncardiac pain.
2. Angina equivalents.
3. Causes of palpitations.
4. Causes of true syncope.
5. Signs of infective endocarditis.
6. Apical impulse—definition and characteristics.
7. First heart sound.
8. Name the diastolic heart sound and give causes for each.
9. List causes for mid-diastolic murmurs.
10. List causes for pansystolic murmurs.
11. List causes for continuous murmurs.
12. Enumerate the signs on cardiac examination of a patient with mitral stenosis.
13. Enumerate the signs on cardiac examination of a patient with aortic stenosis.
14. Enumerate the signs on cardiac examination of a patient with mitral regurgitation.
15. Enumerate the signs on cardiac examination of a patient with aortic regurgitation.

MULTIPLE CHOICE QUESTIONS

1. **Causes of soft first heart sound includes:**
   a. Obesity
   b. Mitral regurgitation
   c. Left sided pleural effusion
   d. All of the above
2. **Erb's area in cardiology refers to:**
   a. Right 2nd intercostal space
   b. Left 2nd intercostal space
   c. Right 3rd intercostal space
   d. Left 3rd intercostal space
3. **Wide fixed split second heat sound occurs in:**
   a. Ventricular septal defect (VSD)
   b. Mitral stenosis
   c. Atrial septal defect (ASD)
   d. Coarctation of aorta
4. **A continuous murmur is heard in all of the following conditions, *except*:**
   a. Patent ductus arteriosus
   b. Coronary AV fistula
   c. Pulmonary AV fistula
   d. Mitral stenosis with mitral regurgitation
5. **Mid-diastolic murmur with presystolic accentuation is typically seen in:**
   a. Mitral stenosis
   b. Mitral regurgitation
   c. Aortic stenosis
   d. Mitral valve prolapse
6. **Pulsatile liver is associated with which valvular disease:**
   a. Aortic stenosis
   b. Tricuspid regurgitation
   c. Pulmonary stenosis
   d. Pulmonary regurgitation
7. **Bell of the stethoscope is used to auscultate which murmur:**
   a. Aortic stenosis
   b. Tricuspid regurgitation
   c. Pulmonary stenosis
   d. Mitral stenosis
8. **Carrey Coombs and Austin Flint murmurs are examples of:**
   a. Early diastolic murmur
   b. Mid-diastolic murmur
   c. Mid-systolic murmur
   d. Pansystolic murmur
9. **Heaving character of cardiac apical impulse is seen in:**
   a. Aortic stenosis
   b. Tricuspid regurgitation
   c. Pulmonary stenosis
   d. Mitral stenosis
10. **Shortness of breath specifically when bending forward, such as when putting on their shoes or socks is called:**
    a. Trepopnea b. Platypnea
    c. Bendopnea d. Orthopnea

ANSWERS

| 1. d | 2. d | 3. c | 4. d | 5. a |
| 6. b | 7. d | 8. b | 9. a | 10. c |

Gastroenterology

CHAPTER OUTLINE

- Symptomatology
- Diseases of the Esophagus
- Dyspepsia
- Dyshagia
- Gastroesophageal Reflux Disease
- GI Bleed
- Diseases of the Stomach and Duodenum
- Peptic Ulcer Disease
- *Helicobacter pylori*
- Diseases of the Intestine
- Malabsorption Syndromes
- Diarrhea
- Inflammatory Bowel Disease

SYMPTOMATOLOGY

Anorexia

Common causes of anorexia are described in **Box 6.1.**

Vomiting

Definition: Vomiting is a *complex reflex and involves both autonomic and somatic neural pathways.*

- *Nausea* is a feeling of wanting to vomit and often precedes actual vomiting.

> **Box 6.1:** Common causes of anorexia.
> - **Infections:** Viral fever and tuberculosis
> - **Endocrine diseases:** Hypothyroidism, hyperparathyroidism, Addison's disease, and panhypopituitarism
> - **Liver disease:** Hepatitis and cirrhosis
> - **Renal disease:** Chronic renal failure
> - **Malignancies:** Any malignant tumors, e.g., carcinoma stomach and pancreas. Leukemias and lymphomas
> - **Psychiatric causes:** Depression and anorexia nervosa

- *Retching* is a strong involuntary unproductive effort to vomit. It is associated with contraction of abdominal muscles but without expulsion of stomach contents through the mouth.

Common Causes of Nausea and Vomiting

Common causes of nausea and vomiting are given in **Table 6.1**.

Complications of Chronic Vomiting

- *Emetic injuries to the esophagus and stomach*
- Mild erythema to *erosions and ulcerations*
- Abrupt retching or vomiting episodes may produce longitudinal mucosal and even transmural lacerations at the level of the gastroesophageal junction. When the lacerations are associated with acute bleeding and hematemesis, the clinical condition is described as the *Mallory–Weiss syndrome*.
- *Boerhaave's syndrome* refers to spontaneous rupture of the esophageal wall, with free perforation and secondary mediastinitis.

Table 6.1: Common causes of nausea and vomiting.

Abdominal causes:	
Mechanical obstruction: Gastric outlet obstruction and small bowel obstruction* Motility disorders: • Functional dyspepsia gastroesophageal reflux disease (GERD)* • Gastroparesis*	Other intra-abdominal causes: Acute appendicitis, acute cholecystitis, acute hepatitis, acute mesenteric ischemia, eosinophilic gastroenteritis, and gastric and duodenal ulcer disease*
Drugs:	
Aspirin and other nonsteroidal anti-inflammatory drugs Antidiabetic agents Antigout drugs Antimicrobials: Acyclovir, antituberculosis drugs, erythromycin, sulfonamides, and tetracycline Cancer chemotherapy: Cisplatin, cytarabine, dacarbazine, etoposide, 5-fluorouracil, and methotrexate	Cardiovascular drugs: Antiarrhythmics, antihypertensives, beta-blockers, calcium channel blockers, digoxin, and diuretics Central nervous system drugs: Antiparkinsonian drugs (levodopa and other dopamine agonists, and anticonvulsants) Others: Theophylline

Contd...

Contd...

Infectious causes:	
Acute gastroenteritis: Viral and bacterial	Nongastrointestinal (systemic) infections
Metabolic and endocrine causes:	
Acute intermittent porphyria, diabetes mellitus, diabetic ketoacidosis, hyperparathyroidism, and other causes of hypercalcemia*	Addison's disease, hyperthyroidism, hyponatremia, hypoparathyroidism, and pregnancy
Central nervous system causes:	
Demyelinating disorders, disorders of the autonomic system, hydrocephalus, meningitis, and migraine headaches*	*Intracerebral lesions with edema (projectile vomiting)*: Abscess, hemorrhage, infarction, and neoplasm*
Labyrinthine disorders:	
• Labyrinthitis* • Motion sickness	Meniere's disease*
Other causes:	
• Anxiety and depression* • Cyclic vomiting syndrome* • Ethanol abuse* • Functional disorders and bulimia nervosa*	*Cardiac disease*: • Congestive heart failure • Myocardial infarction • Myocardial ischemia

*Indicates causes of persistent vomiting.

- *Dental caries* and erosions may result from chronic vomiting.
- *Spasm of the glottis* and aspiration pneumonia
- *Fluid, electrolyte, and metabolic alterations:* Hypochloremic alkalosis, hypokalemia, hypernatremia, and dehydration can occur.
- *Nutritional deficiencies*

Treatment

- **Supportive measure:** *Correction of fluid and electrolyte balance*
- **Medication:**
  - *Phenothiazines and related drugs:* Prochlorperazine 5–10 mg thrice daily
  - *Dopamine antagonists:* Metoclopramide 10 mg 30 minutes before meals and at bedtime. Side effects include drowsiness and extrapyramidal effects. Domperidone (10 mg thrice daily) has no central nervous system (CNS) side effects.
  - *Antihistaminic agents*, e.g., diphenhydramine
  - *Serotonin 5-HT3 receptor antagonists:* Useful in chemotherapy associated emesis. Examples are ondansetron and granisetron.
  - *Neurokinin-1 (NK-1) receptor antagonist*, e.g., aprepitant (oral) and fosaprepitant (parenteral) indicated only in chemotherapy-induced nausea and vomiting.
  - *Motilin receptor agonists:* Erythromycin intravenously in boluses of 200–400 mg every 4–5 hours
  - *Muscarinic receptor agonist:* Bethanechol
  - *Synthetic cannabinoids:* Nabilone and dronabinol
  - *Glucocorticoids:* Especially in raised intracranial tension (ICT), and chemotherapy-induced emesis
  - *Gastric electrical stimulation* in refractory cases

Hiccups

The symptom of hiccups (hiccoughs, singultus) is an involuntary, intermittent, and spasmodic contraction of the diaphragm and intercostal muscles and glottic closure. Its causes are listed in **Table 6.2**.

Table 6.2: Causes of hiccups.

• Hasty ingestion of food and fluids • Hyponatremia • Uremia • Irritation of the phrenic nerve: Due to compression by tumors, esophagitis, pericarditis, mediastinitis, surgery of thorax, and abdomen • Cerebrovascular accidents (especially *lateral medullary syndrome*), encephalitis, and brain tumors	• Diabetic ketoacidosis, renal failure, respiratory failure, and electrolyte imbalance • *Local irritation of the diaphragm*: Due to gaseous distension of stomach and intestines, subphrenic abscess, peritonitis, and acute myocardial infarction • Psychogenic

Symptomatic Treatment

- Advised to drink cold water, swallowing a teaspoon of dry sugar
- Apply pressure over the eyeballs
- Perform Valsalva maneuver
- Rebreathing into a paper bag
- Drugs
- Chlorpromazine 25–50 mg orally or intramuscularly
- Domperidone 10 mg thrice daily
- Metoclopramide 10 mg thrice daily
- Xylocaine viscus 15 mL thrice a day
- Baclofen 5–10 mg thrice a day
- Nifedipine, haloperidol, phenytoin, olanzapine, nefopam, and gabapentin can be used
- Local infiltration of phrenic nerve with procaine
- Acupuncture

Constipation

Definition: Constipation is defined as persistent, difficult, and infrequent passage of hard stools, or seemingly incomplete defecation/evacuation. Many patients may also complain of excessive straining or lower abdominal fullness/discomfort.

> **Box 6.2:** Rome IV criteria for functional constipation.
>
> ❖ *Two or more of the following six must be present**:
>   1. Straining during at least 25% of defecations
>   2. Lumpy or hard stools in at least 25% of defecations
>   3. Sensation of incomplete evacuation for at least 25% of defecations
>   4. Sensation of anorectal obstruction/blockage for at least 25% of defecations
>   5. Manual maneuvers to facilitate at least 25% of defecations (e.g., digital evacuation and support of the pelvic floor)
>   6. Fewer than three defecations/week
> ❖ Loose stools are rarely present without the use of laxatives
> ❖ There are insufficient criteria for IBS

*Criteria fulfilled for the previous three months with symptom onset at least 6 months prior to diagnosis.

(IBS: irritable bowel syndrome)

Criteria for Functional Constipation (Box 6.2)

Risk factors are advanced age, female gender, low level of physical activity, low socioeconomic status, nonwhite ethnicity, and use of certain medications.

Causes of Constipation

Causes of constipation are described in **Box 6.3**:

> **Treatment**
> ❖ Regular exercise and adequate fluid intake
> ❖ Treat the underlying cause or eliminate offending medication
> ❖ **Fiber supplementation:** If there is no secondary cause, increase the fiber content of the diet and fluid intake. A fiber supplement such as wheat bran or psyllium and mucilaginous seeds and seed coats (e.g., ispaghula husk) should be given with water 2–4 times per day.
> ❖ **Laxatives:** They should be restricted to severe cases. Osmotic laxatives act by increasing colonic inflow of fluid and electrolytes by osmotic activity. This softens the stool and stimulates colonic contractility. The stimulatory laxatives act by stimulating colonic contractility and by causing intestinal secretion (**Table 6.3**).

Chronic Blood and Mucus in the Stools

Causes

Common causes of chronic blood and mucus in the stools are described in **Table 6.4**.

> **Box 6.3:** Causes of constipation.
>
> **Primary causes of constipation:**
> *Gastrointestinal disorders:*
> ❖ *Dietary:* Lack of fiber and/or fluid intake
> ❖ *Motility:* Irritable bowel syndrome and slow transit constipation
> ❖ *Structural:* Carcinoma colon, diverticular disease, and Hirschsprung's disease
> ❖ *Defecation:* Anorectal disease, such as Crohn's, fissures, and hemorrhoids
>
> **Secondary causes of constipation:**
> *Medications:*
> ❖ Antacids
> ❖ Anticholinergic agents (e.g., antiparkinsonian drugs, antipsychotics, antispasmodics, and tricyclic antidepressants)
> ❖ Anticonvulsants (e.g., carbamazepine, phenobarbital, and phenytoin)
> ❖ Calcium-channel blockers (e.g., verapamil)
> ❖ Diuretics (e.g., furosemide)
> ❖ Iron supplements
> ❖ Nonsteroidal anti-inflammatory drugs (e.g., ibuprofen)
> ❖ Mu-opioid agonists (e.g., fentanyl, loperamide, and morphine)
>
> *Metabolic and endocrinologic disorders:*
> ❖ Diabetes mellitus
> ❖ Heavy metal poisoning (e.g., arsenic, lead, and mercury)
> ❖ Hypercalcemia
> ❖ Hyperthyroidism
> ❖ Hypokalemia
> ❖ Hypothyroidism
>
> *Neurologic and myopathic disorders:*
> ❖ Amyloidosis
> ❖ Autonomic neuropathy
> ❖ Dermatomyositis
> ❖ Multiple sclerosis
> ❖ Parkinsonism
> ❖ Progressive systemic sclerosis
> ❖ Shy–Drager syndrome
> ❖ Spinal cord injury

Table 6.4: Causes of chronic blood and mucus in the stools.

- **Dysentery:**
  - Amebic dysentery
  - Bacillary dysentery
- **Inflammatory bowel disease:**
  - Ulcerative colitis
  - Crohn's disease
- Intestinal tuberculosis
- *Carcinoma:* Large bowel (rectum, sigmoid, and colon)
- Diverticulitis
- Mesenteric vascular disease
- Necrotizing enterocolitis

Table 6.3: Different types of laxatives.

Bulk laxatives	Emollient laxatives (stool softeners)	Stimulant laxatives (stimulate motility and intestinal secretion)	Osmotic laxatives	Others
• Soluble (ispaghula and psyllium) • Insoluble (methyl cellulose)	• Docusate salts • Mineral oil • Other agents, e.g., polyethylene glycol	• Phenolphthalein • Bisacodyl • Anthraquinones—senna and dantron (only for the terminally ill) • Sodium picosulfate • Castor oil	• Magnesium sulfate • Lactulose/lactitol • Macrogols	• Guanylate cyclase-C receptor agonists (linaclotide and plecanatide) • Lubiprostone (chloride channel activator) • Misoprostol • Colchicine • Prucalopride (5HT4 receptor agonist)

Occult Blood in the Stool

- Stool may appear normal (i.e., no melena) in patients with gastroduodenal bleeding of up to 50–100 mL/day.
- Blood loss in stool of a normal individual varies from 0.5 to 1.5 mL/day. Occult blood tests begin to become positive usually when blood loss is around 2 mL/day.

Conditions with Occult Blood in Stool
Conditions with occult blood in stool are described in **Table 6.5**.

Table 6.5: Conditions with occult blood in stool.

Upper gastrointestinal bleeding	Esophageal varices, esophagitis, peptic ulcer disease, gastritis, and malignancy
Lower gastrointestinal bleeding	Hemorrhoids, malignancy, diverticulitis, inflammatory bowel disease, and celiac sprue
Drugs	Aspirin or steroids (rare)
Others	Hookworm infestation and mesenteric vascular disease

Weight Loss

Common causes of weight loss are described in **Box 6.4**.

> **Box 6.4:** Common causes of weight loss.
>
> **Types of weight loss:**
> - **Physiological:** Due to dieting, exercise, starvation, or decreased nutritional intake (e.g., old age)
> - **Pathological/involuntary:**
>   - *Endocrine and metabolic disorders*: Diabetes mellitus, hyperthyroidism, pheochromocytoma, Addison's disease, and panhypopituitarism
>   - *Gastrointestinal disorders*: Malabsorption, tropical sprue, chronic pancreatitis, inflammatory bowel disease (ulcerative colitis and Crohn disease), and parasitic infestations
>   - *Chronic infections*: Tuberculosis, HIV, fungal infections, and amebic abscess
>   - *Malignancy*: Stomach, colon, pancreas, liver, lung, lymphoma, and leukemia
>   - *Psychiatric illness*: Anorexia nervosa, depression, and schizophrenia
>   - *Renal disease*: Chronic renal failure and infective endocarditis
>   - *Cardiac disorders*: Chronic congestive heart failure
>   - *Respiratory disorders*: Emphysema, empyema, and chronic obstructive pulmonary disease (COPD)
>   - *Rheumatological*: Rheumatoid arthritis
>   - Idiopathic

■ DYSPEPSIA

Dyspepsia is derived from the Greek words *dys and pepse* and literally means "difficult digestion".
- Dyspepsia is a collective description of a variety of gastrointestinal symptoms (**Table 6.6**).
- **Ulcer dyspepsia:** Dyspeptic symptoms associated with peptic ulcer.
- **Nonulcer dyspepsia (functional dyspepsia):** No cause can be found.
- **Flatulent dyspepsia:** Usually due to a functional disorder

Table 6.6: Symptoms of dyspepsia.

Postprandial fullness	Bloating in the upper abdomen
Early satiation	Nausea
Epigastric pain	Vomiting
Epigastric burning	Belching

Symptoms include early satiety, flatulence, bloating, and belching predominate.

Causes
Causes of dyspepsia are described in **Box 6.5**.

Nonulcer Dyspepsia (Functional Dyspepsia, Nervous Dyspepsia; Nonorganic Dyspepsia)

Definition: It is defined as chronic dyspepsia in the absence of organic disease.

It is second most common functional gastrointestinal disorder (after irritable bowel syndrome).

Etiology:
- It is dyspepsia in the absence of organic disease and even on detailed investigation, no cause can be found.
- Etiology is poorly understood but probably due to a spectrum of mucosal, motility, and psychiatric disorders.
- Symptoms are probably due to disturbances in the motor function of the gastrointestinal tract similar to that occurring in the irritable bowel syndrome. Both irritable

> **Box 6.5:** Causes of dyspepsia.
>
> **Luminal gastrointestinal tract:**
> - Chronic gastric or intestinal ischemia
> - Food intolerance
> - Functional dyspepsia
> - Gastroesophageal reflux disease
> - Gastric or esophageal neoplasms
> - Gastric infections (e.g., cytomegalovirus, fungus, tuberculosis, and syphilis)
> - Gastroparesis (e.g., diabetes mellitus, post-vagotomy, scleroderma, chronic intestinal pseudo-obstruction, postviral, and idiopathic)
> - Irritable bowel syndrome
> - Peptic ulcer disease
> - Parasites (e.g., *Giardia lamblia* and *Strongyloides stercoralis*)
>
> **Medications:**
> Acarbose, aspirin, other nonsteroidal anti-inflammatory drugs (including cyclooxygenase-2 selective agents), colchicine, digitalis preparations, estrogens, ethanol, glucocorticoids, iron, levodopa, niacin, narcotics, nitrates, orlistat, potassium chloride, quinidine, sildenafil, and theophylline
>
> **Pancreaticobiliary disorders:**
> - *Biliary pain*: Cholelithiasis, choledocholithiasis, and sphincter of Oddi dysfunction
> - Chronic pancreatitis
> - Pancreatic neoplasms
>
> **Systemic conditions:**
> Adrenal insufficiency, congestive heart failure, diabetes mellitus, hyperparathyroidism, myocardial ischemia, pregnancy, renal insufficiency, and thyroid disease

Table 6.7: Rome IV criteria for functional dyspepsia.

Includes *one* or *more* of the following:
1. Bothersome postprandial fullness
2. Bothersome early satiation
3. Bothersome epigastric pain
4. Bothersome epigastric burning

And

No evidence of structural disease (including at upper endoscopy) that is likely to explain the symptoms.

Subgroups according to Rome IV criteria
- **Epigastric pain syndrome (EPS):** Pain centered in the upper abdomen as the predominant symptom.
- **Postprandial distress syndrome (PDS):** Unpleasant or troublesome nonpainful sensation (discomfort) centered in the upper abdomen is the predominant symptom. This may be accompanied by upper abdominal fullness, early satiety, bloating, and nausea.

Any one of the first two criteria (1 and/or 2, at least 3 days/week) is for PDS while any one of the last two criteria (3 and/or 4, at least 1 day/week) is for EPS.

bowel syndrome and nonulcer dyspepsia often exist together in the same patient.
- *Helicobacter pylori* infection should be excluded, because it may be responsible for symptoms in few patients.

Clinical features:
- It usually occurs in young (<40 years of age) females.
- Symptoms and subtypes are described in **Table 6.7**.
- Morning symptoms of pain and nausea on walking are characteristic.
- Features suggestive of irritable bowel syndrome, such as pellet-like stools and feeling of incomplete evacuation after defecation may be observed.
- History may reveal stress factors such as worries, financial problems, employment, and family affairs.
- On examination, no diagnostic signs, except for inappropriate abdominal tenderness on abdominal palpation
- All the organic causes of dyspepsia, such as peptic ulcer disease, drug ingestion, depression pregnancy, alcohol abuse, etc., should be excluded.
- In older patients, intra-abdominal malignancy should be excluded, which may present with alarming features, such as weight loss, anorexia, dysphagia, and hematemesis or melena.

Investigations:
The history often suggests the diagnosis.
- *Helicobacter pylori* infection should be serologically excluded in all patients.
- *Exclusion of organic causes by following investigations*:
  - Blood count, erythrocyte sedimentation rate (ESR), and occult blood in stools
  - Liver function tests (to exclude alcoholism)
  - Pregnancy test
  - Barium meal
  - Ultrasound scan may detect gallstones.
  - Indications for endoscopy in patients with chronic dyspepsia/*red flags* are listed in **Box 6.6**.

Box 6.6: Indications for endoscopy in patients with chronic dyspepsia/*red flags*.
- Age >60 years
- Dysphagia/previous peptic ulcer disease, odynophagia
- Clinically significant weight loss (>5% usual body weight over 6–12 months)
- Protracted vomiting
- Melena
- Anemia
- Palpable mass
- Jaundice
- Family history of stomach cancer

Management:
- Explanation, reassurance, and lifestyle changes
- Advice to avoid cigarette smoking and alcohol use
- Symptoms, if associated with an identifiable cause of stress, resolve with appropriate counseling.
- Psychological factors influencing on gut function should be explained and may require psychological treatment.
- Idiosyncratic and restrictive diets are not beneficial, but reducing intake of fat and coffee may help.
- If endoscopy is noncontributory, empirical treatment is advised.
  - Prokinetic drugs, such as metoclopramide (10 mg 3 times daily) or domperidone (10–20 mg 3 times daily), may be given before meals for nausea, vomiting, or bloating.
  - Mosapride or itopride may also be tried.
  - H_2-receptor antagonists or proton pump inhibitors (PPIs) may be given, if night pain or heartburn is troublesome.
  - *H. pylori* eradication therapy, if test is positive and may be effective in some patients with functional dyspepsia
  - Selective serotonin reuptake inhibitors may be effective in some patients.
  - Low-dose tricyclic agents (e.g., amitriptyline) may be of help in up to two-thirds.
  - SSRI (selective serotonin reuptake inhibitor) medication is tried in refractory cases.

GASTROINTESTINAL BLEEDING

Upper Gastrointestinal Bleeding

Hematemesis is the bleeding proximal to the duodenojejunal junction (ligament of Treitz).

Etiology: Etiology is described in **Table 6.8 and Figure 6.1**.

Peptic ulcers are the most common cause of upper gastrointestinal (UGI) bleeding (up to about 50%).

Presentation: Patient usually presents with either hematemesis (vomiting of blood or coffee-ground material) and/or melena (black and tarry stool).
- **Hematemesis:** *Color of the vomitus* depends on how long the blood has been in the stomach and the severity of bleeding.
  - *Red* with clots when bleeding is severe and bright red indicates rapid and sizeable bleeding.
  - *Black* ("coffee grounds") when less severe and bleeding is small
- **Melena:** It is the passage of *black, tarry,* and foul-smelling *stools* containing altered blood. The characteristic color and smell are due to the action of digestive enzymes and

Table 6.8: Various causes of upper gastrointestinal (UGI) bleeding.

Esophageal causes:
- Esophageal varices (e.g., due to portal hypertension)
- Erosive esophagitis
- Esophageal carcinoma
- Mallory–Weiss syndrome

Gastroduodenal causes:
- Peptic ulcer (gastric and duodenal) disease
- Erosive gastritis (e.g., after ingestion of NSAIDs and alcohol) or duodenitis
- Stress ulcers occurring with *shock, sepsis, or severe trauma*
- *Curling ulcers* in the proximal duodenum with *severe burns or trauma*
- Carcinoma stomach
- Gastric antral vascular ectasia (GAVE), also described as *watermelon stomach and Dieulafoy's lesion*
- Angiodysplasia or vascular malformations (*Heyde's syndrome* in aortic stenosis)
- Rupture of aortic aneurysm or aortic duodenal fistula following aortic graft. Cushing ulcer associated with elevated intracranial pressure

Other causes:
- Coagulation defects
- *Cameron's lesions:* Linear erosions or ulcerations in the proximal stomach at the end of a large hiatal hernia, near the diaphragmatic pinch
- Hemobilia
- Hemosuccus pancreaticus

(NSAID: nonsteroidal anti-inflammatory drug)

Table 6.9: Differences between hematemesis and hemoptysis.

Features	Hemoptysis	Hematemesis
Definition	Coughing out of blood	Vomiting out of blood
Content and color	Mixed with sputum and bright red in color	Mixed with food particles and coffee-ground in color
Contents	Frothy and associated sputum	No froth, associated food particles
Associated symptoms	Cough and dyspnea	Nausea, vomiting, retching, and abdominal discomfort
Melena	Rare	Common
Reaction	Alkaline (blue litmus remains unchanged)	Acidic (blue litmus remains unchanged)

Table 6.10: Differences between upper and lower gastrointestinal (GI) bleed.

Features	Upper GI tract bleed	Lower GI tract bleed
Site of bleeding	Above ligament of Treitz	Below ligament of Treitz
Clinical presentation	Hematemesis or melena	Hematochezia/rarely melena
Nasogastric aspiration shows	Blood	Clear fluid
Bowel sounds	Hyperactive	Normal
BUN (blood urea nitrogen)/creatinine ratio	Increased	Normal

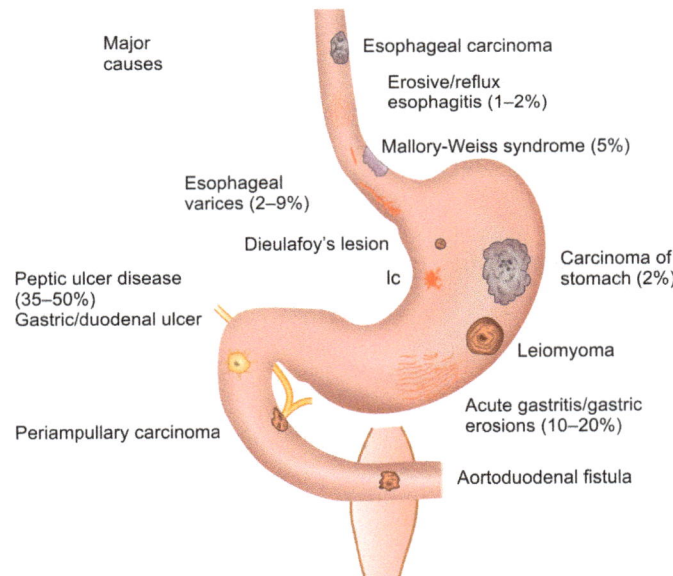

Fig. 6.1: Causes of acute upper gastrointestinal hemorrhage.

bacteria on hemoglobin. It usually occurs when more than 60 mL blood is lost and blood has been present in the upper gastrointestinal tract for at least 14 h (and as long as 3–5 days). Occasionally, it develops due to hemorrhage from the right side of the colon.
- Severe/massive acute upper gastrointestinal bleeding can sometimes cause maroon or bright red stool due to passage of frank blood per rectum (*hematochezia*).
- *Occasionally*, presentation with *symptoms of blood loss only*. These include:
  - *Acute loss with intravascular volume depletion:* Dizziness, extreme pallor, and shock
  - *Chronic loss:* With symptoms of anemia

Differences between hematemesis and hemoptysis are presented in **Table 6.9**.

Differences between upper and lower gastrointestinal (GI) bleed are presented in **Table 6.10**.

Basic investigations:
- **Complete blood count:**
  - Chronic bleeding leads to anemia, but the hemoglobin concentration and the hematocrit level may be normal after sudden, major bleeding until hemodilution occurs.
  - *Low platelet count:* It suggests chronic liver disease, dilution, or hematologic disorder.
- **Blood urea nitrogen (BUN) and creatinine:** The blood urea nitrogen level increases to greater extent than the creatinine level because of increased intestinal absorption of urea after breakdown of blood proteins. An elevated blood urea with normal creatinine concentration implies severe bleeding.
- **Liver function tests:** They may show evidence of chronic liver disease.
- **Prothrombin time:** It may be prolonged in patients with chronic liver disease or in coagulation disorders or patients on anticoagulated therapy.
- **Cross-matching:** Potential infusion of packed red blood cells

Management (Flowchart 6.1)
Medical resuscitation and replenishment of intravascular volume: In case of massive bleeding, resuscitation measures should be initiated simultaneously with the initial assessment.
- *Intravenous access:* The first step is to gain intravenous access using at least one large-bore (14- or 16-gauge) intravenous catheters for essentially all patients so that normal saline can be infused as fast as necessary to maintain hemodynamic stability.
- *Fluid resuscitation:* Adequate resuscitation and hemodynamic stabilization is essential prior to endoscopy (saline). Vasopressors, if persistent hypotension
- *Blood product transfusions:* Initiate blood transfusions, if the hemoglobin is <7 g/dL to maintain the hemoglobin at a level of ≥9 g/dL. Patients with active bleeding and a low platelet count (<50,000/μL) should be transfused with platelets. Patients with a coagulopathy with a prolonged prothrombin time with international normalized ratio (INR) >1.5 should be transfused with fresh frozen plasma (FFP).

Initial clinical assessment:
- *Circulatory status:* Severe bleeding causes tachycardia, hypotension, and oliguria. Closely observe with hourly pulse, blood pressure, postural hypotension urine output, and level of consciousness.
- *Evidence of liver disease:* It may be present in patients with decompensated cirrhosis.
- *Comorbidity*—such as cardiorespiratory, cerebrovascular, or renal—may be worsened by acute bleeding and may also increase the hazards of endoscopy and surgical operations.

Endoscopy:
Pre-endoscopic pharmacotherapy:
For nonvariceal UGIB (upper gastrointestinal bleeding):
- *IV proton pump inhibitor:* 80 mg bolus, 8 mg/h drip (esomeprazole)

Endoscopic hemostasis therapy:
It includes—(1) epinephrine injection, (2) thermal electrocoagulation, and (3) mechanical (hemoclips). Combination therapy is superior to monotherapy.

Nonvariceal UGIB: Postendoscopy management—
- Patients with ulcers requiring endoscopic therapy should receive PPI × 72 hours.
- Determine *H. pylori* status in all ulcer patients.
- Discharge patients on PPI (once to twice daily), duration dictated by underlying etiology and need for NSAIDs/aspirin.
- In patients with cardiovascular disease on low dose aspirin: Restart as soon as bleeding has resolved.

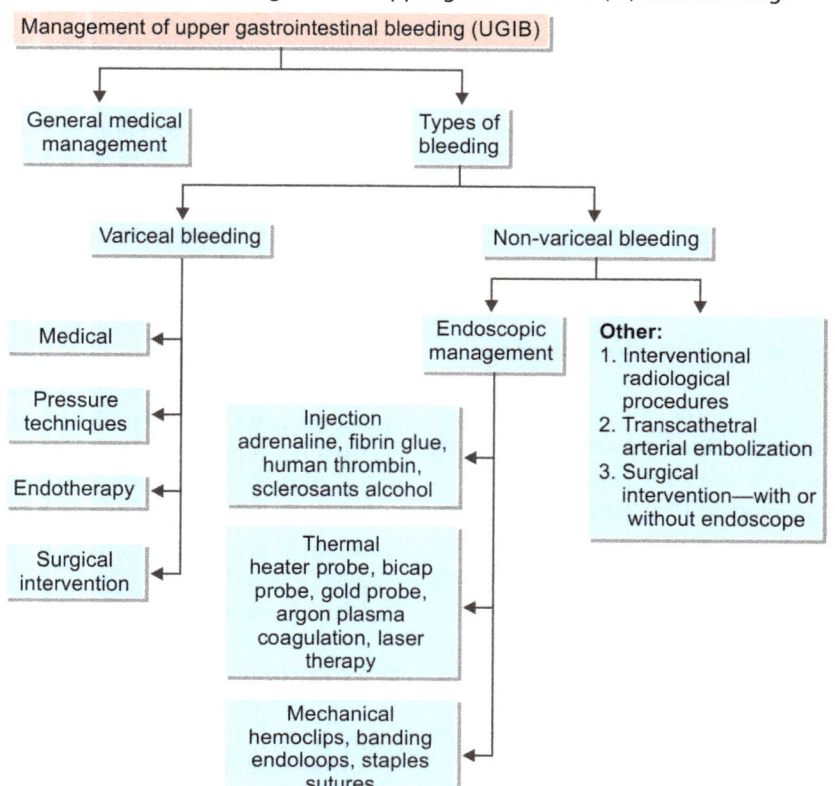

Flowchart 6.1: Management of upper gastrointestinal (GI) tract bleeding.

Variceal Bleeding

It occurs in one-third of patients with cirrhosis. In one-third, initial bleeding episodes are fatal. Among survivors, one-third will rebleed within 6 weeks. Only one-third will survive 1 year or more. Management of variceal bleed is discussed in Chapter 7.

Lower GI Bleeding

Lower gastrointestinal (LGI) bleeding generally signifies bleeding from the colon or anorectum. In patients with severe *hematochezia*, first consider possibility of UGIB. About 10–15% of patients with presumed LGIB are found to have upper GIB.

Etiology

Etiology of LGI bleeding is described in **Table 6.11** and **Figure 6.2**.

Table 6.11: Causes of lower gastrointestinal bleeding.

Diverticulosis (main cause)	Angioectasias
Hemorrhoids anal fissures, ulcer	Colitis (IBD, infectious, and ischemic)
Neoplasms	Postpolypectomy
Dieulafoy's lesion	Radiation colitis and small bowel bleed
	Unknown causes—10%

Management of LGI Bleeding

Management of LGI bleeding is shown in **Flowchart 6.2**:

DIARRHEA (TABLE 6.12)

Definition: Daily bowel movements of three or more times are considered to be abnormal. The upper limit of stool weight is 200 g daily. Although stool weight usually considered as a "scientific definition of diarrhea", diarrhea should not be defined solely in terms of fecal weight.
- *Acute diarrhea* is defined as abrupt onset of increased frequency and/or fluidity of bowel movements.
- *Chronic diarrhea* is defined as passage of loose stools with or without increased stool frequency for more than 4 weeks.

Large-volume versus Small-volume Diarrhea

- Normal rectosigmoid colon functions as a storage reservoir.
- *Left colonic disorders*: Inflammatory or motility disorders involving the left colon compromises this rectosigmoid reservoir capacity and results in *frequent small-volume bowel movements*.
- *Right colonic or small bowel disorders*: In diarrhea due to disorders of the right colon or small bowel and if the rectosigmoid reservoir is intact, individual *bowel movements are less frequent and larger*.

Frequent, small, and painful stools may point to a source in the distal colon, whereas painless large-volume stools suggest a right colonic or small bowel source.

Secretory versus Osmotic Diarrhea

- **Secretory diarrhea:** It results from malabsorption or secretion of electrolytes (secretory diarrhea).
- **Osmotic diarrhea:** It results from intestinal malabsorption of ingested nonelectrolytes.
- Osmotic diarrhea constitutes small number of cases whereas secretory diarrhea forms the much larger number of cases.
- In secretory diarrhea, sodium, potassium, and accompanying anions account almost entire for stool osmolality. In contrast, in osmotic diarrhea, poorly absorbable solutes within the lumen of the intestine account for much of the osmotic activity of stool water.

Watery versus Fatty versus Inflammatory Diarrhea

- **Watery diarrhea:** It implies a defect primarily in water absorption as a result of increased electrolyte secretion or reduced electrolyte absorption (secretory diarrhea) or ingestion of a poorly absorbed substance (osmotic diarrhea).
- **Fatty diarrhea:** It implies defective absorption of fat and perhaps other nutrients in the small intestine.

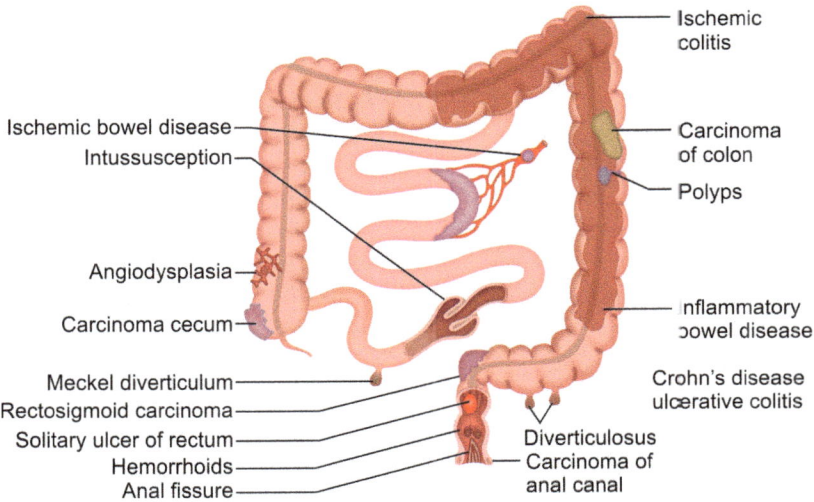

Fig. 6.2: Causes of lower gastrointestinal bleeding (LGIB).

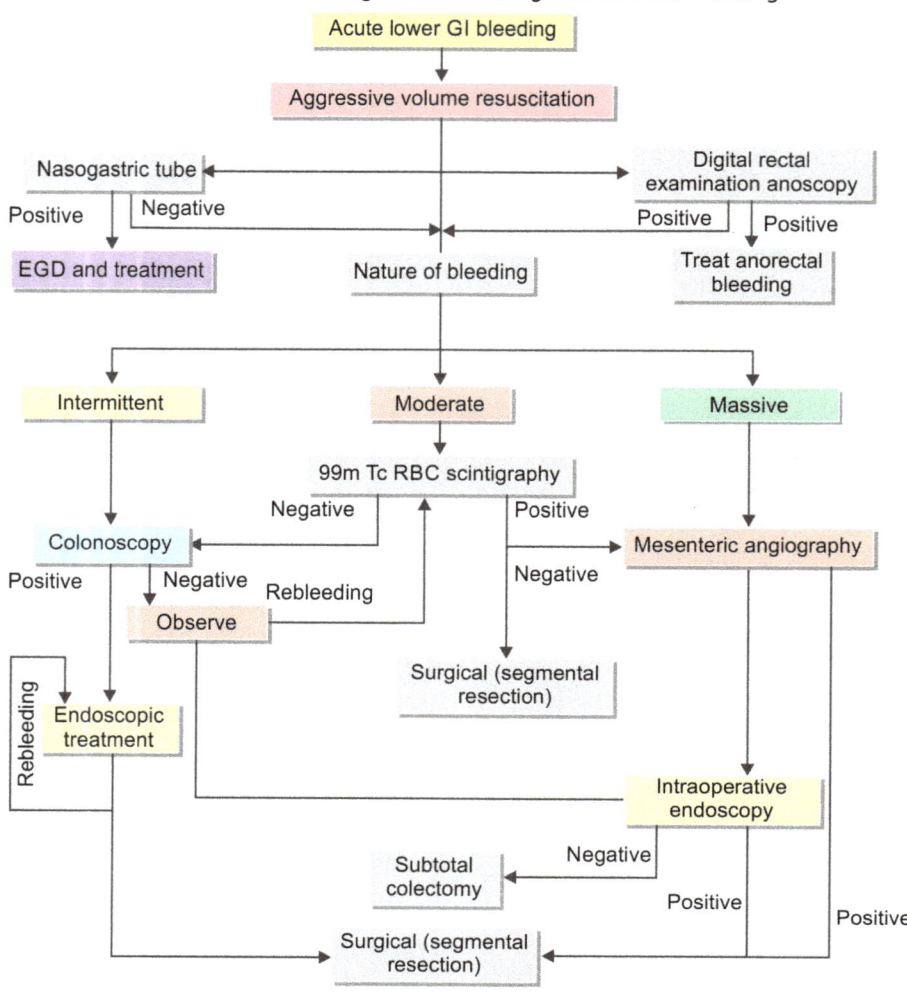

Flowchart 6.2: Management of lower gastrointestinal bleeding.

(EGD: upper endoscopy; GI: gastrointestinal)

Table 6.12: Causes of diarrhea.

Type of diarrhea	Causes	Examples
Secretory diarrhea	Exogenous secretagogues	Enterotoxins (e.g., cholera)
	Endogenous secretagogues	Neuroendocrine tumors (e.g., carcinoid syndrome)
	Absence of ion transporter	Congenital chloridorrhea
	Loss of intestinal surface area	Intestinal resection, diffuse intestinal mucosal disease
	Intestinal ischemia	Diffuse mesenteric atherosclerosis
	Rapid intestinal transit	Intestinal hurry following vagotomy
Osmotic diarrhea	Ingestion of poorly absorbed agent	Magnesium ingestion
	Loss of nutrient transporter	Lactase deficiency

- **Inflammatory diarrhea:** It implies the presence of one of a limited number of inflammatory or neoplastic diseases involving the gastrointestinal tract.

Causes of Chronic Diarrhea

Causes of chronic diarrhea are described in **Table 6.13**.

Approach to the Patient with Acute Diarrhea (Flowchart 6.3)

Physical Examination

- Examine for signs of dehydration to assess the severity of the diarrhea. These include examination of pulse, blood pressure (including postural change), skin turgor, dryness of mucous membranes (e.g., mouth), mental status, and breathing.
- Severity of dehydration **(Table 6.14)**
- *Electrolyte imbalances*: Assess muscle strength and muscle reflexes, which may be reduced in hypokalemia.
- Examination of abdomen to exclude any surgical cause (e.g., intestinal obstruction)

Laboratory Investigations

Laboratory investigations usually do not help in the management acute diarrhea.

Table 6.13: Causes of chronic diarrhea.

Fatty diarrhea	Watery diarrhea

• **Malabsorption syndromes:**
  ▪ Mucosal diseases (celiac disease, Whipple's disease)
  ▪ Mesenteric ischemia
  ▪ Short bowel syndrome
  ▪ Small intestinal bacterial overgrowth
• **Maldigestion:**
  ▪ Inadequate luminal bile acid concentration
  ▪ Pancreatic exocrine insufficiency
	• **Osmotic diarrhea:**
	  ▪ Carbohydrate malabsorption
	  ▪ Osmotic laxatives
	• **Secretory diarrhea**
	  ▪ Bacterial toxins
	  ▪ Congenital syndromes (e.g., congenital chloridorrhea)
	• **Disordered motility, regulation:**
	  ▪ Diabetic autonomic neuropathy
	  ▪ Irritable bowel syndrome
	  ▪ Postsympathectomy diarrhea
	  ▪ Postvagotomy diarrhea

Inflammatory diarrhea	• **Endocrinopathies:** Addison's disease, carcinoid syndrome, gastrinoma, hyperthyroidism, mastocytosis, medullary carcinoma of thyroid, pheochromocytoma, somatostatinoma, and VIPoma • Laxative abuse (stimulant laxatives) • Medications and toxins

• Diverticulitis
• **Infectious diseases:**
  ▪ Invasive bacterial infections (e.g., tuberculosis and yersiniosis)
  ▪ Invasive parasitic infections (e.g., amebiasis and strongyloidiasis)
  ▪ Pseudomembranous colitis (*Clostridium difficile* infection)
  ▪ Ulcerating viral infections (e.g., cytomegalovirus and herpes simplex virus)
• **Inflammatory bowel diseases:** Crohn's disease and ulcerative colitis
• Ischemic colitis
• **Neoplasia:** Carcinoma of colon and lymphoma
• Radiation colitis	

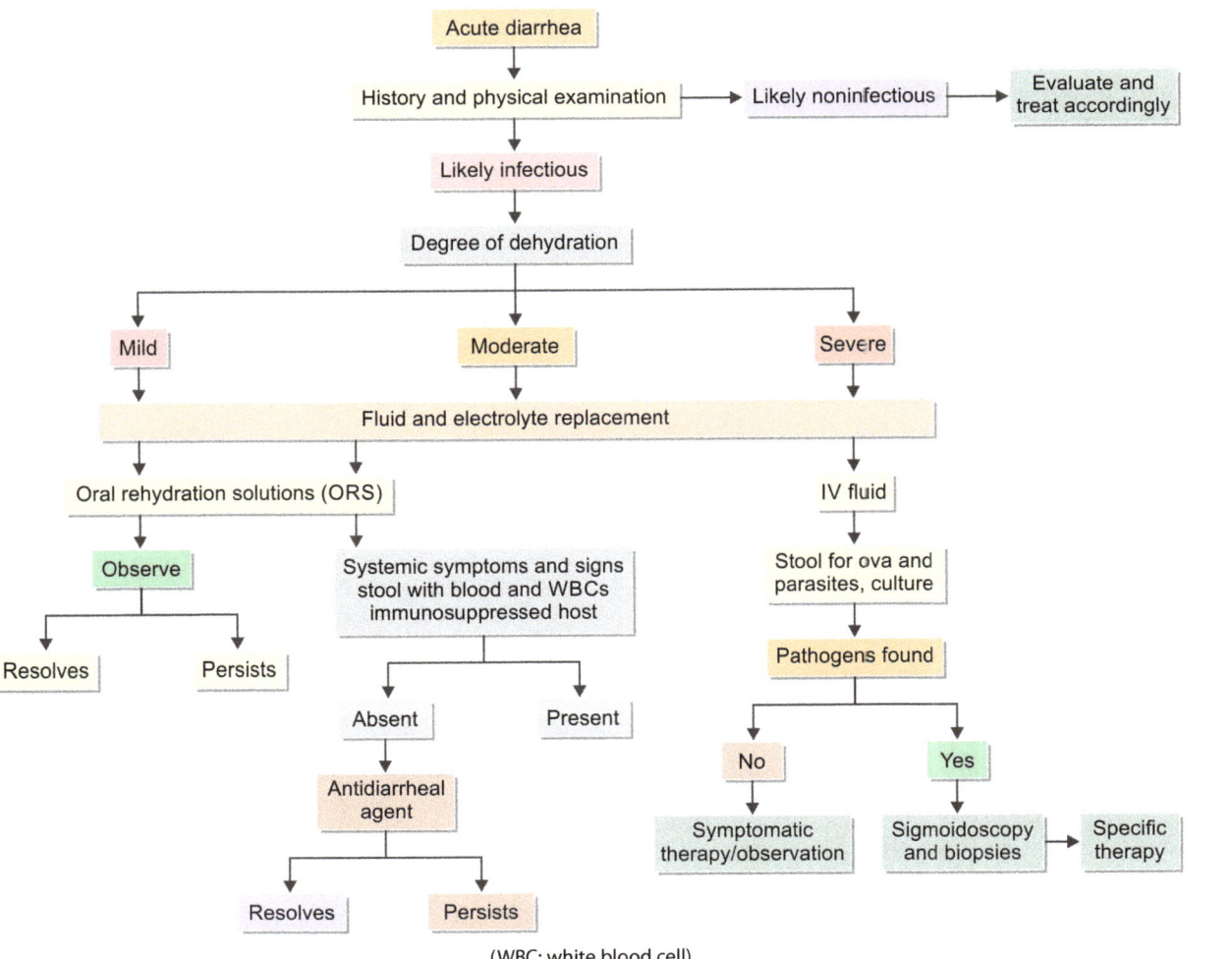

Flowchart 6.3: Approach to the management of acute diarrhea.

(WBC: white blood cell)

Table 6.14: Severity of dehydration.

Features	Mild	Moderate	Severe
Urine output	Decreased	Decreased	Markedly decreased
Physical examination:			
Level of consciousness	Normal	Normal	Depressed
Mental status	Normal/irritable	Lethargic	Comatose
Skin	Normal	Cool	Cool and mottled
Skin turgor	Normal	Reduced with skin tenting	Markedly reduced
Mouth/oral mucosa	Dry	Markedly dry	Parched
Eyes	Normal	Sunken (sunken fontanelle in infants)	Markedly sunken
Pulse rate	Normal or mild increase	Tachycardia and feeble	Marked tachycardia
Blood pressure	Normal	Postural/orthostatic fall	Hypotension and frank shock
Respiration	Normal	Normal	Acidotic
Investigations:			
Urine-specific gravity	<1.020	>1.020	>1.035
Blood urea	Normal	Normal to raised	High

- **Total white blood cell (WBC) count:** Presence of high-leukocyte count with shift to left suggests invasive bacterial infection.
- **Electrolytes and acid–base status:** It should be done in patients with severe dehydration. Severe diarrhea produces metabolic acidosis.
- **Blood cultures:** To be performed when bacteremia or a systemic infection is suspected
- **Stool examination:** Grossly bloody or mucus in the stool suggests an inflammatory process. In severe cases, stool should be examined for the presence of leukocytes, red cells, and cysts or trophozoites/parasites. In cholera, *Vibrio cholerae* shows the characteristic darting motility. Stool with leukocytes considers inflammatory causes (*Shigella, Salmonella, Campylobacter, Escherichia coli, Entamoeba,* and *Clostridium difficile*).
- **Stool culture:** Specific indications for stool cultures include bloody stools, stools that test positive for occult blood or leukocytes, prolonged course of diarrhea that has not been treated with antibiotics, immunocompromised host, or for epidemiologic purposes, such as cases involving food handlers.

Systemic complications of acute diarrheal disease are presented in **Table 6.15**.

Differences between Diarrhea and Dysentery

Differences between diarrhea and dysentery are discussed in **Table 6.16**.

Table 6.15: Systemic complications of acute diarrheal disease.

Complication	Associated organism
Sepsis	*Shigella* species, nontyphoidal *Salmonella enterica*, and *Campylobacter fetus*
Hemolytic–uremic syndrome	*Shigella* species, Shiga toxin-producing *Escherichia coli*
Guillain–Barré syndrome	*Campylobacter jejuni*
Reactive arthritis 0	*Campylobacter* species, *Salmonella* species, and *Shigella flexneri*

Table 6.16: Differences between diarrhea and dysentery.

Diarrhea	Dysentery
Voluminous fluid feces	Scanty sticky feces
No blood in feces	Blood in feces
No mucus in feces	Mucus in feces
Less pus cells	Abundant pus cells
Less straining during defecation	Severe straining during defecation (tenesmus)

Antidiarrheal agents:
Absorbents:
Kaolin absorbs the toxin and may be of use in few patients. However, it does not affect the course of the disease.
Antimotility drugs:
- These are used for symptomatic treatment of toxin-induced diarrhea in adults only. It should not be used in young children and elderly.
- It can be given in inflammatory diarrhea along with antibiotics. These include:
  - *Opiates (e.g., morphine and codeine):* They may cause respiratory depression.
  - *Diphenoxylate/atropine combination:* It may cause respiratory depression and anticholinergic side effects.
  - *Loperamide:* Dose is two tablets of 4 mg each initially, then 2 mg after each unformed stool, not to exceed 16 mg/day for ≤2 days.
  - *Bismuth subsalicylate:* It acts as an antisecretory agent. Dose is one tablet every 30 minutes for a total of 8 doses or 60 mL every 6 hourly.

Antisecretory agents: *Racecadotril—*
- It reduces the hypersecretion of water and electrolytes into the intestinal lumen.
- It inhibits enkephalinase (an enzyme that degrades enkephalins)
- *Dose* is 100 mg thrice daily and to be given to patients with acute, watery diarrhea only.
- *Contraindications:* Renal insufficiency, pregnancy, and breastfeeding

DISEASES OF THE ESOPHAGUS

Dysphagia (Flowchart 6.4)

Dysphagia, from the Greek dys (difficulty, disordered) and phagia (to eat), refers to the sensation that food is hindered in its passage from the mouth to the stomach.

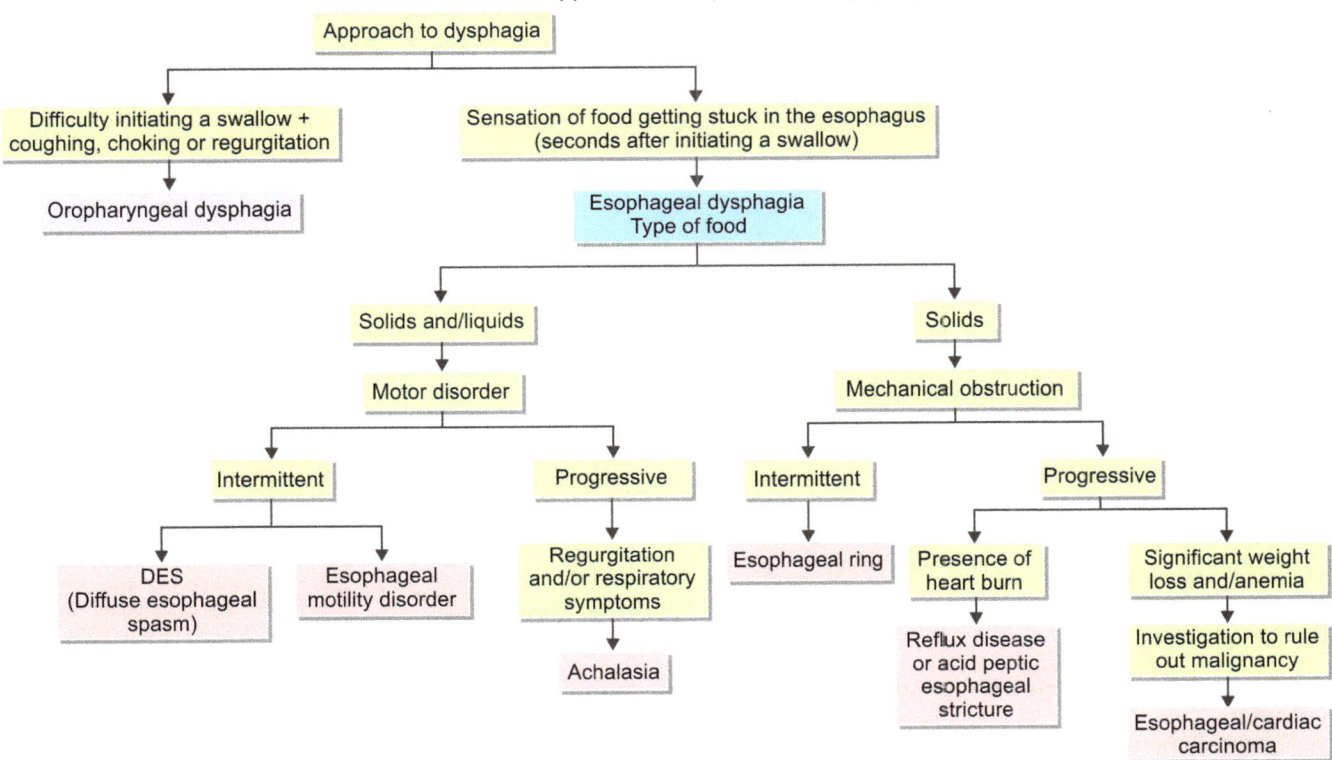

Flowchart 6.4: Approach to the patient with dysphagia.

Causes of Dysphagia

Causes of oropharyngeal and esophageal dysphagia are described in **Tables 6.17 and 6.18**.

Odynophagia

Odynophagia, or painful swallowing, is specific feature for esophageal involvement. It usually reflects an inflammatory process in the esophageal mucosa. Its severity varies. It may be a dull retrosternal ache on swallowing to a stabbing pain with radiation to the back so severe that the patient cannot eat or even swallow their own saliva.

Causes of Odynophagia

Causes of odynophagia are mentioned in **Box 6.7**.

Table 6.17: Causes of oropharyngeal dysphagia.

Neuromuscular causes	Structural causes
• Amyotrophic lateral sclerosis (ALS) • Multiple sclerosis • Muscular dystrophy • Myasthenia gravis • Parkinson's disease • Polymyositis or dermatomyositis • Stroke • Thyroid dysfunction	• Carcinoma • Infections of pharynx or neck • Osteophytes and other spinal disorders • Prior surgery or radiation therapy • Proximal esophageal web • Plummer–Vinson syndrome • Thyromegaly • Zenker's diverticulum

Table 6.18: Common causes of esophageal dysphagia.

Motility (neuromuscular) disorders	Structural (mechanical) disorders
Primary disorders: • Achalasia • Diffuse esophageal spasm • Hypertensive LES • Ineffective esophageal motility • Nutcracker (high-pressure) esophagus	**Intrinsic:** • Carcinoma and benign tumors • Diverticula • Eosinophilic esophagitis • Esophageal rings and webs (other than Schatzki ring) • Foreign body • Lower esophageal (Schatzki) ring • Medication-induced stricture • Peptic stricture
Secondary disorders: • Chagas' disease • Reflux-related dysmotility • Scleroderma and other rheumatologic disorders	**Extrinsic:** • Mediastinal mass • Spinal osteophytes • Vascular compression

GASTROESOPHAGEAL REFLUX DISEASE

Definition

- Gastroesophageal reflux disease (GERD) is a consequence of the failure of the normal antireflux barrier to protect against frequent and abnormal amounts of gastroesophageal reflux (GER; i.e., gastric contents moving retrograde effortlessly from the stomach to the esophagus).
- Spectrum of injury to the esophagus includes *esophagitis, stricture, Barrett's esophagus, and adenocarcinoma*.

> **Box 6.7:** Causes of odynophagia.
>
> **Caustic ingestion:** Acid and alkali
> **Pill-induced injury:**
> - Alendronate and other bisphosphonates
> - Aspirin and other NSAIDs
> - Iron preparations
> - Potassium chloride (especially slow-release form)
> - Tetracycline and its derivatives
> - Quinidine
> - Zidovudine
>
> **Infectious esophagitis:**
> - *Viral*: Cytomegalovirus, Epstein–Barr virus, herpes simplex virus, and human immunodeficiency virus
> - *Bacteria*: Mycobacteria (tuberculosis or *Mycobacterium avium* complex)
> - *Fungal*: *Candida albicans* and histoplasmosis
> - *Protozoan*: *Cryptosporidium* and *Pneumocystis*
> - *Severe reflux esophagitis*
> - *Esophageal carcinoma*

(NSAID: nonsteroidal anti-inflammatory drug)

Pathophysiology

> **Normal defense mechanisms preventing reflux and reflux esophagitis:**
> Several defense mechanisms prevent the reflux of gastric contents into the esophagus.
> - **Antireflux barrier at the gastroesophageal junction (Fig. 6.3):** This consists of—(1) lower esophageal sphincter (LES), at the lower end of esophagus, below the diaphragm, (2) striated muscles of the crural diaphragm, (3) phrenoesophageal ligament, (4) oblique entrance of the esophagus into the stomach (angle of His), (5) attachment of the lower esophageal sphincter (LES) to the crural diaphragm: Intra-abdominal pressure reinforces the LES tone.
> - **Esophageal clearance mechanisms:** Reflux of gastric contents into the esophagus occurs in healthy persons and is normally cleared by esophagus in a two-step process—
>   □ *Volume clearance by peristaltic function:* After acid reflux from stomach, the esophageal peristalsis returns the refluxed fluid to the stomach.
>   □ *Neutralization of acid by bicarbonate in the swallowed saliva:* The small amounts of residual acid refluxed into the esophagus are neutralized by weakly alkaline (bicarbonate) contained in swallowed saliva.
> - **Epithelial defensive factors:** The esophageal mucosa contains mainly three lines of defense—
>   1. *Pre-epithelial barrier:* It consists of (1) small unstirred water layer, (2) bicarbonate from swallowed saliva, and (3) secretions of submucosal glands.
>   2. *Epithelial defense:* It consists of cell membranes and tight intercellular junctions, buffers, and ion transporters.
>   3. *Postepithelial defense:* It consists of the blood supply to the esophagus.

Causes of Disruption of Normal Defense Mechanisms (Fig. 6.3)

- **Defective antireflux barriers:**
  - *Hiatus hernia (sliding type):* This is characterized by sliding of the esophagogastric junction through the diaphragm. This results in increased exposure of the esophagus to acid and may lead to esophagitis, Barrett's esophagus, or peptic strictures.
  - *Abnormalities of lower esophageal sphincter (LES):* Transient relaxation and reduced tone of LES can result in regurgitation, especially when intra-abdominal pressure is increased.
    - Cigarette smoking, chocolate, alcohol, fatty foods, and caffeine cause relaxation and reduction of tone of LES.
    - Cardiomyotomy and vagotomy reduce the efficiency of the LES.
    - Drugs (aminophylline, β-agonists, nitrates, and calcium channel blockers) reduce the tone of LES.
  - Crural diaphragm
  - *Increased the intra-abdominal pressure:* It may occur during pregnancy, obesity, ascites, weight lifting, and straining
- **Prolonged/delayed esophageal clearance of refluxed acid:** It may be due to—(1) impaired peristalsis, (2) reduced salivation, and (3) body position. Poor esophageal clearance leads to increased acid exposure time. Impaired production of saliva may be observed in smokers and Sjogren's syndrome.

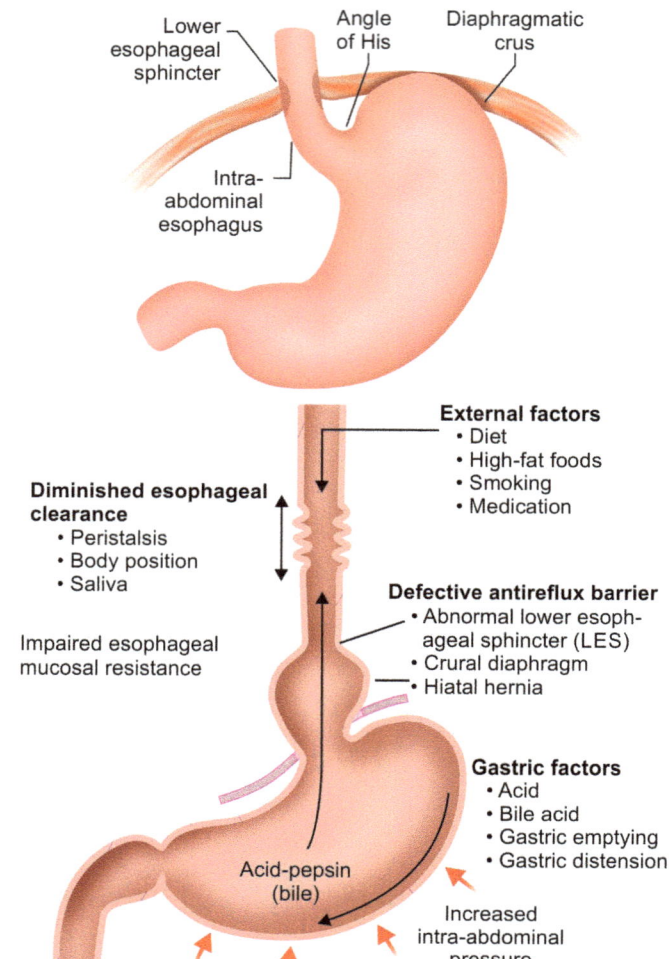

Fig. 6.3: Anatomy of normal antireflux barrier at the lower esophagus and pathophysiological factors associated with the development of gastroesophageal reflux disease (GERD).

- **Defective gastric emptying:** It increases the gastric content available for reflux. It may be due to gastric outlet obstruction, anticholinergic drugs, and fatty food.

Clinical Features

Classical triad of symptoms is—(1) heartburn, (2) acid regurgitation, and (3) epigastric pain.
1. **Heartburn:** It is the classic symptom of GERD. Patients usually complain of a burning feeling, rising from the stomach or lower chest and radiating toward the neck, throat, and occasionally the back. It occurs postprandially, particularly after large meals or after ingesting spicy foods, citrus products, fats, chocolates, and alcohol. The supine position and bending over may exacerbate heartburn.
2. **Acid regurgitation:** Effortless regurgitation of acidic fluid, especially after meals and worsened by stooping or the supine position is highly suggestive of GERD.
3. **Epigastric pain:** Sometimes radiating through to the back

Other Symptoms

- *Odynophagia* (painful swallowing)
- *Dysphagia*: Dysphagia is reported by more than 30% of individuals with GERD. Transient to solids (due to esophageal spasm) or persistent dysphagia to solids (due to strictures).
- Less common symptoms associated with GERD include water brash, burping, hiccups, nausea, and vomiting.
- Iron deficiency anemia may occur due to blood loss.

Extraesophageal Symptoms

- Atypical chest pain, which may be severe and can mimic angina
- **Upper respiratory tract:** Hoarseness, sore throat, sinusitis, otitis media, chronic cough, and laryngitis
- **Pulmonary:** The prevalence of GERD in asthmatics is estimated between 34% and 89%. Other pulmonary diseases associated with GERD include aspiration pneumonia, interstitial pulmonary fibrosis, chronic bronchitis, and bronchiectasis.

Associated conditions: Pregnancy (reducing LES pressure due to the effects of estrogen and progesterone and possibly mechanical factors from the gravid uterus), scleroderma, achalasia cardia, and Zollinger–Ellison syndrome.

Complications of GERD

Complications of GERD are described in **Table 6.19**.

Investigations

Investigations are described in **Box 6.8**.

Table 6.19: Complications of gastroesophageal reflux disease (GERD).

• Esophagitis	• Adenocarcinoma esophagus
• Hemorrhage and bleeding (hematemesis and melena)	• Aspiration pneumonia
	• Iron deficiency anemia
• Esophageal ulceration	• Dental caries
• Esophageal strictures	
• Barrett's esophagus	

Box 6.8: Diagnostic tests for gastroesophageal reflux disease.

Tests for reflux:
- Intraesophageal pH monitoring (catheter or catheter-free system)
- Ambulatory impedance and pH monitoring (nonacid reflux)
- Barium esophagogram

Tests to assess symptoms:
- Empirical trial of acid suppression
- Intraesophageal pH monitoring with symptom analysis

Tests to assess esophageal damage:
- Endoscopy
- Wireless capsule endoscopy
- Esophageal biopsy

Tests to assess esophageal function:
- Esophageal manometry
- Esophageal impedance

Treatment

General measures:
These are lifestyle modifications as listed in **Box 6.9**.

Medical treatment:
Inhibition of gastric acid secretion is the cornerstone of the treatment of acute GERD.

Antacids: Liquid antacids buffer acid and increase LESP. They are used in the dose of 10–15 mL, 1 and 3 hours after meal and at bedtime or as needed. They relieve heartburn in mild cases.

Histamine (H_2)-receptor antagonists: They decrease acid secretion. These drugs include cimetidine (800 mg bid and 400 mg qid) or ranitidine (150 mg qid), or famotidine (20–40 mg bid) daily to be given with meals and before bedtime, for at least 6 weeks (in mild cases).

Proton pump inhibitors (PPIs): They decrease acid secretion and gastric volume. They are superior to histamine (H2)-receptor antagonists. These include omeprazole (20–40 mg/day), lansoprazole (15–30 mg/day), pantoprazole (40 mg/day), esomeprazole (20–40 mg/day), and rabeprazole (10–20 mg/day). Maintenance doses may be necessary for 6–8 months.
- *H. pylori* eradication does not have any therapeutic value.
- Dilatation of esophageal strictures
- Anemia is treated with oral iron or blood transfusion

Surgical treatment:
Indications are (1) failure to respond to medical therapy, (2) patients not willing to take long-term PPIs or intolerant to PPIs, (3) patients with severe symptom, and (4) patients with regurgitation.

Surgical measures:
- *Surgical resection of esophageal strictures*
- *Antireflux surgery*: Laparoscopic fundoplication (additional valve mechanism) yields results comparable to continued PPI therapy.

Box 6.9: Lifestyle modifications in the treatment of gastroesophageal reflux disease (GERD).

- Avoid foods, such as fatty food, alcohol, mint, tomato-based foods, spicy foods, coffee, tea, and acidic foods.
- Avoid late night meals before retiring.
- Avoid weight lifting, stooping, and bending at waist.
- Elevation of the head of the bed in patients with regurgitation or heartburn during night.
- Weight reduction.
- Stop smoking and alcohol.
- Frequents feeds of small volume.

BARRETT'S ESOPHAGUS

Barrett's esophagus is a *premalignant condition*, in which the *normal squamous lining of the lower esophagus is replaced by columnar mucosa* (columnar lined esophagus—CLO). The columnar mucosa may show areas of intestinal metaplasia (with goblet cells). It is an adaptive response to chronic gastroesophageal reflux and is often asymptomatic. The risk of esophageal cancer depends on the severity and duration of reflux and it may be detected when the patient presents with esophageal cancer. It is more common in men, obese and above the age of 50. It is weakly associated with smoking but not with alcohol intake.

Management
Regular endoscopic surveillance should be done to detect dysplasia at an early stage. Currently, recommendations are as follows:
- **Barrett's esophagus with intestinal metaplasia, but without dysplasia:** It should undergo endoscopy at 3–5 yearly intervals, if the length of the Barrett segment is 3 cm and at 2–3 yearly intervals, if the length is >3 cm.
- **Low-grade dysplasia:** Endoscopy should be done at 6-monthly intervals. Treatment is indicated only for symptoms of reflux or complications (e.g., stricture).

Endoscopic therapies, such as radiofrequency ablation or photodynamic therapy, can induce regression. However, they are used only for patients with dysplasia or intramucosal cancer.

High-grade dysplasia or intramucosal carcinoma: Treatment options are either esophagectomy or endoscopic therapy, with a combination of endoscopic resection of any visibly abnormal areas and radiofrequency ablation of the remaining Barrett's mucosa, as an "organ-preserving" alternative to surgery.

HIATUS HERNIA

It is the herniation of elements of the abdominal cavity (part of stomach) through the diaphragm into the thoracic cavity.

Types (Figs. 6.4A to D)
- **Sliding or type I hiatus hernia:** It is the most common type. In this type, the gastroesophageal junction and the fundus of stomach slide upward above the diaphragmatic hiatus.
- **True paraesophageal (rolling) or type II hiatus hernia:** It is uncommon. In this type, location of gastroesophageal junction is in its normal position, but the fundus and parts of the greater curvature of the stomach herniate into the mediastinum alongside the esophagus.
- **Mixed paraesophageal hernia or type III:** In this type, gastroesophageal junction and a large part of the stomach herniate into the mediastinum.

Predisposing factors: These are obesity, pregnancy, and ascites. These occur in 33% of normal adults and 50% of elderly.

Clinical Features
- Majority of hiatus hernias are asymptomatic. Hiatus hernia predisposes to gastroesophageal reflux disease (GERD), and hence, symptoms of GERD may be present.
- *Type I* is usually asymptomatic or presents with symptoms of heartburn or acid regurgitation.
- Type II and III may present with epigastric pain, chest pain, substernal fullness, shortness of breath, nausea, or vomiting.

Management
- Asymptomatic hiatus hernias do not require any treatment. Surgical repair of hernia is required in selected cases with gastroesophageal reflux.
- Symptomatic rolling hiatus hernias require surgical repair because it is potentially liable to undergo volvulus as a dangerous complication.

Surgical treatment:
- Repair of the diaphragmatic defect
- Fixing the stomach in the abdominal cavity (fundoplication) combined with an antireflux procedure.

ACHALASIA OF THE ESOPHAGUS

Achalasia is characterized by *esophageal aperistalsis* and results from progressive degeneration of ganglion cells in the myenteric plexus in the esophageal wall, causing failure of relaxation of the hypertonic lower esophageal sphincter in response to the swallowing wave. Failure of propagated esophageal contraction results in progressive dilatation of the gullet.

Causes
Causes are unknown. Autoimmune, neurodegenerative, and viral etiologies have been suggested. Reduction in nitric oxide synthase containing neurons is detected by

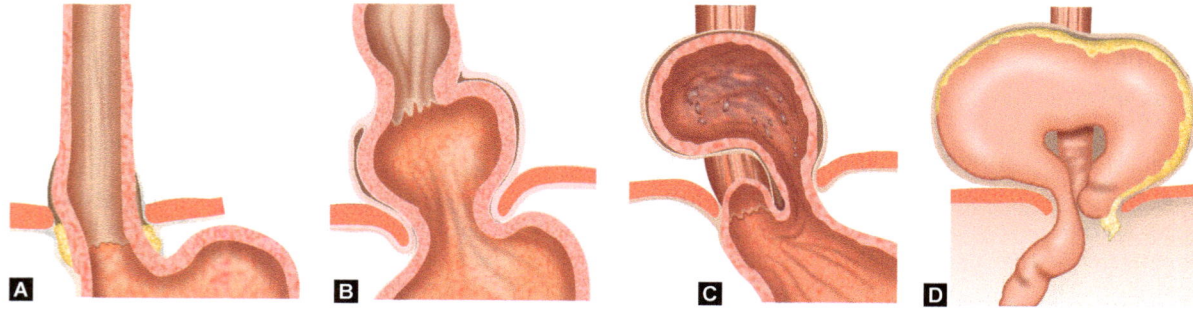

Figs. 6.4A to D: Types of hiatus hernia: (A) Normal esophagus and stomach; (B) Type I (sliding); (C) Type II (paraesophageal/rolling); (D) Type III (mixed paraesophageal) hiatus hernia.

immunohistochemical staining in the lower esophageal sphincter. There is degeneration of ganglion cells within the sphincter and the body of the esophagus. Infection with *Trypanosoma cruzi* in Chagas' disease causes a syndrome that is clinically similar to achalasia.

Clinical Features

- **Age and gender:** Occurs equally in males and females and at all ages but is rare in childhood.
- **Dysphagia:** It develops slowly and is initially intermittent and characteristically for both liquids and solids from the onset (worse for solids). Dysphagia is eased by drinking liquids and by standing and moving around after eating.
- **Episodes of chest pain:** Spontaneous chest pain occurs due to esophageal spasm, which may be misdiagnosed as cardiac.
- **Regurgitation of food from the dilated esophagus:** As the disease progresses, dysphagia worsens and causes poor emptying of the esophagus. This may produce nocturnal pulmonary aspiration and aspiration pneumonia.
- **Heartburn** does not occur because of the closed esophageal sphincter, which prevents gastroesophageal reflux.
- Achalasia *predisposes to squamous carcinoma of the esophagus.*

Investigations

- **Chest X-ray:** It shows a dilated esophagus. Sometimes fluid level may be observed behind the heart. There is *absence of fundic gas shadow.*
- **Barium swallow:** There is absence of peristalsis and often synchronous contractions in the body of the esophagus. There is tapered narrowing of the lower esophagus producing a "*bird's beak*" appearance due to failure of the sphincter to relax.
- **Manometry** shows high-pressure, nonrelaxing lower esophageal sphincter with poor contractility of the esophageal body.
- **Endoscopy:** It should be performed because carcinoma of the cardia can mimic the presentation and radiological and manometric features of achalasia ("pseudoachalasia").

Management

Treatment for achalasia is palliative.

Endoscopic:
- *Endoscopic dilatation of the LES (lower esophageal sphincter)*
- *Endoscopically directed injection of botulinum toxin into the lower esophageal sphincter (intersphincteric injection)*

Surgical:
- *Surgical myotomy (Heller's operation)*
- *Peroral endoscopic myotomy (POEM)*

DISEASES OF THE STOMACH AND DUODENUM

PEPTIC ULCER DISEASE

An ulcer in the gastrointestinal (GI) tract may be defined as a break in the lining of the mucosa, with appreciable depth at endoscopy or histologic evidence of involvement of the submucosa.

Sites of Peptic Ulcer

Any portion of the GI tract exposed to acidic gastric juices:
- **Duodenum:** *More common in the first portion of the duodenum (anterior or posterior wall) than in the stomach.* Occasionally occurs at both anterior and posterior sites ("kissing" ulcers)
- **Stomach:** Lesser curvature near the junction (transitional zone) of the body and antrum—
  - Proximal ulcers: Located in the body of the stomach
  - Distal ulcers: Located in the antrum and angulus of the stomach
- **Gastroesophageal junction of esophagus**
- **Anastomotic site:** Occurs in patients who have undergone a distal gastric resection. Occurs at margins of the gastroduodenal anastomosis/gastrojejunostomy (anastomotic ulcer)
- **Multiple ulcers:** In the duodenum, stomach, and/or jejunum in Zollinger–Ellison syndrome
- *At metaplastic or heterotopic gastric mucosa*, e.g., Meckel diverticulum within an ileum having ectopic gastric mucosa

Incidence

Incidence is ~12% in males and 10% in females.

Etiology

Normal process in the stomach:
Two opposing sets of forces keep stomach in a normal state—(1) damaging forces and (2) defensive forces.

1. **Damaging forces:** Capable of inducing mucosal injury are two gastric secretory products—(1) hydrochloric acid and (2) pepsinogen.
2. **Defensive forces** are a three-level barrier composed of pre-epithelial, epithelial, and subepithelial elements.

Pre-epithelial barrier is a mucus–bicarbonate layer of the stomach.
- **Surface mucus secretion:** Mucin is secreted by surface foveolar cells. Actions of mucus are—(1) mucus layer promotes formation of an "unstirred" protective layer of fluid on the mucosa. (2) It prevents the direct contact of large food particles with the epithelium. (3) It impedes the diffusion of ions and molecules such as pepsin.
- **Bicarbonate secretion into mucus** by surface epithelial cells → diffuses into the unstirred mucus, → buffers the hydrogen ions entering from the luminal aspect, → and results in a pH gradient, ranging from 1 or 2 at the gastric luminal surface, and reaching to a neutrality of 6 to 7 along the epithelial cell surface.

Epithelial barrier: It consists of surface epithelial cells, which act through several factors, such as (1) production of mucus, (2) epithelial cell ionic transporters that maintain intracellular pH, (3) bicarbonate production, and (4) intracellular tight junctions.

Subepithelial barrier:
Rich gastric mucosal blood flow: It provides (1) bicarbonate (HCO^-), which neutralizes the acid generated by parietal cell, (2) an adequate supply of nutrients and oxygen, and (3) removes toxic metabolic byproducts.

Pathogenesis of Peptic Ulcer (Fig. 6.5)

The imbalances between mucosal defensive forces (disruption of any of protective mechanisms) *and damaging forces* (direct

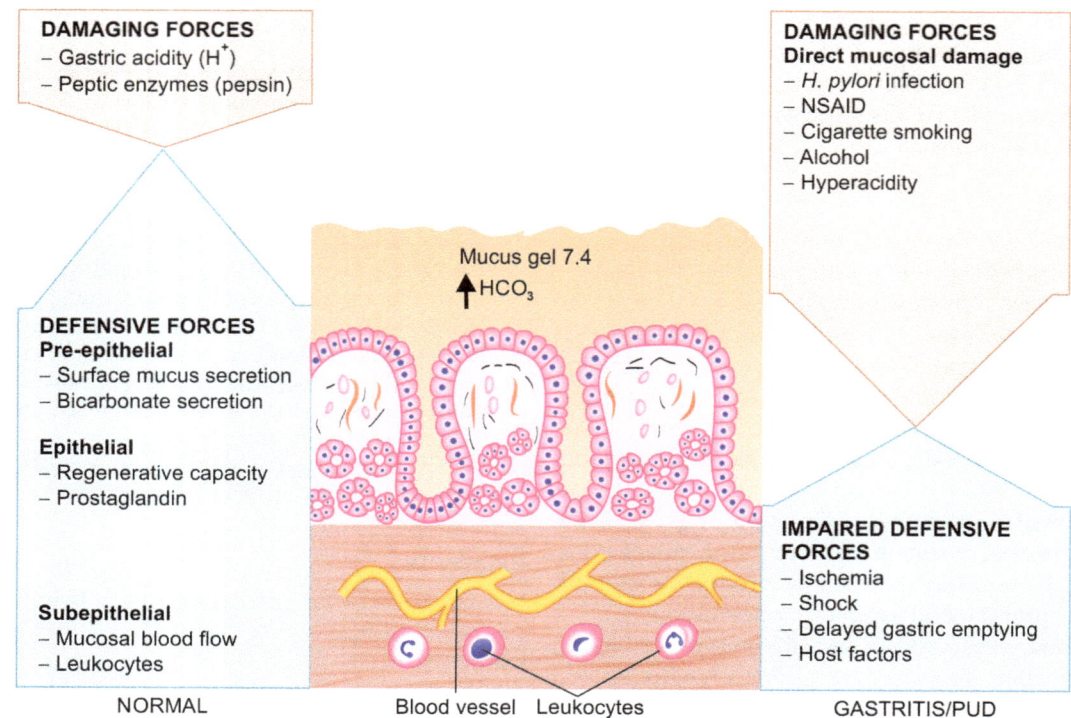

Fig. 6.5: Components involved in mucosal defense and repair in normal (left side) and in acute or chronic gastritis. Gastric mucus barrier consists of viscid mucus (which forms an unstirred layer between the epithelium and the gastric lumen) and bicarbonate.
(NSAID: nonsteroidal anti-inflammatory drug; PUD: peptic ulcer disease)

mucosal injury) *cause chronic gastritis* and also *peptic ulcer disease (PUD)*.

Direct Mucosal Injury/Increased Damage

Majority of PUDs (both gastric and duodenal ulcers) can be attributed to NSAIDs and *H. pylori*.

- ❑ **Helicobacter pylori** is a Gram-negative spiral bacterium with multiple unipolar flagella that allow them to move freely through the gastric mucous layer, where they remain protected from low gastric pH. It is one of the most important, common, and primary causes of PUD. It is associated with ~85–90% of duodenal and ~65% of gastric ulcers. *Helicobacter pylori* infection remains one of the most common chronic bacterial infections in humans; more than 50% of the world's population is infected with the bacterium. *H. pylori* also plays a role in the development of gastric and duodenal ulcer, gastritis, MALT (mucosal-associated lymphoid tissue) lymphoma, and gastric adenocarcinoma.
  - *Mode of spread:* Oral–oral or fecal–oral route either by kissing or ingestion of contaminated vomitus
  - *Lesions produced: H. pylori* may attach to gastric epithelium causing damage to the mucosa. It causes chronic antral gastritis with high acid production, may progress to pangastritis, resulting in multifocal atrophic gastritis and increased risk of gastric adenocarcinoma. Natural history of *H. pylori* infection is shown in **Figure 6.6**.

Nongastric diseases and H. pylori infection: Raynaud's, scleroderma, idiopathic urticaria, acne rosacea, migraines, thyroiditis, and Guillain–Barré syndrome, coronary artery disease, and immune thrombocytopenic purpura

- Mechanism of action by H. pylori:
  - *Flagella:* It makes them motile, allows them to burrow and live beneath the mucus layer above the epithelial surface.
  - *Urease:* It is produced by *H. pylori,* converts urea into ammonia (strong alkali), raises the local gastric pH, acts on the antral G cells, release of gastrin, and hypergastrinemia, and results in hypersecretion of gastric acid.
  - *Adhesion molecule:* It helps to bind to gastric epithelial (surface foveolar) cells.
  - *Enzymes:* These include proteases and phospholipases, which act on the mucous gel and reduce the mucosal defense.
  - *Cytotoxins:* Two genes, namely cytotoxin—associated gene A *(CagA)* and vacuolating agent *(vacA)* gene cause gastritis, peptic ulceration, and cancer.
  - *Cytokine induces inflammatory response:* Normally, *H. pylori* does not invade the cells/tissues. It causes increased production of proinflammatory cytokines [interleukin (IL)-1, IL-6, tumor necrosis factor (TNF), and IL-8] by the mucosal epithelial cells, activation of neutrophils and macrophages (inflammatory response to gastric mucosa), and release of lysosomal enzymes, leukotrienes, and reactive oxygen species, and impairs mucosal defense. The cytokines also stimulate gastrin release and *increased acid production.*
- ❑ **Nonsteroidal anti-inflammatory drugs (NSAID) and aspirin:** These cause (1) direct chemical irritation of

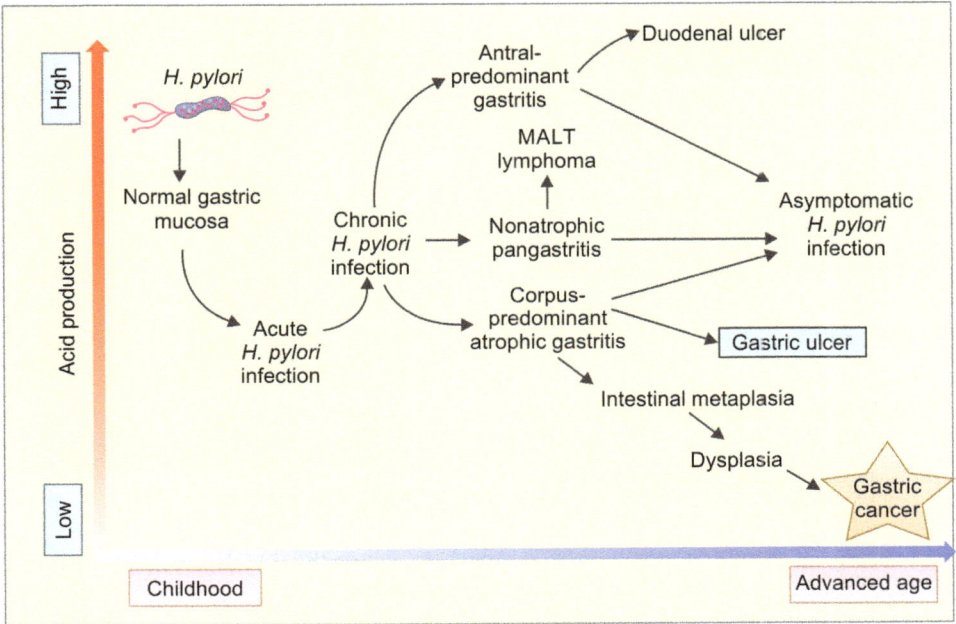

Fig. 6.6: Natural history of *H. pylori* infection.

mucosa, (2) suppress mucosal prostaglandin synthesis, and (3) reduce the bicarbonate secretion.
- **Cigarette smoking** impairs blood flow to the mucosa and healing of mucosal damage.
- **Alcohol, radiation therapy, and chemotherapy:** Direct injury to mucosal cells
- **Ingestion of chemicals**, such as acids or bases, causes direct injury
- **Gastric hyperacidity:** It is induced by *H. pylori* infection, parietal cell hyperplasia, and Zollinger–Ellison syndrome.
- **Others:** High-dose corticosteroids that suppress prostaglandin synthesis and impair healing, other drugs (e.g., bisphosphonates, cocaine, and amphetamines), hypercalcemia psychological stress, duodenal gastric reflux, Crohn's disease, and systemic mastocytosis.

Etiology of Acute and Stress Ulcers

- **Stress ulcers:** They occur with *shock, sepsis, or severe trauma.*
- **Curling ulcers:** They develop in the proximal duodenum with *severe burns or trauma.*
- **Cushing ulcers:** They develop in the stomach, duodenum, and esophagus in patients with *intracranial disease.* They are highly prone for perforation.

Clinical Features

Recurrent episodes of abdominal pain: It is the *most common presentation* and has three notable characteristics:
1. **Localization to the epigastrium:** Pain is referred to epigastrium and the patient will be able to localize the site with one finger (pointing sign). The characteristics of pain are:
   - *Nature:* Usually burning in character or gnawing discomfort
   - *Radiating pain:* May radiate to the back, thorax, and other parts of abdomen
   - *Nocturnal:* Pain in duodenal ulcer occurs 90 minutes to 3 hours after a meal. It may occur at night (most specific) and wakes the patient from sleep between midnight and 3 AM, and is relieved by food, milk, or antacids.
   - *Hunger pain:* Pain occurs on empty stomach (painful hunger) and is relieved by food or antacids.
2. **Relationship to food:**
   - Pain is usually *relieved by food, milk, antacids*, belching, or vomiting in duodenal ulcer.
   - In contrast, in few patients with gastric ulcer, food may precipitate the pain.
3. **Periodicity (episodic pain):**
   - In untreated patients, pain tends to occur in episodes. Each episode consisting of daily pain *lasting 2–8 weeks* is separated by prolonged asymptomatic intervals.
   - Between episodes (periods of remission), patient may be perfectly well and may be able to eat even heavy or spicy meals without apparent discomfort.
   - During the initial stages, the episodes tend to be of short in duration and less frequent. Later, the episodes become longer in duration and more frequent. These are more symptomatic during winter and spring. Relapses are more common in smokers compared to nonsmokers.

Other Symptoms

- Retrosternal burning (heartburn), water brash (excessive salivation), loss of appetite, acidic regurgitation into the throat, and vomiting
- Persistent daily vomiting suggests gastric outlet obstruction, fullness, bloating, anorexia, nausea, and dyspepsia.
- Tarry stools or coffee-ground vomitus indicates bleeding.
- Rarely, with anemia due to chronic blood loss, abrupt hematemesis, acute perforation, or gastric outlet obstruction

Table 6.20: Difference between gastric ulcer and duodenal ulcer.

Features	Gastric ulcer	Duodenal ulcer
Most common site	Along the lesser curvature	First part of duodenum
Incidence	Less common	More common
Age	Beyond 6th decade, M > F	Between 25 and 50 years, M > F
Association with *H. pylori* infection	Less common	Strong association
Acid level	Usually normal	High
Clinical features:		
Relationship of pain to antacids	Relief of pain not consistent	Prompt relief of pain
Relationship of pain to food	Aggravates the pain	Relieves the pain
Night pain	Not observed	Common
Heartburn	Not common	Common
Hematemesis/melena	Hematemesis more common	Melena more common
Vomiting	Common	No vomiting
Weight loss	Present	Absent
Anorexia and nausea	More common	Less common
Duration of episodes of pain	Relatively longer in duration	Relatively shorter in duration
Course of the illness	Less remission	More remission
Complication	Rarely undergo malignant change	No malignant change

Difference between gastric ulcer and duodenal ulcer is discussed in **Table 6.20**.

Complications

Complications are given in **Box 6.10**.

Investigations/Diagnosis

Anatomic diagnosis: Documentation of a peptic ulcer needs either a radiographic (barium study) or an endoscopic examination.
- **Endoscopy (Fig. 6.7):** It is most sensitive and specific for the detection of ulcer disease of the upper GI tract. Typical location of peptic ulcer is duodenal bulb and lesser curvature of stomach. Advantages of endoscopy are:
  - Direct visualization of mucosa (to determine if an ulcer is a source of blood loss) and the ulcer (even lesions are too small to detect by radiographic examination)

Box 6.10: Complications of peptic ulcer.
- Upper gastrointestinal bleeding (20%)
- Perforation of ulcer (6–7%)
- Gastric outlet obstruction (1–2%) (with fluid and electrolyte imbalance), gastrocolic, or duodenocolic fistulas
- Rarely, malignant transformation
- Rarely, pancreatitis due to posterior penetration of ulcer

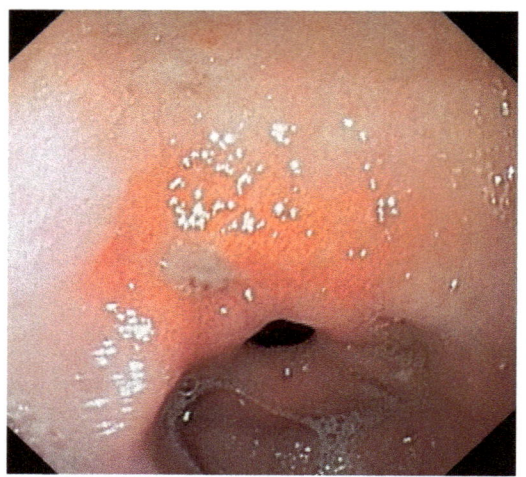

Fig. 6.7: Endoscopic picture of a benign gastric ulcer.

- It is useful for photographic documentation of a mucosal defect
- Biopsy can be taken to rule out malignancy (about 10% of gastric ulcers are malignant) or *H. pylori*.
- **Endoscopic ultrasound:** It may be useful in detecting an unsuspected submucosal component or enlarged lymph nodes (e.g., in gastric malignancies such as lymphoma and linitis plastica).
- **Etiologic diagnosis:** The cause of the ulcer must be established. The major risk factor for peptic ulcers is either *H. pylori* or NSAID.
- Tests for *Helicobacter pylori* are mentioned in **Table 6.21**.
- **Nonsteroidal anti-inflammatory drugs (NSAIDs):** Diagnosis is established based on history of drug use and symptoms of pain.
- **Hypersecretory syndromes:** Zollinger–Ellison syndrome should be considered in patients with multiple ulcers. *Serum gastrin and gastric acid analysis should be* performed in these patients.

Treatment/Management

Treatment may be divided into short-term management and long-term management (intermittent, maintenance, and surgical treatment).

Short-term Management
- **General measures**
- **Acid neutralizing/inhibitory drugs:**
  - *Antacids:* Neutralize the secreted acid and rarely used at present—
    - Mainly used for symptomatic relief of dyspepsia
    - *Preparation*: Tablet or liquid preparations
    - *Dose*: 15–30 mL liquid antacid 1 and 3 hours after food and at bed time for 4–6 weeks
    - *Commonly used antacids*: Combination of aluminum hydroxide and magnesium hydroxide. Others include calcium carbonate and sodium bicarbonate.
    - *Side effects:*
      - Aluminum compounds cause constipation, phosphate depletion, and interfere with the absorption of digoxin and tetracycline

Table 6.21: Diagnostic tests for *Helicobacter pylori* (HP).

	Advantages	Disadvantages
Nonendoscopic tests:		
Serology [qualitative or quantitative immunoglobulin G (IgG)]	Widely available and economical Good NPV (negative predictive value)	Poor PPV (positive predictive value), if HP prevalence is low Not useful after treatment
Urea breath test (^{13}C or ^{14}C)	Detects active infection Accuracy (PPV, NPV) not affected by *H. pylori* prevalence Useful both before and after treatment	Accuracy affected by PPI and antibiotic use, small radiation dose with ^{14}C test
Stool antigen test	Detects active infection Accuracy (PPV, NPV) not affected by *H. pylori* prevalence Useful both before and after treatment (monoclonal test)	Accuracy affected by PPI and antibiotic use
Endoscopic tests:		
Microscopic examination	Excellent sensitivity and specificity, especially with special and immune stains; provides additional information about gastric mucosa	Expensive (endoscopy and histopathology costs), interobserver variability, and accuracy affected by PPI and antibiotic use
Rapid urease test	Rapid results, accurate in patients not using PPIs or antibiotics, and no added histopathology cost	Requires endoscopy, less accurate after treatment or in patients using PPIs
Culture	Specificity 100%, allows antibiotic sensitivity testing	Difficult and tedious to perform; not widely available; and expensive
Polymerase chain reaction (PCR) assay	Excellent sensitivity and specificity, permits detection of antibiotic resistance	Not widely available; technique not standardized; and expensive

- Magnesium compounds cause diarrhea, hypocalcemia, and hypermagnesemia
- Calcium carbonate causes milk-alkali syndrome and sodium bicarbonate produces systemic alkalosis.
- *Histamine H_2-receptor antagonists:*
    - *Drugs:* These include four agents namely cimetidine (400 mg BD or 800 mg at night), ranitidine (150 mg BD or 300 mg at night), famotidine (20 mg BD or 40 mg at night), and nizatidine (150 mg BD or 300 mg at night). All are equally effective.
    - *Mechanism of action:* Inhibit acid and pepsin secretion by blocking H_2-receptors
    - *Duration of treatment:*
        - *Duodenal ulcer:* Usually for 4 weeks. Smokers and patients with recent major complications (e.g., hematemesis and perforation), treatment is prolonged to 6–8 weeks.
        - *Gastric ulcer:* For 6 weeks, followed by endoscopy and further treatment, if necessary
- *Proton pump (H^+/K^+-ATPase) inhibitors (PPIs):*
    - These agents are substituted benzimidazole derivatives that covalently bind and irreversibly inhibit H^+/K^+-ATPase.
    - They include omeprazole (20 mg/d), esomeprazole (20–40 mg/d), lansoprazole (15–30 mg/d), rabeprazole (20 mg/d), and pantoprazole (40 mg/d). All have similar efficacy in the treatment of various acid-peptic disorders.
    - *Mechanism of action:*
        - PPIs are lipophilic compounds that cross the parietal cell membrane and enter the acidic parietal cell canaliculus.
        - Upon entering the acidic parietal cell, the PPIs are protonated and trapped within the acid environment of the tubulovesicular and canalicular system. They become activated and bind covalently with the H^+/K^+ATPase enzyme and potently inhibit all phases of gastric acid secretion by the proton pump.
    - *Side effects:* Side effects are headache, diarrhea, abdominal pain, and nausea. The use of PPI may predispose to an increased risk of *Clostridium difficile* infection, community-acquired pneumonia, hip fracture, and vitamin B_{12} deficiency.
    - *Advantages:* Superior healing rates, shorter healing time, and faster relief of symptom compared to H_2-blockers.
- *Cytoprotective agents:*
    - *Sucralfate:* It is a complex sucrose salt insoluble in water and becomes a viscous paste within the stomach and duodenum. It binds to sites of active ulceration. Sucralfate acts as a protective barrier, over the ulcer and increases the mucosal defense and repair. Standard dose is 1 g qid.
    - *Bismuth-containing preparations:* Colloidal bismuth subcitrate (CBS) and bismuth subsalicylate are used to induce healing of peptic ulcers. Side effects include black stools, constipation, darkening of the tongue, and neurotoxicity. They are commonly used as one of the agents in an anti-*H. pylori* regimen.
    - *Prostaglandin analogs:* They enhance mucosal defense and repair and useful in preventing NSAID-induced mucosal injury. Dose (e.g., misoprostol) is 200 µg qid.
- *Treatment for H. pylori infection*

Table 6.22: First-line treatment of *Helicobacter pylori* infection.

Treatment regimen	Duration	Eradication rate
PPI (omeprazole/lansoprazole/pantoprazole/rabeprazole/esomeprazole), clarithromycin 500 mg, amoxicillin 1,000 mg (each twice daily)	10–14 days	70–85%
PPI, clarithromycin 500 mg, and metronidazole 500 mg (each twice daily)	10–14 days	70–85%
Sequential therapy: PPI, amoxicillin 1,000 mg (each twice daily) for 5 days *followed by* PPI, clarithromycin 500 mg, tinidazole 500 mg (each twice daily) for next 5 days	10 days	90%
Bismuth subsalicylate 525 mg, metronidazole 500 mg, tetracycline 500 mg (each four times daily) *plus* PPI or H_2RA (ranitidine twice daily)	10–14 days	75–90%

(PPI: proton pump inhibitors; H_2RA: histamine H_2-receptor antagonists)

Table 6.23: Rescue treatment for persistent *Helicobacter pylori* infection.

Regimen	Duration	Eradication rate
Quadruple therapy: Bismuth subsalicylate 525 mg, metronidazole 500 mg, tetracycline 500 mg (each four times daily) *plus* PPI or H_2RA (twice daily)	14 days	70%
PPI, amoxicillin 1,000 mg, and levofloxacin 250 mg (each twice daily)	10–14 days	57–91%
PPI amoxicillin 1,000 mg, rifabutin 150 mg (each twice daily)	14 days	60–80%

(PPI: proton pump inhibitors; H_2RA: histamine H_2-receptor antagonists)

- **Indications:** Consensus of opinion is that all patients with proven acute or chronic duodenal ulcer and those with gastric ulcers who are *H. pylori*-positive should be administered drugs against *H. pylori* (even without documenting the presence of bacteria).
- **Advantages:** It reduces the risk of recurrence of ulcer.
- **Type of therapy:** Triple or quadruple therapy **(Tables 6.22 and 6.23)**.

Long-term Management

- **Intermittent treatment:** When the symptoms relapse <4 times a year, 4-week course of one of the ulcer-healing agents is prescribed.
- **Maintenance treatment:**
  - Continuous maintenance treatment is not required after successful eradication of *H. pylori*.
  - If symptoms relapse for more than four times per year or history of complications (e.g., repeated bleeding or perforation) requires the lowest effective dose of PPI.
  - Long-term maintenance is with H_2-receptor antagonists (cimetidine 400 mg at night, ranitidine 150 mg at night, famotidine 20 mg at night, or nizatidine 150 mg at night).

New Treatments

- **Cholecystokinin 2 receptor antagonists (CCK2):** Itriglumide
- **Potassium competitive acid blockers (P-CABs):** Revaprazan
- **Surgical treatment:**
  - Most of peptic ulcers are cured by *H. pylori* eradication therapy and by acid-suppressing drugs. Elective surgery is reserved for the treatment of medically refractory disease (recurrence of ulcer following surgery and gastric outlet obstruction), or urgent/emergency surgery for the treatment of an ulcer-related complication (e.g., perforation and hemorrhage).
  - *Indications for surgery*:
    - *Chronic nonhealing gastric ulcer*: Persistent ulceration despite adequate medical therapy. The procedure of choice is partial gastrectomy with a Billroth I anastomosis, in which the ulcer and the ulcer-bearing area of the stomach are resected.
    - *Gastric outflow obstruction*
    - *Recurrent ulcer following gastric surgery*
    - *Duodenal ulcer*: Most commonly performed procedures are:
      - Vagotomy and drainage (by pyloroplasty, gastroduodenostomy, or gastrojejunostomy)
      - Highly selective vagotomy (which does not require a drainage procedure)
      - Vagotomy with antrectomy
  - As an emergency for complications namely *perforation and hemorrhage*.

DISEASES OF THE INTESTINE

Malabsorption Syndrome

Definition: Malabsorption is defined as defective/diminished intestinal absorption of one or more dietary nutrients.

Classification and Etiology

Classification and etiology are described in **Flowchart 6.5**.

Clinical Features (Fig. 6.8)

- **Onset:** Insidious and gradually progresses
- **General features:** Diarrhea, steatorrhea, abdominal pain, distension, loss of weight, and anemia

Irritable Bowel Syndrome (Flowchart 6.6)

Definition

- Irritable bowel syndrome (IBS) is a functional disorder of the gastrointestinal tract characterized by abdominal pain or discomfort and altered bowel habits in the absence of detectable structural, infective or biochemical abnormalities.
- IBS is benign and chronic, symptom complex of altered bowel habits and abdominal pain.
- Exact cause is not known and pathogenesis of IBS is poorly understood. However, the following factors have been proposed:
  - Gastrointestinal motor abnormalities

Flowchart 6.5: Classification and causes of malabsorption.

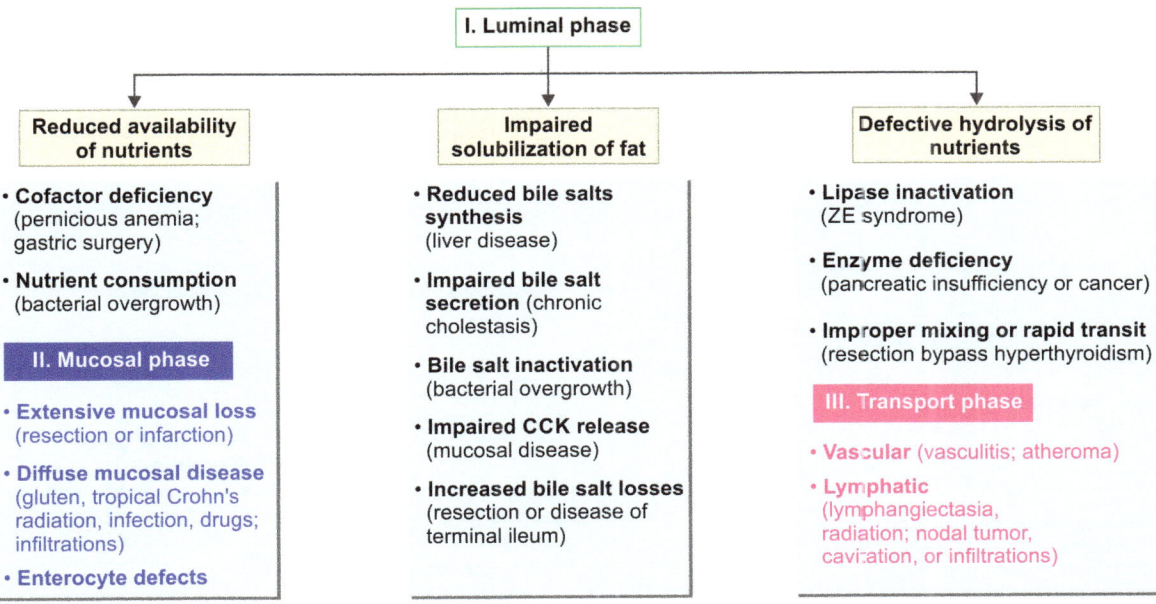

Fig. 6.8: Signs and symptoms of malabsorption.

- Visceral hypersensitivity
- Central neural dysregulation
- Abnormal psychological features
- Bacterial overgrowth
- Abnormal serotonin pathways

Clinical Features

- **Age:** IBS affects all ages. Most patients present before age 45 (20–40 years).
- **Gender:** It is more common in women compared to men (3:1).

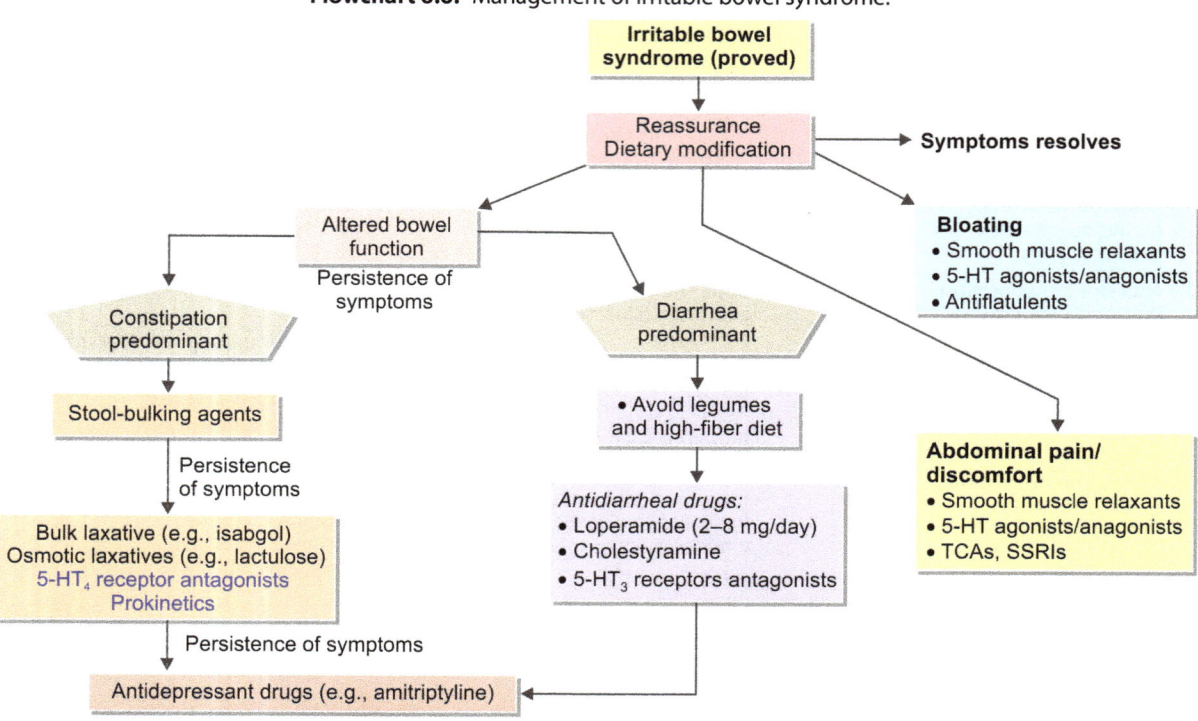

Flowchart 6.6: Management of irritable bowel syndrome.

(5-HT: 5-hydroxytryptamine; TCAs: tricyclic antidepressants; SSRIs: selective serotonin reuptake inhibitors)

- *Abdominal pain* is the most common key symptom (prerequisite clinical feature) for the diagnosis of IBS.
- *Altered bowel habits* are most consistent clinical feature in IBS. Bowel pattern subtypes/*variants* are:
  - *IBS-constipation predominant (IBS-C):* Patient reports that abnormal bowel movements are usually constipation (>25% Bristol stool types 1 or 2; <25% Bristol stool types 6 or 7).
  - *IBS-diarrhea predominant (IBS-D):* Patient reports that abnormal bowel movements are usually diarrhea (>25% Bristol stool types 6 or 7; <25% Bristol stool types 1 or 2)
  - *Mixed IBS (IBS-M):* They have features of alternating diarrhea and constipation (>25% Bristol stool types 1 or 2; >25% Bristol stool types 6 or 7)
  - *IBS-unclassified (IBS-U)*—includes those patients who meet the diagnostic criteria for IBS but cannot be accurately categorized into one of the other three subtypes.

INFLAMMATORY BOWEL DISEASE

Inflammatory bowel disease (IBD) is an immune-mediated chronic intestinal condition. It *results from inappropriate mucosal immune activation*.

These include several conditions:
1. Ulcerative colitis (UC) } Most important
2. Crohn disease (CD)
3. *Others (uncommon) nonspecific inflammatory bowel disease:* Indeterminate colitis (15% patients with IBD) microscopic ulcerative, microscopic lymphocytic and microscopic collagenous colitis.

Ulcerative Colitis (Flowchart 6.7)

Definition
Ulcerative colitis is a severe-ulcerating inflammatory disease. It is limited to large intestine (the *colon and rectum*). It is characterized clinically by recurrent attacks (exacerbations and remissions) of bloody diarrhea. Pathologically, the inflammatory response is found only in the *mucosa and submucosa* of the intestinal wall and shows chronic destruction of crypts.

Pathology
Site: Ulcerative colitis primarily involves the colonic mucosa. Usually, it *involves the rectum* (involved in 95% of cases) and *extends proximally* for a variable distance in a continuous fashion to involve part or the entire colon. Skip lesions are not seen in UC.

- **Pancolitis:** If entire colon is involved by the disease, then it is termed as *pancolitis*.
- **Left-sided colitis:** When disease involves only the left-side of colon.
- **Extensive colitis:** When disease involves colon up to the hepatic flexure.
- **Proctitis/proctosigmoiditis:** When the disease is limited to the rectum alone, then it is known as *ulcerative proctitis*. When the process involves rectum and sigmoid colon, then it is termed as *ulcerative proctosigmoiditis*.
- **Backwash ileitis:** The small intestine is normal. However, in severe cases of pancolitis, mild mucosal inflammation of the distal ileum may be present and is termed as *backwash ileitis*.

Chapter 6: Gastroenterology

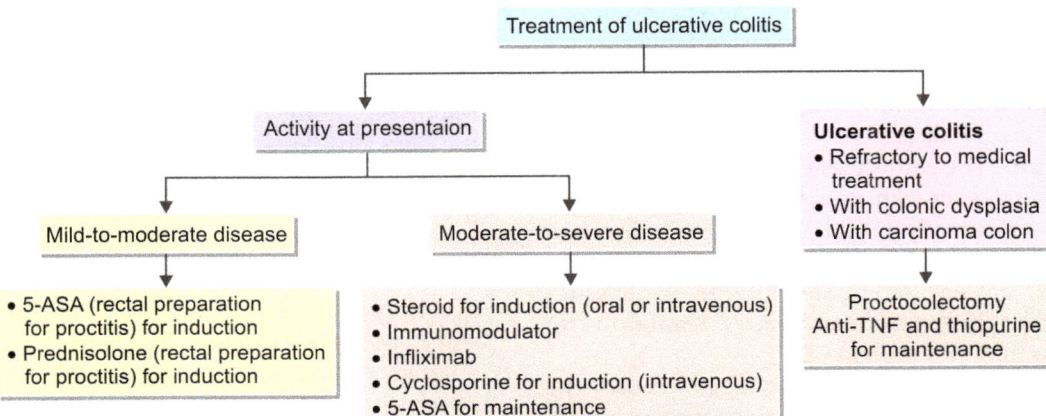

Flowchart 6.7: Algorithm for treatment of ulcerative colitis.

(5-ASA: 5-aminosalicylate agents; TNF: tumor necrosis factor)

Clinical Features of UC

Major symptoms of UC: The first attack is usually the most severe and the disease is later characterized by relapses and remissions.
- *Diarrhea*: Colonic motility is altered due to inflammation. When the disease is severe, patients develop diarrhea and pass liquid stool containing blood, mucus, pus, and fecal matter. Diarrhea is often nocturnal and/or postprandial.
- *Rectal bleeding*: Patients with proctitis usually pass fresh blood. When the disease extends beyond the rectum, blood is usually mixed with stool or grossly bloody diarrhea may be noted.
- *Tenesmus* or urgency with a feeling of incomplete evacuation
- *Passage of mucus*
- *Crampy abdominal pain*: Severe pain is not a prominent symptom, but some patients with active disease may present with vague lower abdominal discomfort or mild central abdominal cramping. Severe cramping and abdominal pain can develop when the attack is severe.
- *Others*: These include anorexia, nausea, vomiting, malaise, fever, and weight loss. There may be symptoms and signs of dehydration and anemia. In severe cases, the patient is toxic with fever, tachycardia, and signs of peritoneal inflammation.

Risk of carcinoma colon: The incidence is high, especially in patients with total colitis and disease of more than 10 years duration and early age of onset.

Signs:
- Tenderness on palpation directly over the colon, especially in the left iliac fossa.
- Signs of proctitis include tender anal canal and blood on rectal examination.
- *Signs of toxic megacolon:* It is a serious complication and its signs include severe pain and bleeding, and signs of peritonitis, if there is associated perforation.

Crohn's Disease

Gross

- **Site (Fig. 6.9):** It can involve any area of the gastrointestinal (GI) tract from mouth to anus. Unlike UC, rectum is spared in CD. Most commonly involved sites are:
  - Terminal ileum and right side of colon (40–55%)
  - *Small intestine/bowel disease alone (30–40%)*: Terminal ileum alone or ileum and jejunum.
  - Colon alone (15–25%)
- **Number of lesions:** Usually, the lesions are *multiple*.
- **Skip lesions:** The intestinal involvement is *discontinuous in which inflamed segments of intestine are* sharply *demarcated/separated by apparently normal* intervening *bowel/intestine* in-between.

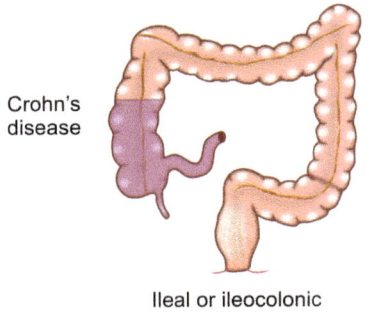

Crohn's disease

Ileal or ileocolonic
40%

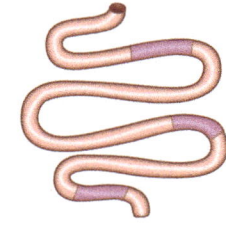

Small intestinal
30–40%

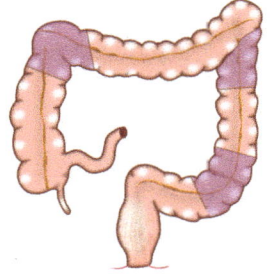

Crohn's colitis
20%

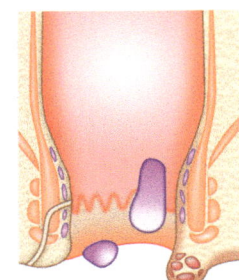

Perianal disease alone
<10%

Fig. 6.9: Patterns of distribution in Crohn's disease.

- **Intestinal wall:** The involved intestinal wall shows *fibrotic thickening and is rubbery* and appears like a hosepipe and produces a characteristic radiological sign known as the *"string sign"*.
- **Transmural inflammation:** Inflammation involves all layers of the bowel wall.
- **Mucosal lesions:** The earliest lesion is the *aphthous ulcer*, which becomes deeper, transmural, and discrete. Multiple lesions may coalesce longitudinally to form linear or *serpentine* (snake-like) ulcers and produces characteristic *"cobblestone"* appearance. Later, the ulcer becomes deeper and form linear clefts or *fissures*. Similar to UC, pseudopolyps may also form in CD.
- **External surface:** The fat may encircle around the antimesenteric serosal surface producing a pattern known as *creeping fat*.
- **Adhesion and fistulae:** Involved loops of bowel are often adherent to each other. *Fissures* frequently develop between mucosal folds. They may extend deeply to become *fistula tracts or sites of perforation*. These fistulas may also penetrate from the bowel into other organs, including the bladder, uterus, vagina, and skin.

Microscopic features:
- **Chronic inflammation** by *lymphocytes, plasma cells, and macrophages*
- *Mucosal ulcerations:* Which are small and superficial (aphthous ulcers)
- *Crypt abscesses:* Clusters of neutrophils within a crypt and are often associated with crypt destruction
- *Noncaseating granulomas*

Clinical Features of Crohn's Disease

Symptoms due to involvement of small intestine or ileum and right colon (ileocolitis). CD presents with one of two patterns of disease—(1) penetrating fistulous pattern or (2) fibrostenotic obstructing pattern. The clinical manifestations depend on the site of disease.
- Crohn's disease is a chronic disease with exacerbations and remissions.
- Major symptoms include abdominal pain (typically in the right lower quadrant), diarrhea, and weight loss (due to malabsorption and patients avoid food because eating provokes pain).
- Ileal Crohn's disease may cause subacute or acute intestinal obstruction and patients present with recurrent episodes of colicky abdominal pain, abdominal distention, nausea, vomiting, and excessive borborygmi.
- Sparing of rectum and the presence of perianal disease are observed in about 30% of patients in the form of fistulas, abscesses, fissures, and skin tags. It presents with pain, discharge, and fever (if there is an abscess).

Physical Examination
- Signs depend on the location and severity of the disease process.
- Abdominal tenderness in the right lower quadrant (classical), accompanied by fullness, guarding or a mass depending on the severity of inflammation
- Palpable mass per abdomen and rectally reflects adherent loops of intestine and abscess
- Features of malabsorption such as weight loss and anemia (iron, folic acid, and vitamin B_{12} malabsorption)
- Sodium, potassium, water, magnesium, and zinc deficiency may develop due to chronic diarrhea.
- Stool usually does not show frank blood, mucus, or pus unless colon is involved.
- Oral ulcers

Treatment approach to Crohn's disease is shown in **Figure 6.10**.

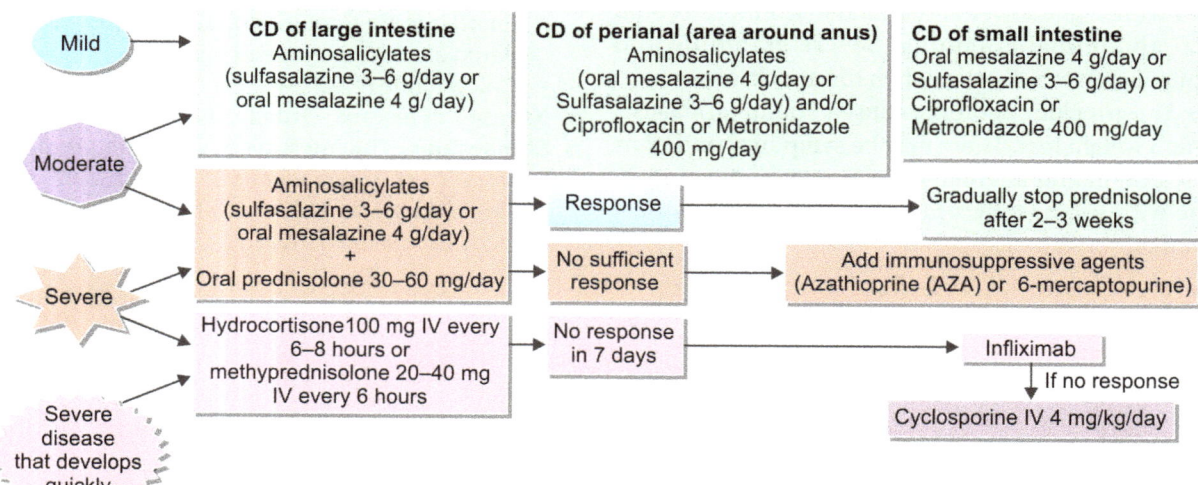

Fig. 6.10: Treatment approach to Crohn's disease.

OBJECTIVE-BASED SELF-EVALUATION

LONG QUESTIONS

1. List the common causes for upper gastrointestinal bleed. Discuss the management of acute nonvariceal upper GI bleed.
2. Define diarrhea. List the common types of diarrhea with examples for each type. How do you asses dehydration status of a patient presents with acute diarrhea?
3. Discuss the pathophysiology, clinical features, and management of gastroesophageal reflux disease.
4. Discuss the etiology, pathophysiology, clinical features, and management of peptic ulcer disease.
5. What are the common causes of malabsorption syndrome. Briefly describe the signs and symptoms of chronic malabsorption.
6. Describe the types, clinical features, complications, and management of inflammatory bowel disease.

SHORT ANSWER QUESTIONS

1. Treatment of *Helicobacter pylori* infection
2. Diagnostic tests for *Helicobacter pylori*
3. Irritable bowel syndrome
4. Difference between gastric ulcer and duodenal ulcer
5. Natural history of *H. pylori* infection
6. Achalasia of the esophagus
7. Hiatus hernia
8. Causes of odynophagia
9. Differences between upper and lower gastrointestinal bleed
10. Causes of oropharyngeal dysphagia
11. Common causes of esophageal dysphagia
12. Causes of lower gastrointestinal bleeding
13. Differences between hematemesis and hemoptysis.
14. Causes of dyspepsia
15. Nonulcer dyspepsia
16. Rome IV criteria for functional constipation

MULTIPLE CHOICE QUESTIONS

1. Which of the following has a well-established association with gastroesophageal reflux?
   a. Chronic sinusitis
   b. Dental erosion
   c. Pulmonary fibrosis
   d. Recurrent aspiration pneumonia.
2. A 36-year-old woman complains of 6 months of epigastric pain that is worst between meals. She also reports symptoms of heartburn. The pain is typically relieved by over-the-counter antacid medications. She undergoes EGD, which demonstrates a well-circumscribed 2-cm duodenal ulcer that is positive for *H. pylori*. Which of the following is recommended initial therapy given these findings?
   a. Pantoprazole plus clarithromycin plus amoxicillin for 14 days
   b. Pantoprazole plus amoxicillin for 21 days
   c. Pantoprazole plus clarithromycin for 14 days
   d. Omeprazole plus bismuth plus tetracycline plus metronidazole for 14 days
3. After a careful history and physical examination, you have diagnosed a young female patient with irritable bowel syndrome. What other condition would you reasonably expect to find in this patient?
   a. Abnormal brain anatomy
   b. Autoimmune disease
   c. History of sexually transmitted diseases
   d. Psychiatric diagnosis
4. *Helicobacter pylori* colonization increases the risk of all of the following conditions, *except*:
   a. Duodenal ulcer disease
   b. Esophageal adenocarcinoma
   c. Gastric adenocarcinoma
   d. Gastric mucosa-associated lymphoid tissue (MALT) lymphoma
5. Heller's operation is done for:
   a. Achalasia cardia
   b. Diffuse esophageal spasm
   c. Peptic ulcer disease
   d. GERD
6. Premalignant condition in which the normal squamous lining of the lower esophagus is replaced by columnar mucosa is called:
   a. Achalasia cardia
   b. Barrett's esophagus
   c. Sjogren's syndrome
   d. Nutcracker esophagus
7. Watery diarrhea is seen in all the following conditions, *except*:
   a. Crohn's disease
   b. Diabetic autonomic neuropathy
   c. Secretory diarrhea
   d. Osmotic diarrhea
8. Abrupt retching or vomiting episodes may produce longitudinal mucosal and even transmural lacerations at the level of the gastroesophageal junction. These are called:
   a. Meniere's disease
   b. Cameron's lesions
   c. Mallory–Weiss syndrome
   d. Dieulafoy's lesion
9. Passage of black, tarry, and foul-smelling stools containing altered blood is called as:
   a. Hematemesis
   b. Melena
   c. Hematochezia
   d. Steatorrhea
10. Pancolitis, proctitis/proctosigmoiditis and Backwash ileitis are patterns of:
    a. Ulcerative colitis
    b. Crohn disease
    c. Indeterminate colitis
    d. Amoebic colitis

ANSWERS

1. b   2. a   3. d   4. b   5. b
6. b   7. a   8. c   9. b   10. a

7 Hepatobiliary Disorders

CHAPTER OUTLINE

- Liver Function Tests
- Jaundice
- Chronic Parenchymal Liver Disease
- Portal Hypertension
- Variceal Bleeding
- Hepatic (Portosystemic) Encephalopathy
- Hepatorenal Syndrome
- Ascites
- Drug and Liver
- Budd–Chiari Syndrome
- Hepatocellular Carcinoma
- Pyogenic Liver Abscess
- Amebic Liver Abscess
- Hereditary Hemochromatosis
- Wilson's Disease

FUNCTIONS OF LIVER

Functions of liver are described in **Box 7.1**.

Box 7.1: Important functions of liver.

- Protein metabolism and urea formation
- **Carbohydrate metabolism:** Including gluconeogenesis, glycogenolysis, and glycogenesis
- Lipid metabolism
- Bilirubin formation from hemoglobin degradation
- Metabolism of vitamin and mineral
- Hormone metabolism
- Drug and alcohol metabolism
- Cholesterol metabolism
- Bile acid formation and bile secretion
- Synthesis of plasma proteins including coagulation factors
- **Immunological function:** Removal of gut endotoxins and foreign antigens
- Maintaining core body temperature
- Maintain pH balance and correction of lactic acidosis

LIVER FUNCTION TESTS

Liver Biochemistry

Serum Bilirubin (Fig. 7.1)

Normal level—1.0 and 1.5 mg/dL (almost all unconjugated)
- Hyperbilirubinemia—conjugated or unconjugated type **(Table 7.1)**

Conjunctival icterus: It is total serum bilirubin level < least 3.0 mg/dL and does not differentiate between conjugated and unconjugated hyperbilirubinemia. Tea- or cola-colored urine may indicate the presence of bilirubinuria and thus conjugated hyperbilirubinemia.
- **Fluctuating hyperbilirubinemia:**
  - Gallstones
  - Carcinoma of ampulla of Vater
  - Chronic hepatitis
  - Hemolytic anemias
  - Gilbert's syndrome

Serum Enzymes

- **Aminotransferases (transaminases):** Aspartate aminotransferase [(AST; serum glutamic oxaloacetic transaminase (SGOT)] and *alanine aminotransferase* [ALT; serum glutamic pyruvic transaminase (SGPT)]
- Present in hepatocytes and leak into the blood with liver cell damage
- **Normal value:** 10–40 U/L
- Poor correlation between the degree of liver cell damage and level of aminotransferases
- **Aspartate aminotransferase (AST):**
  - Mitochondrial and cytoplasmic isoenzymes
  - High concentration also in heart, muscle, kidney, and brain
  - Raised in hepatic necrosis, myocardial infarction, muscle injury, and congestive cardiac failure
- **Alanine aminotransferase (ALT):**
  - Cytosolic enzyme
  - More specific for liver injury

AST:ALT ratio:
- AST:ALT >1 is chronic viral hepatitis and nonalcoholic fatty liver disease.
- AST:ALT ratio >2:1 is suggestive, while a ratio >3:1 is highly suggestive of alcoholic liver disease. A low level of ALT in the serum in alcoholic patients is due to an alcohol-induced deficiency of pyridoxal phosphate.

Causes of elevated serum aminotransferases:
Causes of acute and chronic serum aminotransferases elevation are described in **Tables 7.2 and 7.3**.

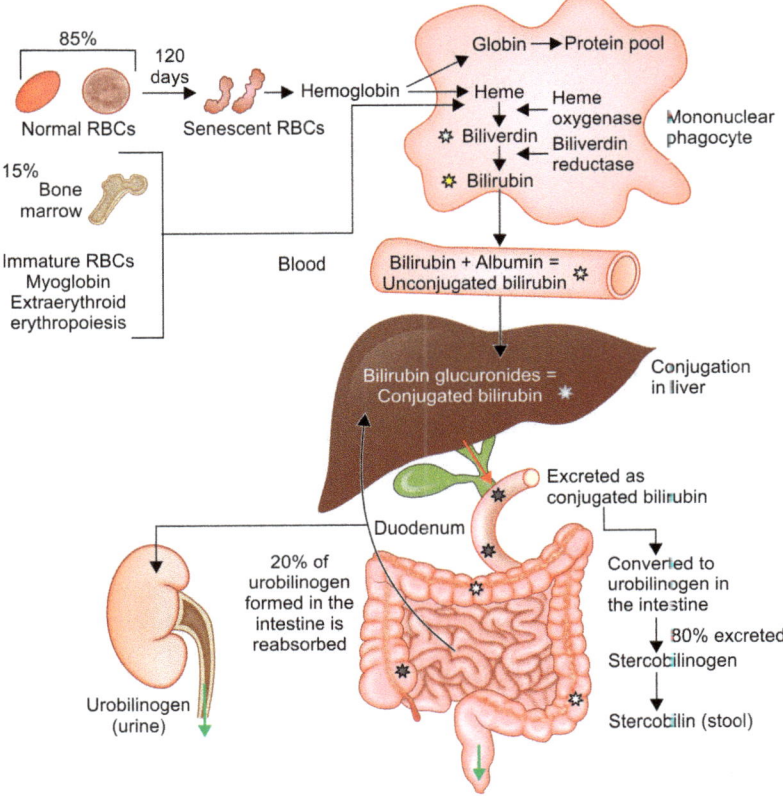

Fig. 7.1: Bilirubin metabolism.

Table 7.1: Types of hyperbilirubinemia.

Type	Bilirubin level	Causes	Bilirubinuria, LFT
Unconjugated hyperbilirubinemia	<6 mg/dL	• Hemolytic anemia • Ineffective erythropoiesis • Gilbert's syndrome	Absent LFT otherwise normal
Conjugated hyperbilirubinemia	Higher levels	• Parenchymal liver diseases • Biliary tract obstructions	Present LFT deranged

(LFT: liver function test)

Enzymes that reflect cholestasis:
- **Alkaline phosphatase (ALP):**
  - Many distinct isoenzymes—liver, bone, kidney, placenta, small intestine, and origin—can be determined by electrophoretic separation.
  - *Normal serum level:* 3–13 KA units (80–240 IU/L)
  - Raised levels of liver-derived ALP are not totally specific for cholestasis.
  - *Low levels:* Wilson's disease, with fulminant hepatitis and hemolysis, possibly because of reduced activity of the enzyme owing to displacement of the cofactor zinc by copper.
  - *Raised serum ALP levels:*
    - *<2.5 times*: Hepatocellular jaundice

Table 7.2: Chronic mild elevations (<150 U/L).

ALT>AST		AST>ALT	
Hepatic	**Nonhepatic**	**Hepatic**	**Nonhepatic**
• α1-antitrypsin deficiency • Autoimmune hepatitis • Chronic viral hepatitis (B, C, and D) • Hemochromatosis • Medications and toxins • Wilson disease • Steatosis and steatohepatitis	• Celiac disease • Hyperthyroidism	• Alcohol-related liver injury • Cirrhosis	• Hypothyroidism • Macro-AST • Myopathy • Strenuous exercise

(ALT: alanine aminotransferase; AST: aspartate aminotransferase)

Table 7.3: Acute severe elevations (>1,000 U/L).

ALT>AST		AST>ALT	
Hepatic	**Nonhepatic**	**Hepatic**	**Nonhepatic**
• Acute bile duct obstruction • Acute Budd–Chiari syndrome • Acute viral hepatitis • Autoimmune hepatitis • Hepatic artery ligation • Ischemic hepatitis • Medications/toxins • Wilson's disease	None	Medications or toxins in a patient with underlying alcoholic liver injury	Acute rhabdomyolysis

- *>4 times*:
  - Obstructive jaundice (intrahepatic or extrahepatic obstruction)
  - Infiltrative liver diseases, e.g., cancer, metastases, and amyloidosis
  - Bone lesions with rapid bone turnover, e.g., Paget's disease
  - Primary biliary cirrhosis
- ϒ-glutamyl transpeptidase (GGT):
  - Microsomal enzymes present in liver, renal tubules, pancreas, and intestine.
  - Identify source of isolated elevation in serum ALP [γ-glutamyl transpeptidase (GGTP) is normal in bone disease)
  - *Screening test for alcoholism*: If ALP is normal, raised serum GGT is a good guide to alcohol intake of more than 60 g/day. Detection and following alcohol abuse in patients who deny it.
  - *Elevated GGT levels*:
    - Biliary obstruction
    - Alcoholism
    - Liver parenchymal damage
    - Nonalcoholic fatty liver
    - *Other causes*: Chronic obstructive lung disease, diabetes mellitus, hyperthyroidism, obesity, and renal failure
    - Patients taking phenytoin, barbiturates, and antiretroviral therapy—non-nucleoside reverse transcriptase inhibitors and abacavir
- 5-nucleotidase (5'-NT):
  - Microsomal enzyme similar significance as that of GGT
  - 5'-NT levels are not increased in bone disease but increased in hepatobiliary disease.

> **Lactic dehydrogenase (LDH):**
> - Not useful in diagnosis of liver diseases
> - *Moderate elevations*: Ischemic hepatitis and hepatic metastasis
> - ALT/LDH ratio >1.5 suggests ischemic hepatitis while ratio <1.5 is seen with paracetamol toxicity

Biosynthetic Function of the Liver
- Plasma proteins:
  - *Serum albumin*:
    - Synthesized exclusively in liver, marker of synthetic function
    - Normal serum albumin level: 4–5.5 g/100 mL
    - *Hypoalbuminemia*: Chronic liver diseases—cirrhosis and chronic hepatitis; reflects severe liver damage and decreased albumin synthesis. Bad prognostic sign
  - *Serum globulins*:
    - Made of ϒ-globulins (immunoglobulins) synthesized by B-lymphocytes and α- and β-globulins synthesized primarily by hepatocytes
    - Normal serum globulin level: 1.5–3.5 g/100 mL
    - Increased in chronic liver disease (e.g., chronic hepatitis and cirrhosis)
  - *Coagulation factors*:
    - Liver produces all the coagulation factors except factor VIII
    - Vitamin K—activation of coagulation factors II, VII, IX, and X
    - Factors have short half-life time, best measure of current hepatic synthetic function for diagnosis and prognosis of acute parenchymal liver disease
  - *Prothrombin time*:
    - *Normal*: 11–12.5 seconds
    - Prothrombin time collectively measures factors II, V, VII, and X.
    - *Prolonged*:
      - *Severe liver damage*: Acute hepatitis (e.g., viral hepatitis) and cirrhosis
      - *Vitamin K deficiency*: Obstructive jaundice, fat malabsorption, poor intake, and antibiotic therapy
      - Disseminated intravascular coagulation
- Marked prolongation of the prothrombin time (>5) seconds above control, if not corrected by parenteral administration of vitamin K, is a poor prognostic sign in acute viral hepatitis and other acute and chronic liver diseases.
- **Ceruloplasmin:**
  - Acute phase reactant synthesized by the liver
  - Major carrier for copper by binding to it in plasma
  - *Normal plasma level*: 20–60 mg/dL
  - *Elevated levels*: Infections, liver diseases, obstructive jaundice, rheumatoid arthritis, and pregnancy
  - *Decreased levels*: Wilson's disease (due to decreased rate of synthesis), neonates, Menke's disease, kwashiorkor, marasmus, protein-losing enteropathy, and copper deficiency

Urine Tests

- **Bilirubin:**
  - Normally, cannot be detected in urine
  - In unconjugated hyperbilirubinemia, urine does not contain bilirubin (acholuric jaundice)
  - In conjugated hyperbilirubinemia, urine contains bilirubin
  - Detected by Fouchet's test
- **Urine urobilinogen:**
  - Normally present in urine in trace amount (1–2 mg/dL), insufficient for significant positive reaction
  - *Increased urobilinogen*:
    - Hemolytic anemias (without bilirubin in urine)—thalassemia, sickle cell anemia, and hereditary spherocytosis
    - Liver diseases (bilirubinuria present)—preicteric phase of infective hepatitis, drugs or toxic hepatitis, and cirrhosis
  - *Cause of absent urobilinogen:* Obstructive jaundice (bilirubinuria present)
  - Detected by Ehrlich's aldehyde test

Alpha-fetoprotein

- Normally produced by fetal liver, levels fall after birth
- Reappearance in increasing and high concentrations in the adult is abnormal
- Causes of elevated levels of alpha-fetoprotein are:
  - Hepatocellular carcinoma (hepatoma)
  - Carcinomas of stomach, pancreas, gallbladder, bile ducts, and lungs
  - Teratomas
- Slightly raised with regenerative liver tissue in patients with:
  - Viral hepatitis
  - Chronic hepatitis
  - Cirrhosis
- Increased concentrations in pregnancy-neural-tube defects of the fetus

Hepatic Elastography

- Hepatic fibrosis—early stage of chronic liver disease and cirrhosis
- Conventional liver tests and imaging studies do not detect hepatic fibrosis
- Noninvasive method for measurement of hepatic fibrosis
- **Methods:**
  - *Ultrasound elastography:* Mild-amplitude and low-frequency (50 H_z) vibration transmitted through the liver. The velocity of wave correlates with tissue stiffness, the wave travels faster through denser fibrotic tissue.
  - *Magnetic resonance elastography:* More reliable than ultrasound elastography

Endoscopic Retrograde Cholangiopancreatography

- Technique used to outline the biliary and pancreatic ducts.
- **Uses:**
  - *Diagnostic procedure:*
    - Biopsy of ampullary carcinoma
    - Administration of brachytherapy for cholangiocarcinoma
    - Direct visualization of the ampulla and common bile duct
    - Placement of stents
    - Sphincterotomy
  - *Therapeutic procedure:*
    - Removal of common bile duct stones
    - Sphincterotomy
    - Dilatation of benign strictures
    - Placement of nasobiliary catheters and biliary stents
    - Obtain samples for culture. Cytology
- **Complications:** The complication rate in diagnostic endoscopic retrograde cholangiopancreatography (ERCP) is 2–3%.
  - Pancreatitis
  - Cholangitis
  - Bleeding
  - Duodenal perforation

Percutaneous Transhepatic Cholangiography

- **Uses:**
  - Identification and localization of the site of obstruction of the biliary tract
  - Preoperative planning of surgery
  - Introduction of stent in malignant strictures
- **Complications:**
  - Bleeding
  - Cholangitis
  - Infection with septicemia
  - Biliary peritonitis

Magnetic Resonance Cholangiopancreatography

- Noninvasive technique largely replacing diagnostic (but not therapeutic) ERCP
- A heavily T2-weighted sequence enhances visualization of the water-filled biliary and pancreatic ducts to produce high-quality images of ductal anatomy.
- **Advantages of magnetic resonance cholangiopancreatography (MRCP) over ERCP:**
  - No need for contrast media or ionizing radiation
  - Images can be acquired faster
  - Less operator dependent
  - No risk of pancreatitis
- **Indications:**
  - Diagnosis of bile duct obstruction and pancreatic duct abnormalities
  - Unsuccessful ERCP or a contraindication to ERCP

Endoscopic Ultrasound

- Gradually replacing diagnostic ERCP
- **Advantages:**
  - High-resolution ultrasound imaging
  - Accurate staging of small, potentially operable pancreatic tumors
  - Offers a less-invasive method for bile duct imaging
- **Uses:**
  - *Diagnostic:*

- Imaging pancreatic and biliary diseases, e.g., choledocholithiasis, pancreatic and biliary cancers, and cystic lesions of the pancreas
- Ampullary carcinoma—to know the local extension, regional nodal metastasis
- Guided fine-needle aspiration from suspicious lesions
- *Therapeutic:* Increasingly used for interventions:
  - Pain relief in unresectable pancreatic carcinoma, injecting bupivacaine and alcohol into celiac ganglia
  - Endoscopic management of pancreatic pseudocysts
- *Disadvantages:* Cost is high, high degree of training required

JAUNDICE (TABLES 7.4 TO 7.7)

- *Jaundice is yellowish pigmentation of skin, mucous membranes, and sclera due to increased levels of bilirubin in the blood.*
- Scleral involvement—rich elastic tissue that has special affinity for bilirubin
- **Normal serum bilirubin level:** 0.3–1.2 mg/dL
- Clinically detected when the serum bilirubin is 2.0–2.5 mg/dL
- Latent jaundice—bilirubin level: 1.2–2.5 mg/dL
- **Carotenemia:** Yellowish pigmentation of skin by carotene but not of sclera

Hemolytic Jaundice

- Increased destruction of red blood cells or their precursors produce increased production of bilirubin.

Table 7.4: Classification of jaundice.

Predominantly unconjugated hyperbilirubinemia	Predominantly conjugated hyperbilirubinemia
Increased production of bilirubin: • Hemolytic anemias • Resorption internal hemorrhage (e.g., GI bleeding and hematomas) • Ineffective erythropoiesis **Reduced hepatic uptake:** • Drugs that interference with membrane carrier systems • Diffuse liver disease (hepatitis and cirrhosis) • Some cases of Gilbert syndrome **Impaired bilirubin conjugation:** • Physiologic jaundice of the newborn • Crigler–Najjar syndrome types I and II • Gilbert syndrome • Diffuse liver disease (hepatitis and cirrhosis)	**Decreased hepatocellular excretion:** • Liver damage or toxicity (e.g., hepatitis) • *Deficiency of membrane transporters*: Dubin–Johnson syndrome and Rotor syndrome **Impaired intra-/extrahepatic bile flow:** • Inflammatory destruction of bile ducts (e.g., primary biliary cirrhosis) • Gallstones • *Carcinoma*: Head of pancreas, periampullary carcinoma, and cholangiocarcinoma

(GI: gastrointestinal)

- Unconjugated bilirubin accumulates in the plasma and results in jaundice.
- It is usually mild, because normal liver can easily handle the increased bilirubin production.

Table 7.5: Classification of jaundice based on the pathological mechanism.

Hemolytic jaundice	
Intracorpuscular defects	*Extracorpuscular defects*
• **Hereditary:** Spherocytosis, sickle cell disease, thalassemia, and G6PD deficiency • **Acquired:** Vitamin B_{12} and folate deficiency	• Autoimmune and alloimmune hemolytic anemias • **Fragmentation syndromes:** Prosthetic valves • Drugs, e.g., sulfasalazine and dapsone • **Infections of RBCs:** Malaria
Hepatocellular jaundice	
• Viral, alcoholic hepatitis • Chronic hepatitis • Cirrhosis—any type • Infiltrations	• Ischemic liver • **Drug-induced hepatitis:** Chlorpromazine, imipramine, INH, rifampicin, erythromycin, amitriptyline, halothane, and methyldopa
Cholestatic (obstructive) jaundice	
Intrahepatic (small duct obstruction):	*Extrahepatic (large duct obstruction):*
• Primary biliary cirrhosis • Primary sclerosing cholangitis • Alcohol, drugs • Viral hepatitis • Cirrhosis • Chronic hepatitis • Secondaries in liver • Severe bacterial infections • Inherited cholestatic liver disease • Pregnancy	• Gallstones in the common bile duct • *Parasitic*: Helminths in the CBD • Carcinoma • Head of pancreas • Ampulla of Vater • Bile duct (cholangiocarcinoma) • Liver metastases • Stricture of bile ducts • Sclerosing cholangitis • Chronic pancreatitis

(CBD: common bile duct; G6PD: glucose 6 phosphate dehydrogenase; RBC: red blood cell)

Table 7.6: Clinical features.

Symptoms	Signs
• Jaundice (gradually progressive/fluctuating)	Deep jaundice with a greenish hue
• Pruritus	Scratch marks
• Pale and clay-colored stools	Xanthelasmas on eyelids
• Dark urine (increased conjugated bilirubin)	Xanthomas over tendons
Depending on the cause: • Fever with chills and rigors (cholangitis) • Weight loss (malabsorption) • Bleeding tendency (vitamin K deficiency) • Bone pains (calcium and vitamin D deficiency) • Abdominal pain (gallstones)	**Depending on the cause:** • Palpable gallbladder in carcinoma head of pancreas • Large hard irregular liver (malignancy) • *Late features*: Secondary biliary cirrhosis and signs of liver cell failure

Table 7.7: Clinical features useful in differentiating different types of jaundice.

Feature	Hemolytic	Hepatocellular	Obstructive
Jaundice:			
• Color	Lemon yellow	Orange yellow	Greenish yellow
• Depth	Mild	Variable	Deep
Pruritus	–	Variable	+
Bleeding tendency	–	+	+ (late)
Anemia	+	–	–
Splenomegaly	+	Variable	Absent (may develop later)
Palpable gallbladder	–	–	May be present
Features of liver cell failure	–	+ (early)	+ (late)

- ❏ **Clinical features**—depend on the cause of anemia.
  - *Pallor*
  - *Mild jaundice* without any signs of liver disease (**Fig. 7.2**)
  - *Hepatosplenomegaly*
- ❏ Gallstones and leg ulcers may be seen depending on the cause of anemia
  - *Dark stools* (stercobilinogen)
  - *Urine turns dark yellow* on standing (increased urobilinogen converted to urobilin)
  - *Investigations:*
    - Hemolysis
    - *Unconjugated hyperbilirubinemia (less than 6 mg%)*
    - *No bilirubin in urine, unconjugated bilirubin—water insoluble (acholuric jaundice)*
    - Urinary urobilinogen is increased (more than 4 mg/24 hours)
    - Other liver function tests are normal

Hepatocellular Jaundice

- ❏ It is a parenchymal liver disease causing inability of liver to transport bilirubin from hepatocytes into bile (**Fig. 7.3**).
- ❏ Defect in bilirubin transport across the hepatocyte may occur at any point between the uptake of unconjugated bilirubin into the hepatocyte and transport of conjugated bilirubin into biliary canaliculi.
- ❏ In hepatocellular jaundice, both unconjugated and conjugated bilirubin level rise in the blood.

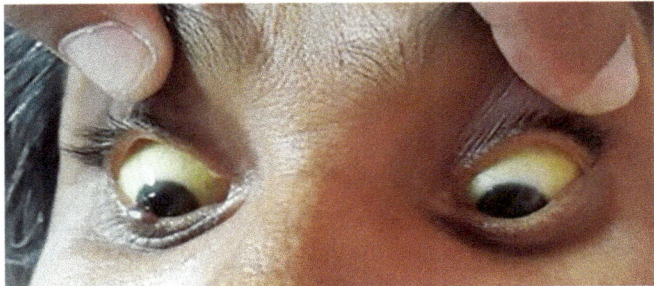

Fig. 7.2: Conjunctiva showing mild jaundice in hemolytic anemia.

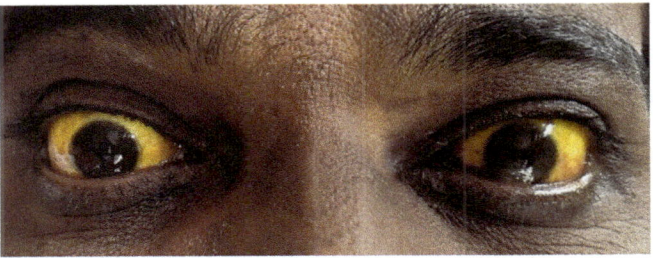

Fig. 7.3: Deep jaundice in viral hepatitis.

- ❏ **Investigations:**
  - Raised AST and ALT
  - Acute jaundice with AST > 1,000 U/L is highly suggestive of an infectious cause (e.g., hepatitis A and B), drugs (e.g., paracetamol), or hepatic ischemia
  - Imaging and liver biopsy

Cholestatic (Obstructive) Jaundice

- ❏ It is failure of bile flow. Its cause may be anywhere between hepatocyte and duodenum.
- ❏ Surgical jaundice, causes require surgical intervention (**Fig. 7.4**).
- ❏ There is retention of bile acids and bilirubin in the liver and blood and deficiency of bile acids in the intestine.
- ❏ **Investigations:**
  - *Serum findings:*
    - Marked conjugated hyperbilirubinemia
    - Serum ALP increased 3–4 times normal
    - Minimal biochemical changes of liver parenchymal damage
  - Antimitochondrial antibody in primary biliary cirrhosis
  - *Urine findings:* Bilirubin present and urobilinogen absent
  - Ultrasonography to detect the underlying cause
  - ERCP or MRCP
  - Percutaneous transhepatic cholangiography (PTC)
  - Liver biopsy performed, if there is evidence of liver cell disease

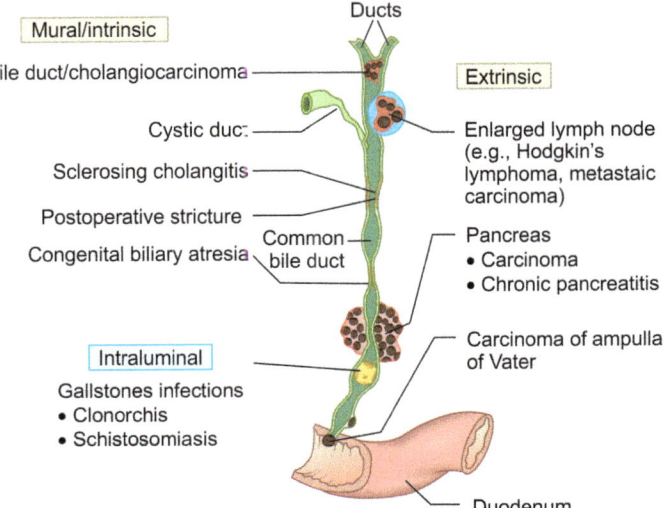

Fig. 7.4: Causes of obstructive jaundice.

Congenital Nonhemolytic Hyperbilirubinemia

Gilbert Syndrome
- It is relatively *common*, autosomal *recessive, harmless,* and inherited disorder.
- **Etiology:** *Mutations in UGT1 gene*—inadequate synthesis of UGT1A1 enzyme (about 30% of normal)
- **Clinical features:**
  - More common in males
  - Usually asymptomatic, jaundice is incidentally detected
  - *Mild, chronic unconjugated fluctuating hyperbilirubinemia*
  - No other functional derangements
  - Depth of jaundice increases with infections, fatigue, exertion, and fasting
  - Physical examination is otherwise normal.
- **Investigations:**
  - Unconjugated hyperbilirubinemia (less than 6 mg%). Raised bilirubin levels during fasting are the most common diagnostic tool.
  - *Urine*: Increased urobilinogen and absent bilirubinuria
  - Peripheral smear, reticulocyte count, and serum haptoglobin: Normal
- **Treatment:** Usually, no treatment is required. Glucuronosyltransferase activity may be increased by administering phenobarbital 60 mg BD.

Crigler–Najjar Syndrome Type I
- It is rare, *autosomal recessive* disorder. It is invariably fatal.
- **Etiology:** Due to *complete absence of hepatic UGT1A1*
- Chronic, severe, *unconjugated hyperbilirubinemia* with severe jaundice, icterus, and *death* secondary to kernicterus *within 18 months* of birth
- *Bile* does contain conjugated into bilirubin; hence, it is *colorless*.
- **Treatment:** *Daily phototherapy* and *liver transplantation*. Phenobarbital has *no effect*.
- *Liver* is *morphologically normal* by light and electron microscopy.

Crigler–Najjar Syndrome Type II
- Less severe, non-fatal disorder, also known as Arias syndrome
- Autosomal recessive inheritance in most cases
- Partial deficiency of UGT1A1 enzyme (<10% of normal)
- Jaundice is milder than type I and does not develop kernicterus
- Treatment includes ultraviolet light therapy and liver transplantation. Phenobarbital treatment can improve bilirubin glucuronidation by inducing hypertrophy of hepatocellular endoplasmic reticulum

Dubin–Johnson Syndrome
- It is benign autosomal recessive disorder.
- **Etiology:** *Complete absence* of the *multidrug-resistance protein 2 (MRP2)*, which is required for secretion of conjugated bilirubin from hepatocytes into canaliculi. This leads to defect in hepatocellular excretion of bilirubin glucuronides across biliary canalicular membrane.
- **Clinical features:** Chronic and recurrent conjugated hyperbilirubinemia, generally after puberty
- **Investigations:**
  - Conjugated hyperbilirubinemia (usually 2–5 mg/dL)
  - Bromsulfthalein clearance—impaired with reflux into blood at 90 minutes
  - Bilirubinuria
  - Gallbladder is usually not visualized on oral cholecystography
  - Liver biopsy: *Dark pigment* in centrilobular hepatocytes, *coarse melanin-like pigmented granules* within the enlarged lysosomes, present in the cytoplasm. Pigment composed of polymers of epinephrine metabolites.
- **No treatment** is required in most cases. Have a normal life expectancy.

Rotor Syndrome
- It is a rare, autosomal recessive, and asymptomatic conjugated hyperbilirubinemia.
- Defects in hepatocellular uptake, intracellular binding, and excretion of bilirubin pigments
- Clinical presentation—mild jaundice
- **Investigations:**
  - Conjugated hyperbilirubinemia
  - Bilirubinuria
  - *BSP clearance test*—impaired without reflux back into blood
  - Gallbladder is visualized on oral cholecystography
- Liver is morphologically normal.

Charcot's Triad
It consists of following in the presence of stones in bile ducts:
- Pain in the right hypochondrium
- Intermittent or persistent jaundice
- Fever with chills and rigors due to acute cholangitis
- *Reynolds pentad* adds mental status changes and sepsis to the triad.

Courvoisier's Law
- In obstruction of common bile duct due to a stone, the gallbladder as a rule is impalpable (no distension), as it is already shriveled, fibrotic, and nondistensible.
- In obstruction from other causes (e.g., carcinoma head of pancreas), distension of the gallbladder is common and hence gallbladder may be palpable.

ACUTE VIRAL HEPATITIS

Acute viral hepatitis can be defined as *infection of hepatocytes* that produces necrosis and inflammation of the liver **(Tables 7.8 and 7.9)**.

Hepatitis A
- **Etiology:** Hepatitis A virus (HAV), nonenveloped, 27-nm, RNA virus, and picornaviridae
- It is most common type, often occurs in epidemics, and affects children and young adults.

Table 7.8: Etiology of viral hepatitis.

Hepatitis caused by common (hepatotropic) viruses		Other viruses
Type of hepatitis:	Causative agent:	Cytomegalovirus
Hepatitis A	Hepatitis A virus (HAV)	Epstein–Barr virus
Hepatitis B	Hepatitis B virus (HBV)	Herpes simplex virus
Hepatitis C	Hepatitis C virus (HCV)	Yellow fever virus
Delta hepatitis	Hepatitis D virus (HDV)	Hepatitis G virus
Hepatitis E	Hepatitis E virus (HEV)	Dengue virus

Table 7.9: Summary of various hepatotropic viruses.

Feature	HAV	HBV	HCV	HDV	HEV
Incubation period in days (range)	30 (15–45)	90 (30–180)	50 (15–160)	90 (30–180)	40 (14–60)
Onset	Acute	Insidious or acute	Insidious	Insidious or acute	Acute
Age group affected	Children and young adults	Young adults, babies, and toddlers	Adults, but any age	Any age (similar to HBV)	Young adults
Mode of transmission	Fecal–oral	Parenteral, sexual contract, and perinatal	Parenteral	Parenteral	Fecal–oral
Clinical:					
Severity	Mild	Occasionally severe	Moderate	Occasionally severe	Mild
Frequency of chronic liver disease	Never	10%	80%	5% with coinfection; ≤70% for superinfection	Never
Carrier state	None	1–30%	1.5–3.2%	Variable	None
Progression to cancer	None	+(Neonatal infection)	+	±	None
Prognosis	Good	Worse	Moderate	Acute, good Chronic, poor	Good
Prophylaxis	Immunoglobulin-inactivated vaccine	Hepatitis B immunoglobulin, recombinant vaccine	None	HBV vaccine (none for HBV carriers)	Vaccine

(HAV: hepatitis A virus; HBV: hepatitis B virus; HCV: hepatitis C virus; HDV: hepatitis D virus; HEV: hepatitis E virus)

- **Source of infection:** Acutely infected person
- Replicates in liver, excreted in bile, then excreted in feces of infected person for 2 weeks before symptoms and for a further 2 weeks or so.
- Maximally infectious just before the onset of jaundice
- **Mode of spread:** *Fecal–oral route*, ingestion of contaminated water or food. It spreads through water, milk, and shellfish. The virus survives on human hands and fomites. Overcrowding and poor sanitation facilitate spread. It is resistant to freezing, detergents, and acids, and inactivated by formalin and chlorine.
- Viremia—transient. No blood-borne transmission
- **Incubation period:** 15-45 days (mean—4 weeks)
- No carrier state
- **Prevention:** Good hygiene and improving social conditions
- Prophylaxis
- **Active immunization:** Formaldehyde-inactivated vaccine is approved for use in above age of 2 years. It probably provides lifelong immunity.
- **Passive immunization:** Normal human immunoglobulin (0.02 mL/kg IM) is used, if exposure to HAV is <2 weeks and protects from infection for 3 months. HAV vaccine should also be administered.

Hepatitis B

- **Etiology:** Hepatitis B virus (HBV), DNA virus, and Hepadnaviridae
- **Structure:** Complete infective virion is called Dane particle. Spherical, 42-nm particle, *double-layered* comprising an inner core or nucleocapsid (27 nm) with an outer envelope of surface protein (HBsAg)
- **Viral genome:** It consists of partially double-stranded circular DNA and has four genes.
  - *HBsAg (S gene):* H*epatitis B surface antigen* is a product of *S gene*, which is secreted into the blood in large amounts. HBsAg is immunogenic. It is also called Australia antigen. It is identified by hemagglutination and radioimmunoassay methods.
  - *HBcAg (C gene):* The *C* gene produces two antigenically different products:
    1. *Hepatitis B core antigen (HBcAg):* Intracellular the hepatocytes and do not circulate in the serum.
    2. *Hepatitis B e antigen (HBeAg):* It is secreted into serum and is a surrogate marker for *high levels of viral replication*. It signifies persistent infection.
  - *HBV polymerase (P gene):* A polymerase (Pol) is a product of *P* gene and DNA polymerase enzyme is needed for virus replication.

- *HBxAg (X gene)*: *HBx protein* is necessary for virus infectivity and has been implicated in the *pathogenesis of liver cancer* in HBV infection.
- **Source:** *Cases* of hepatitis (acute/chronic) *or carriers* are the only source of infection. These are 100 times as infectious as human immunodeficiency virus (HIV) and 10 times as infectious as HCV.
- **Mode of transmission:**
  - *Vertical/congenital transmission*, from mother (HBV carrier) to child, may occur in utero, during parturition, or soon after birth. Not transmitted by breastfeeding
  - *Horizontal transmission:* Dominant mode of transmission
  - *Parenteral*—is the major route of transmission but occasionally nonparenteral.
    - *Percutaneous, mucous membrane* exposure to infectious body fluids, through minor cuts/abrasions. HBV can survive for long periods on household articles may transmit the infection.
    - *Intravenous route*—through transfusion of unscreened infected blood or blood products. This mode of spread is rare now, because of routine screening of all blood donors for HBV and HBC. Intravenous drug abuse with sharing of needles and syringes; tattooing and acupuncture are other ways of developing infection.
  - *Close personal contact*: Spread through body fluids such as saliva, urine, semen, and vaginal secretions. Require close personal contact, unprotected heterosexual or homosexual intercourse.
- **Incubation period:** 30–180 days (mean, 8–12 weeks)
- **Chronic carrier state** can develop with HBV infection (1–20%).
- **Prevention:** Avoiding risk factors—not to share needles, having safe sex, transfuse safe blood and blood products, enforced strict standard safety precautions in laboratories and hospitals to avoid accidental needle punctures and contact with infected body fluids
- **Prophylaxis:**
  - *Active immunization* is by using recombinant vaccines (containing HBsAg). Advised in:
    - *Children*: In India, nonpercutaneous routes of transmission are quite prevalent.
    - *High-risk groups*: Healthcare personnel, hemodialysis patients, injection drug users, hemophiliacs and sexual contacts of HBsAg carriers
  - *Dosage regimen:* Three doses into the deltoid muscle are given at 0, 1, and 6 months; 10 µg (children <10 years) and 20 µg (children >10 years). More frequent, larger doses are required in individuals over 50 years of age or clinically ill and/or immunocompromised.
- **Combined prophylaxis:** This consists of vaccination and immunoglobulin. Advised in:
  - Accidental needle-stick injury, gross personal contamination with infected blood, and exposure to infected blood in the presence of cuts and grazes
  - All newborn babies of HBsAg-positive mothers
  - Regular sexual partners of HBsAg-positive patients, who are HBV-negative
  - *Dosage*: Adults—500 IU of hepatitis B immunoglobulin (HBIG), newborns—200 IU, and the vaccine (I/M) at another site.
- **Treatment:** Pegylated interferon alpha, lamivudine, adefovir, entecavir, telbivudine, or tenofovir may be used as initial therapy but lamivudine and telbivudine are not preferred because of high rates of resistance

Hepatitis C

- It was previously called blood-borne non-A, non-B hepatitis.
- *Etiology:* Small, *enveloped, single-stranded RNA virus,* and Flaviviridae
- *Unstable genomic and antigenic variability*, leading to emergence of an endogenous and newly mutated strain, making producing an *effective HCV vaccine difficult*
- HCV has six genotypes and, in India, most prevalent is HCV 3.
- *Mode of spread:* It spreads through *parenteral route* (*transfusion* of blood, blood products, and drug addicts) as blood-borne infection, *s*exual contact, and perinatal transmission. Not transmitted by breastfeeding
- *Incubation period*: 15–160 days (mean, 7 weeks)
- Nearly 80% develop chronic hepatitis

Hepatitis D (Delta Hepatitis)

- **Etiology:** Hepatitis D virus (HDV or delta virus), defective/incomplete RNA virus, and Deltaviridae. RNA genome is covered by an outer coat/shell of HBsAg.
- No independent existence requires HBV for replication and expression
- Duration of HDV infection is determined by the duration of HBV infection
- Causes *delta hepatitis*, two clinical patterns:
  1. *Acute coinfection:* Simultaneous exposure to serum containing both HDV and HBV. The HBV infection first becomes established and the HBsAg is necessary for development of complete HDV virions.
  2. *Superinfection:* When a chronic carrier of HBV is exposed to a new dose HDV
- **Mode of spread:** Parenteral route and sexual contact
- Fulminant hepatitis can follow both patterns of infection but is more common after coinfection.

Hepatitis E

- It was previously called epidemic or enterically transmitted non-A and non-B hepatitis.
- **Etiology:** Unenveloped, single-stranded RNA, 32–34 nm, and herpes virus genus
- It occurs primarily in young- to middle-aged adults.
- **Source:** *Zoonotic disease* with animal reservoirs, such as monkeys, cats, pigs, rodents, and dogs. Virions are shed in stool during the acute illness
- **Mode of transmission:** *Enterically transmitted, water-borne* infection. Common after contamination of water supplies as after monsoon flooding
- **Incubation period:** 14–60 days (mean, 5–6 weeks)

- **Outcome:**
  - More than 30–60% of cases of sporadic acute hepatitis (similar to hepatitis A) in India
  - Acute self-limiting hepatitis with **high mortality rate (about 20%) among pregnant women**
  - Does not cause chronic liver disease
- **Prevention:** Good sanitation and hygiene. Vaccine has been developed and used successfully in China

Clinical Feature of Viral Hepatitis

Phase 1: *Incubation period:*
- Varies according to the virus

Phase 2: *Symptomatic preicteric phase:*
- Lasts for 1–2 weeks before onset of jaundice
- *Prodromal symptoms*—systemic and variable
- *Constitutional symptoms*—anorexia, nausea, vomiting, poor appetite, fatigue, malaise, headache, etc.
- *Low-grade fever*—more in hepatitis A and E than in hepatitis B or C. Hepatitis B may present with serum sickness-like immunological syndrome consisting of rashes and small joints polyarthritis.
- Upper vague abdominal pain due to stretching of liver capsule
- Dark urine and clay-colored stools

Phase 3: *Symptomatic icteric phase:*
- With the onset of clinical jaundice, the constitutional prodromal symptoms usually diminish.
- Liver becomes enlarged and tender. Pruritus may develop due to bile salt retention.
- Splenomegaly and cervical lymphadenopathy may be observed in about 10–20% of patients.
- Dark urine and pale stool

Phase 4: *Recovery (convalescence) phase:*
- Symptoms disappear, appetite improves, jaundice decreases, stools, urine—normal, and liver size decreases
- Duration is variable, 2–12 weeks. It is more prolonged in acute hepatitis B and C.
- Complete clinical and biochemical recovery within 1–2 months in A and E and 3–4 months in B and C.

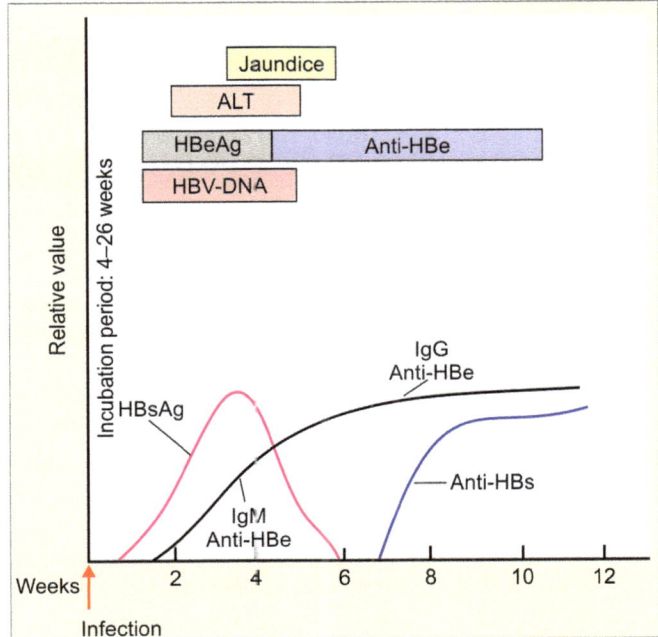

Fig. 7.5: Sequence of serologic markers in acute hepatitis with resolution caused by hepatitis B virus (HBV).

Fulminant hepatitis: It is common in hepatitis B, D, and E, uncommon in C, and rare in A. With hepatitis E, fulminant hepatitis occurs in nearly 20% cases in pregnant females.

Investigations

Investigations for viral hepatitis are summarized in **Table 7.10**.

Serological Markers and Findings for Viral Hepatitis B (Figs. 7.5 and 7.6)

Serological markers and findings for viral hepatitis are described in **Tables 7.11 and 7.12**, respectively.

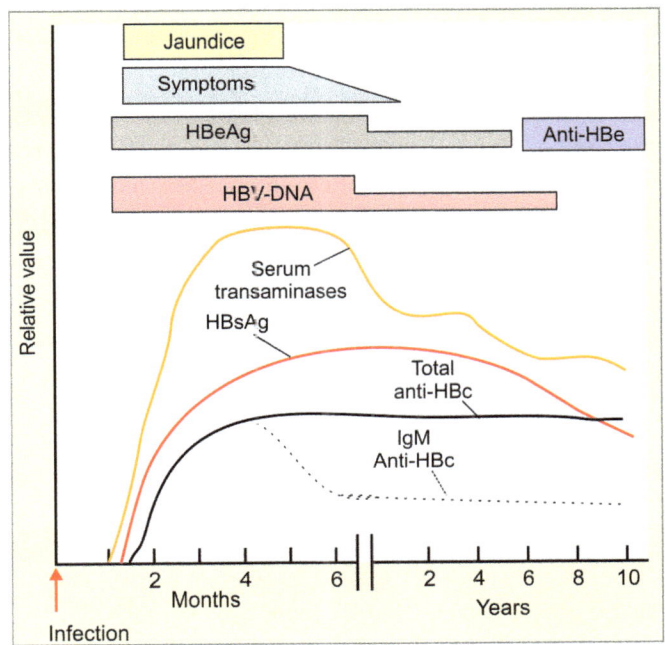

Fig. 7.6: Sequence of serologic markers in chronic hepatitis caused by hepatitis B virus (HBV).

Table 7.10: Investigations for viral hepatitis.

Urine	Blood	Biochemistry
Bilirubinuria (in early stages)	Leukopenia, relative lymphocytosis	AST and ALT—raised, maximum during the prodromal phase, progressively decline during icteric, recovery phase
Increased urinary urobilinogen	PT is prolonged (best prognostic feature)	Conjugated and unconjugated bilirubin levels raised
Slight microscopic hematuria	ESR is raised	ALP—may be raised
Mild proteinuria		*Serum protein:* Normal
		Blood glucose: May be low

(ALP: alkaline phosphatase; ALT: alanine aminotransferase; AST: aspartate aminotransferase; ESR: erythrocyte sedimentation rate; PT: prothrombin time)

Chapter 7: Hepatobiliary Disorders

Table 7.11: Serological markers for viral hepatitis.

Hepatitis A:	
IgM anti-HAV	• Appears at the onset of symptoms, *reliable marker of acute infection*
IgG anti-HAV	• Persists for years, *provides lifelong immunity* against reinfection.
Hepatitis B:	
HBsAg	• *First* marker to appear in serum before symptoms, undetectable in 3–6 months • *Significance*: Presence in acute and chronic hepatitis B indicates *infectious state*. Loss of HBsAg with development of anti-HBs denotes recovery.
Anti-HBs	• Antibody to HBsAg, appears after its disappearance. Present on vaccination • *Significance*: *Protective antibody,* may persist for life providing protection
IgM anti-HBc	• Appears in serum 1–2 weeks after appearance of HBsAg • *Significance*: Earliest antibody marker, indicates recent infection (first 6 months) • High titers in acute hepatitis B and low titers in chronic hepatitis B
IgG anti-HBc	*Significance: Indicates remote infection* (beyond 6 months). Indicates previous infection with HBV even when all the other viral markers are not detectable
HBeAg	• Detected transiently, early in the course • *Significance: Persistence* 6 weeks after the onset *indicates infectivity, severe disease* progressing to *chronic hepatitis*. Absence is a favorable serologic finding.
Anti-HBe	*Significance*: Found in *recovery phase, seroconversion*
HBV-DNA, DNA polymerase	• Found in serum and liver soon after HBsAg • *Significance*: Not helpful in diagnosis of hepatitis B, valuable in *assessing prognosis*, indicates *active viral replication*
Hepatitis C:	
Anti-HCV	• Appears after infection; disappears after recovery; persists in chronic hepatitis C
HCV-RNA	• Appears after exposure
Hepatitis D (delta hepatitis):	
HDV-RNA	Is detectable in the blood and liver before and in the early days of acute disease
Anti-HDV	IgM anti-HDV—most reliable indicator of recent HDV exposure
Hepatitis E:	
HEV-RNA, HEV virions	Before the onset of clinical illness, can be detected in stool and serum
IgM anti-HEV	After the onset of clinical illness, serum aminotransferases rises, and elevated titers also occur simultaneously
IgG anti-HEV	After recovery, the IgM is replaced with a persistent IgG anti-HEV titer

(HAV: hepatitis A virus; HCV: hepatitis C virus; HDV: hepatitis D virus; IgM: immunoglobulin M; HEV: hepatitis E virus; HBsAg: hepatitis B surface antigen; HBeAg: hepatitis B e-antigen)

Table 7.12: Summary of serological findings in hepatitis B virus (HBV).

Antigens		Antibodies			Interpretation
HBsAg	HBeAg	Anti-HBc	Anti–HBs	Anti-HBe	
+	+	IgM	–	–	Acute hepatitis B, highly infectious
+	+	IgG	–	–	Chronic infection, carrier, and high infectivity
+	–	IgG	–	±	Chronic infection, carrier, and low infectivity
–	–	–	+	–	Immunity following HBV vaccine
–	–	+	+		Immune due to natural infection

(HBV: hepatitis B virus; HBsAg: hepatitis B surface antigen; HBeAg: hepatitis B e-antigen)

Complications

Complications of acute viral hepatitis are described in **Table 7.13.**

Treatment

- General measures
- Avoid drugs metabolized in the liver, e.g., sedatives and narcotics
- Avoid alcohol during the acute illness

Table 7.13: Complications of acute viral hepatitis.

Hepatic complications	Extra-hepatic complications
• Fulminant hepatic failure • Cholestatic viral hepatitis • Relapsing hepatitis • Post-hepatitis syndrome • Chronic hepatitis • Cirrhosis • Hepatocellular carcinoma	• Aplastic anemia • Renal failure • Polyarteritis nodosa • Henoch–Schonlein purpura • Myocarditis • Transverse myelitis • Peripheral neuropathy

Chapter 7: Hepatobiliary Disorders

Table 7.14: Extrahepatic manifestations of hepatitis C virus infection.

Proven associations	Possible associations
• Autoimmune thyroiditis	• Chronic polyarthritis
• B-cell non-Hodgkin's lymphoma	• Idiopathic pulmonary fibrosis
• Diabetes mellitus	• Noncryoglobulinemia nephropathies
• Lichen planus	• Sicca syndrome
• Mixed cryoglobulinemia	• Thyroid cancer
• Monoclonal gammopathies	• Renal cell carcinoma
• Porphyria cutanea tarda	• Vitiligo

Table 7.15: Causes for acute hepatitis.

Infectious: Viruses (described earlier), bacterial, parasites, and fungi	Toxin/drugs: Alcohol (described later)	Immunological: Autoimmune hepatitis and primary sclerosing cholangitis
Metabolic or hereditary: • Nonalcoholic fatty liver disease • Hemochromatosis • Wilson's disease	Pregnancy related: • Pre-eclampsia • Acute fatty liver of pregnancy • HELLP syndrome	Ischemic and vascular: • Cardiogenic shock • Hypotension • Cocaine, methamphetamine, and ephedrine • Acute Budd–Chiari syndrome

(HELLP: hemolysis, elevated liver enzymes, low platelet count)

- No specific dietary modifications
- Elective surgery should be avoided, as there is risk of postoperative liver failure
- Liver transplantation performed for complications of cirrhosis due to chronic hepatitis B and C

Manifestations
Extrahepatic manifestations of hepatitis C virus infection are mentioned in **Table 7.14**.

Causes for Acute Hepatitis
Causes for acute hepatitis are summarized in **Table 7.15**.

CHRONIC PARENCHYMAL LIVER DISEASE
It is divided into two part:
1. **Chronic hepatitis:** Chronic persistent hepatitis (CPH), chronic active hepatitis (CAH), and chronic lobular hepatitis (CLH)
2. **Cirrhosis**

Chronic Hepatitis
- It is symptomatic, biochemical, or serologic evidence of hepatic disease for more than 6 months. Microscopically, there should be inflammation and necrosis in the liver.
- **Classification:** To assess response to therapy and prognosis, it is based on:
  - Cause of hepatitis **(Table 7.16)**
  - Histologic activity or grade
  - Degree of progression or stage

Table 7.16: Based on the causes of chronic hepatitis.

Chronic viral hepatitis	Chronic hepatitis B ± hepatitis D, chronic hepatitis C
Drug-associated chronic hepatitis	Methyldopa, isoniazid, ketoconazole, and nitrofurantoin
Autoimmune hepatitis	
Hereditary	Wilson's disease
Unknown cause	Cryptogenic chronic hepatitis
Others	Ulcerative colitis, rarely alcohol

- *Based on the grade of chronic hepatitis*
- Histological assessment of inflammation and necrosis observed on liver biopsy; indicates severity of liver disease
- *Scoring system*: Histologic activity index (HAI) and METAVIR score and can be graded as mild, moderate, and severe.
  - *Interface hepatitis* (piecemeal/periportal necrosis): *Spillover of inflammatory cells* (lymphocytes and plasma cells) from *portal tract into the adjacent* periportal hepatocytes at the limiting plate, with degenerating and apoptosis of periportal hepatocytes.
  - *Bridging necrosis*: Confluent necrosis of hepatocytes observed in severe acute hepatitis; forms bridges between *portal tract to portal tract, central vein to central vein, or portal-to-central* regions of adjacent lobules
  - Degree of hepatocyte degeneration and focal intralobular necrosis
  - Degree of portal inflammation
  - *Fibrosis*: Hallmark of chronic liver damage
- Classification based on stage of chronic hepatitis: Indicates level of progression and based on the degree of hepatic fibrosis **(Table 7.17)**.

Autoimmune CAH (Lupoid)
It is chronic and progressive hepatitis of unknown cause, characterized by unresolving inflammation of liver and by presence of interface hepatitis on histology, hypergammaglobulinemia, and autoantibodies.

Table 7.17: Modified histological activity index—staging.

Degree of fibrosis	Stage
No fibrosis	0
Mild fibrosis of some portal areas	1
Moderate fibrosis of most portal areas	2
Severe fibrosis of most portal areas with occasional portal–portal (P–P) bridging	3
Fibrous expansion of portal areas with marked bridging of P–P and portal–central (P–C)	4
Marked bridging (P–P and/or P–C) with occasional nodules (incomplete cirrhosis)	5
Cirrhosis	6

Clinical features:
- Seen in females, peri- and postmenopausal age group
- Asymptomatic or present with fatigue, anorexia, and jaundice
- Acute hepatitis—jaundice, marked rise of serum aminotransferase, which does not resolve
- *Other autoimmune symptoms*: Fever, polyarthritis, glomerulonephritis, pleurisy, pulmonary infiltration, or fibrosing alveolitis.
- *Other autoimmune diseases*: Hashimoto's thyroiditis, ulcerative colitis, glomerulonephritis, and Sjogren's syndrome
- Jaundice may be mild to moderate
- *Signs of chronic liver disease*: Spider telangiectasia and hepatosplenomegaly

Investigations:
- **Biochemical findings:**
  - *Serum aminotransferases:* High and more than 10 times during relapses
  - *Serum bilirubin:* Mildly raised usually <6 mg/dL
  - *Serum alkaline phosphatase:* Mildly raised
  - *Serum γ-globulins*: High
  - *Serum albumin*: Low
  - *Serum α1-antitrypsin, serum ceruloplasmin, iron, and ferritin levels*: Normal
- **Autoantibodies:** Autoimmune hepatitis may be of three types:
  1. *Type I*: With antibodies to—(1) antinuclear and (2) anti-smooth muscle (anti-actin)
  2. *Type II*: With antibodies to anti-liver/kidney microsomal (anti-LKM). Seen more in girls and young women
  3. *Type III*: With soluble liver antigen (anti-SLP/LP). This behaves as type I.

About 13% of patients do not have above autoantibodies.
- *HBsAg*: Negative
- *Prothrombin time*: Prolonged
- *Liver biopsy*: Chronic hepatitis, variable amounts of interface hepatitis, cirrhosis, and bridging necrosis

Treatment:
- **Prednisolone:** 30 mg given orally daily for 2 weeks. Gradually tapering dose, as LFT improves. Maintenance dose of 10–15 mg daily for at least 2 years after LFT has become normal.
- **Azathioprine:** Dose of 1–2 mg/kg daily, added as a steroid-sparing agent and some patients for sole long-term maintenance therapy or if dose of prednisolone is >10 mg/day.
- **Other immunosuppressive agents:** Mycophenolate, cyclosporine, and tacrolimus for resistant cases
- **Duration of treatment:** Lifelong in most cases
- **Liver transplantation:** If treatment fails

CHRONIC HEPATITIS B
- Follows acute HBV infection (may be subclinical), in about 1–10% of patients
- HBsAg persists for >6 months. May progress to cirrhosis and hepatocellular carcinoma
- Risk of chronic hepatitis depends on:
  - *Age*: More common with neonatal (90%) or childhood (20–50%, <5 years) infection rather than in adults (<10%)
  - *Immune status*: In immunocompetent adults, the incidence of acute hepatitis is high while chronic infection is rare (1–2% of cases)

High-risk Comorbid States
- Down's syndrome
- Lepromatous leprosy
- Leukemias
- Hodgkin's lymphoma
- Polyarteritis nodosa
- Patients on chronic hemodialysis
- Needle using drug addicts—HIV infection

Phases of Infection (Table 7.18)
There are three major phases:
1. **Immune-tolerant phase:**
   - Asymptomatic, may last for decades
   - Active viral replication in liver but little or no evidence of disease activity
   - Associated with HBsAg and HBeAg positive and very high levels of serum HBV DNA
   - Liver without inflammation with normal liver function tests
2. **Immune-active phase (chronic hepatitis):** Progression from immune-tolerant phase. Criteria for chronic HBV hepatitis are:
   - HBsAg positive >6 months

Table 7.18: Phases of hepatitis B.

Phases of chronic hepatitis B infection				
Phase	ALT	HBV DNA	HBeAg	Liver histology
Immune tolerant	Normal	Elevated typically >1 million IU/mL	Positive	Minimal inflammation and fibrosis
HBeAg-postive immune active	Elevated	Elevated ≥20,000 IU/mL	Positive	Moderate-to-severe inflammation or fibrosis
Inactive chronic hepatitis B	Normal	Low or undetectable <2,000 IU/mL	Negative	Minimal necroinflammation but variable fibrosis
HBeAg-negative immune reactivation	Elevated	Elevated ≥2,000 IU/mL	Negative	Moderate-to-severe inflammation or fibrosis

(HBeAg: hepatitis B e antigen; HBV: hepatitis B virus)

- *Liver biopsy*: Chronic hepatitis with moderate-to-severe necroinflammation
- *Evidence of HBV replication*: HBe antigen (HBeAg) and/or anti-HBe and HBV DNA (>20,000 IU/mL) in their serum
- Persistent or intermittent elevation of ALT/AST

3. **Inactive carrier phase with chronic HBV infection:** Incidence varies. Most patients eventually enter inactive carrier phase as they clear HBeAg and develop anti-HBe. Criteria for inactive carrier state are:
   - HBsAg positive in the serum >6 months
   - HBeAg negative and HBe antibody positive
   - Undetectable or low levels (below 400 IU/L) of HBV DNA in the serum
   - Normal aminotransferase (ALT) levels

Liver biopsy does not show any significant hepatitis.
- Liver abnormalities generally do not progress to more severe disease. Low risk for hepatocellular carcinoma
- May be reactivated by severe immunosuppression
- **Age at which infection occurs:**
  1. Infected during adults, adolescents—inactive carriers after they clear HBeAg
  2. Infection during birth, early childhood—prolonged immune-tolerant phase, disease progresses even after disappearance of HBeAg in some. Therefore, lifelong monitoring is necessary
- HBV genotype C (prevalent in India)—increased risk of cirrhosis and hepatocellular carcinoma.

Clinical Features

- Asymptomatic or may develop severe end-stage liver disease
- Fatigue, malaise, anorexia, and persistent or intermittent jaundice
- **In end-stage liver disease:** Symptoms due to complications of cirrhosis
- **Extrahepatic manifestations:** Arthralgias, arthritis, vasculitis, glomerulonephritis, and polyarthritis nodosa
- Mild hepatomegaly
- Long-standing cases may develop hepatocellular carcinoma

Investigations

- **Biochemical investigations:**
  - ALT, AST elevated. ALT > AST (SGOT). Once cirrhosis develops, AST > ALT
  - *Serum bilirubin*: May be normal or raised up to 10 mg/dL
  - *Serum proteins*: Hypoalbuminemia in severe cases and hyperglobulinemia
  - *Prothrombin time*: Prolonged
  - *Serological markers*: Positive HBsAg, positive IgG anti-HBc, negative IgM anti-HBc, positive HBe antigen or rarely, positive anti-HBe, and positive HBV-DNA

Treatment (Flowchart 7.1)

- **Indications:**
  - Serum HBV-DNA above 2,000 IU/mL (about >10,000 copies/mL)
  - Serum ALT level greater than two times normal
  - Moderate-to-severe active necroinflammation and/or fibrosis in the liver biopsy
  - In cirrhosis, oral antiviral agents are recommended, liver transplantation may be necessary.
  - Immunotolerant patients, usually young with normal ALT and high HBV DNA levels, without evidence of liver disease do not need therapy, but be regularly followed-up.
- **Aim of treatment:**
  - Seroconversion. When HBeAg disappears, remission may be attained for several years.
  - Reduction of HBV DNA <400 IU/L
  - Achieve normal levels of serum ALT
  - Histological improvement in inflammation and fibrosis in the liver biopsy.

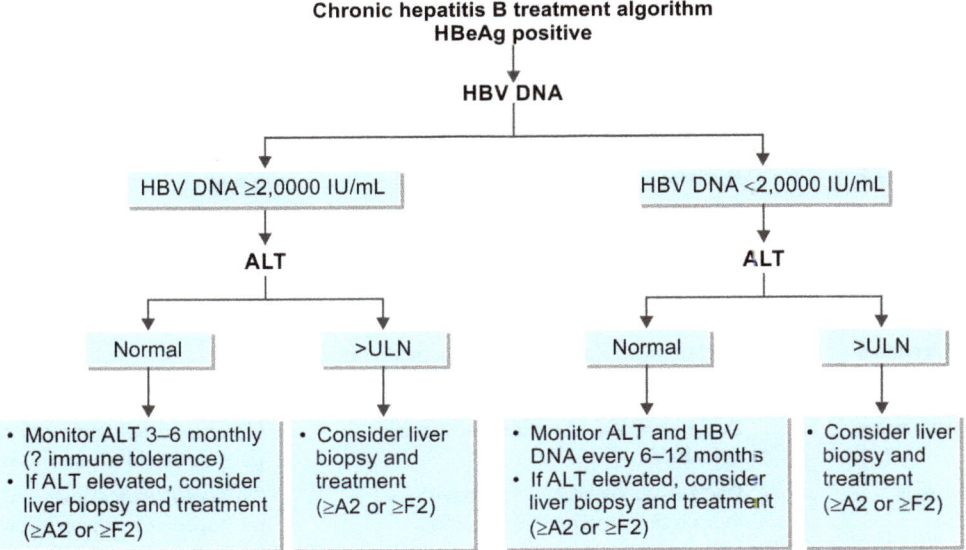

Flowchart 7.1: Treatment algorithm for HBeAg negative and HBeAg positive chronic hepatitis B.

ALT ULN: 19 IU/mL (female) and 30 IU/mL (male)

(ALT: alanine aminotransferase; HbeAg: hepatitis B e antigen; HBV: hepatitis B virus; ULN: upper limit of normal)

Patients usually remain HBsAg positive, but loss of serum HBsAg indicates a good response.

- **Antiviral agents:** Interferon, entecavir, and tenofovir are commonly used.
- **Pegylated α-2a interferon b:** Response occurs in 25–40% of cases. 180 μg given once a week subcutaneously with response in 48 weeks.
- **Side effects:** Acute flu-like symptoms, malaise, headache, depression, reversible hair loss, bone marrow depression, thrombocytopenia, and infection Patients with HIV respond poorly.
- **Oral therapy:**
  - *Entecavir:* Potent, cyclopentyl-guanosine analog, reduces HBV DNA by 48 weeks
  - *Tenofovir:* Cytosine nucleoside analog, very effective, used for HIV–HBV infection
  - *Lamivudine:* Well tolerated, development of resistance (80%) is high and itself may cause hepatitis, and monotherapy—no longer recommended. 100 mg/day orally once a day until HBeAg becomes negative
  - *Adefovir dipivoxil:* It is a nucleotide reverse transcriptase inhibitor. It may be used in patients who develop resistance to lamivudine.
  - *Telbivudine:* L-nucleoside that may cause elevation of creatine phosphokinase (CPK)

Prognosis

- Depends on the age at which infection is acquired
- Development of cirrhosis is associated with a poor prognosis
- Hepatocellular carcinoma is one of the most common carcinomas in HBV-endemic areas

CHRONIC HEPATITIS C

- 70–85% of *individuals infected* by *HCV*.
- *Cirrhosis* develops over 5–20 years in 20–30% of patients; *hepatocellular carcinoma* develops in several patients especially with cirrhosis.
- Accelerate progression in alcoholism, HIV or HBV coinfection, and older age at the time of acquiring the infection.

Clinical Features

- Usually asymptomatic. Detected on routine biochemical tests with mild elevations of ALT.
- Similar to chronic hepatitis B. Most common—fatigue, jaundice—rare
- *Extrahepatic features*: Essential mixed cryoglobulinemia, membranoproliferative glomerulonephritis, uveitis, peripheral neuropathy, non-Hodgkin's lymphoma, lichen planus, Sicca syndrome, and porphyria cutanea tarda

Investigations

- HCV antibody in serum detected—>95% cases
- HCV RNA in all patients
- Liver biopsy, if active treatment is considered. Histological changes—highly variable. Features—chronic hepatitis, with lymphoid follicles in portal tracts, and fatty change
- Other features are similar to chronic hepatitis B

Treatment

- **Indications:**
  - Chronic hepatitis on histology, HCV-RNA in serum and, serum aminotransferases for >6 months
  - Chronic hepatitis with persistently normal aminotransferases
  - Cirrhosis, fibrosis, and moderate inflammation on liver biopsy (biopsy not mandatory)
- Aim of treatment is to eliminate HCV RNA from the serum to prevent progression of active liver disease and development of hepatocellular carcinoma.
- **Combination therapy:** Pegylated interferon (once a week) and ribavirin.
- **Newer drugs (Table 7.19)**
- **Liver transplant**—for patients with decompensated cirrhosis.

Table 7.19: Antivirals for hepatitis C virus (HCV) infection in treatment-naive patients.

	Preferred	Alternative
Genotype 1 without cirrhosis	Daclatasvir/sofosburvir or ledipasvir/sofosbuvir	Simeprevir/sofosbuvir or ombitasvir/paritaprevir/ritonavir/dasabuvir ± ribavirin
Genotype 1 with cirrhosis	Daclatasvir/sofosburvir ± ribavirin or ledipasvir/sofosbuvir ± ribavirin	Simeprevir/sofosbuvir ± ribavirin or ombitasvir/paritaprevir/ritonavir/dasabuvir ± ribavirin
Genotype 2 with and without cirrhosis	Sofosbuvir/ribavirin	Daclatasvir/sofosbuvir
Genotype 3 without cirrhosis	Daclatasvir/sofosburvir or sofosbuvir/ribavirin	
Genotype 3 with cirrhosis	Daclatasvir/sofosburvir ribavirin	Sofosbuvir/pegylated interferon/ribavirin
Genotype 4 without cirrhosis	Daclatasvir/sofosburvir or ledipasvir/sofosbuvir	Simeprevir/sofosbuvir or ombitasvir/paritaprevir/ritonavir/ribavirin
Genotype 4 with cirrhosis	Daclatasvir/sofosburvir ± ribavirin or ledipasvir/sofosbuvir ± ribavirin	Simeprevir/sofosbuvir ± ribavirin or ombitasvir/paritaprevir/ritonavir/ribavirin
Genotype 5 or 6 with and without cirrhosis	Ledipasvir/sofosbuvir	Simeprevir/pegylated interferon/ribavirin

(HCV: hepatitis C virus; IFN: interferon; P: pegylated interferon-alfa 2a or 2b; R: ribavirin; r: ritonavir)

CHRONIC HEPATITIS D (PLUS HEPATITIS B)

- Acute coinfection with hepatitis B or with superinfection in a patient with hepatitis B
- Relatively infrequent chronic hepatitis, spontaneous resolution is rare.
- 60–70% of patients develop cirrhosis and develop more rapidly than with HBV infection.
- **Investigations:** Anti-delta antibody with chronic liver disease with HBsAg-positive. HDV in liver or HDV-RNA in serum by reverse transcription–polymerase reaction
- **Treatment:** Usually supportive. Alpha-interferon at a high dose of 10 M units three times weekly for 12 months gives a poor response. Lamivudine and adefovir are not useful.

FULMINANT HEPATITIS FAILURE

- Rapid development of hepatocellular dysfunction, specifically coagulopathy and mental status changes (encephalopathy) in a patient without known prior liver disease
- Severe hepatic failure (insufficiency) in which encephalopathy develops within 4 weeks (8–28 days) from onset of symptoms in a patient with a previously normal liver
- **Subacute/subfulminant hepatic failure:** If hepatic failure develops at a slower pace (4–12 weeks)
- **Hyperacute hepatic failure:** If encephalopathy develops within 7 days, better prognosis than acute hepatic failure
- **Etiology:** Rare but often life-threatening **(Table 7.20)**

Clinical Features

- **General features:** Jaundice, weakness, nausea, vomiting; right hypochondrial pain, small liver, liver dullness are absent on percussion, ascites and edema develop later
- **Hepatic encephalopathy:**
  - *Mental state*: Mild drowsiness, confusion, and disorientation (grades I and II) to unresponsive coma (grade IV) with convulsions.
  - Fetor hepaticus and flapping tremor (asterixis)
  - Ascites and splenomegaly are rare.
  - Fever, vomiting, hypotension, and hypoglycemia

Table 7.20: Important causes of fulminant hepatic failure.

Viruses: HAV and HBV. Occasionally, HCV and others

Noninfectious causes:

- **Drugs:**
  - Analgesics (e.g., paracetamol)
  - Monoamine oxidase inhibitors
  - Antituberculosis (e.g., isoniazid)
  - Antiepileptic (e.g., valproate)
  - Halogenated anesthetics
  - Social drugs (e.g., "ecstasy")
- **Toxins:** Amanita phalloides (mushroom) poisoning
- **Miscellaneous:**
  - Wilson's disease
  - HELLP syndrome, eclampsia, pre-eclampsia, and acute fatty liver of pregnancy
  - Reye's syndrome
  - Autoimmune hepatitis
  - Budd–Chiari syndrome
  - Shock and ischemic hepatitis
- **Unknown**

(HAV: hepatitis A virus; HCV: hepatitis C virus)

- Spasticity and extension of the arms and legs and plantar responses remain flexor until late.
- **Cerebral edema**—develops in ~80% of patients.
- Bradycardia, intracranial hypertension, and irregular respiration (Cushing's triad)
- **Pupils:** Unequal, abnormally reacting or fixed pupils
- Hyperventilation and hyperreflexia
- Death due to intracranial hypertension and brain herniation

Investigations

- **Serum findings:**
  - Hyperbilirubinemia
  - Serum aminotransferases: Raised, but not useful indicators
  - Decreased levels of clotting factors. Prothrombin time—prolonged
  - Hypoalbuminemia
  - Plasma and urine amino acids are increased
  - Blood ammonia levels: Raised
- **Urine:** Shows protein, bilirubin, and urobilinogen
- Leukocytosis and thrombocytopenia
- **Electroencephalography (EEG):** Grading of encephalopathy
- **Ultrasound:** To detect liver size and for any evidence of underlying liver pathology
- Intracranial pressure is raised, but cerebrospinal fluid (CSF) is normal.

Complications

Complications of fulminant hepatic failure (FHF) are described in **Table 7.21**.

Pathogenesis and Management

Pathogenesis and management of major complications of acute liver failure are described in **Table 7.22**.

General Measures

- Monitor vital signs, urine output, renal functions, central venous pressure, and electrolytes
- Maintain fluid–electrolyte balance
- *Supply of adequate calories*: Glucose (300 g/day) orally, nasogastric tube, and infusion
- Ventilatory support for respiratory failure
- Renal failure is treated with dialysis
- **Drugs:**
  - *Antibiotic prophylaxis*—bacterial and fungal infection and infection treatment
  - H_2-receptor antagonists (omeprazole and pantoprazole): Prevent GI bleeding
  - *Fresh frozen plasma*: If prothrombin time is prolonged more than 1.5 times the normal

Table 7.21: Complications of fulminant hepatic failure.

Encephalopathy	Bacterial and fungal infections
Cerebral edema	Gastrointestinal bleeding, hypotension
Respiratory failure	Hypoglycemia and hypokalemia
Renal failure	Hypothermia
Pancreatitis	Acid–base imbalance
Hypocalcemia	Hypomagnesemia

Table 7.22: Pathogenesis and management of major complications of acute liver failure.

Complication	Pathogenesis	Management
Hypoglycemia	Diminished hepatic glucose synthesis	• Blood glucose monitoring • Intravenous glucose supplementation (10–20% dextrose)
Encephalopathy	Cerebral edema	• ICP monitoring (if stage 3 or 4 encephalopathy) • CT scan (if advanced encephalopathy) • Elevate head of the bed >30° • Consider osmotherapy (mannitol) or barbiturates • Treat other contributing factors • Reduce fever (cooling blankets and antibiotics) • Avoid benzodiazepines and sedative medications • Moderate hypothermia
Infections	• Reduced immune function • Invasive procedures	• Aseptic medical and nursing care • Daily cultures—blood, urine, and sputum • High index of suspicion—bacterial/fungal infection • *Antibiotics*: Gram-negative, anaerobes, and skin flora • Consider antifungal therapy, if patient worsens despite antibacterial coverage
GI hemorrhage	Stress ulceration	• Nasogastric tube placement • Intravenous H_2 receptor antagonist or proton pump inhibitor
Coagulopathy	• Reduced clotting factor synthesis • Thrombocytopenia • Fibrinolysis	• Parenteral vitamin K • Platelet or plasma infusions for bleeding and before procedures • Cryoprecipitate for bleeding with hypofibrinogenemia • Recombinant factor VIIa
Hypotension	• Hypovolemia • Decreased vascular resistance	• Hemodynamic monitoring of central venous pressures • Volume repletion with blood or colloid • α-adrenergic agents
Respiratory failure	ARDS (DAD)	• Hemodynamic monitoring of central venous pressures • Mechanical ventilation
Pancreatitis	Hypoxia	• Supportive care, supplemental oxygen, if needed • Abdominal CT to exclude necrotizing pancreatitis
Renal failure	• Hypovolemia • Hepatorenal syndrome • Acute tubular necrosis	• Hemodynamic monitoring of central venous pressures • Volume repletion with blood or colloid • Avoidance of nephrotoxic agents (e.g., aminoglycosides, NSAIDs, and contrast dye) • Oral *N*-acetylcysteine prior to IV-contrast agent • Hemofiltration and dialysis

(ARDS: acute respiratory distress syndrome; CT: computed tomography; GI: gastrointestinal; ICP: intracranial pressure; NSAID: nonsteroidal anti-inflammatory drug)

- **Encephalopathy:** Supportive therapy
- Protein-restricted diet (starting with 0.5 g/kg/day), suitable antibiotic therapy (e.g., ampicillin, rifaximin, metronidazole, or neomycin), bowel washes, etc.
- **Reduce plasma ammonia level:** Lactulose is catabolized by colonic bacterial flora to short-chain fatty acids that reduce pH of colon. Lowered pH favors formation of nonabsorbable ammonium ion from ammonia, trapping ammonia in the colon, leading to decreased plasma ammonia.
- Avoid sedatives; for restlessness and excitement, intravenous diazepam or midazolam
- **Cerebral edema:**
  - Head elevated at 30°, elective ventilation, in patients with grade 3 or 4 encephalopathy
  - *Raised intracranial pressure*: Mannitol 20% (1 g/kg body weight) is given intravenously over half an hour. Dose may need repetition every 6 hours and maintain the serum osmolarity below 310 mOsm/L.
  - Controlled hyperventilation, so as to maintain $PaCO_2$ between 30 and 35 mm Hg

- **Other measures:**
  - *Coagulopathy*—intravenous vitamin K, platelets, blood, or fresh frozen plasma
  - Steroids, exchange transfusion, and hemodialysis using special membranes—not useful
  - *Liver transplantation* is a major advance in the treatment of FHF.
  - *Prognosis*: Mortality ~80% without liver transplantation, ~35% with transplantation

REYE'S SYNDROME

- Children and adolescents with history of aspirin intake
- Develops following viral infections such as influenza or chickenpox
- Acute presentation with vomiting, lethargy during recovery period of a viral illness followed by encephalopathy and cerebral edema
- Liver shows severe fatty change. Raised ammonia levels and liver enzymes. Usually no jaundice

FATTY LIVER/STEATOSIS

It is abnormal accumulations of triglycerides within cytosol of the parenchymal cells **(Box 7.2)**.

> **Box 7.2:** Causes of fatty liver.
>
> **Alcohol:**
> *Nonalcoholic fatty liver disease/nonalcoholic steatohepatitis*
> - *Drugs:* Glucocorticoids, amiodarone, tetracycline, aspirin, methotrexate, didanosine, zidovudine, tamoxifen, and amiodarone
> - *Nutritional:* Protein–calorie malnutrition, total parenteral nutrition, and rapid weight loss/obesity
> - *Metabolic:* Diabetes, lipodystrophy, and acute fatty liver of pregnancy
> - *Miscellaneous:* Inflammatory bowel disease, HIV infection, chronic hepatitis C, toxic mushrooms (*Amanita phalloides*), Reye's syndrome, obstructive sleep apnea, and Indian childhood cirrhosis

ALCOHOLIC LIVER DISEASE

- Chronic and excessive consumption of alcohol can produce a wide spectrum of liver disease—fatty liver, alcoholic hepatitis, and alcoholic cirrhosis **(Table 7.23)**.
- Effects of alcohol are worse in women compared to men. For women, values should be reduced by 50%.

Alcoholic Fatty Liver

- **Clinical features:**
  - Asymptomatic or may present with discomfort in right upper quadrant, nausea, and jaundice
  - Hepatomegaly
  - Progression to cirrhosis not common
- **Investigations:**
  - *Biochemical findings:* Moderate elevations of aspartate transaminase (AST) and alanine transaminase (ALT). γ-GT level is a sensitive test to determine whether the individual is taking alcohol.
  - *Ultrasound or CT:* Demonstrates fatty liver
  - *Liver biopsy:* Shows accumulation of fat in perivenular hepatocytes and later in entire hepatic lobule
- Cessation of alcohol consumption results in normalization of biochemical findings and histological changes.

Alcoholic Hepatitis

- **Clinical features:**
  - May be asymptomatic or present with fever, rapid onset of jaundice, abdominal discomfort, and proximal muscle wasting
  - Portal hypertension, ascites, and bleeding due to esophageal varices can occur without cirrhosis.
  - Hepatomegaly

Table 7.23: Amount of alcohol consumption and its associated risk of alcoholic liver disease in male.

Amount of ingestion per day	Degree of risk
160 g ethanol (20 single drinks)	High
80 g ethanol (10 single drinks)	Medium
40 g ethanol (five single drinks)	Low

- **Investigations:**
  - *Biochemical findings:*
    - Serum aminotransferase (AST and ALT) raised to 2–7 times of normal (usually <400 IU)
    - AST:ALT ratio is >1 (generally >2)
    - Mildly elevated serum alkaline phosphatase
    - Raised bilirubin
    - Decreased albumin
  - *Hematological findings:* Prolonged prothrombin time and leukocytosis
  - *Liver biopsy:* Ballooning degeneration of hepatocytes with leukocyte infiltration. Mallory bodies are often seen.
- **Prognosis:**
  - Variable. Despite abstinence, disease progresses in many. Conversely, a few patients continue to drink heavily without developing cirrhosis.
  - Mortality high in patients with severe alcoholic hepatitis
  - Poor prognostic factors
    - Prothrombin time >5 seconds of control
    - Anemia
    - Albumin <2.5 g/dL
    - Serum bilirubin >8 mg/dL
    - Progressive encephalopathy
    - Renal failure
    - Presence of ascites
    - Maddrey discriminant function >32
- **Treatment:**
  - Advised to stop alcohol consumption for life, because this is a pre-cirrhotic condition
  - Severe hepatitis needs bed rest.
  - *Nutrition*: Feeding—via a fine-bore nasogastric tube or sometimes intravenously (>3,000 kcal/day; multivitamins mainly vitamins B and C)
  - Treatment for encephalopathy and ascites
  - Corticosteroids—tried in severe cases (discriminant function >32) in the absence of any infection
  - Antibiotics (pentoxifylline) in severe cases (discriminant function >32) and antifungal prophylaxis

NONALCOHOLIC FATTY LIVER DISEASE, NONALCOHOLIC STEATOSIS, NONALCOHOLIC STEATOHEPATITIS

- Disease of affluent societies, prevalence increases proportionately with obesity
- Increasingly recognized and most common cause of chronic liver disease after hepatitis B, C, and alcohol

Classification

- Simple fatty liver disease (nonalcoholic fatty liver, NAFL) with favorable prognosis
- Nonalcoholic steatohepatitis with fibrosis, progression to cirrhosis, and hepatocellular carcinoma

Risk Factors

- Metabolic syndrome
- Obesity, hypertension, type 2 diabetes mellitus, hyperlipidemia, and insulin resistance

- **Rare:** Tamoxifen, amiodarone, and exposure to certain petrochemicals
- *Induced by two steps*—(1) excess fat accumulation and (2) subsequent necroinflammation in the liver

Clinical Features
- Mostly asymptomatic, obesity
- Fatigue, malaise, and sensation of fullness in the upper abdomen
- Hepatomegaly

Diagnosis
- Mild-to-moderately elevated serum transaminases
- No history of alcohol abuse
- Negative chronic liver disease screen

Investigations
- **Mild elevation of AST, ALT with AST:** ALT <1; increases as fibrosis advances; may be only isolated elevation of the GGT; and elevated ALP in about 30% of patients
- Ferritin levels are increased in 20–50% of patients
- Autoantibodies in about 25% patients with more advanced fibrosis
- **Ultrasound and CT features:** Similar to those in alcoholic fatty liver
- **Liver biopsy:** It is best diagnostic tool for confirmation and staging. Microscopic changes are similar to alcohol-induced hepatic injury—steatosis, steatohepatitis, and fibrosis. It is characterized by fat, Mallory bodies, neutrophil infiltration, and pericellular fibrosis

Management
- Weight loss, control of diabetes, and hyperlipidemia
- *Drugs*: Metformin, thiazolidinediones, ursodeoxycholic acid (UDCA), pentoxifylline, and atorvastatin have shown some promise.
- Liver transplantation for end-stage cirrhosis; may recur in graft
- Regular follow-up, particularly for steatohepatitis

▌CIRRHOSIS
- **End stage** of any chronic liver disease, *diffuse process* (entire liver is involved) characterized by *fibrosis* and conversion of normal architecture to structurally *abnormal regenerating nodules* of liver cells.
- Main morphologic characteristics fibrosis, *regenerating nodules,* and *loss of architecture*

- **Pathology and pathogenesis:**
  - Widespread liver cell necrosis
  - Cirrhotic changes affect the whole liver, but not necessarily every lobule
  - Extensive fibrosis causing loss of liver architecture
  - Regenerating nodules due to hyperplasia of surviving liver cells
  - Destruction and distortion of vasculature by fibrosis causing obstruction of blood flow. Vascular reorganization leads to portal hypertension, gastroesophageal varices, and splenomegaly
  - Hepatocellular insufficiency and portal hypertension—ascites and hepatic encephalopathy
  - Hepatocellular damage—jaundice, edema, coagulopathy, and metabolic abnormalities

Alcoholic Cirrhosis
- Safe limits in males—200g and females—140 g per week. 40–80 g/day for men, 20–40 g/day for women for 10 years
- 10 g of alcohol = 30 mL whisky, 100 mL wine, and 250 mL of beer
- 180 g of alcohol/day for 25 years increases, risk of cirrhosis by 25 times
- Cirrhosis is sixfold when consumption is double safety limit
- Hepatitis C infection is an important contributory factor for progression to cirrhosis

Classification (Fig. 7.7)
Tables 7.24 and 7.25 describe the morphological and etiological classification of cirrhosis.

Clinical Features
Table 7.26 describes the clinical feature of alcoholic cirrhosis.

Prognostic Classifications
- The Child–Pugh (CP) scoring was used to risk-stratify patients undergoing shunt surgery. Modifications of Child's grading (A, B, and C) are useful to classify *severity of liver disease and prognosis* in patients with established cirrhosis **(Table 7.27)**.
- **Characteristics of end stage of cirrhosis:** Jaundice; progressive and refractory ascites; worsening of signs of portal hypertension; progressive renal dysfunction; and hepatic encephalopathy.
- **Investigations:** Assess severity and type of liver disease
- **Liver function tests:**
  - *Hyperbilirubinemia:* Conjugated and unconjugated
  - *Serum proteins:* Show reversal of A:G ratio. Hypoalbuminemia—reduced synthesis and hyperglobulinemia—stimulation of reticuloendothelial system
  - Complications of cirrhosis **(Table 7.28)**

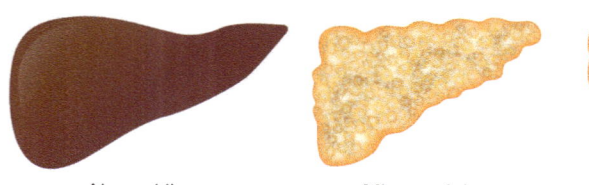
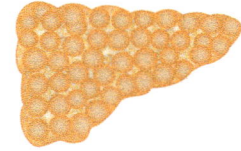
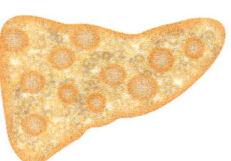

Fig. 7.7: Morphological classification of cirrhosis.

Table 7.24: Morphological classification of cirrhosis.

Micronodular cirrhosis (Laennec's cirrhosis)	Macronodular cirrhosis
• Regular, small nodules <3 mm • Uniform thin regular fibrous connective tissue septa • Involvement of every lobule of whole liver • *Most common cause*: Alcoholic cirrhosis	• Irregular, coarse nodules of variable size, >3 mm • Fibrous connective tissue septa, broad, vary in thickness, liver surface is grossly distorted • *Most common cause*: Chronic viral hepatitis • Increased risk of developing carcinoma of liver

Mixed cirrhosis:
Both micronodular and macronodular cirrhosis

Table 7.25: Etiological classification.

Alcohol	Nonalcoholic fatty liver disease
Chronic viral hepatitis Hepatitis B and hepatitis C Delta hepatitis (hepatitis D) + hepatitis B	*Intra-/extrahepatic biliary obstruction*: Recurrent biliary obstruction (e.g., gallstones)
Autoimmune hepatitis	**Cryptogenic or idiopathic**
Biliary cirrhosis Primary biliary cirrhosis, secondary biliary cirrhosis, and primary sclerosing cholangitis, and autoimmune cholangiopathy	*Inherited metabolic liver disease* Hemochromatosis, Wilson's disease, α_1-antitrypsin deficiency, cystic fibrosis, and glycogen storage disease
Drug-induced cirrhosis: Methotrexate, methyldopa, isoniazid, phenylbutazone, and sulfonamides	*Others*: Indian childhood cirrhosis, cardiac cirrhosis, and chronic venous outflow obstruction

Table 7.26: Clinical features.

Signs	Symptoms
• Jaundice • Hepatomegaly/shrunken liver, ascites • *Circulatory changes*: Spider naevi, palmar erythema • *Endocrine changes*: Loss of libido, diminished body hair and hair loss, gynecomastia, testicular atrophy, impotence in males, irregular menses, and amenorrhea breast atrophy in females • *Hemorrhagic tendency*: Bruises, purpura, and epistaxis • *Portal hypertension*: Splenomegaly, portosystemic collateral vessels, and variceal bleeding • Flapping tremors • Pigmentation, clubbing, cyanosis, and white nails • Dupuytren's contracture and parotid enlargement	• Asymptomatic, diagnosed at ultrasound • *Nonspecific*: Weakness, fatigue, muscle cramps, weight loss, anorexia, nausea, vomiting, and upper abdominal discomfort • Hepatic insufficiency • Portal hypertension, sequelae • *Endocrine changes*: Males—gynecomastia, loss of libido, hair loss; Females: Irregular menses, amenorrhea, and breast atrophy • *Hemorrhagic tendency*: Easy bruising, purpura, epistaxis, menorrhagia, and gastrointestinal bleeding

Table 7.27: Modified Child–Pugh classification or Child–Turcotte–Pugh score.

Parameter	Score		
	1	2	3
Encephalopathy	None	Mild	Marked
Ascites	None	Mild/diuretic controlled	Moderate/severe
Prothrombin time (seconds over normal)	<4	4–6	>6
Serum albumin (g/dL)	>3.5	2.8–3.5	<2.8
Serum bilirubin (mg/dL)	<2	2–3	>3

[CP class A: Points 5–6; CP class B: 7–9; CP class C: >9 (range 5–15)]

Table 7.28: Complications of cirrhosis.

• Portal hypertension and sequelae • Ascites • Spontaneous bacterial peritonitis	• Hepatic encephalopathy • Portal gastropathy • Hepatorenal syndrome • Hepatopulmonary syndrome	• Hepatocellular carcinoma • Bleeding manifestations • Cirrhotic cardiomyopathy • Hepatic hydrothorax

- *Serum transaminases*: AST, ALT—raised, usually <300 units/dL. AST:ALT ratio is more than 2 in alcoholic cirrhosis. AST is disproportionately raised relative to ALT, due to proportionately greater inhibition of ALT synthesis by alcohol. Less than 2 in cirrhosis complicating viral hepatitis
- *Alkaline phosphatase:* May be slightly elevated
- *Prothrombin time:* Prolonged due to reduced synthesis of clotting factors
❑ **Hematological tests:** Peripheral smear shows anemia, acanthocytosis (spur-like projections on RBC), leukopenia, and thrombocytopenia (hypersplenism and bone marrow suppression)
❑ **Serological markers:** For hepatitis B and C
❑ **Serum electrolytes:** Hyponatremia—severe disease due to defect in free water clearance or to excess diuretic therapy, hypokalemia, hypomagnesemia, and hypophosphatemia
❑ **Blood ammonia estimation:** Reliable when hepatic encephalopathy is suspected. Caused due to decreased clearance by liver and shunting of portal venous blood to systemic circulation
❑ **Respiratory alkalosis**—may develop due to central hyperventilation
❑ Glucose intolerance
❑ **Ultrasound:**
  - Changes in size and shape of the liver; nodularity
  - Fatty change and fibrosis produce a diffuse increased echogenicity
  - Distortion of the arterial vascular architecture, patency, and size of the portal and hepatic veins
  - Detect hepatocellular carcinoma
  - Splenomegaly and ascites
❑ **CT scan**—detects hepatosplenomegaly and dilated collaterals. Phase-contrast enhanced CT scan to detect hepatocellular carcinoma
❑ **Endoscopy:** Detecting and treating varices, portal hypertensive gastropathy

- **Liver biopsy:** It is done to confirm diagnosis and assess severity and type of liver disease. Special stains may be necessary for iron and copper. Immunocytochemical stains can identify viruses
- **Special investigations depending on the etiology:**
  - Chemical measurement of iron (serum transferrin saturation level and serum ferritin) and copper (ceruloplasmin) is required to confirm diagnosis of iron overload or Wilson's disease.
  - Serum α-fetoprotein, α1-antitrypsin, antinuclear antibodies, and anti-smooth muscle antibodies, etc., depending on the etiology
- Ascitic fluid examination

PORTAL HYPERTENSION

- It is prolonged elevation of portal venous pressure (more than 30 cm saline).
- Elevation of hepatic venous pressure gradient (HPVG) >7 mm Hg. HVPG more than 10 mm Hg is significant portal hypertension.
- Portal vein is formed by the union of the superior mesenteric and splenic veins. *Normal pressure*: 5–8 mm Hg (or 10–15 cm saline)
- It develops due to combination of two simultaneously occurring hemodynamic processes:
  1. Increased intrahepatic resistance to the blood flow through the liver caused by cirrhosis and regenerative nodules
  2. Increased splanchnic blood flow secondary to vasodilatation within the splanchnic vascular bed

Classification of Portal Hypertension (Fig. 7.8 and Flowchart 7.2)

Sites of obstruction are *prehepatic, intrahepatic, and posthepatic*.

- **Prehepatic:** Obstruction/blockage of portal vein before it ramifies within the liver—portal vein thrombosis, splenic vein thrombosis, and massive splenomegaly (Banti's syndrome)
- **Intrahepatic causes:** Distortion of architecture and may be further divided into *presinusoidal* (schistosomiasis), *sinusoidal* (cirrhosis), and *postsinusoidal* (veno-occlusive syndrome).
- **Posthepatic causes**—due to venous blockage outside the liver and are rare. Examples are severe right-sided heart failure, Budd–Chiari syndrome, constrictive pericarditis, and hepatic vein outflow obstruction.

Clinical Features

Clinical features of portal hypertension are discussed in **Table 7.29.**

Investigations

Diagnosis can be made on clinical grounds.
- **Barium swallow:** Varices as filing defects in lower third of esophagus ("bag of worms appearance")
- **Upper gastrointestinal endoscopy:** It is most reliable method. It appears as blue rounded projections (red spots and red stripes) under submucosa. "Cherry red spots" indicate impending rupture of varices.
- **Ultrasonography:** It detects the size of liver and spleen. Size and patency of portal vein and splenic vein. Presence of collaterals and ascites
- Portal venography is rarely done nowadays
- **Measurement of portal venous pressure:** It is measured by either wedged hepatic venous pressure (WHVP) or transhepatic venous pressure. It is useful for confirmation

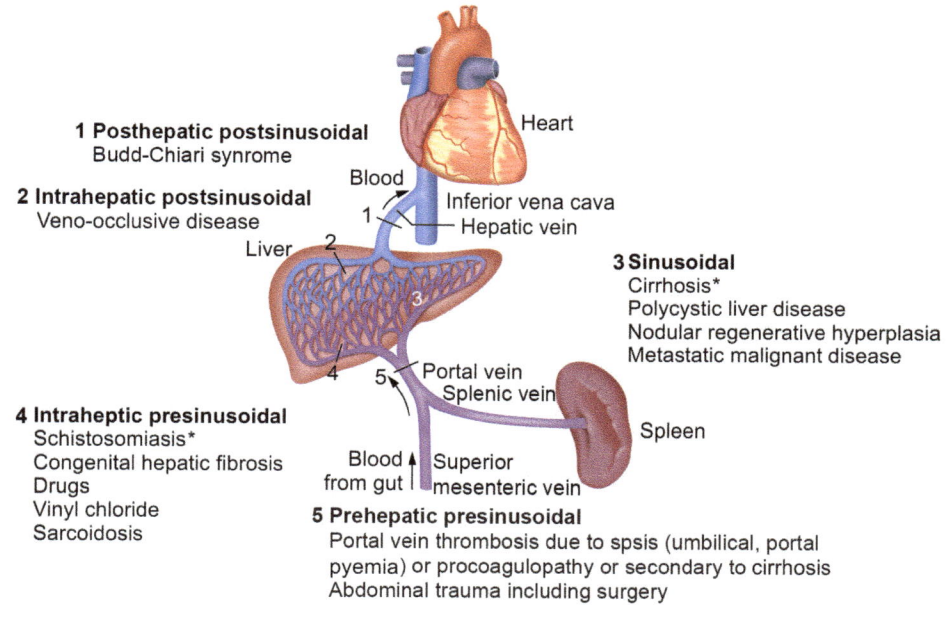

Fig. 7.8: Classification of portal hypertension according to site of vascular obstruction.
*Most common cause.

Flowchart 7.2: Sites of obstruction of portal hypertension.

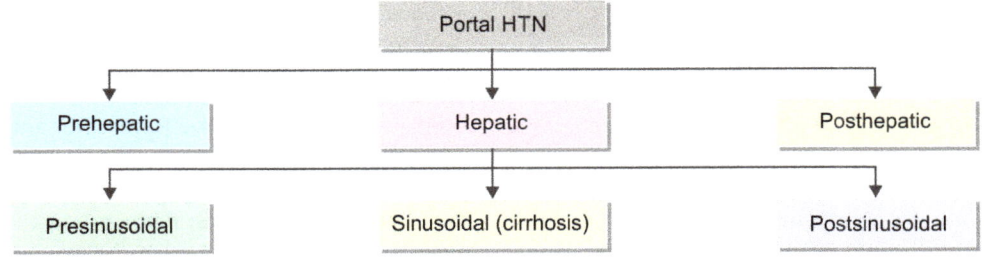

Portal	Nonportal	
Prehepatic • Portal vein thrombosis • Splenic vein thrombosis	**Congenital (mostly pediatric)** • Primary lymphatic hypoplasia • Yellow nail syndrome • Klippel-Trenaunay syndrome • Primary lymphatic hyperplasia • Intestinal lymphangiectasia	**Neoplastic** • Solid organ malignancy (e.g. carcinomas) • Lymphoma (mainly high grade non-Hodgkin B-cell lymphoma) • Lymphangiomyomatosis • Carcinoid tumors • Kaposi sarcoma

Hepatic
• Presinusoidal
  ▪ Schistosomiasis
  ▪ Congenital hepatic fibrosis
• Sinusoidal
  ▪ Cirrhosis
• Postsinusoidal
  ▪ Hepatic veno-occlusive disease
	Inflammatory
	• Radiation
	• Pancreatitis
	• Retroperitoneal fibrosis
	• Sarcoidosis
	• Celiac sprue
	• Whipple disease
		Postoperative
		• Abdominal aneurysm repair
		  ▪ Postliver transplant
		• Retroperitoneal node dissection
		• Inferior vena cava resection

Posthepatic • Budd-Chiari syndrome • Restrictive cardiomyopathy • Constrictive pericarditis • Congestive heart failure	**Infectious** • Tuberculosis • Filariasis • *Mycobacterium avium* itracellulare	**Traumatic** • Blunt abdominal trauma • Penetrating trauma

(HTN: hypertension)

Table 7.29: Clinical features of portal hypertension.

Asymptomatic	History: Alcoholism and hepatitis	Caput medusae
Splenomegaly (required for diagnosis)	Features due to liver cell failure, hepatic encephalopathy	*Hypersplenism*: Leukopenia and thrombocytopenia
Fetor hepaticus: Musty odor of breath due to shunting of blood allowing mercaptans to pass directly to lungs, bypassing liver	• *Bleeding*—esophageal varices or portal gastropathy—hematemesis and melena • *Hemorrhoids*—dilation of rectal veins due to development of collaterals	• Splanchnic arteriovenous fistula—bruit in left or right upper quadrant • Cruveilhier–Baumgarten hum—epigastric venous hum, collateral flow in the falciform ligament
Enlarged or shrunken liver. Small, contracted, and fibrotic liver is found when the portal venous pressure is very high. Soft liver—extrahepatic portal vein obstruction		
Ascites		

of portal hypertension and differentiating sinusoidal from presinusoidal portal hypertension.
- **Proctoscopy and barium enema:** Varices in the rectum and colon
- **Liver function tests**—to confirm the liver diseases

Complications

Complications of portal hypertension are described in **Box 7.3**.
Figure: Major clinical consequences of portal hypertension in cirrhosis.

Treatment

Treatment of underlying disease is discussed in **Table 7.30**.

Box 7.3: Complications of portal hypertension.

❖ **Variceal bleeding:** Esophageal and gastric
❖ Hepatic encephalopathy
❖ Ascites
❖ Renal failure
❖ Congestive gastropathy
❖ Hypersplenism
❖ Iron deficiency anemia

VARICEAL BLEEDING

- 90% patients with cirrhosis develop gastroesophageal varices, but only one-third will bleed.
- The most common site is esophageal varices within 3–5 cm of the esophagogastric junction.

Table 7.30: Treatment of portal hypertension.

Drugs used in the treatment of portal hypertension	
Drugs that decrease portal blood flow	Drugs that decrease intrahepatic resistance
Nonselective β-adrenergic blocking agents	α1-adrenergic blocking agents (e.g., prazosin)
Somatostatin and its analogs	Angiotensin receptor blocking agents
Vasopressin	Nitrates

- Factors that predisposing to rupture of varices are:
  - Large varices
  - "Red sign" on endoscopy suggests imminent rupture
  - It is associated with severe liver disease
  - High portal venous pressure
  - Salicylates and other nonsteroidal anti-inflammatory drugs

Clinical Features

- Painless, mild-massive hematemesis, with or without associated melena
- Depending on amount of blood loss, may vary from mild postural tachycardia to shock
- Features of liver cell failure, ascites, and portal hypertension

Diagnosis (Figs. 7.9 and 7.10)

- **Fiberoptic endoscopy:** Within 8 hours of bleeding reveals bleeding site and the presence of varices
- **Ultrasonography:** Useful to confirm the patency of portal vein

Management

- Management of the active bleeding episode
- Prevention of rebleeding
- Prophylactic measures to prevent the first hemorrhage

Acute variceal bleeding:
General measures:
- Resuscitation
- Immediate hospitalization: Intensive-care nursing. Nil by mouth until bleeding stops.
- Assess pulse and blood pressure, maintain fluid and electrolyte balance
- *Investigations*: Hemoglobin, blood group, urea–creatinine, electrolytes, liver function, and cultures
- Grade cirrhosis by *Child–Pugh* score
- Blood transfusion and avoid saline infusions. Prompt correction of hypovolemia
- Coagulation factor deficiency correction—fresh frozen plasma
- Platelet transfusions and vitamin K IM
- Prevent stress ulcers, give H_2 receptor antagonists or proton-pump inhibitors

Complication prevention:
Prophylactic antibiotics: Reduce infection and mortality—prevent spontaneous bacterial peritonitis
Oral and intravenous quinolones are used (e.g., ciprofloxacin 500 mg twice daily)
Prevent hepatic encephalopathy: Precipitated when the amount of bleeding is large because blood contains protein
Treatment of ascites: Ascitic tap (paracentesis), administration of spironolactone, or amiloride

Monitor for alcohol withdrawal and give thiamine

Urgent endoscopy:
- Confirm diagnosis of esophageal varices. Exclude bleeding from other sites (e.g., gastric ulceration)
- Reduce esophageal ulceration following therapy, sucralfate—1 g four times daily

Local measures:
- *Endoscopic procedures*: Sclerotherapy and variceal banding (endoscopic variceal band ligation—EVBL). They arrest bleeding in 80% of cases and reduce early rebleeding
- Balloon tamponade

Vasoconstrictor therapy:
- Reduce portal pressure for constricting splanchnic vessels and portal inflow of blood
- Terlipressin, somatostatin, octreotide, and vasopressin

- Used for emergency control of bleeding before endoscopy and in combination with endoscopic techniques by reducing portal inflow of blood and pressure by constricting splanchnic vessels
- **Drugs used:**
  - *Terlipressin*: Only drug reduces mortality. 2 mg IV 6-hourly till bleeding stops, 1 mg 4-hourly after 48 hours, if prolonged dosage regimen is used. It is contraindicated in ischemic heart disease. Side effects are abdominal colic, evacuation of bowels, and facial pallor due to generalized vasoconstriction.
  - Somatostatin, octreotide stops bleeding >80% patients, equivalent to vasopressin, endoscopic therapy. Few side effects. Administered as somatostatin infusion of 250–500 µg/h followed by 250 µg/h for 2–5 days;

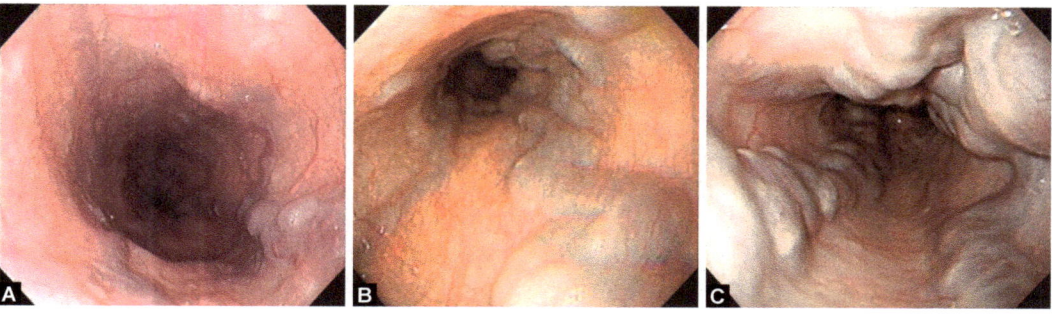

Figs. 7.9A to C: Endoscopy view of esophageal varices (Grade I, II, and III)

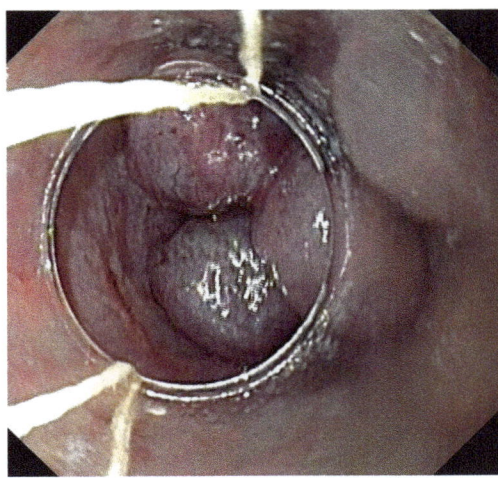

Fig. 7.10: Banding of esophageal varices.

octreotide—50 μg as bolus followed by 50 μg/h for 2–5 days. It is given, if terlipressin is contraindications.

Drugs that are used in the reduction of portal venous pressure: Terlipressin, somatostatin, octreotide, propranolol, nadolol, and nitroglycerin

- *Vasopressin*: It is used in the past but is not commonly used now.

Injection sclerotherapy or variceal banding:
- **Sclerotherapy:** Injection of sclerosing agent into the varices may arrest bleeding by producing thrombosis of vessel. Sclerosants are ethanolamine oleate, sodium morrhuate, absolute alcohol, and sodium tetradecyl sulfate.
- **Banding:** Varices are banded by mounting a band on the tip of the endoscope, sucking the varix just into the end of the endoscope, and dislodging the band over the varix.

Complications of sclerotherapy are:

• 1% mortality	• *Pulmonary complications*: Pain, pleural effusion, mediastinitis, aspiration pneumonia, and acute respiratory failure
• Abdominal pain, fever, and dysphagia	
• *Esophageal complications*: Recurrence of varices, ulceration, perforation, reflux, and stricture formation	• *Anterior spinal artery occlusion*: Spinal paralysis

Balloon tamponade:
- It is indicated in variceal bleeding, if endoscopic therapy or vasoconstrictors fail/contraindicated or exsanguinating hemorrhage. It is useful in initial hours of bleeding in 90% cases.
- Sengstaken-Blakemore tube, Minnesota tube: Four lumens tubes with two balloons esophageal and gastric balloons
- **Complications:** Aspiration pneumonia, esophageal rupture, necrosis, ulcerations of esophageal mucosa, and obstruction to pharynx

Management of an acute rebleed:
- About 30% of patients rebleed within 5 days after a single therapeutic endoscopy

- *Source*—established by endoscopy. Can be due to ulcer from sclerotherapy, difficult to manage
- *Management*: Repeat endoscopic therapy once only to control rebleeding and further sclerotherapy or banding should not be done.

Transjugular intrahepatic portocaval shunt (TIPS):
- It is indicated when bleeding does not stop after two sessions of endoscopic therapy within 5 days.
- *Technique*: Guidewire is passed from the jugular vein into the liver. Expandable metal shunt is forced over it into the liver substance to form a portocaval shunt.
- It reduces hepatic sinusoidal, portal vein pressure without risks of general anesthesia or surgery.
- It has only short-term benefit. If no response, transjugular intrahepatic portosystemic shunt (TIPSS) is useful in most patients.

Emergency surgery:
- It is indicated when other measures fail, TIPS is not available, continued, or recurrent hemorrhage and or bleeding is from gastric fundal varices.
- It is done by esophageal transection and ligation of the feeding vessels to the bleeding varices.
- Infrequently acute portosystemic shunt surgery and esophageal staple transaction

Prevention of variceal bleeding-prophylaxis:
It is described in **Table 7.31**.

HEPATIC (PORTOSYSTEMIC) ENCEPHALOPATHY

- It is chronic neuropsychiatric syndrome (alteration in mental status and cognitive function) secondary to chronic liver disease.
- Acute and potentially reversible, or chronic and progressive.

Etiology

It develops due to spontaneous "shunting" in chronic liver disease with portal hypertension or following a portosystemic shunt procedure, e.g., TIPS or fulminant hepatic failure.

Pathogenesis

Mechanism is unknown, but many factors play a role (**Tables 7.32 and 7.33**). Mechanisms proposed are:
- Gut-derived neurotoxins
- Brain water homeostasis
- Oxidative/nitrosative stress
- Astrocyte dysregulation
- Neurotransmitter dysfunction (decreased glutamine, increased GABA, and serotonin)
- Infection and inflammation

Clinical Features

Clinical features are summarized in **Table 7.34.**

Classification

The different types of hepatic encephalopathy are given in **Table 7.35**.

Table 7.31: Prevention of variceal bleeding–prophylaxis.

Primary prophylactic measures:	
These are useful in patients with cirrhosis and varices, who have not bled.	
Nonselective β-blockers: Propranolol and nadolol: • Reduce chance of upper GI bleeding and cost-effective. Reduce recurrence • Efficacy is similar to prophylactic banding • Act by vasodilatation of splanchnic arterial bed and portal venous system	*Nitrates*: Nitroglycerin, isosorbide dinitrate: Given with β-blockers—reduce risk of variceal bleed Variceal banding is done, if there are contraindications or intolerance to nonselective beta-blockers
Recurrent variceal bleeding (secondary prophylaxis):	
Bleeding recurs in about 60–80% of patients within 2 year after initial bleed.	
Long-term measures	**Surgical portosystemic shunting**
Nonselective beta-blockers—treatment of choice. *Propranolol*: 80–160 mg/day oral, decreases portal pressure, decreases frequency of rebleed (as effective as sclerotherapy or ligation), prevents bleeding from portal hypertensive gastropathy. *Endoscopic treatment*: Injection sclerotherapy or variceal banding. Repeated courses of banding done every 2 weeks until the varices are obliterated. It is superior to sclerotherapy. *Transjugular portosystemic stent shunts*: Reduce rebleeding rates compared to endoscopic techniques but associated with increased rate of encephalopathy. Used if endoscopic or medical therapy fails.	Performed in patients with good liver function (Child-Pugh A, B), when medical therapy, EVBL and sclerotherapy are unsuccessful with very low risk of rebleeding. *Types of portal systemic shunts*: • Nonselective shunt with end-to-side portocaval anastomosis decompresses entire portal venous system, produces significant post-operative hepatic encephalopathy. • Selective distal splenorenal (Warren) shunt—decompresses only varices while maintaining blood flow to liver via superior mesenteric vein, produces less encephalopathy *Complications of portosystemic shunts*: 5% mortality, shunt closure, hepatic encephalopathy due to reduction in portal pressure and hepatic blood flow, postoperative jaundice because of deterioration of liver function. *Esophageal transection*—devascularization procedure that does not produce encephalopathy *Liver transplantation*—treatment of choice when liver function is poor

(EVBL: endoscopic variceal band ligation)

Table 7.32: Toxic substances involved in hepatic encephalopathy.

- Ammonia
- Free fatty acids
- Mercaptans derived from methionine
- γ-aminobutyric acid (GABA)
- Aromatic amino acids—tyrosine and phenylalanine
- Reduced branched-chain amino acids
- Phenol and indole
- False neurotransmitters (octopamine)

Table 7.33: Precipitating factors for portosystemic encephalopathy.

- Increased dietary protein
- Gastrointestinal bleeding
- *Electrolyte disturbance*: Hypokalemia and hyponatremia
- Large volume paracentesis
- Overzealous use of diuretics
- Vomiting and diarrhea
- Constipation
- Acute infections—spontaneous bacterial peritonitis
- Drugs, e.g., sedatives
- Viral/alcoholic hepatitis
- Portosystemic shunt operations
- Development of hepatocellular carcinoma
- Uremia

Table 7.34: Clinical features.

Acute hepatic (portosystemic) encephalopathy:
• Usually has a precipitating factor, patient becomes drowsy and comatose within weeks to months. • Brain edema may occur with severe encephalopathy and may lead to cerebral herniation.
Chronic hepatic (portosystemic) encephalopathy:

Disturbances in consciousness and behavior, which may fluctuate:	Signs:
• Hypersomnia—earliest feature • Reversal of sleep rhythm • Violent and difficult to manage • Very sleepy and difficult to rouse • Irritable, confused, disoriented, and slurred speech • Drowsiness progressing to coma • Change in personality, mood, and intellect • *General features*—nausea, vomiting, and weakness	• Fetor hepaticus (a sweet smell to the breath) • Asterixis or coarse flapping tremor (outstretched hands, head, and trunk). Also seen in uremia, respiratory failure, and severe heart failure • *Fluctuating neurological signs*: Constructional apraxia with the patient being unable to write or draw, hypertonia, hyperreflexia, and decreased mental function

Staging

Staging of hepatic encephalopathy is described in **Table 7.36**.

Diagnosis

It is based on clinical features.
Reitan's number connection test (Fig. 7.11): It is used for >50 years to assess mental function.

Investigations

☐ **Blood ammonia levels:** Raised (upper limit of normal is 0.8–1 μg/mL)

Table 7.35: Types of hepatic encephalopathy.

Type A	Associated with acute liver failure
Type B	Associated with portosystemic bypass with no intrinsic liver disease
Type C	Associated with cirrhosis, portal hypertension, or portosystemic shunts
• *Minimal HE*	
• *Episodic HE*	Persistent, spontaneous, and recurrent
• *Persistent HE*	Mild, severe, and treatment dependent

(HE: hepatic encephalopathy)

Table 7.36: West Haven criteria.

Grade	Consciousness	Intellect and behavior	Neurological findings
0	Normal	Normal	Normal examination or impaired psycho-motor testing
1	Mild lack of awareness	Shortened attention span; impaired addition or subtraction	Mild asterixis or tremor
2	Lethargic	Disoriented, inappropriate behavior	Obvious asterixis, slurred speech
3	Somnolent but arousable	Gross disorientation, Bizarre behavior	Muscular rigidity and clonus Hyperreflexia
4	Coma	Coma	Decerebrate posturing

- **Electroencephalography (EEG):** A decrease in the frequency of the normal α-waves (8-13 Hz) to α-waves of 1.5-3 Hz is seen before coma develops.
- Cerebrospinal fluid—glutamine: Increased; proteins and cell count: Normal
- Visual evoked potential abnormalities may be present during subclinical encephalopathy
- Liver function tests to confirm presence of liver disease

Treatment (Table 7.37)

Treatment is multifactorial.

HEPATORENAL SYNDROME

- It is a form of functional renal failure without renal pathology in patients with advanced cirrhosis or acute liver failure.
- Urine output is low, tubular function is normal, and kidneys are histologically normal.
- 10% of patients with advanced cirrhosis with jaundice and ascites

Pathogenesis

Severe peripheral vasodilatation leads to severe reduction in effective blood volume and hypotension, activating homeostatic mechanisms, renin-angiotensin-aldosterone system leading to vasoconstriction of the renal vessels. Increased preglomerular vascular resistance directs the flow of blood away from the renal cortex. This leads to a reduced glomerular filtration rate. Eicosanoids are also implicated.

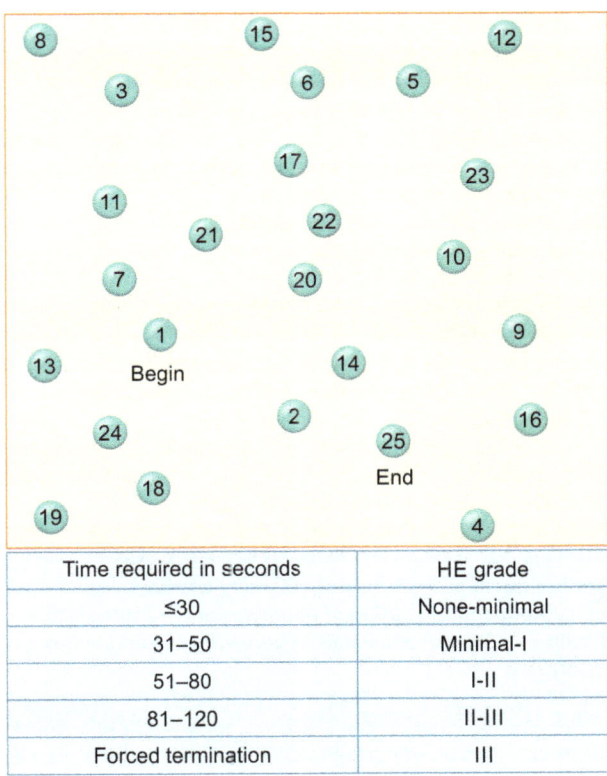

Time required in seconds	HE grade
≤30	None-minimal
31–50	Minimal-I
51–80	I-II
81–120	II-III
Forced termination	III

Fig. 7.11: Number connection test.

Precipitating Factors

Precipitating factors are gastrointestinal bleeding, aggressive paracentesis, diuretic therapy, sepsis including spontaneous bacterial peritonitis, and diarrhea.

Clinical Types

There are two types **(Table 7.38)**.

Clinical Features

- Develops in advanced cirrhosis, almost always with ascites
- Anorexia, weakness, fatigue, oliguria, nausea, vomiting, and thirst
- Terminally coma deepens and hypotension develops

Investigations

- **Urea and creatinine levels:** High
- **Serum sodium:** Less than 120 mEq/L. Urine sodium excretion <10 mEq/day
- **Urinalysis:** Normal. Urine:plasma osmolality ratio is more than 1.5

Diagnosis

- Usually made in the presence of a large amount of ascites in patients who have a stepwise progressive increase in creatinine.

Table 7.37: Treatment of hepatic encephalopathy.

General measures:
- Removal of the precipitating factors. Stop alcohol
- Maintain nutrition with glucose 300 g/day. Maintain hydration and correct electrolyte imbalance
- No restriction of dietary proteins for more than 48 hours. Administer 0.8–1.0 g/kg of proteins daily preferably vegetable protein. Restriction is reserved for resistant cases.
- Zinc supplementation may be helpful.
- Stop or reduce diuretic therapy.
- Treat any infection.

Bowel evacuation:
- Evacuating, sterilizing the bowels of nitrogenous toxins and bacteria.
- *Lactulose*: Nonabsorbable disaccharide, osmotic purgative; metabolized by colonic bacteria—produces colonic acidification. Promotes 2–3 soft stools per day.
- Eliminates nitrogenous waste, limits ammonia absorption, and favors conversion of ammonia to ammonium (poorly absorbed). Lactitol has a similar action, more palatable, and better than lactulose
- *Dose*: 15–30 mL three times orally per day

Poorly absorbed antibiotics:
- Sterilize gut in patients having difficulty with lactulose. Reduce bacterial intestinal ammonia production.
- Alternating administration of neomycin and metronidazole to reduce the individual side effects.
- Rifaximin—550 mg twice daily is very effective and without any side effects of neomycin or metronidazole. It has only 0.4% systemic absorption.

Other measures:
- *Gastrointestinal bleeding*: Ryle's tube aspiration, bowel washes to remove the blood and blood products. It reduces the production of nitrogen in the gut.
- Mannitol and judicious use of intravenous fluids to reduce spontaneous cerebral edema in acute liver failure.

Other drugs tried	Novel treatment strategies
Bromocriptine, L-ornithine L-aspartate (LOLA), branched chain amino acids, probiotics, sodium benzoate, and flunarizine	• L-carnitine, rivastigmine, endocannabinoids, and mGluR1antagonists • MARS—molecular adsorption reversibility system—purifies the blood by removal of albumin bound as well as water-soluble substrates

Liver transplantation

Table 7.38: Clinical types of hepatorenal syndrome.

Type 1 hepatorenal syndrome	Type 2 hepatorenal syndrome
• Progressive oliguria, rapid rise of serum creatinine to >2.5 mg/dL • Very poor prognosis • Precipitated by spontaneous bacterial peritonitis • Without treatment, median survival is <1 month, die within 10 weeks after onset of renal failure	• Reduction in glomerular filtration, moderate, stable increase of serum creatinine (>1.5 mg/dL) • Better prognosis than Type 1 HRS. • Usually occurs in patients with refractory ascites (resistant to diuretics). • Median survival is 3–6 months.

- Diagnostic criteria: All must be present:
  - Cirrhosis with ascites
  - Serum creatinine >1.5 mg/dL, no improvement (decrease to a level of 1.5 mg/dL or less) after at least 2 days of diuretic withdrawal and volume expansion with albumin (1 g/kg body weight/day up to a maximum of 100 g/day)
  - Absence of shock
  - No current or recent treatment with nephrotoxic drugs
  - Absence of parenchymal kidney disease as indicated by proteinuria >500 mg/day, microhematuria (>50 red blood cells per high power field), and/or abnormal renal ultrasonography

Treatment
Liver transplantation is the treatment of choice.

Prevention
- Avoid overvigorous diuretic therapy, slow treatment of ascites
- Early recognition of electrolyte imbalance and hemorrhage. Screen, treat infection (SBP)
- Correct hypovolemia by intravenous plasma protein solution or salt-poor albumin
- Albumin infusions with vasopressin analogues are effective short-term medical therapy
- Currently, midodrine (α-agonist) along with octreotide is also being used.
- TIPSS, if vasoconstrictors fall

ASCITES

It is a condition of accumulation of excess fluid within the peritoneal cavity.

Pathogenesis
Pathogenesis is complex, involving the mechanisms described in **Table 7.39.**

Chapter 7: Hepatobiliary Disorders

Table 7.39: Mechanisms involved in pathogenesis of ascites.

In cirrhosis	Absence of cirrhosis
Portal hypertension: Increase in portal vein hydrostatic pressure, causing extravasation of fluid from plasma into the peritoneal cavity.	**Inflammation of peritoneum:** Peritonitis from bacteria or mycobacteria causes increased vascular permeability and exudation of fluid into peritoneal cavity
Hypoalbuminemia: Decreased synthetic function in cirrhosis reduces plasma oncotic pressure, results in extravasation of fluid (ascites and edema)	**Venous obstruction:** Inferior vena caval (IVC) obstruction increases the hydrostatic pressure, leads to transudation of fluid into peritoneal cavity.
Splanchnic vasodilation: Reduction of arterial blood pressure activates *renin–angiotensin–aldosterone system* causing secondary hyperaldosteronism. Liver fails to metabolize aldosterone increased hyperaldosteronism. Causes *sodium and fluid retention*	**Lymphatic obstruction:** Obstruction of lymphatic flow due to involvement of mesenteric lymph nodes, thoracic duct, and abdominal lymphatic ducts can cause leakage of chyle into peritoneal cavity and can lead to chylous ascites
Percolation of lymph: In cirrhosis, hepatic lymphatic flow exceeds thoracic duct capacity. Excess lymph oozes freely from the surface of cirrhotic liver into the peritoneal cavity causing ascites.	**Rupture of a viscus:** Outpouring of blood, cystic fluid, contaminated material, and favoring ascites. Pancreatic ascites results from leakage of pancreatic enzymes into the peritoneum (pancreatitis).
Combination of portal hypertension, splanchnic arterial vasodilation, and sodium and water retention increases the hydrostatic pressure as well as permeability of interstitial capillaries. It causes extravasation of fluid into the peritoneal cavity.	**Malignancy:** Primary peritoneal malignancies (mesothelioma, sarcoma), abdominal malignancies (gastric, colonic adenocarcinoma), or metastatic disease from breast, lung, or melanoma

Classification of Ascitic Fluid Infection

- Culture-negative neutrocytic ascites
- Monomicrobial non-neutrocytic bacterascites
- Polymicrobial bacterascites
- Secondary bacterial peritonitis
- Spontaneous bacterial peritonitis

Investigations (Fig. 7.12)

- 10–20 mL of ascitic fluid
- *Cell count*: Neutrophil count above 250 cells/mm^3—spontaneous bacterial peritonitis
- *Gram stain and culture*: Bacteria and acid-fast bacilli
- *Protein*: Total ascetic fluid protein >1.5 g/dL—increased risk of spontaneous bacterial peritonitis
- *SAAG (serum ascites albumin gradient)*: Difference between serum albumin and ascitic fluid albumin. Better indicator than simple estimation of protein in the ascetic fluid. A high serum-ascites albumin gradient of >1.1 g/dL suggests portal hypertension, and a low gradient <1.1 g/dL is associated with abnormalities of the peritoneum, e.g., inflammation, infections, and neoplasms.
- *Cytology*: For malignant cells to exclude neoplasms
- *Amylase*: To exclude pancreatic ascites. It is increased in acute pancreatitis
- *Ultrasonography*: Very sensitive, detects small amounts of fluid, and identifies the cause also.
- Paracentesis and evaluation of ascitic fluid
- Laparoscopy and biopsy of peritoneum

Nature of Ascitic Fluid

The ascitic fluid may be transudate or exudate **(Table 7.40)**.

Causes

Various causes of ascites are mentioned in **Table 7.41.**

Examination

Table 7.42 describes the examination of ascetic fluid.

Serum–Ascites Albumin Gradient (Tables 7.43 and 7.44)

- It is useful for differentiating ascites caused by portal hypertension from other causes.
- *Serum albumin concentration*: Ascitic albumin concentration (does not change with diuresis)
- **Significance:**
  - SAAG ≥1.1 g/dL: Portal hypertension, ascites is due to increased pressure in hepatic sinusoids.
  - SAAG <1.1 g/dL: Nonportal hypertensive ascites such as tuberculous peritonitis, peritoneal carcinomatosis, or pancreatic ascites.

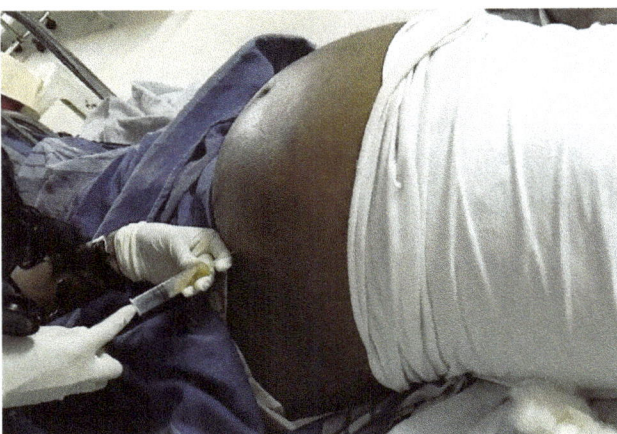

Fig. 7.12: Ascitic tap.

Table 7.40: Difference between transudate and exudate.

Characteristics	Transudate	Exudate
Cause	Noninflammatory process	Inflammatory process
Mechanism	Ultrafiltrate of plasma Increased hydrostatic pressure	Increased vascular permeability
Appearance	Clear and serous	Turbid, chylous, purulent, and hemorrhagic
Color	Straw yellow	Yellow to red
Specific gravity	<1.018	>1.018
Protein	Low, <2 g/dL, mainly albumin	High, >2 g/dL
Clot	Absent	Clots spontaneously (high fibrinogen)
Cell count	Low (<250/µL)	High (>250/µL)
Type of cells	Few lymphocytes and mesothelial cells	• *Acute*: Neutrophils • *Chronic*: Lymphocytes
Bacteria	Absent	Usually present
LDH	Low	High
Edema	Pitting type	No pitting

(LDH: lactate dehydrogenase)

Table 7.41: Various causes of ascites categorized depending on the nature of ascetic fluid.

Transudates:
- Cirrhosis and portal hypertension
- Nephrotic syndrome
- Hypoproteinemia
- Congestive cardiac failure
- Constrictive pericarditis
- Beriberi
- Inferior vena caval (IVC) obstruction

Exudates:
- Tuberculous, bacterial peritonitis
- Malignant peritonitis
- Pancreatic ascites

Miscellaneous (exudate/transudate):
- Meige's syndrome
- Chylous ascites
- Budd–Chiari syndrome

- Depending on the total protein level in the ascitic fluid, it is divided into transudate or exudate. However, many patients with spontaneous bacterial peritonitis (SBP) have a low rather than high total protein in the ascetic fluid, and many patients with portal hypertension secondary to heart failure have a high protein rather than the expected low total protein level in ascetic fluid. In these situations, SAAG is highly sensitive method.
- ❑ **Management:** Produce a net reabsorption of fluid from the ascites into the circulating volume by reducing sodium intake and increasing renal excretion of sodium
- ❑ **General measures:**
  - Hospitalization is necessary, if there is massive ascites
  - Check serum electrolytes, renal function tests at the start and twice a week
  - Measure abdominal girth and weight daily
  - Strict intake output recording
  - Urinary electrolyte determination
- ❑ Bed rest alone induces diuresis in a small proportion of people because renal blood flow increases in the horizontal position, but in practice, is not helpful.

Table 7.42: Examination of ascetic fluid and its interpretation.

Feature	Interpretation
Gross appearance:	
Clear, straw-colored, or light green	Cirrhosis, congestive heart failure, and nephritic syndrome
Hemorrhagic	Malignancy, tuberculosis, and pancreatitis
Cloudy and turbid	Bacterial peritonitis
Milky white (chylous)	Lymphatic obstruction
Biochemistry:	
Specific gravity	Transudates: <1.018; exudates >1.018
Protein	Transudates: <2.5g/dL; exudates >2.5 g/dL
SAAG	Refer below
Glucose	Low in malignancy, tuberculosis, and peritonitis
Amylase activity	More than 1,000 units/L in pancreatitis
Microscopy:	
Polymorphs	<250/mm^3 in cirrhosis >250/mm^3 in bacterial peritonitis
Lymphocytes	Tuberculosis and malignancy
Cytological examination	Malignancy
Special stains:	
Gram's stain	Bacterial peritonitis
Ziehl–Neelsen staining	Tuberculosis
Culture:	
Pyogenic bacteria	Bacterial peritonitis
Mycobacteria	Tuberculosis

Table 7.43: Causes of high and low serum-ascites albumin gradient.

High serum-ascites albumin gradient (>1.1 g/dL)	Low serum-ascites albumin gradient (<1.1 g/dL)
• Portal hypertension, e.g., cirrhosis of liver • Hepatic outflow obstruction • Budd–Chiari syndrome • Hepatic veno-occlusive disease • Right-sided heart failure • Constrictive pericarditis	• Peritoneal tuberculosis • Carcinoma involving peritoneal cavity • Pancreatitis • Nephrotic syndrome

Table 7.44: Causes of ascites according to the nature of ascitic fluid.

Straw-colored	Chylous
• Malignancy (most common cause) • Cirrhosis • *Infective*: Tuberculosis, intra-abdominal perforation • Chronic pancreatitis • *Heart disorders*: Congestive cardiac failure, constrictive pericarditis • Hepatic vein obstruction: Budd–Chiari syndrome • Meigs' syndrome (ovarian tumor) • Hypoproteinemia (e.g., nephrotic syndrome)	• Obstruction of lymphatic duct (e.g., by carcinoma) • Cirrhosis *Hemorrhagic:* • Malignant tumors • Ruptured ectopic pregnancy • Trauma to abdomen • Acute pancreatitis

- Dietary restriction sodium by reducing sodium intake to 40 mmol in 24 h and maintain an adequate protein and calorie intake with a palatable diet.
- Fluid restriction to 1,000–1,500 mL/day, if serum sodium is under 128 mmol/L (hyponatremia)
- **Diuretics:**
    - Aim at producing a net loss of fluid of about 700 mL per day (0.7 kg weight loss in patients with ascites alone or 1.0 kg, if both ascites and peripheral edema is present). The maximum rate at which ascites can be mobilized is 500–700 mL per day. This is to prevent diuretic-induced renal failure and/or hyponatremia.
    - *Aldosterone antagonists*: As there is secondary hyperaldosteronism, diuretics of first choice are aldosterone antagonists (potassium-sparing diuretics), e.g., spironolactone, triamterene, and amiloride. Spironolactone—25 mg QID (100 mg daily), and gradually stepped up every week to a maximum of 400 mg/day (providing there is no hyperkalemia). Chronic administration—gynecomastia. Eplerenone 25 mg once daily does not produce gynecomastia.
    - *Loop diuretics*: When a large dose of spironolactone has failed, add a loop diuretic, such as furosemide 20–40 mg or bumetanide 0.5 mg or 1 mg daily. Usually, spironolactone is combining with furosemide. Disadvantages of loop diuretics include development of hyponatremia, hypokalemia, and volume depletion.
    - Stop all diuretics, if severe hyponatremia (sodium <120 mEq/L), progressive renal failure, or worsening of hepatic encephalopathy occurs.
- **Treatment of refractory ascites:**
    - *Intravenous salt-poor albumin*, 25 g in 3 hours
    - *Large-volume paracentesis* is indicated in refractory ascites, to relieve symptomatic tense ascites, e.g., cardiorespiratory distress due to gross ascites and if there is risk of impending rupture of a hernia.
    - *Complication*: Hypovolemia and renal dysfunction (post-paracentesis circulatory dysfunction) more likely with removal of >5 L and worse liver function.
    - Paracentesis and diuretics usually reduce ascites.
- **Shunts:**
    - *Transjugular intrahepatic portosystemic shunt (TIPS):* It is used for resistant ascites, if there is no spontaneous portosystemic encephalopathy and no disturbance of renal function.
    - *LeVeen shunt:* Peritoneovenous shunt that allows peritoneal fluid to drain directly into the internal jugular vein. Its use has been abandoned in most centers due to a high rate of blockage. It may be considered in patients with refractory ascites who cannot undergo paracentesis, or TIPSS or liver transplant.
    - *Complications:* Infection, thrombosis of superior vena cava, bleeding from esophageal varices, pulmonary edema, and disseminated intravascular coagulation
    - Side-to-side portocaval shunt
- **Liver transplantation**

SPONTANEOUS BACTERIAL PERITONITIS

- It is a common and severe complication of ascites characterized by spontaneous infection of ascetic fluid in the absence of a recognizable intra-abdominal source of peritonitis.
- **Causative agents:** Most commonly due to *Escherichia coli, Klebsiella, Enterococci*, and gut bacteria. Others are streptococci and enterococci.
- **Route of infection:** Infective gut florae traverse the intestine into mesenteric lymph nodes, leading to bacteremia and seeding of ascitic fluid by hematogenous spread.

Clinical Features

- Suspected in any patient with ascites who clinically deteriorates
- Sudden deterioration or hepatic encephalopathy in a cirrhotic patient with ascites
- Fever, abdominal pain or discomfort, rebound abdominal tenderness

Investigations

- **Peripheral blood:** Leukocytosis
- Ascitic fluid
- Cloudy fluid
- **Leukocyte count:** More than 500/mm^3. Neutrophil count >250/mm^3 in ascites, alone sufficient for diagnosis and to start treatment immediately.
- **pH:** Less than 7.3
- **Culture:** Positive. *E. coli* is the most common organism.

Diagnosis

Diagnostic aspiration should always be performed in patients with high clinical suspicion.

Treatment

- **Third-generation cephalosporins:** Cefotaxime and ceftazidime. Modified on the basis of culture results. *Dose of cefotaxime*: 2 g IV 8 hourly for 5 days.
- Alternative therapy in patients without shock or hepatic encephalopathy
- Amoxicillin/clavulanate (1.2 g IV 8 hourly followed by 625 mg orally)
- Ciprofloxacin (200 mg IV 12 hourly followed by 500 mg BD orally)
- Ofloxacin (400 mg twice daily). Quinolones are avoided, if norfloxacin is used for prophylaxis.
- Antibiotic therapy and albumin (1.5 g/kg body weight within 6 hours, 1 g/kg on day 3 reduces risk of type 1 hepatorenal syndrome).

Prophylaxis

Recurrence is common (70% within a year) and prophylaxis is indicated.

- **Acute GI bleed (reduces rate of re-bleed):** Cefotaxime/norfloxacin (400 mg BID for 7 days)
- **Previous episode of SBP and recovered:** Quinolones-norfloxacin (400 mg/day)

- **Low total ascites protein content <1.5 g/dL:** Quinolones-norfloxacin (400 mg/day)
- **Severe liver disease and no prior history of SBP**
- **Alternative and less effective drugs:** Cotrimoxazole (800 mg sulfamethoxazole + 160 mg trimethoprim OD) or ciprofloxacin (750 mg once a week).

DRUG AND LIVER

Common hepatotoxic drugs and toxins with associated morphologic changes are described in **Table 7.45**.

Table 7.45: Common hepatotoxic drugs and toxins with associated morphologic changes.

Cholestasis	Fatty liver	Hepatitis
• Erythromycin estolate • Methimazole • Chlorpromazine • Chlorpropamide • Methyltestosterone • Anabolic steroids • Cyclosporine • Nimesulide • Amoxicillin/clavulanate	• Zidovudine • Amoxicillin • Indinavir • Ritonavir • Methotrexate • Tetracyclines • Valproic acid	• Halothane • Isoniazid • Rifampicin • Phenytoin • Methyldopa • Ibuprofen • Ketoconazole • Zidovudine • Chlorothiazide
Toxic (necrosis)	**Granuloma**	**Hepatic fibrosis:** Methotrexate
• Paracetamol • Carbon tetrachloride • Mushroom (*Amanita phalloides*) • Yellow phosphorus	• Phenylbutazone • Sulfonamides • Carbamazepine • Allopurinol • Quinidine	*Chronic hepatitis:* • Phenytoin • Isoniazid

BUDD–CHIARI SYNDROME (TABLE 7.46)

- Obstruction of hepatic venous outflow owing to occlusion of the hepatic vein.
- Obstruction may be at any level from small hepatic veins to junction of IVC with the right atrium.
- Classically results from thrombosis of one or more hepatic veins at their openings into the inferior vena cava.
- The result is hepatomegaly, pain, ascites, and impaired hepatic function. The ascitic fluid typically has a high serum–ascites albumin gradient.

Table 7.46: Various causes of Budd–Chiari syndrome.

Venous thrombosis	Compression (may also produce thrombosis)
Hypercoagulability states: • *Hematological disorders:* Polycythemia vera, paroxysmal nocturnal hemoglobinuria, antithrombin III, protein C or S deficiencies, antiphospholipid syndrome, sickle cell disease, and leukemia • Pregnancy • Use of oral contraceptive pills	• Hepatic infections • Hydatid cyst • Liver abscess • Obstruction due to tumors • Renal cell carcinoma • Adrenal tumors • Hepatocellular carcinoma • Posterior abdominal wall sarcomas
Radiation injury	*Congenital venous webs*
Trauma to the liver	*Idiopathic (40–50% of cases)*

- **Clinical features:** Triad of abdominal pain, ascites, and hepatomegaly with hepatic histology showing centrilobular sinusoidal distension and pooling.
- **Acute Budd–Chiari** follows sudden venous occlusion (e.g., by renal cell carcinoma, hepatocellular carcinoma, and polycythemia). Acute upper abdominal pain, nausea, vomiting, tender hepatomegaly, marked ascites, and mild jaundice. With total venous occlusion—delirium, coma, and hepatocellular failure
- **Fulminant Budd–Chiari** presents with fulminant hepatic failure in the setting of an additional predisposing factor (e.g., factor V Leiden mutation). It occurs particularly in pregnant women.
- **Chronic Budd–Chiari:** More gradual occlusion presents with pain abdomen, tender hepatomegaly and gross ascites. With the enlarged caudate lobe, the liver becomes palpable. There is splenomegaly with portal hypertension, jaundice is mild or absent. Bilateral pedal edema and distended veins over abdomen, flanks, and back, with IVC obstruction, negative hepatojugular reflux, i.e., pressure over the liver fails to fill the jugular veins. Features of cirrhosis and portal hypertension are seen in patients who survive the acute event. Hepatocellular carcinoma may develop.
- **Investigations:**
  - *Ultrasound:* Enlargement of caudate lobe, intrahepatic collaterals, echogenic areas, and ascites. It also may show compression of the inferior vena cava, if present.
  - *Pulsed Doppler sonography:* Obliteration of hepatic veins, reversed flow or associated thrombosis in the portal vein with high accuracy. Doppler ultrasonography, sensitivity and specificity rates > 80%, is the diagnostic procedure of first choice
  - *CT or MRI:* Occlusion of hepatic veins and inferior vena cava with diffuse abnormal parenchyma on contrast enhancement. It may also demonstrate enlargement of the caudate lobe, which has independent blood supply and venous drainage.
  - *Other investigations:* To identify a cause (e.g., blood tests and coagulation studies).
- **Management:**
  - Predisposing causes should be removed or treated as far as possible.
  - *Acute with recent thrombosis*: Thrombolytic therapy—intrahepatic vein streptokinase (in very early cases of thrombosis), followed by heparin and oral anticoagulation (warfarin).
  - *Short hepatic venous strictures*: Treated with angioplasty
  - *Extensive hepatic vein occlusion*: Insertion of a covered TIPSS followed by anticoagulation may be useful in opening of the hepatic veins.
  - *Ascites*: Initially treated medically with low-salt diet, diuretics, as well as treating the underlying cause (e.g., polycythemia). If not relieved, it may be treated with surgical shunts such as Le Veen shunt and portosystemic shunts.
  - Percutaneous balloon angioplasty for membranous obstruction of the IVC and hepatic vein.

- Congenital web can be treated radiologically or resected surgically.
- Liver transplantation is indicated for chronic Budd-Chiari syndrome and for progressive liver failure, followed by lifelong anticoagulation.
- **Prognosis:** Without transplantation or shunts, acute and fulminant types have poor prognosis.

HEPATOCELLULAR CARCINOMA

- Hepatocellular carcinoma (HCC) is the most common primary malignancy of liver from hepatocytes or their precursors.
- It predominantly presents in males with an M:F ratio of 2.4:1. The number of men and number of women with hepatocellular carcinoma in the absence of cirrhosis are almost equal.
- **Etiology (Table 7.47):**

Table 7.47: Risk factors for hepatocellular carcinoma.

Major risk factors	Minor risk factors	
• Chronic hepatitis B, C viruses • Alcoholic cirrhosis • Aflatoxin B_1 (fungal toxin) • Nonalcoholic steatohepatitis (NASH)	• Hereditary hemochromatosis • Wilson disease • Primary biliary cirrhosis • Tyrosinemia • $α_1$-antitrypsin deficiency • Glycogen storage disease • *Hormones*: Anabolic steroids, estrogens, and androgens	• Oral contraceptives • Cigarette smoking • Betel quid chewing • Thorotrast and arsenic exposure • Obesity • Ataxia telangiectasia • Hypercitrullinemia

- **Clinical features:**
  - Usually develops in patients with underlying cirrhosis
  - Nonspecific symptoms include ill-defined upper abdominal pain in the right hypochondrium, malaise, weakness, anorexia, fatigue, weight loss, and ascites. Rapid development of these symptoms in a patient with cirrhosis is suggestive of HCC.
  - *On examination*: Liver is enlarged, irregular, nodular with pain or tenderness and friction rub or a hepatic bruit over the liver due to vascularity of tumor.
  - *Paraneoplastic syndromes associated with hepatocellular carcinoma*:
    - Carcinoid syndrome
    - Hypercalcemia
    - Hypertrophic osteoarthropathy
    - Hypoglycemia
    - Neuropathy
    - Osteoporosis
    - Polycythemia (erythrocytosis)
    - Polymyositis
    - Porphyria
    - Sexual changes—isosexual precocity, gynecomastia, and feminization
    - Systemic arterial hypertension
    - Thyrotoxicosis
    - Thrombophlebitis migrans
    - Watery diarrhea syndrome
- **Investigations:**
  - *Serum markers:*
    - *Alpha-fetoprotein:* About 50% HCC is associated with high (>500 µg/L) or rising levels of alpha-fetoprotein. However, levels are raised in other neoplastic and nonneoplastic liver diseases and in some extrahepatic disorders.
    - *α-L-fucosidase*—is raised in HCC and also in cirrhosis.
    - *Serum des-γ-carboxy prothrombin* is raised in a majority of hepatocellular carcinoma
    - *Serum alkaline phosphatase*: Very high
  - Ultrasound scans show filling defects
  - CT scan (triple-phase) or MRI abdomen
  - Blood-tinged ascites
  - Hepatic artery angiography shows "tumor blushes". Liver scintigraphic scans
  - Liver aspiration or biopsy particularly under ultrasonic guidance confirms the diagnosis. Microscopy consists of cells resembling hepatocytes.
- **Management:** Treatment is different for patients with cirrhosis and those without. Therapy depends on tumor size, multicentricity, extent of liver disease (Child-Pugh score), and performance status.
  - *Surgical resection.* It is indicated when lesions are 1-3 in number, <5 cm in size; without metastasis; and with child score A. Local or segmental resections are preferred to major resections. After successful resection, tumor recurs in the cirrhotic liver in about 70% of patients after 5 years.
  - *Nonsurgical therapy:* Majority of patients are diagnosed at advanced stage of HCC and cannot be treated by surgical resection
  - *Local ablation strategies:*
    - Radiofrequency ablation (RFA)—uses heat to kill tumor cells. A single electrode inserted into the tumor under CT or ultrasound guidance.
    - *Transarterial embolization (TAE)*: Hepatic artery embolization with Gelfoam and doxorubicin
    - *Transarterial chemoembolization (TACE)*—with drugs such as doxorubicin but is contraindicated in decompensated cirrhosis and when HCC is multifocal.
  - *Local injection therapy*: Percutaneous ethanol injection (PEI) or percutaneous acetic acid injection (PAI). It causes direct destruction of tumor cells, but also destroys normal cells in the vicinity. It usually requires multiple injections (average three) and the maximum size of tumor treated is 3 cm.
  - Conventional chemotherapy and radiotherapy are unsuccessful.
  - *Chemotherapy using intravenous sorafenib*: This drug is a multikinase inhibitor with activity against Raf, vascular endothelial growth factor (VEGF), and platelet-derived growth factor (PDGF) signaling.

- **Liver transplantation:** It is indicated in presence of localized tumor and underlying advanced liver disease. Unfortunately, the underlying liver disease (e.g., hepatitis B and C) may recur in the transplanted liver.

PYOGENIC LIVER ABSCESS (BACTERIAL LIVER ABSCESS)

- It is uncommon.
- **Etiology:**
  - Commonly—echinococcal, amebic infections, less commonly—other protozoans and helminths.
  - Bacterial infections in the liver may be manifested as pyogenic abscess. These develop as a complication of a bacterial infection elsewhere. Commonly, *E. coli*, *Streptococcus milleri*, and *Bacteroides*. Others are *Enterococcus faecalis*, *Proteus vulgaris*, and *Staphylococcus aureus*. Often mixed infection.
- **Route of infection:**
  - *Portal vein:* Intra-abdominal infections (appendicitis, diverticulitis, colitis, and perforated bowel)
  - *Arterial blood supply:* During systemic bacteremia, organism may reach liver via hepatic artery
  - Ascending infection in the biliary tract (ascending cholangitis)
  - Direct invasion of the liver from a nearby source (e.g., subphrenic abscess, perinephric abscess), or a penetrating injury.
- **Clinical features:** Fever, chills, rigors, and right upper quadrant pain radiating to right shoulder. There are weight loss, anorexia, nausea, and vomiting. Pleuritic chest pain and tender hepatomegaly may be present. Mild jaundice may develop when there is extrahepatic biliary obstruction. Respiratory findings at the base of right lung (pleural effusion and crepitations) or a pleural rub.
- **Investigations:** Patients who are not acutely ill, often diagnosed as pyrexia of unknown origin
  - *Serum bilirubin:* Raised in 25% of cases
  - *Serum alkaline phosphatase:* Markedly elevated
  - *Blood cultures:* Positive in only 30% of cases
  - *Normochromic normocytic anemia* with polymorphonuclear leukocytosis
  - *Erythrocyte sedimentation rate (ESR) and C-reactive protein (CRP)* are often raised
  - *Chest radiograph:* Elevation of right dome of diaphragm, and in severe cases right basilar atelectasis and pneumonia or effusion
  - *Ultrasonography*—confirms the diagnosis
  - *CT scan of abdomen*—helpful when ultrasound is normal
  - *Needle aspiration* of pus for culture and sensitivity.
- **Management:**
  - *Antibiotics:* Initiate treatment with antibiotics (combination of ampicillin, gentamicin, and metronidazole) to cover gram-positive, gram-negative, and anaerobic organisms till the causative organism is identified. Later, change the antibiotic according to the culture and sensitivity reports. Duration of treatment is 4–8 weeks.
  - *Ultrasound-guided aspiration of the abscess:* Indications include:
    - Large abscess (>6 cm)
    - Abscess in the left lobe
    - Lack of response within 48–72 hours of medical therapy
    - Ultrasonography suggestive of large abscess impending rupture
  - Surgical drainage via a large-bore needle for those who fail to respond
  - Treat the underlying cause

AMEBIC LIVER ABSCESS

- It is most common extraintestinal complication of amebic dysentery.
- *Entamoeba histolytica* is carried from bowel to the liver in the portal venous system with the development of multiple microabscesses and eventually single or multiple large abscesses.
- Amebic abscess ranges from 8 to 12 cm in diameter, well circumscribed. Cavity contains thick, dark material that has been likened to *anchovy sauce*.
- **Clinical features:**
  - Symptoms are similar to pyogenic abscesses (such as fever, anorexia, weight loss, and malaise)
  - Onset is usually gradual but may be sudden.
  - Past history of dysentery. Jaundice is rare.
  - On examination, patient looks ill, tender hepatomegaly, and signs of an effusion or consolidation in the base of the right side of the chest.
  - Rare complications are intraperitoneal, intrathoracic or pericardial rupture, and multiorgan failure.
- **Investigations:** These are same as for pyogenic abscess, plus:
  - Serological tests for amoeba (e.g., hemagglutination, amebic complement fixation test, ELISA).
  - *Diagnostic aspiration of abscess:* Anchovy sauce
- **Treatment:**
  - Metronidazole, 750 mg TID for 7–10 day orally *or* IV, *or* tinidazole, 2 g orally for 3 days, *followed by* iodoquinol, 650 mg orally TID for 20 days; diloxanide furoate, 500 mg orally TID for 10 days; or aminosidine (paromomycin) 25–35 mg/kg/d orally in three divided doses for 7–10 days
  - If an amebic abscess continues to grow, it may rupture into the peritoneal cavity, where it produces peritonitis, a complication associated with a mortality rate as high as 40%. The amebae may also invade the blood, in which case abscesses of the brain and lung may ensue.

HEREDITARY HEMOCHROMATOSIS

- It is an inherited disease characterized by abnormal (excessive) accumulation of iron in various parenchymal organs leading to eventual fibrosis and functional organ failure.

- **Etiology:**
  - *HFE* gene (chromosome 6) regulates intestinal absorption of dietary iron. *HFE* gene product along with proteins hemojuvelin (HJV) and transferrin receptor 2 (TfR2) regulates iron metabolism through hepcidin. *Hepcidin* synthesized in the liver is the central regulator of iron homeostasis. It controls iron absorption and storage. When hepcidin levels rise, iron gets stored within enterocytes forming mucosal ferritin and is shed with the cells.
  - *Mutations* in *HJV, TfR2,* and *HFE* lead to absence of hepcidin, causing absorption of iron even when there is substantial *elevation of body iron stores*. The free iron produces reactive oxygen metabolites, which cause cell injury and fibrosis.
  - Most are inherited as autosomal recessive genetic disorder, associated with HLA-B3, B7, and B14 histocompatibility antigens.
  - 90% patients are males. Unlikely in females due to loss of iron—menstruation and pregnancy.
- **Pathology:** Excess iron is deposited in liver, joint, heart, pancreas, endocrine glands, and skin.
- **Clinical features:**
  - Develop due to toxic damage of cells by accumulated iron and consequent fibrosis.
  - Muscle aches, weakness, abdominal, and/or joint pain.
- **Classic triad:** Bronze skin pigmentation (melanin deposition in exposed parts, axillae, groin, and genitalia), hepatomegaly, and diabetes mellitus (bronzed diabetes) in patients with gross iron overload.
- **Late features:** Loss of libido, testicular atrophy, cardiac complaints (heart failure and cardiac arrhythmias), hepatosplenomegaly, spiders, loss of body hair, jaundice, and ascites.
- Cirrhosis (disease and scarring of the liver)
- **Cardiac manifestations:** Heart failure and arrhythmias are in younger patients. Hypogonadism, related to involvement of pituitary gland and genitalia
- **Complications:** Chondrocalcinosis (asymmetrical deposition of calcium pyrophosphate in both large and small joints and leads to an arthropathy), hepatocellular carcinoma, and multiorgan failure.
- **Investigations:**
  - *Serum iron profile*:
    - *Serum iron* is elevated (>30 µmol/L)
    - *Total iron-binding capacity (TIBC)*—reduced
    - *Transferrin saturation of >45%*—highly sensitive for diagnosis
    - *Serum ferritin* is elevated (usually >500 µg/L or 240 nmol/L): Less sensitive than transferring saturation in screening for hemochromatosis because it is also increased in alcoholic liver disease, hepatitis C infection, and nonalcoholic steatohepatitis.
- Acute phase reactant and increased in other inflammatory and neoplastic conditions.
  - *Biochemical tests for liver function are* often normal, even with established cirrhosis
  - *Genetic testing*—is performed, if iron studies are abnormal.
  - *CT scan*—shows increased density of liver due to deposits of iron.
  - *Magnetic resonance imaging (MRI)*: Sensitive to detect liver iron content
  - *Liver biopsy*—shows iron deposition and hepatic fibrosis leading on to cirrhosis.
- **Management:** Started before permanent organ damage occurs due to iron toxicity. Excess iron should be removed as rapidly as possible and prolongs life and may reverse tissue damage.
  - *Venesection*: Venesection of 500 mL blood (removes 250 mg of iron) is performed twice weekly until the serum iron is normal. Takes 2 years or more. Thereafter, reaccumulation of iron can be prevented by 3 or 4 venesections per year to keep the serum ferritin normal range. Blood removed can be utilized for routine transfusion.
  - *Chelation therapy*: Rarely, in patients who cannot tolerate venesection because of severe cardiac disease or anemia, chelation therapy with desferrioxamine (40-80 mg/kg/day subcutaneously) can be used. It removes about 10-20 mg of iron/day.
  - Treatment of diabetes, congestive heart failure, and cardiac arrhythmias
  - *Treatment of cirrhosis*: There is a risk of malignancy, if cirrhosis is present

WILSON'S DISEASE (HEPATOLENTICULAR DEGENERATION)

- **Normal copper metabolism:** Copper in the diet is absorbed from the stomach and upper small intestine is transported to the liver, loosely bound to albumin in the blood. In the liver, copper is incorporated into proceruloplasmin and forms ceruloplasmin (a glycoprotein synthesized in the liver) and secreted into the blood. Remaining copper is excreted in the bile and excreted in stool.
- **Wilson's disease** is a very rare inborn error of copper metabolism characterized by increased total body copper. Excess copper gets deposited in the liver, basal ganglia of the brain, cornea, kidneys, and skeleton. It is a potentially treatable condition. Excessive accumulation of copper in the body due to failure of incorporation of copper into proceruloplasmin and leads to low serum ceruloplasmin and failure of biliary copper excretion, causing its accumulation in the body.
- **Etiology:** Autosomal recessive disorder due to a molecular defect within a copper-transporting ATPase encoded by a gene (*ATP7B*) located on chromosome 13. More than 300 mutations have been identified. Rare in India and Asia. Consanguinity is risk factor.
- **Pathology:** Microscopic features are not diagnostic and vary from that of chronic hepatitis to macronodular cirrhosis. Stains for copper show a periportal distribution of copper

- **Clinical features:**
  - *Presents* between 5 and 30 years. Children—with hepatic problems. Young adults—with more neurological problems
  - *Liver involvement*: Varies from acute hepatitis, fulminant hepatic failure, and chronic hepatitis to cirrhosis.
  - *Brain involvement*: Tremor, dysarthria, involuntary movements (especially resting and intention tremors, wing beating), and eventually dementia
  - *Psychiatric manifestations*—phobia, depression, and compulsive behavior
  - *Features of eye involvement—Kayser-Fleischer rings*:
    - Characteristic sign due to deposition of copper in the Descemet's membrane of cornea.
    - Greenish-brown or golden-brown ring at the corneoscleral junction, appearing first at the upper periphery, best identified by slit-lamp examination.
    - Absent in young children and disappears with treatment
    - May be associated with "sunflower cataracts"
    - Not specific for Wilson disease; found occasionally with other types of chronic liver disease, with a prominent cholestatic component, such as primary biliary cirrhosis, primary sclerosing cholangitis, or familial cholestatic syndromes
- **Other manifestations:** Renal tubular damage, osteoporosis, and arthropathy
- **Investigations:**
  - *Slit-lamp examination* of the eyes for Kayser-Fleischer ring
  - *Serum copper*—reduced but can be normal
  - *Serum ceruloplasmin levels*: Low and less than 29 mg/dL
  - *Urinary copper:* Increased 100–1,000 μg in 24 h (1.6–16 μmol)
  - *Liver biopsy:* Diagnosis—dependent on amount of copper in liver (>250 μg/g dry weight)
  - *Hemolysis and anemia* may be found.
- **Treatment and management:** Started early, improvement seen—clinically and biochemically.
  - *Chelating drugs*:
    - Penicillamine—pyridoxine (1–1.5 g daily)—should be given lifetime, effectively chelates copper.
    - Asymptomatic cases, maintenance therapy (after maximal improvement with penicillamine)—Trientine dihydrochloride—in the dose of 1.2–1.8 g/day. *Zinc acetate*: Dose 150 mg/day; blocks absorption of copper from intestine. However, it should not be administered with penicillamine or trientine as both chelate zinc
  - For severe neurologic involvement, who do not improve with penicillamine or trientine, may be treated with—(1) intramuscular dimercaprol, or (2) ammonium tetrathiomolybdate.
  - Liver transplantation—in fulminant hepatic failure and decompensated/advanced cirrhosis
  - All siblings and children of the patient should be screened for Wilson's disease and treated even if they are asymptomatic, and if there is evidence of copper accumulation.

OBJECTIVE-BASED SELF-EVALUATION

LONG QUESTIONS

1. Define jaundice. List the types with clinical differentiating features and examples.
2. List the etiology of acute hepatitis. Discuss the clinical features and complications of acute viral hepatitis.
3. Discuss the modes of transmission, clinical features, serological markers and management of chronic hepatitis B.
4. Discuss the modes of transmission clinical features, serological markers and management of chronic hepatitis C.
5. List the etiology, clinical features and complications of cirrhosis of liver.
6. Discuss the pathogenesis, precipitating features, clinical features and management of hepatic encephalopathy.
7. Discuss bilirubin metabolism. Add a note on NAFLD.
8. Define portal hypertension. What are the common causes and clinical features you see in a patient with portal hypertension?
9. Discuss the pathogenesis of ascites. Define spontaneous bacterial peritonitis. Discuss the management of ascites in a patient with cirrhosis.
10. List the complications of cirrhosis. Discuss the types and management of hepatorenal syndrome.
11. Discuss the pathogenesis, clinical features and management of amoebic liver abscess.

SHORT ANSWER QUESTIONS

1. Functions of the liver
2. Congenital hyperbilirubinemia
3. Obstructive jaundice
4. Liver enzymes
5. NASH
6. Management of acute variceal bleed
7. List common drugs causing liver injury
8. Budd-Chiari syndrome
9. Wilsons's disease
10. SAAG
11. Grading of hepatic encephalopathy
12. Child-Pugh score
13. Classify etiology of portal hypertension
14. Portocaval anastomosis
15. Alpha fetoprotein
16. Fatty liver
17. Liver abscess
18. Fulminant hepatic failure
19. List viruses causing hepatitis
20. List causes of tender hepatomegaly

MULTIPLE CHOICE QUESTIONS

1. Which of the following is the most common symptom or sign of liver disease?
   a. Fatigue
   b. Itching
   c. Jaundice
   d. Nausea

2. Micronodular cirrhosis is commonly seen in all, *except*:
   a. Chronic hepatitis B
   b. Alcoholic liver disease
   c. Hemochromatosis
   d. Chronic extrahepatic biliary obstruction

3. Raised unconjugated bilirubin is seen in?
   a. Gilbert's syndrome
   b. Dubin Johnson syndrome
   c. Drug-induced hemolysis
   d. Hepatocellular necrosis

4. Ascitic tap of a child reveals SAAG <1.1 g/dL. The probable diagnosis is:
   a. Cirrhosis
   b. Portal hypertension
   c. Congestive cardiac failure
   d. Nephrotic syndrome

5. In Budd-Chiari syndrome the site of venous thrombosis is?
   a. Hepatic veins
   b. Portal veins
   c. Splenic vein
   d. Superior mesenteric vein

6. 5' nucleotidase activity is increased in?
   a. Bone disease
   b. Prostrate cancer
   c. Chronic renal failure
   d. Cholestatic disease

7. All the following are used for treatment of chronic hepatitis B, *except*:
   a. Entecavir
   b. Telbivudine
   c. Zidovudine
   d. Lamivudine

8. A 44-year-old male presents with fatigue and tea colored urine for 5 days. Physical examination reveals jaundice and tender hepatomegaly, Laboratories are remarkable for an aspartate aminotransferase (AST) of 2400 U/L and an alanine aminotransferase (ALT) of 2640 U/L. Alkaline phosphatase is 210 U/L. Total bilirubin is 8.6 mg/dL. Which of the following diagnoses is most likely?
   a. Acute hepatitis A infection
   b. Cirrhosis of liver
   c. Drug-induced hemolysis
   d. Acute renal failure

9. Which of the following viral causes of acute hepatitis is most likely to cause fulminant hepatitis in a pregnant woman?
   a. Hepatitis A
   b. Hepatitis B
   c. Hepatitis C
   d. Hepatitis E

10. All of the following are associated with an increased risk for cholelithiasis, *except*:
    a. Chronic hemolytic anemia
    b. Female sex
    c. High-protein diet
    d. Obesity

ANSWERS

1. a   2. a   3. a   4. d   5. a
6. d   7. c   8. a   9. d   10. c

Respiratory System

CHAPTER OUTLINE

- Bronchial Asthma
- Chronic Obstructive Pulmonary Disease
- Pulmonary Tuberculosis
- Suppurative Lung Disease
- Bronchiectasis
- Lung Abscess
- Pleural Effusion
- Empyema Thoracis
- Pneumothorax
- Pneumonia
- Occupational Lung Diseases
- Respiratory Failure
- Acute Respiratory Distress Syndrome
- Allergic Bronchopulmonary Aspergillosis
- Hemoptysis
- Pulmonary Eosinophilic Syndromes

BRONCHIAL ASTHMA

Definition

Asthma is a *chronic inflammatory disorder* of the airways (bronchial tree) in which *breathing is periodically rendered difficult* by *widespread narrowing of the bronchi* (reversible bronchoconstriction).

It is *clinically characterized by recurrent episodes* (paroxysms) *of wheezing, breathlessness* (dyspnea), *tightness of the chest, and cough*.

Global Initiative for Asthma (GINA)—2015 definition of asthma: "Asthma is a heterogeneous disease, usually characterized by chronic airway inflammation. It is defined by the history of respiratory symptoms, such as wheeze, shortness of breath, chest tightness, and cough that vary over time and in intensity, together with variable expiratory airflow limitation." *These episodes are usually associated with widespread but variable airflow obstruction that is often reversible either spontaneously or with treatment.*

Characteristics of Asthma

- **Airflow narrowing:** It is due to combination of muscle edema and viscid bronchial secretion. It is generally reversible spontaneously or with treatment.
- **Airway hyper-reactivity (AHR)/bronchial hyper-responsiveness (BHR):** It is characterized by increased tendency for airway (tracheobronchial tree) narrowing in response to triggers (stimuli) that have little or no effect in normal individuals.
- **Bronchial inflammation:** Inflammation of the bronchial walls by T lymphocytes, mast cells, eosinophils with associated plasma exudation, edema, smooth muscle hypertrophy, mucus plugging, and epithelial damage.

Classification

Classification of asthma is described in **Box 8.1**.

Box 8.1: Classification of asthma.

According to type of antigen:
- Early-onset asthma (*atopic*/allergic/extrinsic)
- Late-onset asthma (*nonatopic*/intrinsic/idiosyncratic) without evidence of allergen sensitization

According to the agents or events that trigger bronchoconstriction:
- Seasonal
- Exercise-induced
- Drug-induced (e.g., aspirin)
- Occupational asthma
- Asthmatic bronchitis in smokers
- Cough variant asthma (CVA) in which cough is the only asthma symptom

Differentiating features of early-onset asthma and late-onset asthma is presented in **Table 8.1**.

Risk Factors and Triggers

Risk factors and triggers involved in asthma are described in **Table 8.2**.

Risk Factors (Fig. 8.1)
Endogenous factors

- **Genetic predisposition:** Major etiological factor in atopic asthma is genetic predisposition to *type I hypersensitivity (atopy) reaction* and exposure to environmental trigger. *One of the susceptibility loci is on the chromosome 5 (5q)* → several genes involved in regulation of IgE synthesis and mast cell and eosinophil growth and differentiation.
- **Atopy:** Atopic individuals tend to *have higher serum IgE levels*, and a positive family history of allergy is found in 50% of atopic individuals. Patients with asthma commonly suffer from other atopic diseases (e.g., allergic rhinitis, atopic dermatitis/eczema).
- **Airway hyperresponsiveness:** It is an abnormality in which there is *excessive tendency for airways to contract*

Table 8.1: Differentiating features of early-onset asthma and late-onset asthma.

Features	Early-onset (atopic) asthma	Late-onset (nonatopic) asthma
Onset	Early age (usually begins in childhood)	Late age
Individuals	Atopic individuals	Nonatopic individuals
Role of external allergens	Have strong role	No role
Family history	Positive history of asthma or allergic diseases (e.g., eczema, urticaria, or hay fever)	Less common or absent
Triggering events	Environmental allergens (e.g., dusts, pollens, animal dander, and foods)	Respiratory infections due to viruses (e.g., rhinovirus, parainfluenza virus) inhaled air pollutants (e.g., smoke and fumes)
Serum level of IgE	Increased	Normal
Skin hypersensitivity test to common inhalant allergens	Positive	Negative
Response to provocation tests	Positive	Negative

Table 8.2: Risk factors and triggers involved in asthma.

Risk factors	
Endogenous factors: • Genetic predisposition • Atopy • Airway hyperresponsiveness • Gender and age • Ethnicity • Obesity • Early viral infections	**Environmental factors:** • Allergens (indoor/outdoor) • Occupational sensitizers • Respiratory infections
Triggers	
• Inhaled allergens • Upper respiratory tract viral infections • Air pollution (e.g., sulfur dioxide, irritant gases) • Passive smoking (tobacco smoke)	• Drugs (β-blockers, aspirin) • **Physical factors:** Exercise, cold air, and hyperventilation • Emotional stress • Irritants (household sprays paint fumes)

(bronchoconstrictor) too easily in response to multiple inhaled triggers that usually does not have any effect on normal individuals.

☐ **Gender and age:** More common in boys than girls and, after puberty, women slightly more commonly than men. Most cases *begin before the age of 25 years*.

Environmental factors
Hygiene hypothesis proposes that individuals with *lack of infections in early childhood* are more prone to asthma than children brought up on farms who are exposed to a high level of endotoxin. Intestinal parasite infection may also be associated with a decreased risk of asthma. Conversely, early childhood in a "dirtier" environment (exposure to inhaled and ingested products of microorganisms) may allow the immune system to avoid developing allergic responses.

Pathogenesis (Pathophysiology) of Asthma
Airway Inflammation
☐ **Inflammation** is chronic and involves many cell types and inflammatory mediators.

☐ **Strong T_H2 response:** *Genetic predisposition* with susceptibility genes makes individuals prone to develop strong T_H2 (type of T lymphocytes) *reactions against environmental antigens* (allergens).

☐ **T_H2 cells secrete cytokines:** Which promote allergic inflammation and *stimulate B cells to produce IgE*.

Cells involved in the inflammatory response
Important cells involved in asthma are—*mast cells, eosinophils, dendritic cells (macrophages), and lymphocytes*.

☐ **Mast cells:**
- *Early reaction* is characterized by *bronchoconstriction, increased mucus production*, and *vasodilation with increased vascular permeability* (causes edema).
- *Late phase reaction*: It is characterized by *inflammation and airway remodeling*.

☐ **Eosinophils:**
- *Mediators released from eosinophils*: LTC_4, and basic proteins, such as major basic protein (MBP), eosinophil cationic protein (ECP), and eosinophils peroxidase (EPX). They are toxic to epithelial cells.
- Corticosteroid rapidly decreases the number and reduces the activation of eosinophils.
- Sputum eosinophilia is of diagnostic help and is a biomarker of response to therapy.

☐ **Dendritic cells and lymphocytes**
They release prostaglandin, thromboxane, LTC_4, LTB_4, and platelet-activating factor (PAF).

Airway Remodeling
Airway remodeling is the *group of structural* and *functional changes in the bronchial wall due to repeated bouts of inflammation* observed in chronic asthma.

☐ An *increase in size and number* (hypertrophy/hyperplasia) of the *submucosal glands*
☐ *Hypertrophy and/or hyperplasia of the bronchial wall smooth muscle*
☐ *Increased vascularity*
☐ *Deposition of subepithelial collagen* accompanied by fibrosis and thickening of the basement membrane.

Pathogenesis of asthma is summarized in **Figures 8.2A and B.**

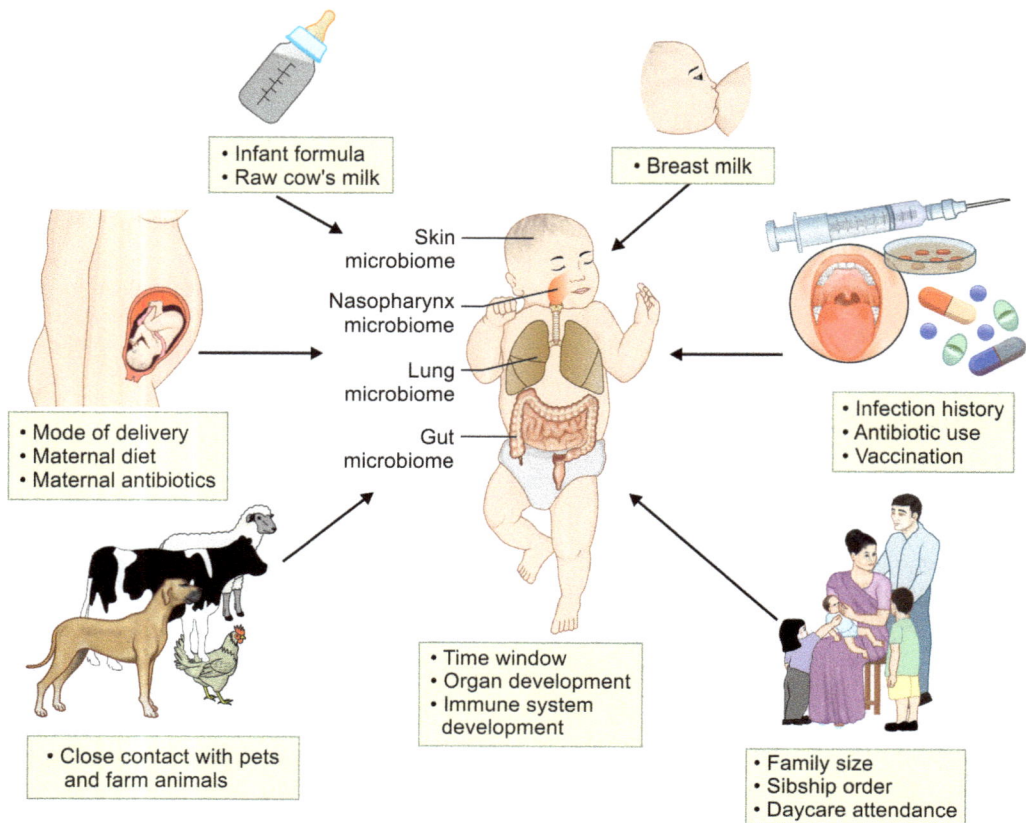

Fig. 8.1: Risk factors for asthma.

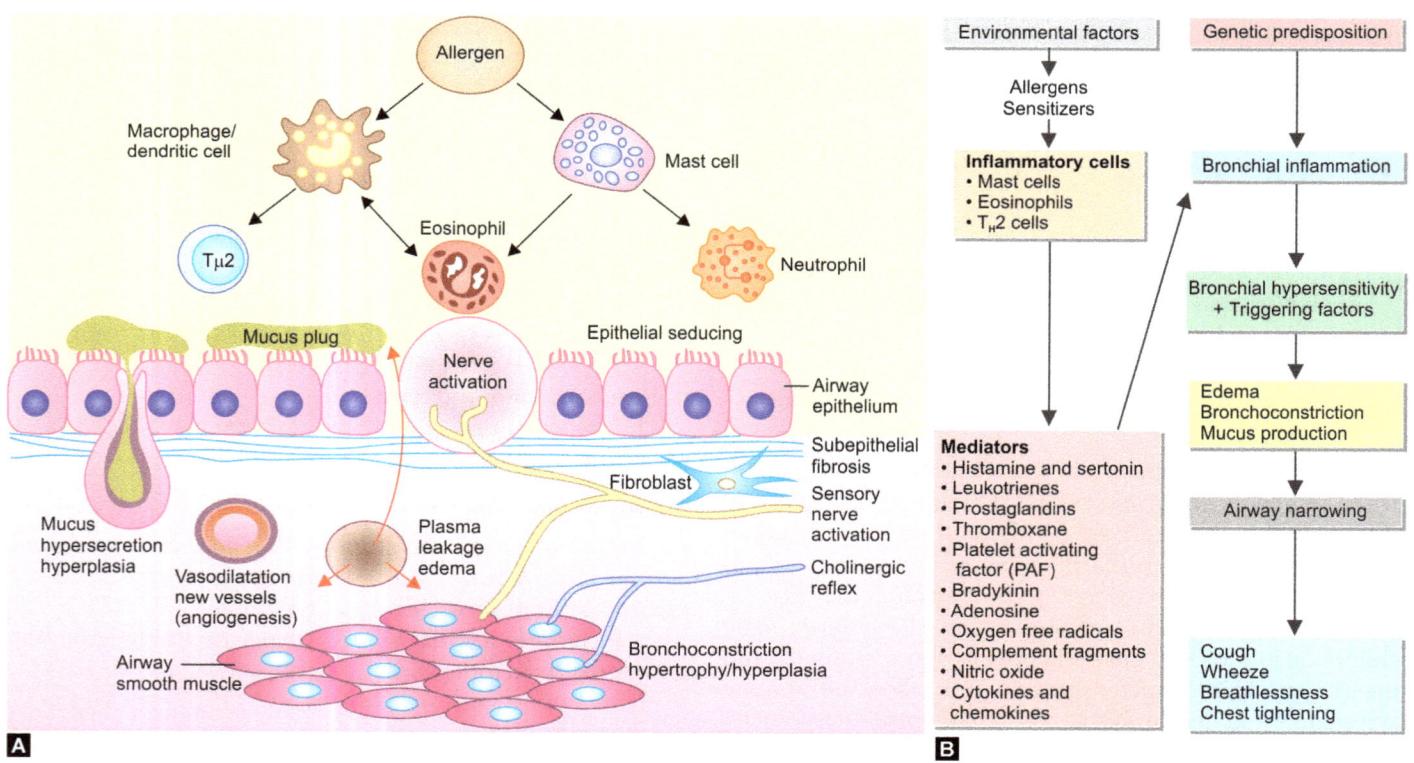

Figs. 8.2A and B: Pathogenesis of asthma.

Clinical Features

- Clinical features are divided into three headings, namely (1) episodic, (2) severe acute (status asthmaticus), and (3) chronic asthma.
- Usually, atopic individuals develop episodic asthma and nonatopic individuals develop chronic asthma.

Episodic Asthma

- Occurs as episodes with asymptomatic period between asthmatic attacks.
- Frequency and duration of attacks vary.
- Present with relatively sudden onset of paroxysms of *wheezing and dyspnea*.
- May develop spontaneous or triggered by allergens, exercise, or viral infections.
- It may be mild to severe and may last for hours, days, or even weeks.

Severe Acute Asthma (Status Asthmaticus)

- It is the *most severe form of asthma* in which the severe acute paroxysm persists for days and even weeks.
- Presents with severe dyspnea and unproductive cough.
- During this attack, patients prefer an upright position fixing the shoulder girdle to assist the accessory muscles of respiration.
- Physical signs include sweating, central cyanosis, tachycardia, and pulsus paradoxus. The *bronchoconstriction* and asthmatic symptoms *do not respond* despite the initial administration of standard *acute asthma therapy*.
- It may cause *severe airflow obstruction leading to severe cyanosis and even death*.

Chronic Asthma

- It has chronic persistent symptoms and includes chest tightness, wheeze, and breathlessness on exertion.
- It is characterized by episodes of spontaneous cough and wheeze, worst during the night.
- Chronic productive cough with mucoid sputum, punctuated by recurrent attacks of purulent expectoration from frank infection. They are prone to repeated attacks of "severe acute asthma". Features sometimes resemble those of chronic bronchitis.

Physical Signs

- **During an attack:**
  - *Inspection*: Increased respiratory rate with use of accessory muscles for respiration.
  - *Percussion:* Hyper-resonant percussion note over the lungs.
  - *Auscultation*:
    - Breath sounds are vesicular with prolonged expiration.
    - High-pitched polyphonic expiratory and inspiratory rhonchi.
    - Very severe attacks may result in a silent chest, which is an ominous sign.
- **In-between the attacks:** Chest may not reveal any abnormal physical signs.
- **Chronic asthmatics:** Usually reveal few scattered rhonchi.

Global Initiative for Asthma (GINA) Severity Grades (Table 8.3)

Severe Asthma (Table 8.4)

- It is an asthma, which requires treatment with high dose inhaled corticosteroids and long-acting β_2-agonist and/or leukotriene receptor antagonists for the previous year or systemic corticosteroids for $\geq 50\%$ of the previous year to prevent from becoming uncontrolled asthma.
- Asthma, which remains uncontrolled despite this therapy.

Investigations (Table 8.5)

The diagnosis is mainly clinical and based on a characteristic history. There is no single satisfactory diagnostic test for asthma.

Lung Function Tests

Pulmonary function tests useful in asthma are forced expiratory volume in 1 second (FEV_1), vital capacity (VC), and peak expiratory flow rate (PEFR).

- **Spirometry:** It is useful, especially in assessing reversibility. Simple spirometry is useful in confirming the airflow limitation with a reduced FEV_1, FEV_1/FVC ratio, and PEF. Asthma can be diagnosed, if there *is greater than 15% improvement in FEV_1 or PEFR following the inhalation of a bronchodilator*.
- **Peak expiratory flow rate (PEFR):** It is useful in demonstrating the variable airflow limitation. PEFR measurements to be done on waking, prior to taking a bronchodilator and before bed after a bronchodilator. The diurnal variation in PEFR of more than 20% (the lowest values typically being recorded in the morning) is considered diagnostic. It also provides good measure of disease severity.
- **Carbon monoxide (CO) transfer test:** Increased in asthma
- **Exercise tests:** It is used in the diagnosis of asthma in children. The child is asked to run for 6 minutes on a treadmill (heart rate should be above 160 beats per minute). A negative test does not rule out asthma.
- **Airway responsiveness (AHR):** AHR is sensitive but nonspecific.
- **Histamine or methacholine bronchial provocation test**
- **Indirect challenge tests**—release of endogenous mediators that causes the contraction of airway smooth muscle. These include exercise eucapnic voluntary hyperpnea (EVH), ultrasonically nebulizer hypertonic saline, and dry-powder mannitol.

Imaging

- **Chest X-ray:**
  - Usually normal between attacks without any diagnostic features.
  - During an acute episode or in chronic severe disease, there may be hyperinflated lungs (overinflation)
  - May be helpful in excluding complications, such as pneumothorax, lobar collapse (if mucus occludes large bronchus) or in detecting the pulmonary infiltrates associated with allergic bronchopulmonary aspergillosis.

Table 8.3: Classification of asthma severity and initiating treatment in persons >12 years of age.

Components of severity		Classification of asthma severity (>12 years of age)			
		Intermittent	Persistent		
			Mild	Moderate	Severe
Impairment Normal FEV_1/FVC: 8–19 years: 85% 20–39 years: 80% 40–59 years: 75% 60–80 years: 70%	Symptoms	≤2 days/week	>2 days/week but not daily	Daily	Throughout the day
	Nighttime awakenings	≤2×/month	3–4×/month	>×/week but not nightly	Often 7×/week
	Short-acting beta$_2$-agonist use for symptom control	≤2 days/week	>2 days/week but not daily, and not more than 1× on any day	Daily	Several times per day
	Interference with normal activity	None	Minor limitation	Some limitation	Extremely limited
	Lung function	• Normal FEV_1 between exacerbations • FEV_1 >80% predicted • FEV_1/FVC normal	• FEV_1 >80% predicted • FEV_1/FVC normal	• FEV_1 >60% but <80% predicted • FEV_1/FVC reduced 5%	• FEV_1 <60% predicted • FEV_1/FVC reduced >5%
Risk	Exacerbations requiring oral systemic corticosteroids	0–1/year	←——————————— ≥2/year ———————————→ ←—— Consider severity and interval since last exacerbation ——→ Frequency and severity may fluctuate over time for patients in any severity category Relative annual risk of exacerbations may be related to FEV_1		
Recommended step for initiating treatment		Step 1	Step 2	Step 3	Step 4 or 5
				And consider short course of oral systemic corticosteroids	
		In 2–6 weeks, evaluate level of asthma control that is achieved and adjust therapy accordingly			

(FEV: forced expiratory volume; FVC: forced vital capacity)

Table 8.4: Assessment of asthma control.

Characteristics	Controlled asthma	Partly controlled asthma	Uncontrolled asthma
Daytime symptoms more than twice/week	No	Any 1 or 2 characteristics present	Any 3 or more characteristics partly controlled asthma
Limitation of activities due to asthma	No		
Nocturnal symptoms/awakening due to asthma	No		
Need for reliever/rescue medicine more than twice/week	No		

- **High-resolution computed tomography (CT):** It may show areas of bronchiectasis (complication) and thickening of the bronchial walls, but these changes are not diagnostic of asthma.

Measurement of Allergic Status
- **Skin prick tests (SPT):** SPT is performed by intradermal injections of common allergens (house dust mite, cat fur, and grass pollen) and checking the development of a wheal and flare reaction. They are positive in allergic asthma and negative in intrinsic asthma.
- **Elevated serum IgE levels:** Measurement of total and allergen-specific IgE in serum may be seen.

Blood and Sputum Tests
Patients with asthma may show increased numbers of eosinophils (eosinophilia) in peripheral blood (>0.4 × 10^9/L) but sputum eosinophil is a more specific diagnostic finding. Sputum examination may reveal Curschmann spirals, Creola bodies, and Charcot–Leyden crystals. *Serum periostin* is also a marker of T_H2-associated airway inflammation and a better predictor of airway eosinophilia than blood eosinophil counts or fraction of exhaled nitric oxide (FeNO).

Fraction of Exhaled Nitric Oxide (FeNO)
It is used as a noninvasive test to measure airway inflammation and as an index of efficacy of corticosteroid response in children (demonstration of insufficient response to anti-inflammatory therapy).

Trial of Corticosteroids
Patients with severe airflow limitation should be given a formal trial of corticosteroids. Prednisolone 30 mg orally/day is given for 2 weeks with lung function measured before and immediately after the course. A substantial improvement in FEV (>15%) confirms the presence of a reversible airflow obstruction and indicates that the administration of inhaled steroids will be beneficial to the patient.

Arterial Blood Gas Analysis
- Hypoxia and hypocarbia during acute attack
- Hypercarbia during severe acute asthma

Table 8.5: Differences between bronchial asthma and cardiac asthma.

Features	Bronchial asthma	Cardiac asthma
Pathology	Bronchospasm	Pulmonary edema
Age	Young	Elderly (above 50–60 years)
Sex/gender	Both genders	Mostly male
Past history	Of eczema, urticaria (allergy) susceptibility to cold, allergy to pollen, groundnuts, and eggs	No history of allergy, history of left ventricular failure, and right ventricular failure
Family history	Other family members may have similar disease	Hypertension may run in families
Personal history	Highly sensitive individual	Nil
Onset	Acute, usually in early hours of morning or late hours of night	Acute usually at midnight (very specific) 2–3 hours after sleep
Symptoms		
Dyspnea	Expiratory dyspnea	Both expiratory and inspiratory dyspnea
Expectoration	Scanty and mucoid sputum	Profuse and frothy sputum
Palpitation	Absent	Present
On examination		
Respiratory	Expiratory wheeze present	Basal crepitations and sweating present
Cyanosis	Present during acute severe asthma	Cyanosis present
Pulse rate	May be high	Very high (may be pulsus alternans)
Blood pressure	Normal or slightly more systolic	BP usually high
Heart sounds	Heart sounds are distant	S3, Gallop rhythm may be present

Management

Management is discussed under following headings.

Avoid Identified Aggravating Factors/Allergens

- This is important in the management of occupational asthma and atopic asthma.
- Avoid causative allergens, such as pets, moulds, and certain foodstuffs particularly in childhood.
- If it is due to single allergen, it is easy to reduce or avoid the exposure. However, when multiple allergens are responsible, avoidance is difficult.

Control of Risk Factors Causing Exacerbation

The rapid identification and removal of extrinsic causes of asthma and risk factors that exacerbate asthma should be done.

- Active and passive smoking should be avoided.
- Control, if there is associated rhinitis and gastroesophageal reflux disease (GERD).
- Control obesity
- Individuals intolerant to aspirin should avoid nonsteroidal anti-inflammatory drugs (NSAIDs)
- Avoid inadequate use of inhaled corticosteroids
- Avoid overuse of inhaled short acting β-agonists (e.g., more than one canister of 200 doses/month)
- Follow proper inhalation techniques

Drug Therapy (Table 8.6)

Drug therapy is used to control or suppress clinical manifestations.

Table 8.6: Drugs useful in asthma.

Relievers	Controllers
• Short-acting inhaled beta2-agonist bronchodilators (SABA) • Low-dose ICS-formoterol • Short-acting anticholinergics	• Inhaled corticosteroids (ICS) • ICS and long-acting beta-2 agonist (LABA), bronchodilator combinations (ICS-LABA) • Leukotriene modifiers • Chromones
Add-on controller medications	

• **Long-acting anticholinergic** (at Step 4 or 5 with a history of exacerbations despite ICS ± LABA)
   ▪ Tiotropium
• **Anti-IgE** (with severe allergic asthma uncontrolled on high dose ICS-LABA)
   ▪ Omalizumab
• **Anti-IL5 and anti-IL5R** (severe eosinophilic asthma uncontrolled on high-dose ICS-LABA)
   ▪ Mepolizumab and reslizumab
   ▪ Benralizumab
• **Anti-IL4R** (severe eosinophilic asthma uncontrolled on high-dose ICS-LABA, or requiring maintenance OCS)
   ▪ Dupilumab
• **Systemic corticosteroids:**
   ▪ Prednisolone
   ▪ Hydrocortisone
   ▪ Methylprednisolone	

The drugs useful in asthma can be divided into bronchodilators (rapidly relieve of symptoms through relaxation of airway smooth muscle), and controllers (inhibit the underlying inflammatory process).

Miscellaneous

❏ **Proton pump inhibitor (PPI)** may be used in patients with symptomatic gastroesophageal reflux disease and suboptimally controlled asthma.
❏ **Desensitization or immunotherapy:** Desensitization is performed by repeated subcutaneous injections of gradually increasing doses of the extracts of allergen(s). However, its benefit is doubtful. GINA, 2017 recommends adding *sublingual immunotherapy (SLIT)* in adult house dust mite (HDM)—sensitive patients with allergic rhinitis who have exacerbations despite ICS treatment, provided FEV_1 is 70% predicted.
❏ **Bronchial thermoplasty:** It is an invasive procedure for severe asthma. In this therapy, controlled thermal energy is delivered to the airway wall during a series of bronchoscopies. It results in a prolonged reduction in airway smooth muscle mass. But, patient still needs to use their asthma-maintenance medications after the procedure.

Stepwise Management of Chronic Asthma

Stepwise management of chronic asthma is discussed in **Table 8.7 and Figure 8.3.**

Step-down Therapy

Once asthma is controlled, the dose of inhaled (or oral) corticosteroid should be reduced to the lowest dose at which effective control of asthma is maintained **(Table 8.8)**.

Treatment of Severe Acute Asthma (Status Asthmaticus) (Flowchart 8.1)

Acute severe asthma is the term used for an exacerbation of asthma that has not been controlled by the use of standard medication.

Treatment at Home

❏ **Give high concentrations of oxygen (40–60%)** through a mask, if available.
❏ **Bronchodilator therapy:** Any one of the following should be given—
  • Nebulized *salbutamol* 5 mg or *terbutaline* 10 mg every 20 minutes for three doses.
  • Salbutamol/terbutaline through metered-dose inhalers (four to eight puffs with a spacer every 20 minutes for 3 doses), followed by 4–8 puffs every 2–4 hours.
❏ **Corticosteroids:**
  • Give IV hydrocortisone sodium succinate 200 mg
  • Give oral prednisolone 60 mg
❏ **Admit to hospital, if there is no response** within 1 hour or if patient becomes drowsy.

Management in Hospital

Initial assessment: Take brief history, perform rapid examination of the patient, and assess the severity **(Table 8.9)**. Administer high concentration of oxygen (40–60%).

Treatment of Mild-to-Moderate Exacerbation

❏ $β_2$-agonists (via inhaler or nebulizer) every 20 minutes for 3 doses (as mentioned above)
❏ Oral corticosteroids, if there is no immediate response.
❏ Patient is reassessed every hour.

Treatment of Severe Exacerbation

❏ **Give high concentration of oxygen (40–60%)**
❏ **Bronchodilators:**
  • Administer *nebulized (in oxygen) salbutamol* (5 mg) or terbutaline (10 mg) or levosalbutamol (1.25–2.5 mg) immediately and may be repeated after a few minutes, if there is no response.

Table 8.7: Stepwise management of chronic asthma.

Step	Management
Step 1 (only for intermittent/less frequent symptoms)	Short-acting inhaled $β_2$-agonist as required (required in all steps)
Step 2: Daily symptoms	**Regular inhaled preventer therapy:** • Low-dose inhaled corticosteroids up to 800 µg daily • Leukotriene receptor antagonists (LTRA), (if patient develops side effects to inhaled corticosteroids), SLIT (sublingual immunotherapy)
Step 3: Severe symptoms	**Inhaled corticosteroids and long-acting inhaled $β_2$-agonist:** • Continue low-dose inhaled corticosteroids plus long-acting $β_2$-agonist • Medium- or high-dose inhaled corticosteroids • Low-dose inhaled corticosteroids plus leukotriene receptor antagonists (LTRA) • Low-dose inhaled corticosteroids plus sustained-release oral theophylline
Step 4: Severe symptoms uncontrolled with high-dose inhaled corticosteroids	**High-dose inhaled corticosteroid and regular bronchodilators:** • Medium- or high-dose inhaled corticosteroids (up to 2,000 µg daily) plus long-acting $β_2$-agonist • May add leukotriene receptor antagonists (LTRA) • May add sustained-release theophylline
Step 5: Severe symptoms deteriorating	**Regular oral corticosteroids:** • Add oral corticosteroids (prednisolone 40 mg daily) • Consider anti-IgE treatment (omalizumab) • Anti-IL5: Reslizumab (IV) added to mepolizumab (SC) for ≥18 years
Step 6: Severe symptoms deteriorating in spite of prednisolone	Hospital admission

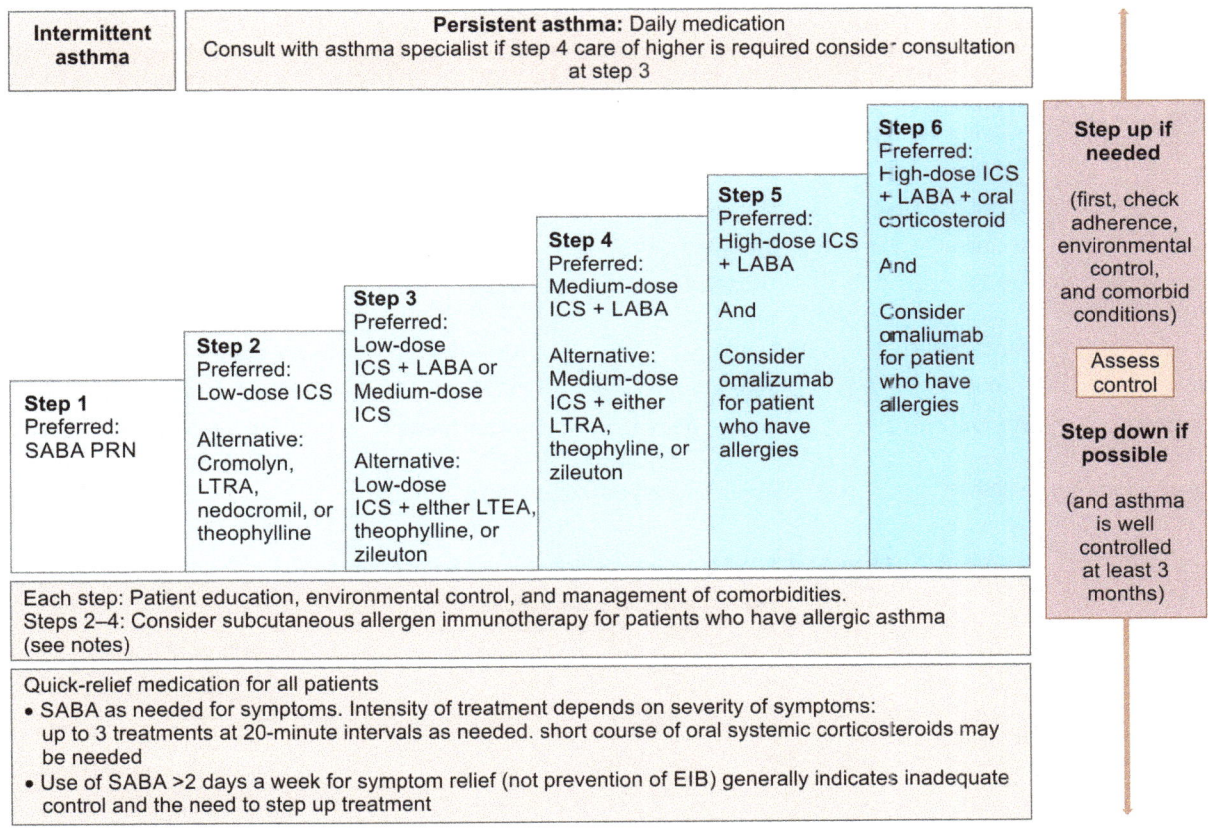

Fig. 8.3: Stepwise management of asthma in adults.
(LABA: long-acting inhaled β$_2$-agonist; LTRA: leukotriene receptor antagonists; SR: sustained-release; SABA: short-acting β$_2$-agonist; EIB: exercise induced bronchoconstriction)

Table 8.8: New phenotype/endotype-based therapy to treat severe asthma.

Asthma phenotype	Characterized by difficult-to-treat asthma plus	Targeted treatment
Allergic asthma (IgE)	Total serum IgE = 30–700 IU/mL and demonstrated IgE-mediated hypersensitivity to a perennial allergen	Add anti-IgE biologic • Omalizumab
Eosinophilic	Blood eosinophils >300 cells/μL and 2 or more exacerbations requiring OCS in past year or ≥150 cells/μL and 3 or more exacerbations requiring OCS in past year	Add anti-IL-5 biologic • Mepolizumab • Reslizumab • Benralizumab Add anti-IL-4/IL-13 biologic • Dupilumab
Neutrophilic	Sputum neutrophils in patients who do not respond to high-dose corticosteroids and do not have other type 2 markers	Consider adding a macrolide antibiotic
Airway smooth muscle (ASM) hypertrophy	Patient who does not qualify for other targeted therapies and/or has tried and failed targeted therapies for which he/she might be eligible and obstruction by bronchodilator reversibility	Consider bronchial thermoplasty, an outpatient medical procedure, in addition to regular treatment

(IL: interleukin)

- *β$_2$-agonists (subcutaneously or intravenously)* are indicated in patients with excessive cough, too weak to inspire adequately or moribund.
- *Terbutaline* is administered subcutaneously (0.25–0.5 mg) or intravenously (0.1–10 μg/kg/min).
- *Epinephrine (adrenaline)* may be administered in children and young adults. Adult dose is 0.2–0.5 mg as 1:1,000 solution subcutaneously every 20 minutes.
- *Add nebulized ipratropium bromide* 0.5 mg to nebulized salbutamol 5 mg/terbutaline 10 mg to those patients who do not respond within 15–30 minutes. It can be repeated every 20 minutes for three doses.
- *Aminophylline* can be given intravenously to those patients who do not respond to nebulized bronchodilators. Give a loading dose of 5 mg/kg/hr as an infusion.
- **Corticosteroids:** In severely ill patients, *hydrocortisone sodium succinate 100 mg* is administered intravenously at presentation and then repeated 4–6 hourly for 24 hours.
- **Antibiotics** are indicated only, if there is respiratory infection.
- Role of magnesium sulfate either intravenously or by nebulization is not clear.

Table 8.9: Assessment of severity of asthma.

	Mild	Moderate	Severe	Respiratory arrest imminent
Breathless	• Walking • Lying down possible	• Talking • Sitting preferred	• At rest • Hunched forward	
Talking in	Sentences	Phrases	Words	
Alertness	Possibly agitated	Usually agitated	Usually agitated	Drowsy or confused
Respiratory rate	Increased	Increased	Often >30/min	
Accessory muscles/suprasternal retractions	Usually not	Usually	Usually	Paradoxical thoracoabdominal movement
Wheeze	Moderate	Loud	Usually loud	Absent
Pulse/min	<100	100–120	>120	Bradycardia
Pulsus paradoxus	Absent	May be present	Often present	Possibly absent due to muscle fatigue
PEF after bronchodilator	>80%	Approximately 60–80%	<60%	

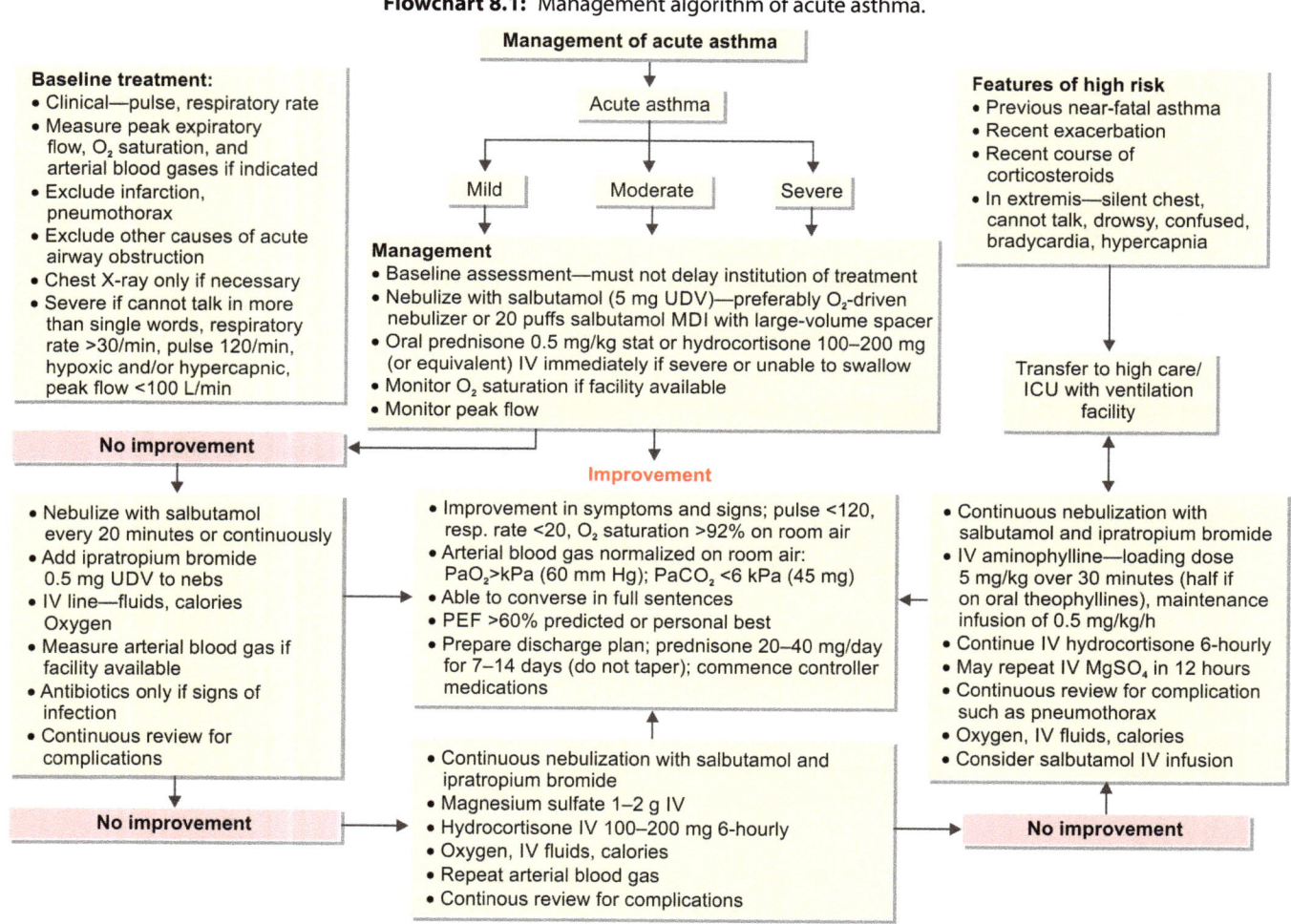

Flowchart 8.1: Management algorithm of acute asthma.

(UDV: unit dose vial; PaO_2: partial pressure of oxygen; PEF: peak expiratory flow)

- **If no improvement** with above measures, perform *endotracheal intubation* and *mechanical ventilation.*
  - *Indications for intubation:* Cardiac or respiratory arrest, severe hypoxia (PaO_2 <60 mm Hg), hypercapnia ($PaCO_2$ >50 mm Hg), acidosis (pH <7.3), exhaustion, or deterioration in mental status.
- **Noninvasive ventilation (NIV)** using continuous positive pressure of BiPAP (bi-level positive airway pressure) machines and tight fitting face mask reduces the work of breathing without intubation. It is useful in assisting breathing. It is used in a cooperative and alert patient who has impending respiratory failure but does not require immediate intubation.

- Treatment with 70–80% helium with oxygen may be useful, since it reduces airway resistance and improves efficacy of bronchodilators.
- Assessment of response to treatment is done by noting the patient distress, respiratory rate, FEV_1, heart rate, presence of pulsus paradoxus, and serial arterial blood gas (ABG) studies.
- More severe cases should remain in hospital for 2–5 days with regular monitoring of oxygen saturation and peak flow rates. Bronchial thermoplasty may be beneficial for moderate-to-severe persistent asthma. This reduces the mass of airway smooth muscle, reducing bronchoconstriction.

Occupational Asthma

Triggering occupational agents include—fumes (epoxy resins and plastics), organic and chemical dusts (wood, cotton, and platinum), gases (toluene diisocyanate), animal allergens, plants and plant products (flours and cereals) and other chemicals (formaldehyde and penicillin products). *Work-exacerbated asthma* is defined as pre-existing or concurrent asthma that subjectively worsens in the workplace.

Management

- Primary prevention (e.g., avoiding sensitizer agent)
- Secondary prevention (e.g., medical surveillance program)
- Tertiary prevention (e.g., appropriate treatment), i.e., treatment as per asthma severity

Drug-induced Asthma

Drugs Implicated

- Most commonly due to *aspirin [aspirin-induced asthma, (AIA)] followed by ibuprofen, indomethacin, naproxen, phenylbutazone,* and *mefenamic acid*. About 10% of asthma patients are aspirin sensitive.
- *Drugs that can cause bronchospasm*: Adenosine, prostaglandin analogs, BBs (beta-blockers), cholinergic drugs, streptomycin, pentazocine, and penicillin.
- *Nonpharmaceutical agents*: Tartrazine (coloring agent) and sulfating agents (preservatives in food/medicines).

CHRONIC OBSTRUCTIVE PULMONARY DISEASE

Introduction

Chronic obstructive pulmonary disease (COPD) is also known as chronic obstructive lung disease (COLD), chronic obstructive airway disease (COAD), chronic airflow limitation (CAL), and chronic obstructive respiratory disease (CORD).

Definition

- COPD is a *preventable and treatable pulmonary disease* associated *with* some *significant extrapulmonary effects* that may contribute to the severity in individual patients.
- Pulmonary disease is characterized by *airflow limitation*, which is *not fully reversible*.
- The airflow limitation is usually progressive and associated with an abnormal inflammatory response of the lung to various noxious particles or gases.

Conditions Included under COPD

Disease is considered COPD, only if chronic airflow obstruction occurs.
- **Emphysema:** An anatomically defined condition characterized by abnormal and permanent enlargement of the airspaces distal to the terminal bronchioles. It is accompanied by destruction of the airspace walls, without obvious fibrosis (i.e., there is no fibrosis visible to the naked eye).
- **Chronic bronchitis:** It is defined as a chronic productive cough for 3 months in each of two successive years in a patient in whom other causes of chronic cough (e.g., bronchiectasis) have been excluded.
- **Small airways disease:** A condition in which small bronchioles are narrowed.

Pathogenesis

- *Major physiologic change* in the COPD is *airflow limitation*. It can develop due to both small airway obstruction and emphysema. The small airways may become narrowed by cells (hyperplasia and accumulation), mucus, and fibrosis.
- Activation of transforming growth factor-β (TGF-β) contributes to airway fibrosis, whereas absence of TGF-β may produce parenchymal inflammation and emphysema. The mechanism involved in emphysema is better understood than small airway obstruction.

Chronic Bronchitis

Various risk factors for COPD are described in **Box 8.2**.

Incidence

- **Age and gender:** Occurs during *middle and late adult life*. It is more common in *males than in females*.
- More common *in smokers than in nonsmokers*. Also more often develops in urban than in rural dwellers.

Types of Chronic Bronchitis

- Simple chronic bronchitis
- Chronic mucopurulent bronchitis
- Chronic asthmatic bronchitis
- Chronic obstructive bronchitis

Box 8.2: Risk factors for chronic obstructive pulmonary disease (COPD).

Environmental:
- Tobacco smoke
- Indoor air pollution. Cooking with biomass fuels
- *Toxic industrial inhalants*: Occupational dust exposure (e.g., coal dust, silica, and cadmium)
- *Respiratory infections*: Recurrent infection; HIV infection (associated with emphysema), previous tuberculosis
- Low birth weight and bronchopulmonary dysplasia
- *Lung growth*: Childhood infections or maternal smoking may affect growth of lung during childhood
- Low socioeconomic status, antioxidant deficiency
- Cannabis smoking

Host factors:
- *Genetic factors*: α1-antiproteinase deficiency TGF-beta1 polymorphism, *Serpine2* gene expression
- Airway hyper-reactivity

Etiology

Smoking and COPD:

- **Cigarette smoking:** It is the most important risk factor for the development of COPD. The risk of developing COPD relates to both the amount and the duration of smoking. However, only about 15–20% of smokers develop clinically significant COPD. This suggests that genetic predisposition and environmental factors play a role in the pathogenesis.
- **Second-hand smoke:** Environmental tobacco smoke that is inhaled involuntarily or passively by someone who is not smoking.
- **Environmental tobacco smoke** is generated from the *sidestream* (the burning end) of a cigarette, pipe, or cigar or from the exhaled *mainstream* (the smoke puffed out by smokers) of cigarettes, pipes, and cigars.
- **Abnormalities due to smoking:** Cigarette smoking is associated with a variety of abnormalities of the respiratory system that predispose to the development of chronic bronchitis. These include:
  - Sluggishness of movement of cilia
  - Bronchoconstriction due to constriction of smooth muscle
  - Hypertrophy and hyperplasia of mucous-secreting glands. *The ratio of the thickness of the mucous gland layer* to the *thickness of the bronchial wall* between the base of the surface epithelium and the inner limit of the cartilage plates is called *Reid index*. It is useful for detecting the increase in the size and number of the mucous glands. Reid index (normally 0.44 ± 0.094) is increased in chronic bronchitis (>0.51). There is a direct correlation between the value of Reid index and the volume of daily sputum production by the patient.
  - Release of proteolytic enzymes from polymorphonuclear leukocytes and release of inflammatory mediators in lungs.
  - Inhibits the function of alveolar macrophages
  - Adverse effect on surfactant and favors overdistension of the lungs

Pathogenesis (Flowchart 8.2)

Major physiologic change in COPD is airflow limitation. It can result from both small airway obstruction and emphysema.

- Irritants cause inflammation → infiltration by $CD8^+$ T-lymphocytes, macrophages, and neutrophils.
- **Hypersecretion of mucus:**
  - *Hyperplasia/hypertrophy of the submucosal glands in large airways (trachea and bronchi)*: It develops as response to inhaled *environmental irritants* and *proteases released from neutrophils* (e.g., elastase and cathepsin). This leads to *hypersecretion of mucus*.
  - *Marked increase of goblet cells in small airways (small bronchi and bronchioles)*: They produce excessive mucus → Mucus plugging of bronchial lumen → inflammation and fibrosis of bronchial wall → *leads to airway obstruction*

Clinical Features

History: Most common three symptoms in COPD are impressive history of cough, sputum production, and exertional dyspnea (breathlessness).

- **Cough:** Initially, the cough is present only in the winter seasons (often referred as "winter cough" or "smoker's cough"), especially in the mornings ("morning cough"). Later, cough increases in frequency, severity, and duration.
- **Sputum:** Usually *scanty, mucoid,* and more in the mornings. It may be occasionally blood-stained (hemoptysis) or frankly purulent ("mucopurulent relapse").
- **Breathlessness:** It is *relatively insidious in onset* and is due to airflow obstruction. It is aggravated by infection, excessive smoking, and adverse atmospheric conditions. Breathlessness severity can be assessed by the modified MRC dyspnea scale.

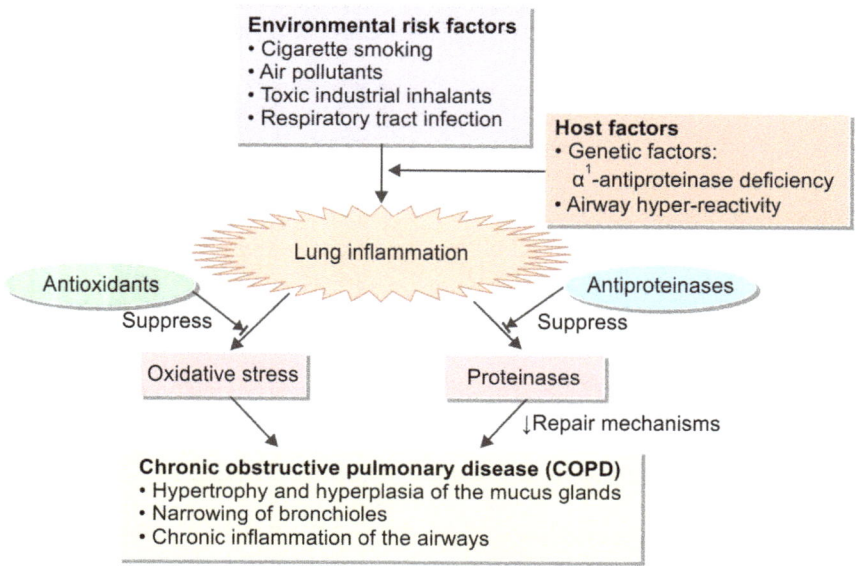

Flowchart 8.2: Pathogenesis of chronic obstructive pulmonary disease.

Other symptoms: Fever during mucopurulent relapses, wheezing, and tightness in the chest.

Physical signs:
- Patient is usually overweight.
- In the early stages, patients are entirely normal on physical examination. At rest, there is no respiratory distress, respiratory rate is normal and accessory muscles of respiration are not acting.
- **Auscultation:** (1) Vesicular breath sounds with prolonged expiration; (2) inspiratory and expiratory rhonchi; and (3) crepitations that either disappear or change in location and intensity after coughing; (4) forced expiratory time >4 seconds.

Associated comorbidities in COPD **(Box 8.3)**: Although COPD affects the lungs, it is associated with comorbidities probably a part of a generalized systemic inflammatory process.

Investigations
- **Radiological examination:**
  - *Chest X-ray:* May assist in the classification of the type of COPD. There is no reliable radiographic signs that indicate the severity of airflow limitation.
    - *Features of emphysema:* Presence of bullae, paucity of parenchymal markings, or hyperlucency
    - *Features of hyperinflation:* Increased lung volumes and flattening of the diaphragm
    - *Chronic bronchitis:* No characteristic abnormality
    - Essential *to identify complications,* such as cardiac failure, other complications of smoking (e.g., lung cancer)
  - *High-resolution CT scan (HRCT):* It is useful in detection, characterization, and quantification of emphysema.
- **Pulmonary function tests:**
  - Reduced FEV_1, FEV_1/FVC (less increased RV, FRC, and TLC than 0.7), FVC, and PEF
  - *Gas transfer* may be normal or mildly reduced
- **Arterial blood gases (ABG) study:** To demonstrate resting or exertional hypoxemia. It is important in the evaluation of patients with exacerbation.
- **Measurement of lung volumes:** It assesses hyperinflation and is usually performed by using the helium dilution technique.

Box 8.3: Common comorbidities in chronic obstructive pulmonary disease (COPD).

Cardiovascular disorders:
- Pulmonary hypertension
- Right heart failure and cor pulmonale
- *Vascular disease:* Coronary artery disease, cerebrovascular disease, and peripheral vascular disease
- Systemic hypertension

Nutritional disorders: Cachexia
Musculoskeletal disorders:
- Muscle dysfunction
- Osteoporosis

Cancer: Lung cancer
Other: Sleep disorders, sexual dysfunction, diabetes, depression, anxiety, anemia, osteoporosis, peptic ulcer, and glaucoma

---

- **Exercise testing:** 6-minute walk test is used to assess exercise tolerance, response to bronchodilator therapy, disability, and effectiveness of pulmonary rehabilitation.
- **Blood:**
  - *Hemoglobin* level and *PCV* may be elevated due to persistent hypoxemia (secondary polycythemia). In patients with normal kidney function, an elevated serum bicarbonate may indirectly identify chronic hypercapnia.
  - α_1-*antiproteinase*: It should be assayed in younger patients with predominantly basal emphysema.
- **Electrocardiography:** It is often normal. In advanced cases, it may show features of right atrial and ventricular hypertrophy (tall P waves-P-Pulmonary; right bundle branch block; RSR pattern in V_1).

BODE (body mass index, airflow obstruction, dyspnea, and exercise capacity) index:
- A multidimensional prognostic index. Takes into account several indicators of COPD prognosis *[body mass index (BMI), obstructive ventilatory defect severity, dyspnea severity, and exercise capacity].*
- The components are derived from measures of the body mass index (weight in kg/height m²), FEV_1 percent predicted, the modified Medical Research Council dyspnea and 6-minute walk test.
- A BODE score greater than 7 is associated with a 30% 2-year mortality
- A score of 5–6 is associated with 15% 2-year mortality
- If score is less than 5, the 2-year mortality is less than 10%

Complications of COPD
- **Mucopurulent relapses:** It may develop due to secondary bacterial infection by *Streptococcus pneumoniae, Haemophilus influenzae,* or *Moraxella catarrhalis.* It presents with fever and increased production of purulent sputum.
- **Carbon dioxide narcosis:** Persistent retention of CO_2 (hypercarbia: high $PaCO_2$) manifests as clouding of consciousness, altered behavior, drowsiness, headache, and papilledema.
- **Respiratory failure:**
  - *Type 1 respiratory failure (low PaO_2 normal $PaCO_2$):* In mild-to-moderate COPD.
  - *Type II respiratory failure*: Acute or chronic in severe COPD.
- **Secondary polycythemia:** Due to hypoxemia, which stimulates erythropoiesis
- Pulmonary hypertension and right ventricular failure (cor pulmonale)
- Pneumonia
- Tuberculosis
- Lung cancer
- Pneumothorax (emphysema)
- Deep vein thrombosis
- Pulmonary embolism

Management
General measures:
- Regular exercises and management of nutritional status.
- Weight loss, if the patient is obese.

- *Reduce exposure to noxious particles and gases that cause bronchial irritation*
- **Smoking cessation:** Complete smoking cessation and this may be aided by bupropion (a noradrenergic antidepressant) nicotine replacement therapy (by gum, transdermal patch lozenge inhaler or nasal spray) or varenicline [partial agonist of the nicotinic acetylcholine receptor (nAChR) subtype α4β2].
- **Reduce smoke:** Reducing the risk from indoor and outdoor air pollution. Reduce exposure to smoke from biomass fuel, particularly among women and children.
- **Avoid:** Dusty and smoke-laden atmospheres.

Drug therapy (Table 8.10)

It is used both for short-term management of exacerbations and for long-term relief of symptoms. However, none of the medications for COPD reduce the rate of decline of lung functions.

- **Bronchodilators:** They are central to the management of breathlessness.
  - β_2-*adrenergic agonists*: The inhaled route is preferred.
    - *Mild disease:* Short-acting agents namely salbutamol 200 μg or terbutaline 500 μg 6 hourly.
    - *Moderate-to-severe disease:* Long-acting agents, such as salmeterol 50 μg twice daily or formoterol (12 μg powder inhaled twice daily) or indacaterol (150–300 μg daily) achieve bronchodilation and also reduce the incidence of infective exacerbations. LABAs include salmeterol, formoterol, arformoterol, indacaterol, vilanterol, and olodaterol; all are β-2 selective.
  - *Antimuscarinic (anticholinergic) drugs:* More prolonged and greater bronchodilatation is achieved by adding ipratropium bromide (40–80 μg 6 hourly) or tiotropium bromide (18 μg once a day) or oxitropium (200 μg twice daily) in severe disease.
  - Oral long-acting theophylline or doxophylline may be beneficial in selected cases. Umeclidinium, aclidinium, and glycopyrronium are newer long-acting anticholinergic drugs available.
- **Phosphodiesterase type-4 inhibitors:** Roflumilast is an inhibitor with anti-inflammatory properties. It may be used as an adjunct to bronchodilators. Weight loss is a significant side effect.
- **Corticosteroids:**
  - Inhaled corticosteroids (ICS) reduce the frequency and severity of exacerbations, and are used in moderately severe COPD. These include beclomethasone, budesonide, fluticasone, ciclesonide, flunisolide, and beclametasone.
  - Oral corticosteroids are useful during exacerbations and should be avoided as a maintenance therapy, because it may lead to osteoporosis and impaired skeletal muscle function.

Respiratory infections:

- **Treatment of infection:** Bacterial infection precipitates exacerbations. Azithromycin (has both anti-inflammatory and antimicrobial properties) administered daily to subjects with a history of exacerbation in the past 6 months may reduce the exacerbation. If patient develops purulent (yellow or green) sputum, oral tetracycline or ampicillin 250 mg 6 hourly or cotrimoxazole 960 mg 12 hourly for 10 days should be given. If there is no response, sputum culture and sensitivity are done and the antibiotic is changed accordingly.
- **Prevention of infection:** Patients with COPD should receive *vaccination with polyvalent pneumococcal and influenza vaccines.*

Symptomatic measures:

- **Antimucolytic agents:** They reduce viscosity of sputum and can reduce the number of acute exacerbations and total number of days of disability. Mucolytic agents include bromhexine, N-acetylcysteine carbocysteine, ambroxol, and erdosteine can be tried.
- **Antitussives:** Regular use of antitussives to control cough in stable COPD is not recommended.
- **Chest physiotherapy**

Pulmonary rehabilitation:

- It is an individually designed treatment program consisting of education and cardiovascular conditioning (reverse muscular and cardiovascular dysfunction).
- Program includes breathing technique, chest physiotherapy, postural drainage, activities of daily living (work simplification and energy conservation) and exercise conditioning (upper and lower extremity).

Oxygen therapy:

Long-term domiciliary oxygen therapy (LTOT):

- *Aim of therapy*: To increase the PaO_2 to at least 8 kPa (60 mm Hg) or SaO_2 to at least 90%. It is administered through nasal cannulae for at least 15 hours per day at a low-dose (2 L/minute)
- *Indications*: In COPD patient with exertional hypoxemia or nocturnal hypoxemia
- Daytime $PaO_2 \leq 55$ mm Hg at rest or oxygen saturation $\leq 88\%$ with or without hypercapnia during a period of clinical stability OR
- Daytime PaO_2 between 56 and 59 mm Hg or oxygen saturation >88% in the presence of secondary polycythemia,

Table 8.10: Drug therapy in chronic bronchitis.

• **β2-agonists:**
  ▪ Short-acting β2-agonists (SABA)
  ▪ – Long-acting β2-agonists (LABA)
	• *Methylxanthines*
	• *Inhaled corticosteroids (ICS)*
	• *Combination long-acting beta2-agonists + corticosteroids in one inhaler*

• Anticholinergics/muscarinic antagonists
  ▪ Short-acting anticholinergics (SAMA)
  ▪ Long-acting anticholinergics (LAMA)
	• *Systemic corticosteroids*
	• *Phosphodiesterase-4 inhibitors*

• *Combination short-acting β2-agonists + anticholinergic in one inhaler*	• **Acebrophylline**: An airway mucoregulator and anti-inflammatory agent

nocturnal hypoxemia, peripheral edema, or evidence of pulmonary hypertension.
- *Benefits*: LTOT has significant benefits and reduces mortality rates in selected patients. It decreases pulmonary hypertension and prolongs life in hypoxemic COPD patients with right heart failure. It also reduces polycythemia, pulmonary artery pressures, dyspnea, and hypoxemia during sleep and reduces nocturnal arrhythmias.

Treatment of pulmonary hypertension is by long-term oxygen therapy, sildenafil, bosentan, and synthetic prostacyclin (epoprostenol). Pharmacologic therapy in COPD depending on severity is presented in **Figure 8.4**.

Surgical treatments:
Lung volume reduction surgery (LVRS) is more efficacious than medical therapy among patients with upper-lobe predominant emphysema and low exercise capacity.

In appropriately selected patients with very severe COPD, *lung transplantation* has been shown to improve quality of life and functional capacity.

Acute Exacerbations of COPD
- **Definition:** "An event in the natural course of COPD characterized by a change in patient's baseline dyspnea, cough, and/or sputum that is beyond normal day-to-day variations. It is acute in onset, and may warrant a change in regular medication in a patient with underlying COPD."
- **Causes of exacerbation:** (1) Infection of the tracheobronchial tree, and (2) air pollution. In about one-third of cases, no cause can be identified.
- **Trigging factors:** Infections by bacteria, viruses, or a change in air quality.

Treatment of Severe Acute Exacerbations
Oxygen
- Adequate oxygenation (i.e., to achieve an oxygen saturation of 88–92%) must be assured.
- *Method of administration*: By nasal catheter or through a facemask equipped to control the inspired oxygen fraction. Venturi masks are preferred because they permit a precise fraction of inspired oxygen (FiO_2).

Exacerbations in the prior year	Symptoms	
	Fewer	More*
Fewer <2 outpatient	**Group A** Bronchodilator [usually a short-acting beta agonist (SABA) or short-acting antimuscarinic antagonist (SAMA)]	**Group B** Long-acting beta agonist (LABA) or Long-acting antimuscarinic antagonist (LAMA)
More ≥2 outpatient or ≥1 hospitalization	**Group C** LAMA ↓ LAMA + LABA	**Group D** LABA + LAMA ↓ LABA + LAMA + inhaled corticosteroid (ICS)

Fig. 8.4: Pharmacotherapy based on severity of chronic obstructive pulmonary disease (COPD).

Bronchodilators:
Nebulized short-acting β2-agonists (salbutamol 2.5 mg every 20 minutes for initial 1–2 hours) and/or anticholinergic agent (ipratropium bromide 0.5 mg) should be given. Intravenous aminophylline may be added, if the patient fails to respond to the above treatment.

Antibiotics:
- **Indications:** Patients with—(1) increase in sputum purulence, sputum volume, or (2) breathlessness (dyspnea), or (3) those requiring mechanical ventilation.
- **Most common organisms during exacerbations:** *S. pneumoniae, H. influenzae,* and *M. catarrhalis*. Risk factors for *P. aeruginosa* infection include recent hospitalization, frequent antibiotics use, and severe exacerbation.
- **Antibiotics used:**
  - *Outpatient*: Doxycycline, cotrimoxazole, or amoxicillin-clavulanate can be given. Patients older than 65 years are treated with newer fluoroquinolones (levofloxacin, gemifloxacin, and moxifloxacin).
  - *Hospitalized patients*: Intravenous antibiotics (azithromycin or fluoroquinolone or a third-generation cephalosporin—like ceftriaxone or cefotaxime).
  - *Severe exacerbations*: Third-generation cephalosporin plus a fluoroquinolone or an aminoglycoside.

Corticosteroids:
Intravenous or oral corticosteroids shorten the recovery time, improve lung functions (FEV_1), and hypoxemia.

Diuretics:
These are given to patients with gross right ventricular failure.

Respiratory stimulants:
These may be used when there is no response to the conventional agents. Doxapram in the dose of 1.5–4 mg/minute as infusion is the most often used agent. Other respiratory stimulants are almitrine, nikethamide, medroxyprogesterone, and acetazolamide.

Mechanical ventilatory support:
- **Noninvasive positive airway pressure ventilation (NIPPV):** NIPPV is by using tight-fitting facemask to deliver BiPAP.
- **Invasive (conventional) ventilation:** It is administered via an endotracheal tube.

Management of Associated Comorbidities
It is necessary to manage comorbidities because they are responsible for mortality and hospitalization.

GOLD staging for severity of COPD and management (Fig. 8.5): It is used for both chronic bronchitis and emphysema.

Emphysema
The word "emphysema" literally means inflation or distension with air.

Definition: Emphysema (pulmonary) is a *chronic lung disease* characterized by abnormal *irreversible* (permanent) *dilatation of the airspaces distal to the terminal bronchiole*. This is associated with destruction of their walls but without obvious fibrosis.

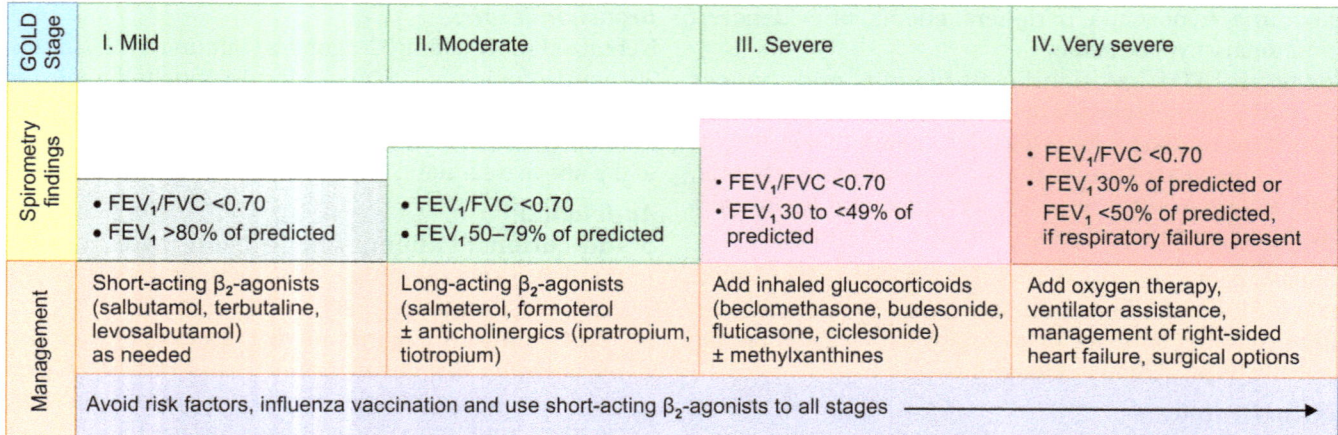

Fig. 8.5: GOLD staging for severity of COPD and management.

Types of Emphysema/Classification (Figs. 8.6A and B)

Emphysema is *classified according to its anatomic distribution* (location of the lesions) within the lobule into *four major types*—(1) centriacinar, (2) panacinar, (3) paraseptal, and (4) irregular.

Etiology and Pathogenesis (Fig. 8.7)

The *major event* in emphysema is *destruction of alveolar wall*.
- **Mechanism that checks the destruction of alveolar wall:** These include—(1) *anti-elastases* (e.g., α_1-antitrypsin) and (2) *antioxidants*. If these two mechanisms are defective, these result in (1) *protease-antiprotease imbalance* (e.g., α_1-antitrypsin deficiency) and (2) *imbalance between oxidants and antioxidants*.

- *Unchecked inflammation and proteolysis*: It develops due to deficiency of the above protective mechanism.
- **Genetic factors:**
  - *Deficiency of α_1-antitrypsin*: It is inherited as *autosomal recessive*, which exhibits polymorphism → tendency to develop emphysema. α_1-antitrypsin *is a major inhibitor of proteases* (particularly elastase). It is normally present in serum, tissue fluids, and macrophages and a balance is maintained between protease and antiproteases. During inflammation, protease (proteolyic enzyme) is secreted by neutrophils and digests the connective tissue of the lung. α_1-antitrypsin is a protease inhibitor (antiprotease), preventing this proteolytic digestion. Hence, a deficiency or absence of α_1-antitrypsin results

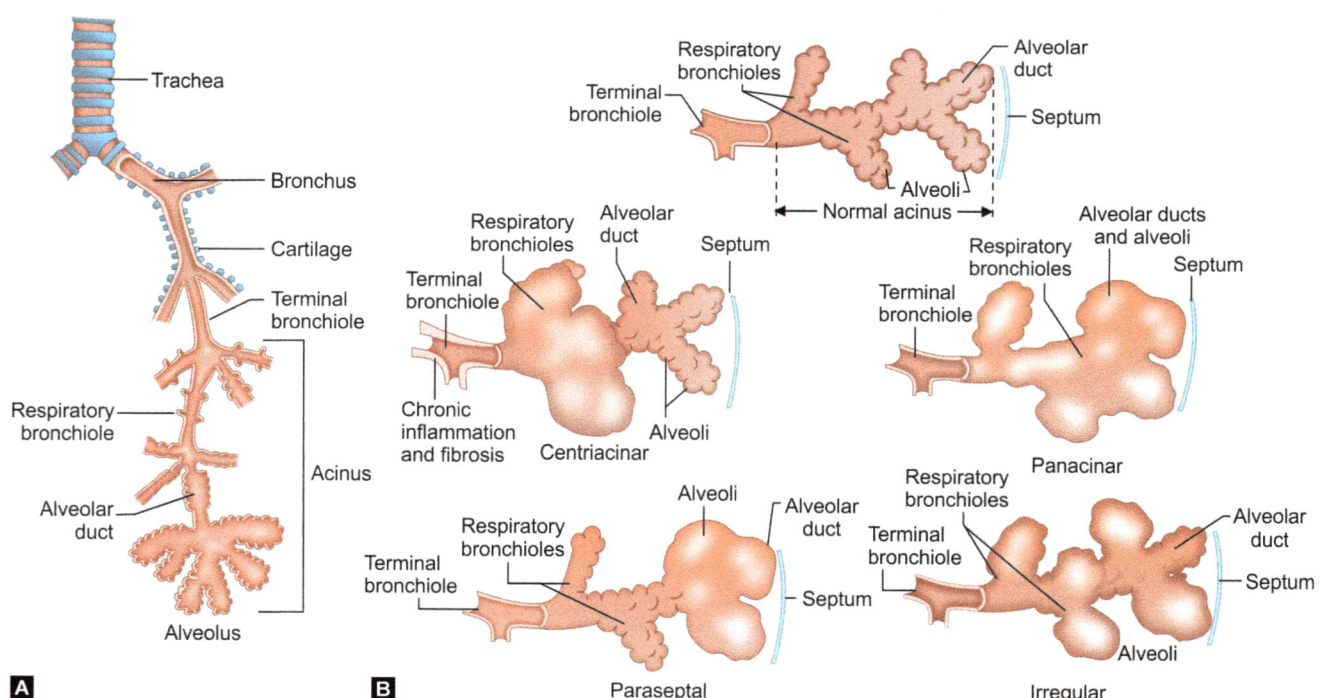

Figs. 8.6A and B: (A) Normal components of respiratory tree; (B) Types of emphysema.

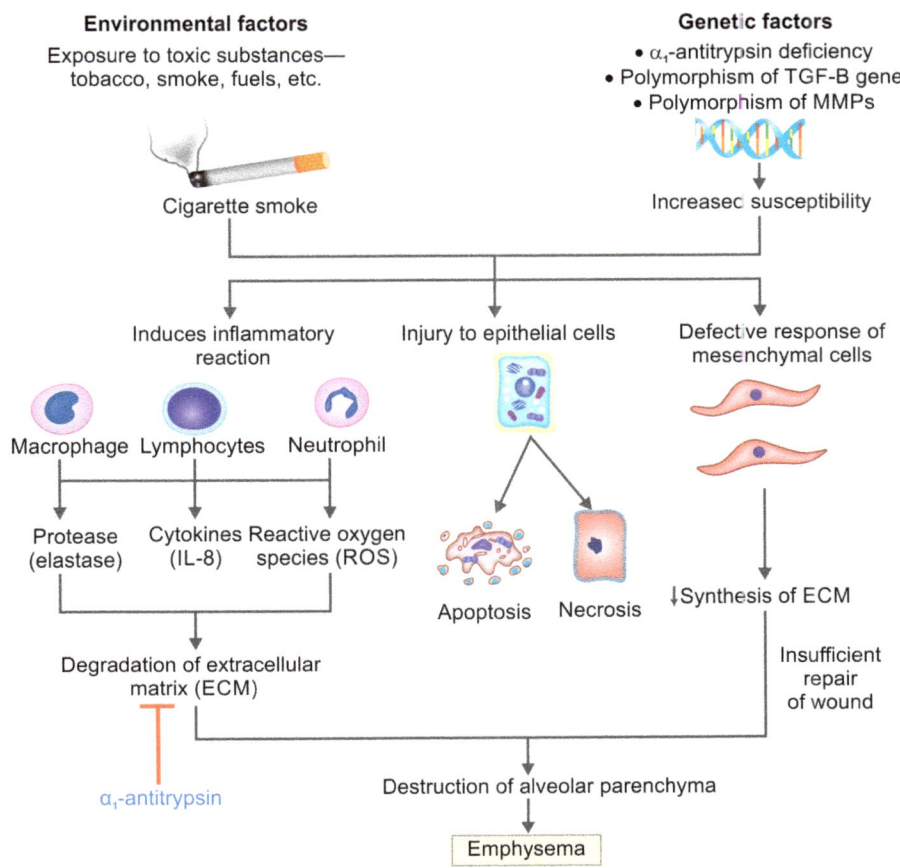

Fig. 8.7: Pathogenesis of emphysema. Exposure to environmental toxins (e.g., cigarette smoke) causes inflammatory reaction, cell death, and proteolysis of extracellular matrix (ECM). α₁-antitrypsin (α₁-AT) deficiency also results in increased degradation of ECM.
(IL-8: interleukin-8; TNF: tumor necrosis factor)

in the proteolyic destruction of lung. These patients develop severe panacinar emphysema.

Clinical Features

Manifestations appear late, until, at least one-third of the functioning pulmonary parenchyma is damaged.
- *Dyspnea* is the most striking feature that begins insidiously and steadily progresses, ultimately ending in breathlessness on trivial exertion and even at rest.
- *Cough and expectoration* of scanty mucoid sputum.
- *Weight loss,* weakness, anorexia, and lethargy are common with advanced disease.

Physical findings:
General: Body build is asthenic, short, and thick neck; neck veins may appear distend during expiration and collapse during inspiration. Patient leans forwards, extending the arms to brace himself during sitting posture.

Respiratory:
- **Inspection:**
  - Patient appears *distressed* and *tachypneic, hypertrophy of accessory muscles of respiration* (sternomastoid and scalene muscles), length of the trachea above the suprasternal notch is reduced, and apical impulse is invisible or feeble.
  - *During inspiration*: *Exaggerated tracheal descent* (Campbell's sign), excavation of the suprasternal and supraclavicular fossae, and *indrawing of the costal margins*.
  - *Expiration*: *Prolonged through pursed lips* (purse-lip breathing) and beginning of expiration with a *grunting sound*.
  - *Chest*: Cylindrical or barrel like (*barrel-shaped chest*), anteroposterior diameter of the chest is markedly increased. Whole chest is in a fixed state of full inspiration. Ribs are placed more horizontally and widely. Chest expansion diminished symmetrically. Thoracic kyphosis is exaggerated and the subcostal angle is widened.
  - *Dahl sign*: Above the knee, patches of hyperpigmentation or bruising caused by constant "tenting" position of hands or elbows.
  - *Hoover's sign*: Briefly, during inspiration a paradoxical medial movement of the chest. The "subcostal angle" is the angle between the xiphoid process and the right or left costal margin. Normally, during inhalation, the chest expands laterally, increasing this angle. When the diaphragms are flattened (as in COPD), inhalation paradoxically causes the angle to decrease.
  - *Harrison's sulcus*: A horizontal grove where the diaphragm attaches to the ribs; associated with chronic asthma, COPD, and rickets.

- **Percussion:** Hyper-resonant percussion note over the lungs, reduced cardiac dullness, and liver dullness is pushed down or absent. Tidal percussion is negative.
- **Auscultation:** Diminished intensity of the breath sound, breath sounds are vesicular with prolonged expiration. Scattered, faint, high-pitched, and end-expiratory rhonchi may be audible.

Investigations
- **Chest X-ray (Fig. 8.8):**
  - *Posteroanterior (PA) view:* Features include low set, flat diaphragm, translucent lung field, long and narrow heart ("tubular heart"), loss of peripheral vascular markings, and prominent pulmonary artery shadows at the hilum and bullae.
  - *Lateral view:* Large retrosternal translucency.

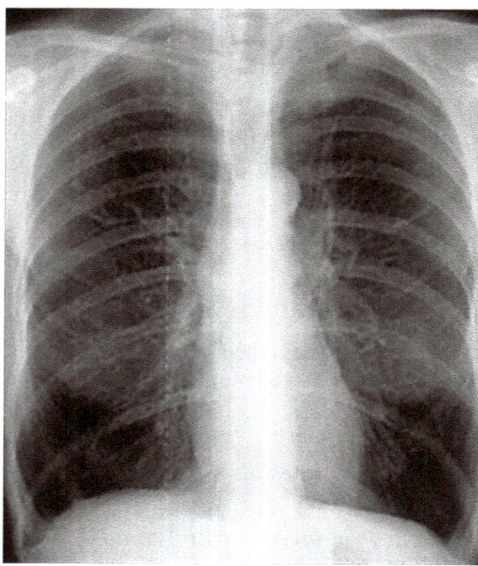

Fig. 8.8: Chest X-ray of emphysema. Posteroanterior (PA) view showing low set, flat diaphragm, translucent lung field, long and narrow heart ("tubular heart"), loss of peripheral vascular markings, prominent pulmonary artery shadows at the hilum.

- **Computed tomography:** It can identify emphysema with certainty.
- **Pulmonary function tests:**

Reduced: FEV_1, FVC, FEV_1:FVC ratio, and PEF	Increased: TLC, RV, and RV:TLC

GAS transfer factor for carbon monoxide (diffusion) is reduced.

Arterial blood gas studies: Slightly reduced PaO_2 and normal or mildly elevated $PaCO_2$.

Complications
Emphysema progresses steadily and gradually.
- **Pulmonary bullae:**
  - *Complications:* A subpleural bulla may rupture producing spontaneous pneumothorax. Large bullae can interfere with pulmonary ventilation.
- **Respiratory failure:** Type 1 and type II respiratory failure can occur.
- **Pulmonary hypertension and right heart failure (cor pulmonale):** These are late complications and right ventricular failure in emphysema is usually a terminal event.
- **Severe weight loss:** Leading to emaciation

> **Treatment:** Treatment similar as described for COPD
> - No specific treatment for established case of emphysema. Bronchodilators and steroids may be helpful in few patients.
> - **Prevention of progression:** Cessation of smoking and avoidance of occupational exposure.
> - **Treatment of aggravating factors and complications:** Treatment of infections, respiratory failure, and right heart failure.
> - **Physiotherapy**
> - **Surgical therapy:** *Ablation of giant bullae,* lung volume reduction surgery reduced hyperinflation of one or both lungs and/or laser resection.
> - **Heart and lung transplantation:** In young patients with severe emphysema due to α1-antitrypsin deficiency.

Blue Bloaters (Fig. 8.9A)
It is a distinctive clinical pattern seen in chronic bronchitis, the characteristics of which are:

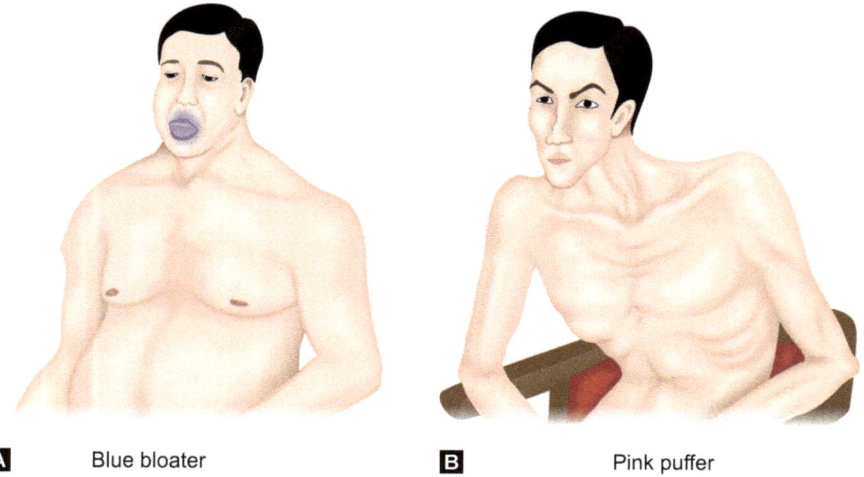

Figs. 8.9A and B: (A) Blue bloater (in chronic bronchitis) versus; (B) Pink puffer (in emphysema).

- Marked/heavy cyanosis ("blue") and peripheral edema ("bloated") and secondary polycythemia.
- Current evidence demonstrates that most patients have elements of both bronchitis and emphysema and by physical examination cannot reliably differentiate "blue bloaters" from "pink puffers".

Pink Puffers (Fig. 8.9B)

- It is a distinctive clinical pattern seen in emphysema of lung.
- Patients are thin and noncyanotic at rest (hence "pink").
- They have marked dyspnea ("puffer") and have prominent use of accessory muscle. They develop steadily progressive dyspnea.

Differences between Emphysema and Chronic Bronchitis

Table 8.11 describes the differences between emphysema and chronic bronchitis.

Differentiating Features of Asthma and Chronic Obstructive Pulmonary Disease

Table 8.12 describes the differentiating features of asthma and chronic obstructive pulmonary disease.

Cigarette Smoking

Cigarette smoke is a complex aerosol-containing gaseous and particulate compound.

Components of Cigarette Smoke

It consists of mainstream smoke and sidestream smoke.
- **Mainstream smoke:** It is produced by inhalation of air through cigarette. It is the primary source of smoke exposure in smokers.
- **Sidestream smoke:** It is produced from emitting of smoke between cigarette puffs and is the main source of environmental smoke or second-hand smoke.

Chemical Constituents of Cigarette Smoke

It contains about 2,000–4,000 chemical substances and more than 60 carcinogens. About 95% of the weight of the mainstream smoke is derived from 400 gaseous compounds and about 5% of the weight is made up of about 3,500 particulate components.

Tobacco addiction is due to nicotine present in cigarette smoke and is the total particulate matter responsible for carcinogenesis.
- **Carcinogens:** Tar, polycyclic aromatic hydrocarbons, benzo[a]pyrene, and nitrosamine
- **Others:**
  - Nicotine causes ganglionic stimulation and depression; tumor promotion
  - Phenol causes tumor promotion; mucosal irritation
  - Carbon monoxide impairs oxygen transport and utilization
  - Formaldehyde produces toxicity to cilia; mucosal irritation

Table 8.11: Differences between emphysema and chronic bronchitis.

Feature	Emphysema	Chronic bronchitis
Clinical features		
Dyspnea	Severe	Mild-to-moderate
Cough	Develops after dyspnea starts	Frequent, develops before dyspnea starts
Sputum—amount and nature	Scanty and mucoid	Copious and purulent
Frequency of mucopurulent relapses	Less	More
Cyanosis	Absent	Present
Pulmonary hypertension	Late and mild	Early and severe
Right ventricular failure and respiratory failure	Late and often terminal	Repeated episodes
Mechanism of airway obstruction	Loss of elastic recoil	Decreased airway lumen due to mucus and inflammation
Investigations		
Hematocrit (PCV)	Normal	Increased
PaO_2	Normal to low "pink puffer"	Low "blue bloater"
$PaCO_2$	Normal mildly increased	High (>40)
FEV_1	Decreased	Decreased
Diffusing capacity	Reduced	Normal
Chest X-ray	Features of hyperinflation, bullae, and tubular heart	Increased bronchovascular markings and cardiomegaly
Elastic recoil	Decreased	Normal
Airway resistance	Normal to slightly increased	Increased
Cor pulmonale	Late and mild	Early and marked
Prognosis	Good	Poor

Table 8.12: Differentiating features of asthma and chronic obstructive pulmonary disease.

Characteristics	Bronchial asthma	COPD
Age of onset	Usually children and young adults	Usually older individuals
Risk factors	Family history of allergy, exposure to allergens, and occupational sensitizers	Smoking, atmospheric pollution, occupational exposure, and α1-antitrypsin deficiency
Respiratory symptoms:		
Main symptoms	Wheezing, cough, and dyspnea	Chronic dyspnea and productive cough
Nature of symptoms	Vary from time to time and even over hours and days	Usually continuous symptoms
Triggers	Exercise, dust or exposure to allergens	Unrelated to triggers
Recovery of symptoms	Symptoms improve spontaneously or with treatment	Slowly progressive despite therapy
Comorbidities	Generally absent	Often present (cardiovascular diseases, metabolic syndrome, depression, osteoporosis, and muscle wasting)
Chest X-ray	Normal	Hyperinflation
Spirometry	Reversibility of airway obstruction and normal between symptoms	$FEV_1/FVC <0.7$ and persistent airflow limitation

(COPD: chronic obstructive pulmonary disease; FEV: forced expiratory volume; FVC: forced vital capacity)

- Nitrogen oxides produces toxicity to cilia; mucosal irritation

Diseases caused by smoking are listed in **Table 8.13**.

Asthma COPD Overlap Syndrome

Major criteria for ACOS:
- Asthma COPD overlap syndrome (ACOS) is characterized by persistent airflow limitation with several features usually associated with asthma and several features usually associated with COPD.
- History or evidence of atopy (e.g., hay fever and elevated total IgE)
- Age 40 years or more
- Smoking >10 pack-years, post-bronchodilator FEV_1 <80% predicted and FEV_1/FVC <70%

A ≥15% increase in FEV_1 or ≥12% and ≥200 mL increase in FEV_1 postbronchodilator treatment with albuterol would be a minor criterion.

Table 8.13: Diseases caused by smoking.

System	Diseases produced
General	Cancers of lung, oropharynx, esophagus, stomach, pancreas, bladder, kidney, cervix, colon, and acute myeloid leukemia
Respiratory	COPD, chronic cough, and infections
Cardiovascular	Coronary artery disease, cerebrovascular disease, peripheral artery disease, and abdominal aortic aneurysm
Reproductive	Miscarriage, prematurity, low birth weight, ectopic pregnancy, and SIDS
Gastrointestinal	Gastroesophageal acid reflux, peptic ulcer, and Crohn's diseases
Others	Poor oral and skin health, cataract, fire-related injuries, osteoporosis, and macular degeneration

(COPD: chronic obstructive pulmonary disease; SIDS: sudden infant death syndrome)

PULMONARY TUBERCULOSIS

Mycobacteria

Classification

Mycobacteria are classified into three groups:
1. *Mycobacterium tuberculosis* complex (*M. tuberculosis*, *M. bovis*, and *M. africanum*)
2. *Mycobacterium leprae*
3. Atypical mycobacteria or nontuberculous mycobacteria (NTM) or mycobacteria other than tuberculosis (MOTT).

- MOTT or NTM are ubiquitous in the environment. They occur in soil and water and are *not usually pathogenic* due to their lack of virulence. Therefore, their isolation from a site that is not normally sterile (e.g., sputum, skin, or urine) does not constitute proof of disease. Groups of atypical *Mycobacterium* are listed in **Box 8.4**.
- *Patients with NTM lung disease* often *have predisposing disease of the lung* (e.g., COPD, bronchiectasis, cystic fibrosis, pneumoconiosis, etc.).
- **Mycobacterium avium** intracellulare:
  - Also known as MAC (*Mycobacterium avium* complex)
  - Most common nontuberculous mycobacterial infection associated with AIDS

Box 8.4: Groups of atypical *Mycobacterium*.

Slow growing:
- *Group I*: Photochromogens (P): Pigment producers in the presence of light, e.g. *Mycobacterium kansasii, M marinum, Mycobacterium simiae*
- *Group II*: Scotochromogens (S)—pigment producers in the absence of light, e.g., *Mycobacterium scrofulaceum, Mycobacterium szulgai,* and *Mycobacterium gordonae*
- *Group III*: Non-photochromogens (N)—do not produce any pigment, e.g., *Mycobacterium malmoense, Mycobacterium xenopi,* and *M. avium* intracellulare)

Fast growing:
- *Group IV*: Fast growers (3–5 days), e.g., *Mycobacterium fortuitum, Mycobacterium chelonae,* and *Mycobacterium abscessus*

- Symptoms include fever, swollen lymph nodes, diarrhea, fatigue, weight loss, and shortness of breath
- May develop into pulmonary MAC
☐ *Mycobacterium marinum* causes infections of skin and swimming pool granuloma.
☐ *Mycobacterium ulcerans* causes skin infections.
☐ *Mycobacterium kansasii* causes lung disease.

Tuberculosis

Tuberculosis (also called Koch's disease) is a *communicable, chronic granulomatous disease* caused by *Mycobacterium tuberculosis*.

Tuberculosis (TB) is caused by four main *Mycobacterial* species collectively termed as *Mycobacterium tuberculosis complex (MTb)*—(1) Mycobacterium tuberculosis (reservoir human), (2) Mycobacterium bovis (reservoir cattle), (3) Mycobacterium africanum, and (4) Mycobacterium microti. These are obligate aerobes and facultative intracellular pathogens, which usually infect mononuclear phagocytes.

☐ Majority of tuberculosis are due to Mycobacterium tuberculosis hominis (human strain). The source of infection is patients suffering from active open case of tuberculosis.
☐ Oropharyngeal and intestinal tuberculosis can be due to drinking milk contaminated by *M. bovis* (bovine strain) from infected cows. Routine pasteurization has almost eliminated this source of infection.
☐ *M. avium* and *intracellulare* are nonpathogenic to normal individuals. They cause infection in patients *suffering from AIDS*.

Characteristics of Mycobacteria

☐ It is an aerobic, slender, and rod-shaped bacterium. It measures 2–10 µm in length.
☐ It has a high-lipid content in the cell wall, which makes it difficult to stain, but *once stained, it resists decolorization by acids and alcohol*. Hence, it is termed as acid-fast bacilli (AFB), because once stained by carbol fuchsin (present in *Ziehl–Neelsen stain*), it is not decolorized by acid and alcohol.

Epidemiology

Tuberculosis is common in India. High incidence of tuberculosis is observed with poverty, overcrowding, and chronic debilitating illness. An estimated 1.7 million people died from TB, including nearly 400,000 people who were coinfected with HIV.

☐ *Diseases associated with increased risk* of tuberculosis include diabetes mellitus, Hodgkin lymphoma, malnutrition, immunosuppression, alcoholism, chronic lung disease (e.g., silicosis), and chronic renal failure.
☐ *HIV is the most important risk factor*.
☐ **NRAMP-1 gene:** *NRAMP-1 is a transmembrane protein* (a product of *NRAMP-1* gene), which *inhibits microbial growth* and it determines the susceptibility to tuberculosis.

In individuals with *polymorphisms in the NRAMP-1* (*n*atural *r*esistance-*a*ssociated *m*acrophage *p*rotein-*1*) *gene, tuberculosis may progress due to the absence of an effective immune response*.

Mode of Transmission

☐ **Inhalation:** It is the *most common mode* of transmission. *Source of organisms is an active open case of tuberculosis to a susceptible individual.* Infection spreads by inhalation of respiratory droplet from other infected patients.
☐ **Ingestion:** Tuberculosis may be transmitted by drinking nonpasteurized milk from infected cows contaminated with *M. bovis*. It causes oropharyngeal and intestinal tuberculosis. Nowadays, the ingestion mode of transmission occurs when a patient with open case of tuberculosis swallows the infected sputum resulting in tuberculosis of intestine.
☐ **Inoculation:** It *is extremely rare* and may develop during postmortem examination through cuts resulting from handling tuberculous infected organs.

Primary Tuberculosis

Initial infection that occurs on first exposure to the organism (*Mycobacterium tuberculosis*) *in an unsensitized* (previously unexposed tuberculin-negative) *individual* is known as primary tuberculosis. First infection of the lung caused by the tubercle bacillus is termed as primary pulmonary tuberculosis.

Primary infection usually occurs during childhood. Many patients give a history of contact with a case of active pulmonary tuberculosis. About 5% of newly infected people develop clinically significant disease. Source of the organism is always exogenous.

Sites of Primary Tuberculosis

The sites of primary tuberculosis are lung, intestine, tonsil, and skin (very rare).

Primary tuberculosis of lung:

It is the *most common site* of primary tuberculosis. Primary pulmonary tuberculosis develops when the bacillus is inhaled and lodged in the alveoli of the lung.

Ghon lesion/focus:

Following inhalation, tubercle bacilli reach distal airspaces.
☐ **Site of deposit:** Lower part of the upper lobe or upper part of the lower lobe near the pleural surface (subpleural) is the usual site of deposit.
☐ **Ghon focus:** About 2–4 weeks after the infection, a circumscribed *gray-white area of* about *1–1.5 cm develops in the lung* known as the Ghon focus, the center of which undergoes caseous necrosis.
☐ **Regional lymphadenitis:** Tubercle bacilli (free or within macrophages) are carried along the lymphatics to the regional draining nodes, which often show caseous necrosis.

Ghon complex:
It is the combination of subpleural parenchymal lung lesion (*Ghon focus*) and *regional lymph node* involvement.

Fate of Ghon complex:
- **Healing:** In *majority* (about 95%), cell-mediated immunity controls the infection and primary tuberculosis *heals*.
  - The *hallmark of healing is fibrosis*. Ghon complex may undergo progressive fibrosis and calcification. It is radiologically detected as a small calcified nodule (***Ranke complex***) in caseous material and very rarely undergoes ossification.
  - In the majority of individuals infected by *Mycobacterium*, the immune system contains the infection and the patient develops cell-mediated immune memory to the bacteria. This is termed as *latent tuberculosis*.
- **Spread:** Lymphatic and hematogenous spread to other organs or parts of the body occurs during the first few weeks.
  - *Progressive pulmonary tuberculosis:* In few patients, primary lesion in the lung may progress from the beginning (progressive pulmonary tuberculosis or progressive primary pulmonary tuberculosis).
  - *Bronchial spread:* Tuberculous lymph node may rupture/ulcerate through the bronchial wall and discharge caseous material into the bronchial lumen. This results in spread of infection to the related lobe or segment through bronchi.
  - *Hematogenous spread:* In some patients, the tubercle bacilli may enter the blood and produce tuberculous lesions in different parts of the body. The hematogenous spread can be of two types:
    1. *Acute form*: It is more likely to occur in infants or young children and results in *miliary tuberculosis* or tuberculous meningitis.
    2. *Chronic form*: It is characterized by tuberculosis in the lungs, bones, joints, liver, and kidneys. These lesions may develop months or even years after primary infection. The infection in these secondary foci may remain dormant for years.
  - *Lymphatic spread:* In some cases, the infection may be carried by lymphatics from mediastinal lymph nodes to pleura or pericardium resulting in tuberculous pleurisy with effusion or tuberculous pericarditis with effusion.

Other sites of primary tuberculosis:
- **Intestine:** Primary focus always involves the small intestine (usually ileal region) and is associated with mesenteric lymphadenitis.
- **Tonsils:** Primary focus in the pharynx and tonsil with cervical lymph node enlargement.
- **Skin:** Primary focus in the skin associated with regional lymphadenopathy

Bronchial Complications
- **Middle lobe syndrome:** Enlarged mediastinal lymph nodes of primary complex may compress a bronchus causing collapse of the lung. Compression of middle lobe bronchus may lead to collapse–consolidation and bronchiectatic changes. This may be present later as the *"middle lobe syndrome, Brock's syndrome"*.
- An unusual phenomenon in primary tuberculosis is obstruction of bronchus by lymph nodes referred to as *epituberculosis* resulting in some clinical signs, e.g., localized wheeze or bronchial breathing.
- **Obstructive emphysema:** Rarely, the compression of bronchus may result in a valve action with air trapping. This leads to obstructive emphysema.
- **Broncholith:** Calcification in a Ghon focus or regional lymph node may be extruded into a bronchus leading to "broncholith" or present as hemoptysis.

Clinical Features: Pulmonary Disease
Primary pulmonary TB:
Symptoms:
- Majority are asymptomatic.
- A few patients may present with self-limiting febrile illness, which may lasts no more than 7–14 days. It occurs at the time of tuberculin conversion.
- Clinical disease only occurs, if there is progressive infection. If the infection is severe or the host resistance is low, child may present with reduced appetite and failure to gain weight. Slight dry cough may be occasionally present.

Physical signs:
- Majority of patients does not reveal any abnormal physical signs.
- *General features*: If the lesion is severe or extensive, signs of general debility may be present. Child is thin, pale, and fretful with less glossy hair and less elastic skin.
- *Respiratory system*: Usually, no abnormal physical signs detected in the chest. Sometimes, few crepitations may be heard over lung parenchyma involved by the primary complex. More extensive physical signs in the chest may be produced when there are complications. Rarely, pleural effusion can be seen.
- *Erythema nodosum*: It may accompany primary pulmonary tuberculosis. They are bluish-red, raised, tender, and skin lesions commonly seen on the shins and less commonly on the thighs. In few, it may be associated with fever and polyarthralgia.

Diagnosis
- **History of contact:** With a case of active tuberculosis.
- **Tuberculin test:** It is very valuable in children. A positive test in a previously non-sensitized/immunized child strongly indicates the disease. A negative test makes the diagnosis of tuberculosis very unlikely.
- **Chest radiograph:** Primary complex may appear as a peripheral parenchymal lung lesion and an enlarged hilar lymph node.
  - *In children:* Enlargement of (e.g., hilar) lymph node of the primary complex is more prominent than the pulmonary component.
  - *In adults:* Pulmonary component (peripheral parenchymal lesion) of the complex is more obvious than the lymph node component.

- **Bacteriological examination:**
  - Sputum examination—for AFB is preferable.
  - Alternatively, three laryngeal swabs or fasting gastric washings can be examined.
  - Detection of the tubercle bacilli either in the direct smear or culture confirms the diagnosis.

Postprimary (Secondary) Tuberculosis

(Synonyms: Postprimary tuberculosis, reactivation tuberculosis)
- *Tuberculosis* developing *in a previously sensitized* individual (by earlier exposure) is known as secondary tuberculosis.
- It may develop shortly or after many years following primary tuberculosis, when resistance host is reduced.

Source of Infection
- **Endogenous:** Most common source is *reactivation of a latent infection*.
  - Direct progression of a primary tuberculous lesion
  - Reactivation of a dormant primary lesion
  - Hematogenous spread to the lungs
- **Exogenous:** Rarely exogenous new infection (reinfection)
Any location may be involved in secondary tuberculosis, but lungs are by far the most common site.

Morphology
Gross:
- **Site:** In the lungs, postprimary (secondary) tuberculosis usually involves the *apex of the upper lobes* of one or both lungs, *within 1–2 cm of the apical pleura*. It commonly involves apical and posterior segments of the upper lobe or apical segment of the lower lobe. This predilection may be due to good ventilation, decreased blood and lymphatic supply of these regions in the erect posture, and the oxygen tension that favors survival of the strictly aerobic tubercle bacilli.
- **Appearance:** *Initially small focus (less than 2 cm in diameter) of consolidation,* sharply circumscribed, firm, and *gray-white to yellow* in color. The central caseated liquefied material of a tuberculous primary lesion may be discharged into a bronchus and forms a tuberculous cavity in the lung.
- Regional lymph node involvement is not as prominent as that seen in primary tuberculosis.

Fate of Secondary Tuberculosis (Fig. 8.10)
Healing: In immunocompetent individuals, localized, apical focus may *heal with fibrosis and calcification but* rarely ossification.

Progress: It may occur along several different pathways.
- **Progressive pulmonary tuberculosis:** It occurs mainly in the elderly and immunosuppressed. Apical lesion may expand into surrounding lung and may erode into bronchi and vessels.
  - *Erosion into bronchi*: It leads to release of the central area of caseous necrosis, resulting in a ragged, irregular *apical cavity* surrounded by fibrous tissue. This

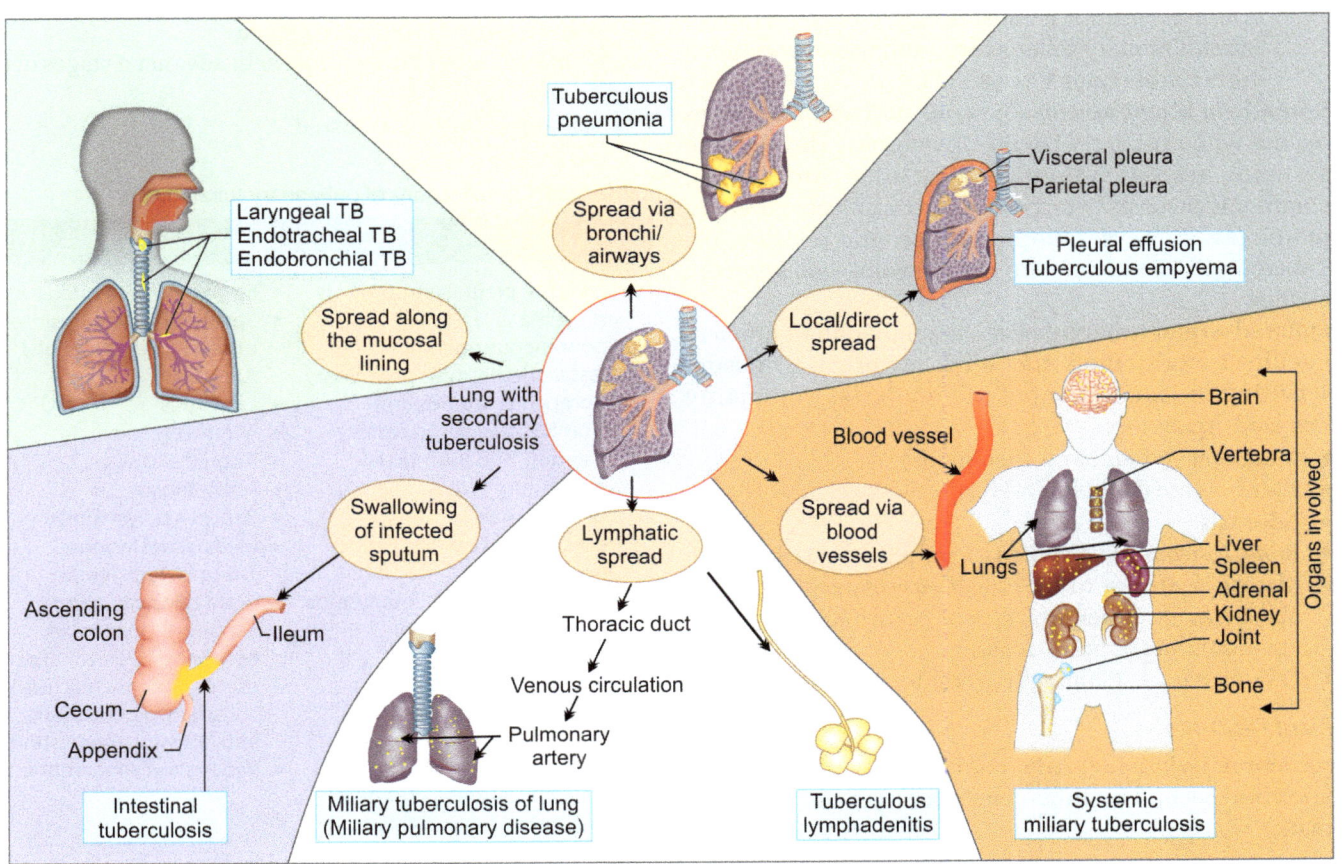

Fig. 8.10: Progress and complications of secondary tuberculosis of lung.

produces an *important source of infection*, because when the patient coughs, sputum contains bacteria.
- *Erosion of blood vessels*: It may result in hemoptysis.
❒ **Spread of infection:** If the treatment is inadequate or if host defenses are impaired, the infection may spread via—(1) airways, (2) lymphatics, or (3) blood vessels.
  - *Local/direct spread:* Tuberculosis can directly spread to the surrounding tissue. In the lung, local spread to the pleura may result in serous *pleural effusions, tuberculous empyema,* or *obliterative fibrous pleuritis*.
  - *Spread through bronchi/airways:* It may produce tuberculous pneumonia.
  - *Spread along mucosal lining*: Spread through lymphatic channels or along the mucosal lining from mycobacteria present in the expectorated infectious material may lead to *endobronchial, endotracheal, and laryngeal tuberculosis*. In the past, intestinal tuberculosis was due to drinking of contaminated unpasteurized milk. However, this is rare following pasteurization of milk. Nowadays, it is caused by the *swallowing of coughed-up infective material* in patients with open case of advanced pulmonary tuberculosis. It *mainly develops in the ileum*.
  - *Lymphatic spread*: Spread through lymphatic channels mainly reach regional lymph nodes. It may also cause disseminated disease.
    - *Miliary pulmonary disease*: It is the disseminated form of tuberculosis. If the dissemination is only limited to the lungs, it is termed as miliary pulmonary disease.
    - *Lymphadenitis*: It is most frequent presentation of extrapulmonary tuberculosis, and usually occurs in the cervical region ("scrofula").
❒ **Spread via blood vessels:** *Systemic miliary tuberculosis* occurs when tubercle bacilli disseminate through the systemic arterial system. Miliary tuberculosis most commonly involves liver, bone marrow, spleen, adrenals, meninges, kidneys, fallopian tubes, and epididymis. Tuberculosis can involve any organ *except nail, hair, and enamel*.
❒ **Isolated-organ tuberculosis:** Dissemination of tubercle bacilli through blood may seed any organ or tissue, resulting in isolated organ tuberculosis. Commonly involved organs are:
  - Meninges (tuberculous meningitis)
  - Kidneys (renal tuberculosis)
  - Adrenals
  - *Bones (osteomyelitis)*: When it involves the vertebrae, the disease is referred to as *Pott's disease*. Paraspinal "cold" abscesses may track along tissue planes and present as an abdominal or pelvic mass.
  - Fallopian tubes (salpingitis)/orchitis

Clinical Features
Symptoms of pulmonary tuberculosis:
❒ Localized secondary tuberculosis may remain asymptomatic.
❒ Many patients are symptom free, and may be detected on routine radiography.
❒ Onset is usually insidious or gradual, with symptoms developing slowly over weeks or months.
❒ **Nonspecific:** Malaise, anorexia, loss of appetite and weight, and tiredness.
❒ **Low-grade fever:** It is *remittent* (appearing late each afternoon and then subsiding—commonly known as *evening rise of temperature*), and *night sweats*.
❒ **Others:** Amenorrhea.

Respiratory symptoms:
❒ **Chronic cough:** It is the most consistent symptom. If a patient has cough of more than 3 weeks, he/she should be investigated for pulmonary tuberculosis.
❒ **Hemoptysis:** It is a classical symptom. *Hemoptysis is present in 50% of cases of pulmonary tuberculosis*.
❒ **Sputum:** It may be mucoid, purulent, or blood stained. Classical sputum is described as *"numular"*.
❒ **Pain in the chest:** Pain may be due to pleurisy, intercostals myalgia, or cough fracture.
❒ **Unresolved pneumonia:** It may be another mode of presentation.
❒ **Breathlessness** may be a feature observed in advanced and extensive disease or due to pleural effusion.
❒ Localized wheeze may be observed due to local ulceration and narrowing of a major bronchus.
❒ Recurrent cold may be also a presenting symptom.
❒ **Presentation due to complications:** Very occasionally, it may present with one of the complications **(Table 8.14)**.

Physical signs:
❒ Fever, tachycardia, and tachypnea
❒ Pallor and cachexia may be seen in advanced stages of the disease.
❒ Clubbing of finger is unusual.

Table 8.14: Complications of pulmonary tuberculosis.

Pulmonary	Nonpulmonary
• Exudative pleural effusion/empyema • Spontaneous pneumothorax • Massive hemoptysis pulmonary or bronchial arteritis and thrombosis, bronchial artery dilatation, and Rasmussen aneurysm) • Cor pulmonale • Persistence of cavities even after treatment • Pulmonary fibrosis/emphysema • Atypical mycobacterial infection • Aspergillus → aspergilloma • Lung/pleural calcification • Obstructive airways disease **Airway lesions:** These include bronchiectasis, tracheobronchial stenosis, and broncholithiasis • Bronchopleural fistula • Bronchogenic carcinoma	• Empyema necessitans • Spread of tuberculosis to other organs (especially Addison's) • Laryngitis • Enteritis • Anorectal disease • Amyloidosis • Poncet's polyarthritis • Mediastinal lesions: These include lymph node calcification and extranodal extension, esophagomediastinal or esophagobronchial fistula, constrictive pericarditis, and fibrosing mediastinitis. • Venous thromboembolism

Chest:
- Often, there are no abnormal signs detected.
- **Fine crepitations:** Most common sign is fine crepitations in the upper part (apices) of one or both lungs. They are better heard particularly on taking a deep breath after coughing *(post-tussive crepitations)*.
- Classical physical signs of consolidation (dullness to percussion), cavitation, fibrosis, bronchiectasis, pleural effusion, or pneumothorax may be present.
- *Cavernous bronchial breathing* with *post-tussive suction* may be heard, if there is a superficial collapsible cavity.
- There may be bronchial breathing in the upper part and localized wheeze due to local tuberculous bronchitis or pressure by a lymph node on a bronchus may be heard. In chronic tuberculosis, when accompanied with fibrosis, it may show evidence of volume loss and mediastinal shift.

Extrapulmonary manifestations depend on the organ/system involved.

Conditions/diseases that favor reactivation/reinfection of tuberculosis are presented in **Table 8.15**.

Investigations

Presence of an unexplained cough for more than 2–3 weeks, particularly in regions where TB is prevalent, or typical chest X-ray changes, should prompt for further investigation.

Blood examination:
- **Anemia:** Moderate degree
- **White cell count:** Usually normal or below normal
- **Erythrocyte sedimentation rate (ESR):** Usually raised
- **Other findings:**
  - *Serum electrolytes:* Hyponatremia and hyperkalemia may be observed in severe disease.
  - *Liver function tests:* Occasionally may be impaired.

Radiological examination:
For practical purposes, a normal chest radiograph excludes the diagnosis of pulmonary tuberculosis (**Fig. 8.11**).

Radiological features of pulmonary tuberculosis (Table 8.16): For all practical purposes, a normal chest radiograph excludes the diagnosis of pulmonary tuberculosis.
- **Radiological findings:** It shows ill-defined opacification in one or both of the upper lobes. As the disease progresses, features of consolidation, collapse, and cavitation develop to varying degrees **(Fig. 8.11)**. It is often difficult to distinguish between active from quiescent form of tuberculosis on radiological criteria alone, but the presence of a miliary pattern or cavitation favors active disease.
- In extensive disease, collapse may cause significant displacement of the trachea and mediastinum.

Table 8.15: Condition/diseases that favor reactivation/reinfection of tuberculosis.

• Immunosuppression: HIV, anti-tumor necrosis factor (TNF) therapy, high-dose corticosteroids, cytotoxic agents • Malnutrition • Diabetes mellitus • Hemophilia • Chronic kidney disease	• Silicosis • Malignancies (e.g., lymphoma and leukemia) • Gastrointestinal disease associated with malnutrition (gastrectomy, jejunoileal bypass, cancer of the pancreas, malabsorption) • Deficiency of vitamin D or A

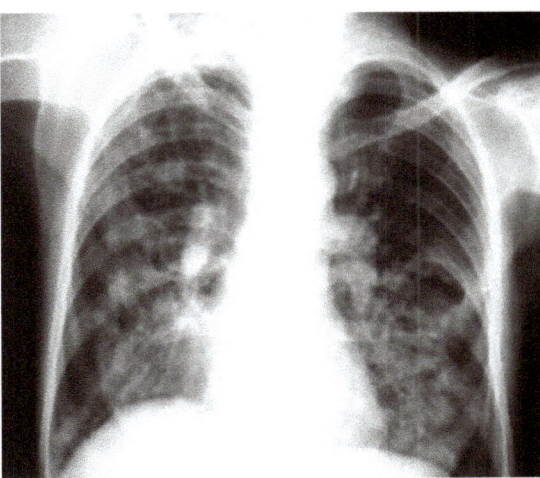

Fig. 8.11: Chest X-ray of tuberculosis showing bilateral infiltrates and thin-walled cavities.

Table 8.16: Radiological features of tuberculosis of lung.

Radiological shadows that strongly suggest tuberculosis	Radiological shadows that may be due to tuberculosis
• Patchy or nodular shadows in the upper zone (on one or both sides) • Cavitation (especially if more than one) • Calcified lesion • Pleural effusion/thickening	• Oval or round single shadow (tuberculoma) • Hilar and mediastinal shadows (due to enlarged lymph nodes) • Diffuse small nodular shadows (miliary tuberculosis)

Occasionally, a caseous lymph node may drain into an adjoining bronchus, resulting in tuberculous pneumonia.
- **CT chest:** It may be useful in evaluating parenchymal and lymph node lesions. It may show *tree in bud appearance*.
- ^{18}F-FDG PET (positron emission tomography) scans and ^{11}C-choline PET scans may be done in few selected patients.

Sputum examination:
- **Direct microscopic examination of sputum:** It remains the most important first step investigation in pulmonary TB. Three specimens of sputum should be examined and if two of these smears are positive, diagnosis of TB is certain.
  - *A first spot specimen:* Obtained when the patient presents himself.
  - *An early morning specimen:* When the patient returns with an early morning specimen.
  - *A second spot specimen:* When the patient returns with an early morning specimen.
- **Revised WHO definition of a new sputum smear-positive case of pulmonary tuberculosis:** Presence of at least one acid fast bacillus in at least one sputum sample in countries with a well-functioning external quality-assurance system. Presently, WHO recommends that the number of sputum specimens to be examined for screening of tuberculosis cases can be *reduced from three to two*—in places (1) where a well-functioning external quality-assurance system exists, (2) where the workload is very high, and (3) human resources are scarce.
- **Stain:** Rapid identification of the presence of tubercle bacilli by immediate stains is essential and should be done within 24 hours. The most effective stains are the

Ziehl–Neelsen and rhodamine–auramine. Auramine–rhodamine staining is more sensitive (though less specific) than Ziehl–Neelsen.

Culture of sputum:
- A *positive sputum smear is sufficient for the presumptive diagnosis of TB* but definitive diagnosis requires culture of tubercle bacillus. Smear-negative sputum should also be cultured.
- **Culture medias:** It may be—
  - *Liquid/broth culture (Middlebrook 7H12) or the nonradiometric mycobacteria growth indicator tube (MGIT)):* Faster growth (1–3 weeks) occurs in liquid media. *The BACTEC radiometric growth detection method detects mycobacterial growth by measuring the liberation of $^{14}CO_2$ following metabolism of ^{14}C-labeled substrate present in the medium. The growth can be detected in 4–8 days.*
  - *Solid media (Löwenstein–Jensen slopes):* MTb grows slowly and may take between 4 and 6 weeks.
- **Drug sensitivity testing:** It should be done in selected cases. It is important in patients with a previous history of TB, treatment failure or chronic disease, and in those who are resident in or have visited an area of high prevalence of resistance, or who are HIV-positive. Using liquid culture in the presence of antimycobacterial drugs (usually first line therapy initially) establishes the drug sensitivity for that strain and usually takes approximately 3 weeks.
- **Nucleic acid amplification (NAA) tests:** The *amplified Mycobacterium tuberculosis direct (MTD) test and the Gene Xpert MTb/RIF test*. NAA is more sensitive than smear but less sensitive than culture; as few as 1–10 organisms/mL may give a positive result. Resistance to rifampin can be detected by Xpert MTB/RIF or MTBDRplus; resistance to isoniazid can be detected by MTBDRplus.

Other investigations:
- Laryngeal swab, early morning gastric lavage, and bronchoalveolar lavage samples can be used for detecting AFB.
- **Tuberculin test:** It is used for diagnosis but is less valuable. However, this test may be negative in patients with active tuberculosis associated with malnutrition or other diseases. It may be positive in patients without active tuberculosis. Strongly positive test favors tuberculosis, whereas a negative test does not exclude tuberculosis.
- **Interferon gamma release assays (IGRAs):**
  - IGRAs are *in-vitro* tests of cellular immunity. These assays measure cell-mediated immune response by quantifying interferon gamma (IFNγ) released by T cells in response to stimulation by *Mycobacterium tuberculosis*-specific antigens. These specific antigens include early secretory antigenic target-6 (ESAT-6) and culture filtrate protein-10 (CFP10).
  - The test does not differentiate between active and latent infection. This test requires high cost and trained personnel.
- **Other methods of diagnosis:**
  - *MGIT (mycobacteria growth indicator tube) method*: In this method, growth is detected by a nonradioactive detection system using fluorochromes for detection and drug screening.
  - Identification by mycolic acids using high-pressure liquid chromatography
  - *ELISA testing for IgM and IgA:* It is commonly used but has low specificity.
  - Mycobacterial-specific phages (reporter phages) to detect luciferase gene. It can be used to detect drug-resistant isolates.

Causes of Hemoptysis in Pulmonary Tuberculosis

- **Hemoptysis from a pulmonary cavity:**
  - *Rasmussen's aneurysm:* Blood vessels traversing a tuberculous cavity can undergo changes due to inflammatory and necrosis. Over a period of time, these vessels may develop aneurysmal dilatation (Rasmussen's aneurysm). These aneurysms may rupture resulting in hemoptysis.
  - *Allergic response of vessel:* Occasionally, intense allergic response to antigens of tubercle bacilli can damage the walls of the blood vessels in and around the tuberculous cavities leading to hemoptysis.
- **Hemoptysis from endobronchial tuberculosis:**
  - *Tuberculosis of endobronchial region* may be surrounded by vessels with small aneurysmal dilatation. Rupture of these aneurysms can produce hemoptysis.
  - Occasionally, sloughing of the part of the granuloma may result in hemoptysis.
- **Hemoptysis as a sequel of pulmonary tuberculosis:**
  - *Open-healed cavities:* A tuberculous cavity may persist as sequelae following chemotherapy, which are designated as "open-healed cavities"/INH cysts. The aneurysmal dilations of vessels may also persist in these open-healed cavities, which can rupture producing hemoptysis.
  - *Post-tuberculous bronchiectasis:* The upper lobe bronchiectasis is common sequelae of pulmonary tuberculosis. This may be characterized by repeated attacks of hemoptysis without sputum production (bronchiectasis sicca or dry bronchiectasis).
  - *Broncholith:* Calcification in a primary/Ghon focus or lymph node may be extruded into a bronchus as a "broncholith" and can cause hemoptysis. Hemoptysis may also result from the broncholith eroding through blood vessels.
  - *Aspergilloma:* Treated and healed tuberculous cavities may sometimes remain open and can be infected by the fungus *Aspergillus fumigatus*. This may produce a fungal ball (aspergilloma) in the cavity and can present as severe hemoptysis.
  - Hemoptysis due to scar carcinoma.

Tuberculin Skin Test

First infection with mycobacteria leads to development of delayed hypersensitivity to *M. tuberculosis* antigens (tuberculin) and this is detected by the tuberculin skin test.

Tuberculin: There are two commonly used tuberculins in present use:

1. PPD-S has been adopted as the international standard for purified protein derivative (PPD) of mammalian tuberculin.
2. PPD-RT23 is widely used in epidemiological studies throughout the world.

Mantoux test (Fig. 8.12): It is ideal to begin the test with 5 IU PPD-S or 1 or 2 IU PPD-RT23.

Method:
- Select an area of skin at the junction of the mid and upper thirds of flexure surface of the left forearm.
- Skin is cleaned with soap and water and allowed to dry.
- Using a tuberculin syringe and an intradermal needle, inject 0.1 mL of the tuberculin solution strictly intradermally. It should result in papule in the skin measuring 5–6 mm in diameter.

Reading and Interpreting the Result
- The test is read after 48–72 hours
- If a reaction has taken place, there will be an area of erythema (redness) and an area of induration (thickening) of the skin. Measure the diameter of induration across the transverse axis of the arm. The reaction is considered positive, if an area of *induration* of the skin *of 10-mm diameter or more* at the site of injection of PPD. The amount of erythema (redness) present is not important. Induration ≥5 mm is considered as positive in patients with HIV infection (or risk factors for HIV infection, but unknown status), recent close contact to person with known active TB, patients with chest X-ray consistent with prior TB, patients with organ transplants, and other immunosuppressed patient.

Significance
- **Positive tuberculin test:** It indicates T-cell-mediated *immunity* to mycobacterial antigens. A strongly positive test is particularly valuable in children, especially in very young children, and favors the diagnosis of tuberculosis.
- **False-negative reactions:** If the diameter of induration is below 10 mm, the test is considered negative. But a negative test does not exclude tuberculosis. It is seen in certain viral infections, sarcoidosis, malnutrition, Hodgkin lymphoma, immunosuppression, and overwhelming active tuberculous disease, HIV infection, measles, chickenpox, glandular fever (infectious mononucleosis), cancer, corticosteroids, and similar drugs.

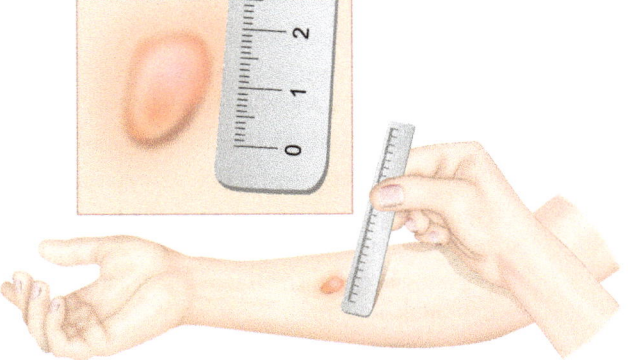

Fig. 8.12: Mantoux test.

- **False-positive reactions:** It is seen in infection by *atypical mycobacteria* or prior *vaccination with BCG (bacillus Calmette–Guerin)* or lymphoma. Most infants immunized with BCG at birth have a negative tuberculin test by 1–2 years. In infants immunized after 1 year, the tuberculin reaction often remains positive for some years. It may also be positive in nontuberculous mycobacteria (NTM) infections.

Latent Tuberculosis
- In the majority of individuals infected by *Mycobacterium tuberculosis*, the immune system contains the infection and the patient develops cell-mediated immune memory to the bacteria. These individuals do not currently have active tuberculosis disease. This is termed as latent tuberculosis.
- Individuals with latent tuberculosis are at risk of progression to active tuberculosis. About 5–10% is at the lifetime risk of progression. The increased risk of progression from latent tuberculosis to active tuberculosis is during the first 2 years after infection. Groups of individuals at high risk of tuberculosis infection are listed in **Table 8.17**.

Groups at increased risk of progression to active tuberculosis are listed in **Table 8.18**.

Screening for Latent Tuberculosis
- Tuberculin skin test
- T-cell IGRAs

Antituberculous Drugs
Classification of Antituberculous Drugs—First-Line Antituberculous Drugs
Tables 8.19 and 8.20 describe the classification of antituberculous drugs and tuberculous foci and the drugs acting on them.

Table 8.17: Groups of individuals at high-risk of tuberculosis infection.

- Employees working at long-term care facilities, hospitals, and medical laboratories
- Individuals having close contact with patients with active tuberculosis
- Residents and employees of congregate living facilities (e.g., prison and jails, nursing homes, hospitals, and homeless shelters

Table 8.18: Groups at increased risk of progression to active tuberculosis.

- Children younger than 5 years of age
- History of tuberculous infection:
  - Individuals infected with *Mycobacterium tuberculosis* within the past 2 years
  - Past history of untreated or inadequately treated tuberculosis
- Associated conditions:
  - Individuals with HIV infection
  - Silicosis
  - IV drug users
  - Immunocompromised conditions
  - Long-term use of corticosteroids or other immunosuppressants (including anti-TNF-α)
  - Chronic renal failure
  - Diabetes mellitus
  - Malignancy

Table 8.19: Classification of antitubercular drugs.

First-line antituberculous drugs	
• Isoniazid (H) • Rifampin (R) • Pyrazinamide (Z)	• Ethambutol (E) • Streptomycin (S)
Second-line antitubercular drugs	
• Thiacetazone (Tzn) • Paraaminosalicylic acid (PAS) • Ethionamide (Etm) • Cycloserine (Cys) • Kanamycin (Kmc) • Amikacin (Am) • Capreomycin (Cpr)	• Newer antitubercular drugs • Bedaquiline • Delamanid and pretomanid • Sutezolid • Ciprofloxacin • Ofloxacin • Moxifloxacin • Clarithromycin • Azithromycin • Rifabutin

Table 8.20: Tuberculous foci and the drugs acting on them.

Tuberculous foci	Drugs acting on them
Extracellular, in alkaline medium	Streptomycin
Rapidly metabolizing mycobacteria (in a cavity)	Rifampicin
Less actively multiplying bacilli in acidic and closed lesions	Isoniazid
Dormant bacilli (that cause a relapse)	Pyrazinamide

Side Effects of the Commonly Used Antituberculous Drugs

Side effects of the commonly used antituberculous drugs are mentioned in **Table 8.21**.

Antituberculous Chemotherapy

Short-course chemotherapy:

☐ Short-course chemotherapy (SCC) is regimens of 6–9 months duration, which are highly effective and widely accepted as the treatment of choice for tuberculosis.
☐ **All the short course regimens have two phases:** An initial intensive (bactericidal) phase and a continuation (sterilizing) phase
  • *Initial phase*: It lasts for 2–3 months and aimed to rapidly kill majority of mycobacteria. The symptoms resolve, sputum becomes negative, and the patient becomes noninfectious.
  • *Continuation phase*: It lasts for 4–6 months during which the remaining bacilli are eliminated, so that relapse does not occur.

Categories of Diagnosis and Treatment

Treatment regimen for tuberculosis is presented in **Table 8.22**.

Directly Observed Treatment, Short Course

☐ Directly observed treatment, short course is an *intermittent method* of administering potent antituberculous regimens to a patient with tuberculosis *under direct supervision*.
☐ Daily chemotherapy is excellent. However, it is expensive and not possible to supervise therapy and hence compliance rate is low and relapse rate is high.

Drug-resistant TB

☐ **Multiple drug resistance or multidrug-resistant TB:**
  • Multidrug-resistant tuberculosis (MDR-TB) is a form of TB that is *resistance to at least both of INH and rifampicin,*

Table 8.21: Side effects of the commonly used antituberculous drugs.

Drug (daily dosages)	Adverse reactions	
	Major	Less common (rare)
Isoniazid (H) (5–10 mg/kg)	• Hepatitis • Peripheral neuropathy (preventable and treatable with pyridoxine) • Cutaneous hypersensitivity	Giddiness, seizures, optic neuritis, mental symptoms, hemolytic anemia, aplastic anemia, agranulocytosis, lupoid reactions, arthralgia, and gynecomastia
Rifampicin (R) (10 mg/kg)	Febrile reactions ("flu" syndrome; more common with intermittent therapy), hepatitis, cutaneous reactions, and gastrointestinal disturbances	Shortness of breath, shock, hemolytic anemia, interstitial nephritis, and thrombocytopenia
Pyrazinamide (Z) (20 mg/kg)	Anorexia, nausea, flushing, hepatitis, gastrointestinal disturbance, and hyperuricemia	Hepatitis (dose related), vomiting, arthralgia, cutaneous hypersensitivity, and gout
Ethambutol (E) (15 mg/kg)	Retrobulbar neuritis (dose related), arthralgia	Peripheral neuropathy, rash
Streptomycin (S) and other aminoglycosides (15–20 mg/kg)	8th nerve damage, cutaneous hypersensitivity, giddiness, numbness, and tinnitus	Vertigo, ataxia, deafness, hypokalemia, renal damage, aplastic anemia, and agranulocytosis
Ethionamide (Etm) (10–20 mg/kg)	Anorexia and vomiting	Serious neurologic reactions and hepatitis
Cycloserine (Cys) (10–20 mg/kg)	Headache and somnolence	Psychosis, seizures, and peripheral neuropathy
Quinolones (7.5–15 mg/kg)	GI intolerance and skin rashes	Phototoxicity (with sparfloxacin), dizziness, headache, and insomnia
Thiacetazone (Tzn) (2.5 mg/kg)	Gastrointestinal reactions, cutaneous hypersensitivity, vertigo, and conjunctivitis	Hepatitis, erythema multiforme, exfoliative dermatitis, and hemolytic anemia
Paraaminosalicylic acid (PAS) (8–12 g/day)	Gastrointestinal reactions, hepatitis, cutaneous hypersensitivity, and hypokalemia	Acute renal failure, hemolytic anemia, thrombocytopenia, and hypothyroidism

Table 8.22: Treatment regimen for tuberculosis.

A. DOTS (directly observed treatment, short course)	Regimen
1. New: • New smear-positive patients • New smear negative pulmonary TB with extensive parenchymal invasion • Severe concomitant HIV disease; or • New cases of severe forms of extrapulmonary TB • New cases of smear negative pulmonary TB with limited parenchymal involvement	2 months (HRZE) + 4 months (HRE) *Duration: 6 months*

2. Previously treated:
• Includes previously treated sputum smear-positive pulmonary TB:
  – Relapse
  – Treatment after interruption
  – Treatment failure
	2 months (HRZES) followed by 1 month (HRZE), followed by 5 months (HRE)
	Duration: 8 months

B. DOTS-Plus	
Includes MDR and chronic TB cases (still sputum-positive after supervised retreatment)	6–9 months (KM LVX, ETO CS, Z, E) followed by 18 months (LVX, ETO, CS, and E) *Duration: 24–27 months*
Extensively drug-resistant TB (XDR-TB)	6–12 months intensive phase followed by 18 months continuation phase (Capreomycin, PAS, moxifloxacin, clofazimine, linezolid, amoxicillin/clavulanate, clarithromycin, and thiacetazone) *Duration: 24–30 months*
C. Non-DOTS	
Rare TB patients may need non-rifampicin and non-pyrazinamide regimen	2 SHE + 10 HE or 12 HE

Note: Since 2017, the thrice weekly regimen has been changed daily regimen.
(H: isoniazid; R: rifampin; Z: pyrazinamide; E: ethambutol; S: streptomycin; KM: kanamycin; LVX: levofloxacin; ETO: ethionamide; CS: cyclosporine; PLHIV: people living with HIV)

with or without other drug resistance. Hence, a patient should not be classified as multidrug-resistant disease, if the patient has an infection with a bacterium susceptible to rifampicin but resistant to many other drugs.
- MDR-TB can rarely be observed in new cases. It is more common in individuals in retreatment cases (prior history of TB, particularly if treatment has been inadequate, and those with HIV infection). It is a man-made phenomenon.
- Chronic cases and MDR-TB cases are not synonymous. Chronic patients probably have MDR-TB because they have previously received at least two full courses of treatment with essential antituberculous drugs.
☐ **Extensive drug-resistance TB (XDR-TB):**
  - Extensively drug-resistance TB is a form of TB that is resistant to at least four of the core anti-TB drugs. These drugs include most important (core) anti-TB drugs—(1) isoniazid and (2) rifampicin and (3) injectable second-line aminoglycoside drugs (amikacin, capreomycin, or kanamycin) + (4) fluoroquinolone (such as ofloxacin or moxifloxacin).
☐ **Totally drug-resistant TB or (extremely XXDR, TDR):**
  - Totally drug-resistant tuberculosis (TDR-TB) is a form of TB strains that shows in vitro resistance to all first- and second-line drugs tested (isoniazid, rifampicin, streptomycin, ethambutol, pyrazinamide, ethionamide, para-aminosalicylic acid, cycloserine, ofloxacin, amikacin, ciprofloxacin, capreomycin, and kanamycin).
  - It was first reported in 2003 from Italy. In early January 2012, twelve cases had been diagnosed in Mumbai and in all cases, the strain of TB was resistant to all first- and second-line antitubercular drugs.

Indications for Treatment with Steroids
☐ Severely ill patients, e.g., TB meningitis with decreased consciousness, neurological defects, or spinal block or severe pulmonary TB.
☐ Severe hypersensitivity reaction to anti-TB drugs
☐ To prevent exudation, its organization and stricture formation:
  - TB pericarditis with effusion or constriction
  - Large TB pleural effusion with severe symptoms
  - Meningeal tuberculosis
  - Renal tract TB to prevent ureteric scarring
  - TB laryngitis with life-threatening airway obstruction
☐ Hypoadrenalism (tuberculosis of adrenal glands)
☐ Massive lymph node enlargement with pressure effects
☐ In AIDS patient with severe manifestations of tuberculosis

Extrapulmonary Tuberculosis
Extrapulmonary sites of tuberculosis and their presentation are summarized in **Table 8.23 and Figure 8.13**.

Miliary or Disseminated TB
Miliary TB is the disseminated form of tuberculosis. The lesions are usually yellowish granulomas 1–2 mm in diameter. These lesions resemble millet seeds (hence termed miliary).

Table 8.23: Extrapulmonary sites of tuberculosis and their presentation.

Extrapulmonary site	Presentation
Pleural	Pleural effusion and pleuritis
Lymph nodes	Tuberculous lymphadenopathy (including mediastinal) nonhealing sinuses
Skeletal system	Tuberculous osteomyelitis, cold abscess, vertebral tuberculosis, and pyarthrosis
Nervous system	Tuberculous meningitis tuberculous arteritis and cerebral tuberculoma
Gastrointestinal	Ulcerations of the tongue, intestinal tuberculosis, and tuberculous peritonitis
Pericardium	Pericardial effusion and tamponade and constrictive pericarditis
Genitourinary	Renal tuberculosis, salpingitis, tubal abscess, and tuberculous epididymitis
Miscellaneous	Addison's disease (tuberculous adrenalitis), skin tuberculosis (scrofuloderma, lupus vulgaris, and tuberculids), phlyctenular keratoconjunctivitis, choroiditis, iritis, and erythema nodosum

Route of Spread

Miliary TB results from widespread hematogenous dissemination of tubercle bacilli. The tubercle bacilli may enter the bloodstream either hematogenous or lymphatic route.

Types

Clinically, the miliary TB patients may be divided into three different types—(1) classical (acute) miliary tuberculosis, (2) cryptic (obscure) miliary tuberculosis, and (3) nonreactive miliary tuberculosis.

1. **Classical (acute) miliary tuberculosis:**
   - *Age:* Can occur at any age, but more commonly affects children and young adults.
   - *Onset:* Sudden or gradual. It is usually present with insidious onset of fever, malaise, and weight loss over weeks.
   - *Other symptoms:*
     - Systemic symptoms include high-grade fever, drenching night sweats, and progressive pallor.
     - Cough and breathlessness are occasionally present.
   - *Signs:*
     - There may not be any abnormal physical signs in the lungs. Widespread crepitations may be heard late in the disease.
     - Hepatosplenomegaly may be seen.
     - *Choroidal tubercles* on ophthalmoscopy—diagnostic
2. **Cryptic (obscure) miliary tuberculosis:**
   - *Age:* Usually in the elderly
   - *Symptoms:*
     - Prolonged low-grade pyrexia is common presenting manifestation
     - Lassitude, weight loss, and general debility
   - *Signs:*
     - Hepatosplenomegaly may occur
     - Chest is usually normal
     - Choroidal tubercles are rare
3. **Nonreactive miliary tuberculosis:**
   - Rare and usually develops in elderly with disease reactivation
   - Acute severe form of tuberculous septicemia, resulting in necrotic lesions without granulomatous reaction containing numerous bacilli
   - Patients are extremely ill and die rapidly.

Diagnosis

- **Chest radiograph (Fig. 8.14):** If it shows the characteristic miliary shadows (miliary mottling), it is virtually diagnostic. Miliary mottling appears as diffuse small shadows of 1–2 mm diameter and evenly distributed throughout both lung fields. Upper zones are always involved. The early lesions

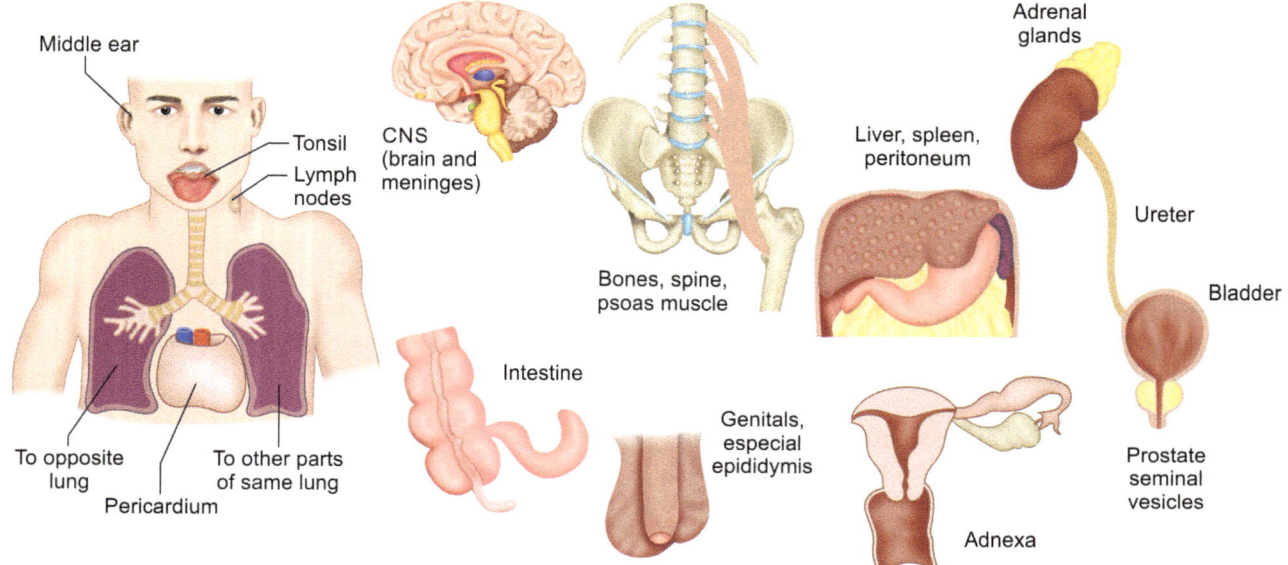

Fig. 8.13: Various extrapulmonary sites of tuberculosis.

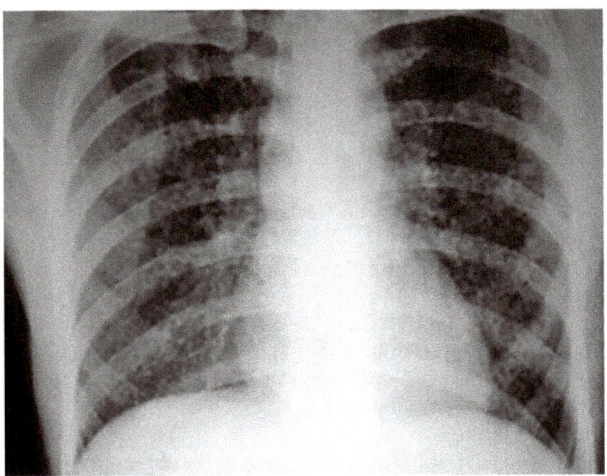

Fig. 8.14: Chest X-ray showing miliary mottling.

may be difficult to appreciate. These lesions are better visualized by—(1) an overpenetrated (dark) radiograph and a bright light behind the outer rib spaces, (2) lateral chest film, (3) underpenetrated anteroposterior radiograph, or (4) high-resolution CT of chest.
- **Positron emission tomography CT (PET-CT):** Use of radiopharmaceutical ^{18}F labeled 2-deoxy-D-glucose (FDG) may show "hot" spots. It can determine the activity of lesion, guide biopsy, and detect occult foci.
- **Sputum** smear is usually negative but bronchoalveolar lavage and bronchial biopsy are likely to be positive.
- **Culture:** Confirmation of diagnosis should be done by culture of sputum, urine, or bone marrow.
- **Hematological abnormalities:** These include anemia, leukopenia, neutrophilic leukocytosis, and leukemoid reaction. Rarely, disseminated intravascular coagulation (DIC) can develop.
- Elevation of alkaline phosphatase and other liver enzymes may be observed in patient with severe liver involvement.
- Hyponatremia may develop in about 50% cases.
- **Bone marrow biopsy:** It may show miliary tubercles/bacilli on histology. Part of the specimen should be sent for culture for tubercle bacilli.
- **Liver biopsy:** May show miliary tubercles.
- **Tuberculin test:** Only of limited value in miliary tuberculosis.

Management
- **Acute and cryptic miliary tuberculosis:** Standard antituberculous chemotherapy. In severely ill patients, prednisolone is given along with chemotherapy. It reduces life-threatening toxicity and gives time for antituberculous drugs to act.
- **If the diagnosis is not proved (e.g., cryptic miliary tuberculosis):** Therapeutic trial of antituberculous chemotherapy.

Tuberculous Pleural Effusion
- **Age group:** Tuberculous pleural effusion usually occurs in *younger individuals*.
- **Underlying pulmonary tuberculosis:** *Only one-third* of patients show simultaneous pulmonary tuberculosis.

Pleural Fluid Analysis
- **Color:** Fluid is usually straw/amber colored, but sometimes hemorrhagic.
- **Exudative in nature:** Characteristically fluid is an exudate, with a high-protein content (>3 g/dL) >50% of that in serum (usually 4–6 g/dL), a normal to low glucose concentration, a pH of –7.3 (occasionally <7.2) and raised white blood cells (usually 500–6,000/µL).
- **Cells:** *Predominant lymphocytosis*. Neutrophils may predominate in the early stage (less than 2 weeks), but lymphocytosis is the typical finding later. Mesothelial cells are usually rare or absent. If the pleural fluid shows more than 10% eosinophils, diagnosis of tuberculous effusion is unlikely unless the patient has a pneumothorax or had previously undergone thoracocentesis.
- **Smear for AFB:** Smears prepared from the centrifuged deposit may rarely show the tubercle bacilli (<10% of immunocompetent cases).
- **Culture for *M. tuberculosis*:** Positive in approximately 25–50% of patients and are more common among post-primary/secondary cases.
- **Determination of the pleural concentration of adenosine deaminase (ADA):** It is a useful screening test, and TB can be excluded, if the value is very low.
  - It is a T-lymphocyte enzyme.
  - In majority of cases, the levels of *ADA in the pleural fluid are elevated* (>40 IU/L) and is probably due to increased activity of T lymphocytes (CD4+) in the pleural fluid.
  - Other causes with high ADA include rheumatoid arthritis, lymphoma, chronic lymphatic leukemia, empyema, and mesothelioma. However, because the incidence of tuberculosis far exceeds than any other cause of a lymphocytic pleural effusion (like in India), high ADA level has a predictive value.
  - Specificity of raised levels of ADA in diagnosing tuberculous effusion is nearly 0.83 and the reported sensitivity is 77–100%. Specificity increases when pleural fluid lymphocytes/polymorph ratio is greater than 3.
  - ADA is not useful in HIV patients with TB.
  - There are two isoenzymes of ADA namely ADA1 and ADA2. ADA1 isoenzyme is found in all cells and they are high in lymphocytes and monocytes. ADA2 isoenzyme is present only in monocytes. In *tuberculous pleural effusion, ADA2 isoenzyme* is mainly responsible for high ADA concentration.
- **Interferon-gamma (INF-γ):** It is produced by lymphocytes specifically sensitized to PPD. Its level above 140 pg/mL is suggestive of TB and is elevated irrespective of immune status. It is more expensive than ADA.
- **Other tests on pleural fluid:** These include raised lactate dehydrogenase (LDH), raised lysozymes, marked elevation in the levels of soluble interleukin-2 (IL-2) receptors, and polymerase chain reaction (PCR) for DNA of *M. tuberculosis*. Nucleic acid amplification technology has low sensitivity.

- **Pleural biopsy:** Closed pleural biopsy shows noncaseating granulomas in 80% of patients. It should be stained with Z-N stain and cultured for mycobacteria. Diagnostic yield increases to 90% with pleural biopsy and biopsy cultures for AFB.

Management
- *Therapeutic aspiration of pleural fluid*: It may be required in patients with severe symptoms.
- *Antituberculous chemotherapy*
- *Corticosteroid*: It may reduce the symptoms of toxemia. However, they do not reduce the incidence of pleural fibrosis. Prednisolone is administered in the dose of 0.75 mg/kg/day for up to 4 weeks with gradual reduction over an additional 2–4 weeks.

SUPPURATIVE LUNG DISEASE

Bronchiectasis

Definition: Bronchiectasis is defined as an *irreversible* (permanent), *abnormal dilation of the cartilage-containing airways bronchi or bronchioles.*

Classification (Box 8.5)
- **According to the shape of the bronchial dilation (Figs. 8.15A to C)** and based on the bronchographic appearance (Reid's classification)
- **According to the extent of involvement:**
  - **Diffuse (generalized) bronchiectasis:** It is *characterized by* widespread bronchiectatic changes throughout the lung. It is *usually bilateral* and commonly affects the *lower lobes. Left lobe is more commonly involved than the right.* It is most severe in distal bronchi and bronchioles.
  - **Focal (localized) bronchiectasis:** Bronchiectatic change is *restricted to a* localized area of the lung *(single segment of the lung)* and usually occurs in association with obstruction of the airway (parenchymal tumor or aspiration of foreign bodies).
- **According to the underlying disease/mechanism:**
  - Congenital/acquired
  - Cystic fibrosis (CF) associated and non-CF bronchiectasis
  - *Associated with post-fibrosis*: Traction bronchiectasis
  - *Without much expectorant*: Dry bronchiectasis

Clinical Features
- **Severe persistent (chronic) productive cough:** It is the most common symptom. Cough is chronic, daily, and persistent. *Paroxysms of cough develop when the patient rises in the morning* because the postural changes drain the collections of pus and secretions into the bronchi. Sputum production varies with posture.
- **Sputum:** It is *foul-smelling* (due to anaerobic infections), thick, copious, tenacious, and continuously purulent, sometimes bloody.
- **Hemoptysis:** Streaks of blood are common with exacerbations of infection and are commonly recurrent.

Box 8.5: Causes of bronchiectasis.

Congenital:
- Cystic fibrosis (CF)
- **Ciliary dysfunction syndromes:**
  - Primary ciliary dyskinesia (immotile cilia syndrome) and Young's syndrome
  - Kartagener's syndrome (sinusitis and transposition of the viscera)
- Primary hypogammaglobulinemia, alpha-1 antitrypsin deficiency
- *Others*: Bronchial cysts, cul-de-sacs, bronchomalacia, atopic bronchial asthma, pulmonary sequestration, Mounier–Kuhn syndrome, or tracheobronchomegaly, Williams–Campbell syndrome (bronchomalacia)

Acquired: Children—
- Pneumonia (complicating whooping cough or measles)
- Primary tuberculosis
- Inhaled foreign body

Acquired: Adults—
- Pulmonary tuberculosis, *M. avium* complex (MAC)
- Suppurative pneumonia
- Allergic bronchopulmonary aspergillosis complicating asthma (ABPA)
- **Postobstructive bronchiectasis:** Partial or total obstruction of the bronchial lumen, e.g., endobronchial tumors or foreign bodies, enlarged hilar lymph nodes or tumor masses, and bronchostenosis following endobronchial tuberculosis
- Autoimmune diseases, e.g., rheumatoid arthritis, Sjögren's syndrome, systemic lupus erythematosus, and inflammatory bowel disease
- **Others:** Repeated aspiration of gastric juice, inhalation of toxic gas (ammonia), HIV infection, interstitial lung fibrosis (traction bronchiectasis), radiation fibrosis, sarcoidosis, chronic hypersensitivity pneumonitis, and bronchiolitis obliterans after lung transplantation

Proximal bronchiectasis: In which dilatation involves larger airways:
- Allergic bronchopulmonary aspergillosis (ABPA)
- **Brock's syndrome/middle lobe syndrome:** Primary TB/foreign body/tumor compressing main bronchus
- **Lady Windermere syndrome:** These women have the habit of voluntarily suppressing cough. It results in inability to clear the secretions from the right middle lobe and lingual leading to infection and later bronchiectasis.

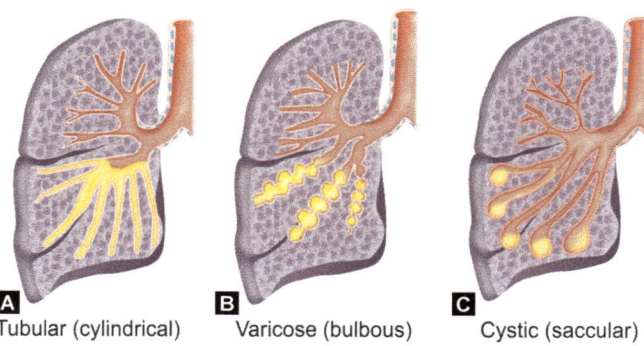

Figs. 8.15A to C: Morphological types of bronchiectasis: (A) Cylindrical type; (B) Fusiform type; (C) Saccular.

Rarely massive hemoptysis occurs. Hemoptysis occurs due to rupture of the thin-walled blood vessels present on the walls of dilated bronchi.
- **Pleuritic (chest) pain:** It may be caused due to infection of pleura, or due to segmental collapse caused by retained secretions.
- **Infective exacerbation:** Increased sputum volume with fever, malaise, and anorexia is precipitated by upper respiratory tract infections.
- **General debility:** In severe/widespread bronchiectasis, the patient presents with difficulty maintaining weight, anorexia, exertional breathlessness/dyspnea, wheezing, and orthopnea.
- **Bronchiectasis sicca/dry bronchiectasis:** Occasionally, the patient is asymptomatic or has nonproductive cough. It is termed as bronchiectasis sicca and commonly follows tuberculosis of upper lobe. Only manifestation will be hemoptysis.
- Situs inversus is found in 50% cases of ciliary dyskinesia.

Physical findings:
General examination: It may reveal anemia, *pandigital clubbing* (7% cases), fever, weight loss, night sweat, weakness, *halitosis* (may accompany purulent sputum), and sinusitis. Signs and symptoms of lung infection, such as fever, may not be present.

Respiratory system:
- Nasal polyps and signs of chronic sinusitis may be present.
- Signs may be unilateral, but are usually bilateral and basal. In dry bronchiectasis, no abnormal physical signs may be found.
- *Auscultation*: It reveals *crackles* and wheezing. Presence of large amounts of secretion is responsible for the characteristic *"bilateral, coarse, and leathery crepitations"* of bronchiectasis, which may be palpable (tactile fremitus).

Investigations
- **Blood:** Anemia, raised ESR, and leukocytosis indicating suppuration. Arterial blood gas (ABG) studies may show respiratory alkalosis or hypoxemia.
- **Sputum examination:**
  - If sputum is collected in a conical flask and allowed to stand, it forms three layers (*"three-layered sputum"*), top mucoid layer, middle mucopurulent layer, and purulent layer at the bottom.
  - Stain the sputum by Gram's stain, Ziehl–Neelsen stain for acid fast bacilli
  - *Culture and sensitivity*: Culture usually grows organism in the normal nasopharyngeal flora or *Pseudomonas*.
- **Chest radiograph (Fig. 8.16):** It lacks sensitivity. Signs on chest X-ray (CXR) include the identification of parallel linear densities, tram-track opacities, or ring shadows reflecting thickened and abnormally dilated bronchial walls.
- **Chest computed tomography (CT):** It is more specific and sensitive, and is the imaging modality of choice for confirmation for bronchiectasis. High-resolution computed tomography *(HRCT) findings* **(Fig. 8.17)** are:

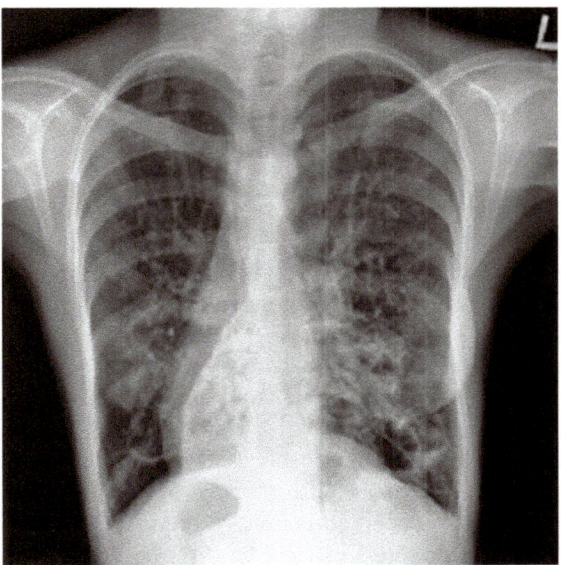

Fig. 8.16: Chest X-ray showing bilateral bronchiectasis with dextrocardia with situs inversus.

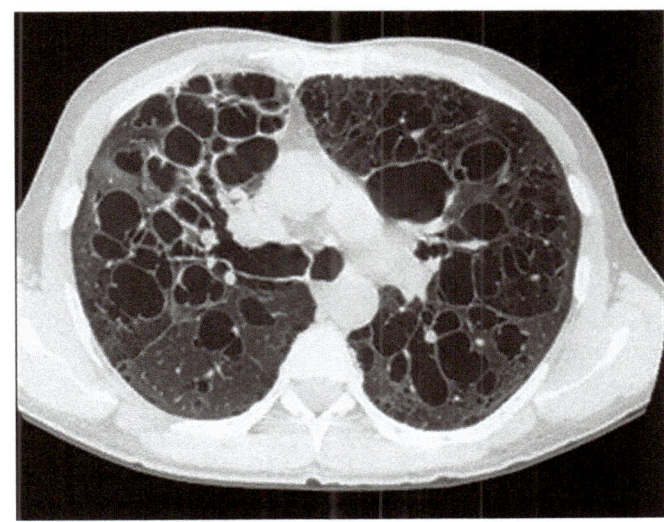

Fig. 8.17: High-resolution computed tomography (HRCT) image of bronchiectasis.

- *Specific criteria:*
  - Thickened, dilated airways (parallel "tram tracks" or as the "signet ring sign"). Internal diameter of the bronchus is minimum 1.5 times more than that of the nearby vessel.
  - Absence of bronchial tapering in the periphery of the chest (presence of tubular structures within 1 cm from the pleural surface)
- *Other findings:* Inspissated secretions (e.g., the "tree-in-bud pattern") or cysts arising from the bronchial wall (in cystic bronchiectasis).
- May suggest the etiology of bronchiectasis (e.g., proximal bronchiectasis suggests ABPA).
- **Sinus X-rays:** About 30% of patients have rhinosinusitis.
- **Bronchoscopy:** It does not establish the diagnosis.
  - Indications are: (1) to identify the source of secretions, (2) to identify the site of bleeding in patients with

hemoptysis, (3) therapeutically to remove secretions, and (4) localized bronchiectasis.
- **Bronchography:** It is rarely indicated.
- **Pulmonary function tests:** It may detect mild-to-moderate airflow obstruction, but a restrictive pattern evolves with advanced disease.
- **Urine examination:** In advanced and chronic cases, proteinuria may develop due to renal amyloidosis.
- **Electrocardiogram:** Usually normal, but right ventricular hypertrophy may be detected when cor pulmonale develops.
- **Sweat electrolytes:** Measurement of sodium and chloride concentrations in sweat is useful in cystic fibrosis.
- **Serum immunoglobulins:** Up to 10% of adults with bronchiectasis have antibody class or subclass deficiency (mainly IgA). Its estimation is also useful when primary hypogammaglobulinemia is suspected.
- **Patients suspected of ciliary dysfunction syndrome:** Assessment of ciliary function may be done by several ways:
  - *Mucociliary clearance (nasal clearance of saccharin*

Complications of Bronchiectasis
- Hemoptysis
- Pneumonia
- Lung abscess
- Empyema
- Cor pulmonale
- Septicemia
- Meningitis
- Osteomyelitis
- Metastatic abscesses (e.g., brain abscess)
- Generalized edema (100 mL sputum/4-5 g protein)—protein-losing pneumopathy
- Generalized amyloidosis
- Aspergilloma
- Respiratory failure
- Microbial resistance to antibiotics

Management
Improvements in secretion clearance and bronchial hygiene:
- Bronchial hygiene so as to reduce the microbial load within the airways and minimize the risk of repeated infections.
- Many methods are used to increase secretion clearance in bronchiectasis. These include chest physiotherapy (e.g., postural drainage), hydration, and mucolytic administration, aerosolization of bronchodilators, and hyperosmolar agents (e.g., hypertonic saline).
- **Postural drainage:** Postural drainage is valuable and consists of adopting a position in which the affected lobe(s) to be drained is uppermost. Patients must be trained by physiotherapists and this should be performed at least three times daily for 5-10 minutes. Lying over the side of the bed with head and thorax down is effective in most patients. Gentle mechanical chest percussion through hand clapping to the chest helps to dislodge the sputum.
- Bronchoscopic removal of inspissated secretions is rarely necessary.

Antibiotic therapy:
Antibiotics for eradication of bacteria:
For *Pseudomonas*: Oral ciprofloxacin (500-750 mg twice daily) or ceftazidime by intravenous injection or infusion (1-2 g three times daily) for 7-10 days.

Suppressive antibiotics:
- After resolution of an acute infection in patients with recurrences, the use of suppressive antibiotics may minimize the microbial load and reduce the frequency of exacerbations.
- Inhaled antibiotics are safe and effective, e.g., tobramycin and gentamicin.

Antibiotics for exacerbation:
- Choice of the antibiotic depends on the results of culture and sensitivity of sputum.
- If no specific pathogen is identified and the patient is not seriously ill, oral agents, such as amoxicillin, ampicillin, cotrimoxazole, tetracycline, one of the fluoroquinolones or a fixed combination of amoxicillin, and clavulanic acid are recommended.
- More seriously ill patients with pneumonitis require parenteral antibiotics.
- **Duration of therapy:** Usually, a 7-10-day course is sufficient. Few patients may need prolonged therapy for several weeks.

Anti-inflammatory therapy:
- Control of the inflammatory response may be of benefit in bronchiectasis.
- Inhaled or oral steroids can reduce the rate of progression of bronchiectasis.
- **Macrolide antibiotics:** They have immunomodulatory action.

Reversal of airflow obstruction:
- Bronchodilators (β-adrenoreceptor agonists, anticholinergics) improve obstruction and help in clearance of secretion. They are useful in patients with demonstrable airflow limitation.
- Inhaled corticosteroids may be useful in some patients.

Surgical treatment:
- It can be considered only in refractory cases.
- The procedure involved is excision of bronchiectatic areas. It is usually done in cases where the bronchiectasis is restricted to a single lobe or segment on CT.
- **Indications of surgery:**
  - Children or young adults with localized lesions who fail to respond to medical treatment
  - Recurrent hemoptysis
  - Recurrent localized pneumonias
- Lung transplantation is considered in patients with advanced disease and respiratory failure.
- **Treatment of the hemoptysis:** Bed rest and antibiotics. Blood transfusion is given, if necessary. Occasionally, fiberoptic bronchoscopy is needed to detect the source of bleeding. If the hemoptysis continues, embolization of bronchial artery is the treatment of choice. Surgical resection may be needed, if embolization fails.

Other measures:
- **General management:** Graded exercise, routine deep breathing, and maintenance of good nutrition
- Vaccination
- Promptly treat episodes of sinusitis
- Treat complicated ABPA with prednisolone and itraconazole
- Mucolytic dornase (DNase) is recommended in cystic fibrosis (CF)-related bronchiectasis. It reduces viscosity of sputum by breaking down DNA released from neutrophils.

Bronchiectasis Sicca (Dry Bronchiectasis)
- Usually bronchiectasis presents with copious sputum.
- *Bronchiectasis sicca* is a condition where bronchiectasis presents with repeated episodes of hemoptysis without sputum production.
- It usually occurs in bronchiectasis of upper lobe following tuberculosis.

ATELECTASIS
- Atelectasis refers either to *incomplete expansion of the lungs* (neonatal atelectasis) or to the *complete collapse* of previously inflated lung parenchyma.
- It produces areas of relatively airless pulmonary parenchyma.

Classification
Main types of acquired atelectasis are:
1. **Obstructive atelectasis (absorption atelectasis):**
   - It is most common type
   - *Mechanism:* Complete obstruction (intrabronchial) of an airway causes obstruction of communication between the alveoli and major airways. This leads to absorption of air from the dependent alveoli, diminished lung volume, shifting of the mediastinum toward the atelectatic lung.
   - *Causes:* Due to complete obstruction (intrabronchial) of an airway.
     - Exogenous, e.g., foreign body aspiration, or recurrent aspiration of either gastric or oral contents due to a swallowing disorder
     - Endogenous, e.g., excessive secretions (e.g., mucus plugs) or exudates within smaller bronchi, (e.g., in bronchial asthma, chronic bronchitis, bronchiectasis, and postoperative states), bronchial tumors
2. **Nonobstructive atelectasis:**
   - *Compression atelectasis:*
     - Develops due to compression of lung
     - *Causes:* It develops from any space-occupying lesion of the thorax (e.g., tumors, cysts, enlarged lymph nodes, and cardiomegaly). It can also occur with chest wall defects (e.g., scoliosis), neuromuscular diseases, and compression by emphysematous bulla.
     - In compression atelectasis, the mediastinum shifts away from the affected lung.
   - *Relaxation or passive atelectasis:*
     - Contact between visceral and parietal pleura is lost resulting in passive atelectasis of lung
     - *Causes:* Significant volumes of fluid (transudate, exudate, or blood) or air (*pneumothorax*) accumulation within the pleural cavity.
   - *Fibrotic or cicatrisation or contraction atelectasis:* It occurs when focal or generalized pulmonary or pleural fibrosis prevents full expansion of lung.
3. **Atelectasis due to surfactant deficiency or dysfunction:**
   - Surfactant deficiency or dysfunction causes increased alveolar surface tension and failure to maintain small airway patency.
   - *Causes:* ARDS (particularly in preterm neonates and meconium aspiration), and pneumonia in elderly.

Clinical Features
- Depend on the underlying cause, the degree of volume loss within the lung, and rate of volume loss.
- No symptoms may develop when atelectasis develops slowly.
- Chronic atelectasis may be a nidus of chronic purulent infection. This may damage bronchial wall leading to bronchiectasis.
- **Physical examination:**
  - Reduced chest movement during breathing on the involved region.
  - Deviation of trachea and apex beat toward affected side.
  - Dullness over the involved region
  - Absence of breath sounds over involved region. There are no added sounds.

Investigations
- **Chest radiograph (Fig. 8.18) and CT chest findings:**
  - Homogenous opacification of the *atelectatic region*
  - Displacement of fissure
  - Loss of volume and shift of trachea and mediastinum
- Bronchoscopy to identify obstructive lesions and is also useful in removing the mucus plug.
- Arterial blood gas may reveal hypoxemia. Hypocapnia may develop due to tachypnea.

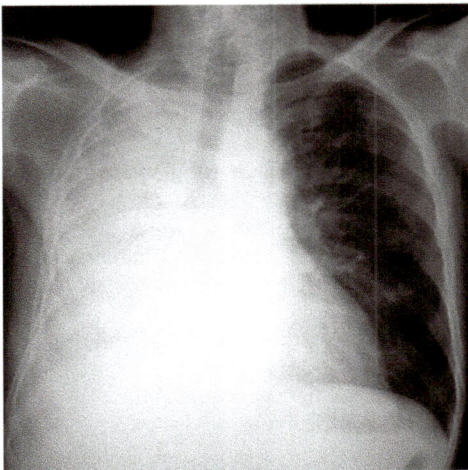

Fig. 8.18: Chest X-ray shows collapse of the right lung.

Treatment of Collapse

- Emergency bronchoscopy and removal of mucus plug and foreign body
- Treatment of underlying cause

LUNG ABSCESS

Definition: Lung (pulmonary) abscess is defined as a severe, *local suppurative process within the lung* associated with cavity formation. It is characterized by necrotic area of lung parenchyma containing *pus accompanied by the destruction of lung tissue. Necrotizing pneumonia*: It is often used to describe similar pathologic process with multiple small (<2 cm) cavities in contiguous areas of the lung.

Classification

- **Duration of symptoms prior to diagnosis:** Acute <1 month, and chronic >1 month
- **Primary or secondary**

Etiology (Box 8.6)

- **Infectious causes:** Any pathogen can produce lung abscess
- **Noninfectious causes**

Box 8.6: Causes of lung abscess.

A. **Infectious causes:**
 1. *Bacteria:*
    - *Usual*: Mouth flora anaerobes, most frequently isolated anaerobes—Peptostreptococcus, Fusobacterium nucleatum, and Prevotella melaninogenica
    - *Less common*: Staphylococcus aureus, Streptococcus pyogenes, Pseudomonas aeruginosa, Klebsiella pneumoniae, Streptococcus pneumoniae, gram-negative bacilli, such as E. coli, Haemophilus influenzae type B, Legionella, and Nocardia asteroides. Mixed infections occur when lung abscess develops due to inhalation of foreign material
    - *Mycobacteria*: M. tuberculosis, M. avium complex, M. kansasii, and other mycobacteria
 2. *Fungi*: Aspergillus species, Histoplasma capsulatum, Pneumocystis jirovecii, Coccidioides immitis, Blastocystis hominis, and Cryptococcus
 3. *Parasites*: Entamoeba histolytica, Paragonimus westermani, and Strongyloides stercoralis (postobstructive)

B. **Noninfectious causes:**
 1. *Neoplasms:* Primary lung cancer, metastatic carcinoma, and lymphoma
 2. *Pulmonary infarction:* Due to bland embolus (may be secondarily infected in <5%)
 3. *Septic embolism:* Tricuspid endocarditis due to S. aureus and others (typically with positive blood cultures), jugular venous septic phlebitis due to Fusobacterium necrophorum (Lemierre syndrome)
 4. *Vasculitis*: Wegener's granulomatosis and rheumatoid lung nodule
 5. *Developmental:* Pulmonary sequestration
 6. *Airway disease:* Bullae, blebs, or cystic bronchiectasis (usually thin-walled)
 7. *Other:* Sarcoidosis, transdiaphragmatic bowel herniation giving appearance of cavity with air fluid level

---

Clinical Features

Lung abscess may present either as an acute (symptoms less than 1 month) or chronic (symptoms more than 1 month).

- **Acute:**
  - Majority present acutely with dry *cough*, high-grade *fever*, chills, rigors, and pleuritic chest pain
  - After a few days, when the abscess ruptures into a patent bronchus, the patient suddenly starts expectorating *large amounts of foul-smelling purulent or sanguineous sputum*. The sputum may often be blood-tinged and expectoration *varies with posture.*
- **Chronic:** Lung abscess secondary to aspiration often presents as chronic, insidious in onset with low-grade fever, malaise, weight loss, anorexia, and a deep-seated chest *pain*/discomfort.

Physical Findings

- **General examination:** Anemia, fever, *clubbing of the fingers and toes* (may develop rapidly), *halitosis,* and oronasal sepsis.
- **Respiratory system examination:**
  - *Early stages*: May be normal
  - *Later*:
    - *Signs of consolidation:* Dullness of percussion, increased vocal fremitus and vocal resonance, bronchial breathing, crepitations, and pleural rub.
    - *Signs of cavitation:* Once the abscess opens into a bronchus, signs of cavitation, such as cavernous or amphoric bronchial breathing and coarse post-tussive crepitations are heard on auscultation.

Investigations

- **Blood:** Normocytic anemia and/or raised inflammatory markers (ESR/CRP), leukocytosis, and raised ESR.
- **Sputum:**
  - Gram's stain, Ziehl–Neelsen staining for acid-fast bacilli
  - *Culture and sensitivity*: For aerobic and anaerobic
  - *Cytological examination*: For malignant cells
- **Chest radiograph (Fig. 8.19):** It reveals radiolucency in an opaque area of consolidation. The wall of the abscess cavity completely surrounds the radiolucent area. An air-fluid level may be seen in the abscess cavity.

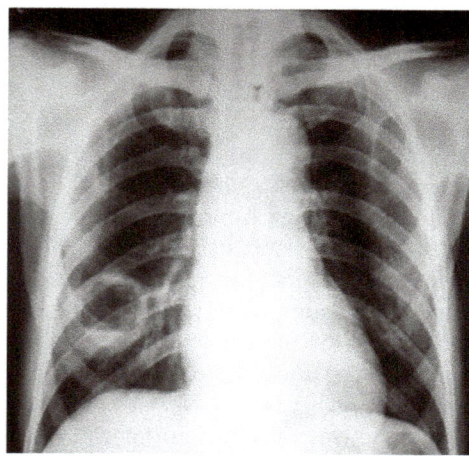

Fig. 8.19: Chest X-ray shows lung abscess in right lower zone.

- **CT scan of thorax:** It shows lung abscess.
- **Bronchoscopy:** It is indicated (1) to exclude malignancy, (2) to obtain specimens for studies, and (3) for removal of secretions.

Complications

Complications of lung abscess:
- *Extension of the infection into the pleural cavity*: Leading to empyema/pneumothorax/pyopneumothorax/bronchopleural fistula/pleural effusion/pleurocutaneous fistula
- Hemorrhage into the abscess cavity
- Hemoptysis
- Septic emboli may cause metastatic brain abscesses or meningitis
- Secondary amyloidosis (type AA)
- Aspergilloma
- Residual fibrosis and bronchiectasis

Treatment

- **Postural drainage** (refer bronchiectasis) and chest physiotherapy.
- **Antibiotic therapy:** Choice of drug depends on culture and sensitivity result. Broad guidelines include:
  - *Aspiration abscess:* Antibiotic therapy is similar to that of aspiration pneumonia.
  - *Oral treatment:* Majority respond to oral treatment with ampicillin 500 mg four times daily or cotrimoxazole 960 mg twice daily or clindamycin 300 mg thrice daily.
  - *Anaerobic bacterial infection*, e.g., patients with foul-smelling sputum, oral metronidazole 400 mg 8 hourly should be combined with the above oral treatment. It should not be used alone.
  - *Parenteral antibiotic therapy:* It is required in seriously ill patients and consists of β-lactamase inhibitor [e.g., ampicillin-sulbactam 3 g intravenously (IV) every 6 hours] or a carbapenem (e.g., imipenem and meropenem) with clindamycin and metronidazole.
- **Duration of antibiotic therapy:** It is usually given for 4–6 weeks. Antibiotic treatment should be continued until the chest radiograph has shown either the resolution of lung abscess or the presence of a small stable lesion. There is a risk of relapse with shorter antibiotic regimen.
- **Large lung abscess:** Aspiration and placement of pigtail catheters may be useful.
- **Resectional surgery:** It is indicated in few cases. These include:
  - Massive hemoptysis
  - Lung abscess associated with symptomatic bronchiectasis
  - Lung abscess associated with localized malignancy
  - Persistent lung abscess cavity

The surgical procedure is either lobectomy or pneumonectomy. Consider lobectomy/pneumonectomy with large cavities (>8 cm), resistant organisms, such as *Pseudomonas*, obstructing neoplasm, or massive hemorrhage.

CYSTIC FIBROSIS

Cystic fibrosis is a fatal multisystem genetic disorder because of abnormal ion transport function causing inability to adequately hydrate mucus.

Genetics and Pathogenesis

It is transmitted as an autosomal-recessive disorder and characterized by mutation in a gene on the long arm of chromosome 7. This gene codes for a chloride channel known as cystic fibrosis transmembrane conductance regulator (*CFTR*). This influences salt and water movement across epithelial cell membranes.

CFTR Protein

- It is normally present in epithelia and functions as cAMP-regulated chloride ion channel and as inhibitor of Na^+ channels.
- Mutation in *CFTR* gene causes intracellular degradation of CFTR. Thus, epithelial membranes are unable to secrete chloride ion in response to cAMP-mediated signals.

Clinical Features

- Most patients present in infancy. Earliest presentation is *meconium ileus*. Pancreatic and intestinal manifestations occur early.
- Pulmonary manifestations occur late. After the neonatal period, maximum morbidity and mortality are due to pulmonary disease.

Respiratory Tract

- **Upper respiratory tract:** Chronic sinusitis, rhinorrhea, and nasal polyps
- **Lower respiratory tract:**
  - Earliest functional abnormality is small airways disease and earliest symptom is cough. Final expression is bronchiectasis. Earliest and most severe changes in *right upper lobe*.
  - Persistent cough → viscous, purulent sputum. Intermittent exacerbations → increased cough, increased sputum volume, decrements in pulmonary function, weight loss. As exacerbations become more frequent, lung function deteriorates → eventually, respiratory failure.
  - *Pathogens*: In newly diagnosed patients include *H. influenzae* and *S. aureus* and in established diseases *Pseudomonas aeruginosa* (mucoid form).
  - *Chest X-ray*: Earliest manifestation is hyperinflation later bronchiectatic changes.
  - *Pulmonary function tests*: Obstructive pattern with partial bronchodilator response.
  - *Complications*: Pneumothorax, hemoptysis, clubbing, respiratory failure, and cor pulmonale.

Gastrointestinal Tract

- Most common is *exocrine pancreatic insufficiency*: Steatorrhea, azotorrhea → consequent malnutrition. Recognized only when secretion of amylase and lipase falls below 90%.
- Endocrine pancreatic insufficiency occurs in 10% much later
- *Others*: Intestinal obstruction, appendicitis, and recurring acute or chronic pancreatitis
- Increased incidence of GI malignancy

Genitourinary Tract

- Late onset of puberty in both males and females
- 95% azoospermic, 20% women infertile, and 90% completed pregnancies produce viable infants; breastfeeding normal.
- Retardation of bone age and heat stroke

Treatment

- **Lung disease:**
  - *Clear secretions:* By breathing exercises, flutter valves, chest percussion, and recombinant human DNAse.
  - *Infection:* Long courses of culture and sensitivity-guided antibiotic therapy; higher doses required; oral/IV/aerosolized.
  - *Inhaled β-agonists/anticholinergics:* Short-term benefit. O_2 and medical management are temporary measures.
  - Long-term high dose NSAID (some patients)
  - *The only effective therapy for respiratory failure in CF:* Lung transplantation
- **Gastrointestinal:**
  - Pancreatic enzyme replacement (microsphere formulation)
  - Replacement of fat-soluble vitamins
  - **Treatment of acute obstruction:** Enema of hypertonic radio-contrast material (megalodiatrizoate)
- **Reproductive:** Assisted reproductive technology

PLEURAL EFFUSION

Definition: Excessive accumulation of serous fluid within the pleural cavity/space (between parietal pleura and visceral pleura). It can be detected on X-ray when ≥300 mL of fluid is accumulated and clinically, when a minimum of 500 mL is present.

- **Empyema:** Accumulation of purulent fluid (frank pus) within the pleural cavity/space.
- **Hydrothorax:** Passive transudation of fluid into the pleural cavity. It occurs in congestive heart failure, nephrotic syndrome, cirrhosis of liver, severe malnutrition, etc.
- **Hemothorax:** Accumulation of blood within the pleural cavity/space
- **Chylothorax:** Accumulation of chyle within the pleural cavity/space

Classification and Causes

Table 8.24 describes the normal composition of pleural fluid.

Table 8.24: Normal composition of pleural fluid.

Feature	Normal value
Volume	0.1–0.2 mL/kg
Cells	1,000–5,000/mm³
• Mesothelial cells	3–70%
• Monocytes	30–70%
• Lymphocytes	2–30%
• Granulocytes	~10%
• Eosinophils	0%
Protein	1–2 g/dL
Albumin	50–70%
Glucose	~Plasma level
LDH	<50% plasma level

(LDH: lactate dehydrogenase)

Table 8.25: Classification and causes of pleural effusion.

Types of effusion	Causes	
Transudative effusion	• Cardiac failure • Hypoproteinemia (e.g., nephrotic syndrome, cirrhosis of liver, and severe malnutrition) • Constrictive pericarditis	• Hypothyroidism • Meigs syndrome (benign ovarian tumors with ascites and pleural effusion) • Peritoneal dialysis
Exudative effusion	• Tuberculosis • Bacterial pneumonia • Malignancy • Pulmonary infarction • Autoimmune diseases (e.g., rheumatoid arthritis, systemic lupus erythematosus) • Acute pancreatitis • Postmyocardial infarction syndrome (Dressler's syndrome)	• Drug-induced effusion • Benign asbestos-related effusion • Intra-abdominal abscess • Meigs' syndrome (can be transudative as well) • Ruptured amebic liver abscess, chylous pleural effusion • Acute rheumatic fever

Table 8.25 describes the classification and causes of pleural effusion.

Clinical Features

- **Symptoms (pain on inspiration and coughing) and signs of pleurisy (a pleural rub):** They often precede the development of a pleural effusion.
- **Breathlessness:** It may be the only symptom and its severity depends on the size and rate of accumulation of fluid.

Physical Findings in the Chest

- **Inspection:** *Tachypnea.* Shift of trachea to opposite side
- **Palpation:**
  - *Shift of trachea and mediastinum* (shift of apex beat) to the opposite side
  - *Reduced chest movements* on the affected side, bulging of the intercostal spaces, fullness of the affected chest, and markedly reduced vocal fremitus
  - *Measurements*: Diminished chest expansion, increase in the size of the affected hemithorax, and an increase in spinoscapular distance
- **Percussion:**
  - *Stony dullness* over the fluid. Upper level of the dullness is highest laterally in the axilla and is lower anteriorly and posteriorly (*Ellis-S-Shaped curve*).
  - *Small effusions*: When there is a small effusion, it may be detected as follows—
    - *Left-sided* small pleural effusion may be detected only by the obliteration of Traube's space on percussion.
    - *Right-sided* small effusion may be detectable only by tidal percussion.
  - *Moderate-to-large effusions*: Percussion reveals a triangular area of dullness or impaired note over the

> **Box 8.7:** Causes of left-sided pleural effusion.
>
> - Pancreatitis
> - Pericardial inflammation
> - Rupture of esophagus
> - Left-sided subdiaphragmatic abscess
> - Thoracic duct involvement above D_3 level

back of chest on the contralateral side or opposite side of the effusion. It may be due to shift of the posterior mediastinum to the opposite side by effusion.

Causes of pleural effusion without tracheal mediastinal shift are listed in **Box 8.7**.

- **Auscultation:**
  - *Breath sounds: Intensity is markedly diminished* or absent over the fluid
  - *Vocal resonance: Markedly diminished* over the fluid
  - Bronchial breathing at the level of pleural effusion
  - *Occasional findings*: Egophony and enhanced breath sounds can often be appreciated at the superior border of the effusion because of underlying atelectatic lung tissue.

Investigations

- **Radiological investigations:**
  - *75 mL of pleural fluid*: Subpulmonic space without spillover can obliterate the posterior costophrenic sulcus.
  - *Upright chest radiograph*:
    - 175 mL is required to obscure the lateral costophrenic sulcus
    - 500 mL of fluid will obscure the diaphragmatic contour
    - 1,000 mL of effusion reaches the level of the fourth anterior rib.
- **Decubitus radiographs and CT scans:** Less than 10 mL (even as little as 2 mL) can be identified.
  - Small effusions are thinner than 1.5 cm, moderate effusions are 1.5–4.5 cm thick, and large effusions exceed 4.5 cm.
  - Effusions thicker than 1 cm are usually large enough for sampling by thoracentesis, since at least 200 mL of liquid are already present.
  - A significant pleural effusion is large enough to produce a pleural fluid strip >10 mm wide on lateral decubitus radiographic views.

  Radiological features of pleural effusion in an erect chest film are shown in **Figure 8.20**.
- **Ultrasonography:** More accurate than plain chest X-ray for detection of pleural effusion and it can detect as little as 5 mL of effusion.
- Pleural aspiration and fluid analysis

Interpretation of Pleural Fluid Parameters

Light's criteria:

- Light's criteria are used to differentiate exudative from transudative pleural effusion by measuring the lactate dehydrogenase (LDH) and protein levels in the pleural fluid. Exudative pleural effusions must meet at least one of the following criteria, whereas transudative pleural effusions meet none (**Box 8.8 and Tables 8.26 and 8.27**).
- In general, Light's criteria occasionally misidentify a transudative effusion as an exudative effusion as in cardiac failure with diuretic therapy.

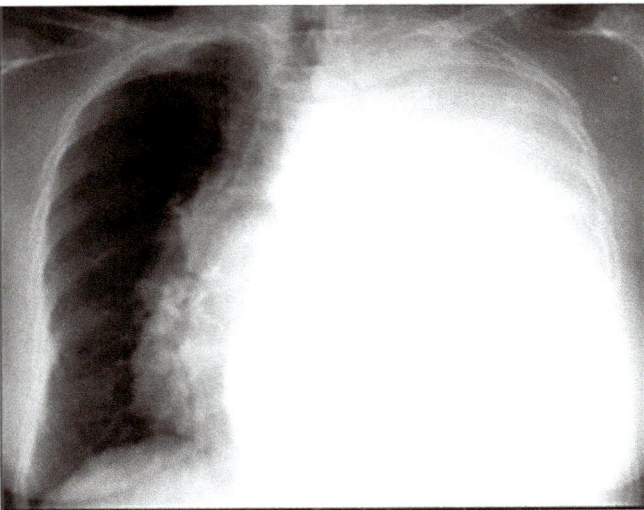

Fig. 8.20: Chest X-ray shows left-sided massive pleural effusion.

> Clinically, if a patient should have a transudative effusion, but meets Light's criteria for an exudative effusion, measure serum-pleural fluid albumin gradient, or measure the serum-pleural protein gradient *(Roth's criteria)*:
> - Serum effusion albumin gradient of >1.2 g/dL—transudative
> - Serum effusion protein gradient >3.1 g/dL—transudative

- **Pleural biopsy is indicated in undiagnosed cases**
- **Other investigations in pleural effusion:**
  - *Pleural fluid tumor markers:* Carcinoembryonic antigen (CEA), cancer antigen 125 (CA-125), cancer antigen 15-3 (CA 15-3), and cytokeratin 19 fragments (CYFRA). They are not used in routine investigations of pleural effusion.
  - *Blood examination*: Total and differential leukocyte counts, ESR, proteins, sugar, LDH, amylase, rheumatoid factor, and antinuclear factor
  - *Sputum examination:* For tubercle bacilli and malignant cells
  - *Mantoux test*

> **Box 8.8:** Modified Light's criteria for distinguishing pleural transudate from exudate.
>
> **Pleural fluid is an exudate if one or more of the following criteria are met:**
> Pleural fluid
> - Serum protein ratio >0.5
> - Serum LDH ratio >0.6
> - LDH >2/3 upper limit of normal serum LDH
> - Protein >30 g/L
>   If only one of the above criteria is met, then calculate the fluid to serum albumin gradient
> - If the albumin gradient >12 g/L, consider a transudate
>
> (LDH: lactate dehydrogenase)

Table 8.26: Differentiation of transudative from exudative effusion.

Characteristics	Transudative effusion	Exudative effusion
Cause and mechanism	Noninflammatory process. Ultrafiltrate of plasma, due to increased hydrostatic pressure or decreased serum oncotic pressure with normal vascular permeability	Inflammation process and is rich in proteins due to increased vascular permeability
Appearance	Clear and serous	Cloudy/purulent/hemorrhagic/chylous
Color	Straw yellow	Yellow to red
Specific gravity	<1.018	>1.018
Protein		
• Absolute value	Low, <2 g/dL, mainly albumin	High, >2 g/dL
• *Pleural fluid*: Serum ratio	<0.5	>0.5
Clot	Absent	Clots spontaneously because of high fibrinogen
Leukocytes		
• Total leukocytes	<1,000/mm^3	>1,000/mm^3
• Type of cells Differential leukocytes	>50% lymphocytes or mononuclear cells and mesothelial cells	>50% lymphocytes (tuberculosis, malignancy) >50% polymorphs (acute inflammation)
• Erythrocytes	<500/mm^3	Variable
Bacteria	Absent	Usually present
Lactate dehydrogenase (LDH)		
Absolute value	<200 IU/L	200 IU/L
Pleural fluid LDH: Serum LDH ratio	<0.6	>0.6
Glucose	>60 mg/dL (usually same as in blood)	<60 mg/dL (variable)

(LDH: lactate dehydrogenase)

Table 8.27: Interpretation of pleural fluid parameters.

Parameter	Interpretation
Appearance of pleural fluid	Putrid odor (anaerobic empyema), food particles (esophageal rupture), bile stained (chylothorax/biliary fistula), milky (chylothorax/pseudo-chylothorax), and anchovy sauce-like fluid (ruptured amebic abscess)
Pleural fluid glucose concentration	
Low-glucose concentration (<60 mg/dL)	Suggests empyema, malignancy, or tuberculosis
Very low-glucose concentration (<15 mg/dL)	Empyema and rheumatoid effusions
Pleural fluid eosinophilia (>10% of all cells)	May be observed in resolving infections, pneumothorax, hydropneumothorax, hemothorax and asbestos-related pleural effusion, dantrolene, bromocriptine, nitrofurantoin, paragonimiasis, or Churg–Strauss syndrome
Pleural fluid erythrocyte counts >100,000/mm^3	Most often in malignancy or pulmonary infarction/embolism, but may result from a traumatic tap
Low pH of pleural fluid <7.2	Complicated parapneumonic effusion, esophageal rupture, rheumatoid pleuritis, tuberculous pleuritis, malignant pleural disease, hemothorax, systemic acidosis, paragonimiasis, lupus pleuritis, and urinothorax
Raised pleural fluid amylase	Pancreatic diseases and esophageal rupture. However, routine amylase estimation is not recommended unless the clinical features suggest either of the two diseases
Pleural fluid antinuclear antibody titers or rheumatoid factor	No diagnostic significance and is not indicated in most cases
Mesothelial cells	*Absent*: Tuberculosis *Markedly increased*: Pulmonary embolism

- *Repeat radiograph:* When effusion is massive, a repeat radiograph after removal of a large volume of fluid may reveal an underlying parenchymal lesion.
- Biopsy or fine-needle aspiration of scalene lymph nodes
- Bronchoscopy and biopsy
- Thoracoscopy and biopsy

Approach to the Diagnosis of Pleural Effusions

Approach to the diagnosis of pleural effusions is outlined in **Flowchart 8.3**.

Causes of hemorrhagic pleural effusion	
Malignancy	Tuberculosis (very rare)
Pulmonary infarction	Postcardiac injury effusion
Asbestos-related pleural effusion	

Chylous Pleural Effusion (Chylothorax)

- **Definition:** It is the accumulation of chyle in the pleural cavity.
- **Mechanism:** A chylothorax results from leakage of chyle from the thoracic duct into the pleural space.
- **Causes:** Most common cause is trauma (most frequently during thoracic surgery). It may also result from lymphomas, lung cancer with mediastinal spread, mediastinal fibrosis, and tumors.
- **Presentation:** Dyspnea and a large pleural effusion on chest X-ray.

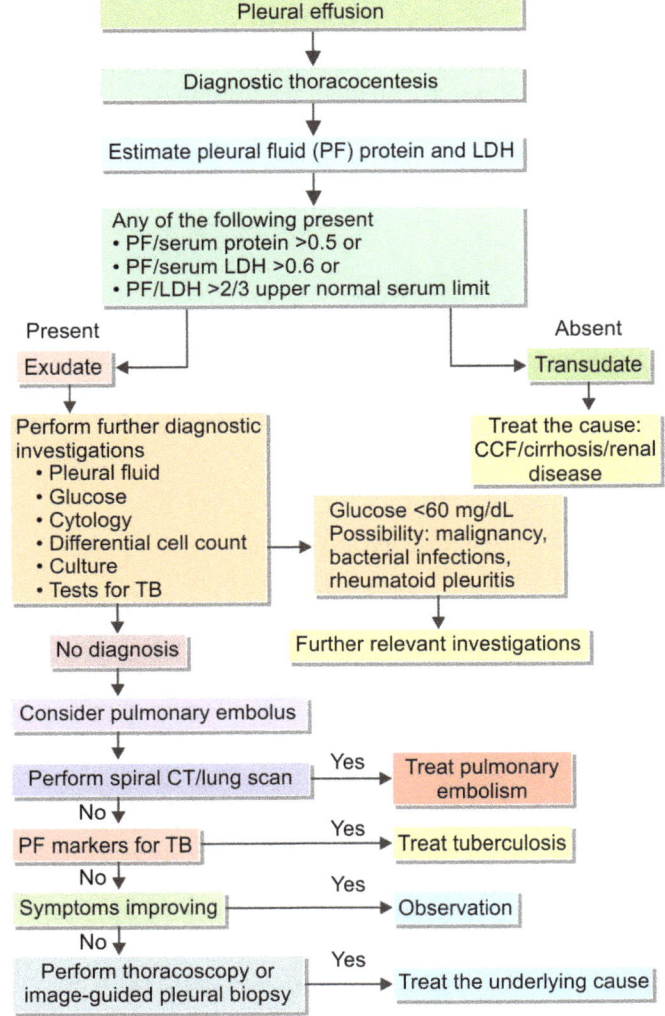

Flowchart 8.3: Approach to the diagnosis of pleural effusions.

(CCF: congestive cardiac failure)

- **Pleural fluid findings:**
  - Appears milky and shows the characteristics of exudates.
  - Total triglyceride level is >110 mg/dL. The cholesterol level is very low. Sudan III staining shows fat globules.

EMPYEMA THORACIS

Definition
- Empyema thoracis is defined as collection of pus in the pleural space/cavity. It may be as thin as serous fluid or so thick that it is impossible to aspirate, even with a wide-bore needle. Microscopically, it shows numerous neutrophil leukocytes.
- It usually involves whole pleural space/cavity and unilateral. If only a part of the pleural space is involved, it is termed encysted or loculated empyema.

Etiology
- **Spread of infection from neighboring structures:** For example, bacterial pneumonias, bronchiectasis, lung abscess, rupture of subphrenic abscess through the diaphragm, esophageal perforation, and infection of hemothorax following trauma or surgery
- **From distant source:** For example, bacteremia
- **Direct infection from external source:** For example, penetrating chest injury, chest tube placement, and thoracic surgery

Common organisms: *Pneumococcus, Streptococcus, Staphylococcus, Pseudomonas, M. tuberculosis, H. influenzae,* and anaerobes

Clinical Features
Box 8.9 describes the clinical features of empyema.

Investigations
- **Blood:** Polymorphonuclear leukocytosis and high CRP (C-reactive protein)
- **Chest X-ray:** Findings may be similar to those of pleural effusion. However, pleural adhesions may produce a "D"-shaped shadow against the inside of the chest wall (**Fig. 8.22**). If air is present along with pus (pyopneumothorax), a horizontal "fluid level" mark is detected at the air/liquid interface.
- **Ultrasound:** It shows the position of the fluid, the extent of pleural thickening, and whether fluid is collected as a single locule or multiloculated.

Box 8.9: Clinical features of empyema.

Systemic features:
- High-grade, remittent fever
- Chills, rigors, sweating, malaise, and weight loss

Respiratory symptoms: Pleuritic chest pain, breathlessness and dry cough. Copious, purulent sputum develops when the empyema ruptures into a bronchus (bronchopleural fistula)

Physical examination: Clinical signs of pleural effusion PLUS intercostals tenderness, digital clubbing, and edema of the chest wall

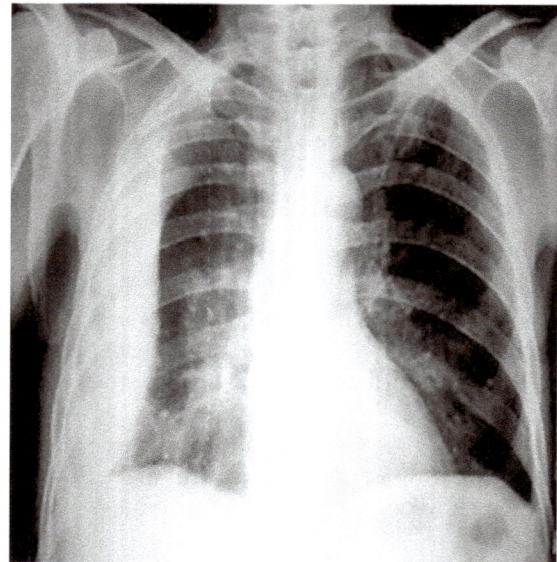

Fig. 8.22: Chest X-ray of loculated effusion—D sign.

- **Computed tomography:** It gives information regarding the pleura, underlying lung parenchyma, and patency of the major bronchi. Ultrasound or CT is used to detect the optimal site for aspiration.
- **Aspiration of empyema**—exudative with frank pus. AFB—culture can be performed.

Management of Empyema Thoracis

1. **Nontuberculous empyema:**
   Acute:
   - *Antibiotics*: It should be given depending on the culture and sensitivity report.
   - *Drainage of pus*: The pus in the pleural cavity should be drained.
     - *Aspiration*: In early and small empyema with thin fluid, daily aspiration of the fluid with a wide-bore needle is attempted.
     - *Tube drainage* is necessary in most cases.
     - *Limited thoracotomy*: If tube drainage fails or pus is thick or loculated, limited thoracotomy is performed. It involves resection of a small segment of the rib, clearing the empyema cavity, breaking down any adhesions, and introducing a wide-bore tube (for prolonged drainage).
     - Intrapleural administration of fibrinolytic agents (e.g., streptokinase) is of no benefit.
   Chronic:
   - *Surgery*:
     - Surgical "decortication" of the lung may be necessary when there is gross thickening of the visceral pleura, which is preventing re-expansion of the lung in chronic empyema. It involves stripping of the whole grossly thickened visceral pleura in order to allow the lung to re-expand.
     - Surgery is also required, if a bronchopleural fistula develops.
2. **Tuberculous empyema:**
   - *Antituberculous chemotherapy*
   - *Repeated aspiration*: Through a wide-bore needle or tube-drainage
   - Rarely, surgical treatment may be required

PNEUMOTHORAX

Definition

Presence of air/gas in the pleural cavity/space is known as pneumothorax.

Pneumothorax may be localized (if there is a prior disease causing adhesion of visceral pleura to parietal pleura) or generalized (if there are no pleural adhesions).

Classification

Classification of pneumothorax is summarized in **Flowchart 8.4**.

Etiology

Spontaneous Pneumothorax

- **Primary (simple) spontaneous pneumothorax:** It occurs in the absence (no evidence) of overt lung disease.
  - Occurs in individual without any underlying lung disease or any trauma.
  - *Age*: Commonly occurs between the age group of 20 and 40 years.
  - *Risk factors*: Smoking, tall stature, and the presence of apical subpleural blebs, mostly familial.

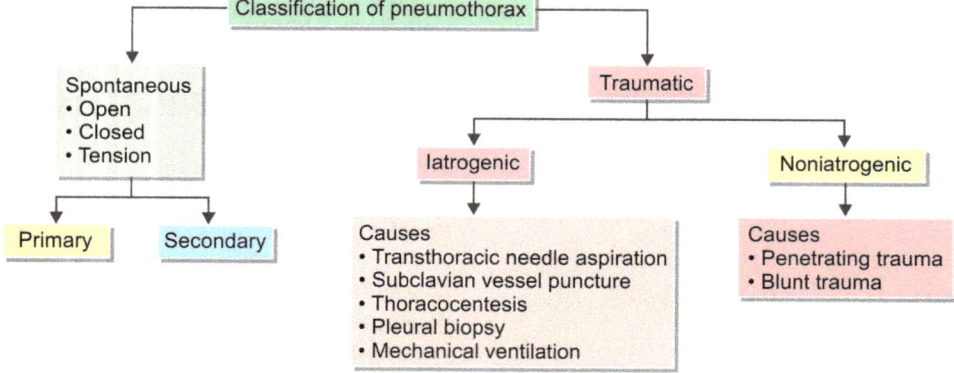

Flowchart 8.4: Classification of pneumothorax.

- About 50% of patients will have a recurrence. Both lungs are affected with equal frequency.
- **Secondary spontaneous pneumothorax** occurs in the presence of an underlying lung disease.
  - *Causes*: Most common causes are *COPD* (chronic bronchitis and emphysema) *and* cavitary active pulmonary *tuberculosis. It occurs* due to rupture of emphysematous bullae and subpleural tuberculosis focus. Other causes include bronchial asthma, suppurative diseases of lung and pleura, cystic fibrosis, and *Pneumocystis jirovecii* pneumonia.

Traumatic pneumothorax results from penetrating or nonpenetrating injuries to the chest.
- **Iatrogenic:** Following diagnostic or therapeutic interventions. These include transthoracic and transbronchial needle aspiration/biopsy (24%), subclavian vessel puncture (22%), thoracocentesis (22%), pleural biopsy (8%), and mechanical ventilation (7%).
- **Noniatrogenic:** Blunt and penetrating injuries to the chest wall, bronchi, lung, or esophagus.

Clinical Features

A small pneumothorax may be asymptomatic without any abnormal physical signs in the chest.
- Most common symptoms are *sudden onset unilateral pleuritic chest pain* and *breathlessness* (dyspnea).
- Severity depends on—(1) extent of lung collapse and (2) amount of pre-existing lung disease.
- **Tension pneumothorax:** Distressed with rapid labored respiration, cyanosis, marked tachycardia, and profuse diaphoresis.

Physical Signs

General examination: Patient will be cyanosed and tachypneic, peripheral pulses may be feeble, and hypotension may be present.

Respiratory system:
- **Inspection and palpation:**
  - *Accessory muscles of respiration in action, trachea, and mediastinal* (apex beat) *shift to the opposite side.*
  - *On the affected side*: Fullness of the chest, diminished chest movements, increase in the size and diminished expansion of the hemithorax, increased spinoscapular distance, and markedly diminished vocal fremitus. Subcutaneous emphysema may be present.
- **Percussion:** Hyper-resonant note over the affected hemithorax.
- **Auscultation:**
  - *On the affected side*: Markedly diminished/absent of breath sounds and vocal resonance, and absence of adventitious sounds. Open pneumothorax with a bronchopleural fistula, there may be amphoric bronchial breathing.

Investigations

Radiological findings on chest radiograph (Fig. 8.23):
Standard erect chest X-ray in inspiration is recommended for

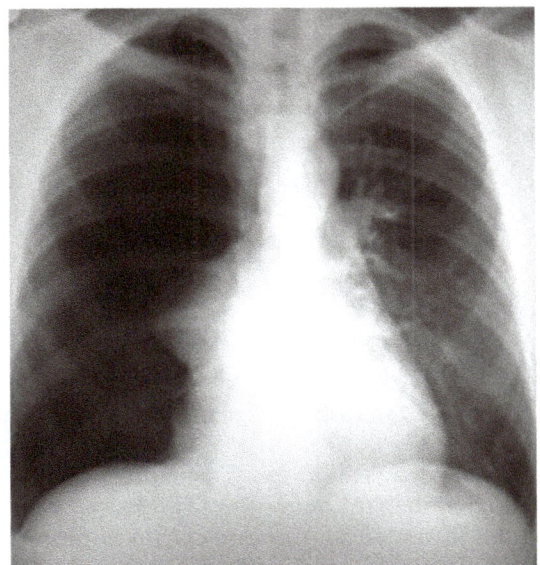

Fig. 8.23: Chest X-ray shows right sided pneumothorax.

the initial diagnosis of pneumothorax rather than expiratory films. Following features are observed:
- Sharply defined edge of the deflated lung
- Complete translucency and absence of bronchovascular markings (no lung markings) in the area between the edge of the lung and chest wall. A clear *visceral pleural line/ collapsed lung margin* can be seen.
- Mediastinal shift/displacement to the opposite side

It may also reveal the presence or absence of pleural fluid, complicating empyema, or underlying lung lesion. CT is used in difficult cases.

Computed tomography scanning is done, if accurate size estimates are required.
- It is recommended only in difficult cases, such as patients in whom the lungs are obscured by overlying surgical emphysema.
- To differentiate a pneumothorax from suspected bulla in complex cystic lung disease.

Ultrasonography (USG) signs of pneumothorax are: (1) loss of lung sliding, (2) loss of comet tails, (3) loss of seashore sign (M mode), and (4) stratosphere sign or bar code sign (M mode).

Types of Spontaneous Pneumothorax

There are three types namely—(1) closed spontaneous pneumothorax, (2) open spontaneous pneumothorax, and (3) tension (valvular) pneumothorax **(Figs. 8.24A to C)**.

Tension (Valvular) Pneumothorax

In tension pneumothorax, the pressure in the pleural space is positive throughout the respiratory cycle.
- It is a condition of pneumothorax where communication between pleura and lung persists. This is due to formation of a valvular mechanism (one way valve through) in which air is sucked into the pleural space during inspiration (coughing, sneezing, and straining) but not expelled during expiration. Large quantity of air gets "trapped" in the

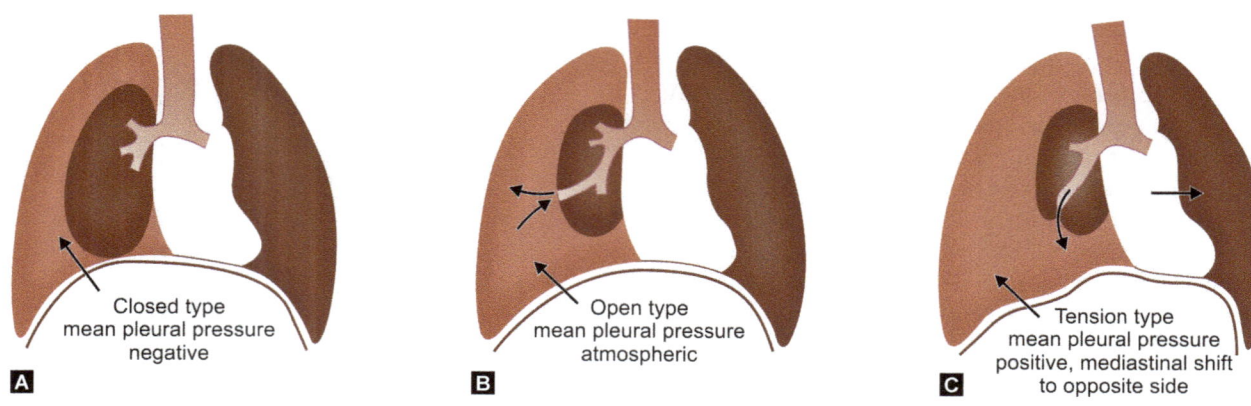

Figs. 8.24A to C: Types of spontaneous pneumothorax: (A) Closed type; (B) Open type; (C) tension (valvular) type.

pleural space/cavity and raises the intrapleural pressure much higher than the atmospheric pressure.
- The high intrapleural pressure causes compression of the underlying lung and shifts the mediastinum to the opposite side with consequent compression of the opposite lung also. It also decreases venous return to the heart by compressing the vena cava resulting in reduced cardiac output.

Clinical features: Rapidly progressive breathlessness, central cyanosis, rapid thread pulse, and signs of peripheral circulatory failure. Signs of pneumothorax are present.

Treatment:
- Tension pneumothorax should be treated as an *acute medical emergency*.
- **Emergency treatment:** *Insertion of a large-bore needle into the pleural space through the second anterior intercostal space*. The diagnosis is confirmed, if large amounts of air escape through the inserted needle. The needle should be left in place till a thoracostomy tube can be inserted. Cover the open end of the needle with a glove finger. Other methods are:
  - Insertion of wide-bore plastic cannula. The opposite end is attached to long rubber tubing, the end of which is placed underwater in a bottle.
  - *Introduction of an intercostals catheter* connected to a water-seal drainage system.
  - If above methods cannot be performed, simple stab on chest wall to release pressure.

Treatment of Pneumothorax

- **Goals:** (1) To promote lung expansion, (2) to eliminate the pathogenesis, and (3) to decrease recurrence of pneumothorax.
- **Treatment options according to**—(1) classification of pneumothorax, (2) pathogenesis, (3) pneumothorax frequency, (4) the extension of lung collapse, (5) severity of disease, and (6) complication and concomitant underlying diseases.
  1. *Primary spontaneous pneumothorax (PSP):* Observation—small, closed, and mildly symptomatic spontaneous pneumothoraces do not require hospital admission. Patient is asked to return to hospital in the event of developing breathlessness.
  2. *Secondary spontaneous pneumothorax (SSP):*
     - *Hospitalization and observation:* Small SSP of <1 cm depth or isolated apical pneumothoraces in asymptomatic patients, supplemental high-flow (10 L/min) oxygen inhalation of high concentration oxygen may reduce the total pressure of gases in pleural capillaries by reducing the partial pressure of nitrogen. This should increase the pressure gradient between the pleural capillaries and the pleural cavity, thereby increasing absorption of air from the pleural cavity. The rate of resolution/reabsorption of spontaneous pneumothoraces is 1.25–1.8% of volume of hemithorax/24 hours.

Active intervention: All other cases will require active intervention (aspiration or chest drain insertion).
- **Simple aspiration:**
  - It is recommended as first-line treatment for all PSP requiring intervention.
  - Less likely to succeed in secondary pneumothoraces and in such cases, it is only recommended as an initial treatment in small (<2 cm) pneumothoraces in minimally breathless patients under the age of 50 years.
- **Repeated and catheter aspiration:** It is reasonable for primary pneumothorax when the first aspiration has been unsuccessful. A volume of <2.5 L has been aspirated on the first attempt.
- **Intercostal tube and under water seal drainage:** Suction to an intercostal tube should not be applied directly after tube insertion. But it can be added after 48 hours for persistent air leak or failure of a pneumothorax to re-expand. High-volume, low-pressure (–10 to –20 cm H_2O) suction systems are recommended.
- **Chemical pleurodesis:**
  - *Goals:* (1) To prevent pneumothorax recurrence and (2) to produce inflammation of pleura and adhesions.
  - *Indications:* Persistent air leak and repeated pneumothorax, bilateral pneumothoraces, those complicated with bullae, and occupations where pneumothorax should not occur (e.g., drivers and pilots).
  - *Sclerosing agents: Tetracycline, minocycline, doxycycline, talc,* and *erythromycin*

- The instillation of sclerosing agents into the pleural space should lead to an aseptic inflammation with dense adhesions.
- **Other types of pleurodesis:**
  - Biological pleurodesis using *Corynebacterium parvum*
  - Physical pleurodesis *mechanical abrasions*

Surgical Treatment

- **Indications:** No response to medical treatment, persistence of air leak, hemopneumothorax, bilateral pneumothoraces, recurrent pneumothorax, tension pneumothorax failed to drain, thicken pleura making lung unable to re-expansion, and multiple blebs or bullae.
- *Open thoracotomy and pleurectomy* remain the procedure with the lowest recurrence rate for difficult or recurrent pneumothorax.
- Minimally invasive procedures, thoracoscopy (VATS), pleural abrasion, and surgical talc pleurodesis are all effective alternative strategies.

Hydropneumothorax

Similar findings as pneumothorax, *except the following findings:*
- Percussion note is hyper-resonant over the upper air-containing part and stony dull over the lower fluid-containing part.

❖ Straight line dullness. *Shifting dullness* can be elicited
❖ *Amphoric bronchial breathing* in case of bronchopleural fistula
❖ *Coin test* is positive over the upper air-containing part
❖ *Succussion splash* can be elicited on the affected side

PNEUMONIA

Definition

Pneumonia is as an acute respiratory illness, defined as inflammation with exudative solidification of the lung parenchyma. It causes the alveoli to be filled with inflammatory exudates and usually results in consolidation (solidification) of lung.
- **Pathological definition:** It is defined as infection of the alveoli, distal airway, and interstitium of the lung. It is characterized by increased weight, replacement of the normal sponginess by the consolidation. Alveoli are filled by the WBC, RBC, and fibrin.
- **Clinical definition:** It is defined as constellation of symptoms and signs (fever, chills, cough, pleural chest pain, sputum, bronchial breathing, egophony, crackles, wheeze, and pleural friction rub) with at least one opacity on chest X-ray PA view.

Classification of Pneumonia

Pneumonias can be classified in different ways (**Box 8.10**).
- **Classification depending on the anatomic distribution:**
  - *Lobar pneumonias (alveolar or air space pneumonia):* The organism causes inflammatory exudates involving many contiguous alveoli (e.g., pneumococcal pneumonia). This radiologically appears as nonsegmental consolidation.

Box 8.10: Classification of pneumonia.

❖ **Classification depending on the anatomic distribution:**
  - Lobar pneumonia
  - Bronchopneumonia
  - Interstitial pneumonia
❖ **Etiological classification:**
  - Primary
  - Secondary
  - Suppurative
❖ **Clinical setting in which the infection occurs (if no pathogen can be isolated):**
  - Community-acquired acute pneumonia
  - Community-acquired atypical pneumonia
  - Nosocomial pneumonia or hospital-acquired pneumonia
  - Pneumonia in immunocompromised host
  - Healthcare-associated pneumonia

- *Bronchopneumonia:* Inflammation involving conducting airways, especially terminal and respiratory bronchioles, and the surrounding alveoli (e.g., staphylococcal pneumonia).
- *Interstitial pneumonia:* The inflammation is confined to interalveolar septa. X-ray chest gives a reticular pattern (e.g., *Mycoplasma pneumoniae, Pneumocystis jirovecii,* and viruses).
- **Etiological classification:**
  - *Primary pneumonia:* It is caused by a specific pathogenic organism and there is no pre-existing abnormality of the respiratory system. The causative organisms are listed in **Table 8.28**.
  - *Secondary pneumonia (including aspiration pneumonia)* (discussed earlier)
  - *Suppurative pneumonia (necrotizing pneumonia)* (discussed earlier)
- **Clinical setting in which the infection occurs (if no pathogen can be isolated):** Pneumonia is classified by the setting in which the person has contracted their infection.

Table 8.28: List of organism causing primary pneumonia.

Common	Less common
• *Streptococcus pneumoniae* (most common) • *Haemophilus influenzae* • *Moraxella catarrhalis* • *Staphylococcus aureus* • *Legionella pneumophila* • *Mycoplasma pneumonia*	• Enterobacteriaceae (*Klebsiella pneumoniae*) and *Pseudomonas* species • *Streptococcus pyogenes* • *Pseudomonas aeruginosa* • *Coxiella burnetii* (Q-fever) • *Chlamydia* species (*C. pneumoniae, C. psittaci,* and *C. trachomatis*) • **Viruses:** Respiratory syncytial virus, H1N1 influenza virus, seasonal influenza virus, parainfluenza virus, and human metapneumovirus (children); influenza A and B (adults); adenovirus (miliary recruits); coronavirus producing severe acute respiratory syndrome (SARS) • *Actinomyces israelii*

- *Community setting or community-acquired pneumonia (CAP)*: It is defined as an acute pulmonary infection in a patient who is not hospitalized or living in a long-term care facility 14 days or more before presentation and does not meet the criteria for healthcare-associated pneumonia (HCAP). This category includes both immunocompetent and immunocompromised patients, as causative agents are almost similar in both the conditions.
- *Nosocomial pneumonia or hospital-acquired pneumonia*:
  - *Definition*: Hospital-acquired pneumonias are pulmonary infections acquired in the course of a hospital stay (development of pneumonia after more than 48 hours of hospitalization).
  - Most of this pneumonia occurs outside intensive care units. However, the highest risk is observed in patients on mechanical ventilation [ventilator associated pneumonia (VAP)].
  - *Etiology*: Predisposing factors include severe underlying disease, immunosuppression, and prolonged antibiotic therapy, patients on mechanical ventilation or invasive access devices, such as intravascular catheters. The hospital-acquired pneumonias are serious and may be life threatening. The various causative organisms causing hospital-acquired pneumonia are:

Various etiological agents causing hospital-acquired pneumonia:
- Gram-negative rods, Enterobacteriaceae (*Klebsiella* species, *Serratia marcescens*, and *Escherichia coli*) and *Pseudomonas* species
- *Staphylococcus aureus* (penicillin and usually methicillin-resistant *Staphylococcus aureus*)

- *Pneumonia in immune compromised host:* This is a type of pneumonia found in patients whose immune system is compromised, through either genetic defect, immunosuppressive medication, or acquired immunodeficiency, such as HIV infection and malignancies.
  - It may be caused by classical organisms, atypical organisms, *Mycobacterium tuberculosis*, or *Pneumocystis jirovecii*.
  - Usually symptoms are more than the signs.
- *Healthcare-associated pneumonia (HCAP)*:
  - *Definition*: Hospital-acquired pneumonias are pulmonary infections acquired in the course of a hospital stay. It occurs:
    - Within 90 days of a 2 day or longer hospitalization. In a nursing home or long-term care residence
    - Within 30 days of receiving intravenous antibacterial therapy, chemotherapy, or wound care or after a hospital or hemodialysis clinic visit; or in any patient in contact with a multidrug resistant pathogen.
  - Features of HCAP more closely resemble nosocomial pneumonia and may require treatment accordingly.

Noninfective Pneumonias
- **Lipid/lipoid pneumonia:**
  - Aspiration of fatty/oily material into lungs
  - *Decreasing order of severity of manifestations*: Mineral oil >animal oil >vegetable oil (because vegetable oil to some extent, animal oils can be hydrolyzed in the body)
- **Radiation pneumonitis:** Dose is >25 Gy. Risk depends on radiation dose and volume of lung irradiated.
- **Chemical pneumonitis:** If aspirated fluid: pH <2.5 and volume >0.3 mL/kg results in chemical pneumonia (Mendelson syndrome)—ARDS/secondary bacterial infection.

Community-acquired Pneumonia
- Community-acquired pneumonia affects all ages, but is commoner at extremes of age.
- Most cases are spread by droplet infection.
- CAP may occur in previously healthy individuals. However, several factors may impair the effectiveness of local defenses and predispose to CAP (**Box 8.11**).
- Pneumonia can be classified either according to the organism responsible for infection or anatomical distribution of infection.
- *Streptococcus pneumoniae (Pneumococcus)* is the most common cause. Viral infections are important causes of CAP in children (**Table 8.29**).
- Depending upon the anatomical distribution of infection, it may be classified as lobar pneumonia (localized with the whole of one or more lobes affected) or bronchopneumonia (diffuse in which lobules of the lung are mainly affected, often due to infection centered on the bronchi and bronchioles) (**Table 8.30**).

Clinical Features of CAP
- The clinical features vary according to the immune status of the patient and the infecting agent.
- **Systemic features:** Pneumonia (especially lobar pneumonia) usually presents as an acute illness. Sudden onset

Box 8.11: Predisposing conditions for community-acquired pneumonia.
- Extremes of age
- Upper respiratory tract infections
- *Comorbidities*: For example, congestive heart failure, diabetes, chronic kidney disease, and recent influenza infection and malnutrition
- Cigarette smoking
- Alcohol
- Corticosteroid therapy
- Congenital or acquired immune deficiencies, e.g., HIV
- Decreased or absent splenic function, e.g., sickle cell disease or postsplenectomy (risk for infection with encapsulated bacteria)
- *Other respiratory conditions*: Cystic fibrosis, bronchiectasis, COPD, obstructing lesion (endoluminal cancer and inhaled foreign body)
- Indoor air pollution

(COPD: chronic obstructive pulmonary disease)

Table 8.29: Causative agent and salient feature of community-acquired acute pneumonia.

Microorganism	Features
Streptococcus pneumonia or Pneumococcus	Most common cause
Haemophilus influenzae	Most common bacterial cause in COPD
Moraxella catarrhalis	Elderly
Staphylococcus aureus	Secondary bacterial pneumonia following viral respiratory illnesses
Enterobacteriaceae (*Klebsiella pneumoniae*)	In debilitated and malnourished people
Pseudomonas aeruginosa	Common in patients with neutropenia
Legionella pneumophila	Organ transplant recipients

Table 8.30: Types of presentations of community-acquired pneumonia (CAP).

Classical	Atypical
• Sudden onset of CAP • High fever, shaking chills • Pleuritic chest pain, sudden onset of breathlessness • Productive cough • Rusty sputum and blood tinge • Poor general condition • High mortality up to 20% in patients with bacteremia • **Causes:** *S. pneumoniae*	• Gradual and insidious onset • Low-grade fever • Dry cough, no blood tinge • Low mortality 1–2%; except in cases of legionellosis • **Causes:** *Mycoplasma, Chlamydiae, Legionella,* rickettsiae, and viruses • Systemic manifestations present

of fever, rigors, shivering, and malaise are predominant symptoms and delirium may be present. The appetite is lost and there may be headache. Fever can be as high as 39.5–40°C. Swinging fevers often indicates empyema.

☐ **Pulmonary symptoms:**
- *Cough*: First, it is characteristically short, painful, and dry. Later, it is productive with expectoration of mucopurulent sputum. Characteristically, rusty sputum may be seen in patients with *Streptococcus pneumoniae* (pneumococcal pneumonia) and the occasional hemoptysis can occur.
- *Chest pain*: It is commonly pleuritic chest pain and may be a presenting feature. It is due to inflammation of the pleura. A pleural rub may be heard. Occasionally, pain may be referred to the shoulder or anterior abdominal wall. Upper abdominal tenderness is sometimes apparent in patients.
- *Breathlessness*: The alveoli become filled and inflammatory exudate impairs gas exchange producing breathlessness.
- *Other features*: CAP can present with confusion or nonspecific symptoms in the elderly. When symptoms have been present for several weeks or have failed to respond to standard antibiotics, the possibility of tuberculosis should always be considered.

Table 8.31: Extrapulmonary features of community-acquired pneumonia.

Extrapulmonary symptoms	Infectious agent
Myalgia, arthralgia, and malaise	*Legionella* and *Mycoplasma*
Myocarditis and pericarditis	*Mycoplasma pneumoniae*
Headache, abdominal pain, diarrhea, and vomiting	*Legionella pneumoniae*
Labial herpes simplex reactivation	Pneumococcal pneumonia
Skin rashes: Erythema multiforme and erythema nodosum	*Mycoplasma pneumoniae*

☐ **Extrapulmonary features:** They are more common in certain infections and sometimes give a clinical clue to the etiology **(Table 8.31)**.

Examination

☐ **Fever:** About 80% are febrile, although this finding is frequently absent in older patients. This is a helpful diagnostic clue, if present.
☐ Respiratory and pulse rate may be raised and the blood pressure may be low and this may be the most sensitive sign in the elderly.
☐ **Tachycardia** is common. However, relative bradycardia is a characteristic feature of Legionnaire's pneumonia. There may be delirium.
☐ Oxygen saturation on air may be low, and the patient is cyanosed and distressed.
☐ **Chest examination:**
- Chest signs vary, depending on the phase of the inflammatory response.
- *During consolidation phase:* Lung is typically dull to percussion and, as conduction of sound is enhanced, auscultation reveals tubular bronchial breath sounds over areas of consolidated lung bronchophony and whispering pectoriloquy. Coarse crackles are heard throughout on auscultation, due to consolidation of the lung parenchyma.

Investigations in CAP

Table 8.32 describes the investigations in community-acquired pneumonia.

Complications of Community-acquired Pneumonia

General complications of community-acquired pneumonia:

- ❖ Respiratory failure acute respiratory distress syndrome (ARDS)
- ❖ **Bacteremic dissemination (bacteremia):** It *can cause*—
  - ☐ Endocarditis (heart valves)
  - ☐ Pericarditis (pericardium)
  - ☐ Meningitis (meninges)
  - ☐ Suppurative arthritis (joint)
  - ☐ Metastatic abscesses in kidneys or spleen
  - ☐ Sepsis—multisystem failure

Local complications:

☐ **Lung abscess**
☐ **Organization:** Delayed and incomplete resolution can cause *ingrowth of granulation tissue into the alveolar*

Table 8.32: Investigations in community-acquired pneumonia (CAP).

Investigation	Significance
Complete blood count:	
• Very high (>20 × 10^9/L) or low (<4 × 10^9/L) WBC count	• Marker of severity • In viral and atypical pneumonias, total leukocyte count is often less than 5,000/mm^3
• Neutrophilic leukocytosis >15 × 10^9/L	Suggests bacterial pneumonia
• Hemolytic anemia	Occasionally complicates *Mycoplasma*
Urea and electrolytes:	
• Urea >7 mmol/L (~20 mg/dL)	Marker of severity
• Hyponatremia	Marker of severity may occur in patients with Legionnaire's disease
Liver function tests:	
• Abnormal transaminitis, raised bilirubin	When basal pneumonia inflames liver, or in atypical pneumonia
• Hypoalbuminemia	Marker of severity
Erythrocyte sedimentation rate/C-reactive protein	Nonspecifically elevated
Blood culture	Bacteremia is a marker of severity. Causative organism may be grown (e.g., pneumococcal pneumonia). However, blood cultures are recommended only in hospitalized patients
Serological and antigen detection tests	• Pneumococcal antigens can be detected in the serum or urine in pneumococcal pneumonia • Acute and convalescent titers for *Mycoplasma, Chlamydia, Legionella,* and viral infections
Cold agglutinins	Positive in 50% of patients with *Mycoplasma*
Arterial blood gases	Measure when SaO$_2$ <93% or when severe clinical features to assess ventilatory failure or acidosis
HIV testing	Since pneumonia is a common in previously undiagnosed HIV infection, a test should be offered to all patients with pneumonia
Sputum: It can be distinguished from saliva by microscopic examination. Sputum contains alveolar macrophages	Gram stain, culture, antimicrobial sensitivity testing, and Ziehl–Neelsen staining
Oropharynx swab	PCR for *Mycoplasma pneumoniae* and other atypical pathogens
Urine	• Pneumococcal and/or *Legionella* antigen • Hematuria may occur in patients with Legionnaire's disease
Chest X-ray	Essential for the confirmation of diagnoses, follow-up, and detection of complications, such as parapneumonic effusion and empyema
• Lobar pneumonia	• Patchy opacification evolves into homogeneous consolidation of affected lobe • Air bronchogram (air-filled bronchi appear lucent against consolidated lung tissue) may be present
• Bronchopneumonia	Patchy and segmental shadowing
• Complications	Parapneumonic effusion, intrapulmonary abscess, or empyema
• *Staphylococcus aureus*	Multilobar shadowing, cavitation, pneumatoceles, and abscesses
• *Mycoplasma*	Usually one lobe is involved but infection can be bilateral and extensive
• *Legionella*	There is lobar and then multilobar shadowing, with the occasional small pleural effusion. Cavitation is rare.
Aspiration	• Percutaneous transtracheal aspiration of secretions • Percutaneous transthoracic needle aspiration, preferable under CT guidance
Fiberoptic bronchoscopy with BAL and brushings	Gram stain, AFB stain, culture, and cytology
Biopsy	A transbronchial biopsy of the lung tissue for culture and histopathology may be done in selected cases. Diagnostic open-lung biopsy, which carries a high risk, is reserved for selected patients
Pleural fluid	Aspirate and culture when present in more than trivial amounts, preferably with ultrasound guidance

(AFB: acid-fast bacilli; BAL: bronchoalveolar lavage; PCR: polymerase chain reaction; SaO$_2$: arterial oxygen saturation)

exudate. The intra-alveolar plugs of granulation tissue are known as organizing pneumonia. Gradually, *increased alveolar fibrosis leads to a shrunken and firm lobe and is called as cornification.*
- **Spread of infection to the pleural cavity:** It may result in—
  - *Pleuritis*
  - *Parapneumonic pleural effusion*
  - *Pyothorax*: Which may lead to fibrothorax
  - *Pneumothorax*, especially in *Staphylococcus pneumoniae* due to pneumatocele rupture

Management Guidelines for CAP
- Rational use of microbiology laboratory
- Pathogen-directed antimicrobial therapy whenever possible
- Prompt initiation of antibiotic therapy
- Decision to hospitalize based on prognostic criteria CURB-65

Severity: The need to hospitalize (severity) a patient is commonly assessed by CURB-65 or the CRB-65 score (**Box 8.12**). The CRB-65 score is used in the community where the serum urea level is not usually available. Other severity score available is Pneumonia Severity Index (PSI), which combines several clinical and laboratory features and comorbid conditions.

General management (treatment) of CAP:
- Check the airway, breathing, and circulation. The most important aspects are—oxygenation, fluid balance, and antibiotic therapy.
- **Oxygen:** Oxygen is indicated in all patients with tachypnea, hypoxemia, hypotension, or acidosis. The aim is to maintain saturations between 94 and 98%. In patients with known COPD, high concentrations (35% or more), preferably humidified oxygen, should be used to maintain a saturation between 88 and 92%. If hypoxia continues or patient develops increasing hypercapnia, ventilate the patient mechanically.
- **Intravenous fluids:** These are required in patients with severe illness, older patients, and those who are vomiting. Treat shock (hypotensive showing any evidence of volume depletion) with intravenous fluids initially. Otherwise, an adequate oral intake of fluid is enough.

Box 8.12: CURB-65 rule.

- **Confusion:** New mental confusion
- **Urea** >7 mmol/L (mg/dL)
- **Respiratory rate** >30 breaths per minute
- **Blood pressure:** Diastolic BP <60 mm Hg or systolic blood pressure <90 mm Hg
- **Age** ≥65 years of age (1 point for each)
- **Group 1:** 0 or 1 of the above—mortality low—1.5%. Likely suitable for treatment at home
- **Group 2:** 2 of the above—mortality—9.2%. Hospitalization for treatment
- **Group 3:** 3 or more of the above—mortality—22%. Likely requires admission to ICU

(ICU: intensive care unit)

New treatment paradigm:
Hit hard early with antibiotics and de-escalate:
- *Antibiotics:* Administer antibiotics as soon the diagnosis of CAP is established preferably within 4 hours of presentation in hospital and treatment should not be delayed while investigations are awaited. Prompt administration of antibiotics improves the outcome. Empiric regimens and antibiotic treatment are described in **Tables 8.33 and 8.34**.

Duration of therapy: Duration is minimum of 5 days (usually 7–10 days). It is afebrile for at least 48–72 hours. Duration is 10–14 days for patients with *Mycoplasma* and *Chlamydia pneumonia*. Patients initially treated with intravenous antibiotics can be switched to oral agents when they become febrile. Longer duration of therapy is needed, if initial therapy was not active against the identified pathogen or complicated by extrapulmonary infection.
- *Mild analgesics for pleuritic pain:* Pleural pain may prevent the patient from breathing normally and coughing efficiently resulting in sputum retention, atelectasis, or secondary infection. Hence, it is relieved by simple analgesia, such as paracetamol, codeine, or NSAIDs.

Table 8.33: Empiric regimens for pneumonia.

Setting	Therapeutic options
Ambulatory, not requiring hospitalization, and age under 60 years	Oral macrolide (erythromycin or azithromycin)
Ambulatory, not requiring hospitalization, and comorbidity or age over 60 years	Oral β-lactam/β-lactamase inhibitor + macrolide *or* oral antipneumococcal fluoroquinolone
Requiring hospitalization	β-lactam (cefoperazone or ceftriaxone) + macrolide or antipneumococcal fluoroquinolone
Aspiration pneumonia requiring hospitalization	β-lactam/β-lactamase inhibitor alone (ampicillin/sulbactam, piperacillin/tazobactam)

Table 8.34: Antibiotic treatment for community-acquired pneumonia (CAP).

Antibiotic	Dosage, route, frequency, and duration
Doxycycline	100–200 mg PO/IV BID for 7–10 days
Azithromycin	500 mg OD IV—3 days + 500 mg OD PO for 7–10 days
Clarithromycin	250–500 mg BID PO for 7–14 days
Telithromycin	800 mg PO OD for 7–10 days
Levofloxacin	750 mg PO/IV OD for 5 days
Gatifloxacin	400 mg PO or IV OD for 5–7 days
Moxifloxacin	400 mg PO or IV OD for 5–7 days
Gemifloxacin	320 mg PO OD for 5–7 days
Amoxiclav	2 g of amoxicillin + 125 mg of clavulanic acid PO BID for 7–10 days
Ceftriaxone	2 g IV BID for 3–5 days
Ertapenem	1 g OD IV or IM for 7–14 days

(PO: per oral; IV: intravenous; IM: intramuscular; OD: once daily; BID: twice daily)

- *Nonresolving pneumonia* is defined as a clinical syndrome in which focal infiltrates begin with some clinical association of acute pulmonary infection and despite a minimum of 10 days of antibiotic therapy, patients either do not improve or worsen or radiographic opacities fail to resolve within 12 weeks.
- Causes of unresolved/slow resolving pneumonia are described in **Table 8.35**.

Pneumococcal Pneumonia (Lobar Pneumonia)

Definition: Lobar pneumonia is characterized by *diffuse inflammation* affecting the *part or entire lobe, usually the lower lobes.*

Etiology

- **Causative organism:** It is most common form of pneumonia and is caused by *Streptococcus pneumoniae* (e.g., *Pneumococcus*, a gram-positive, lancet-shaped *diplococcus*).
- **Mode of infection:** By droplet infection

Risk factors for pneumococcal pneumonia:
- **Age:** Younger than 2 years or older than 65 years
- **Strongest independent risk factor for invasive pneumococcal disease:** *Cigarette smoking*
- **Strongest independent risk factor for CAP:** *Alcoholism*

Table 8.35: Causes of unresolved/slow resolving pneumonia.

Incorrect microbiological diagnosis (e.g., tuberculosis instead of classical organisms) or incomplete antimicrobial treatment	• Underlying antibiotic resistance • Inadequate dose/duration • Nonadherence • Malabsorption
Complication of CAP (community-acquired pneumonia)	• Parapneumonic pleural effusion (exudative), empyema, and lung abscess
Underlying neoplastic lesion or other lung disease	• Bronchial obstruction causing partial or complete obstruction, bronchoalveolar cell carcinoma, and bronchiectasis
Alternative diagnosis	• Pulmonary thromboembolic disease, cryptogenic organizing pneumonia, eosinophilic pneumonia, and pulmonary hemorrhage
Host factors	• Age especially >50 • *Comorbid illness*: Diabetes, COPD (chronic obstructive pulmonary disease) • Others, e.g., alcoholism, immunosuppressive/cytotoxic therapy
Superinfection	• Fungi and *Mycobacterium tuberculosis*
Defects in defense	• For example, impaired cough (sedatives, neuromuscular illness, and stroke), impaired mucociliary transport (chronic bronchitis), immune deficiency states—primary and secondary (B-cell and T-cell)

Alcoholism, leukopenia, pneumococcal sepsis (ALPS): Mortality rate 80%

- Poverty and overcrowding
- **Lowered systemic resistance of the host:** It may be due to—
  - *Chronic diseases:* Diabetes mellitus, severe liver disease, and chronic lung disease
  - *Immunological deficiency:* Defects in innate immunity and humoral immunodeficiency (complement or immunoglobulin), defects in cell-mediated immunity (congenital and acquired), and HIV infection
  - *Treatment with immunosuppressive agents*
  - *Leukopenia*
  - *Asplenia or hyposplenia*
- **Impaired local defense mechanisms:**
  - *Loss or suppression of the cough reflex:* For example, coma, anesthesia, drugs, chest pain, or neuromuscular disorders. It may lead to aspiration of gastric contents into the lung.
  - *Damage or injury to the mucociliary apparatus:* It may be due to cigarette smoke, viral diseases, inhalation of hot or corrosive gases, or genetic defects of ciliary function (e.g., the immotile cilia syndrome).
  - *Accumulation of secretions:* Cystic fibrosis and bronchial obstruction
  - *Interference with the phagocytic or bactericidal action of alveolar macrophages:* It may be due to alcohol intoxication, tobacco smoke, anoxia, or oxygen intoxication. Antecedent influenza
  - *Pulmonary congestion and edema*

Clinical Features

- These are *sudden onset of high fever, chills and rigors, coughs, and vomiting.* Fever is usually high grade (39–40°C). Convulsions may occur in children.
- Cough is initially short, painful, and dry, but soon becomes productive with *mucopurulent sputum*. Rust-colored sputum (*"rusty" sputum*) is characteristic but occasionally may be frankly blood stained.
- Nonspecific symptoms include loss of appetite, headache, and pains in the body and limbs.
- Localized pleuritic chest pain develops at an early stage due to fibrinosuppurative pleuritis. It may be referred to the shoulder or abdominal wall. It may be companied by pleural friction rub. Breathing is rapid and shallow due to pleuritic pain.
- Other features are tachycardia, hot and dry skin, herpes labialis, and flushed face.

Physical signs in the chest:
Q. Write short note on signs of consolidation.
- **First 2 days:** The physical signs are minimal and include diminished respiratory movements, slight impairment of percussion note, and pleural rub. In early stages, numerous fine crepitations are audible.
- **After 2 days:** Frank signs of consolidation appear **(Box 8.13)**.

Investigations

- **Blood:**
  - Severe neutrophil leukocytosis
  - Blood culture may show *Streptococcus pneumoniae*

> **Box 8.13:** Signs of consolidation.
> - Diminished respiratory movements
> - Dull percussion note
> - No mediastinal shift
> - Markedly increased vocal fremitus and vocal resonance
> - High-pitched tubular bronchial breathing
> - Bronchophony, egophony, and whispering pectoriloquy may be present
> - During resolution, coarse crepitations
> - If parapneumonic effusion develops, additional signs of pleural effusion

- **Sputum:**
  - Gram staining of the sputum may show pneumococci, which appear as gram-positive, lancet-shaped diplococci
  - Sputum culture may show *Streptococcus pneumoniae*
  - Assays on sputum are based on detecting nucleic acids for pneumococci
- **Serological tests:** They can detect pneumococcal antigen in serum, urine, and sputum. Detection of C-polysaccharide (part of pneumococcal cell wall) in urine by an immunochromatography assay is quite sensitive. Urinary antigen remains positive for weeks after onset of severe pneumococcal pneumonia. However, it is often negative in mild pneumococcal pneumonia.
- **Chest radiograph (Figs. 8.25A and B):**
  - Involved lobe or segment appears homogeneous radiopaque with air bronchograms.
  - Associated parapneumonic effusion or empyema can also be detected.
- **Others:** In rare instances, fiberoptic and bronchoscopic aspiration or transthoracic needle aspiration may be necessary.

Treatment

General measures:
- Administration of oxygen in high concentration to all hypoxemic patients
- Treatment of pleuritic pain with mild analgesics, such as paracetamol and NSAIDs. However, few may require pethidine 50–100 mg or morphine 10–15 mg intramuscularly or intravenously.

Antibiotic therapy (discussed earlier)

Vaccine: *Two types—*
1. **Pneumococcal polysaccharide vaccine (PPV):** It consists of 23 most common capsular serotypes that produce invasive pneumococcal disease. However, it has poor protection in individuals at greatest risk for severe pneumococcal disease namely elderly, immunocompromised, and infants younger than 2 years.
2. **Polysaccharide-protein conjugate pneumococcal vaccine (pneumococcal conjugate vaccine—PCV):** It targets seven serotypes responsible for most of pneumococcal infections in children. Hence, it is used mainly in children younger than 2 years.

Staphylococcal Pneumonia

- It produces bronchopneumonia that is characterized by *widespread* focal/*patchy areas* of *acute suppurative inflammation*.
- They are *centered on bronchioles and bronchi* with subsequent spread to surrounding alveoli. The involved alveoli show *consolidation*.
- **Causative agent:** *Staphylococcus aureus*. Methicillin-resistant *Staphylococcus aureus* (MRSA) is an important pathogen in nosocomial pneumonia. Recently, community-acquired MRSA (CA-MRSA) infections (skin and soft tissue infections and necrotizing pneumonia) developing in previously healthy persons have emerged as a serious clinical condition.
- **Predisposing factors:** These are common following influenza, in debilitated patients in hospital, and patient with cystic fibrosis.
- **Characteristic features:**
  - Abscess formation is very common. These abscesses are multiple and often bilateral.
  - Abscesses may rupture into pleura leading to pneumothorax or pyopneumothorax.

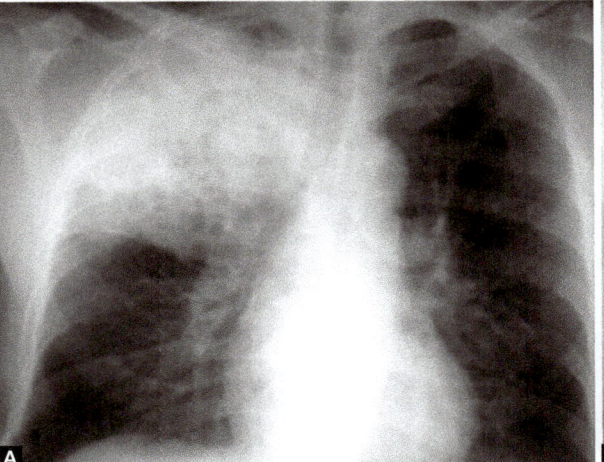 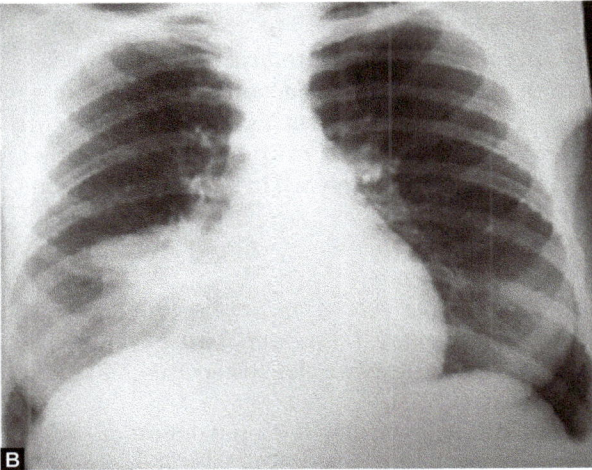

Figs. 8.25A and B: Chest X-ray: (A) Shows right upper lobe pneumonia; (B) Shows right middle lobe pneumonia.

- **Chest radiograph** shows bronchopneumonia. It is often bilateral, with multiple thin-walled cyst-like lesions (*pneumatoceles*).
- Sputum smear shows gram-positive *Staphylococcus aureus* in clumps.

Treatment
- Drug of choice is penicillin
- Methicillin-sensitive *Staphylococcus aureus*: Oxacillin or flucloxacillin
- Methicillin-resistant *Staphylococcus aureus*: Vancomycin and teicoplanin
- Ceftaroline and ceftobiprole, new fifth generation cephalosporins
- Drugs used in treatment of resistant *Staphylococcus* are discussed earlier.

Klebsiella pneumoniae (Friedlander's Pneumonia)
- **Causative agent:** *Klebsiella pneumoniae* (Friedlander's bacillus)
- **Predisposing factors:** Common in alcoholics and diabetics
- **Characteristics:**
  - Severe illness with a high mortality rate
  - Massive consolidation of one or more lobes. The *upper lobes are* most often affected.
  - Abscess formation and pleural effusion are common.

Investigations
- **Sputum:**
  - It may be viscid, jelly-like, and blood stained *(red-current-jelly sputum)*. Sometimes, it may be purulent or rusty.
  - Sputum smear shows gram-negative *Klebsiella pneumoniae*. *Klebsiella pneumoniae* can be cultures from the sputum.
- **Chest radiograph:**
  - It shows air space pneumonia, usually in one of the upper lobes, with abscess formation and pleural effusion.
  - *Bulging interlobar fissure* is a characteristic finding.

Treatment
Antibiotic therapy:
- Gentamicin, ceftazidime, or ciprofloxacin for 2–3 weeks
- *Severe cases*: Piperacillin + tazobactam or meropenem
- *Extended-spectrum β-lactamases (ESBL)-producing organisms*: Meropenem (or imipenem + cilastatin), amikacin, and tigecycline. Polymyxin B for highly resistant strains

Atypical Pneumonias
- **Causes:** *Mycoplasma pneumoniae, Legionella pneumophila, C. pneumoniae, C. burnetii*, viruses [influenza, adenovirus, RSV, measles, varicella-zoster virus (VZV), and cytomegalovirus (CMV)]
- Evolve much more slowly than bacterial pneumonias
- Symptoms >>signs
- They tend to have a slower onset, often with more prominent extrapulmonary symptoms and complications.

> **Parameters that favor the diagnosis of atypical pneumonias:**
> ❖ Age 60 years
> ❖ Absence of any underlying comorbid condition
> ❖ Paroxysmal cough
> ❖ No expectoration
> ❖ Few clinical signs on examination of chest
> If total WBC count 10,000/mm³ is added to the above five parameters, then presence of 4 features indicates a strong likelihood of atypical pneumonia.

Acute Bronchopneumonia
- *Bronchopneumonia* is characterized by *patchy* (scattered solid foci) *area of consolidation in the same or several lobes* of the lung.
- It is a type of secondary pneumonia and invariable proceeded by bronchial infection. It is common in patients with chronic bronchitis.
- Bronchopneumonia is characterized by *widespread* focal/*patchy areas* of *acute suppurative inflammation*. They are *centered on bronchioles and bronchi* with subsequent spread to surrounding alveoli. The involved alveoli show *consolidation*. The *consolidated areas are larger and more numerous in lower lobes* (because of the tendency of secretions to gravitate into the lower lobes) and *frequently bilateral.*
- **Predisposing factors:**
  - *In children:* As a complication of *measles or whooping cough*
  - *In adults:* As a complication of *acute bronchitis or influenza*
  - *In elderly or debilitated patients:* As *hypostatic pneumonia*
- Viral pneumonias and "atypical" pneumonias may also present as bronchopneumonia.

Clinical Features
- High fever, severe cough with purulent expectoration, breathlessness, tachypnea, tachycardia, and central cyanosis
- *Physical signs in the chest*: In early stage, signs of acute bronchitis, and in later stage, bilateral crepitations appear.
- **Investigations:**
  - *Chest X-ray:* Bilateral mottled opacities, predominantly in the lower zones **(Fig. 8.26)**
  - *Blood:* Neutrophilic leukocytosis is common.

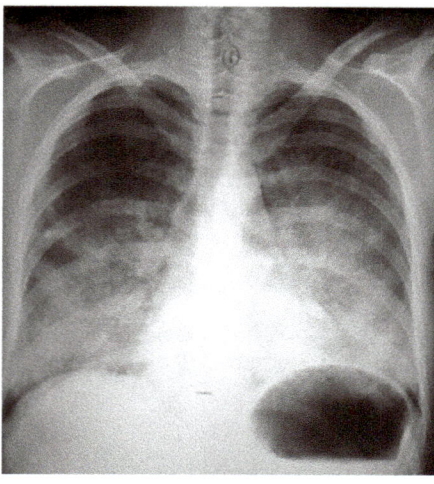

Fig. 8.26: Chest X-ray of bronchopneumonia.

Treatment

Antibiotic therapy:
- **Mild cases:** Ampicillin or cotrimoxazole given orally is effective.
- **Serious cases:** Third generation cephalosporin along with a macrolide

OCCUPATIONAL LUNG DISEASES

Table 8.36 describes the occupational exposure and associated lung diseases.

Asbestos-related Lung and Pleural Diseases

Asbestos-related Diseases
- Asbestosis (progressive pulmonary fibrosis)—highest dose is required to cause asbestosis
- Benign localized pleural fibrous plaques—calcification of parietal pleura more pronounced on the diaphragm and mediastinum
- Benign pleural effusions
- Carcinoma of lung
- Malignant mesothelioma of pleura and mesothelioma of peritoneum (rare)
- Laryngeal carcinomas

Table 8.36: Occupational exposure and associated lung diseases.

Occupational exposure	Disease associated with chronic exposure
Diseases due to inorganic (mineral) dusts: Common Pneumoconiosis	
• Coal • Silica • Asbestos • Beryllium • Iron oxide • Tin dioxide	Coal-worker's pneumoconiosis (CWP) Silicosis Asbestos-related diseases Berylliosis Siderosis *Stannosis*
Diseases due to organic dusts:	
• Cotton, flax, or hemp dust • Moldy hay, grain, and straw • Mold malting • Contaminated bagasse (sugar cane)	Byssinosis Farmer's lung Malt worker's lung Bagassosis
Diseases due to gases and fumes:	
• Irritant gases, isocyanates cadmium • Platinum salts	Occupational asthma, bronchitis, and ARDS Occupational asthma
Diseases due to biological substances:	
Proteolytic enzymes, allergens from animals and insects (excreta), contaminated grain dust	Occupational asthma and bronchitis
Diseases due to chemicals and radioactive substances:	
Polycyclic hydrocarbons and radon	Bronchial carcinoma

(ARDS: acute respiratory distress syndrome)

Silicosis

Associated risk: Silicosis is associated with increased risk of tuberculosis (silicotuberculosis), lung cancer, and COPD. The increased risk is lifelong even if exposure ceases. Chemoprophylaxis using INH for 9 months is recommended, if latent tuberculosis is diagnosed with a positive tuberculin test. Other diseases that can develop in silicosis include chronic renal insufficiency and autoimmune diseases (e.g., scleroderma, rheumatoid arthritis, and Wegener's granulomatosis).

RESPIRATORY FAILURE

Definition
- Respiratory failure is the term used when pulmonary gas exchange fails to maintain normal arterial oxygen and carbon dioxide levels.
- Respiratory failure is a syndrome of inadequate gas exchange due to dysfunction of one or more essential components of the respiratory system:
  - Chest wall (including pleura and diaphragm)
  - Airways
  - Alveolar-capillary units
  - Pulmonary circulation
  - Nerves
  - Central nervous system (CNS) or brainstem
- **Criteria:** Respiratory failure is present when PaO_2 is 60 mm Hg (8.0 kPa) and/or $PaCO_2$ is 50 mm Hg (6.5 kPa).
- **Features of respiratory failure:** These are (1) breathlessness at rest, (2) central cyanosis, (3) raised respiratory rate, and (4) drowsiness, confusion, or unconsciousness. In such patients, arterial blood gas analysis to be done.

Classification

It can be classified in different ways—(1) type I, II, III, and IV, (2) acute and chronic type I respiratory failure; acute and chronic type II respiratory failure, and (3) type I (hypoxemic) respiratory failure and type II (hypercapnic) respiratory failure.

Type I or Hypoxemic (PaO_2 <60 at Sea Level): Failure of Oxygen Exchange
- **Increased shunt fraction (Q_S/Q_T):**
  - Due to alveolar flooding
  - Hypoxemia refractory to supplemental oxygen

Type II or Hypercapnic ($PaCO_2$ >45): Failure to Exchange or Remove Carbon Dioxide
- Decreased alveolar minute ventilation (V_A)
- Often accompanied by hypoxemia that corrects with supplemental oxygen

Type III Respiratory Failure: Perioperative Respiratory Failure
- Increased atelectasis due to low functional residual capacity (FRC) in the setting of abnormal abdominal wall mechanics
- Often results in type I or type II respiratory failure

Table 8.37: Causes of acute and chronic type I respiratory failure.

Acute type I respiratory failure	Chronic type I respiratory failure
• Pneumonia • Pulmonary edema • Acute asthma • Pulmonary embolism • Acute respiratory distress syndrome (ARDS) • Pneumothorax	• Diseases with widespread pulmonary fibrosis • Chronic pulmonary edema • Chronic disorders of chest wall or neuromuscular diseases • Chronic pulmonary thromboembolism

Box 8.14: Causes of acute and chronic type II respiratory failure.

Acute type II respiratory failure:
- *Respiratory depressant drugs*, e.g., diazepam, opiates, and alcohol
- *Severe obstruction to the airflow*, e.g., severe acute asthma, laryngeal and tracheal obstruction, and acute exacerbation of chronic obstructive pulmonary disease (COPD)
- *Disorders of respiratory muscles*, e.g., acute polymyositis
- *Injuries to chest*, e.g., tension pneumothorax, massive hemothorax, and flail chest
- *Brainstem damage*, e.g., stroke, encephalitis, and trauma
- *Disorders of spinal cord, nerves, and neuromuscular transmission*, e.g., spinal trauma, transverse myelitis, acute GB syndrome, poliomyelitis, myasthenia gravis, and botulism

Chronic type II respiratory failure:
- COPD (most common)
- Chest wall abnormalities, e.g., marked kyphoscoliosis and marked obesity
- Amyotrophic lateral sclerosis and muscular dystrophy
- Central hypoventilation

(COPD: chronic obstructive pulmonary disease; GB: Guillain–Barre)

Table 8.38: The Berlin definition of acute respiratory distress syndrome (ARDS).

The Berlin definition of acute respiratory distress syndrome (ARDS)	
Timing	Within 1 week of a known clinical insult/new/worsening respiratory symptoms
Chest X-ray	Bilateral opacities—not fully explained by effusions, lobar/lung collapse or nodules
Origin of edema	• Respiratory failure not fully explained by cardiac failure or fluid overload • Need objective assessment (e.g., echocardiography) to exclude hydrostatic edema, if no risk factor is present
Oxygenation	
Mild	200 mm Hg <PaO_2/FiO_2 ≤300 mm Hg with PEEP or CPAP >5 cm H_2O
Moderate	100 mm Hg <PaO_2/FiO_2 ≤ 200 mm Hg with PEEP >5 cm H_2O
Severe	PaO_2/FiO_2 ≤100 mm Hg with PEEP >5 cm H_2O

(CPAP: continuous positive airway pressure; PEEP: positive end-expiratory pressure; PaO_2: arterial oxygen partial pressure; FiO_2: fractional inspired oxygen)

The Berlin definition of ARDS (Table 8.38): It is an acute, diffuse, and inflammatory lung injury that leads to increased pulmonary vascular permeability, increased lung weight, and a loss of aerated tissue.

Acute respiratory distress syndrome and ALI are serious diseases characterized by damage to alveolar epithelium and pulmonary capillary endothelium. Alveoli become filled with edema fluid of high protein content and inflammatory cells.

Etiology of ARDS and ALI

Acute respiratory distress syndrome may develop due to diffuse lung injury from many medical and surgical disorders. The lung injury may be direct (e.g., toxic inhalation) or indirect (e.g., in septicemia) **(Table 8.39)**.

Pathophysiology of Acute Respiratory Distress Syndrome

Pathophysiology of acute respiratory distress syndrome is described in **Flowchart 8.5**.

Clinical Features

- Development of *acute dyspnea and hypoxemia within hours to days* of an inciting event
- *Tachypnea, tachycardia,* cyanosis, and the need for a high fraction of inspired oxygen (FiO_2) to maintain oxygen saturation
- Febrile or hypothermic
- Sepsis—hypotension and peripheral vasoconstriction with cold extremities

- Can be ameliorated by anesthetic or operative technique, posture, incentive spirometry, postoperative analgesia, and attempts to lower intra-abdominal pressure

Type IV Respiratory Failure: Shock

Type IV describes patients who are intubated and ventilated in the process of resuscitation for shock.

Acute Type I and Chronic Type I Respiratory Failure

Causes of acute and chronic type I respiratory failure are described in **Table 8.37**.

Acute Type II and Chronic Type II Respiratory Failure

Causes of acute and chronic type II respiratory failure are described in **Box 8.14**.

ACUTE LUNG INJURY AND THE ACUTE RESPIRATORY DISTRESS SYNDROME

Definition

Acute respiratory distress syndrome (ARDS) is a sudden and progressive form of acute respiratory failure in which the alveolar capillary membrane becomes damaged and more permeable to intravascular fluid resulting in severe dyspnea, hypoxemia, and diffuse pulmonary infiltrates.

Table 8.39: Disorders commonly associated with ARDS.

Direct lung injury	
Pulmonary infections	Pneumonia (viral, bacterial, fungal *Pneumocystis jirovecii*, and *Mycoplasma*)
Aspiration	Aspiration of gastric contents (vomitus)
Inhalation of toxic gas	Ammonia, chlorine, nitrogen dioxide, ozone, oxygen, and smoke
Blunt chest trauma	Pulmonary contusion
Near drowning	
Indirect lung injury	
Systemic disorders	Shock, septicemia, uremia, and eclampsia
Severe trauma	Multiple bone fractures (fat embolism), flail chest, head trauma, and burns
Blood	Multiple transfusions
Drug overdose:	
• Narcotic overdose	Heroin, methadone, morphine, and dextropropoxyphene
• Nonnarcotic drugs	Barbiturates, thiazides, and nitrofurantoin
Others	Acute pancreatitis, cardiopulmonary bypass, trauma, Goodpasture's syndrome, and SLE

(ARDS: acute respiratory distress syndrome; SLE: systemic lupus erythematosus)

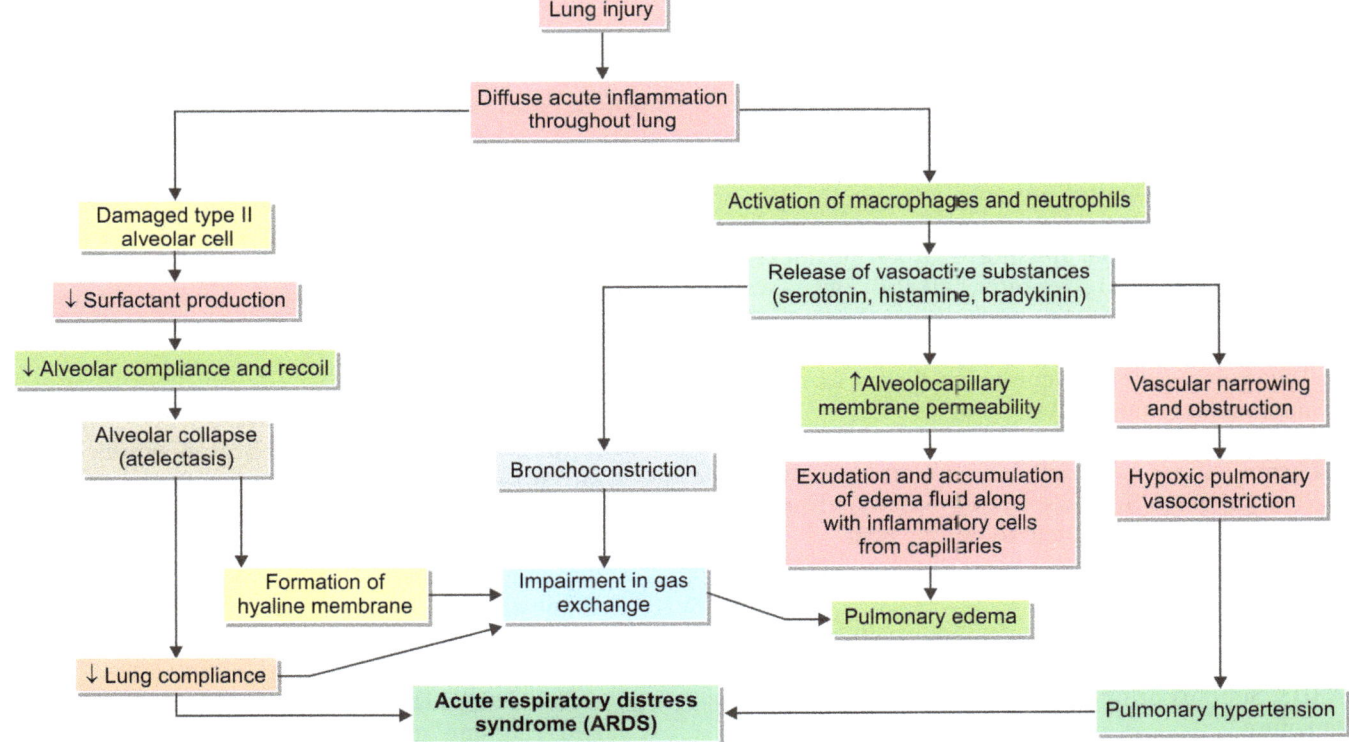

Flowchart 8.5: Pathophysiology of acute respiratory distress syndrome.

- Bilateral rales/crepitations
- Manifestations of the underlying cause
- Because cardiogenic pulmonary edema must be distinguished from ARDS, carefully look for signs of congestive heart failure or intravascular volume overload, including jugular venous distension, cardiac murmurs and gallops, hepatomegaly, and edema.

Investigation

- Chest radiograph (Fig. 8.27): Diffuse, bilateral alveolar infiltrates consistent with pulmonary edema—

- *Early stage*: Infiltrates associated with ARDS *may be variable*—mild or dense, interstitial or alveolar, and patchy or confluent.
- Initially, the *infiltrates* may have a *patchy peripheral distribution*, but soon they progress to *diffuse bilateral involvement with ground glass changes or frank alveolar infiltrates*.
- *Cardiogenic edema*: Increased heart size, increased width of the vascular pedicle, vascular redistribution toward upper lobes, the presence of septal lines, or a perihilar ("bat's wing") distribution of the edema.

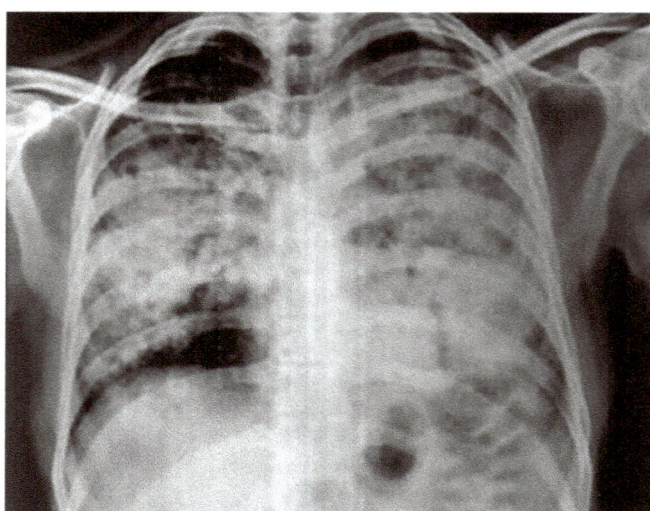

Fig. 8.27: Bilateral alveolar shadows in acute respiratory distress syndrome (ARDS) on chest X-ray.

Lack of these findings, in conjunction with patchy peripheral infiltrates that extend to the lateral lung margins, suggests ARDS.

- **Arterial blood gas analysis:**
  - PaO_2/FiO_2 ratio and severity (**Table 8.40**)
  - In addition to hypoxemia, arterial blood gases often initially show a respiratory alkalosis.
  - However, in ARDS occurring in the context of sepsis, a metabolic acidosis with or without respiratory compensation may be present.
  - As the condition progresses and the work of breathing increases, the partial pressure of carbon dioxide (PCO_2) begins to rise and respiratory alkalosis gives way to respiratory acidosis.
- **To exclude cardiogenic pulmonary edema:**
  - *Echocardiogram*: Left ventricular ejection fraction, wall motion, and valvular abnormalities
  - Plasma B-type natriuretic peptide (BNP) value
- **CT scan:** Diffuse consolidation with air bronchograms, bullae, pleural effusions, pneumomediastinum, and pneumothorax. Later, it may show lung cysts.

Management

- Treatment of respiratory system abnormalities
- Diagnose and treat the precipitating/initiating cause of ARDS. Support or treat other organ system dysfunction or failure.

Maintaining adequate oxygenation: Mechanical ventilation using limited tidal volumes.

Table 8.40: ARDS severity and PaO_2/FiO_2.

ARDS severity	PaO_2/FiO_2
Mild	200–300
Moderate	100–200
Severe	<100

(ARDS: acute respiratory distress syndrome; PaO_2: arterial oxygen partial pressure; FiO_2: fractional inspired oxygen)

Prone positioning ventilation: About two-thirds of patients with ARDS improve their oxygenation after being placed in a prone position.

Adjuncts to lung-protective mechanical ventilation: Inhaled nitric oxide, inhaled prostacyclin, tracheal gas insufflation, extracorporeal membrane oxygenation (ECMO), or extracorporeal CO_2 removal ($ECCO_2R$).

BRONCHOPULMONARY ASPERGILLOSIS

Bronchopulmonary aspergillosis is the term used for the bronchopulmonary diseases caused by fungus *Aspergillus* species, the most common being *Aspergillus fumigates*. Others fungus in *Aspergillus* species include *A. clavatus, A. niger, A. flavus,* and *A. terreus*.

Allergic Bronchopulmonary Aspergillosis (ABPA—Asthmatic Pulmonary Eosinophilia)

Allergic bronchopulmonary aspergillosis (ABPA) occurs due to hypersensitivity reaction against germinating fungal spores in the wall of the airway. Usually, hypersensitivity reactions are seen to *A. fumigatus* and rare cases are due to other Aspergilli and other fungi.

- It can complicate bronchial asthma or cystic fibrosis.
- It is one of the causes of pulmonary eosinophilia.

Clinical Features

- Fever, breathlessness, coughing up of thick sputum casts, and worsening of asthmatic symptoms
- Aspergillus may grow in the walls of proximal bronchi and may produce *proximal bronchiectasis*. It may cause repeated episodes of eosinophilic pneumonia, which manifests as wheeze, cough, fever, and expectoration with sputum-containing fungal mycelia.

Investigations

- **Radiological signs on chest X-ray:**
  - Radiographically show infiltrates, which may be mistaken for pneumonia. Segmental or lobar collapse on chest X-rays in patients where asthma symptoms are stable, suggestive of ABPA.
  - Repeated pneumonic episodes may show fleeting shadows of infiltrates on chest radiographs. Other findings include transient area of opacification (due to mucoid impact in of the airways), band-like opacities with rounded distal margin (gloved finger appearance), and "ring sing" and "tram lines" (due to thickened and inflamed bronchi). Eventually, it may result in central bronchiectasis and progressive pulmonary fibrosis.
- Other relevant investigations and diagnostic features of allergic bronchopulmonary aspergillosis are mentioned in **Table 8.41**.

Management

- **Corticosteroids:** Oral prednisolone 30 mg daily for 7–10 days causes rapid clearing of the pulmonary infiltrate. Prednisolone should be gradually tapered to a maintenance dose of 5–10 mg/day for long term. Asthma responds to inhaled corticosteroids.

Table 8.41: Diagnostic features of allergic bronchopulmonary aspergillosis.

Rosenberg–Patterson criteria	
Major criteria (ARTEPICS)	**Minor criteria**

A = Asthma (bronchial)
R = Roentgenographic fleeting pulmonary opacities
T = Skin test positive (immediate wheal-and-flare response) for *Aspergillus* (type I)
E = Eosinophilia—in peripheral blood (>1000/mm^3)
P = Precipitating antibodies (IgG) in serum
I = IgE in serum elevated (>1,000 IU/mL)
C = Central/proximal bronchiectasis (inner two-thirds of chest CT field)
S = Serum *A. fumigatus*-specific IgG and IgE (more than twice the value of pooled serum samples from patients with asthma who have *Aspergillus* hypersensitivity)
	• Sputum
	  ▪ Fungal hyphae of *A. fumigates* and eosinophils on microscopic examination of sputum
	  ▪ Expectoration of brownish black mucus plugs in sputum
	  ▪ Culture of *A. fumigatus* from sputum
	❖ Delayed skin reaction to *Aspergillus* antigen (type III)
	• Presence of 6 of 8 major criteria makes diagnosis almost certain

- **Antifungal agents:** Oral itraconazole; dose is 200 mg BID for 16 weeks then once a day for 16 week or voriconazole should be used in patients on high doses of steroids. It reduces exacerbations and requirement of steroids.
- **Humanized monoclonal antibody against IgE:** Omalizumab is under trial.
- **Bronchoscopic extraction of the casts:** If there is persistent lobar collapse, bronchoscopic (usually under general anesthesia) removal of impacted mucus and casts may result in reinflation of the collapsed lobe.

Aspergilloma

Aspergilloma is the growth of *Aspergillus* fungus within previously damaged lung tissue and forms a ball of fungus (mycelium) within lung cavities. Most commonly, the fungal ball is produced by *Aspergillus fumigatus* and rarely by other fungi (e.g., Zygomycetes and Fusarium).

Clinical Features

- Simple aspergilloma is usually asymptomatic.
- Occasionally, it may cause recurrent scanty to *massive hemoptysis*. The source of hemoptysis is usually bronchial blood vessels. It may be due to local invasion of blood vessels lining the cavity, endotoxins released from the fungus, or mechanical irritation of the vessels inside the cavity during rolling of the fungus ball.
- Nonspecific systemic features, such as lethargy and weight loss may be present.

Invasive Pulmonary Aspergillosis

Invasive pulmonary aspergillosis (IPA) is invasion of previously healthy lung tissue by *Aspergillus fumigatus* and usually develops as a complication in patients who are immunocompromised (with profound neutropenia) either by drugs (especially immunosuppressants) and/or disease.

Management

- Treatment should not be delayed because IPA has a high mortality rate. It requires aggressive antifungal therapy and immunosuppression should be reduced, if possible.
- *Voriconazole and liposomal amphotericin B* allow a safer and more effective treatment of invasive aspergillosis when compared with amphotericin B-deoxycholate.
- *First-line agents*: The treatment of choice is intravenous voriconazole (6 mg/kg every 12 hours for two doses and then 4 mg/kg twice a day). It is better tolerated and more effective than amphotericin B. Antifungal therapy with amphotericin (1.0–1.5 mg/kg/day) with or without flucytosine is equally effective.
- *Second-line agents*: Intravenous echinocandin derivatives, such as caspofungin, micafungin, and anidulafungin are used in refractory cases or if the patient cannot tolerate first-line agents.
- In less immunosuppressed patients, oral itraconazole (200 mg twice a day) may be given.

HEMOPTYSIS

Definition

- Hemoptysis is defined as coughing of blood originating from below the vocal cords.
- Hemoptysis can range from blood-streaking of sputum to the presence of gross blood in the absence of any accompanying sputum.
- Life-threatening (or) massive hemoptysis is defined as coughing of blood >150 mL/time (or) >600 mL/24 hours.
- Only 5% of hemoptysis is massive but mortality is 80%.
- Clinical definition of massive hemoptysis is any bleeding that results in a threat to life because of airway or hemodynamic compromise due to bleeding.

Causes

Causes of hemoptysis are mentioned in **Tables 8.42 and 8.43**.

Differences between True and False Hemoptysis

Differences between true and false hemoptysis are described in **Table 8.44**.

Differences between Hemoptysis and Hematemesis

Differences between hemoptysis and hematemesis are described in **Table 8.45**.

PULMONARY EOSINOPHILIC SYNDROMES

Heterogeneous group of pulmonary disorders is characterized by pulmonary parenchymal or peripheral blood eosinophilia.
- **Loeffler's syndrome (simple pulmonary eosinophilia):**
  - It is a clinical syndrome characterized by:
    ▪ Mild respiratory symptoms
    ▪ Peripheral blood eosinophilia
    ▪ Transient and migratory pulmonary infiltrates
  - Affects all ages
  - *Immune hypersensitivity to Ascaris lumbricoides* is the likely cause. Other parasites, such as *Necator, Ancylostoma, Dirofilaria*, etc., can be associated.

Table 8.42: Causes of hemoptysis.

Structure involved	Common causes	Uncommon causes
Bronchial disease	Bronchial carcinoma, bronchiectasis, acute and chronic bronchitis	Bronchial adenoma and foreign body
Parenchymal disease of lung	Pulmonary tuberculosis (Rasmussen's aneurysm—dilation of a pulmonary artery in a tuberculous cavity), lung abscess, pneumonia (particularly *Klebsiella*), fungal infections (aspergilloma and invasive aspergillosis, and pulmonary contusion/laceration (traumatic)	Parasites (e.g., hydatid disease and flukes), trauma, actinomycosis, and mycetoma
Vascular diseases of lung	Pulmonary infarction	Goodpasture's syndrome, polyarteritis nodosa, idiopathic, pulmonary hemosiderosis, and primary pulmonary hypertension
Cardiovascular disease	Acute left ventricular failure	Mitral stenosis, aortic aneurysm, and pulmonary thromboembolism
Hematological disorders		Leukemia, hemophilia, anticoagulants, and hemorrhagic diathesis

Table 8.43: Causes of massive hemoptysis.

Pulmonary tuberculosis	Cystic fibrosis	Mitral stenosis
Pulmonary infarction	Lung abscess	Pulmonary arteriovenous malformation
Bronchiectasis	Necrotizing pneumonia	
Bronchogenic carcinoma		

Table 8.44: Differences between true and false hemoptysis.

True hemoptysis	False hemoptysis (spurious)
Below vocal cords	Above vocal cords
Persists as blood-tinged sputum	Does not persist
May be mixed with sputum	Not mixed with sputum
History of cardiopulmonary disease	Obvious by ENT examination
Chest X-ray may be abnormal	Normal chest X-ray

Table 8.45: Differences between hemoptysis and hematemesis.

Hemoptysis	Hematemesis
Coughing of blood Cough precedes hemoptysis	Vomiting of blood Nausea and vomiting precede hematemesis
History of cardiopulmonary disease	History of gastrointestinal disease
Bright red in color	Dark brown in color
Sputum remains blood stained after the attack for few days	Usually followed by melena
Mixed with sputum	Mixed with gastric contents
Blood is frothy due to admixture of air	Airless and not frothy
Alkaline	Acidic
Sputum contains hemosiderin laden macrophages	No
Melena absent	Melena present

- *Chest X-ray*: Transient, migratory, nonsegmental interstitial, and alveolar infiltrates (often peripheral or pleural based).
- *Pulmonary function test*: It typically reveals mild-to-moderate restrictive ventilatory defect with a reduced diffusing capacity of the lungs for carbon monoxide (DLCO).

☐ **Drug and toxin-induced pulmonary eosinophilic syndromes:**
  - *Onset*: Acute or subacute
  - *Respiratory symptoms*: Vary wide in severity
    - Mild Loeffler's-like illness with dyspnea, cough, and fever
    - Severe fulminant respiratory failure
  - Drugs implicated are acetyl salicylate, nitrofurantoin, bleomycin, methotrexate, minocycline, sulfa drugs, gold salts, INH, etc.

☐ **Idiopathic acute eosinophilic pneumonia:**
  - It is more common in younger men (mean age about 30 years).
  - It occurs commonly in previously healthy persons. It is also seen in persons with history of chronic myeloid leukemia (CML), HIV infection, recent commencement of smoking, etc.
  - *Diagnostic criteria*:
    - Acute onset of febrile respiratory manifestations (≤1 month duration before consultation)
    - Bilateral diffuse infiltrates on chest X-ray
    - Hypoxemia, with PaO_2 on room air <60 mm Hg, and/or PaO_2/FiO_2 ≤300 mm Hg, and/or oxygen saturation on room air <90%.
    - Lung eosinophilia, with >25% eosinophils in BAL (or eosinophilic pneumonia at lung biopsy)
    - Absence of infection or of other known causes of eosinophilic lung disease (especially exposure to drug known to induce pulmonary eosinophilia)
  - *Treatment*:
    - Initial doses of methylprednisolone are used in the range from 60 to 125 mg every 6 hours.
    - After resolution of respiratory failure, oral prednisolone (in doses of 40–60 mg per day) may be continued for 2–4 weeks with a subsequent slow taper over the next several weeks.

- Idiopathic acute eosinophilic pneumonia (AEP) carries an excellent prognosis.
□ **Tropical pulmonary eosinophilia:**
  - Tropical pulmonary eosinophilia (TPE) was first described in the early 1940s by Weingarten, in India. It is seen mainly in South and South-east Asia and Africa.
  - *Definition*: Tropical pulmonary eosinophilia is an occasional atypical host response (hypersensitivity reaction) of an individual to a mosquito-borne filarial infection by tissue-dwelling human nematode (microfilariae) *Wuchereria bancrofti* and *Brugia malayi*.
  - *Pathogenesis*: When filarial parasites are destroyed, the antigens released initiate an immediate IgE-mediated reaction.
  - There is dense inflammatory reaction with eosinophils, which over time progresses to granuloma formation and fibrosis. In children, marked enlargement of lymph nodes and spleen (*Meyers–Kouwenaar syndrome*) may be evident. In adults, symptoms are predominantly due to lung involvement. Microfilariae are trapped in the pulmonary capillaries and produce symptoms of lung involvement.
□ **Clinical features:**
  - Paroxysmal dry cough, fever, malaise, anorexia, weight loss, dyspnea or wheeze/nocturnal bronchospasm (asthma-like symptoms), and miliary pulmonary infiltrates (*Weingarten syndrome or tropical pulmonary eosinophilia*)
  - Tropical pulmonary eosinophilia is a complication seen mainly in India. If untreated, it may progress to chronic interstitial lung disease. Spontaneous resolution over several weeks
  - *Other features*:
    - Presentation can be similar to status asthmaticus
    - Chest pain, muscle tenderness, pericardial and CNS involvement
    - Rarely, patients remain asymptomatic
  - *Chest examination*: Coarse crackles and rhonchi
  - Generalized lymphadenopathy and hepatosplenomegaly may be present.
□ **Diagnosis:**
  - *History* of long period of residence in an endemic area
  - *Peripheral blood*:
    - Absence of microfilariae in the despite repeated examinations
    - Marked peripheral blood *eosinophilia* in excess of 3,000/mL
  - Chest X-ray—miliary mottling
  - *Serological findings*:
    - High titers of antifilarial antibodies
    - Elevated levels of total IgE (at least 1,000 units/mL)
  - *Therapeutic response to DEC* (6 mg/kg/day for 3 weeks) within 7–10 days of initiating therapy
□ **Treatment:** Diethylcarbamazine in a dose of 2 mg/kg orally three times a day for 14–21 days or for as long as 4 weeks. It is directly filaricidal to both adult worms and microfilariae.

□ **Chronic eosinophilic pneumonia:**
  - Typically subacute presentation
  - Symptoms present for several months before diagnosis
  - Common presenting complaints include—low-grade fevers, drenching night sweats, moderate (10 to 50-pound) weight loss, and cough.
  - History of atopy, allergic rhinitis, or nasal polyps may be found.
  - *About two-thirds develop adult-onset asthma*: Preceding or concurrent with the occurrence of CEP.
  - No major extrapulmonary manifestations
  - *Chest X-ray*: Bilateral opacities in upper and mid zone. Photographic negative of pulmonary edema
  - Corticosteroids are the mainstay of therapy for CEP. Dramatic clinical, radiographic, and physiological improvements
□ Allergic bronchopulmonary aspergillosis (discussed earlier)
□ **Churg–Strauss syndrome:** It is a form of necrotizing vasculitis in several organs, associated with eosinophilic tissue inflammation and extravascular granulomas. It occurs in asthmatics and presents with fever and peripheral hypereosinophilia.
□ **Idiopathic hypereosinophilic syndrome:**
  - *Several names*: Eosinophilic leukemia, Loeffler's fibroblastic endocarditis, and disseminated eosinophilic cardiovascular disease
  - *Clinical features*: Often nonspecific and include—
    - Weakness, fatigue, low-grade fevers, myalgias, cough, angioedema, rash, retinal lesions, and dyspnea
    - Can affect every organ system
    - Cough is nocturnal, either nonproductive or productive of small quantities of nonpurulent sputum
    - Wheezing and dyspnea without evidence of airflow obstruction on spirometry
    - Pulmonary hypertension, ARDS, and pleural effusions
    - Progressive chronic heart failure due to eosinophilic myocarditis and endocarditis, intracardiac thrombi, and endocardial fibrosis.
    - Encephalopathy with neuropsychiatric dysfunction and thromboembolic events, such as hemiparesis. Peripheral neuropathy is extremely common in IHS.
    - Hepatosplenomegaly and lymphadenopathy.
  - *Investigations*:
    - Anemia and thrombocytopenia
    - Elevated vitamin B_{12} levels
    - *Bone marrow*: Universally affected with a striking eosinophilia (up to 25–75% of the differential count)

Treatment:
- Glucocorticoids are the first-line therapy in all patients without *FIP1L1/PDGFRA* mutation.
- *Patients with FIP1L1/PDGFRA mutation*: Imatinib is the drug of choice with a very good response rate.
- Other drugs include—hydroxyurea, vincristine, interferons, anti-interleukin-5 (IL-5) monoclonal antibody (e.g., mepolizumab) and an anti-CD52 antibody (alemtuzumab).

Chapter 8: Respiratory System

OBJECTIVE-BASED SELF-EVALUATION

LONG QUESTIONS

1. Define asthma. Discuss the pathogenesis of atopic asthma. Describe the Global Initiative for Asthma (GINA) severity grades of asthma.
2. List the risk factors of bronchial asthma. Discuss the clinical features and management of status asthmaticus.
3. Define COPD. What are the types of COPD. Discuss the management of acute exacerbation of COPD.
4. Define emphysema and list its types. Discuss GOLD staging for severity of COPD and management.
5. Discuss the clinical features, complications, and management of post-primary tuberculosis.
6. Discuss antitubercular drugs—classification, dosage, side effects and regimen.
7. Discuss the clinical features, diagnosis, and management of right-sided tubercular pleural effusion.
8. Discuss the clinical features, diagnosis, and management of bronchiectasis.
9. Discuss the clinical features, diagnosis, and management of right upper lobe collapse.
10. Discuss the etiology, clinical features, diagnosis, and management of lung abscess.
11. Discuss the clinical features, diagnosis, and management of right-sided empyema.
12. List the types of pneumothorax. Discuss the clinical features, diagnosis, and management of left-sided pneumothorax.
13. Discuss the etiology, clinical features, diagnosis, and management of community acquired pneumonia.
14. Define ARDS. List the common causes. Discuss the clinical features and management of ARDS.
15. Discuss the clinical features, diagnosis, and management of pneumococcal pneumonia.

SHORT ANSWER QUESTIONS

1. Differences between bronchial asthma and cardiac asthma
2. List the drugs useful in asthma
3. Phenotypes of asthma
4. Examination findings in a patient with emphysema
5. Differences between emphysema and chronic bronchitis
6. Differentiating features of asthma and chronic obstructive pulmonary disease
7. Mantoux test
8. DOTS
9. Define MDRTB and XDRTB
10. Extrapulmonary tuberculosis—manifestations
11. Complications of bronchiectasis
12. Bronchiectasis sicca
13. Lights criteria
14. Clinical features of hydropneumothorax
15. Predisposing conditions for community-acquired pneumonia
16. List causes of hemoptysis
17. Types of respiratory failure
18. Loeffler's syndrome
19. Allergic bronchopulmonary aspergillosis
20. List common pneumoconiosis
21. Complications of pneumonia
22. CURB-65 rule
23. BODE index
24. Complications of COPD
25. Classification of pneumonia

MULTIPLE CHOICE QUESTIONS

1. **With respect to the definition of COPD all the following terms are correct, *except*:**
   a. Enhanced chronic inflammatory response
   b. Preventable and treatable
   c. Progressive
   d. Reversible airflow limitation

2. **All the following are components of CURB-65 criterion, *except*:**
   a. Altered conscious levels
   b. Chest pain
   c. Hypotension
   d. Increased respiratory rate

3. **A 36-year-old lady presents to the OPD complaining of cough since 15 years. It is more on lying down on the right side. The cough is the worst when the patient wakes up in the morning. Cough is productive and she brings out copious sputum. It is yellowish green in color and is aggravated by the same factors as cough. She also gives multiple episodes of blood in the sputum. What is the most likely diagnosis in this patient?**
   a. Bronchiectasis
   b. Lung abscess
   c. Chronic bronchitis
   d. Tuberculosis

4. **All of the following causes transudative pleural effusions, *except*:**
   a. Acute renal failure
   b. Cirrhosis
   c. Congestive cardiac failure
   d. Tuberculosis

5. **Hyperuricemia is an adverse effect of the following anti TB drug:**
   a. Ethambutol
   b. Rifampicin
   c. Isoniazid
   d. Pyrazinamide

6. **A young male presents with high fever, agonizing left pleuritic pain and cough with rusty sputum. On examination, the man appears acutely ill with rapid shallow respiration. What clinical finding will you expect?**

a. Decreased movements in left hemithorax with increased vocal resonance
b. Increased movements in left hemithorax with decreased vocal resonance
c. Decreased movements in left hemithorax with decreased vocal resonance
d. Increased movements in left hemithorax with increased vocal resonance

7. According to Lights criteria a patient is considered to have an exudative effusion when:
   a. Ratio of pleural fluid protein to serum protein is higher than 0.5
   b. Ratio of pleural fluid LDH to serum LDH higher than 0.6
   c. Pleural fluid LDH higher than 2/3rd of upper limit of normal range
   d. Any of the above

8. Which of the following associations correctly pairs clinical scenarios and community-acquired pneumonia (CAP) pathogens?
   a. Aspiration pneumonia: *Streptococcus pyogenes*
   b. Heavy alcohol use: Atypical pathogens and *Staphylococcus aureus*
   c. Poor dental hygiene: *Chlamydia pneumoniae, Klebsiella pneumoniae*
   d. Structural lung disease: *Pseudomonas aeruginosa, S. aureus*

9. The most common cause of a pleural effusion is:
   a. Cirrhosis
   b. Left ventricular failure
   c. Malignancy
   d. Pneumonia

10. Determination of the pleural concentration of adenosine deaminase (ADA) is a useful screening test for diagnosis of:
    a. Bronchogenic carcinoma
    b. Tuberculosis
    c. Pneumonia
    d. Bronchial asthma

───── ANSWERS ─────

1. d 2. b 3. a 4. d 5. d
6. a 7. d 8. d 9. b 10. b

Cardiology

CHAPTER OUTLINE

- Ischemic Heart Disease
- Acute Coronary Syndrome
- Hypertension
- Acute Rheumatic Fever
- Valvular Heart Disease
- Infective Endocarditis
- Heart Failure
- Pulmonary Edema
- Cardiac Arrhythmias
- Cardiomyopathy
- Congenital Heart Diseases
- Cardiac Arrest
- Syncope
- Cor Pulmonale
- Circulatory Failure: Shock
- Deep Venous Thrombosis
- Pulmonary Embolism
- Hyperlipidemia

ISCHEMIC HEART DISEASE

Definition

Ischemic heart disease (IHD) is a group of heart diseases in which there is an imbalance between myocardial blood supply and its oxygen demand. IHD is the *leading cause of death* in both males and females.

Etiology

- **Coronary arterial occlusion is the main cause of myocardial ischemia:** It is mostly due to coronary atherosclerosis and its complications. Coronary atherosclerosis narrows one or more of the epicardial coronary arteries and decreases the coronary blood flow in about 90% of cases. Hence, IHD is often known as coronary artery disease (CAD) or coronary heart disease.
- **Other rare causes:** Emboli, vasculitis, coronary vasospasm, and hematologic disorders such as sickle cell disease and diminished availability of blood or oxygen (lowered systemic blood pressure as in shock).

Risk Factors for Atherosclerosis

The risk factors may be broadly classified as modifiable, nonmodifiable, and additional **(Box 9.1)**.

Pathogenesis of Atherosclerosis

Atherosclerosis is a progressive inflammatory disorder of the arteries characterized by focal deposits of lipids in the intima. It may be clinically silent until they become large enough to reduce tissue perfusion, or until ulceration and disruption of the atheromatous lesion lead to thrombotic occlusion or distal embolization of the vessel.

> **Box 9.1:** Risk factors for atherosclerosis.
>
> A. **Modifiable major risk factors:** Hyperlipidemia, hypertension, cigarette smoking, and diabetes mellitus
> B. **Nonmodifiable risk factors:** Increasing age (men ≥45 years and females ≥55 years), male gender, family history, genetic abnormalities (e.g., familial hypercholesterolemia)
> C. **Additional risk factors:** Inflammation, raised CRP level, hyperhomocystinemia, metabolic syndrome, lipoprotein (a), raised procoagulant levels, inadequate physical activity, stressful lifestyle, obesity, and alcohol

Early Atherosclerosis

- **Fatty streaks** may be the earliest or precursor lesions of atherosclerosis. Endothelial injury and dysfunction leads to adhesion of leukocyte (mainly monocyte) to endothelium, increased vascular permeability, platelet adhesion, and movement of low-density lipoproteins (LDL) across the endothelium into the intima. This initiates the atheroma formation. Lipid accumulated in the intima is engulfed by the macrophages and forms foam cells. This is followed by migration and proliferation of smooth muscle cells into the intima. Lipids accumulate both intracellularly (within macrophages and smooth muscle cells) and extracellularly. This results in formation of atheromatous plaque.
- **Atheromatous plaque (Figs. 9.1A to E):** It consists of three regions—(1) superficial fibrous cap (formed by fibrous tissue synthesized by smooth muscle cells around the lipid core), (2) lipid-rich necrotic core (formed by lipid-laden foam cells that have undergone apoptosis), and (3) shoulder. Some atheromatous plaques bulge into the lumen of the coronary artery and narrow its lumen. This

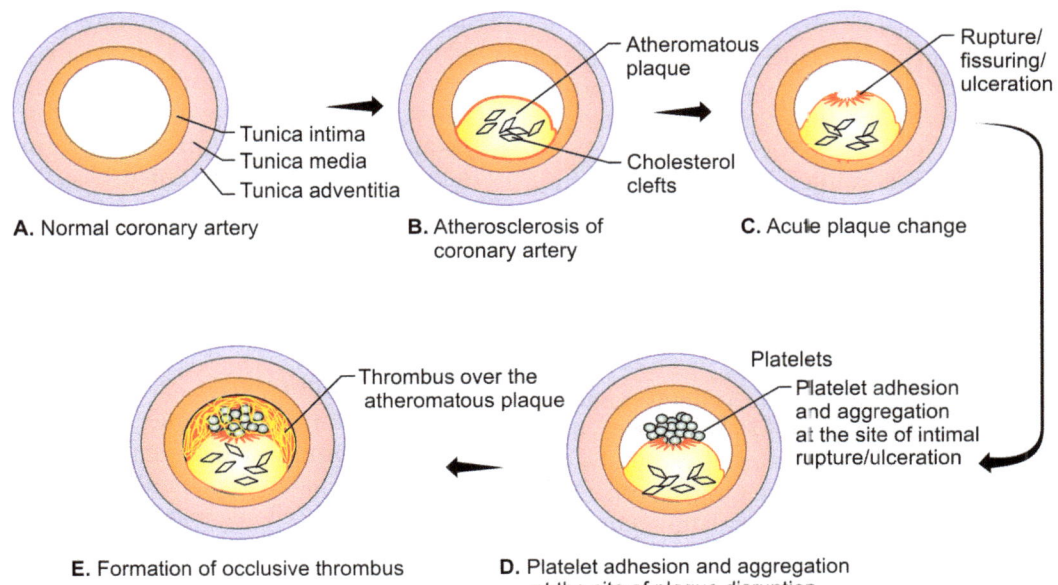

Figs. 9.1A to E: Sequential changes in coronary artery atherosclerosis causing occlusion of lumen in ischemic heart disease.

may limit the blood flow, particularly during increased myocardial demand leading to ischemic symptoms. Depending on the structure of plaque, they can be divided into stable and vulnerable (unstable) plaques:
- *Stable plaques*: They have dense collagenous and thick fibrous caps with minimal inflammation and negligible underlying atheromatous necrotic core. These are less likely to undergo rupture.
- *High-risk or vulnerable plaque*: They have core with many foam cells and abundant extracellular lipid (large lipid core). The fibrous cap is thin with few smooth muscle cells or groups of inflammatory cells (high density of macrophages and T lymphocytes) and increased inflammation. These are likely to undergo rupture.
- *Advanced atherosclerosis/complicated plaques*: Atherosclerotic plaques can undergo clinically important changes
- **Rupture, ulceration, or erosion:** Plaque protrudes into the lumen and can disturb the blood flow, resulting in turbulent flow of blood, which can damage the endothelium and cause rupture, ulceration, or erosion of the intimal surface of plaques.
- **Hemorrhage into a plaque:** It may occur due to rupture of the fibrous cap of the plaque or of the thin-walled vessels formed due to neovascularization.
- **Thrombosis and embolism:** Ulceration/erosion/rupture of endothelial surface exposes the blood to highly thrombogenic subendothelial collagen, favors *thrombus formation*, can partially or completely occlude the lumen (depending on the size of the lumen), and lead to ischemia. The thrombus may become organized or fragmented to form thromboemboli.
- **Atheroembolism:** Plaque rupture, discharge atherosclerotic debris into the bloodstream, and results in atheroemboli.
- **Aneurysm formation:** Atherosclerosis even though an intimal disease may cause pressure or ischemic atrophy of the underlying media. It may also damage the elastic tissue and cause weakening the wall, and result in aneurysmal dilation, which may rupture.
- **Calcification:** It may occur in the central necrotic area of the plaque (dystrophic calcification).

CORONARY ARTERY DISEASE

Angina Pectoris

Definition: Angina pectoris is a clinical syndrome that presents as *paroxysmal* and *recurrent attacks of substernal or precordial chest discomfort* due to *transient myocardial ischemia*, which falls short of inducing necrosis of myocardial cell.
- **Cause:** Transient myocardial ischemia is due to—(1) obstruction of coronary flow by atherosclerosis, (2) coronary arterial spasm, or (3) thrombosis of coronary artery. Others include embolus, coronary ostial stenosis, and coronary arteritis [e.g., in systemic lupus erythematosus (SLE)].
- **Precipitate factors for angina:** These include factors that either increase the oxygen requirement of myocardium or reduce blood supply to the myocardium **(Table 9.1)**.

Table 9.1: Factors precipitating angina.

Factors that increase oxygen demand or cardiac work	Factors that decrease oxygen supply or coronary blood flow
• Exercise and tachycardia • Hypertension, anemia, and pregnancy • Left ventricular hypertrophy • Emotional stress (anger, fright, and excitement) • Hyperthyroidism and arrhythmias • Aortic stenosis or regurgitation	• Decreased oxygenation due to anemia or reduced oxygen saturation • Duration of diastole (coronary blood flow occurs mainly in diastole) • Coronary perfusion pressure (aortic diastolic pressure minus coronary sinus or right atrial diastolic pressure)

Stable Angina Pectoris

❏ Coronary autoregulation is modified by coronary atherosclerosis, left ventricular hypertrophy, and alterations in autonomic nerve function and endothelial function.
❏ Coronary atherosclerosis reduces the lumen of the coronary arteries. It cannot increases in perfusion when the demand for flow is increased (e.g., during exertion or excitement). This leads to a situation where when the demand for blood flow is increased (e.g., during exertion or excitement), there cannot be a corresponding increase in perfusion due to the atheroma.
❏ Stable angina is due to transient myocardial ischemia. Stable angina shows a fixed reduction of at least 70% in the diameter of coronary arteries, which cause reduction in coronary blood flow. Inability to increase oxygen extraction or reduced coronary blood flow, together with increased myocardial demand, leads to angina.

Clinical Features
History
Diagnosis of angina is mainly depends on the clinical history.

Classical or stable or exertional angina pectoris
It is characterized by:
❏ **Chest pain:** Constricting discomfort/squeezing/tightening/heaviness/aching in the front of the chest. Pain may radiate to left arm, neck (throat), jaw (chin), or less commonly to right arm, back, and epigastrium. Typical chest pain lasts 2–5 minutes. *Levine's sign* (clenched fist held over the chest) may be positive.
❏ **Brought on by physical exertion**, such as after meals and in cold, windy weather or by anger or excitement/emotion
❏ **Relieved** (usually within minutes) with *rest or sublingual glyceryl trinitrate*. Occasionally, it may disappear with continued exertion ("walking through the pain"). Pain seldom lasts more than 20 minutes.

Typical angina has all the three features mentioned above. Atypical angina has two out of the three, and nonanginal chest pain (Table 9.2) *one or less of these features. Many patients with angina may have silent episodes of angina, i.e., without any symptoms.*

❏ **Variant (Prinzmetal/vasospastic) angina:** Pain occurs without exertion and usually at rest. It is due to spasm of coronary artery and is more frequent in women. Characteristically, it is associated with transient ST segment elevation on the ECG during the pain. Provocation tests (e.g., hyperventilation, cold pressure testing, or ergometrine challenge) may be needed for establishing the diagnosis. Prognosis is usually better than those with fixed and significant obstructive lesions. Usually, the response to beta-blockers may be poor. Calcium channel blockers are used for the treatment.
❏ Severity of angina is classified by New York Heart Association Classification/Canadian Cardiovascular Society functional classification of angina.

Physical Examination
❏ Usually no abnormal findings in angina. Occasionally, a third/fourth heart sound may be detected during an angina episode, dyskinetic cardiac apex, mitral regurgitation, and even pulmonary edema may be appreciated.
❏ Physical examination should include a careful search for evidence hyperlipidemia (e.g., xanthelasma and tendon xanthoma) valve disease (particularly aortic stenosis characterized by slow rising carotid impulse and ejection systolic murmur radiating to the neck), important risk factors (e.g., hypertension and diabetes mellitus), left ventricular dysfunction (cardiomegaly and gallop rhythm), manifestations of arterial disease (carotid bruits and peripheral vascular disease) and unrelated conditions that may exacerbate angina (anemia and thyrotoxicosis), and obesity. Check the blood pressure to identify coexistent hypertension.

Investigations
Electrocardiography (ECG)
Resting ECG and ECG in-between attacks is normal in most patents (even in patients with severe coronary artery). ECG may show evidence of previous MI and there may be T-wave flattening or inversion in some leads, due to myocardial ischemia or damage. The most convincing ECG evidence of myocardial ischemia is the demonstration of reversible ST segment depression or elevation, with or without T-wave inversion, during the attack of pain (whether spontaneous or induced by exercise testing such as treadmill testing or bicycle ergometry).

Exercise ECG: An exercise tolerance test (ETT) is usually done by using a standard treadmill or bicycle ergometer protocol (recording of ECG before, during, and after exercise). During this process, patient's ECG, BP, and general condition are monitored.
❏ **Indications:**
  • Two sets of cardiac enzymes at 4-hour intervals should be normal.
  • No significant abnormality in 12-lead ECG at the time of arrival and pre-exercise
  • Absence of ischemic chest pain at the time of exercise testing
❏ **Interpretation:** Planar or down-sloping ST segment depression of 1 mm or more indicates ischemia. Up-sloping ST depression is less specific and often found in normal individuals (modified Bruce protocol is followed)

Table 9.2: Differentiating features of chest pain of ischemic and nonischemic origin.

	Favors ischemic origin	Against ischemic origin
Character	Constricting, squeezing, burning, and heaviness	Dull ache, knife-like, sharp, jabs, and pleuritic
Location	Substernal, anterior thorax, arms, shoulders, neck, teeth, and interscapular	Left submammary area and left hemithorax
Provoking factors	Exertion, excitement, cold, meals, and stress	Pain after completion of exercise and pain with movement

Other forms of stress testing
- **Myocardial perfusion scanning:** It is performed using radioactive isotopes. The scintiscans of the myocardium are obtained at rest and during stress (either exercise testing or pharmacological stress, such as a controlled infusion of dipyridamole, adenosine or dobutamine), after the administration of an intravenous radioactive isotope, such as thallium (^{201}thallium) or technetium (^{99}technetium sestamibi). The radioactive isotopes are taken up by viable perfused myocardium. If there is a perfusion defect during stress but not at rest, it indicates evidence of reversible myocardial ischemia, whereas a persistent perfusion defect seen during both phases is usually indicative of previous MI.
- **Stress echocardiography:** It is an alternative to myocardial perfusion scanning and has similar predictive accuracy. On transthoracic echocardiography, the ischemic segments show reversible defects in contractility during exercise or pharmacological stress, whereas infarcted regions do not contract at rest or during stress.

Coronary angiography: It gives detailed anatomical information about the extent and nature of coronary artery disease. It is usually done with a view to coronary artery bypass graft (CABG) surgery or percutaneous coronary intervention (PCI). It is done under local anesthesia and requires specialized radiological equipment, cardiac monitoring, and an experienced team.

Laboratory Tests
- Fasting lipid profile
- Fasting glucose and/or glycated hemoglobin (HbA1c) level, if available; additional oral glucose tolerance test (OGTT), if both are inconclusive
- Complete blood count (CBC) and hematocrit
- Creatinine level with estimation of glomerular filtration rate (GFR)
- Biochemical markers of myocardial injury (Troponin T or I), if clinical evaluation suggests an acute coronary syndrome (ACS).
- Thyroid function tests
- Liver function tests early after beginning statin therapy
- **Newer modalities:** These include multiple-slice spiral computed tomographic coronary angiography (CTCA), intravascular ultrasound, magnetic resonance coronary angiography (MRCA), and positron emission tomography (myocardial viability is assessed using glucose metabolism).

Management of Angina Pectoris
Management can be discussed under three headings—(1) general measures, (2) drug treatment, and (3) surgical treatment.

General measures
- Careful explanation about the nature of their condition (disease process)
- Evaluate the risk factors and steps to correct them where possible.
- Correction of precipitating underlying conditions, e.g., anemia, hyperthyroidism, valvular disease, and arrhythmias should be treated.
- **Management of coexistent conditions:** Identification and treatment of aggravating conditions such as aortic stenosis, hypertrophic cardiomyopathy, control of hypertension, and diabetes (ACE inhibitors are useful in these patients).
- **Lipid management:** Identify hypercholesterolemia (hyperlipidemia) and treat with diet and drugs (with the goal of reducing LDL <100 mg dL; goal of <70 mg/dL in very high-risk patients)
- **Lifestyle modification:**
  - *Healthy diet*: Increase polyunsaturated fatty acid consumption, mainly from oily fish: *2 to 3 servings of oily fish per week* may help to prevent cardiovascular disease (CVD).
  - Saturated fatty acids must comprise less than 10% of the total energy intake. Protein with low saturated fats should replace those high in these harmful fats.
  - Limit salt intake to less than 5 g per day.
  - Consume 30–45 g of fiber/day (e.g., wholegrain products, fruits, and vegetables). Avoid simple carbohydrates with high glycemic load.
  - Consume 200 g of vegetables and 200 g of fruits per day.
  - Limit consumption of alcoholic beverages.

Anti-anginal drug treatment
Anti-angina drugs can be divided into five groups. They are used to relieve or prevent the symptoms of angina. These include—(1) nitrates, (2) β-blockers, (3) calcium antagonists, (4) potassium channel activators, and (5) I_f channel antagonist.

1. **Nitrates:**
   - Short-acting [glyceryl trinitrate (GTN), nitroglycerine] or long-acting (isosorbide dinitrate and isosorbide mononitrate)
     - *Mechanism of action*: Nitrates directly act on smooth muscle in the walls of blood vessels and produce dilatation of arteries and veins. This lowers blood pressure, reduces venous return to heart, and produces dilatation of coronary blood vessels. Nitrates cause reduction in myocardial oxygen demand (lower preload and afterload) as well as an increase in myocardial oxygen supply (coronary vasodilatation) predominantly by perfusing the subendocardial region.
     - *Indications*: Prophylaxis and treatment of angina. Prophylactically to use the drug before taking exercise that is liable to produce pain. Prophylactic use of glyceryl trinitrate (GTN) should be encouraged because physical activity promotes the formation of collateral vessels. For predominant nocturnal angina, long-acting nitrates can be given at the end of the day.
     - *Contraindications*: Nitrates should not be given along with phosphodiesterase type-5 (PDE-5) and inhibitors (e.g., sildenafil, tadalafil, and vardenafil) within the same 24 hours period because these may produce sever hypotension. Other contraindications include obstructive hypertrophic cardiomyopathy, severe aortic stenosis, constrictive pericarditis, mitral stenosis, and closed-angle glaucoma.

- **Glyceryl trinitrate (GTN):**
  - *Preparations*: (1) Metered-dose aerosol (400 µg per spray) or (2) as a tablet (300 or 500 µg)
  - *Action*: Sublingual GTN has a short duration of action will relieve an attack of angina in 2–3 minutes.
- **Isosorbide dinitrate** (10–20 mg 2–3 times daily) has prolonged action and is given by mouth. Headache is a common side effect but tends to diminish, if the patient perseveres with the treatment. Tolerance can develop with continuous nitrate therapy, which can be avoided by a 6–8-hour nitrate-free period. Hence, doses are given in the morning and afternoon.
- **Isosorbide mononitrate** (20–60 mg once or twice daily) also can be given by mouth.

2. **β-blockers:**
   Mechanism: These drugs lower oxygen demand of myocardium by reducing heart rate, blood pressure, and myocardial contractility. They inhibit apoptosis by inhibiting beta adrenoceptors, and have antioxidant and antiproliferative properties. They also counteract the direct adverse effects of catecholamines and have antiarrhythmic action. They are useful to control tachycardia, hypertension, and continued angina.
   - *Cardioselective* β-blockers: These include slow-release *metoprolol* 50–200 mg daily, *bisoprolol* 5–15 mg daily, and *atenolol* (50–200 mg/day). They have fewer peripheral side effects.
   - *Non-selective* β-blockers: *Propranolol* is started in a small initial dose (20 mg thrice daily) and gradually increased to 80–120 mg three times daily. They may aggravate coronary vasospasm by blocking the coronary artery β2-adrenoceptors.
   - *Carvedilol* (3.125–25 mg twice a day) has additional advantage of having antiarrhythmic effects.

3. **Calcium channel antagonists (calcium channel blockers):**
   - *Dihydropyridine calcium antagonists* [e.g., nifedipine, amlodipine (dihydropyridines), felodipine, and nicardipine]: They produce coronary and peripheral arterial dilatation, and negative inotropy. They often cause a reflex tachycardia.
     - *Nifedipine*: It is a powerful coronary and systemic arteriolar dilator. This can cause marked reflex tachycardia. Short-acting nifedipine are not used because it can increase mortality due to myocardial infarction. Long-acting preparations are given usually along with a β-blocker. Dose is 5–20 mg 3 times daily.
     - *Amlodipine*: Dose is 2.5–10 mg daily. Side effects are ankle edema and reflex tachycardia.
   - *Nondihydropyridine calcium antagonists*, e.g., verapamil (phenyl alkylamines), diltiazem (benzothiazepine). They produce coronary and peripheral arterial dilatation and negative inotropy, and also reduce conductivity. Because of their negative inotropic effect, they should be avoided in patients with impaired ventricular function (uncompensated heart failure).
     - *Verapamil*: Dose is 40–80 mg thrice daily. It has useful anti-arrhythmic properties. Common adverse effect is constipation.
     - *Diltiazem*: Dose is 60–120 mg 3 times daily. It has similar anti-arrhythmic properties to verapamil.
     - β-blockers reduce mortality after myocardial infarction. Hence, it is reasonable to start a β-blocker and then add a calcium channel blocker, if needed. However, β-blockers should not be combined with verapamil, because of their synergistic effect on heart rate and myocardial contractility.

4. **Second-line anti-anginal drugs:**
   - *Potassium channel activators/openers*: Nicorandil is given in the dose of 10–30 mg twice daily orally.
   - I_f *channel antagonist*: Ivabradine selectively inhibits inward sodium-potassium current [important pacemaking current in the cells sinus (SA) node]. This slows the rate of diastolic depolarization and induces bradycardia ("bradycardic" drug).
   - *Ranolazine*: It inhibits late sodium channels in cardiac cells. It does not affect heart rate and blood pressure. Dose is 500–1000 mg twice a day. Side effects include constipation, dizziness, and prolongation of QT interval.
   - *Trimetazidine*: Dose is 20 mg three times daily. It is associated with greater improvements in time to onset of angina, and the mean weekly number of anginal episodes.
   - *Fasudil*: It is an inhibitor of Rho kinase that is involved in the vascular smooth muscle contractile response, and is of benefit in patients with stable and microvascular angina (angina with normal coronary arteries).

   Indications and contraindications of various antianginal drugs are given in **Table 9.3**.

5. **Antiplatelet therapy:**
   Anti-anginal drugs ameliorate only symptoms but may not reduce mortality. To reduce the risk of adverse events such as MI, antiplatelet drugs are given.
   Aspirin:
   - Aspirin inhibits the synthesis of prostaglandins namely thromboxane A_2, which is a potent vasoconstrictor and platelet activator.
   - *Dose*: Low-dose therapy in the dose of 75–150 mg/day.

   P2Y12 antagonists:
   - *Clopidogrel:*
     - It is a thienopyridine, which inhibits ADP-dependent activation of the GPIIb/IIIa complex and prevents platelet aggregation.
     - It is an equally effective antiplatelet agent that can be used in patients who cannot tolerate aspirin.
     - It may have a synergistic effect when combined with aspirin in patients following acute coronary syndrome or implantation of a drug-eluting stent. The benefit of its combination with aspirin was not found chronic stable angina.
     - *Dose* is 75 mg daily.
   - *Prasugrel and ticagrelor* are new P2Y12 antagonists have higher platelet inhibition compared to clopidogrel.

Table 9.3: Indications and contraindications of various antianginal drugs.

Drug	Indication	Contraindication
β-blockers	• Postmyocardial infarction • CHF (compensated) • Ventricular tachycardia • Supraventricular tachycardia (SVT) • Systemic hypertension • Hyperthyroidism	• Decompensated HF • Severe bradycardia or AV block • Severe depression • Symptomatic PAD • Raynaud's phenomenon • Severe COPD
DHP-CCB	• Systemic hypertension • Raynaud's phenomenon • Prinzmetal angina • Severe bradycardia or AV block	Hypotension
Non DHP-CCB	• SVT • Systemic hypertension	• Severe bradycardia • Significant AV block • LV dysfunction or HF
Nitrates	LV dysfunction or HF	• Severe aortic stenosis • PDE-5 inhibitor use
Ivabradine	Increased resting heart rate	• Bradycardia • Second degree AV block
Ranolazine	• Bradycardia or AV block • Low blood pressure • LV dysfunction • Possible diabetes	• Treatment with QT prolonging Agents • Moderate or severe Hepatic dysfunction
Nicorandil	Refractory angina	• Severe aortic stenosis • PDE5 inhibitor use

(AV: atrioventricular; CCBs: calcium channel blockers; COPD: chronic obstructive pulmonary disease; DHP: dihydropyridine calcium antagonists; LV: left ventricular; PAD: peripheral artery disease; PDE-5 inhibitor: phosphodiesterase type-5 inhibitor)

6. **Statins:** Irrespective of the LDL or cholesterol levels, proprotein convertase subtilisin/kexin type 9 (PCSK9) inhibitors confer a mortality benefit to patients with IHD whose LDL levels remain >70 mg/dL despite high-intensity statins.

Invasive (Surgical) Treatment: Revascularization

Percutaneous Coronary Intervention (PCI)

❏ Percutaneous coronary interventions include angioplasty [percutaneous transluminal coronary angioplasty (PTCA)] or stent placement in the coronary artery. It is the process to maximize and maintain dilatation of a stenosed coronary artery. A coronary stent is a piece of coated metallic "scaffolding" (fine guidewire) that can be deployed on a balloon. In this process, a small inflatable balloon and metallic coronary stent introduced percutaneously into the arterial circulation via an arterial catheter through the femoral, radial, or brachial artery under radiographic control. It is passed across the coronary stenosis and balloon is inflated to dilate the stenosis. Dilatation can be repeated, if symptoms recur.

❏ **Types of stents:** Two types, namely—*(1) bare-metal stents and (2) drug-eluting stents*. The drug-eluting stents are coated stents lined with substances (e.g., sirolimus and pacliltaxel) that prevent neointimal hyperplasia and reduce the risk of coronary artery reocclusion. Recent data suggest both types of stents to be equally effective over long-term follow-up.

❏ **Indications for percutaneous coronary interventions (PCI):**
  • Ideal for single-vessel or two-vessel coronary disease without significant lesions in the proximal left anterior descending artery (LAD), with normal LV function, with high risk on noninvasive testing and a large area of viable myocardium.
  • Undergone prior PCI with either recurrence of stenosis or high risk on noninvasive testing
  • Failure of medical therapy and with acceptable risk for PCI. Treatment of choice for unstable angina (UA) when rest pain recurs in spite of full medical treatment
  • Lesion suitable for PCI
  • No diabetes

Coronary artery bypass grafting (CABG):

❏ In coronary artery bypass grafting, autologous veins (reversed segments of the patient's own saphenous vein) or arteries (internal mammary artery/radial artery/gastroepiploic arteries) are anastomosed to the ascending aorta at one end and to the native coronary arteries distal to the area of occlusion/stenosis at the other end.

❏ It is usually done under cardiopulmonary bypass but, in few cases, it can be done in the beating heart ("off-pump" surgery). Aspirin (75–150 mg daily) and clopidogrel (75 mg daily) both improve graft patency, and one or other should be given indefinitely.

❏ **Indications:**
  • Significant left main coronary disease
  • Triple vessel disease/two blood vessel disease with reduced left ventricular function (left ventricular ejection fraction is <50%)
  • Two vessel disease with significant proximal left anterior descending artery disease and either left ventricular ejection fraction (LVEF) <50% or demonstrable ischemic on noninvasive testing.
  • Failure of medical therapy and with acceptable risk for CABG
  • Diabetes
  • Prior CABG, PCI (percutaneous coronary interventions) with recurrent restenosis
  • Abnormal stress test

Flowchart 9.1 shows scheme for the investigation and management of stable angina.

ACUTE CORONARY SYNDROME

Ischemic heart disease (IHD) forms a spectrum of diseases (**Flowchart 9.2**) and consists of stable angina and acute coronary syndromes [includes ST-segment elevation myocardial infarction (STEMI), non-ST segment elevation myocardial infarction (NSTEMI), and unstable angina].

Flowchart 9.1: Scheme for the investigation and management of stable angina.

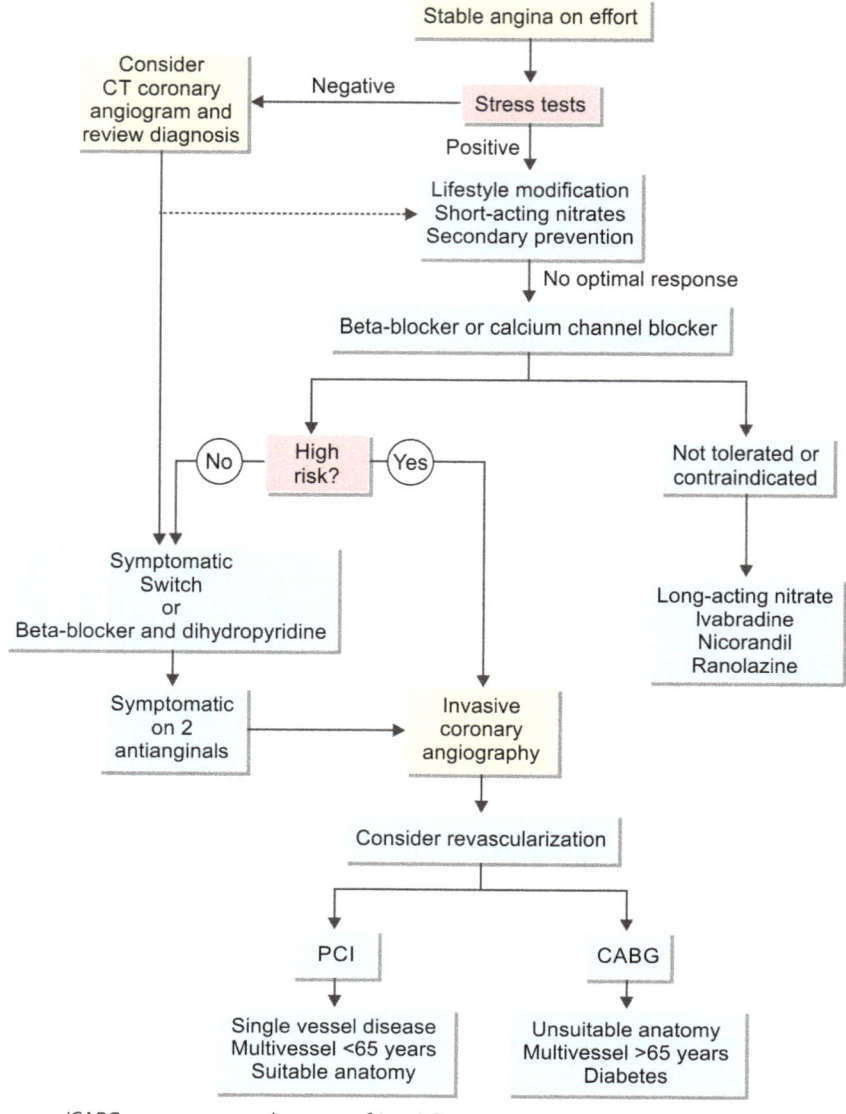

(CABG: coronary artery bypass grafting; PCI: percutaneous coronary intervention)

Flowchart 9.2: Spectrum of ischemic heart disease.

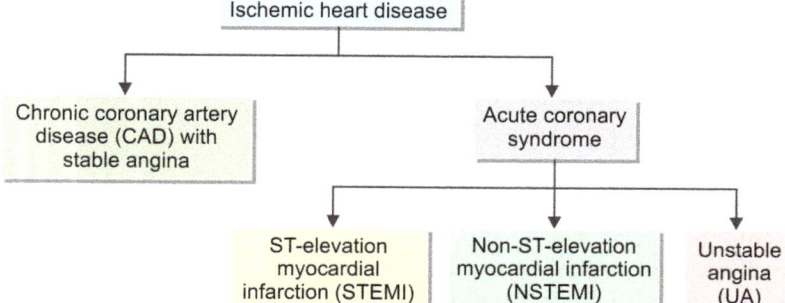

Acute coronary syndrome (ACS) is a term used for spectrum of clinical presentations due to acute myocardial ischemia. It includes:
- **ST-elevation myocardial infarction (STEMI) (Flowchart 9.3):** Majority of STEMI has Q-wave MI (QwMI).
- **Non-ST elevation myocardial infarction (NSTEMI):** A small percentage of STEMI and majority of NSTEMI have non-Q-wave MI (NQwMI, previously known as subendocardial infarction). However, the terms Q-wave or non-Q-wave infarctions are not used at present.
- **Unstable angina (UA):** Includes patients with acute coronary syndrome but with normal ECG, without elevation of cardiac injury markers and no ST elevation in the ECG. Management of unstable angina and NSTEMI is similar.

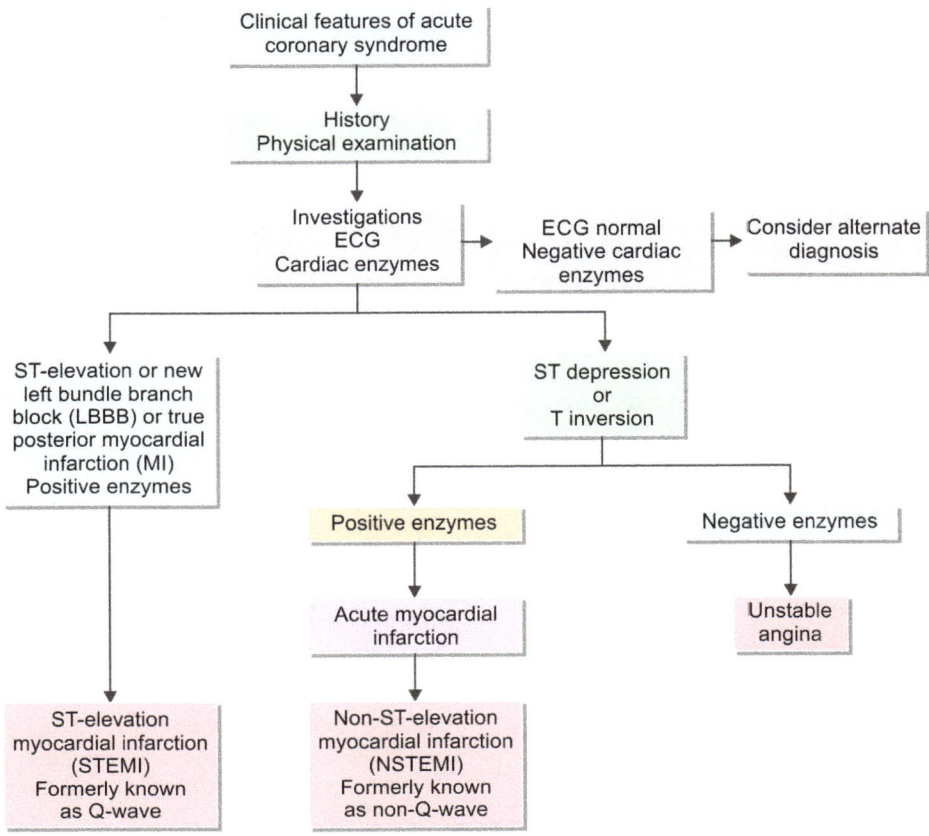

Flowchart 9.3: New classification scheme of acute coronary syndrome.

Pathophysiology

Pathophysiology of acute coronary syndrome is described in **Table 9.4**.

ST Elevation Myocardial Infarction

- STEMI is due to the *formation of an occlusive thrombus at the site of rupture of an atheromatous plaque* in a coronary artery. Usually, there is minimal prior narrowing of coronary lumen.
- **Other causes:** These are coronary spasm, rarely coronary emboli as well as by ostial narrowing due to aortitis, hypercoagulable state, and use of cocaine. Congenital anomalies such as the origin of the left anterior descending coronary artery from the pulmonary artery may cause myocardial ischemia in infancy, but this cause is very rare in adults.
- Limitation of the ability to increase flow to meet increased myocardial demand occurs with 50% coronary stenosis, while 80% coronary stenosis causes myocardial ischemia at rest or with minimal stress.

Non-ST Elevation Myocardial Infarction

Causes:

- It is most commonly caused by an imbalance between oxygen supply and oxygen demand. This imbalance results from a partially occluding thrombus forming on a disrupted atherothrombotic coronary plaque or on eroded coronary artery endothelium.
- Severe ischemia or myocardial necrosis may develop due to the reduction of coronary blood flow caused by the partially occluding thrombus and by downstream embolization of platelet aggregates and/or atherosclerotic debris.
- **Other causes:** More than one of the following processes may be involved:
  - Dynamic obstruction (e.g., coronary spasm, as in Prinzmetal variant angina)
  - Severe mechanical obstruction due to progressive coronary atherosclerosis
  - Increased myocardial oxygen demand produced by conditions such as fever, tachycardia, and thyrotoxicosis in the presence of fixed epicardial coronary obstruction.

Table 9.4: Pathophysiology of stable angina and acute coronary syndrome.

Stable angina	Unstable angina	NSTEMI	STEMI
Progressive narrowing of coronary lumen Stable fibrous cap	Progressive narrowing Acute worsening of coronary lumen due to thrombus formation	Acute worsening of coronary lumen due to thrombus formation Subocclusive/transient coronary thrombus with myocardial necrosis	Minimal prior narrowing of coronary lumen Acute rupture of thin fibrous cap Occlusive thrombus formation Acute injury pattern Myocardial necrosis

(STEMI: ST-segment elevation myocardial infarction; NSTEMI: non-ST segment elevation myocardial infarction)

Diagnosis of NSTEMI:

- *Clinical presentation*: Diagnosis of NSTEMI is largely based on the clinical presentation. Typically, chest discomfort is severe and has at least one of three features:
  1. Occurs at rest (or with minimal exertion) lasting for >10 minutes
  2. Relatively recent onset (i.e., within the prior 2 weeks) and/or
  3. Occurs with a crescendo pattern (i.e., distinctly more severe, prolonged, or frequent than previous episodes)
- *Evidence of myocardial necrosis*: Diagnosis of NSTEMI is established, if a patient with the above clinical features shows the evidence of myocardial necrosis, as reflected in abnormally elevated levels of biomarkers of cardiac necrosis.

Clinical Features of Acute Coronary Syndrome

Symptoms (Table 9.5)

- **Prolonged cardiac pain:** Myocardial ischemia causing chest discomfort is termed as angina pectoris. Thus, classic manifestation of ischemia is angina, which is usually described as a heavy chest pressure or squeezing, a burning feeling, or difficulty breathing.
- The discomfort often radiates to the left shoulder, neck, or arm. It typically builds in intensity over a period of a few minutes.
- The pain may begin with exercise or psychological stress, but ACS most commonly occurs without obvious precipitating factors.
- Pain may be absent in patients with prior cardiac, prior stroke, age >75 years, and diabetes mellitus. Painless MI is more common in females compared to males.
- Any patient with severe chest pain that lasts for more than 20 minutes may be suffering from a myocardial infarction. This pain is usually does not respond to sublingual GTN.
- **Other features:** These include anxiety and fear of impending death, nausea and vomiting, breathlessness, and collapse/syncope.

Table 9.5: Symptoms and signs of acute myocardial infarction.

Cause of signs	Sign
Tissue damage	Mild fever
Sympathetic activation	Pallor, sweating, and tachycardia
Impaired myocardial function	Hypotension, oliguria, cold peripheries, narrow pulse pressure, raised JVP, third heart sound, soft first heart sound, diffuse apical impulse, and basal crepitations in the lung
Vagal activation	Vomiting and bradycardia
Complication	Systolic murmur due to mitral regurgitation or uncommonly due to VSD, pericardial friction rub due to pericarditis

Complications of Acute Coronary Syndrome

Various signs of acute coronary syndrome and its causes are described in **Table 9.6**.

Table 9.6: Various signs of acute coronary syndrome and its causes.

Type	Complication
Ischemic	Infarct extension, reinfarction, and angina
Mechanical	Cardiogenic shock, cardiac failure, mitral regurgitation, ventricular aneurysm, and cardiac rupture (papillary muscle, ventricular septum, and cardiac wall)
Arrhythmic	Atrial or ventricular arrhythmia, dysfunction of sinus or atrioventricular node
Thromboembolic	Left ventricular mural thrombus, CNS embolism (e.g., stroke), and peripheral embolism
Inflammatory	Pericarditis

(CNS: central nervous system)

Investigations

Electrocardiogram

The 12-lead ECG is central to confirming the diagnosis and should be done and interpreted within 10-minute of arrival. The initial ECG may be normal or nondiagnostic in about 30% of cases. Repeated ECGs are needed, especially where the diagnosis is uncertain or the patient has recurrent or persistent symptoms.

Changes in ECG: Characteristic changes are observed in leads that "face" the ischemic or infracted area (e.g., anteroseptal, anterolateral, strict anterior, inferior, and posterior wall infarction) (**Fig. 9.2**).

- **STEMI:** *ST-segment deviation* is the earliest ECG change. With proximal occlusion of a major coronary artery, ST-segment elevation (or new bundle branch block) is observed initially. Later, there is diminution in the size of the R wave and, in transmural (full-thickness) infarction, there is development of a Q wave. Subsequently, the T wave becomes inverted and persists after the ST segment has returned to normal.
- **NSTEMI and unstable angina:** It is due to partial occlusion of a major vessel or complete occlusion of a minor vessel, causing unstable angina or partial-thickness (subendocardial) MI. They usually produce ST-segment depression and T-wave changes. When infarction is present, there may be some loss of R waves in the absence of Q waves.

Plasma Cardiac Biomarkers (Biochemical Markers of Cardiac Injury)

- **Unstable angina:** There is no detectable rise in cardiac biomarkers or enzymes in unstable angina and the initial diagnosis is made from the clinical history and ECG only.
- **Myocardial infarction:** It causes arise in the plasma concentration of enzymes and proteins that are normally concentrated within cardiac cells. These include creatine kinase (CK), aspartate aminotransferase (AST), lactate dehydrogenase (LDH), myoglobin, and troponins (troponin I and troponin T). These markers leak from the necrotic myocardial cells into the blood circulation.
- **Cardiac creatine kinase (CK):** It is a *nonspecific enzyme marker* and it is present in brain, myocardium, and skeletal muscle. It has two isoforms designated "M" and "B".

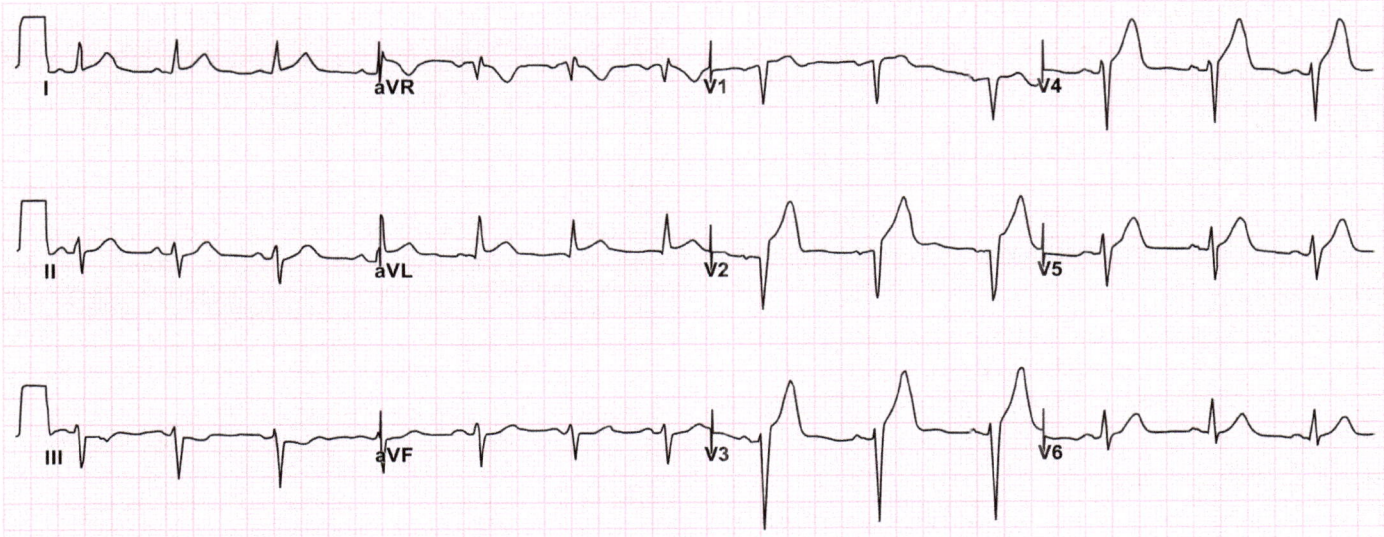

Fig. 9.2: Electrocardiogram (ECG) showing acute anterolateral ST-elevation myocardial infarction (STEMI).

MB heterodimers are chiefly in cardiac muscle (lesser amounts in skeletal muscle).
- MB form of creatine kinase (CK-MB) is sensitive but not specific, because it is also raised with skeletal muscle injury.
- CK-MB levels rise within 4–6 hours of the onset of MI, peaks at 12 hours, and returns to normal within 72 hours.
- Total CK is also raised elevated in diseases of skeletal muscle (e.g., polymyositis and muscular dystrophies), hypothyroidism, and stroke.

☐ **Lactate dehydrogenase (LDH):** It is not specific marker. It *starts rising* after *24–48 hours*. It remains *for many days* and *returns to normal in 7–14 days*. An elevated LDH_1 (an isoenzyme of LDH) is a more sensitive indicator of myocardial infarction than total LDH.

☐ **Myoglobin:** It is an oxygen-carrying respiratory protein found only in skeletal and cardiac muscle. It is an *earliest marker of MI*; the level rises within 1–3 hours, *peaks in about 8–12 hours*, and returns to normal in about 24–36 hours.

☐ **Cardiac troponins:** These are proteins involved in heart muscle contraction. *Increased plasma levels establish the diagnosis of myocardial infarction*. Cardiac-specific proteins are of two types namely cardiac *Troponins I (cTnI) and T (cTnT)*. They are *most sensitive and specific markers* of myocardial infarction. Levels begin to *rise at 4–6 hours* and *peaks at 48 hours*. The elevated troponin levels may *remain for 7–10 days* after acute MI and, therefore, this assay is particularly useful in the evaluation of patients who present sufficiently long after their episode of chest pain. Further, about one-third of patients with unstable angina also have elevated cTn, which classifies these groups of patients to non-ST elevation MI.

☐ **Aspartate aminotransferase:** It starts to rise by about 12 hours and reaches a peak on the 1st or 2nd day.

☐ **Other enzymes:** (1) Ischemia-modified albumin, (2) N-terminal proBNP, (3) suPAR (soluble urokinase-type plasminogen activator receptor), and (4) glycogen phosphorylase isoenzyme BB

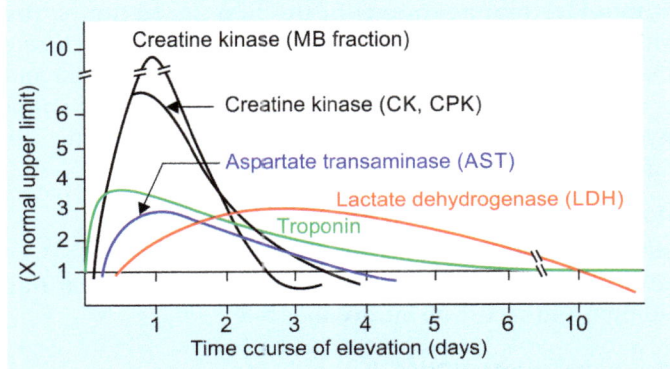

Fig. 9.3: Various enzyme levels following acute myocardial infarction.

Table 9.7: Characteristics of plasma biomarkers for acute myocardial infarction (AMI).

Marker protein	Elevation in plasma after AMI (h)	Peak plasma concentration (h)	Normalization of plasma level (days)
Myoglobin	2–3	6–12	1–2
Cardiac troponin I	3–8	12–24	7–10
Cardiac troponin T	3–8	12–24	7–10
Creatine kinase MB	2–6	12–24	2–3

Various enzyme levels in acute coronary syndrome are shown in **Figure 9.3** and **Table 9.7**.

Other Blood Tests
☐ Leukocytosis with a peak on 1st day
☐ *Erythrocyte sedimentation rate (ESR)*: Raised and may remain so for days
☐ *C-reactive protein*: Elevated
☐ *Heart-type fatty acid-binding protein (H-FABP)* as a plasma marker for the diagnosis of patients presenting with chest

pain suggestive of myocardial infarction, especially in the early hours (within 2 hours) after onset of symptoms. However, their use as a diagnostic tool for MI is limited.

Chest X-ray
- It may show evidence of pulmonary edema that is not evident on clinical examination.
- Heart size is usually normal but there may be cardiomegaly due to previous myocardial damage or pericardial effusion.

Echocardiography
It is useful for assessing ventricular function and for detecting complications (e.g., mural thrombus, cardiac rupture, ventricular septal defect, mitral regurgitation, and pericardial effusion).

Radionuclide Scanning
It is used to detect the site of necrosis and the extent of damage to ventricular function.

Management
Immediate management: In the first 24–48 hours, the patients should be admitted immediately to hospital. During first 24–48 hours, the risk for fatal arrhythmia is highest and as a result, there is a significant risk of death or recurrent myocardial ischemia. Patients are best treated in an intensive coronary care unit.

Management of Acute Myocardial Infarction
Initial Treatment
Admit in intensive coronary care unit, attach a cardiac monitor, and secure an intravenous line.

> General treatment (**"MONAC"**):
> - **M**orphine 2–4 mg q 5–10 minute to control chest pain.
> - **O**xygen 4 L/minute: Hypoxemia in uncomplicated MI is usually due to ventilation–perfusion abnormalities and may be exacerbated by CHF. Therefore, oxygen is given to patients suspected of having an acute coronary syndromes and oxygen saturation <90%.
> - **N**TG (nitroglycerine) sublingual or spray, followed by infusion for persistent chest pain
> - **A**spirin 160–325 mg chew and swallow or/and
> - **C**lopidogrel 300 mg oral
> - *Specific therapy*:
>   - Thrombolysis or percutaneous coronary interventions
>   - Treat complications (arrhythmias, congestive failure, and shock)

Control of pain by analgesics:
- Proper control of pain is necessary not only to relieve distress but also to lower adrenergic drive, which reduces vascular resistance, BP, infarct size, and susceptibility to ventricular arrhythmias.
- *Intravenous opiates*: Initially, morphine in the dose of 2–4 mg or diamorphine 2.5–5 mg is administered along with antiemetics (metoclopramide 10 mg) should be administered, and repeated until the patient is comfortable.
- β-*blockers*, nitroglycerine, and thrombolysis may also help in reducing the pain.

Table 9.8: Various antiplatelet agents and their dosage.

Oral antiplatelets	
Aspirin	Initial dose of *325 mg* nonenteric formulation followed by *75–100 mg/day* of an enteric or a nonenteric formulation
Clopidogrel	Loading dose of *300–600 mg* followed by *75 mg/day*
Prasugrel	Pre-PCI: Loading dose *60 mg* followed by *10 mg/day*
Ticagrelor	Loading dose of *180 mg* followed by *90 mg twice daily*
Intravenous antiplatelet therapy	
Abciximab	0.25 mg/kg bolus followed by infusion of 0.125 μg/kg per min (maximum 10 μg/min) for 12–24 hours
Eptifibatide	180 μg/kg bolus followed 10 min later by second bolus of 180 μg with infusion of 2.0 μg/kg per min for 72–96 hours following first bolus
Tirofiban	5 μg/kg per min followed by infusion of 0.15 μg/kg per min for 48–96 hours
Others	*Phosphodiesterase inhibitors*—cilostazol

Antiplatelet therapy
Various antiplatelet agents and their dosage are mentioned in **Table 9.8**.

Anticoagulants (antithrombin therapy)
Prophylactic anticoagulants are given to prevent deep vein thrombosis and pulmonary embolism in patients who do not receive fibrinolytic agents. They reduce the risk of thromboembolic complications and prevent reinfarction in the absence of reperfusion therapy or after successful thrombolysis.

Preparations
- **Unfractionated heparin:** It is given as an initial bolus dose of 60 IU/kg (with a maximum dose of 4,000 units) followed by an initial infusion of 12 IU/kg/h (maximum 1,000 units/h). The dose is adjusted to attain the activated partial thromboplastin time at 1.5–2 times control. Heparin is given before the completion of infusion of rt-PA or tenecteplase or patients receiving STK.
- **Low-molecular weight heparin:** It is used as an adjunct to thrombolytics. It produces higher re-perfusion rate and lower re-occlusion rate compared to unfractionated heparin. Dose of 5,000 units is given twice a day subcutaneously.
- **Direct thrombin inhibitors:** These appear better than the unfractionated heparin in patients undergoing PCI. These include hirudin and bivalirudin. Pentasaccharides (subcutaneous fondaparinux 2.5 mg daily) are safe and effective. However, fondaparinux is not be used as sole agent and contraindicated, if PCI is planned.

Statins
High-dose statins are recommended in all patients during the first 24 hours of admission for STEMI, irrespective of the patient's cholesterol concentration, if there is no contraindication (e.g., allergy and active liver disease). They are recommended during the early phase of therapy up to at least 4 weeks. Patient on statin therapy presenting with STEMI should continue statin.

Flowchart 9.4: Management of acute coronary syndrome.

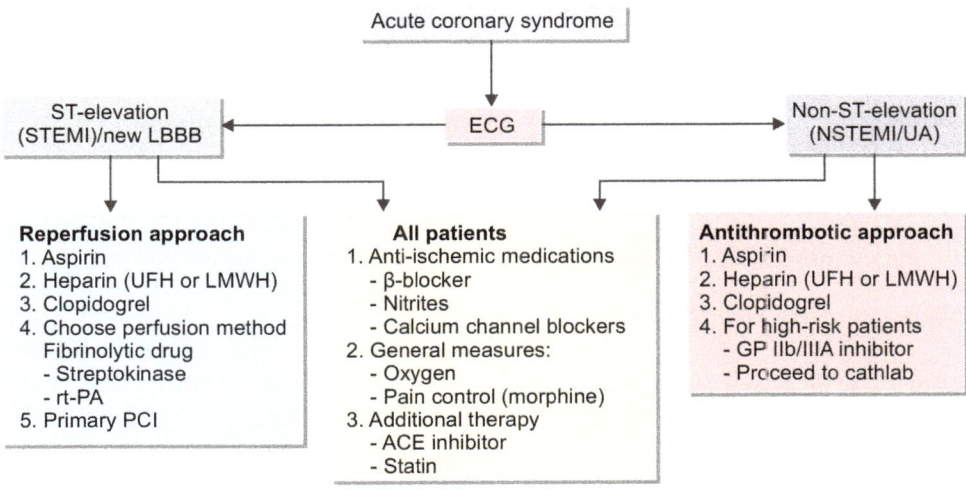

(ACE: angiotensin-converting enzyme; UFH: unfractionated heparin; LBBB: left bundle branch block; LMWH: low-molecular-weight heparin; PCI percutaneous coronary intervention)

Statins lower cholesterol, direct effects on endothelial function, oxidative stress, inflammation, thrombosis, as well as plaque stabilization. High-dose atorvastatin (40–80 mg) or rosuvastatin (20–40 mg) therapy before emergency percutaneous coronary intervention has following advantages.

Management of acute coronary syndrome is indicated in **Flowchart 9.4.**

Thrombolytic (or Fibrinolytic) Therapy in Acute Coronary Syndrome

Indications for thrombolysis in acute myocardial infarction are described in **Box 9.2.**

Fibrinolytic therapy should be initiated within 30 minutes (door-to-needle time or first medical contact-to-needle time).

Thrombolytic agents: These include plasminogen activators, i.e., streptokinase (STK), urokinase (UK), human tissue plasminogen activator (tPA-alteplase), recombinant plasminogen activator (rPA-reteplase), tenecteplase, anisoylated plasminogen streptokinase activator complex (APSAC, anistreplase), and single-chain urokinase plasminogen activator (scu-PA) **(Table 9.9).**

Mechanism of action: Thrombolytic or fibrinolytic agents lyse thrombi/clot to recanalize the occluded vessels (mainly coronary arteries) by the activation of plasminogen to form plasmin. They are curative rather than prophylactic.

Box 9.2: Indications for thrombolysis in acute myocardial infarction.

Thrombolysis: Definitely beneficial—
* ST-segment elevation of more than 0.1 mV in two or more contiguous leads, with time to therapy 12 hours or less
* Left bundle-branch block (LBBB) obscuring ST-segment analysis and history of acute myocardial infarction for less than 12 hours

Thrombolysis: Some benefit—
* ST-segment elevation with time to therapy 12–24 hours

Thrombolysis: Not indicated—
* ST-segment depression only (unless leads V_1-V_4 show ST depression related to posterior wall myocardial infarction)
* Time to therapy >24 hours

Table 9.9: Various thrombolytic agents and their dosage.

Thrombolytic agent	Dose
Alteplase (tissue plasminogen activator-tPA)	15 mg bolus followed by 50 mg intravenously over the first 30 minute, followed by 35 mg over the next 60 minutes
Streptokinase (STK)	1.5 million units (MU) intravenous infusion over 1 hour
Tenecteplase (TNK)	Given as a single weight-based intravenous bolus of 0.53 mg/kg over 10 seconds
Reteplase (rPA)	Double-bolus regimen consisting of a 10-MU bolus given over 2–3 minutes, followed by second 10-MU bolus 30 minutes later

❑ *Fibrin-specific fibrinolytics:* They generate fibrin-specific fibrinolytics at the site of thrombus/clot. Examples include rPA (reteplase), tenecteplase (TNK), and scu-PA. They have lower mortality rate compared with STK and also lack the significant acute side effects of hypotension and allergy caused by STK.

❑ *Generation plasmin in the systemic circulation:* These agents generate plasmin in systemic circulation producing a systemic lytic state. This leads to a reduction in blood viscosity, and produces strong anticoagulant and antiplatelet effects. Examples include streptokinase (STK) and urokinase (UK). STK use is associated with lower incidence of intracranial hemorrhage, especially in older individuals.

Thrombolytic therapy is not recommended for patients with NSTEMI and unstable angina (**Box 9.3**).

Complications of thrombolytic therapy
❑ **Hemorrhage:** It is the major complication. The most common site is in the region of puncture sites, genitourinary system, and intracranial hemorrhage (in about 0.5% of patients).
❑ **Allergic reactions:** These may develop with use of STK and APSAC.
❑ **Hypotension:** It may develop, if STK is infused rapidly.

> **Box 9.3: Contraindications to thrombolytic therapy.**
>
> *Absolute:*
> - History of cerebrovascular hemorrhage anytime in life
> - History of nonhemorrhagic stroke or other cerebrovascular event within the past 1 year
> - Uncontrolled marked hypertension (systolic BP >180 mm Hg, diastolic BP >110 mm Hg). However, STK can be given
> - Suspected aortic dissection
> - Active internal bleeding (excluding menses)
> - Known intracranial aneurysm/AV malformation/neoplasm (primary or metastatic)
> - Intracranial/spinal surgery within last 3 months
>
> *Relative:*
> - Current use of anticoagulants (INR ≥2)
> - Recent (<2 weeks) invasive or surgical procedure, prolonged (>10 min) CPR
> - Known bleeding diathesis
> - Recent trauma (including traumatic resuscitation)
> - Pregnancy
> - Hemorrhage ophthalmic condition
> - Active peptic ulcer disease
> - History of severe hypertension that is currently controlled

Percutaneous Coronary Intervention

Percutaneous coronary intervention (PCI) is the treatment of choice, provided it is performed promptly by a qualified interventional cardiologist in an appropriate facility.

Indications: Patients with STEMI with following features—
- Symptoms of ischemia of less than 12 hours duration
- Symptoms of ischemia of less than 12 hours duration who have contraindications to fibrinolytic therapy, irrespective of the time delay from first medical contact
- Cardiogenic shock or acute severe heart failure (HF), irrespective of time delay from MI onset
- May be recommended, if there is clinical and/or ECG evidence of ongoing ischemia between 12 and 24 hours after symptom onset. *Maximum acceptable delay* for primary PCI from presentation to balloon inflation is 60 minutes, if a patient presents within 1 hour of symptom of onset or 90 minutes, if a patient present later.

Types of PCI: These include primary PCI, rescue PCI, and facilitated PCI.
- **Primary PCI:** In which PCI is used solely in acute MI. It is indicated in cardiogenic shock, and in patients in whom thrombolytic therapy is contraindicated.
- **Rescue PCI:** It is combination of PCI with thrombolytic therapy and PCI is performed within 12 after failed thrombolysis/fibrinolysis for patients with continuing or recurrent myocardial ischemia.
- **Facilitated PCI:** In this type, PCI is done following initial pharmacological regimen aimed at improving patency of coronary arteries before PCI.

Coronary Artery Bypass Grafting
Recommended in:
- Failed PCI with persistent pain or hemodynamic instability in patients with coronary anatomy suitable for surgery.
- Persistent or recurrent ischemia refractory to medical therapy in patients who have coronary anatomy suitable for surgery, and are not candidates for PCI or fibrinolytic therapy.
- Patients with STEMI at the time of operative repair of mechanical defects.

Aftercare and Rehabilitation
- **Physical activities:** To be restricted for 4–6 weeks because replacement of infarct by fibrous tissue takes 4–6 weeks. Advised gradual mobilization and return to work over 6 weeks. Exercise and sexual activity within the limits.
- **Complications:** Patients who had complications, the regimen depends on the type of complication.
- **Lifestyle and risk factor modification:** Control of risk factors, such as obesity by regular exercises, cessation of smoking, lifestyle modifications, and control of plasma lipids by diets and drugs.
- **Secondary prevention drug therapy:**
  - *Aspirin and clopidogrel*: Low-dose aspirin (75–150 mg daily) is given unless there is any contraindication. Clopidogrel (75 mg daily) is given for up to 12 months, particularly after stent implantation. It may be given as an alternative when aspirin is contraindicated, or in combination with aspirin particularly in patients with unstable angina or recurrent cardiac events.
  - β-blocker: Oral β-blockers are continued indefinitely (unless any contraindications). Carvedilol, bisoprolol, or metoprolol (extended release) is given to patients with heart failure. Role of β-blockers in the secondary prevention in unstable angina is not known.
  - ACE inhibitor is given early after an acute coronary syndrome. Long-term treatment with an ACE inhibitor (e.g., enalapril 10 mg twice daily or ramipril 2.5–5 mg twice daily) is found to counteract ventricular remodeling, prevent the onset of heart failure, and reduce recurrent MI.
  - *Statin therapy* is started in the hospital for all patients with coronary artery disease.
  - *Warfarin* after myocardial infarction is given to patients having a high risk of systemic thromboembolism due to atrial fibrillation, mural thrombus, congestive heart failure, or previous embolization.
  - *Nitrates*: Short-acting nitrates are given for chest pain. Long-acting nitrates are given for relief of symptom when β-blocker alone is unsuccessful or is contraindicated.
  - *Aldosterone antagonist* (e.g., eplerenone) is given early after myocardial infarction to patients who have LVEF ≤40%, despite optimum dose of ACE inhibitors and β-blockers, and have either CHF or diabetes.
- **Device therapy:** Implantable cardiac defibrillators can prevent sudden cardiac death in patients who have severe left ventricular impairment (ejection fraction ≤30%) after MI.

Non-ST Segment Elevation Acute Coronary Syndrome
- It includes unstable angina (UA) and non-ST elevation myocardial infarction (NSTEMI).
- Both are caused by coronary artery spasm, progression of the underlying coronary artery disease (CAD), or hemorrhage into a nonoccluding atheromatous plaque with

subsequent thrombosis producing coronary obstruction over a period of few hours. The difference between UA and NSTEMI is that the NSTEMI shows an occluding thrombus, which leads to myocardial necrosis and a rise in serum troponins or CKMB (creatine kinase-myocardial band).

Non-ST elevation MI

- It is usually shows ST depression and T inversion in the ECG along with elevation in serum troponins or CKMB.
- Myocardial function (as shown by ejection fraction) in NSTEMI is less deranged when compared to STEMI. However, in NSTEMI, early as well as late reinfarction rates are higher than in STEMI.

Unstable Angina

Three principal presentations include:
1. **Rest angina:** Angina occurring at rest and prolonged, usually >20 minutes.
2. **New-onset angina:** New-onset angina of at least CCS Class III severity.
3. **Increasing angina:** Previously diagnosed angina that has become distinctly more frequent, longer in duration, or lower in threshold (i.e., increased by >1 CCS) class to at least CCS Class III severity.
Classification of risk categories in NSTEMI/UA and its management are mentioned in **Table 9.10**.

Table 9.10: Risk categories in non-ST elevation myocardial infarction (NSTEMI)/unstable angina (UA).

Category	Management

High risk (12–30%):
• Prolonged chest pain (>20 minutes or ongoing), plus
  ▪ ECG: (1) Transient ST changes, (2) sustained ST depression, and (3) deep T wave inversion (>5 leads)
  ▪ *Biochemical markers:* Troponin/CKMB abnormal
• Recurrent ischemia
• Acute MI in last 4 weeks
• Hemodynamic compromise
	• Aspirin + heparin/low molecular weight heparin (LMWH)
	• GP IIb/IIIa antagonist
	• Early percutaneous coronary intervention (PCI)

Intermediate risk (4–8%):
• No high-risk features but ≥1 of:
  ▪ Ongoing chest pain
  ▪ Crescendo angina
  ▪ Borderline positive troponin I (0.4–2.0)
  ▪ *Previous intervention:* PCI or CABG
  ▪ Increased baseline risk (diabetes mellitus, elderly)
	• Aspirin ±clopidogrel
	• Unfractionated heparin (UFH) or low molecular weight heparin (LMWH)
	• PCI

Low-risk (<2%): • No high or intermediated features • Chest pain, single episode, exertional • *ECG:* Normal or nonspecific or unchanged • May include previous history of CAD or risk factors	• Aspirin • No heparin • Observe

(CABG: coronary artery bypass graft; CAD: coronary artery disease; PCI: percutaneous coronary intervention)

Prinzmetal Variant Angina

It is syndrome of severe ischemic pain that usually occurs at rest and is associated with transient ST-segment elevation.

Etiology

- **Focal spasm of an epicardial coronary artery** is the cause of Prinzmetal variant angina (PVA) and leads to severe transient myocardial ischemia and occasionally infarction.
- The cause of the spasm is not well defined, but it may be related to hypercontractility of vascular smooth muscle due to adrenergic vasoconstrictors, leukotrienes, or serotonin.

Clinical Features

- Pain occurs without exertion and usually at rest. It is more frequent in women.
- It is associated with migraine, Raynaud's phenomenon, and aspirin-induced asthma. Younger patients with history of cigarette smoking

Investigation

- Characteristically, it is associated with transient ST segment elevation on the ECG during the pain.
- Coronary angiography is gold standard for diagnosis. Focal spasm commonly accompanied by *stenosis within 1 cm of spasm* is the hallmark (most commonly in right coronary artery).
- Provocation tests (e.g., hyperventilation, cold pressor testing, or ergometrine or intracoronary acetylcholine challenge) may be needed for demonstration of focal spasm and establishing the diagnosis.

Management

- Nitrates and calcium channel blockers are the main therapeutic agents. Aspirin may actually increase the severity of ischemic episodes, possibly as a result of the sensitivity of coronary tone to modest changes in the synthesis of prostacyclin.
- The response to β-blockers is variable but usually poor. Prazosin can be useful.
- Coronary revascularization may be helpful in patients with discrete, flow-limiting, and proximal fixed obstructive lesions.

Prognosis

- Many patients pass through an acute, active phase, with frequent episodes of angina and cardiac events during the first 6 months after presentation.
- Prognosis is better in patients with no or mild fixed coronary obstruction than patients with severe, fixed, and significant obstructive lesions. Survival at 5 years is excellent (90–95%).
- Nonfatal MI occurs in up to 20% of patients by 5 years. Patients with PVA who develop serious arrhythmias during spontaneous episodes of pain are at a higher risk for sudden cardiac death. In most patients, who survive an infarction or the initial 3- to 6-month period of frequent episodes, there is a tendency for symptoms and cardiac events to diminish over time.

HYPERTENSION

Hypertension is a hemodynamic disorder and about 15% of the general population can be regarded as hypertensives.

Hypertension is defined arbitrarily at levels above generally accepted normal (Joint National Committee—JNC-7/8 recommendations), which are presented in **Table 9.11**. Other guidelines for classification of hypertension are summarized in **Table 9.12 and Figure 9.4**.

Classification and Causes (Box 9.4)

- **Primary or essential hypertension:** It constitutes about 85% of the cases in which it is not possible to define a specific underlying cause. About 70% of these patients give a positive family history.
- **Secondary hypertension:** It constitutes remaining 15% of the cases and is due to a specific disease or abnormality.

Etiology

Genetic factors: Blood pressure tends to run in families and this may be partly due to environmental influences.

Environmental factors: Several environmental factors may be involved and these include salt intake, obesity, occupation, alcohol intake, family size, and crowding.
- *Obesity*: Higher blood pressures are seen in obese individuals compared to thin individuals. Sleep disordered breathing/obstructive sleep apnea often observed with obesity may be an additional risk factor.
- *Alcohol intake*: There is close relationship between the consumption of alcohol and blood pressure level.
- *Sodium intake*: Higher sodium intakes may be associated with an increase in blood pressure. A high-potassium diet can have protective role against the effects of a high sodium intake. About 60% of hypertensives are salt sensitive. Primary aldosteronism, bilateral renal artery stenosis, renal parenchymal disease, and low-renin essential hypertension are all salt sensitive.

Table 9.11: Systolic and diastolic values used in the classification of hypertension (JNC7/8).

Classification	Systolic BP (mm Hg)		Diastolic BP (mm Hg)
Normal	<120	AND	<80
Prehypertension	120–139	OR	80–89
Stage 1 Hypertension	140–159	OR	90–99
Stage 2 hypertension	≥160	OR	≥100
Isolated systolic hypertension	>140	AND	<90

Table 9.12: Current classification of high blood pressure.

SBO (mm Hg)		DBP (mm Hg)	ESH/ESC 2018	AHA/ACC 2017	Position of the DHL, 2017	NICE 2016
<120	and	<80	Optimal	Normal	Optimal	Optimal
120–129	and	<80	Normal	Elevated	Normal	Normal
130–139	or	80–89	Upper range of normal	Grade I hypertension	Upper range of normal	Upper range of normal
140–159	or	90–99	Grade I hypertension	Grade II hypertension	Grade I hypertension	Grade I hypertension (>135/85 mm Hg)*
160–179	or	100–109	Grade II hypertension	Grade II hypertension	Grade II hypertension	Grade II hypertension (≥150/95 mm Hg)*
≥180	or	≥110	Grade III hypertension	Grade II hypertension	Grade III hypertension	Severe hypertension

A comparison of the new definitions of normal blood pressure and the different grades of high blood pressure by the American Heart Association (AHA) and American College of Cardiology (ACC) with the definitions by the European Society of Cardiology (ESC) and European Society of Hypertension (ESH), as well as the most recent position of the German Hypertension League (Deutshce Hochdruckliga, DHL) and the National Institute for Health and Care Excellence (NICE) of the United Kingdom.

The lowering of cutoff values led to an increase in the prevalence of hypertension in the USA from 32% to 46%.

*The value refers to further measurements in the outpatient setting or at home.

(DBP: diastolic blood pressure; SBP: systolic blood pressure)

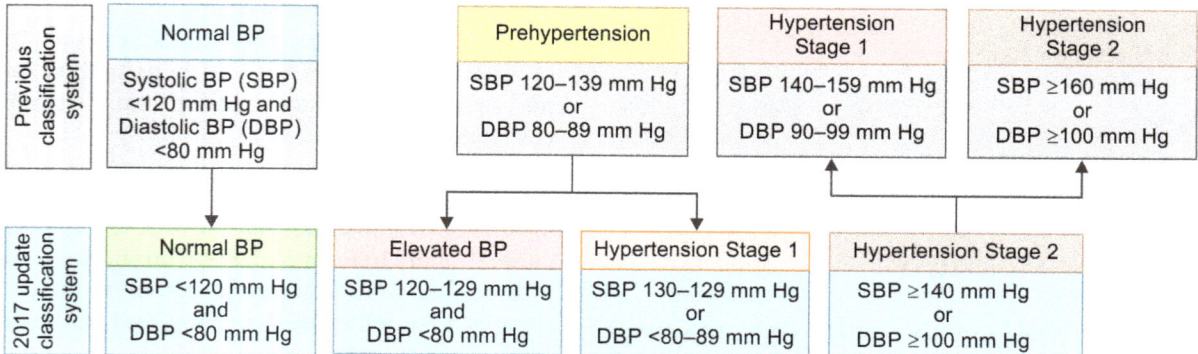

Fig. 9.4: Classification of hypertension.

> **Box 9.4:** Major causes of hypertension (systolic and diastolic).
>
> **Primary/essential hypertension** (~ 85% of case)
> **Secondary hypertension** (~15% of case)
> - **Renal:**
>   - *Renal parenchymal disease* (most common cause of secondary hypertension): Acute glomerulonephritis, polycystic kidney disease, chronic nephritis, diabetic nephropathy, and hydronephrosis (obstructive uropathy)
>   - Renal artery stenosis (renovascular hypertension) and renin-producing tumors
> - **Endocrine:**
>   - *Adrenal disorders*: Cushing's syndrome, primary aldosteronism, primary adrenal hyperplasia, and pheochromocytoma
>   - *Others*: Hypothyroidism (myxedema), hyperthyroidism (thyrotoxicosis), hypercalcemia, acromegaly, carcinoid, and exogenous hormones
> - **Cardiovascular:** Coarctation of aorta and polyarteritis nodosa
> - **Neurologic:** Psychogenic, porphyria, lead poisoning, primary dysautonomia (Riley–Day syndrome), increased intracranial pressure, and GB syndrome
> - **Obstructive sleep apnea**
> - **Preeclampsia/eclampsia**
> - **Medications and toxins:**
>   - High-dose estrogens, alcohol, and drugs—oral contraceptives, anabolic steroids, corticosteroids, decongestants, nonsteroidal anti-inflammatory drugs (NSAIDs), COX-2 inhibitors, carbenoxolone, sympathomimetics, cyclosporine, sibutramine, bromocriptine, and erythropoietin
> - **Stress:** Postoperative pain, burns, hypoglycemia, alcohol withdrawal, and hypoglycemia
>
> **Causes of isolated systolic hypertension:** Atherosclerosis, aortic regurgitation, patent ductus arteriosus, thyrotoxicosis, and coarctation of aorta

- *Stress*: Acute pain or stress is associated with raised blood pressure. However, the relationship between chronic stress and blood pressure is not known.

Humoral mechanisms: The autonomic nervous system, the renin-angiotensin, natriuretic peptide, and kallikrein–kinin system play a role in the physiological regulation of short-term changes in blood pressure. They may also be probably involved in the pathogenesis of essential hypertension.
- *A low-renin, salt-sensitive, and essential hypertension,* in which patients have renal sodium and water retention, has been found.
  Low renin hypertension is more common in elderly and diabetics. These patients are salt-sensitive and diuretic responsive.
- *Normal renin hypertension* (nonmodulators) is more common in males and postmenopausal females. They are salt sensitive.
- *High-renin hypertension* is characterized by high plasma renin activity and responsiveness to angiotensin II antagonists.
- Low calcium intake has been associated with an increase in blood pressure in epidemiologic studies.
  Insulin resistance is responsible for essential hypertension in majority of the patients.
- *Metabolic syndrome*: It is characterized by hyperinsulinemia, glucose intolerance, reduced levels of HDL cholesterol, hypertriglyceridemia, and central obesity (all related to insulin resistance). Metabolic syndrome is associated with hypertension and is a major risk factor for cardiovascular disease.

Fetal factors: Impaired intrauterine growth resulting in low birth weight is associated with subsequent development of high blood pressure.

Approach to Newly Diagnosed Hypertension

Hypertension is usually asymptomatic and the diagnosis is usually made at routine examination or when a complication arises. A routine BP checkup is necessary every 5 years in adults.

Goals of the initial evaluation with high BP are to:
- Obtain accurate BP measurements
- Identify contributing factors, and risk factors, and any underlying cause (secondary hypertension)
- Quantify cardiovascular risk
- Detect any complications (target organ damage)
- Identify comorbidity that may influence the choice of antihypertensive therapy

Ambulatory Blood Pressure Monitoring

Ambulatory blood pressure monitoring (ABPM) is the preferred method for confirming the diagnosis of hypertension. High-quality data suggest that ABPM predicts target-organ damage and cardiovascular events better than office blood pressure readings. ABPM records the blood pressure at preset intervals (usually every 15–20 minutes during the day and every 30–60 minutes during sleep).

Uses of ambulatory blood pressure monitoring:
- Confirm white coat and masked hypertension
- Suspected episodic hypertension (e.g., pheochromocytoma)
- Determining therapeutic response (i.e., blood pressure control) in patients who are known to have a substantial white coat effect
- Hypotensive symptoms while taking antihypertensive medications
- Resistant hypertension
- Autonomic dysfunction

White coat hypertension: It is a transient increase in blood pressure in normal individuals when blood pressure is recorded either in a hospital or in a physician's clinic.

Isolated ambulatory or masked hypertension:
- It is reversal of white coat hypertension in which individuals have normal blood pressure (<140/90 mm Hg) in a hospital or in a physician's clinic but have increased ambulatory or home blood pressure values.
- These individuals have increased prevalence of organ damage, with an increased prevalence of metabolic risk factors.

History
- Record family history, lifestyle (exercise, salt intake, and smoking), other risk factors, history of drug intake or alcohol.

Table 9.13: Findings and specific investigations in various secondary hypertension.

Findings	Disease suspected	Specific investigation
Paroxysmal hypertension, palpitations, headache, and diaphoresis	Pheochromocytoma	Urine VMA, metanephrine, and plasma metanephrine
Fatigue, weight gain, menstrual irregularities, and diastolic hypertension	Hypothyroidism	Serum thyroid-stimulating hormone (TSH)
Weight loss, tachycardia, tremors, heat intolerance, and systolic hypertension	Hyperthyroidism	Serum TSH
Depression, muscle weakness, kidney stones, and osteoporosis	Hyperparathyroidism	Serum calcium and parathormone (PTH)
Headaches, fatigue, visual disturbances, enlarged tongue, and enlarged extremities	Acromegaly	Growth hormone (GH)
Weight gain, muscle weakness, striae, obesity, amenorrhea, and moon facies	Cushing's syndrome	Serum cortisol
Obesity, snoring, and daytime somnolence	Obstructive sleep apnea (OSA)	Polysomnography
Enlarged palpable kidneys and family history positive	Autosomal dominant polycystic kidney disease (ADPKD)	Ultrasound abdomen
Proteinuria, elevated serum creatinine, edema, and anemia	Chronic kidney disease (CKD)	Ultrasound
Abdominal/renal bruit	Renovascular cause	MR angiogram
Fatigue, hypokalemia, hypernatremia	Aldosteronism	Plasma renin to aldosterone ratio, MRI abdomen

(VMA: vanillylmandelic acid)

- Symptoms of causes of secondary hypertension (**Table 9.13**) or complications such as coronary artery disease (e.g., angina and breathlessness).

Clinical Features

Clinical features of hypertension may be due to hypertension itself and the underlying cause of hypertension. Clinical features due to hypertension per se:
- Majority of patients are asymptomatic and hypertension is usually detected during routine examination.
- Acute hypertension may produce transient headache and polyuria.
- Long-standing hypertension may cause left ventricular hypertrophy and heaving apical impulse, accentuation of the aortic component of the second heart sound (A2), a fourth heart sound (S4), and very short early diastolic murmur and fundal changes.

Target Organ Damage (Complications of Hypertension)

Target organ damage in hypertension can be clinically detected.

Central Nervous System Complications
- **Transient ischemic attacks (TIAs):** Carotid atheroma and TIAs are more common in patients with hypertension.
- **Cerebrovascular accident (stroke)** is a common complication of hypertension and may be due to cerebral hemorrhage or infarction (due to cerebral atherothrombosis)
- **Subarachnoid hemorrhage** is also a complication of hypertension
- **Hypertensive encephalopathy** is a rare complication characterized by very high blood pressure, neurological manifestations (include transient disturbances in speech and vision, paresthesias, seizures, disorientation, and loss of consciousness), and papilledema.

Ophthalmic (Retinal) Complications
Hypertensive retinopathy (**Box 9.5 and Fig. 9.5**)

> **Box 9.5:** Grading of hypertensive retinopathy—Keith–Wagener–Barker classification.
>
> *Grade 1*: Mild narrowing of the arterioles—"copper wire"
> *Grade 2*: Moderate narrowing—copper wire and AV nicking, changes associated with long-standing essential hypertension
> *Grade 3*: Severe narrowing—silver wire changes, hemorrhage, cotton wool spots, and hard exudates
> *Grade 4*: Grade 3 + papilledema. Grade 3 and 4 highly correlated with progression to end-organ damage and decreased survival

(AV: arteriovenous)

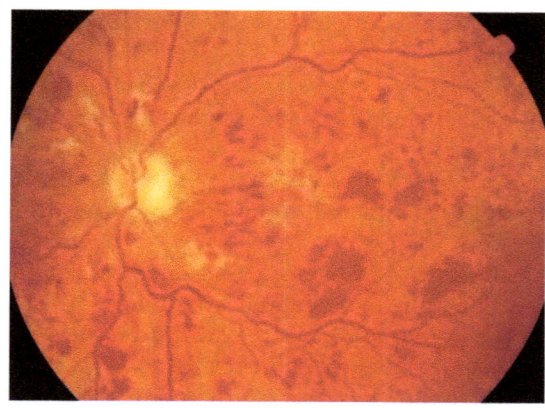

Fig. 9.5: Fundus image of hypertensive retinopathy.

Cardiovascular Complications

- **Coronary artery disease (angina and myocardial infarction):** Increased cardiac mortality and morbidity associated with hypertension are chiefly due to a higher incidence of coronary artery disease. High BP may produce left ventricular hypertrophy with a forceful apex beat and fourth heart sound. ECG or echocardiography is useful in risk assessment.
- **Left ventricular failure and pulmonary edema:** It may develop with severe hypertension.
- *Atrial fibrillation* is common and may be due to diastolic dysfunction caused by left ventricular hypertrophy or the effects of coronary artery disease.

Blood Vessels

Larger arteries show thickening of the internal elastic lamina, hypertrophy of smooth muscle, and deposition of fibrous tissue. Smaller arteries show hyaline arteriosclerosis in the wall, narrowing of the lumen, and aneurysm. *Atherosclerosis* may develop in coronary and cerebral blood vessel. Hypertension is a major risk factor involved in the pathogenesis *of aneurysm of aorta* and dissecting hematoma of aorta *(aortic dissection).*

Renal Complications

Long-standing hypertension may cause damage of the renal vasculature and produce (1) proteinuria, (2) hematuria, and (3) progressive renal failure.

Investigations

Basic investigations in all patients:
- **Urinalysis:** For protein, blood, and glucose
- **Blood urea and creatinine:** To assess renal function
- **Serum electrolytes:** For hypokalemia (is usually due to diuretic therapy) and alkalosis in hyperaldosteronism
- **Fasting and postprandial blood glucose:** For hyperglycemia
- **Lipid profile:** Serum total cholesterol and HDL cholesterol
- **Electrocardiogram:** 12-lead ECG for left ventricular hypertrophy and coronary artery disease

Secondary Investigations in Selected Patients

- **Chest radiograph:** For detecting the cardiac size, evidence of cardiac failure and aortic dilatation, coarctation of the aorta
- **Ambulatory BP recording:** To detect borderline, masked hypertension or "white coat" hypertension
- **Echocardiogram:** To detect or quantify left ventricular hypertrophy and function
- **Renal ultrasound:** To detect renal disease
- **MRI, renal isotope scan, and renal angiography:** To detect or confirm renal artery stenosis
- **Urinary catecholamines:** To detect pheochromocytoma
- **Urinary cortisol and dexamethasone suppression test:** To detect Cushing's syndrome
- **Thyroid function tests:** To detect hypothyroidism or hyperthyroidism
- **Serum calcium and parathyroid hormone level:** To detect hyperparathyroidism
- **Plasma renin activity and aldosterone:** To detect possible primary aldosteronism
- **Growth hormone:** To detect acromegaly

Treatment

- **Objective of antihypertensive therapy:** To reduce the incidence of adverse cardiovascular events (e.g., coronary artery disease), stroke, and heart failure
- **Target blood pressure:** For most patients, a target is <140 mm Hg systolic blood pressure and ≈85 mm Hg diastolic blood pressure. For patients with diabetes, renal impairment or established cardiovascular disease the target is <130/80 mm Hg.

Management of hypertension can be studied under three headings:
1. General measures
2. Antihypertensive drug therapy
3. Treatment of underlying cause (in secondary hypertension)

1. General measures:

- **Lifestyle modifications:** Recommended for all patients with hypertension and pre-hypertension. A reduction in systolic blood pressure of 5 mm Hg has been associated with about 10% reduction in mortality caused by stroke and heart disease:
  - *Control of obesity*: Maintain normal body weight (BMI 20–25 kg/m^2)
  - *Diet*: Dietary approaches to stop hypertension or *DASH* eating plan.
    - Restrict salt in the diet (<100 mEq sodium or <6 g NaCl or <2.4 g Na/day)
    - Reduce intake of fat and saturated fat
    - Increase consumption of diet rich in fruit vegetables (≥5 portions of fresh fruit and vegetables/day) and potassium
    - Limit/reduce alcohol consumption to ≤3 units/day men and ≤2 units/day women
- **Cardiovascular risk reduction:** Stop/avoid cigarette smoking and increase intake of oily fish
- **Regular aerobic/physical exercises:** Perform ≥30 min brisk walk most days of the week. Relaxation classes, meditation, and biofeedback.

2. Antihypertensive drug therapy (Fig. 9.6):

- Various antihypertensive drugs are described in **Table 9.14**.
- Individualizing antihypertensive therapy is described in **Table 9.15**.
- Newer antihypertensive agents are listed in **Table 9.16.**

"Malignant" or "Accelerated" Phase Hypertension

- It is a rare condition that may complicate hypertension of any etiology. It occurs when blood pressure rises rapidly with severe hypertension (diastolic blood pressure >120 mm Hg). Histologically, it is characterized by fibrinoid necrosis in the walls of small arteries and arterioles and intravascular thrombosis.
- **Diagnosis:** Presence of high BP and rapidly progressive end-organ damage, such as retinopathy (grade 3 or 4 with flame-shaped hemorrhages, cotton wool spots, hard exudates and papilledema), renal dysfunction (e.g., proteinuria and hematuria), and/or cerebral edema and

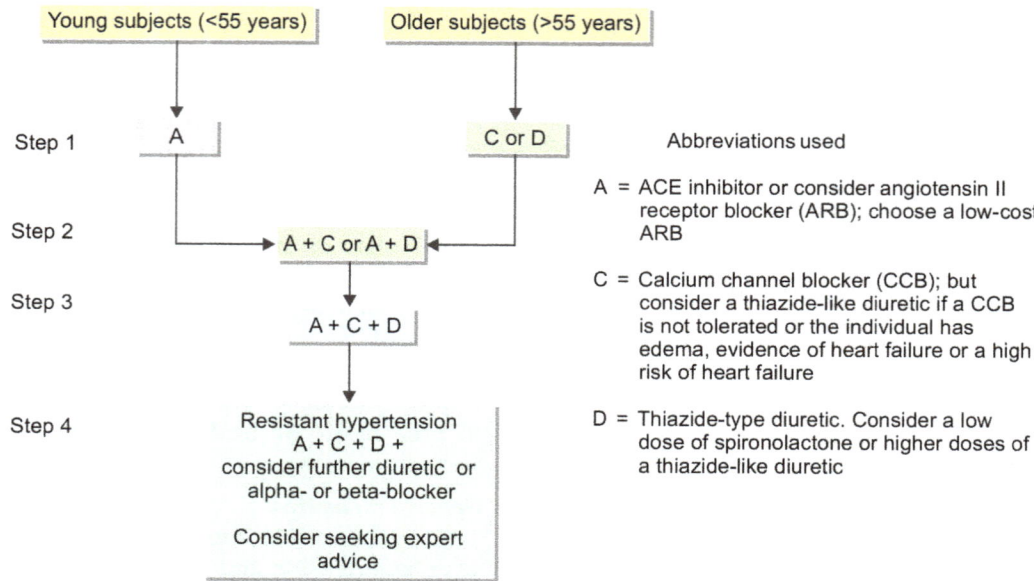

Fig. 9.6: Choosing antihypertensive drug and its combinations for patients newly diagnosed with hypertension.

Table 9.14: Various antihypertensive drugs (dose).

Drugs by class	Properties	Initial dose	Dosage range (mg)
β-adrenergic antagonists			
Atenolol	Selective	50 mg PO daily	25–100
Betaxolol	Selective	10 mg PO daily	5–40
Bisoprolol	Selective	5 mg PO daily	2.5–20
Metoprolol	Selective	50 mg PO bid	50–450
Metoprolol XL	Selective	50–100 mg PO daily	50–400
Nebivolol	Selective with vasodilatory properties	5 mg PO daily	5–40
Nadolol	Nonselective	40 mg PO daily	20–240
Propranolol	Nonselective	40 mg PO bid	40–240
Propranolol LA	Nonselective	80 mg PO daily	60–240
Timolol	Nonselective	10 mg PO bid	20–40
Pindolol	ISA	5 mg PO daily	10–60
Labetalol	α- and β-antagonist properties	100 mg PO bid	200–1,200
Carvedilol	α- and β-antagonist properties	6.25 mg PO bid	12.5–50
Carvedilol CR	α- and β-antagonist properties	10 mg PO daily	10–80
Acebutolol	ISA and selective	200 mg PO bid, 400 mg PO daily	200–1,200
Calcium channel antagonists:			
Amlodipine	DHP	5 mg PO daily	2.5–10
Diltiazem		30 mg PO qid	90–360
Diltiazem LA		180 mg PO daily	120–540
Diltiazem CD		180 mg PO daily	120–480
Diltiazem XR		180 mg PO daily	120–540
Diltiazem XT		180 mg PO daily	120–480
Isradipine	DHP	2.5 mg PO bid	2.5–10
Nicardipine	DHP	20 mg PO tid	60–120
Nifedipine	DHP	10 mg PO tid	30–120
Nifedipine XL (or CC)	DHP	30 mg PO daily	30–90

Contd...

Contd...

Drugs by class	Properties	Initial dose	Dosage range (mg)
Nisoldipine	DHP	20 mg PO daily	20–40
Verapamil		80 mg PO tid	80–480
Verapamil SR		120 mg PO daily	120–480
Angiotensin-converting enzyme inhibitors:			
Benazepril		10 mg PO bid	10–40
Captopril		25 mg PO bid–tid	50–450
Enalapril		5 mg PO daily	2.5–40
Fosinopril		10 mg PO daily	10–40
Lisinopril		10 mg PO daily	5–40
Moexipril		7.5 mg PO daily	7.5–30
Quinapril		10 mg PO daily	5–80
Ramipril		2.5 mg PO daily	1.25–20
Trandolapril		1–2 mg PO daily	1–4
Perindopril		4 mg PO daily	2–16
Angiotensin II receptor blockers:			
Azilsartan		40 mg PO daily	40–80
Candesartan		8 mg PO daily	8–32
Eprosartan		600 mg PO daily	600–800
Irbesartan		150 mg PO daily	150–300
Olmesartan		20 mg PO daily	20–40
Losartan		50 mg PO daily	25–100
Telmisartan		40 mg PO daily	20–80
Valsartan		80 mg PO daily	80–320
Direct renin inhibitor:			
Aliskiren		150 mg PO daily	150–300
Diuretics:			
Chlorthalidone	Thiazide diuretic	25 mg PO daily	12.5–50
Hydrochlorothiazide	Thiazide diuretic	12.5 mg PO daily	12.5–50
Hydroflumethiazide	Thiazide diuretic	50 mg PO daily	50–100
Indapamide	Thiazide diuretic	1.25 mg PO daily	2.5–5
Methyclothiazide	Thiazide diuretic	2.5 mg PO daily	2.5–5
Metolazone	Thiazide diuretic	2.5 mg PO daily	1.25–5
Bumetanide	Loop diuretic	0.5 mg PO daily (or IV)	0.5–5
Ethacrynic acid	Loop diuretic	50 mg PO daily (or IV)	25–100
Furosemide	Loop diuretic	20 mg PO daily (or IV)	20–320
Torsemide	Loop diuretic	5 mg PO daily (or IV)	5–10
Amiloride	Potassium-sparing diuretic	5 mg PO daily	5–10
Triamterene	Potassium-sparing diuretic	50 mg PO bid	50–200
Eplerenone	Aldosterone antagonist	25 mg PO daily	25–100
Spironolactone	Aldosterone antagonist	25 mg PO daily	25–100
α-adrenergic antagonists:			
Doxazosin		1 mg PO daily	1–16
Prazosin		1 mg PO bid–tid	1–20
Terazosin		1 mg PO at bedtime	1–20

Contd...

Contd...

Drugs by class	Properties	Initial dose	Dosage range (mg)
Centrally acting adrenergic agents:			
Clonidine		0.1 mg PO bid	0.1–1.2
Clonidine patch		TTS 1/week (equivalent to 0.1 mg/day release)	0.1–0.3
Guanfacine		1 mg PO daily	1–3
Guanabenz		4 mg PO bid	4–64
Methyldopa		250 mg PO bid–tid	250–2,000
Direct-acting vasodilators:			
Hydralazine		10 mg PO qid	50–300
Minoxidil		5 mg PO daily	2.5–100
Miscellaneous:			
Reserpine		0.5 mg PO daily	0.01–0.25

(DHP: dihydropyridine)

Table 9.15: Individualizing antihypertensive therapy.

Compelling indications (major improvement in outcome independent of blood pressure):	
Diabetes mellitus	ACE inhibitor or ARB
Heart failure with reduced ejection fraction	ACE inhibitor or ARB, β-blocker, diuretic, aldosterone antagonist
Postmyocardial infarction	ACE inhibitor or ARB, β-blocker, and aldosterone antagonist
Proteinuric chronic kidney disease (nondiabetic)	ACE inhibitor or ARB
Angina pectoris	β-blocker and calcium channel blocker
Atrial fibrillation/flutter rate control	β-blocker, non-dihydropyridine calcium channel blocker
Previous CVA/TIA	ACE inhibitor ± diuretic
Antihypertensive agents with a favorable effect on symptoms in comorbid conditions:	
Benign prostatic hyperplasia	α-blocker
Essential tremor	β-blocker (non cardioselective)
Hyperthyroidism	β-blocker
Migraine	β–blocker and calcium channel blocker
Osteoporosis	Thiazide diuretic
Raynaud phenomenon	Dihydropyridine calcium channel blocker
Contraindications:	
Angioedema	Do not use an ACE inhibitor
Peripheral vascular disease	Avoid β-blocker
Bronchospasm	Do not use a nonselective β-blocker
Liver disease	Do not use methyldopa
Pregnancy	Do not use an ACE inhibitor, ARB, or renin inhibitor
Second- or third-degree heart block	Do not use a β-blocker, non-dihydropyridine calcium channel blocker unless a functioning ventricular pacemaker
Bilateral renal artery stenosis	Avoid ACE inhibitors/ARB/renin inhibitor
Drug classes that may have adverse effects on comorbid conditions:	
Depression	Avoid β–blocker and central alpha-2 agonist
Gout	Avoid loop or thiazide diuretic
Hyperkalemia	Avoid aldosterone antagonist, ACE inhibitor, ARB, and renin inhibitor
Hyponatremia	Avoid thiazide diuretic
Renovascular disease	Avoid ACE inhibitor, ARB, or renin inhibitor

(ACE: angiotensin-converting enzyme; ARB: angiotensin receptor blocker)

Table 9.16: Newer antihypertensive agents.

Direct renin inhibitor	Aliskiren
Protein kinase C inhibitors	Staurosporine
Calcium channel blocker	Cilnidipine, azelnidipine, and clevidipine
Nonselective β-blocker and weak β-blocker	Bucindolol
Chymase inhibitors	SPF-32629A
Prostacycline analog	Treprostinil
Serotonin receptor antagonist	Ketanserin
Endothelin receptor antagonist	Ambrisentan, sitaxsentan, bosentan, and darusentan
Advanced glycation end product (AGE) cross-link breaker	Alagebrium
Phosphodiesterase type-5 (PDE5) inhibitor	Sildenafil

hemorrhage with resultant hypertensive encephalopathy. Left ventricular failure may develop.
- If this is untreated, it may lead to death within months from progressive renal failure, heart failure, aortic dissection, or stroke.

Hypertensive Emergencies

Reason includes renovascular disease, pheochromocytoma, nonadherence to antihypertensive medication, hyperaldosteronism, erythropoietin administration, acute glomerular nephropathy, and eclampsia.

Hypertensive Urgency

- Severe elevation in BP >180/120 mm Hg without symptoms or signs of acute target organ involvement
- Adequate treatment of these conditions, a BP lowering within 24 hours by administration of oral drugs
- Intensive care unit (ICU) admission is usually not required

> **Treatment:** Treatment requires an immediate BP reduction in few minutes to hours in an ICU care and brought by IV drugs.

Various hypertensive emergencies and their treatment are presented in **Table 9.17**.

Drugs used in hypertensive emergencies and their dosage, action, and adverse effects are presented in **Table 9.18**.

Resistant Hypertension

Definition

Resistant hypertension is defined as blood pressure above goal (>140/90 mm Hg; >130–139/80–85 mm Hg in patients with diabetes mellitus; and >130/80 mm Hg in chronic kidney disease), despite treatment with ≥3 antihypertensive drugs of different classes, including a diuretic, at optimal doses.
- Resistant hypertension is observed in about 10–20% of patients with hypertension.
- Almost 50% of these patients experience an adverse cardiovascular event compared with patients with blood pressure controlled by three or fewer antihypertensive agents. Non-compliance to medication is an important cause.
- Diagnosis requires exclusion of both pseudoresistance and reversible or organic causes.

Treatments for Resistant Hypertension

- **Nonpharmacologic intervention:** Reinforce lifestyle changes
- **Drug intervention:** Look for drug compliance and optimize doses. Add drugs from other classes.

Table 9.17: Various hypertensive emergencies and their treatment.

Diagnosis	Suggested drugs	Targets	Remarks
Acute aortic dissection	Esmolol/labetelol + nitroprusside would be a better combination	Reduce SBP as rapidly as possible down to 100–110 mm Hg, simultaneously control tachycardia due to the sympathetic activation	Avoid volume depletion Use β-blockers before vasodilators Hydralazine is contraindicated
Acute pulmonary edema	Nitroglycerine infusion, IV enalaprilat, nitroprusside infusion, and IV furosemide	Reduce blood pressure by 20–30%	Hypotension may develop with enalaprilat
Acute coronary syndrome	Nitroglycerine infusion β-blockers (metoprolol or labetalol)	Reduce blood pressure by not more than 20–30%	Beware of hypotension in right ventricular infarction Avoid hypotension
Acute renal failure	Labetalol IV, nicardipine infusion, and dialysis	Reduce blood pressure not more than 20–30%	Avoid nitroprusside and ACE inhibitors
Subarachnoid hemorrhage	Labetalol bolus and infusion Esmolol bolus and infusion Nicardipine infusion	Systolic pressure <160 mm Hg or mean arterial pressure <130 mm Hg (to reduce recurrence)	Control of pain will help in BP control
Intracranial bleed	Labetalol and infusion Nitroglycerine infusion Nimodipine	To prevent rebleeding and reduce edema formation May benefit from gradual 20–25% reduction in BP	Avoid lowering blood pressure by more than 10–15% in 24 hours
Hypertensive encephalopathy	IV sodium nitroprusside is the drug of choice and rapid onset of action). IV labetalol, nicardipine, and hydralazine	Mean BP should be reduced by 20% within 1st hour	

Table 9.18: Drugs used in hypertensive emergencies.

Drug	Administration	Onset	Duration of action	Dosage	Adverse effects and comments
Fenoldopam	IV infusion	<5 min	30 min	0.1–0.3 µg/kg/min	Tachycardia, nausea, and vomiting
Sodium nitroprusside	IV infusion	Immediate	2–3 min	0.5–10 µg/kg/min (initial dose, 0.25 µg/kg/min for eclampsia and renal insufficiency)	Hypotension, nausea, vomiting, and apprehension; risk of thiocyanate and cyanide toxicity is increased in renal and hepatic insufficiency, respectively; levels should be monitored; must shield from light
Diazoxide	IV bolus	15 min	6–12 h	50–100 mg q5–10 min, up to 600 mg	Hypotension, tachycardia, nausea, vomiting, fluid retention, hyperglycemia; may exacerbate myocardial ischemia, heart failure, or aortic dissection
Labetalol	IV bolus	5–10 min	3–6 h	20–80 mg q5–10 min, up to 300 mg	Hypotension, heart block, heart failure, bronchospasm, nausea, vomiting, scalp tingling, paradoxical pressor response; may not be effective in patients receiving α- or β-antagonists
	IV infusion			0.5–2 mg/min	
Nitroglycerin	IV infusion	1–2 min	3–5 min	5–250 µg/min	Headache, nausea, and vomiting. Tolerance may develop with prolonged use
Esmolol	IV bolus	1–5 min	10 min	500 µg/kg/min for first 1 minute	Hypotension, heart block, heart failure, and bronchospasm
	IV infusion			50–300 µg/kg/min	
Phentolamine	IV bolus	1–2 min	3–10 min	5–10 mg q5–15 min	Hypotension, tachycardia, headache, angina, and paradoxical pressor response
Hydralazine (for treatment of eclampsia)	IV bolus	10–20 min	3–6 h	10–20 mg q20 min (if no effect after 20 mg, try another agent)	Hypotension, fetal distress, tachycardia, headache, nausea, vomiting, and local thrombophlebitis Infusion site should be changed after 12 h
Methyldopa (for treatment of eclampsia)	IV bolus	30–60 min	10–16 h	250–500 mg	Hypotension
Nicardipine	IV infusion	1–5 min	3–6 h	5 mg/h, increased by 1.0–2.5 mg/h q15min, up to 15 mg/h	Hypotension, headache, tachycardia, nausea, and vomiting
Clevidipine	IV infusion	2–4 min	5–15 min	1–2 mg/h, double dose every 90 seconds up to 16 mg/h	Hypotension and reflex tachycardia
Enalaprilat	IV bolus	5–15 min	1–6 h	0.6255 mg q6h	Hypotension

- **Device therapy:** Two techniques
  - Percutaneous transluminal radiofrequency sympathetic denervation of the renal arteries
  - Carotid baroreflex activation
- **Medical therapy:** Aldosterone antagonist, angiotensin-converting enzyme (ACE) inhibitors, and angiotensin II receptor blockers (ARBs) plus chlorthalidone
- Percutaneous angioplasty with/without stent placement
- Surgical revascularization or nephrectomy in unilateral cases

ACUTE RHEUMATIC FEVER

Definition

Rheumatic fever (RF) is an *acute, post-streptococcal, immune-mediated, and multisystem inflammatory disease.*

It occurs as a sequel to group A streptococcal pharyngitis.
- Multisystem disease affecting connective tissue particularly of the heart, joints, brain, cutaneous, and subcutaneous tissues.

Two Major Phases

1. **Acute rheumatic fever (ARF):** It frequently manifests as acute rheumatic carditis.
2. **Chronic rheumatic heart disease (RHD)** is the permanent heart valve damage resulting from one or more attacks of ARF. About 40–60% of patients with ARF will develop RHD. The most common valve affected is the mitral followed by aortic, in that order. However, all four valves can be affected. The deforming fibrotic valvular lesions are the principal/key features of chronic RHD.

Epidemiology and Incidence

- **Age group:** Most common in children between 5 and 15 years. It is rare <3 years of age.
- **Sex:** Both sexes are equally affected. However, certain clinical manifestations, such as mitral stenosis and Sydenham chorea, have a female preponderance after puberty.

- **Socioeconomic conditions:** Rheumatic fever is a worldwide disease and it is prevalent in regions with poor economic conditions, overcrowding, and substandard housing. Incidence and mortality rate of RF and RHD have markedly decreased over the past century, due to improved socioeconomic conditions and rapid diagnosis and treatment of streptococcal pharyngitis. In India, the annual incidence is 0.18–0.3 per 1,000 school children.
- **Poor economy and overcrowding:** It is a predisposing factor in developing countries. It is a major cause of death and disability in children and adolescents in socioeconomically deprived regions.

Etiology
- Acute rheumatic fever is a post-streptococcal disease.
- It develops after a latent period of 2–6 weeks after an episode of pharyngitis (sore throat) or tonsillitis by group A β-hemolytic streptococci. It occurs most often in children.
- Rheumatogenic potential of various serotypes of group A streptococci varies. M-protein is one of the well-defined determinants of bacterial virulence. M-type 5 is commonly responsible for rheumatic fever and other rheumatogenic serotypes include 1, 3, 5, 14, 18, 19, and 24. M-type 12 is highly prevalent, but usually does cause rheumatic fever.
- Recently, virus (Coxsackie B-4) has been suggested as causative agent with streptococcus acting as conditioning agent.

Pathogenesis (Fig. 9.7)
Immunologically mediated disease: Exact pathogenesis of rheumatic fever is not known. Streptococcal infection introduces the streptococcal antigens into the body and may activate both antibody and T cell-mediated reactions against streptococci.

Molecular Mimicry
- Antibodies may be produced by B-lymphocytes against various antigenic components of the *Streptococcus*.
- These antibodies cross-react with human tissues because of the antigenic similarity between streptococcal components and human connective tissues (molecular mimicry). One of them produced against the M-proteins of streptococci seems to cross-react with certain similar self-antigens in the myocardial cells and glycoproteins of the valves in the heart. This may be the mechanism for pancarditis in acute rheumatic fever.
- Immunologically mediated inflammation and damage (autoimmune) to human tissues, which have antigenic similarity with streptococcal components—such as heart, joint, and brain connective tissues.

Streptococcal Super Antigens
Super antigens are glycoproteins synthesized by bacteria and viruses. They can bridge class II major histocompatibility complex molecules to specific T-cell receptors, simulating antigen binding and activation of *CD4+ T-cells*. These T-cells along with antibodies *cross-react with self-proteins in the heart*. These reactions produce cytokines leading to activation of macrophages, which are seen in lesions of rheumatic fever.

Host Factors
- Rheumatic fever occurs in a susceptible host and only 0.3–3% of individuals with acute streptococcal pharyngitis develop rheumatic fever.
- In India, HLA-DR3 is associated more frequently in patients with rheumatic fever and rheumatic fever has low frequency of HLA-DR2.

Clinical Manifestations
Acute rheumatic fever is a multisystem disorder. It usually presents with fever, anorexia, lethargy, and joint pain.
Previous history of sore throat: Only two-thirds of patients remember having any upper respiratory symptoms (episode of streptococcal pharyngitis) in the past 2–3 weeks.

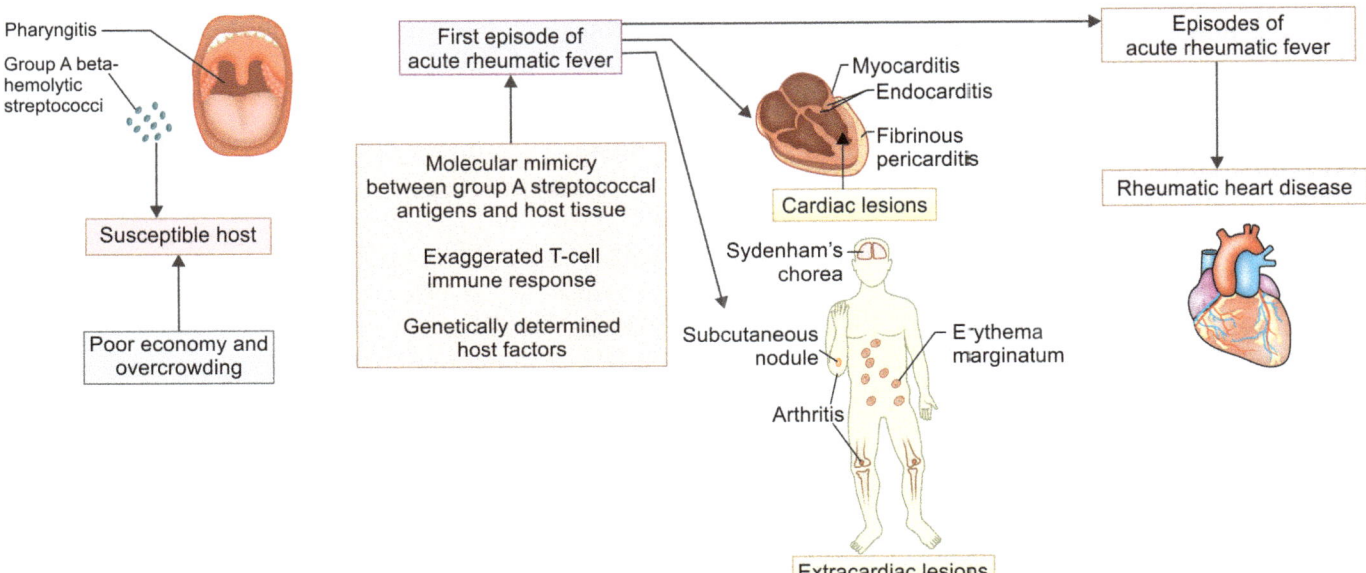

Fig. 9.7: Pathogenesis of rheumatic fever and rheumatic heart disease.

Migrating Polyarthritis

- It is most common major manifestation. It occurs early when streptococcal antibody titers are high in about 75–90% of patients.
- It is acute, painful, migratory, and asymmetric and is of short duration (*fleeting and flitting*). Usually >5 joints are affected and mainly involves large joints (knees, ankles, wrists, elbows, and shoulders). The joints are involved in quick succession. Small joints and cervical spine are less commonly involved.
- Involved joints show signs of inflammation (red, swollen, and tender) with or without effusion. Pain and swelling develop quickly and subside within 5–7 days. Arthritis does not progress to chronic disease and over a period of time involved joints heal without any residual deformity (licks the joints).
- Excellent response of high dose aspirin (salicylates) and NSAIDs.
- *Jaccoud's arthritis* is a rare deformity of the metacarpophalangeal joints following repeated attacks of rheumatic fever.
- In children below 5 years, arthritis is usually mild but carditis is more prominent.

Carditis

- It is an early and most serious manifestation that occurs in 60–70% of patients.
- It manifest as pancarditis involving all three layers of the heart (*endocardium, myocardium, and pericardium*). On microscopic examination, myocardium shows *Aschoff body* that is pathognomonic of rheumatic myocarditis. *Rheumatic endocarditis* may involve valvular (valvular endocarditis) or mural endocardium (mural endocarditis). Rheumatic pericarditis produces pericardial effusion and thick fibroserous exudates.
- Carditis leaves a sequela and permanent damage to the organ (bites the heart).
- Valvular damage is the hallmark of RF. Chronic phase is characterized by fibrosis, calcification, and stenosis of heart valves (fish-mouth valves).
- It is more common in younger children, and may be asymptomatic. It is detected only on echocardiograph.

Manifestations of carditis
Pancarditis involves the endocardium, myocardium, and pericardium. Incidence of carditis decreases with increasing age. It ranges from 90% at 3 years to around 30% in adolescence.

- **Myocarditis:**
  - *Tachycardia*: It is disproportionate to fever and persists during sleep.
  - *Features of congestive heart failure*: Breathlessness (due to heart failure or pericardial effusion). Cardiac failure may be either caused by dysfunction of myocardium or valvular regurgitation.
  - Physical examination may reveal third heart sound (S_3), fourth heart sound (S_4), or a summation gallop.
  - Arrhythmias, prolongation of PR interval being the most common.

- **Endocarditis:** Murmurs are most commonly observed during acute rheumatic fever. It may be a new or changed murmur and includes:
  - Apical pansystolic murmur is a high-pitched, blowing-quality murmur of mitral regurgitation that radiates to the left axilla.
  - Apical soft mid-diastolic murmur (also known as a *Carey–Coombs murmur*) is heard during active carditis due to valvulitis with nodules forming on the mitral valve leaflets. It accompanies severe mitral insufficiency.
  - It is an early diastolic murmur of aortic regurgitation and is high-pitched, blowing, decrescendo, and heard best along the right upper and mid-left sternal border after deep expiration while the patient is leaning forward.

- **Pericarditis:**
  - Chest/pericardial pain (due to pericarditis or pancarditis)
  - Pericardial friction rub and precordial tenderness
  - Pericardial effusion (uncommon and always small). Rheumatic pericarditis never causes constriction.

Other clinical features of acute rheumatic carditis: These include palpitations, cardiac enlargement (cardiomegaly), and syncope due to conduction defects.

Skin Lesions
Subcutaneous nodules
- These occur in 9–20% of cases and are often associated with carditis.
- It appears as a small (0.5–2.0 cm), painless, and mobile hard nodules beneath skin appears 4 weeks after onset of RF. Thus, it helps to confirm rather than make the diagnosis.
- It is most common along extensor surfaces of joint-knees, elbows, wrists, and also on bony prominences, tendons, dorsum of feet, and occipital or cervical spine.
- Delayed manifestation, disappears: Leaves no residual damage.

Erythema marginatum
- It occurs in <7% and often associated with chronic carditis and is evanescent
- Unique, transient, and serpiginous-looking lesions of 1–2 inches in size
- Pink/red macules clear centrally and serpiginous spreading edge. More on trunks and limbs, non-itchy and almost never on the face. The resulting red rings or "margins" may coalesce or overlap.
- Worsens with application of heat.

Chorea
It is also known as *Sydenham's chorea, Saint Vitus dance*, St Johannis' chorea, *chorea minor*, or rheumatic chorea.

Definition: Rheumatic chorea is a syndrome characterized by chorea, muscle weakness, and emotional instability.

Etiology
Triggering factor is pharyngeal infection by group A β-hemolytic streptococci.

Clinical features
- **Age and gender:** Occur in 5–10% of cases, mainly in girls of 1–15 years of age.

- **Onset of chorea:** Rheumatic chorea is a late neurological manifestation of acute rheumatic fever. It usually occurs 3–8 months after the triggering infection by A β-hemolytic streptococci when all the other signs may have disappeared. If there is no previous rheumatic manifestation, the term pure chorea is used.
- **First sign:** Emotional lability, difficulty walking, talking, and writing which is observed in 30% of patients with acute rheumatic fever (ARF).
- It is characterized by spasmodic, brief, purposeless (unintentional), involuntary, and jerky movements. Choreiform movements particularly affect the head/face (darting movement of tongue) upper limb hands or feet. Speech may be affected and may be explosive and halting and fidgety. It can be unilateral (hemichorea) or bilateral.
- **Mild forms** may be difficult to diagnose and following signs are helpful in these cases
- **Milkmaid's grip:** When the patient is asked to squeeze the examiner's fingers, a squeezing and relaxing motion (such as milking a cow) occurs. This is described as milkmaid's grip and is due to inability to maintain muscular contraction.
- **Bag-of-worms appearance** is due to asynchronous contractions of the lingual muscles.
- **Jack-in-the-box sign:** When the patient is asked to keep the tongue protruded out, it retracts involuntarily.
- **Pronator sign:** Holding the arms outstretched may elicit "spooning" (hyperextension of the fingers with dorsiflexion of the wrist)
- **Severe forms:** Patients are unable to get up or sit, and have violent continuous jerks that may cause physical injury.
- Additional features include hypotonia, pendular knee jerks, and mild generalized muscular weakness.

Others
- Epistaxis, arthralgia, tender lymph nodes, scarlet fever rash, abdominal pain, tonsillar exudates in older children, etc.
- Systemic manifestations are rare and include pleurisy, pleural effusion, and pneumonia.

Laboratory Investigations

Investigations for Evidence of Preceding Streptococcal Infection (Specific)
- **Isolation of group A streptococci/throat swab culture:** Group A β-hemolytic streptococci are usually in only 10–25% of cases. It can be done also in family members and contacts. However, serologic tests are usually done to show the evidence of streptococcal infection.
- **Streptococcal antibody tests (serologic tests)**
- Serological tests usually confirm a recent group A β-hemolytic streptococcal infection
- Raised streptococcal antibody levels are found in the early stages of acute rheumatic fever. However, in two situations, their levels may be low.
- When the interval between the streptococcal pharyngitis and detection of rheumatic fever in more than 2 months (e.g., chorea).
- **In patients with rheumatic carditis only:** Common serologic tests
- **Antistreptolysin O antibodies (ASO titers):** Rising titers, or levels of >200 U (adults) or >300 U (children). This test is positive in 80% of cases. ASO titers are normal in 20% of adult cases of rheumatic fever and most cases of chorea.
- Anti-DNase B
- Antihyaluronidase (AH)
- Antistreptozyme test (ASTZ) is a very sensitive indicator of recent streptococcal infection and is also helpful in ruling out rheumatic fever. Titers more than 200 units/mL are considered positive.

The above four tests when combined together help in conforming the diagnosis in 95% of cases.

Investigations for Evidence of a Systemic Illness (Nonspecific)
- **Acute phase reactants:** These tests confirm the presence of an inflammatory process, but are nonspecific.
  - Erythrocyte sedimentation rate (ESR) is raised
  - Raised C-reactive protein (CRP) in the blood
- **Other tests confirming an inflammatory reaction:**
  - *Peripheral blood*: Polymorphonuclear leukocytosis and anemia (due to suppression of erythropoiesis)
  - *Serum*: Increase in serum complements, and increase in serum mucoproteins, and α_2 and γ globulin levels.

Investigations for Evidence of Carditis
- **Chest radiography:** Chest X-ray may show evidences of cardiac failure, cardiomegaly, and pulmonary congestion
- **Electrocardiogram:** ECG changes commonly include:
  - Most consistent change is a prolongation of the PR interval and T-wave inversion
  - Other findings are rarely second-degree AV block features of pericarditis and reduction in QRS voltages
- **Echocardiography:** It can detect myocardial dysfunction, cardiac dilatation, valvular abnormalities, and pericardial effusion.

Diagnosis of Acute Rheumatic Fever
- Diagnosis of acute rheumatic fever (ARF) is made by the presence of combination of typical clinical features together with evidence of the precipitating group A streptococci (GAS) infection. This uncertainty led Dr T Duckett Jones in 1944 to develop a set of criteria known as Jones Criteria to aid diagnosis.
- **Modified Jones criteria:** Presently, diagnosis is based on modified Jones criteria (**Table 9.19**).

Exceptions to Jones Criteria
- Chorea alone, if other causes have been excluded.
- Insidious or late-onset carditis (indolent carditis) with no other explanation.
- Patients with documented RHD or prior rheumatic fever, one major criterion, or of fever, arthralgia or high CRP suggests recurrence.

Table 9.19: World Health Organization criteria (2002–2003) for the diagnosis of rheumatic fever and rheumatic heart disease (based on the 1992 revised Jones criteria).

Diagnostic categories	Criteria
Primary episode of rheumatic fever	Two major or one major and two minor manifestations plus evidence of preceding group A streptococcal infection
Recurrent attack of rheumatic fever in a patient without established rheumatic heart disease	
Recurrent attack of rheumatic fever in a patient with established rheumatic heart disease	Two minor manifestations plus evidence of preceding group A streptococcal infection
Rheumatic chorea	Other major manifestations or evidence of group A streptococcal infection not required
Insidious onset rheumatic carditis	
Chronic valve lesions of rheumatic heart disease (patients presenting for the first time with pure mitral stenosis or mixed mitral valve disease and/or aortic valve disease)	Do not require any other criteria to be diagnosed as having rheumatic heart disease
Major manifestations	*Minor manifestations*
• Carditis • Polyarthritis • Chorea • Erythema marginatum • Subcutaneous nodules	• *Clinical*: Fever and polyarthralgias • *Laboratory*: Elevated erythrocyte sedimentation rate or leukocyte count • *Electrocardiogram*: Prolonged P-R interval

Supporting evidence of a preceding streptococcal infection within the last 45 days:
- Elevated or rising antistreptolysin O or other streptococcal antibody
- A positive throat culture
- Rapid antigen test for group A *Streptococcus*
- Recent scarlet fever

Management of Acute Rheumatic Fever

- **Step I:** Primary prevention (eradication of streptococci)
- **Step II:** Anti-inflammatory treatment (aspirin and steroids)
- **Step III:** Supportive management and management of complications
- **Step IV:** Secondary prevention (prevention of recurrent attacks)

Step I: Primary Prevention (Eradication of Streptococci)

- Primary prevention is accurate diagnosis and treatment of group A β-hemolytic streptococcal pharyngeal infection.
- Antistreptococcal therapy/primary prevention is mentioned in **Table 9.20**.

Table 9.20: Antistreptococcal therapy for primary prevention.

Drug	Dose	Mode and duration
Benzathine penicillin G *or*	600,000 U for patients <27 kg 1,200,000 U for patients >27 kg	Intramuscular once
Penicillin V (phenoxymethylpenicillin) *or*	*Children*: 250 mg 2–3 times daily or adolescents and adults: 500 mg 2–3 times daily	Oral for 10 days
Procaine penicillin	Daily 600,000 units	Intramuscular for 10 days
Erythromycin	20–40 mg/kg/day 2–4 times daily (maximum 1 g/day)	Oral for 10 days

Step II: Anti-inflammatory Treatment

- **Arthritis only:**
  - *Aspirin* usually rapidly relieves the symptoms of arthritis within 24 hours and also helps to confirm the diagnosis. Aspirin is given in the dose of *75–100 mg/kg body weight/day* divided into 4 doses for 6 weeks (attain a body level 20–30 mg/dL). It should be continued till the ESR has fallen. It produces mild toxicity such as nausea, tinnitus, and deafness and serious toxicity as vomiting, tachypnea, and acidosis.
  - Carditis or severe arthritis
- **Corticosteroids** produce more rapid symptomatic relief compared to aspirin. They are indicated in patients with carditis or severe arthritis. However, their long-term use is not found to be beneficial.
- **Prednisolone given in the dose of 1.0–2.0 mg/kg per day** in divided doses for 4–6 weeks (until the ESR is normal) and then to be tapered off.

Step III: Supportive Management and Management of Complications

- **Bed rest** is important, because it reduces joint pain and cardiac workload.
- **Patients without carditis:** Advice bed rest until temperature and ESR are normal.
- **Patients with carditis:** Bed rest to be continued for 2–6 weeks after the ESR and temperature has returned to normal. Avoid strenuous exercise in patients who had carditis.
- **Treatment of congestive cardiac failure:** Digitalis and diuretics
- **Treatment of chorea:** Diazepam or haloperidol
- Rest to joints and supportive splinting

Step IV: Secondary Prevention of Rheumatic Fever (Prevention of Recurrent Attacks)

- Patients with acute rheumatic fever are susceptible to further attacks of rheumatic fever, if another streptococcal infection occurs.
- Secondary prevention is directed at preventing acute group A β-hemolytic streptococcal (GABHS) pharyngitis in patients at substantial risk of recurrent acute rheumatic fever by long-term prophylaxis. Duration of prophylaxis is controversial and its broad outlines are provided in **Table 9.21**.
- Regimens for secondary prevention of rheumatic fever are mentioned in **Table 9.22**.

Management of Rheumatic Chorea

- Rule out other causes of chorea such as systemic lupus erythematosus, Huntington's disease, and Wilson's disease.
- **Rest:** Complete mental and physical rest. Keep the patient in a quiet room.
- Padded sideboards for beds to prevent physical injury.
- **Drugs:** Haloperidol or sodium valproate with diazepam. Steroids may be needed in severe cases.

VALVULAR HEART DISEASE

Mitral Stenosis

Mitral stenosis (MS) is a valvular heart disease and is characterized by the narrowing of the orifice of the *mitral* valve due to structural abnormality of the *mitral* valve apparatus.

Table 9.21: Categories of rheumatic fever and duration of prophylaxis.

Category	Duration
Rheumatic fever without carditis	At least for 5 years or until age 21 year, whichever is longer
Rheumatic fever with carditis but without residual heart disease (no valvular disease)	At least for 10 years or well into adulthood, whichever is longer
Rheumatic fever with carditis and residual heart disease (persistent valvular disease) and post-valve surgery cases	At least 10 years since last episode and at least until age 40 years; sometime lifelong

Table 9.22: Regimens for secondary prevention of rheumatic fever.

Drug	Dose	Route
Penicillin G benzathine	600,000 U for children, <27 kg and 1.2 million U for children >27 kg, every 3 week	Intramuscular
Penicillin V	250 mg, twice a day	Oral
Sulfadiazine or sulfisoxazole	0.5 g, once a day for patients <60 lb; 1.0 g, once a day for patients >60 lb	Oral
For individuals who are allergic to penicillin and sulfonamide drugs		
Macrolide or azalide (erythromycin and azithromycin)	Variable	Oral

Etiology (Table 9.23) and Pathology

- Rheumatic fever is the most common cause of mitral stenosis. It develops secondary to previous rheumatic fever due to infection with group A β-hemolytic *Streptococcus*
- Mitral stenosis is more common in females
- The latent period from the first attack of rheumatic fever and the development of onset of symptoms due to mitral stenosis is usually as short as 1–2 years in India, compared to long in Western countries. This may due to repeated attacks of severe carditis in India.
- Clinical manifestation in *juvenile mitral stenosis*/malignant mitral stenosis develops below the age of 19 years and is common in India. Pediatric mitral stenosis manifests below the age of 12 years.

Rheumatic Mitral Stenosis

In rheumatic mitral stenosis (MS), chronic inflammation produces:
- Diffuse thickening of the mitral valve leaflets due to fibrosis and/or calcification
- Fusion of commissures and cusp
- Fusion and shortening of the chordae tendineae

The above morphological changes progress and cause rigidity of mitral valvular cusps, which in turn lead to narrowing at the apex of the funnel-shaped ("fish-mouth") mitral valve → severe narrowing (stenotic) of valve orifice and progressive immobility of the valve cusps.

Clinical Features

Symptoms

- **Dyspnea on exertion** is due to pulmonary hypertension and is slowly progressive.
  - It precipitated by severe exertion, excitement, fever, anemia, sexual intercourse, pregnancy, thyrotoxicosis, and atrial fibrillation.
- **Fatigue on exertion:** It is due to pulmonary hypertension and low cardiac output. It is slowly progressive.
- **Hemoptysis**
- Rupture of bronchial veins or of pulmonary vein or bronchial vein collaterals—pulmonary apoplexy
- Rupture of pulmonary capillaries during pulmonary edema

Table 9.23: Causes of mitral stenosis.

- Rheumatic fever (leading cause)
- Congenital mitral stenosis (parachute mitral valve, Shone complex)
- Metastatic carcinoid tumor to the lung, or primary bronchial carcinoid
- Calcification of mitral valve apparatus
- Systemic lupus erythematosus
- Rheumatoid arthritis (extremely rare)
- Endomyocardial fibrosis
- Gout
- Methysergide treatment
- Lutembacher's syndrome (combination of acquired mitral stenosis and an atrial septal defect)
- Mucopolysaccharidosis—Hurlers syndrome and Hunters
- Whipple's disease
- Infective endocarditis with large vegetations

Mimics of MS:
- Myxoma
- Ball valve thrombus
- Cor triatriatum

(MS: mitral stenosis)

- Pulmonary congestion, embolism, and infarction
- Winter bronchitis
- Pulmonary hemosiderosis due to chronic recurrent pulmonary edema
- Anticoagulant use
- **Chest pain:** Develops in about 15% patients due to—(1) right ventricle enlargement, right ventricular hypertrophy, and pulmonary hypertension, (2) coexistent coronary artery disease (CAD), (3) coronary embolism, and (4) angina due to decreased cardiac output.
- Palpitations develop when there are atrial fibrillations (AF), chamber enlargement (right ventricle and pulmonary artery).
- **Systemic thromboembolism:** Paroxysmal AF results in embolism most commonly to the cerebral vessels resulting in stroke, but mesenteric, renal, and peripheral emboli (e.g., ischemic limb) can also develop.
- **Syncope:** PAH, arrhythmias, and ball valve thrombus
- **Hoarseness of voice—La Ortner's syndrome:** Due to compression of the left recurrent laryngeal nerve due to the dilated pulmonary artery or giant left atrium.
- Right heart failure
- **Orthopnea and paroxysmal nocturnal dyspnea:** Due to left atrial failure.
- **Winter bronchitis:** Patients with MS are susceptible to recurrent attacks of bronchitis, especially during the winter.

Physical signs
General examination:
- **Mitral facies** is characterized cyanotic lips and face, malar flush (dusky pink discoloration over the upper cheeks due to arteriovenous anastomoses and vascular stasis), and mild jaundice. It may develop when MS is very severe with low cardiac output and peripheral vasoconstriction.
- Peripheral edema and ascites when right heart failure develops.
- Pulse
- Pulse in low volume and peripheral pulse may be absent, if embolism develops.
- Pulse rhythm is irregularly irregular and varying volume in atrial fibrillation.
- **Blood pressure:** May be mildly reduced. Mean of 3 readings to be taken, if atrial fibrillation is present
- Jugular veins
- **Jugular venous pressure** is raised when congestive heart failure develops.
- **Jugular venous pulse:** (1) Prominent a waves (due to vigorous right atrial systole) observed when there is pulmonary hypertension without atrial fibrillation, (2) absence of waves in atrial fibrillation, and (3) prominent v waves (c-v waves) and rapid y descent when there is development of functional tricuspid regurgitation.

Inspection and Palpation of Precordium
- *Apex beat* is not shifted and is tapping character of S_1 at apex (closing snap). Apex beat is shifted when there is coexistent of MS with mitral regurgitation (MR)/aortic stenosis (AS)/systemic hypertension/ischemic heart disease (IHD)/myocarditis
- *Diastolic thrill* at apex
- *Palpable pulmonary component of second heart sound* (P_2), if there is pulmonary arterial hypertension.
- *Left parasternal heave:* Present when there is right ventricular hypertrophy or left atrial enlargement.
- *Epigastric pulsations* of right ventricular type.
- Precordial bulge in juvenile/malignant MS

Other findings: Right heart failure is associated with peripheral edema, tender hepatomegaly, and ascites.

Auscultation
- **Loud first heart sound:**
  - In mitral stenosis, the forces that open and close the mitral valve increase as left atrial pressure increases. Hence, the first heart sound (S_1) is loud and can be palpable (tapping apex beat) in mitral stenosis.
  - When associated with atrial fibrillation, the intensity of first heart sound varies.
  - A low intensity of the first heart sound in MS may be due to—(1) calcification of the mitral valve, (2) congenital MS, and (3) dominant associated mitral/aortic regurgitation.
- **Loud second heart sound:** It is a sign of pulmonary hypertension. The second heart sound is closely split and the pulmonary component of the second heart sound (P_2) is loud.
- **Mitral opening snap:**
  - OS is a sharp, snappy sound heard during early diastole, following the sound of aortic valve closure (A_2) by 0.05–0.12 s.
  - Opening snap (OS) is produced due to the sudden (abrupt) opening of the dome of the stenosed mitral valve with the force of the increased left atrial pressure during diastole. It is the most important auscultatory sign of valvular involvement in MS. Absent OS indicates the calcification of body of the leaflets.
  - The time interval between A_2 and OS is inversely proportional to the severity of the MS.
  - *Best heard*: During expiration, just medial to the cardiac apex with the diaphragm of the stethoscope.
- **Murmur of mitral stenosis:**
  - *Mid-diastolic/presystolic murmur*: Turbulent blood flow through stenosed mitral valve produces the characteristic *low pitched, rumbling, mid-diastolic murmur* and sometimes accompanied by a thrill. Murmur is best heard with the bell of the stethoscope held lightly at the apex with the patient lying on the left side.
    - To increase intensity of MDM: Left lateral position using bell of stethoscope, while holding expiration auscultate after walking (isotonic exercise), and squatting (increased peripheral resistance in these procedures contribute to the increased murmur).
- In the early phase of mitral stenosis, a *presystolic murmur* may be the only auscultatory abnormality. Mechanism of presystolic murmur—(1) atrial contraction, (2) persistent atrioventricular gradient, and (3) left ventricular contraction in presystole-reducing mitral funnel.

- **Presystolic accentuation of the murmur:** Atrial contraction contributes to increased gradient in presystole. Hence, mid-diastolic murmur is accentuated by exercise. In patient with sinus rhythm, the murmur becomes louder during atrial systole and during long R-R interval in atrial fibrillation is termed as *presystolic accentuation*.
  - *Systolic murmur:* When *pulmonary hypertension* develops, it will lead to right ventricular hypertrophy and dilatation with secondary tricuspid regurgitation. This produces a systolic murmur and giant "*v* waves" in the venous pulse.
    - If MS coexists with mitral regurgitation, it produces a loud pansystolic murmur that radiates toward the axilla and is heard at the lower left sternal border. Functional tricuspid regurgitation produces a pansystolic murmur. It is accentuated during inspiration (de Carvallo's sign).
  - *Murmur of pulmonary regurgitation (Graham–Steell murmur):* It is a high-pitched early diastolic decrescendo murmur heard along the left sternal border and indicative of severe pulmonary hypertension.

Diagrammatic representation of timing of heart sounds and murmur in mitral stenosis are shown in **Figure 9.8**.

Clinical judgment of the severity of mitral stenosis:
Following features suggest severe MS:
- Presence of pulmonary hypertension
- More closeness of the opening snap to the second heart sound (short A2-OS interval)
- Lengthy mid-diastolic murmur

Investigations
Radiological features of mitral stenosis (chest X-ray) are shown in **Figure. 9.9**.

Electrocardiogram
It can confirm enlargement of left atrium ("P" mitrale), right ventricular hypertrophy, tall R waves in V_1-V_3, P mitrale, and atrial fibrillation.

Echocardiogram
- It can reveal thickening of mitral valve area, valvular leaflet, thickening and shortening chordae tendinae, fusion of commissures, calcification of leaflets and chordae, and diastolic doming (due to commissural fusion).
- **Wilkins score (4–16):** Four points each for leaflet thickness, leaflet mobility, leaflet calcification, and chordal involvement.

Transesophageal echocardiography (TEE)
To assess mitral regurgitation (MR) severity and to rule out left atrial appendage (LAA) thrombus

Doppler
It provides definite evaluation of MS. It shows pressure gradient across mitral valve, pulmonary artery pressure, and left ventricular function.

Complications of Mitral Stenosis
Complications of mitral stenosis are described in **Table 9.24.**

Management
Mild mitral stenosis may not require any treatment other than treatment of attacks of bronchitis.
- **Medical management:** MS with minor symptoms are treated medically.
  - Rheumatic fever prophylaxis to be given. However, infective endocarditis prophylaxis is not necessary.
  - *Indications for anticoagulation*: (1) Atrial fibrillation (persistent or paroxysmal), (2) embolic events, (3) left trial thrombus, (4) left atrial diameter >55 mm, and (5) spontaneous echo contrast.

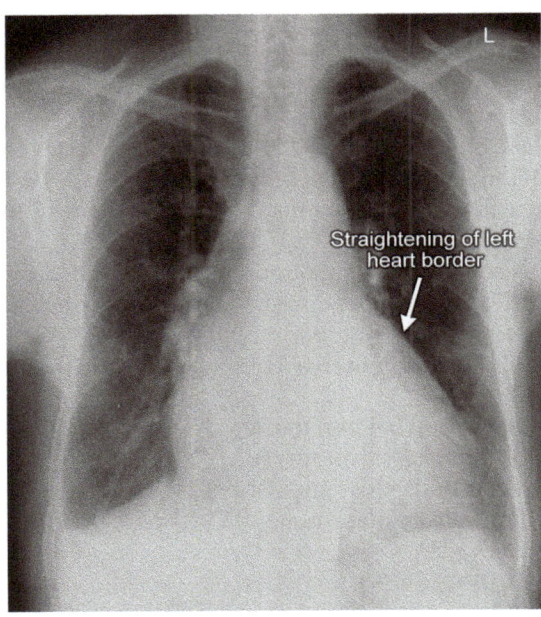

Fig. 9.9: X-rays of mitral stenosis showing double atrial shadow and straightening of left heart border.

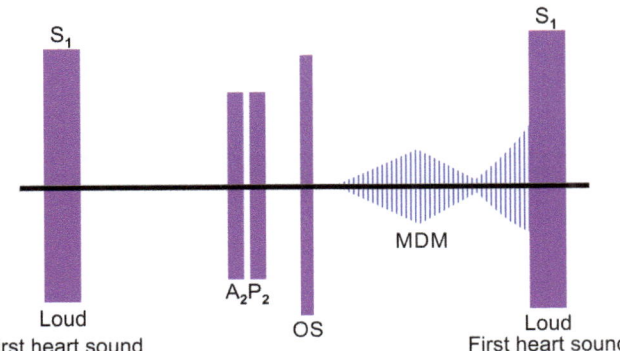

Fig. 9.8: Diagrammatic representation of timing of heart sounds and murmur in mitral stenosis features are loud first heart sound, an opening snap (OS), mid-diastolic murmur (MDM) with presystolic accentuation.

Table 9.24: Complications of mitral stenosis.

• Atrial fibrillation	• Ortner's syndrome	• Pulmonary edema
• Thrombus formation	• Hemoptysis	• Pulmonary infarction
• Systemic embolization	• Dysphagia	
• Pulmonary hypertension	• Lower lobe pneumonia	• Cardiac cirrhosis
• Infective endocarditis	• Right heart failure	• Pulmonary hemosiderosis

- Restrict/decrease sodium intake
- *Diuretics*: Early symptom such as mild dyspnea (due to pulmonary congestion) is usually treated with low doses of diuretics.
- Beta-blockers or non-dihydropyridines (DHP) calcium channel blockers (e.g., verapamil or diltiazem) to reduce heart rate (even in sinus rhythm, more useful in atrial fibrillation).
- Digoxin, if atrial fibrillation with right heart failure. Atrial fibrillation also needs anticoagulation to prevent atrial thrombus and systemic embolization.

❑ **Surgical management:** Four operative measures are available:
1. Trans-septal balloon mitral valvotomy (BMV)
2. Closed mitral valvotomy (CMV)
3. Open mitral valvotomy (OMV)
4. Mitral valve replacement (MVR)

Mitral Regurgitation

Mitral regurgitation (MR) or mitral insufficiency (MI) or mitral incompetence is a disorder of the heart in which the mitral valve does not close properly.

Etiology (Box 9.6)

Lesion in any one of five components of mitral valve apparatus namely—(1) valve leaflets, (2) the annulus, (3) the chordae tendineae or (4) papillary muscles, or (5) the left ventricle can produce mitral regurgitation (MR).

Clinical Features

Symptoms

❑ **Acute mitral regurgitation:** Usually presents dyspnea due to acute pulmonary edema.
❑ **Chronic mitral regurgitation:** It may be asymptomatic for many years. It may become symptomatic only after the onset of irreversible LV dysfunction.
- *Palpitation* is the most common symptom due to increased stroke volume or atrial fibrillation.

> **Box 9.6: Causes of mitral regurgitation.**
>
> **Causes of acute mitral regurgitation:** *Infective endocarditis, rupture of a papillary muscle* (e.g., acute myocardial infarction and mitral valve prolapse), chest trauma, cardiac surgery, acute rheumatic carditis, and dysfunction of prosthetic valve.
>
> **Causes of chronic mitral regurgitation:**
> ❖ **Damage to valve leaflets:** *Rheumatic heart disease*, myxomatous degeneration, mitral valve prolapse (MVP), *infective endocarditis,* and SLE
> ❖ **Damage to annulus:** Abscess (IE), *annular calcification,* and dilated cardiomyopathy
> ❖ **Damage to chordae tendineae:** Myxomatous degeneration (MVP, Marfan syndrome, and Ehlers–Danlos syndrome), infective endocarditis, and acute rheumatic fever
> ❖ **Damage to papillary muscles:** Coronary artery disease [ischemia, myocardial infarction (MI), rupture, and dilated cardiomyopathy]
> ❖ **Damage to left ventricle:** Ischemia and dilated cardiomyopathy

Note: Major causes are highlighted in bold letter
(SLE: systemic lupus erythematosus)

- *Dyspnea and orthopnea*: Due to pulmonary venous hypertension and left ventricular failure occur late in the course of mitral regurgitation
- *Fatigue and lethargy*: Due to reduced cardiac output
- *Symptoms of right heart failure*: Develop in the late stages and lead to congestive cardiac failure
- Cardiac cachexia
- *Thromboembolism*: Less common than in mitral stenosis. However, subacute infective endocarditis is more common.

❑ Other symptoms and complications are similar to mitral stenosis.

Signs

❑ **Pulse:** Volume is high and in severe mitral regurgitation, it may be mildly collapsing.
❑ Irregular rhythm and varying volume, if there is atrial fibrillation.

Jugular veins

❑ **Uncomplicated mitral regurgitation:** Jugular venous pressure (JVP) is normal.
❑ **With atrial fibrillation:** Disappearance of "a" waves
❑ **With pulmonary hypertension:** Prominent "a" waves
❑ **With right ventricular failure and functional tricuspid regurgitation:** Jugular venous pressure is raised and very prominent v waves.

Blood pressure: In severe mitral regurgitation, wide pulse pressure. Three recordings are necessary, if patient has atrial fibrillation (AF). Pulsus alternans in acute MR

Inspection and palpation:
❑ Hyperdynamic precordium
❑ **Apex beat:** Shifted to the left (due to left ventricular dilatation), forceful (feels active and rocking), and diffuse (hyperdynamic) in character due to left ventricular volume overload.
❑ **Cardiomegaly:** In chronic MR. Acute MR does not produce cardiomegaly.
❑ Systolic thrill (if MI is severe) at the apex.
❑ Left parasternal heave and palpable P_2.
❑ Epigastric pulsations of right ventricular type.

Auscultation (Fig. 9.10)

❑ **Soft first heart sound (S_1):** Because of the incomplete apposition of the mitral valve cusps and partial closure

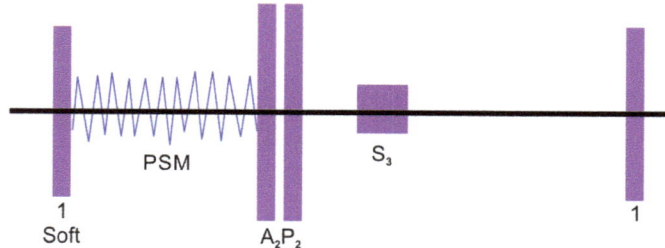

Fig. 9.10: Diagrammatic representation of timing of heart sounds and murmur in mitral regurgitation. Features are normal or soft first heart sound, pansystolic murmur (PSM), extending to the second heart sound (A_2 and P_2). A third heart sound (S_3) may develop with severe mitral regurgitation.

of these valve cusps when ventricular systole begins. It is loud, if there is coexistent MS, mitral valve prolapse–mitral regurgitation (MVP-MR), or papillary muscle dysfunction MR.
- **Widely split second heart sound (S_2)** is due to aortic valve closure (A1) occurring early but the split is mobile.
- **Pulmonary component (P_2) of S_2** is loud and palpable in pulmonary hypertension and also due to anterior displacement of pulmonary artery caused by dilated LA.
- **Left ventricular third heart sound (S_3):** It indicates severe mitral regurgitation.
- S4 is a sign of acute MR, as left atrium is not dilated in acute MR.
- Pulmonary ejection sound in pulmonary hypertension.

Murmur of mitral regurgitation
- **Apical pansystolic murmur:** The typical features of murmur in mitral regurgitation are:
- High pitched, blowing and usually holosystolic/pansystolic loudest at the apex.
- Plateau shaped best heard with diaphragm of stethoscope
- Commonly radiates widely over the precordium and into the axilla and left interscapular area (if anterior leaflets involved as in rheumatic) or radiating to base (if posterior leaflets involved).
- It is produced due to the mitral regurgitant jet occurring throughout the whole of systole.
- It may be accompanied by a thrill.
- **Short mid-diastolic flow murmur:** Sometimes, a short, rumbling mid-diastolic murmur may be detected at the apex in severe cases due to an increased flow across the mitral valve. It may follow the third heart sound.
- **Other murmurs:**
  - Ejection systolic murmur or early diastolic murmur at pulmonary area when there is pulmonary hypertension.
  - Pansystolic murmur at lower left sternal border when there is functional tricuspid regurgitation.
  - Opening snap can be heard in 10% patients with MR.

Investigations
- **Electrocardiogram (ECG):** It can reveal—
  - Enlargement/hypertrophy of left atrium (if not in atrial fibrillation)
  - Dilatation and hypertrophy of left ventricle
  - Hypertrophy of both left and right ventricle in pulmonary hypertension
  - Atrial fibrillation
- **Chest X-ray:** May show the following abnormalities—all signs as described for MS:
  - Enlargement of left atrium (more than in MS) and left ventricle
  - Pulmonary venous congestion
  - *Pulmonary edema:* Interstitial edema in acute MR, chronic decompensated MR, or with coexistent MS.
  - Annular calcium appears as a C-shaped opacity in posterior third of heart in lateral or RAO (right anterior oblique) view.

> **Box 9.7:** Complications of mitral regurgitation.
> - Progressive heart failure is the most common cause of death
> - **Less frequent:** Sudden death, stroke, and fatal endocarditis
> - Atrial fibrillation, infective endocarditis, and left ventricular failure
> - Pulmonary hypertension (late) and right ventricular failure (very late)
> - Rarely systemic embolism

- **Echocardiogram:**
  - It shows a dilated left atrium and left ventricle.
  - Structural abnormalities of mitral valve, e.g., prolapsed, chordal, or papillary muscle ruptures, if present.
- **Doppler echocardiogram:**
  - Detects and assesses the severity of regurgitation (quantification of regurgitation)
  - Mitral annular calcification between mitral valve apparatus and posterior wall
- **Transesophageal echocardiography (TEE):** It is useful to identify structural valve abnormalities and can be helpful before surgery especially in MVP. Intraoperative TEE helps in the assessment of the efficacy of valve repair. MVP is defined as more than 2 mm systolic displacement of mitral leaflet into left atrium (LA).

Complications of mitral regurgitation are listed in **Box 9.7**.

Management
Medical management
- **Acute MR:** Afterload reduction with nitroprusside
- **Chronic MR:** In mitral regurgitation, high afterload may worsen the degree of regurgitation, and hypertension is treated with vasodilators, e.g., ACE inhibitors and nifedipine are used.
- Diuretics
- **Treatment of AF:** Digoxin and anticoagulants
- Anticoagulation
- Infective endocarditis prophylaxis
- Rheumatic fever prophylaxis

Surgery—mitral valve replacement

Mitral Valve Prolapse (MVP)
- Mitral valve prolapse (MVP) is an abnormal movement of one or both of the mitral valve leaflets >2 mm beyond annular plan into the left atrium during systole with or without mitral regurgitation.
- **Barlow's syndrome:** It involves the posterior leaflet and cusps. *Reads syndrome*/floppy valve syndrome is considered as a variant of Barlow that affects both mitral cusps as well-other valves like aortic valve.
- *Cobb's syndrome* selectively affects the anterior mitral cusp.
- MVP syndrome is also called as *systolic click-murmur syndrome*.
- MVP is one of the more common causes of mild mitral regurgitation.

Symptoms

- **Age and gender:** More common in females between 15 and 30 years. But, severe mitral regurgitation caused by prolapsed mitral valve is more common in older males compared to young females.
- May be asymptomatic or present with anxiety neurosis.
- Symptoms include atypical chest pain (precordial stabbing), palpitation, syncope or presyncope, and fatigue.
- **Rarely:** Symptoms of left ventricular failure (exertional dyspnea, orthopnea, and paroxysmal nocturnal dyspnea) in patients with mitral regurgitation, sudden death, and transient ischemic attacks.

Signs

- Asthenic built, straight back/pectus excavatum
- **Mid-systolic click:** In mildest forms, the valve is competent but bulges back into the atrium during systole, causing a mid-systolic click occur >0.14 seconds after S_1 without any murmur.
- **Late systolic murmur:** When there is mitral regurgitation, the click is followed by a late systolic murmur apical murmur (rarely "whooping" or "honking"). Its length increases as the regurgitation becomes more severe. The systolic murmur of mitral valve prolapse increases during standing and Valsalva maneuver, but decreases during squatting and isometric exercise.

Aortic Stenosis

- Aortic stenosis is a chronic progressive disease and characterized by obstruction to the left ventricular stroke volume.
- Normal aortic valve area 3–4 cm² without any gradient across it. Critical aortic stenosis develops when an aortic valve area becomes less than 0.8 cm² or a gradient of more than 50 mm Hg.

Classification and Etiology of Aortic Stenosis
See **Box 9.8**.

Clinical Features
Usually asymptomatic aortic stenosis is moderately severe (aortic orifice reduced to one third of its normal size). It is commonly diagnosed in asymptomatic patients during routine clinical examination.

Symptoms
- **Age of onset of symptoms:** Bicuspid aortic valve between 50 and 70 years, calcific aortic stenosis >70 years, and rheumatic aortic stenosis between 40 and 50 years of age.
- **Symptomatic triad of aortic stenosis:** Three cardinal symptoms are (1) breathlessness (dyspnea), (2) angina, and (3) syncope.
- **Exercise intolerance:** Most common initial presentation. Dyspnea with exertion due to cardiac decompensation or fatigue with exertion due to inadequate rise of cardiac output with exertion.
- **Angina** is typical exertional and is due to mismatch in myocardial oxygen demand-supply ratio, or coexistent coronary artery disease (CAD).

Box 9.8: Classification and etiology of aortic stenosis.

Valvular aortic stenosis:
- **Acquired:** *Rheumatic aortic stenosis* (young adults, middle-aged, and elderly), *calcific aortic valvular disease* (CAVD—in middle aged to elderly), systemic lupus erythematosus (SLE), Fabry's disease, chronic kidney disease, Paget's disease of bone, rheumatoid arthritis, infective endocarditis, senile degenerative aortic stenosis (middle-aged to elderly), previous radiation exposure, homozygous familial hypercholesterolemia, and ochronosis
- **Congenital:** Congenital aortic stenosis (infants, children, and adolescents), bicuspid aortic valve (BAV), calcification and fibrosis of congenitally *bicuspid aortic valve* (young adults to middle-aged)

Subvalvular aortic stenosis:
- Membranous diaphragm
- Hypertrophic cardiomyopathy
- Congenital subvalvular aortic stenosis (infants, children, and adolescents)

Supravalvular aortic stenosis:
- Hourglass constriction of aorta
- Congenital supravalvular aortic stenosis (infants, children, and adolescents)
- Williams' syndrome

Williams' syndrome: It is characterized by Elfin facies, supravalvular aortic stenosis, idiopathic hypercalcemia, mental retardation, and behavioral profile. On examination, the right upper limb blood pressure may be a higher than the left upper limb and the pulse volume on the right arm better than left. This is called *Coanda effect*.

Shone's complex: It is a rare combination of four left-sided congenital cardiac anomalies including parachute mitral valve, supravalvular ring, coarctation of the aorta, and subaortic obstruction

---

- **Exertional syncope (or presyncope):** Due to failure of cardiac output to rise to meet demand, leading to a fall in BP.
- **Heart failure:** Orthopnea and paroxysmal nocturnal dyspnea (PND).
- Infective endocarditis
- Embolism
- Gastrointestinal bleed due to angiodysplasias (Heyde syndrome) and acquired von Willebrand syndrome.

If untreated, the approximate time interval from the onset of symptoms to death is 1.5–2 years for heart failure (Dyspnea, PND), 3 years for syncope, and 5 years for angina.

Signs
- **Appearance:** Severe AS produces "Dresden China" look-asthenic appearance with pale skin.
- **Pulse:**
  - *Parvus and tardus pulse:* Slow rising, late peaking, and low amplitude.
  - Pulsus bisferiens, if AS is associated aortic regurgitation (AR)
  - Anacrotic pulse and apicocarotid delay in severe AS
- Blood pressure
- Low systolic and pulse pressures. Systolic decapitation (SBP <120 mm of Hg)

- **Carotid shudder:** Thrill in carotids
- **Jugular venous pressure (JVP):** Prominent a waves (*Bernheim effect*).
- **Apex beat:** Thrusting/heaving LV type apex beat due to LV pressure overload. It is not usually displaced because hypertrophy (as opposed to dilatation) does not produce significant cardiomegaly.
- Palpable LV S4

Auscultation (Fig. 9.11)
- S_1 is normal. If loud, suspect coexistent MS.
- S_2-A_2: Soft (single S_2) in rheumatic AS, loud in BAV, normal in sub-/supravalvular AS. In severe AS paradoxical (reversed) split of second heart sound A_2 (splitting on expiration).
- Systolic ejection click in bicuspid aortic valve (BAV)
- **Ejection mid-systolic murmur:** Harsh/rough, radiates to the neck (to carotids arteries) and also the precordium with late peaking in severe AS. Best heard in the base of heart (aortic area). Murmur is likened to a saw cutting wood and especially in older patients may have a musical quality like the "mew" of a seagull. It is diamond-shaped (crescendo decrescendo). The murmur is usually longer in severe AS. The intensity of the murmur should not be correlated with the severity of AS because it is less intense when the cardiac output is reduced. In severe AS, it may not be audible. In calcific AS, high-frequency components radiate to apex producing a long systolic murmur at apex—*Gallavardin phenomenon*/hour-glass conduction due to periodic wake phenomenon. With LV failure, murmur intensity decreases and murmur may disappear.

Treatment
Asymptomatic patients: Irrespective of the severity of AS, asymptomatic patients have a good immediate prognosis. Hence, they should be managed conservatively with regular review for assessment of symptoms and echocardiography.

Medical treatment
- Avoid vigorous physical activity in patients with severe AS.
- **Diuretics** decrease dyspnea but may also reduce cardiac output.
- **ACE inhibitors:** To be used with caution and given only if there is LV failure.
- **Avoid β-blockers:** Because they produce LV failure.
- **Vasodilators for other purposes such as angina:** Be careful in titration, as there will be no compensatory increase in cardiac output.
- **Atrial fibrillation:** Cardioversion can be tried.
- Infective endocarditis prophylaxis for those who have undergone valvular replacement.
- Rheumatic fever prophylaxis.

Surgical treatment
Surgical procedures:
- Balloon dilatation (valvuloplasty)
- Aortic valve replacement
- Percutaneous valve replacement
- Transcatheter aortic valve replacement (TAVR) or transcatheter aortic valve implantation (TAVI) is a procedure for select patients with severe symptomatic aortic stenosis.

Bicuspid Aortic Valve Disease
- Bicuspid aortic valve (BAV) is the most common congenital heart disease found in 1–2% of live births.
- Male to female ratio is 3:1.
- Some cases are inherited as autosomal dominant and *NOTCH1* gene mutation is found in some cases.
- **Associated conditions:** Other congenital cardiac diseases (e.g., dilatation of proximal ascending aorta secondary to abnormalities of the aortic media), coarctation of aorta, ventricular septal defect (VSD), and atrial septal defect (ASD). Calcification is common in adults with bicuspid aortic valve.
- **Auscultatory findings:** Ejection click best heard at the apex and may be associated murmurs of aortic stenosis or aortic regurgitation.

Aortic Regurgitation
Aortic regurgitation (AR) is incompetency of the aortic valve, which causes backflow (reflux) of blood from the aorta through the aortic valve into the left ventricle during diastole.

Etiology
See **Box 9.9**.

Clinical Features
Symptoms
Age and gender: About three-fourths of patients with pure or predominant valvular AR are males. Females with primary valvular AR have associated rheumatic mitral valve disease. Chronic AR usually begins during late 50s. Usually, the prevalence and severity of AR increase with age.

Acute AR
- Sudden, severe shortness of breath
- Chest pain, if myocardial perfusion pressure is decreased or an aortic dissection is present
- Rapidly developing heart failure, pulmonary edema, and cardiogenic shock

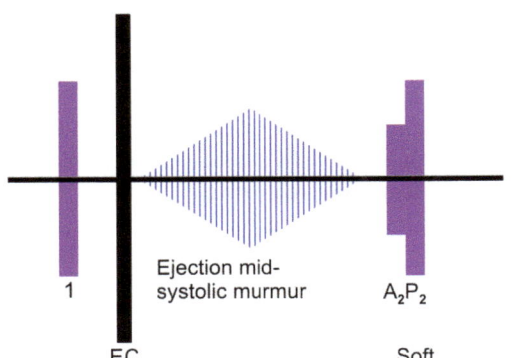

Fig. 9.11: Diagrammatic representation of timing of heart sounds and murmur in aortic stenosis. Features are diamond-shaped ejection mid-systolic murmur. An ejection click (EC) may be present in young patients with a bicuspid aortic valve. Soft second heart sound (A_2 and P_2).

> **Box 9.9: Causes of aortic regurgitation.**
> **Acute aortic regurgitation:**
> - Infective endocarditis
> - Aortic dissection
> - Acute rheumatic fever
> - Ruptured sinus of Valsalva aneurysm
> - Failure of prosthetic valve
> - Trauma
>
> **Chronic aortic regurgitation:**
> - **Congenital:** Bicuspid aortic valve or disproportionate cusps
> - **Acquired:**
>   - Rheumatic heart disease
>   - Infective endocarditis
>   - Trauma
>   - Aortic dilatation, e.g., aneurysm and dissection
>   - Arthritides, e.g., ankylosing spondylitis
>   - Rheumatoid arthritis
>   - Syphilitic aortitis
>   - Hypertension
>   - Connective tissue disorders, e.g., Marfan syndrome, and Ehlers–Danlos syndrome
>   - Osteogenesis imperfecta and methysergide

- Chronic AR
- Relatively asymptomatic for 10–15 years and significant symptoms occur late. Symptoms may not develop until left ventricular failure occurs.
- Palpitations, especially on lying down, may persist for many years. Sinus tachycardia, during exertion or with emotion, may produce palpitations as well as head pounding.
- **Exertional dyspnea:** Usually, it is the first symptom of diminished cardiac reserve. It depends on the extent of left ventricular dilatation and dysfunction. It is followed by orthopnea, paroxysmal nocturnal dyspnea, and excessive diaphoresis.
- **Angina pectoris:** Anginal chest pain develops even in the absence of coronary artery disease (CAD) at rest as well as during exertion. Nocturnal angina may be accompanied by marked diaphoresis. These episodes of angina can be prolonged and usually do not respond satisfactorily to sublingual nitroglycerine. Mechanisms of angina in AR:
- Associated CAD
- Low-aortic diastolic pressure leading to decreased myocardial perfusion (because coronary flow occurs mainly in diastole)
- Increased myocardial oxygen demand due to myocardial hypertrophy
- Congestive heart failure
- Sudden cardiac death
- Arrhythmias are not common

Signs
Peripheral signs of aortic regurgitation (Table 9.25):

Pulses
- **Peripheral pulses:** Prominent, large-volume (bounding) or collapsing.
- **Low diastolic and increased/wide pulse pressure:** Pulse pressure is the difference between the systolic and diastolic blood pressures. In aortic regurgitation, there is increased/wide pulse pressure. **Table 9.25** shows list of (rare) signs of wide pulse pressure that indicates a hyperdynamic circulation in aortic regurgitation.

Inspection and palpation
- Prominent neck pulsations and thrill in the carotids
- **Apex beat:** Displaced inferiorly and toward the axilla. The point of maximal impulse may be diffuse or hyperdynamic
- Presystolic impulse
- **Diastolic thrill:** It may be palpable along the left sternal border in patients with thin-chest (Erb's maneuver).
- **Prominent systolic thrill:** It may be palpable in the suprasternal notch and transmitted upward along the carotid arteries.

Auscultation
- **First heart sound (S_1):** May be soft
- **A_2 component of second heart sound (S_2):** Soft in rheumatic aortic regurgitation and loud and *"tambour"* such as in syphilitic AR. Narrowly split, single, or paradoxically split second heart sound.
- S_3 gallop and third heart sound (S_3), if left ventricular dysfunction is present.
- Fourth heart sound (S_4) prominent in left ventricular hypertrophy
- Murmurs
- **Early diastolic murmur:** Early holodiastolic murmur, immediately after A_2, usually as a high-pitched blowing sound that is loudest at the left sternal border, and decrescendo. It is best heard in at end of expiration, in sitting, and leaning forward position. The duration of the murmur correlates better with the severity of AR than does the loudness of the murmur.
- **Cole-Cecil murmur:** It is the term used for the diastolic murmur of AR when well or predominantly heard in the left axilla.
- If the murmur is musical (cooing dove murmur), it signifies eversion or perforation of an aortic cusp.
- **Harvey sign:** When regurgitation is caused by primary valvular disease, the diastolic murmur is heard best along the left sternal border in the 3rd and 4th intercostal space. When murmur is caused mainly by dilation of the ascending aorta, the murmur is more readily audible along the right sternal border.
- A functional systolic flow murmur may also be present because of increased stroke volume, although concurrent AS may also be present.
- **Austin–Flint murmur:** It may be audible at the cardiac apex in severe AR. It is a low-pitched, mid-diastolic rumbling murmur caused due to:
  - AR jet impinges on anterior mitral leaflet (AML), which forces it down and reduces the mitral orifice.
  - Turbulence produced when AR jet meets mitral inflow jet
  - AML fluttering due to AR jet
  - LV endocardial vibrations due to AR jet
  - The auscultatory features of AR are intensified by strenuous and sustained handgrip (increases systemic vascular resistance).

Table 9.25: Signs of wide pulse pressure in aortic regurgitation.

Sign	Feature
Light house sign/Morton and Mahon sign	Alternate flushing and blanching of forehead
Landolfi's sign	Change in pupillary size in synchronous with cardiac cycle
Becker's sign	Retinal artery pulsations
De Musset's sign	Head nodding with each heart beat/pulse
Muller's sign	Systolic pulsations of uvula
Quincke's sign	Capillary pulsations in the lip or nail bed. Detected by pressing a glass slide on patients lip or nail bed
Corrigan's sign	Dancing carotids
Locomotor brachii	Prominent pulsation of brachial artery
Watson's water hammer pulse/collapsing pulse	Bounding and forcible, rapidly increasing and subsequently collapsing pulse
Pulsus bisferiens	Double peaking in single systole
Pistol shot femorals or Traube's sign	Sharp bang heard on auscultation over the femoral arteries in time with each a heart beat
Duroziez's sign	To and fro murmur heard when the femoral artery is auscultated with pressure applied distally
Hill's sign	Popliteal cuff systolic pressure exceeds brachial cuff pressure by >20 mm Hg (Mild AR: 20–40 mm Hg, moderate AR: 40–60 mm Hg, and severe AR: > 60 mm Hg)
Drummond sign	Systolic expulsion of air from nose when mouth is closed
Mayan's sign	When arm is raised, diastolic BP drops by more than 15 mm Hg
Rosenbach's sign	Pulsations of liver
Gerhardt's sign	Pulsations of spleen
Ashrafian sign	Pulsatile pseudoproptosis
Bozzolo sign	Pulsatile nasal mucosa
Palmar click	Pulsating palm
Dennison/Shelley sign	Pulsatile cervix
Lincoln sign	Popliteal pulsation
Sherman sign	Dorsalis pedis prominent pulsation in age of 75 years or more

Treatment
- Underlying causes of AR, such as dissection, endocarditis, and syphilis, have to be treated.
- **Prophylaxis:** Rheumatic fever prophylaxis is needed, if due to rheumatic. Infective endocarditis prophylaxis is not required.
- **Acute severe AR:** Surgical intervention is usually needed, but the patient may be medically supported with *dobutamine* to augment cardiac output and shorten diastole and *sodium nitroprusside* to reduce afterload in hypertensive patients.
- **Chronic severe AR**

Medical treatment
- Vasodilator therapy may be used in selected conditions to reduce afterload in patients with systolic hypertension to reduce wall stress and optimize LV function. In normotensive patients, vasodilator therapy may not be useful because it does not reduce regurgitant volume (preload) significantly.
- The acute administration of sodium nitroprusside, hydralazine, nifedipine, or felodipine reduces PVR and results in an immediate augmentation in forward cardiac output and a reduction in regurgitant volume. Nitroprusside and hydralazine induced acute hemodynamic changes lead to a consistent decrease in end-diastolic volume (EDV) and an increase in ejection fraction (EF).

Surgical treatment
AR usually requires replacement of the diseased valve with a prosthetic valve, although valve-sparing repair is available like *transcatheter aortic valve replacement/implantation (TAVR/TAVI)*.

Tricuspid Stenosis
Tricuspid stenosis is a *narrowing of the tricuspid valve* opening. Uncommon valve lesion that is more common in females than males.

Etiology
See **Box 9.10**.

Clinical Features
Symptoms
- Usually, symptoms are due to associated left-sided rheumatic valve lesions (e.g., mitral stenosis).
- Tricuspid stenosis may produce symptoms of right heart failure—abdominal pain/hepatic discomfort (due to hepatomegaly), peripheral edema, and ascites.
- Little or no dyspnea and fatigue are common.

> **Box 9.10: Causes of tricuspid stenosis.**
> - **Rheumatic** (frequently associated with mitral and/or aortic valve disease)
> - **Carcinoid syndrome:** Tricuspid stenosis and regurgitation are found in carcinoid syndrome
> - **Congenital**
> - **Infective endocarditis**
> - **Anorectics:** Fenfluramine
> - **Fabry's disease**

Signs
- **Jugular venous pressure (JVP):** JVP is raised with prominent a waves (giant a waves) and slowly descent due to the loss of normal rapid right ventricular filling.
- **Mid-diastolic murmur:** It is loud first heart sound and a rumbling mid-diastolic murmur (higher-pitched than the murmur of mitral stenosis) with presystolic accentuation, best heard at the lower left sternal border, and increases/louder during inspiration (*De-Carvallo's sign*).
- **Tricuspid opening snap (OS):** It is occasionally heard.
- **Right heart failure:** Hepatomegaly with presystolic pulsation felt over the liver, ascites, and peripheral edema.

Investigations
- **Chest X-ray:** May show a prominent right atrial bulge
- **ECG:** Enlarged right atrium
- **Echocardiogram:** May reveal thickened and immobile tricuspid valve

Treatment
- **Medical management:** Diuretic therapy and salt and fluid restriction
- **Surgical treatment:** Tricuspid valve replacement

Tricuspid Regurgitation

In tricuspid regurgitation (TR), tricuspid valve does not close properly, causing blood to flow backward (leak) into the right atrium.

Etiology
Tricuspid regurgitation is common. Most commonly, it is functional secondary to right ventricular dilatation.

Causes of Tricuspid Regurgitation
- **Primary/organic:** Rheumatic heart disease, endocarditis (IV drug abuse), Ebstein's congenital anomaly, and carcinoid syndrome
- **Secondary:**
  - *Functional tricuspid regurgitation:* Right ventricular dilatation due to chronic left heart failure
  - Right ventricular infarction and inferior wall infarction
  - Pulmonary hypertension (e.g., cor pulmonale)
  - Cardiomyopathy

Clinical Features
- Symptoms are usually nonspecific. Tiredness due to reduced forward flow.
- Valvular regurgitation increases the right atrial and systemic venous pressure. Patients may develop of right heart failure, i.e., edema, ascites, and hepatomegaly with systolic pulsations due to venous congestion.
- **Jugular venous pressure (JVP):** Raised with most prominent "giant" v wave in the jugular venous pulse (a *cv* wave replaces the normal *x* descent).
- **Earlobe pulsations** *(Lancisi's sign)*
- **Blowing pansystolic murmur:** At the lower-left sternal border that is increased during inspiration and reduced during expiration (De-Carvallo's sign).
- P_2 may be loud (due to pulmonary hypertension) and RV S_3 is heard.
- **Severe TR:** Right jugular venous thrill and an RV impulse at the left lower sternal border. Long-standing severe TR may lead to RV dysfunction-induced heart failure and atrial fibrillation (AF).
- **Echocardiogram:** It shows dilated right ventricle and thickened valve.

Treatment
- **Functional tricuspid regurgitation** due to right ventricular dilatation usually disappears with treatment of the underlying cause of right ventricular overload. Treatment consists of with diuretic and vasodilator treatment of congestive cardiac failure.
- **Organic tricuspid regurgitation:** TR is usually well tolerated when there is normal pulmonary artery pressure. Severe organic tricuspid regurgitation may require operative repair of the tricuspid valve by annuloplasty or plication or valve repair, or occasionally tricuspid valve replacement. In drug addicts with infective endocarditis of the tricuspid valve, surgical removal of the valve is recommended to eradicate the infection.

INFECTIVE ENDOCARDITIS

Infective endocarditis (IE) is an *infection of the endocardium of heart valves or the mural endocardium.*

Definition
Infective endocarditis is defined as an endovascular infection of cardiovascular structures by microbes. These structures include heart valves, atrial and ventricular endocardium, large intrathoracic vessels, and intracardiac foreign bodies (e.g., prosthetic valves, pacemaker leads, and surgical conduits).
- The causative organism may be bacterium, fungus, Chlamydia, or Rickettsia. Majority of cases are due to infection by streptococci and staphylococci.
- **Consequences of infective endocarditis:** Valvular dysfunction, localized or generalized sepsis and source for embolism.

Classification
- **According to the clinical course:** Acute, subacute, and chronic
- **According to the causative organism:** Bacterial, viral, rickettsial, or fungal
- **According to the nature of valve or device:** Native or prosthetic

- **According to the side affected:** Left-sided or right-sided infective endocarditis
- **According to the side affected and nature of valve/device:** (1) Left-sided infective endocarditis, (2) left-sided prosthetic infective endocarditis, (3) right-sided infective endocarditis, and (4) device-related (permanent pacemaker and implantable cardioverter defibrillator) infective endocarditis.

Differences between acute endocarditis and subacute endocarditis are described in **Table 9.26**.

Predisposing Factors

Underlying heart disease:
- About 72% of patients have a pre-existing structural cardiac abnormality.
- Congenital isolated aortic valvular stenosis is most often associated with infective endocarditis (IE). Other congenital heart diseases include ventricular septal defect (VSD), tetralogy of Fallot (TOF), idiopathic subaortic stenosis, and atrial septal defect (uncommon).
- When IE involves valves, it commonly involves mitral valve followed by aortic valve and uncommonly tricuspid valve (1%).
- Major risks for IE are cardiac prosthetic valves and parenteral narcotic drug abuse.
- *Impaired host defense mechanism*: It may occur in diabetes mellitus, malignancies (e.g., leukemias and lymphomas), cytotoxic therapy, and neutropenia.
- **Conditions with bacteremia:** Most important predisposing factors to the development of endocarditis are conditions that lead to bacteremia. Transient bacteremia from any cause may lead to infective endocarditis and include the following surgical procedures from different sources.

- **Respiratory tract:** Tonsillectomy and/or adenoidectomy, surgical operations (incision or biopsy) involving respiratory mucosa and any invasive procedure of the respiratory tract used to treat an established infection (e.g., drainage of an abscess or empyema).
- **Oral cavity:** All dental procedures in which there is handling of gingival tissue or the periapical region of teeth or perforation of the oral mucosa (e.g., dental extractions, suture removal, placement of orthodontic band, and root canal treatment).
- **Gastrointestinal tract (GIT):** Procedures done in an established GIT infection.
- **Genitourinary tract:** Procedures performed in an established infection (e.g., cystoscopy during known enterococcal urinary tract infection—UTI).
- **Skin and musculoskeletal system:** Procedures involving infected tissue.

Common Organisms for Infective Endocarditis (Table 9.27)
More than 75% of infective endocarditis is caused by streptococci or staphylococci.

Postoperative Endocarditis or Prosthetic Valve Endocarditis

- It develops after cardiac surgery and may affect native or prosthetic valves and other prosthetic materials.
- Depending on the time of development of endocarditis following surgery, it can be divided into early, intermediate, and late endocarditis.
- Early (within 60 days of surgery) endocarditis is caused by intraoperative or hospital-acquired infections. The most common organism is a coagulase-negative *Staphylococcus* (*Staphylococcus epidermidis*), which is a normal commensal in the skin and followed by fungi (*Candida* and *Aspergillus*).

Table 9.26: Differences between acute and subacute endocarditis.

Characteristic	Acute infective endocarditis	Subacute infective endocarditis
Onset	Acute	Insidious
Condition of valve	Infection of normal heart valve as well as damaged valves	Infection of structurally abnormal/deformed valves or at sites where the endothelium is damaged by a high pressure jet of blood
Virulence of organisms	Highly virulent (suppurative) and invasive organisms	Low virulent
Source of infection or portal of entry	Often evident	Common sources of infection are periodontal infections (dental treatment), gastrointestinal tract infections, and urinary tract infections
Lesions	Vegetations are more florid. Affected valve is rapidly destroyed. Abscess (local and metastatic) formation is more common	Less destructive. Formation of vegetations, embolic episodes, mycotic aneurysms, valve regurgitation, splenic and renal infarcts, and immune glomerulonephritis
Clinical features	Of acute infection	Of complications
Course	Fulminant course, death within 6 weeks	Protracted course of weeks
Complications	Acute heart failure or overwhelming sepsis	Infectious complications are uncommon
Causative organisms	• *Staphylococcus aureus* • *Pseudomonas* • *Candida* • *Streptococcus pneumoniae* • *Neisseria gonorrhoeae*	*Streptococcus viridans* (*S. sanguis* and *S. mitis*), *Streptococcus milleri*, *Streptococcus bovis*, *Enterococcus faecalis*, and *Staphylococcus aureus* HACEK Group*

(*HACEK: H = *Haemophilus parainfluenzae*, *Haemophilus aphrophilus*, *Haemophilus paraphrophilus*, *Haemophilus influenzae*; A = *Actinobacillus actinomycetem comitans*; C = *Cardiobacterium hominis*; E = *Eikenella corrodens*; K = *Kingella kingae* and *Kingella denitrificans*)

Table 9.27: Organisms causing infective endocarditis.

Native valves	%	Narcotic addicts	%	Prosthetic valves	%
Streptococcus viridians	30–40	*Staphylococcus aureus*	50–60	*Staphylococcus epidermidis*	20–30
Staphylococcus aureus	10–30	Streptococci	8–15	*Staphylococcus aureus*	15–20
Staphylococcus epidermidis	1–3	*Staphylococcus epidermidis*	2–5	*Streptococcus viridans*	5–20
Enterococci	5–15	Enterococci	8–10	Enterococci	5–10
Other streptococci	15–20	Other streptococci	10–15	Other streptococci	1–5
Gram negative bacilli	2–10	Gram negative bacilli	4–8	Gram negative bacilli	10–20
Fungi	2–4	Fungi	4–5	Fungi	5–15
Culture negative	5–10	Culture negative	5–8	Culture negative	<5

- Late (after 1 year) endocarditis is caused by infection with community-acquired organisms. The causative organism is the same with those causing acute and subacute endocarditis of native valve.
- Endocarditis developing between 60 days and 1 year is due to a mixture of hospital-acquired episodes caused by less virulent organisms' community-acquired episodes. The organisms include *Streptococcus viridans* and enterococci.

Right-sided Endocarditis
It develops in intravenous drug users and is mainly caused by organisms found on the skin (e.g., *Staphylococcus aureus* and *Candida*). It usually presents with acute endocarditis and affects mainly tricuspid valve.

Culture-negative Endocarditis (Box 9.11)
- It is defined as endocarditis without etiology following inoculation of at least three independent blood samples in a standard blood culture system with negative cultures after 7 days of incubation and subculturing.
- They constitute 5–10% of cases of endocarditis.

Pathogenesis
Mechanism by which virulent organisms infect apparently normal valves is poorly understood.

The probable sequence of events, which occur with the infection of a damaged valve by less-virulent organisms, is as follows:
- **Endocardial damage/injury and denudation**
- **Formation of sterile thrombus**
- **Adherence of the microorganisms:** Transient bacteremia → microorganisms gain access to the circulation and adhere and get deposited to the sterile vegetations (infection of thrombi).

> **Box 9.11:** Causes of culture-negative endocarditis.
> - It is usually due to prior antibiotic therapy
> - Inadequate quantity of blood taken for culture
> - Anaerobic infection
> - Some may be due to a variety of fastidious organisms that do not grow in normal blood cultures. These include *Coxiella burnetii* (cause of Q fever), *Chlamydia* species, *Bartonella* species (cause trench fever and cat scratch disease), and *Legionella*
> - Right-sided endocarditis
> - Noninfective endocarditis

- **Proliferation of microorganisms within vegetations**
- **Formation of emboli:** The vegetation may get detached and forms infective emboli → causes spread of infection to visceral organs such as kidney, spleen, and brain. They may result in infarction or abscess. Septic emboli cause arteritis with weakness of arterial wall leading to mycotic aneurysms.
- **Deposition of immune complexes:** *Antigen and antibody may form immune complexes and can produce* focal glomerulonephritis and microscopic hematuria, diffuse glomerulonephritis, and vasculitis of cerebral vessels leading to cerebrovascular accidents and perisplenitis.

Clinical Features
- The clinical features of infective endocarditis depend on the causative organism and the presence of predisposing cardiac conditions.
- Endocarditis may be acute or a more insidious "subacute" form. However, there is overlap between the two because the clinical pattern depends not only on the causative organism, but also depends on the site of infection, prior antibiotic therapy, and the presence of a valve or shunt prosthesis.

Subacute Endocarditis
Clinical suspicion of subacute endocarditis (SBE) is necessary when a patient with congenital or valvular heart disease develops certain features. These include:

Evidence of infection
- Vague symptoms such as unusual tiredness, fatigue, lassitude, loss of appetite, and loss of weight.
- Persistent or intermittent low-grade or high-grade *fever* (84%) with night sweats, chills, and rigors.
- *Clubbing* (**Fig. 9.12A**) in fingers is a late sign and is found only in 10–20% of patients.
- **Splenomegaly:** Spleen is frequently palpable and the liver may also be enlarged.
- Brownish pigmentation of face and limbs

Evidence of new valve lesion (regurgitant)/murmurs or change of murmur
- **New murmur:** Particularly, a diastolic murmur is the diagnostic feature. It is detected in about 15% of patients during initial period. However, most patients develop a murmur during the course of the disease.

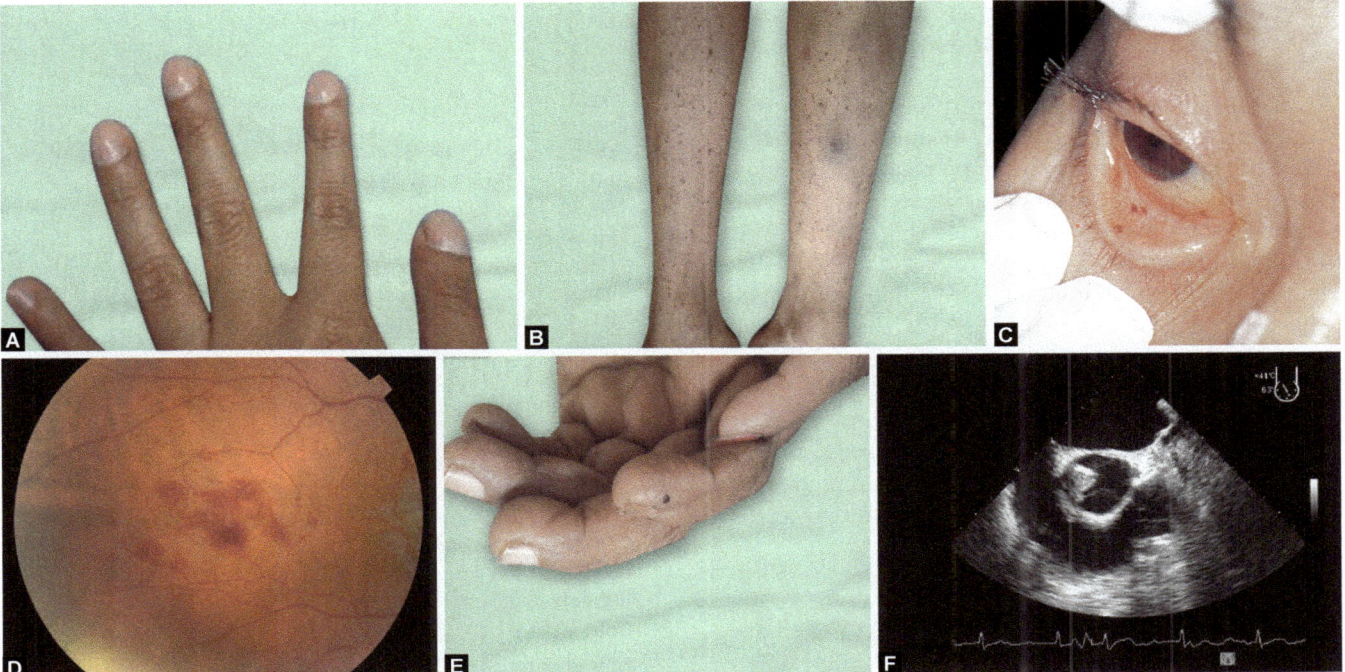

Figs. 9.12A to F: Signs of infective endocarditis: (A) Clubbing; (B) Petechiae; (C) Subconjunctival hemorrhage; (D) Roth spots; (E) Osler's nodes; and (F) Echocardiography showing vegetation.

- **Changing murmurs:** Apart from integrity of valves, factors such as change in cardiac output, temperature, and hematocrit may be responsible for change of murmurs. However, new regurgitant murmur developing in acute sepsis is almost diagnostic of endocarditis.

Evidence of embolism
- **Cutaneous manifestations:** These include the following:
  - *Purpura and petechiae* (20–40%) (**Fig. 9.12B**), subconjunctival splinter (**Fig. 9.12C**), or subungual splinter hemorrhages due to microthromboemboli.
  - *Janeway lesions:* Erythematous, non-tender nodules on palms or soles
  - *Ocular manifestations:* Roth spot (**Fig. 9.12D**) are flame-shaped hemorrhages, which may occasionally appear like cotton wool spots.
  - *Septic infarcts/abscess:* Spleen (painful splenomegaly), kidney (loin pain, hematuria, and renal failure), brain (convulsions, hemiplegia, aphasia, loss of vision, and cerebellar disturbances), peripheral arteries (claudication, absence of peripheral pulses, and gangrene), or lungs (pulmonary infarction, pleurisy, and pleural effusion due to right-sided endocarditis)
  - *Mycotic aneurysms*

Evidence of immunological phenomena
- **Osler nodes (Fig. 9.12E):** Tender, small, painful, swollen, and purplish/erythematous subcutaneous papules/nodules in pulp of distal fingers due to hypersensitive angiitis. Cultures are negative and persist for hours to several days.
- **Roth spots (Fig. 9.12D)** are circular retinal hemorrhages with white or pale centers spots composed of fibrin.
- **Focal segmental glomerulonephritis:** It develops due to deposition of antigen-antibody complexes in glomeruli. Grossly, the outer surface of kidney develops a flea-bitten appearance due to patchy hemorrhagic foci involving the glomeruli. Patients develop *microscopic hematuria*.

Investigations

Aim of investigations: (1) To confirm the diagnosis of infective endocarditis, (2) to identify the causative organism for appropriate therapy, and (3) to assess the patient's response to therapy.

Microbiological Investigations

- **Blood cultures** are the crucial investigations in infective endocarditis—(1) to identify the causative microorganism and (2) guide antibiotic therapy. At least three sets of blood samples for cultures should be taken from different venipuncture sites over 24 hours before commencing therapy. Aseptic technique should be followed and the risk of contaminants should be minimized. Blood samples for cultures should not be obtained from an in-dwelling line. Both aerobic and anaerobic cultures are needed.
- **Serological tests** are useful, if there is suspicion of diagnosis and the cultures are negative. Culture-negative cases may be due to organisms, which will not grow in blood cultures such as *Coxiella, Bartonella, Legionella,* and *Chlamydia*.
- **Electrocardiogram:** ECG will help to detect complications such as conduction abnormalities (AV block) and occasionally myocardial infarction due to emboli. PR prolongation/heart block is associated with aortic root abscess.
- **Chest X-ray:** It may show evidence of cardiac failure, cardiomegaly, pulmonary edema in left-sided disease, and pulmonary emboli/abscess in right-sided disease.
- **Echocardiography:** It plays a key role to identify the presence and size of vegetations (**Fig. 9.12F**), assess valve damage, abscess formation, detect intracardiac

complications, and assess cardiac function. However, if vegetations are not detected, the diagnosis of endocarditis cannot be excluded.

- **Transthoracic echocardiography (TTE):** It is a first-line noninvasive imaging test with sensitivity of 60–75% and high specificity for demonstrating vegetations, valvular dysfunction, ventricular function, and abscesses. Vegetations as small as 2–4 mm can be detected (**Fig. 9.12F**).
- **Transesophageal echocardiography (TOE):** It is a second-line invasive imaging test with greater sensitivity (>90%) and specificity than TTE. It can detect vegetations even smaller ones (1–1.5 mm), aortic root abscess, and prosthetic valve endocarditis.
- **Complete blood counts:** These may show normocytic normochromic anemia (reduced hemoglobin) and increased WBC counts and increased or reduced platelets.
- **Urea and creatinine:** These may be increased due to glomerulonephritis.
- **Liver biochemistry:** Serum alkaline phosphatase may be increased.
- **Inflammatory markers:** Increased erythrocyte sedimentation rate (ESR) and C-reactive protein are observed. CRP also helps in monitoring response to therapy; it is reduced in response to therapy and increased with relapse.
- **Urine:** Proteinuria and hematuria occur frequently.

Modified Duke Criteria for the Diagnosis of Infective Endocarditis (Box 9.12)
- Diagnosis by these guidelines requires either pathologic or clinical criteria.
- **If clinical criteria are used:**
  - Definite endocarditis, two major or one major + three minor or five minor criteria are required for diagnosis.
  - Possible endocarditis = One major and one minor or three minor criteria.

Complications

Cardiac Complications

These are *due to direct valvular damage* and *consequences of local invasion*. The infection may spread locally from valve into the valve ring, adjacent mural endocardium, or chordae tendineae.
- **Ring abscess:** Vegetations may erode the *underlying myocardium* and produce an *abscess,* which is known as ring abscess.
- **Perforation and rupture:** May involve valve leaflets, aorta, or interventricular septa (depending on the site of infection)
- *Myocardial abscess* usually due to *S. aureus*
- *Suppurative pericarditis*
- **Valvular dysfunction and heart failure:** Stenosis or insufficiency. Heart failure is most common and is due to valvular regurgitation
- Prosthetic dehiscence
- Valvular distortion/destruction chordal rupture
- Conduction abnormalities
- Purulent pericarditis

Box 9.12: Modified Duke criteria for the diagnosis of infective endocarditis (IE).

Clinical criteria:
Major:
Positive blood cultures for IE (one of the following): Typical microorganisms consistent with IE from two separate blood cultures:
- *Staphylococcus aureus*
- *Viridans streptococci*
- *Streptococcus gallolyticus (formerly S. bovis),* including nutritional variant strains (*Granulicatella* species and *Abiotrophia defectiva*)
- HACEK group: *Haemophilus* species, *Aggregatibacter* (formerly *Actinobacillus actinomycetemcomitans*), *Cardiobacterium hominis, Eikenella* species, and *Kingella kingae*
- Community-acquired enterococci, in the absence of a primary focus

Persistently positive blood culture:
- *For organisms that are typical causes of IE*: At least two positive blood cultures from blood samples drawn >12 hours apart
- *For organisms that are more commonly skin contaminants*: Three or a majority of >4 separate blood cultures (with first and last drawn at least one hour apart)

Single positive blood culture for *Coxiella burnetii* or phase I IgG antibody titer >1:800

Evidence of endocardial involvement (one of the following): Echocardiogram positive for IE:
- Vegetation (oscillating intracardiac mass on a valve or on supporting structures, in the path of regurgitant jets, or on implanted material, in the absence of an alternative anatomic explanation)
- Abscess
- New partial dehiscence of prosthetic valve

New valvular regurgitation:
Increase in or change in preexisting murmur not sufficient
Minor:
- Fever >38°C (100.4°F)
- *Predisposition*: Predisposing heart lesion or intravenous drug use
- *Vascular phenomena*: Arterial petechiae, subungual/splinter hemorrhages, emboli, septic pulmonary infarcts, mycotic aneurysm, intracranial hemorrhage, conjunctival hemorrhages, and Janeway lesions
- *Immunological phenomena*: Focal segmental glomerulonephritis, Osler nodes, and Roth spots
- Microbiologic evidence, including a single culture positive but not meeting a major criterion, or for an unusual organism that can cause infective endocarditis

Pathologic criteria: Demonstration of microorganisms by culture or histologic examination in:
- Vegetation
- Embolus from a vegetation
- Intracardiac abscess

Histological confirmation of active endocarditis in vegetation or intracardiac abscess

---

Renal Complications

At least in four forms—(1) prerenal due to low cardiac output, (2) microabscess formation secondary to septic emboli, (3) glomerular dysfunction as a result of circulating immune complexes, and (4) renal failure as a result of antibiotics.

Embolic events (discussed under evidence of embolism—subacute endocarditis):

- **Embolic complications (due to septic emboli):** Emboli contain large numbers of virulent organisms → abscesses develop at the sites of arrest of the emboli. Septic emboli from left side of the heart—they enter systemic circulation and their consequences are:
  - Septic infarcts (e.g., spleen, kidney, or brain)
  - Mycotic aneurysms
  - Small emboli (microthromboemboli) may produce—(1) splinter or subungual hemorrhages and (2) Janeway lesions
  - *Septic emboli from right side of the heart*: They enter pulmonary circulation → lead to pulmonary abscess.
- **Immunological phenomena:**
  - *Focal segmental glomerulonephritis:* It develops due to deposition of antigen-antibody complexes in glomeruli. Grossly, the outer surface of kidney develops a flea-bitten appearance due to patchy hemorrhagic foci involving the glomeruli.
  - *Osler nodes:* They are small, tender subcutaneous nodules in the pulp of the digits and persist for hours to several days.
  - Roth spots are retinal hemorrhages with white or pale centers composed of fibrin.

Management

Medical Treatment

- Blood should be collected for cultures before starting the empirical antibiotic therapy. However, this should not delay therapy in unstable patients.
- If source of infection is identified, it should be removed as soon as possible (e.g., tooth with an apical abscess should be extracted).
- **Empirical treatment regimen:** Penicillins are fundamental to the therapy of bacterial endocarditis. Empirical treatment regimen depends on the mode of presentation, the suspected organism, and whether the patient has a prosthetic valve or penicillin allergy (**Table 9.28**).

Prognosis: It is fatal in about 20% patients and higher in those with prosthetic valve endocarditis and those infected with antibiotic-resistant organisms.

Surgical Treatment (Box 9.13)

Decisions to carry out surgical intervention in patients with infective endocarditis should take into account the (1) patient-specific features such as age, noncardiac morbidities, and presence of prosthetic material or cardiac failure and (2)

Table 9.28: Antimicrobial treatment of common causative organisms in infective endocarditis.

Organism	Antimicrobial treatment with dose and duration
Infective endocarditis awaiting culture report, no suspicion of staphylococci	Benzylpenicillin IV 1.2 g 4 hourly, 4–6 weeks *Plus* Gentamicin IV 80 mg 12 hourly, 2–6 weeks *Or* Amoxicillin/clavulanate 12 g/day in four divided doses plus gentamicin 1 mg/kg thrice a day for 4–6 weeks
Suspected staphylococcal endocarditis (IVDU, recent intravascular devices or cardiac surgery, and acute infection)	Vancomycin IV 1 g 12 hourly (30 mg/kg/day—(not to exceed 2 g/day) for 6 weeks *Plus* Gentamicin IV 80–120 mg 8 hourly for 1–2 weeks. In prosthetic valve endocarditis, add rifampicin 20 mg/kg/day in two divided doses
Streptococci highly sensitive to penicillin	Benzylpenicillin IV 1.2 g 4 hourly for 4 weeks *Or* Ceftriaxone IV 2 g once a day for 4 weeks *Or* Benzylpenicillin or ceftriaxone for 2 weeks plus gentamicin 3 mg/kg once a day for 2 weeks Vancomycin 30 mg/kg/day in two divided doses (not to exceed 2 g/day) for 4 weeks in penicillin-sensitive patients
Streptococci less sensitive to penicillin	Benzylpenicillin IV 1.2 g 4 hourly or ceftriaxone IV 2 g for 4–6 weeks and gentamicin 3 mg/kg/day (as single infusion) for at least 2 weeks
Anaerobic streptococci	Benzylpenicillin IV 1.2 g 4 hourly and metronidazole
Staphylococcal endocarditis (methicillin-sensitive)	Cloxacillin 2 g 4 hourly *or* cefazolin 2 g 8 hourly, vancomycin 1 g 12 hourly, *or* flucloxacillin 2 g 4 hourly *or* benzylpenicillin 1.2 g 4 hourly for 4–6 weeks *Plus* Gentamicin 80–120 mg (1 mg/kg) three times a day for 3–5 days
Enterococcal endocarditis	Ampicillin/amoxicillin 2 g 4 hourly for 4–6 weeks *or* vancomycin 1 g twice daily *plus* gentamicin 1 mg/kg three times a day for 6 weeks
Candida	Amphotericin B 1 mg/kg QID 2 weeks maximum up to 4 weeks. Do not exceed 50 mg/day Flucytosine 150 mg/kg oral for 4 days
Coxiella burnetii	Doxycycline 100 mg twice daily with either hydroxychloroquine 600 mg daily *or* rifampin (900 mg/day) for 18–24 months
Bartonella	Doxycycline (100 mg PO or IV twice daily) *plus* gentamicin (1 mg/kg IV every eight hours) for 14 days

> **Box 9.13:** Indications for surgical treatment in infective endocarditis.
>
> - Endocarditis of prosthetic valve
> - Large vegetations:
>   □ Left-sided large vegetation (10 mm) with an episode of embolization
>   □ Very large (15 mm) and mobile vegetation (high-risk of embolism)
> - Progressive cardiac failure due to valvular damage
> - Active infection persisting, i.e., fever and evidence of bacteremia for more than 7–10 days in spite of adequate antibiotic treatment
> - Abscess formation, perivalvular involvement, *Staphylococcus Aureus*, and fungal endocarditis

> **Box 9.14:** Infective endocarditis prophylaxis.
>
> *High-risk group:*
> - Prosthetic heart valves
> - Prior bacterial endocarditis
> - Complex cyanotic congenital heart disease
> - Surgically constructed systemic pulmonary shunts
> - Repaired shunts within 6 months
> - Valvulopathy after cardiac transplantation
>
> *Moderate-risk group:*
> - Congenital cardiac malformations (other than those listed in other 2 groups)
> - Acquired valvular dysfunction (e.g., rheumatic heart disease)
> - Hypertrophic cardiomyopathy
> - Mitral valve prolapse with valvular regurgitation, thickened leaflets, or both
>
> *Negligible-risk group:*
> - Isolated secundum atrial septum defect
> - Surgical repair of atrial septal defect, ventricular septal defect, or patent ductus arteriosus
> - Previous coronary artery bypass graft surgery
> - Mitral valve prolapse without valvular regurgitation
> - Physiologic, functional, or innocent heart murmurs
> - Previous Kawasaki syndrome without valvular dysfunction
> - Previous rheumatic fever without valvular dysfunction
> - Cardiac pacemakers (intravascular and epicardial) and implanted defibrillators

infective endocarditis features, such as causative organism, size of vegetation, presence of perivalvular infection, and systemic embolization.

Cardiac surgery consists of debridement of infected material and valve replacement. Antimicrobial therapy should be started before surgery.

Bacterial Endocarditis Prophylaxis

Prophylaxis is not needed for routine local anesthetic injections through noninfected tissue, placement of removable prosthodontic or orthodontic appliances, shedding of deciduous teeth, vaginal delivery, and hysterectomy or tattooing, bronchoscopy, laryngoscopy, endotracheal intubation, cystoscopy, colonoscopy, or skin suturing.

Indications

Cardiac lesions: For which antibiotic prophylaxis is advised are listed in **Box 9.14**.

□ **Procedures:** Endocarditis prophylaxis is advised in patient at high or moderate risk for endocarditis. These include following procedures:
- *Dental procedures*: Extraction, periodontal procedures, implant placement, root canal instrumentation, and intraligamentary injections (anesthetic)
- *Respiratory procedure*: Bronchoscopy with rigid bronchoscope operations involving the mucosa
- *Gastrointestinal procedures*: Sclerotherapy of esophageal varices, stricture dilation, ERCP, biliary tract surgery, and surgery involving mucosa
- *Genitourinary procedures*: Urethral dilation, prostate or urethral surgery, or cystoscopy.

□ **Antibiotic regimen** for prophylaxis of endocarditis in adults at moderate or high risk.

Oral Cavity, Respiratory Tract, or Esophageal Procedures

□ **Standard regimen:** *Amoxicillin 2.0 g PO 1 hour before procedure.*
□ **Inability to take oral medication:** Ampicillin 2.0 g IV or IM within 30 minutes of procedure.
□ Penicillin allergy
□ Clarithromycin 500 mg PO 1 hour before procedure
□ Cephalexin or cefadroxil 2.0 g PO 1 hour before procedure
□ Clindamycin 600 mg PO 1 hour before procedure or IV 30 minutes before procedure

□ **Inability to take oral medication:** Cefazolin 1.0 g IV or IM 30 minutes before procedure.

> **Note:** For patients at high-risk, administer of half-dose 6 hours after the initial dose.

Genitourinary and Gastrointestinal Tract Procedure

□ **High-risk patients:** Ampicillin 2.0 g IV or IM plus gentamicin 1.5 mg/kg IV or IM within 30 minutes of procedure. Repeat ampicillin, 1.0 g IV or IM or amoxicillin 1.0 g PO 6 hours later.
□ **High-risk penicillin-allergic patients:** Vancomycin 1.0 g IV or IM over 1–2 h plus gentamicin 1.5 m/kg IV or IM within 30 minutes before procedure, no second dose recommended.
□ **Moderate-risk patients:** Amoxicillin 2.0 g PO 1 hour before procedure or ampicillin 2.0 g IV or IM 30 minutes before procedure.
□ **Moderate-risk, penicillin-allergic patients:** Vancomycin 1.0 g IV inferred over 1–2 hours and completed within 30 minutes of procedures.

Noninfective Endocarditis

It is characterized by the formation of sterile platelet and fibrin thrombi on cardiac valves and adjacent endocardium.

□ It develops in response to trauma, circulating immune complexes, vasculitis, or a hypercoagulable state.
□ Symptoms are caused due to systemic arterial embolism.
□ Diagnosis is by echocardiography and negative blood cultures.

Marantic Endocarditis (Nonbacterial Thrombotic Endocarditis—NBTE)

- NBTE is often encountered in a number of conditions. These include debilitated patients with cancer or sepsis, hence previously termed as *marantic endocarditis* (root word *marasmus*, relating to malnutrition). It frequently develops concomitantly with deep venous thrombosis, pulmonary emboli, or underlying systemic hypercoagulable state and advanced malignancy. There is a striking association with mucinous adenocarcinomas, potentially relating to the procoagulant effects of tumor-derived mucin or tissue.
- Other less common causes include systemic lupus erythematosus, antiphospholipid syndrome, rheumatic heart disease, rheumatoid arthritis, and burns.

Libman–Sacks Endocarditis

- Libman–Sacks endocarditis (otherwise known as verrucous endocarditis) is characteristic cardiac manifestation of the autoimmune disease, such as systemic lupus erythematosus.
- **Pathogenesis:** It is produced due to circulating immune complexes.
- **Endocarditis:** It is characterized by small or medium-sized vegetations on either side of the valve leaflets. They appear mulberry-like clusters of verrucae and consist of accumulations of immune complexes and mononuclear cells.

HEART FAILURE

Definition

Heart failure or cardiac failure is the pathophysiological process in which the heart as a pump is unable to meet the metabolic requirements of the tissue for oxygen and substrates despite the venous return to heart is either normal or increased.

It is a complex syndrome that can result from any structural or functional cardiac disorder. In heart failure, *heart is unable to pump blood at a rate of sufficient to meet the metabolic demands of the tissues* or can do so only at an elevated filling pressure.

Types of Heart Failure

Depending on Output

- **Low-output heart failure:**
  - *Systolic heart failure:* It is characterized by decreased cardiac output and decreased left ventricular ejection fraction.
  - *Diastolic heart failure:* It is characterized by elevated left and right ventricular end-diastolic pressures and may have normal left ventricular ejection fraction.
- **High-output heart failure:** It is characterized by failure of the heart to maintain sufficient circulation despite an increased cardiac output (defined as cardiac output >8 L/min or a cardiac index >3.9 L/min/m^2). Examples include cardiac failure associated with hyperthyroidism, anemia, pregnancy, arteriovenous fistulae, beriberi, and Paget's disease.

Diastolic and Systolic Dysfunction

- **Systolic dysfunction:** Systolic heart failure is characterized by an abnormality of *ventricular contraction*. The ejection fraction is usually below 40%. Causes include coronary artery disease, hypertension, and valvular heart disease.
- **Diastolic dysfunction:** It is characterized by an impaired *ventricular relaxation* and increased ventricular stiffness resulting in reduced filling (diastolic dysfunction). Causes include hypertension, coronary artery disease, hypertrophic obstructive cardiomyopathy (HOCM), and restrictive cardiomyopathy.

Acute and Chronic Heart Failure

- **Acute heart failure** is characterized by sudden development of heart failure. This suddenly reduces cardiac output and systemic hypotension without peripheral edema. Examples include acute myocardial infarction and rupture of a cardiac valve. Acute left heart failure may develop either de novo or as an acute decompensated episode, on a background of chronic heart failure (acute-on chronic heart failure).
- **Chronic heart failure** is characterized by gradual development of heart failure and systemic arterial pressure is well maintained, but edema develops. Examples include dilated cardiomyopathy and multivalvular disease.
- **Compensated heart failure** is the term used to describe the condition of those with impaired cardiac function, in whom adaptive/compensatory changes have prevented the development of overt heart failure. Severe overt or acute heart failure may precipitated by minor insult such as an infection or development of atrial fibrillation.

Left-sided, Right-sided and Biventricular Heart Failure

The left side of the heart consists of the functional unit of the left atrium, left ventricle, mitral and aortic valves. The right side of the heart consists of the right atrium, right ventricle, and tricuspid and pulmonary valves.

- **Left-sided (left ventricular) heart failure is characterized by:**
  - Reduction in left ventricular output
  - *Increase in left atrial and pulmonary venous pressure*: An acute increase in left atrial pressure produces pulmonary congestion or pulmonary edema (e.g., myocardial infarction). A more gradual increase in left atrial pressure leads to reflex pulmonary vasoconstriction, which prevents the development pulmonary edema (e.g., in mitral stenosis and aortic stenosis). This increases pulmonary vascular resistance and leads to pulmonary hypertension, which in turn can impair the function of right ventricle.
- **Right-sided (right ventricular) heart failure is characterized by:**
  - Reduction in right ventricular output
  - Increase in right atrial and systemic venous pressure
  - Causes of isolated right heart failure, e.g., chronic lung disease (cor pulmonale), multiple pulmonary embolism and pulmonary valvular stenosis.
- **Biventricular heart failure** is characterized by failure of the ventricles of the left and the right heart.

Table 9.29: Causes of heart failure (HF).

Reduced ejection fraction (<40% HFrEF)	
• *Coronary artery disease:* Myocardial infarction and myocardial ischemia	• *Chronic pressure overload:* Hypertension, obstructive valvular disease (e.g., mitral/tricuspid stenosis), and endomyocardial fibrosis
• *Chronic volume overload of ventricle:* Regurgitant valvular disease (e.g., mitral/aortic regurgitation), left-to-right shunt (e.g., ventricular septal defect, patent ductus arteriosus, atrial septal defect)	• *Chronic lung disease:* Cor pulmonale and pulmonary vascular disorders
• *Nonischemic dilated cardiomyopathy*	• Chagas' disease
• *Toxic/drug-induced damage*	
Preserved ejection fraction (>40–50%):	
Pathologic hypertrophy, aging, and restrictive cardiomyopathy	
High-output states	
• Metabolic disorders: Thyrotoxicosis	• Chronic anemia
• Nutritional disorders (beriberi)	

(HFrEF: heart failure with reduced ejection fraction)

- Dilated cardiomyopathy or ischemic heart disease affects both ventricles
- Disease of the left heart leads to chronic elevation of the left atrial pressure, pulmonary hypertension, and leads to right heart failure.

Forward and Backward Heart Failure

- Forward heart failure is characterized by decreased cardiac output and inadequate perfusion of organs that cause poor tissue perfusion. Reduced renal perfusion activates renin-angiotensin-aldosterone system resulting in excessive absorption of sodium by renal tubules.
- Backward heart failure is characterized by a normal cardiac output, severe salt and water retention, and venous congestion in the pulmonary and systemic circulation. Causes of heart failure are listed in **Table 9.29**.

In practice, the most common causes of heart failure are ischemic heart disease, hypertensive heart diseases.

Risk factors for heart failure: Hypertension, diabetes mellitus, use of cardiotoxic substances (e.g., alcohol, tobacco, and cocaine), hyperlipidemia, and coronary artery disease.

Clinical Manifestations of Heart Failure

Clinical manifestations of heart failure are described in **Table 9.30**.

Investigations in Heart Failure

- **Chest X-ray:** It may reveal cardiomegaly. Other findings include phantom tumor (fluid in horizontal or oblique fissures of lungs, which disappears after treatment with diuretics), bat's wing appearance (hazy opacification spreading from the hilar regions on both sides and pleural effusion (bilateral or unilateral).
- **Electrocardiography:** It may reveal previous MI, active ischemia, ventricular hypertrophy (e.g., due to hypertension), atria abnormality, arrhythmias, and conduction abnormalities (e.g., arrhythmia).
- **Echocardiography** is very useful to—(1) determine the etiology, (2) detect any unsuspected valvular heart disease

Table 9.30: Symptoms and signs of heart failure.

Symptoms	Signs	
Left ventricular failure		
Dyspnea • Exertional dyspnea • Orthopnea • Paroxysmal nocturnal dyspnea • Acute pulmonary edema Cough Fatigue Decreased urine output	*Cardiac sign* • Pulsus alternans • Enlargement of LV • Gallop rhythm S_3 • Systolic murmur in apex *Pulmonary sign:* • Crepitations • Pleural effusion	*Think FACES* Fatigue, Activities limited, Chest congestion, Edema or ankle swelling, and Shortness of breath
Right ventricular failure		
Leg swelling Anorexia and oliguria Pain in right hypochondrium Dyspnea	Raised JVP Hepatojugular reflux positive Hepatomegaly Edema Pleural fluid and ascites	

(JVP: jugular venous pressure)

(e.g., occult mitral stenosis), (3) identify patients who will benefit from long-term drug therapy (e.g., ACE inhibitors), (4) assess cardiac chamber dimension (size and shape), ejection fraction, valvular functions, cardiomyopathies, and regional wall motion abnormalities, and (5) differentiate between systolic and diastolic heart failure.

- **Stress echocardiography:** It helps in assessing the viability in dysfunctional myocardium. Dobutamine stress identifies contractile reserve in stunned or hibernating myocardium.
- **Nuclear cardiology:** Radionucleotide angiography (RNA) is useful for quantify ventricular ejection fraction, single photon emission computed tomography (SPECT) or positron emission tomography (PET) can reveal myocardial ischemia and viability in dysfunctional myocardium.
- **CMR (cardiac MRI):** It helps to assess the viability in dysfunctional myocardium with the use of dobutamine

- **Cardiac catheterization:** It is useful in the diagnosis of ischemic heart failure (and suitability for revascularization), measurement of pulmonary artery pressure, left atrial (wedge) pressure, and left ventricular end diastolic pressure.
- **Cardiac biopsy:** It is useful in the diagnosis of cardiomyopathies (e.g., amyloid) and follow-up of cardiac transplanted patients to assess rejection.
- **Cardiopulmonary exercise testing:** Peak oxygen consumption (VO) is useful in predicting hospital admission and death in heart failure.
- **Ambulatory 24-hour ECG monitoring (Holter):** May be necessary in patients with suspected arrhythmia. It may be useful in severe heart failure or inherited cardiomyopathy to decide the necessity of defibrillator.
- **Brain natriuretic peptide (BNP) or N-terminal portion of proBNF (NPproBNP)** is elevated in heart failure and highly sensitive for the diagnosis of its diagnosis. It is a marker of risk *(>100 pg/mL) and* is useful in the investigation of patients with breathlessness or peripheral edema (to differentiate cardiac from respiratory cause of acute dyspnea).
- **Blood tests:** Full blood count, liver function tests, serum urea, creatinine and electrolytes, cardiac enzymes in acute heart failure, and thyroid function may help to establish the nature and severity of the underlying heart disease and detect any complications.
- **Invasive hemodynamic monitoring:** It is useful in selected patients with acute heart failure who have persistent symptoms in spite of empiric standard therapies.

Complications in Advanced Heart Failure

- **Renal failure:** *Cardiorenal syndrome* (poor renal perfusion caused by low cardiac output) may be worsened by therapy [e.g., diuretics, angiotensin-converting enzyme (ACE) inhibitors, and angiotensin receptor blockers].
- **Hypokalemia:** Due to the result of treatment with potassium-losing diuretics or hyperaldosteronism produced by activation of the renin–angiotensin system and impaired aldosterone metabolism due to congestion of liver.
- **Hyperkalemia:** Due to the effects of drugs, which promote renal resorption of potassium (e.g., combination of ACE inhibitors or angiotensin receptor blockers, and mineralocorticoid receptor antagonists).
- **Hyponatremia:** It may develop in severe heart failure and is a poor prognostic sign. It may be due to diuretics, inappropriate retention of water (due to high ADH secretion), or failure of the cell membrane ion pump.
- **Hepatic dysfunction:** Due to hepatic venous congestion and poor arterial perfusion.
- **Thromboembolism:** Deep vein thrombosis and pulmonary embolism may develop due to the effects of a low cardiac output and immobility. Systemic emboli may develop in patients with atrial fibrillation or flutter, or with intracardiac thrombus complicating conditions such as mitral stenosis, MI, or left ventricular aneurysm.
- **Atrial and ventricular arrhythmias:** These are very common and include atrial fibrillation (20%), sudden death (50%) due to a ventricular arrhythmia, ventricular ectopic beats, and nonsustained ventricular tachycardia. They may be due to electrolyte changes (e.g., hypokalemia and hypomagnesemia), the underlying heart disease, and the pro-arrhythmic effects of sympathetic activation.

Management of Heart Failure

Aim of treatment: (1) Relief of symptoms, (2) prevent and control of disease causing cardiac dysfunction and heart failure, (3) retard disease progression, and (4) improve quality and length of life.

General Lifestyle Advice/Measures

- **Education of patients and their relatives:** Explanation of nature of disease, about the causes and treatment of heart failure.
- **Measures to prevent heart failure:** Cessation of smoking and illicit drugs, control of hypertension, diabetes and hypercholesterolemia, and pharmacological treatment following myocardial infarction. Identify and treat any factor that aggravates the heart failure.
- **Treatment of the underlying cause of heart failure (e.g., coronary artery disease):** Wherever possible to prevent progression to heart failure.
- **Dietary modifications:** Good general nutrition and maintain desired weight and body mass index. Avoid large meals, foods rich in salt or added salt. Diet low in fat, rich in fruit and vegetables, and increase fiber. Fluid restriction (limited to 1.5 liters) is needed only when heart failure is severe. Alcohol has a negative inotropic effect and should be avoided. Omega-3 polyunsaturated fatty acids reduce mortality and admission.

Physical activity, exercise, and emotional rest:

- **Physical activity and exercise:** Regular low level endurance exercise (e.g., 20–30 minutes walking 3 or 5 times/week at 70–80% of peak heart rate) reverses "deconditioning" of peripheral muscle metabolism and is advisable in patients with compensated heart failure. Avoid strenuous isometric activity.
- **Bed rest:** It reduces the demands on the heart. Bed rest for a few days is for patients with exacerbations of congestive cardiac failure. However, prolonged bed rest may predispose to deep vein thrombosis. This can be avoided by daily leg exercises, low-dose subcutaneous heparin, and elastic support stockings.

Drug Therapy/Management

- **Diuretic therapy:**
  - Loop diuretics (e.g., furosemide 20–40 mg once or twice) and thiazide diuretics (e.g., hydrochlorothiazide 25 mg once or twice, or metolazone 2.5–5 mg OD) are given to patients with fluid overload.
  - In severe heart failure, the combination of a loop and thiazide diuretic may be needed. Regular monitoring

of serum electrolytes and renal function is necessary because of risk of hypokalemia and hypomagnesemia.
- Mineralocorticoid receptor antagonists, such as spironolactone (12.5–25 once or twice), are potassium-sparing diuretics and are beneficial in patients having heart failure with severe left ventricular systolic dysfunction.

☐ **Angiotensin-converting enzyme inhibitors (ACEI) therapy:**
- *Drugs and dosage:* Captopril (6.25 mg thrice till 50 mg thrice a day), enalapril (2.5 mg twice to 10–20 mg twice a day), lisinopril (2.5–5 mg once to 20–40 mg once a day), and ramipril (1.25–2.5 mg once till 10 mg once a day).

☐ **Angiotensin II receptor antagonists (ARA)/blockers therapy:**
- *Drugs and dosage:* Losartan (25–50 mg once till 50–150 mg once a day), valsartan, telmisartan, and olmesartan (20–40 mg twice till 160 mg twice).

☐ **Beta-adrenoceptor blocker therapy:**
- *Indications:* To all patients with current or prior HF and a LVEF ≤40% (HFrEF) in the absence of a contraindication.
- Drugs and dosage bisoprolol (1.25–2.5 mg once till 10 mg once), carvedilol (3.125 twice till 50 mg twice), and metoprolol succinate (12.5 once till 200 mg once).

☐ **Aldosterone receptor antagonists:**
- *Indications*: New York Heart Association (NYHA) II–IV, EF <35%, no contraindication (GFR >30, creatinine: 2.5 mg/dL male and 2.0 mg/dL female, and K < 5 mg/dL). They improve survival in patients with heart failure.
- *Dose*: Spironolactone 12.5–25 mg once till 50 mg daily.
- *Monitoring:* Stop all K+ supplements, check K+ and creatinine 2–3 days after starting then 1 week and every month for 3 months and every 3 month and when clinically indicated.
- *Side effects*: Increase K+ (10–15%), gynecomastia, or breast pain.

☐ **Digoxin (cardiac glycoside):** Digoxin is a cardiac glycoside that is used in patients in atrial fibrillation with heart failure. It can be used as add on therapy in symptomatic heart failure patients already receiving ACEI and beta-blockers. No mortality benefit, only decrease frequency of hospitalizations.

☐ **Vasodilators and nitrates (hydralazine nitrate combination):**
- The combination of hydralazine and nitrates reduces afterload and preload. Their use is limited by pharmacological tolerance and hypotension.
- *Indication*: African–American origin, NYHA III–IV, low EF on ACEI and BB, and patients intolerant or contraindication of ACEI or ARA (e.g., in severe renal failure).
- *Dose*: 37.5 mg hydralazine and 20 mg and isosorbide dinitrate start one tablet TID to increase till 2 tablets TID.

☐ **Ivabradine:**
- Ivabradine acts on I_f (inward current) in the SA node and reduces the heart rate. It reduces hospital admission and mortality rates in patients with heart.
- It is best given to patients who cannot take β-blockers or in whom the heart rate remains high despite β-blockade. It is not useful in patients with atrial fibrillation.

☐ **Anticoagulation therapy** is indicated in patients with heart failure who are at risk for thromboembolism. These include patients with atrial fibrillation, valvular heart disease, documented left ventricular thrombus, or a history of embolic stroke.

Nonpharmacological Treatment of Heart Failure
Device therapy

☐ **Implantable cardioverter defibrillator (ICD):** Patients with symptomatic ventricular arrhythmias and heart failure have a very bad prognosis. Irrespective of their response to anti-arrhythmic drug therapy, implantation of a cardiac defibrillator improves survival of all these patients. It is indicated in nonischemic or ischemic heart disease (at least 40 days post-MI) with LVEF of <35% with NYHA class II or III symptoms or NYHA 1 with EF <30% on chronic medical therapy, who have reasonable expectation of meaningful survival for more than 1 year.

☐ **Cardiac resynchronization therapy (CRT):**
- It is indicated for patients who have LVEF of 35% or less, sinus rhythm, left bundle-branch block (LBBB) with a QRS duration of 150 ms or greater, and NYHA class II, III, or ambulatory IV symptoms.
- In this, both the LV and RV are paced simultaneously to generate a more coordinated left ventricular contraction and improve cardiac output. It improves symptoms and survival.

☐ **Coronary revascularization:** Coronary artery disease is the most common cause of heart failure. Patients with angina and left ventricular dysfunction have a higher mortality from surgery (10–20%), but most patients' symptoms and prognosis are improved. Coronary artery bypass surgery or percutaneous coronary intervention may improve function in region of the myocardium that is "hibernating" because of inadequate blood supply. The "hibernating" myocardium can be identified by stress echocardiography and specialized nuclear or MR imaging. Before recommending for surgery, factors such as age, symptoms, and evidence for reversible myocardial ischemia must be considered.

☐ **Hibernating myocardium and myocardial stunning:**
- *Hibernating myocardium* is the reversible left ventricular dysfunction with decreased myocardial perfusion, which is just sufficient to maintain viability of the heart muscle. It is due to an underlying chronic coronary artery disease. Myocardial hibernation is produced due to repetitive episodes of cardiac stunning, which may occur, e.g., with repeated exercise in a patient with coronary artery disease. It responds positively to inotropic stress and indicates the presence of viable heart muscle that may recover after revascularization.
- *Myocardial stunning* is reversible ventricular dysfunction that persists following an episode of ischemia when the blood flow has returned to normal. This is due to a mismatch between flow and function.

- **Heart (cardiac) transplantation:**
  - Cardiac transplantation is an established and successful treatment of choice for younger patients with severe intractable heart failure, whose life expectancy is <6 months.
  - *Indications*: Usually reserved for young patients with severe symptoms despite optimal therapy. Most common indications are coronary artery disease and dilated cardiomyopathy.
  - *Contraindication:* Patients with pulmonary vascular disease due to long-standing left heart failure, complex congenital heart disease (e.g., Eisenmenger's syndrome) or primary pulmonary hypertension.
- **Ventricular assist devices (VADs):** There is limited supply of donor organs and VADs takes over pumping for the ventricles. Hence, VADs are used as—(1) a bridge to cardiac transplantation, (2) potential long-term therapy, and (3) short-term restoration therapy following a potentially reversible insult (e.g., viral myocarditis).

Newer Agents in Heart Failure Management
- Nesiritide (recombinant analog of BNP)
- *Endopeptidase inhibitor (ACE + neutral peptidases)*, e.g., omapatrilat
- **Calcium sensitizer:** For example, levosimendan. *Levosimendan* is a novel agent with inotropic properties developed specifically for the management of ADHF (acute decompensated heart failure). It acts by sensitizing troponin C to calcium.
- **Endothelin receptor antagonist:** For example, bosentan and tezosentan. Effective in acute coronary syndromes, acute renal failure, and acute heart failure. Indirectly improve contractility while decreasing pulmonary capillary wedge pressure.
- **Vasopressin antagonists (V2 RA):** For example, tolvaptan, lixivaptan, and conivaptan. It can be used as adjuvant to diuretic in advanced heart failure.
- **Enoximone:** Type 3 phosphodiesterase inhibitor.
- **Angiotensin receptor–neprilysin inhibitor:** Sacubitril-valsartan for NYHA class II to IV heart failure with reduced ejection fraction.
- Management of heart failure based on symptoms, cardiac output, and pulmonary capillary wedge pressure is depicted in **Figures 9.13 and 9.14**.

PULMONARY EDEMA

Definition
Pulmonary edema is a condition characterized by accumulation of excess fluid in interstitium and alveoli of the lung as a result of an alteration in one or more of starling forces.

Classification and Causes of Pulmonary Edema (Table 9.31)
Pulmonary edema can result from hemodynamic disturbances (hemodynamic or cardiogenic pulmonary edema) or from direct increases in capillary permeability (noncardiogenic pulmonary edema due to microvascular injury). Based on underlying cause it can be classified as:
- **Cardiogenic pulmonary edema** is defined as a high pulmonary capillary hydrostatic pressure (as estimated clinically from the pulmonary capillary wedge pressure—PCWP) is responsible for abnormal fluid accumulation in alveoli of the lung.
- **Noncardiogenic pulmonary edema** is caused by various disorders in which factors other than elevated pulmonary capillary pressure are responsible for protein and fluid accumulation in the alveoli.
- **Clinical features of left heart (acute ventricular) failure:** Extreme breathlessness, shortness of breath orthopnea, and paroxysmal nocturnal dyspnea, anxiety, and feelings of drowning. Cough and pink frothy sputum.

Physical findings
- Tachypnea and tachycardia
- Hypertension
- Cool extremities may indicate low cardiac output
- Auscultation reveals fine, crepitations, or wheezes
- *CVS findings*: S_3, accentuation of pulmonic component of S_2, and jugular venous distention
- Patients with (RV) failure may present with hepatomegaly, sustained hepatojugular reflux, and peripheral edema. Change in mental status, caused by hypoxia or hypercapnia.

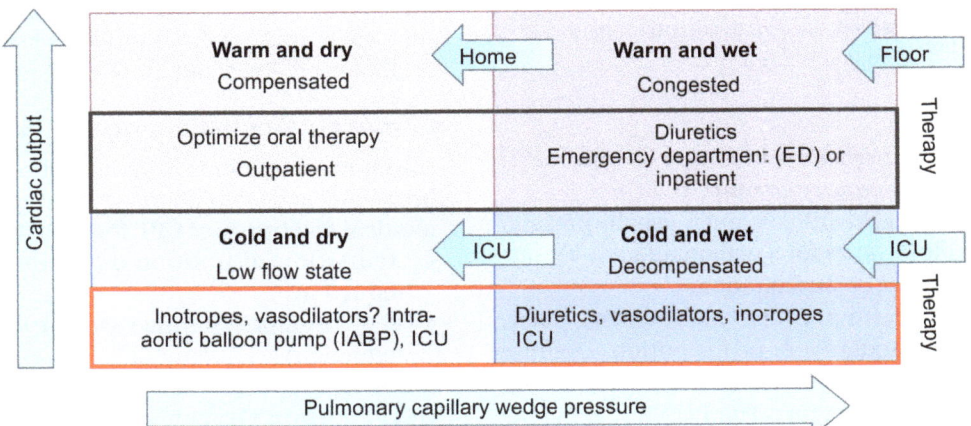

Fig. 9.13: Management of heart failure based on symptoms, cardiac output, and pulmonary capillary wedge pressure.
(ICU: intensive care unit)

```
Mechanical circulatory support depending on cause:
Intra-aortic balloon pump (IABP) therapy,
ventricular assist devices (VADs),
Device therapy-permanent,
implantable VAD, transplant/artificial heart
```
```
All the measures of Stage A, B and C
temporary intravenous inotropic support
```
Stage D: End stage disease, refractory symptoms requiring special intervention

```
Aldosterone receptor antagonists
Depending on the cause revascularization, mitral valve surgery
```
```
Device therapy: Cardiac resynchronization therapy (CRT) if there is bundle branch block
Implantable cardioverter defibrillator (ICD)
```
```
Dietary restriction of sodium, diuretics and digoxin
```
```
ACE inhibitors and beta blockers in all patients. All measures of stage A and B
```
Stage C: Have symptoms (previous/current) and structural heart damage

```
Care measures as in Stage A along with ACE inhibitors or ARBs in all patients,
beta blockers in selected patients and spironolactone (if LVEF <40%)
Surgical consultation for coronary artery revascularization and
valve repair/replacement (as appropriate)
```
Stage B: Asymptomatic but have signs of structural heart damage

```
Risk factor control: Control of BP and diabetes, weight reduction,
quit smoking, lipid management, atrial fibrillation
ACE inhibitors and ARAs in some patients
Education of patients and their relatives
```
Stage A: Asymptomatic with no heart damage but have high-risk factors for heart failure

Fig. 9.14: American College of Cardiology (ACC)/American Heart Association (AHA) guidelines (four stages of heart failure and treatment options for systolic heart failure).

Table 9.31: Various causes of pulmonary edema.

Cardiogenic pulmonary edema (CPE)	Noncardiogenic pulmonary edema (NCPE) [other name of NCPE = ARDS (acute respiratory distress syndrome)]
Cardiac disorders: Atrial outflow obstruction, LV systolic dysfunction, LV diastolic dysfunction *Dysrhythmias:* • LV hypertrophy and cardiomyopathies • LV volume overload • Myocardial infarction • LV outflow obstruction	*Direct injury to lung:* Chest trauma, pneumonia, and pulmonary embolism *Indirect injury to lung:* Sepsis, multiple transfusions, cardiopulmonary bypass, pancreatitis, and toxins *Lung injury plus increased hydrostatic pressure:* Neurogenic pulmonary edema, high altitude pulmonary edema, re-expansion pulmonary edema

(LV: left ventricle)

Differences between cardiogenic pulmonary edema (CPE) and noncardiogenic pulmonary edema (NCPE):

- **CPE:** A history of an acute cardiac event is usually present. Physical examination shows an S_3 gallop, jugular venous distention, and crackles on auscultation.
- **NCPE:** They have a warm periphery, a bounding pulse, and no S_3 gallop or jugular venous distention. Definite differentiation is based on pulmonary capillary wedge pressure (PCWP) measurements. The PCWP is generally >18 mm Hg in CPE and <18 mm Hg in NCPE.

Unusual Type Pulmonary Edema

- **Neurogenic pulmonary edema:** It is seen in patients with central nervous system disorders and without apparent preexisting LV dysfunction.
- **Re-expansion pulmonary edema:** It develops after removal of air or fluid that has been in pleural space for some time, post-thoracocentesis. Patients may develop hypotension or oliguria resulting from rapid fluid shifts into lung.
- **High altitude pulmonary edema:** It occurs in young individuals who have quickly ascended to altitudes above 2,700 m (8,000 feet) and who then engage in strenuous physical exercise at that altitude, before they have become acclimatized. Reversible in less than 48 hours.

Treatment of Acute Cardiogenic Pulmonary Edema

- **Initial management:** ABCs of resuscitation, i.e., airway, breathing, and circulation
- **Medical treatment of CPE focuses on three main goals:**
  - Reduction of pulmonary venous return (preload reduction)
  - Reduction of systemic vascular resistance (afterload reduction)
- Inotropic support
- **Oxygenation:** Oxygen should be administered to all patients to keep oxygen saturation at greater than 90%.

Methods of oxygen delivery include the use of a face mask [noninvasive ventilation which includes bi-level positive airway pressure (BiPAP) and continuous positive airway pressure (CPAP)], and intubation and mechanical ventilation. Oxygen corrects hypoxia and positive pressure raises intra-alveolar pressure reducing transudation of fluid.

- **Preload reduction** decreases pulmonary capillary hydrostatic pressure and reduces fluid transudation into the pulmonary interstitium and alveoli. *Nitroglycerin* oral or IV 10–100 µg/min
- **Diuretics:** They reduce the circulating blood volume and hasten the relief of pulmonary edema. *Intravenous furosemide* has a venodilator action by which it reduces venous return. This effect occurs within a few minutes while diuresis may take 30 minutes.
- **Morphine sulfate:** Morphine 2–5 mg intravenously slowly, and repeated if necessary, reduces anxiety and reduces venous return.
- **Afterload reduction** increases cardiac output and improves renal perfusion, which allows for diuresis in the patient with fluid overload.
- **ACE inhibitors:** Enalapril 1.25 mg IV or captopril 25 mg sublingually.
- Angiotensin II receptor blockers.
- Nitroprusside for 3–4 µg/kg/min IV infusion
- **Inotropic agents:** Dobutamine and dopamine
- **Intra-aortic balloon pumping (IABP):**
  - The IABP is inserted percutaneously through the femoral artery to descending aorta using a modified technique. Fluoroscopy may be used for correct positioning of the balloon, and Helium gas is used to inflate the balloon.
  - The IABP decreases afterload as the pump deflates; during diastole the pump inflates to improve coronary blood flow.
- **Ultrafiltration** is a fluid removal procedure that is particularly useful in patients with renal dysfunction and expected diuretic resistance.
- Correction of precipitating causes, e.g., infection or arrhythmias
- Treatment of underlying cause

CARDIAC ARRHYTHMIAS

Definition
An abnormality (disturbance) of either rate or electrical rhythm of contraction of the heart is called a cardiac arrhythmia.
- Arrhythmias are usually due to structural disease of the heart but may also occur because of abnormal conduction or depolarization in an otherwise healthy heart.

Main Types of Arrhythmia
- **Bradyarrhythmia:** The heart rate is slow and less than 60/min during the day or less than 50/min at night.
- **Tachyarrhythmia:** The heart rate is fast and more than 100/min.

Classification
Classification of cardiac arrhythmias is described in **Table 9.32**.

Ventricular Tachycardia (Fig. 9.15)

Etiology
Etiology of ventricular tachycardia is described in **Table 9.33**.

Clinical Features
Clinical features of ventricular tachycardia are described in **Table 9.34**.
- If the patient is hemodynamically unstable in the form of hypotension, angina, heart failure or altered sensorium, immediate cardioversion in synchronized mode is required.
- If the patient is stable, amiodarone and lidocaine are the drugs of choice.

Table 9.32: Classification of cardiac arrhythmias.

Disturbances of impulse formation	Disturbances of impulse conduction
❖ *Disturbances of sinus mechanism:* ▫ Sinus tachycardia ▫ Sinus bradycardia ▫ Sinus arrhythmia ❖ *Disturbance of atria:* ▫ Atrial premature contraction ▫ Atrial fibrillation ▫ Atrial flutter ▫ Paroxysmal supraventricular tachycardia (PSVT) ❖ *Disturbance of atrioventricular (AV) node:* ▫ Junctional ectopics ▫ Junctional tachycardia ❖ *Disturbance of ventricles:* ▫ Ventricular ectopics ▫ Ventricular tachycardia ▫ Ventricular fibrillation (VF)	❖ Sinoatrial blocks ❖ *AV nodal blocks:* ▫ First degree block ▫ Second degree block ▫ Wenckebach (Mobitz type 1) block ▫ Mobitz type II block ▫ Complete or third degree block ❖ *Bundle blocks:* ▫ Right bundle branch block ▫ Left bundle branch block ▫ Left anterior hemiblock ▫ Left posterior hemiblock

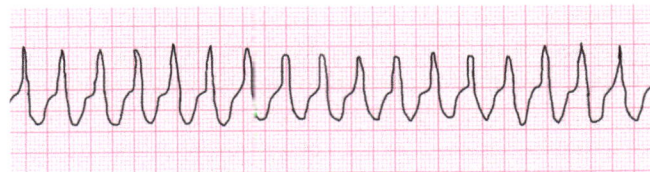

Fig. 9.15: Ventricular tachycardia.

Table 9.33: Causes of ventricular tachycardia.

• Ischemic heart disease Acute MI, after chronic infarction • Dilated cardiomyopathy • Hypertrophic cardiomyopathy • Post-CABG and post-TOF surgery • Idiopathic • Specific etiology—genetic	*Reversible causes of VT:* • Hypoxia • Hyperthyroidism and catecholamines • *Electrolyte abnormalities:* Hypokalemia, hypomagnesemia, hypocalcemia, and metabolic acidosis • Drugs, alcohol, and starvation

(CABG: coronary artery bypass graft; TOF: tetralogy of Fallot)

Table 9.34: Clinical features of ventricular tachycardia.

- Asymptomatic
- May have palpitations—transient/sustained
- Chest pain: Angina
- Syncope/dizziness
- Presyncope
- Cannon a waves
- Absent pulse
- Hypotension
- Variable S_1

☐ Amiodarone 150 mg intravenously over 10 minutes, then 1 mg/minute for 6 hours and then 0.5 mg/minute for next 18 hours.
☐ Lidocaine 1–1.5 mg/kg IV over 1 minute followed by infusion at 10–40 µg/kg/minute.

Torsade De Pointes (Fig. 9.16)

☐ It is type of VT characterized by gradual changing of QRS axis so that it appears around the isoelectric line.
☐ It is usually due to prolonged Q-T interval.
☐ It can result from ingestion of certain drugs such as quinidine, procainamide, antidepressants and phenothiazines, and the trolyte imbalances such as hypokalemia and hypocalcemia.
☐ Magnesium in a dose of 2–4 kg IV over a period of 30 minutes is quite effective in terminating an episode and preventing its recurrence.

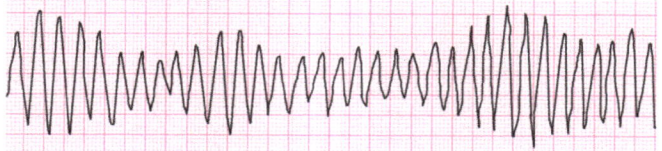

Fig. 9.16: Torsade de pointes.

Atrial Fibrillation

It is disorganized and multiple atrial foci fire impulses at a rate of 350–600/minute. The ventricles respond at irregular intervals, usually at a rate of 100–140/minute.

☐ **Atrial fibrillation can be:**
- Paroxysmal atrial fibrillation means that episodes terminate without intervention in lesser than 7 days.
- Persistent atrial fibrillation means that episodes lasting longer than 7 days or require an intervention
- Permanent atrial fibrillation means that the arrhythmia is continuous, and interventions to restore sinus rhythm have either failed or not been attempted.

Etiology

Etiology of atrial fibrillation is described in **Table 9.35**.

Table 9.35: Etiology of atrial fibrillation.

- Rheumatic heart disease (especially mitral valvular disease)
- Ischemic heart disease (especially acute myocardial infarction)
- Hypertension
- Thyrotoxicosis
- Congenital heart diseases (especially atrial septal defect)
- Cardiomyopathy
- Pericardial diseases
- Other rare causes—alcohol, pulmonary embolism, exercise, and chronic lung diseases
- Lone atrial fibrillation—elderly patients without underlying heart disease

Symptoms

Usual symptoms include palpitations, fatigue, syncope, and angina.

Signs

☐ Irregularly irregular pulse
☐ Varying volumes of pulse
☐ Pulse deficit (apex pulse deficit) > 10
☐ Varying intensity of the first heart sound
☐ Absence of a waves on JVP

Classification

Table 9.36 describes the clinical classification of atrial fibrillation and choice of treatment.

Electrocardiogram (Fig. 9.17)

☐ An irregularly irregular rhythm of QRS complexes
☐ Absent P waves
☐ Small, irregular waves (fibrillary waves)

Complications

☐ Syncope
☐ **Thromboembolism:**
- Risk of stroke in atrial fibrillation: A risk index (CHA_2DS_2-VASc score) has been developed to determine the risk of stroke due to thromboembolism in patients with atrial fibrillation (**Table 9.37**).
- Warfarin is recommended, if score >2.

Table 9.36: Clinical classification of atrial fibrillation (AF) and choice of treatment.

Terminology	Clinical features	Treatment
Initial event (first detected episode)	Symptomatic/asymptomatic. Onset unknown	Rhythm/rate control
Paroxysmal (may be vagotonic AF or adrenergic AF)	Intermittent episodes that stops spontaneously (self-termination) within 7 days and most often <48 hours	Rhythm control. Vagotonic AF responds to digitalis, disopyramide while beta-blockers are helpful for adrenergic AF
Persistent	Prolonged, not self-terminating, lasting >7 days, which requires termination by electrical or chemical cardioversion	Rhythm/rate control
Permanent ("accepted")	Not spontaneously terminated or terminated but relapsed, no cardioversion attempt	Rate control

Note: Atrial fibrillation may be asymptomatic and the first detected episode should not be considered as the true onset.

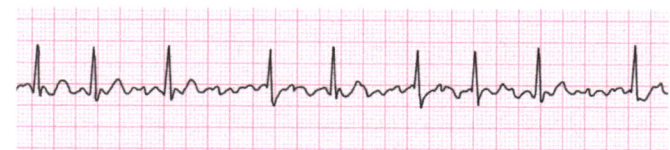

Fig. 9.17: Electrocardiogram of atrial fibrillation.

Table 9.37: CHA$_2$DS$_2$-VASc stroke risk scoring system for nonvalvular atrial fibrillation.

Risk factor	Score	
C: Congestive heart failure	1	**0 points: Low risk** (no prophylaxis required)
H: Hypertension	1	**1–2 points: Moderate risk** (oral anticoagulant or aspirin recommended)
A: Age >75 years	2	
D: Diabetes mellitus	1	
S$_2$: Prior stroke or TIA	2	**≥3 points: High risk** (oral anticoagulant recommended)
V: Vascular disease	1	
A: Age 65–74 years old	1	
Sc: Sex category (female)	1	

- Precipitation/worsening of cardiac failure
- Angina
- Hypotension

Treatment
- If the patient's clinical status is severely compromised à synchronized DC cardioversion is the treatment of choice.
- **If the patient's clinical status is not severely compromised, treatment is in two steps:**
  1. Slowing the ventricular rate with verapamil, diltiazem, propranolol, esmolol, or digoxin.
  2. Converting rhythm to normal sinus rhythm Pharmacological cardioversion to sinus rhythm with quinidine, ibutilide, flecainide, propafenone, or amiodarone
- Chronic anticoagulation includes warfarin and dabigatran

Atrial Flutter
- It is a regular, rapid atrial rate of 250–350/minute, where ventricles responded to every second, third, or fourth beat (2:1, 3:1, or 4:1 AV block).
- **Electrocardiographic feature:** Characteristic flutter waves are seen as regular sawtoothed waves ("F" waves) (**Fig. 9.18**).
- **Management:** Same as atrial fibrillation

Paroxysmal Supraventricular Tachycardia
- It is usually paroxysmal and recurrent, and has a rate of 140–220 beats/minute with 1:1 conduction.
- It usually results from re-entry of an atrial ectopic in the AV node (AV nodal re-entry tachycardia-AVNRT or [AV re-entry tachycardia (AVRT)].
- **Causes:**
  - Idiopathic in health individuals
  - Excessive coffee, tea, alcohol, or tobacco
  - Anxiety
  - Hyperthyroidism
  - Organic heart disease (ischemic, valvular, or congenital)

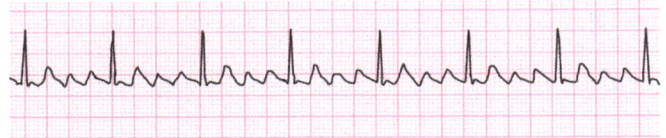

Fig. 9.18: Electrocardiogram of atrial flutter.

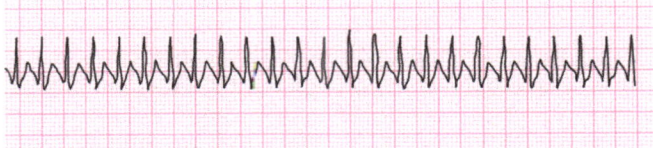

Fig. 9.19: Electrocardiogram of paroxysmal supraventricular tachycardia.

- Clinical features
- The onset and termination of the arrhythmia are sudden
- Patients most commonly complain of palpitations, an odd feeling in the chest, and on occasion, lightheadedness, or pain.
- Some patients have polyuria and experience diuresis during or after paroxysmal supraventricular tachycardia (PSVT).

Electrocardiogram
The P wave is usually buried in the QRS complex or occurs slightly before or after the QRS complex (**Fig. 9.19**).

Treatment
- Vagal maneuvers such as carotid sinus massage, Valsalva maneuver, and gag reflex
- Adenosine is administered as in initial bolus of 6 mg rapidly over 1–3 seconds followed immediately by 20 mL of saline.
- Propranolol, esmolol, verapamil, diltiazem, and adenosine.
- Synchronized cardioversion is performed, if patient is hemodynamically compromised
- Long-term control can be achieved by radiofrequency ablation of the re-entrant pathway.

Wolff–Parkinson–White Syndrome
- **Cause:** Presence of an abnormal band of atrial tissue (bundle of Kent) connecting the atria and ventricles and bypassing the AV node.
- **ECG:** Short PR interval (<0.12 seconds), a delta wave in the beginning of ORS and prolonged QRS complex (>0.12 seconds)
- Acts as a re-entry pathway and the patient may develop supraventricular tachycardia.

Treatment
- Disopyramide, quinidine, flecainide, and amiodarone to increase the refractory period and reduce the conducting rate through the bypass tract.
- Radiofrequency ablation of the bypass tract can be done.

Sick–Sinus Syndrome
- It includes sinus bradycardia, sinus arrest, combinations of sinoatrial and AV blocks, and supraventricular tachycardias
- The abnormalities are usually due to ischemia, fibrosis, drug-induced or autonomic dysfunction
- **Clinical features:** Many patients are asymptomatic.
- Treatment of recurrent symptomatic bradycardia or prolonged pauses requires implantation of a permanent pacemaker.

Brugada Syndrome

- ST segment elevation (>2 mm) in right precordial leads (V1 to V3), incomplete or complete right bundle branch block
- Susceptibility to ventricular tachyarrhythmia (particularly polymorphic ventricular tachycardia) and sudden cardiac death
- Treatment involves implantable cardioverter defibrillator

Sudden Cardiac Death

It is an unexpected, nontraumatic death due to cardiac causes occurring in a short time period in a person with known or unknown cardiac disease in whom no previously diagnosed fatal condition is apparent.

Causes

Causes of sudden cardiac death are described in **Table 9.38**.

Table 9.38: Causes of sudden cardiac death.

• Coronary artery disease	• Brugada syndrome
• Ischemic cardiomyopathy	• Wolff–Parkinson–White syndrome
• Non-ischemic cardiomyopathy	• Electrolyte abnormalities
• Hypertrophic cardiomyopathy	• Cocaine
• Valvular heart disease	• Myocarditis
• Congenital heart disease	• Long QT syndrome

Cardiac Arrest

- Cardiac arrest is defined as an abrupt loss of cardiac pump function, which may be reversible by a prompt intervention, but will lead to death in its absence.
- Cardiac arrest may result from one of the following four mechanisms—(1) VF, (2) pulseless ventricular tachycardia, (3) asystole, and (4) pulseless electrical activity (PEA).

Causes

Causes of cardiac arrest are described in **Table 9.39**.

Table 9.39: Causes of cardiac arrest.

Six Hs:	Six Ts:
• Hypoxia	• Tamponade, cardiac
• Hypovolemia	• Tension pneumothorax
• Hypothermia	• Toxins/tablets
• Hydrogen ions (acidosis)	• Thrombosis, coronary (myocardial infarction)
• Hypokalemia/hyperkalemia	• Thrombosis, pulmonary embolism
• Hypoglycemia	• Trauma

Management

Cardiopulmonary resuscitation (CPR)

Atrioventricular Blocks

First-degree Block

In the ECG, the P-R interval is prolonged to more than 0.20 seconds. All the P waves are conducted and the QRS is normal as the delay is most often in the AV mode (**Fig. 9.20**).

Second-degree Block

- It can be subdivided into Mobitz type I and Mobitz type II blocks.
- **Mobitz type I (Wenckebach) second-degree AV block:** The ECG typically shows progressive prolongation of successive PR intervals until one P wave is not conducted. The QRS is usually normal (**Fig. 9.21**).
- **Mobitz type II second-degree AV block:**
  - The block is characterized by a constant P-R interval with intermittent failure of atrial impulses to conduct to the ventricles (**Fig. 9.22**)
  - Patients generally require a pacemaker.

Third-degree or Complete AV Block

- Regular and slow pulse (30–40/minute)
- High-volume pulse
- Irregular cannon waves on JVP
- Varying intensity of first heart sound
- Stokes–Adams attacks
- The ECG shows constant P-P and R-R intervals but with complete AV dissociation, i.e., the atria and ventricles beat independently and there is no relation between the P waves and the QRS complexes (**Fig. 9.23**).

Management

Implantation of a permanent pacemaker

Adams–Stokes Attacks (Stokes–Adams–Morgagni Attacks)

- An episode of syncope caused by bradycardia related to AV block is called Stokes–Adams–Morgagni syndrome. These commonly occur due to an underlying Mobitz type II block or complete heart block in distal conduction system. Even though VT can also produce loss of consciousness, it is not typically included under Adams–Stokes attack.
- **Clinical features:**
  - Some patients describe a prodrome preceding the attack.
  - Rapid loss of consciousness and the patient may fall, followed by rapid recovery.
  - Convulsions and later death may result, if the asystole or severe bradycardia is prolonged to more than 10 seconds.

CARDIOMYOPATHY

Cardiomyopathies are a heterogeneous group of diseases of the myocardium that affects the mechanical or electrical function of the heart.

The term cardiomyopathy should be restricted to the conditions, which primarily affect the myocardium. It does not include myocardial involvement due to congenital, acquired valvular, hypertensive, and coronary arterial or pericardial abnormalities.

Etiology

They can be genetic/inherited or have infective and toxic causes or idiopathic.

Classification (Fig. 9.24)

Cardiomyopathies may be classified according to a variety of criteria, including the underlying genetic basis of dysfunction. Two fundamental forms of cardiomyopathy (**Box 9.15**) are:

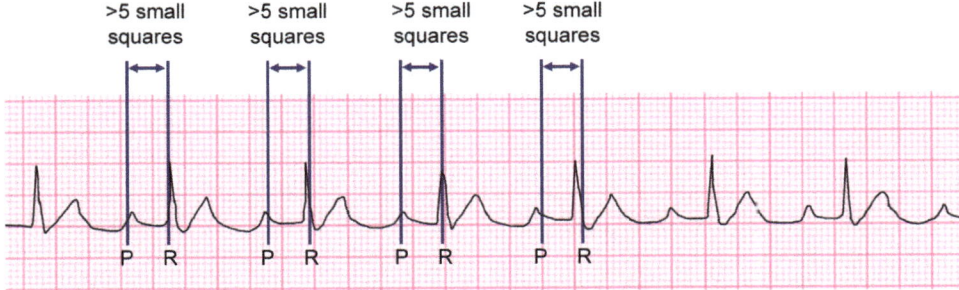

Fig. 9.20: Electrocardiogram of first-degree atrioventricular blocks.

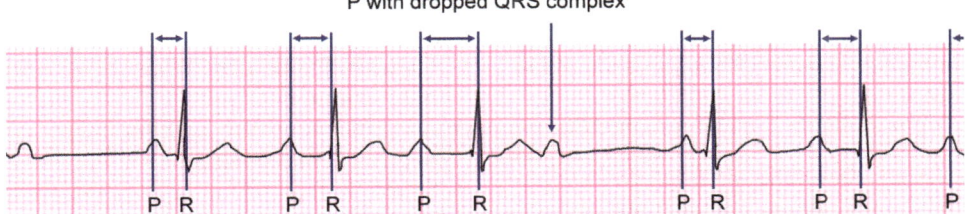

Fig. 9.21: Electrocardiogram of Mobitz type I (Wenckebach) second-degree atrioventricular block.

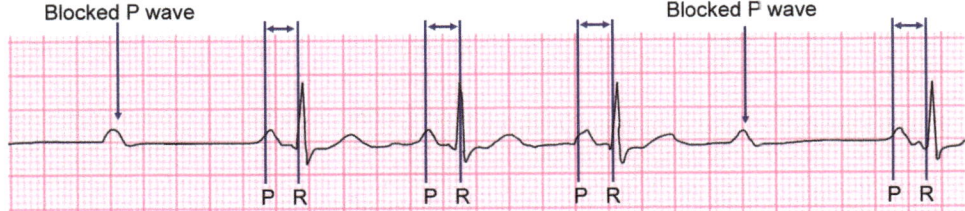

Fig. 9.22: Electrocardiogram of Mobitz type II (Wenckebach) second-degree atrioventricular block.

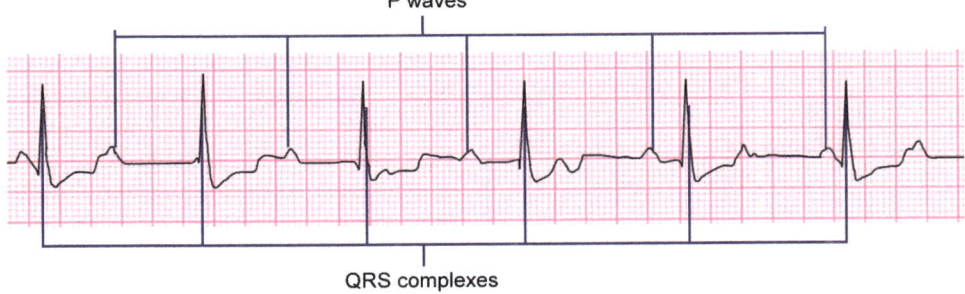

Fig. 9.23: Electrocardiogram of third-degree or complete atrioventricular block.

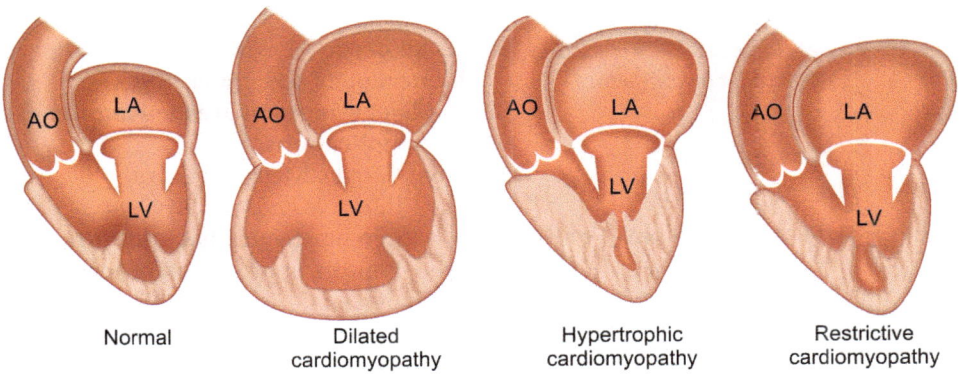

Fig. 9.24: Clinical classification of cardiomyopathy.
(AO: aorta; LA: left atrium; LV: left ventricle)

> **Box 9.15:** Etiologic classification of cardiomyopathy.
>
> *Primary cardiomyopathy:*
> - Idiopathic (D, R, and H)
> - Familial (D, R, and H)
> - Eosinophilic endomyocardial fibrosis (R)
> - Endomyocardial fibrosis (R)
>
> *Secondary cardiomyopathy:*
> - *Infective (D):* Viral, bacterial, fungal, protozoal, metazoal, rickettsial, and spirochetal myocarditis
> - *Metabolic (D):* Familial storage disease (D and R): Glycogen storage disease, mucopolysaccharidosis, hemochromatosis, and Fabry's disease
> - *Deficiency (D):* Electrolytes and nutritional
> - *Autoimmune disease:* Systemic lupus erythematosus, polyarteritis nodosa, and rheumatoid arthritis
> - *Infiltrations and granulomas diseases (R and D):* Amyloidosis, sarcoidosis, and malignancy
> - *Neuromuscular:* Muscular dystrophy, myotonic dystrophy, and Friedrich's ataxia (H and D)
> - *Sensitivity and toxic reaction (D):* Alcohol, drugs, and radiation
> - *Peripartum heart disease:* Takotsubo (stress) cardiomyopathy

(D: dilated cardiomyopathy; H: hypertrophic cardiomyopathy; R: restrictive cardiomyopathy)

1. **Primary cardiomyopathy:** It consists of heart muscle disease predominantly involving the myocardium and/or of unknown cause.
2. **Secondary cardiomyopathy:** It consists of myocardial disease of unknown cause or cardiomyopathy associated with systemic disease (e.g., chronic alcohol use and amyloidosis).

CONGENITAL HEART DISEASES

Classification of congenital heart diseases is described in **Table 9.40**.

Congenital heart disease (CHD) is the most common group of structural malformations in children. CHD occurs in 8 per 1,000 infants. About 1 in 10 stillborn infants have a cardiac anomaly.

Atrial Septal Defect

- Ostium secundum defects (75–85% of ASDs) are located in the region of the mid-septum (fossa ovalis).

Table 9.40: Classification of congenital heart diseases.

Acyanotic	Cyanotic
With (left to right) shunts	**With (right to left) shunts**
Ventricular septal defect	Tetralogy of Fallot
Atrial septal defect	Tricuspid atresia
Patent ductus arteriosus	Ebstein's anomaly
	Transposition of great vessels
	Truncus arteriosus
Without shunts (obstructive lesions)	**Without shunts (obstructive lesions)**
Aortic stenosis	Pulmonary stenosis
Coarctation of aorta	

- Ostium primum (atrioventricular septal) defects (10–15%) are located in the lower portion of the atrial septum.
- **Sinus venosus defects:**
  - *Superior sinus venosus type defect (5–10%)*: Defects are located in the superior part of the septum near the orifice of the superior vena cava (SVC).
  - *Inferior sinus venosus (IVC) type defect (1%)*: Defects are located on the inferior part of the septum near the inferior vena cava (IVC) entry point.
- Coronary sinus (1%) septal defect (in which a defect between the coronary sinus and the left atrium allows a left-to-right shunt to occur through an "unroofed" coronary sinus)

Signs
- **S2-wide fixed split:** Wide, fixed splitting of the second heart sound (S2)
- A systolic flow murmur over the pulmonary valve not due to atrial septal defect.
- Diastolic flow murmur over the tricuspid valve may be heard in children with a large shunt.

Ventricular Septal Defect

Congenital ventricular septal defect are due to incomplete septation of the ventricles. Embryologically, the interventricular septum has two portions namely—(1) a membranous and (2) a muscular portion (which is further divided into inflow, trabecular, and outflow portions).

Pansystolic murmur in left lower sternal border is pathognomonic.

Complications include congestive heart failure, pulmonary hypertension, Eisenmenger's syndrome, right ventricular outflow tract obstruction, infective endocarditis.

Persistent Ductus Arteriosus (PDA)

About 50% of the left ventricular output is recirculated through the lungs, with a consequent increase in the work of the heart. PDAs may occur as an isolated anomaly (about 90%), or associated with other abnormalities such as VSD, coarctation of the aorta, or pulmonary or aortic valve stenosis.

Patent ductus arteriosus produces a characteristic continuous harsh murmur known as "machinery-like"/Gibson's murmur.

Coarctation of Aorta

It can occur anywhere from distal part of arch of aorta to bifurcation of abdominal aorta.
- **Major symptoms are the symptoms related to four major complications:**
  - Congestive heart failure
  - Infective endocarditis
  - Cerebral hemorrhage due to rupture of Berry aneurysm
  - Rupture or dissection of aorta
- Hypertension in the upper limbs with low or normal pressure in lower limbs (difference >20 mm Hg)
- Weak and delayed femoral pulses (radiofemoral delay)
- "Suzman's ring" is dilated, tortuous, and pulsatile arteries seen around the scapulae and intercostals regions in the

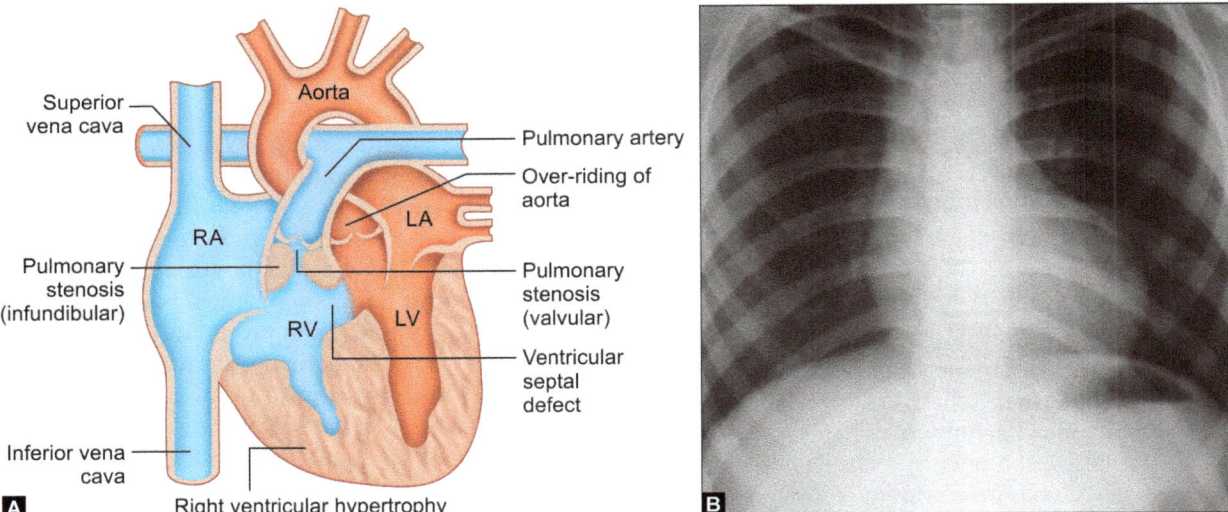

Figs. 9.25A and B: (A) Diagrammatic representation of tetralogy of Fallot. Four components are—(1) ventricular septal defect (VSD); (2) subpulmonic stenosis/pulmonary valvular stenosis; (3) aorta overriding the VSD, and (4) right ventricular hypertrophy; (B) X-ray shows an abnormally small pulmonary artery, large right ventricle, and a "boot-shaped" heart.
(LA: left atrium; LV: left ventricle; RV: right ventricle; RA: right atrium)

back. It is better seen with the patient bent forwards and hands hanging down.
- "Cork-screw"-shaped retinal arteries.

Tetralogy of Fallot

It is the most common congenital cyanotic heart disease in adults (75%).
- Ventricular septal defect usually large and similar in aperture to the aortic orifice.
- **Pulmonary stenosis:** Right ventricular outflow tract obstruction mostly subvalvular (infundibular) but may be valvular, supravalvular, or a combination of these.
- Overriding of dextroposed aorta
- Right ventricular hypertrophy
  Presence of ASD along with TOF is known as pentalogy of Fallot (**Figs. 9.25A and B**).

Eisenmenger's Syndrome

- Eisenmenger's syndrome is the consequence of the reversal of a left-to-right shunt to a right-to-left shunt.
- It occurs in patients with congenital heart disease, especially PDA, VSD, and ASD.

Clinical Features

- Dyspnea, cyanosis, fatigue, dizziness, and syncope.
- Central cyanosis and clubbing occur from mixing of deoxygenated blood with oxygenated blood.
- It is generalized to ASD and VSD reversal, while it is differential (only lower limbs) in PDA with reversal.
- S2 is loud with palpable P2
- S2 fixed but narrowly split in ASD with reversal
- S2 single in VSD with reversal
- S2 mobile but narrowly split in PDA with reversal
- Eventually, patient dies of right heart failure.

Treatment

- Vasodilator therapy using calcium-channel blockers may be detrimental, as systemic vasodilatation may further increase right-to-left shunt.
- Long-term oxygen inhalation may improve symptoms.
- Phlebotomy in patients with hyperviscosity syndrome due to erythrocytosis.
- The only curative treatment is heart–lung transplantation.
- Prostanoids (epoprostenol, iloprost, and treprostinil), endothelin receptor antagonists (bosentan), and phosphodiesteraase-5 inhibitors (sildenafil and tadalafil) may improve symptoms.

CARDIAC ARREST

Definition

Cardiac arrest is a sudden loss of cardiac pump function, which can be reversed by a prompt intervention, without which it leads to death.

Causes of Cardiac Arrest (Box 9.16)

Diagnosis of cardiac arrest (TRIAD): (1) Loss of *consciousness*, (2) loss of apical and central *pulsations* (carotid and femoral), and (3) apnea.

Box 9.16: Causes of cardiac arrest (6 H and 4 T).

- Hypoxia
- Hypotension
- Hypothermia
- Hypoglycemia
- Acidosis (H^+)
- Hyperkalemia (electrolyte disturbance)
- Cardiac *Tamponade*
- Tension pneumothorax
- Thromboembolism (pulmonary and coronary)
- Toxicity (e.g., digoxin, local anesthetics, and insecticides)

ECG: Three basic patterns:
1. **Ventricular tachyarrhythmia:** Ventricular fibrillation (VF)/sustained type of pulseless ventricular tachycardia.
2. Ventricular asystole or a bradyasystolic rhythm with an extremely slow rate.
3. Pulseless electrical activity (PEA) previously referred to as electromechanical dissociation.

Management

Chain of Survival

It refers to the sequence of events that is required to maximize the chances of survival in a patient with cardiac arrest. Survival is most likely, if all links in the chain are strong. The chain of survival consists of following links namely:
- Immediate identification of cardiac arrest and activation of the emergency response system (ERS) by a trained individual.
- Immediate CPR with chest compressions.
- Quick defibrillation.
- Effective advanced life support (ALS).
- Integrated post-cardiac arrest care.

Immediate Identification and Activation of Emergency Response System

- **Immediate identification of cardiac arrest:** Assessment is of crucial importance. It includes—(1) unresponsiveness (check the individual for a response, gently shake shoulders and ask 'are you all right?'), (2) no breathing or no normal breathing (i.e., only gasping), and (3) no pulse felt within 10 seconds.
- **Activation of ERS:** After activation of the ERS, all rescuers should immediately begin CPR.
- **Cardiopulmonary Resuscitation (CPR):** It provides artificial ventilation and perfusion to the vital organs, particularly heart and brain until spontaneous cardiopulmonary function is restored. It consists of both basic life supports (BLS) and advanced life support (ALS). BLS provides adequate oxygen and perfusion to322 vital organs (brain and heart) until advanced cardiac life support is available **(Table 9.41)**.
Basic life support (BLS) consists of maneuver purpose of which is to maintain a low level of circulation until more definitive treatment with advanced life support can be provided.
- **Change from A-B-C to C-A-B:** CPR includes four sequential: *C*irculation, *A*irway, and *B*reathing (CAB) and defibrillation. Previously, the sequence used to be *A*irway, *B*reathing, and *C*irculation (ABC).

Table 9.41: Cardiopulmonary resuscitation.

Phases	Steps
Phase 1: Basic life support (BLS)	C = Circulation, A = Airway, B = Breathing
Phase 2: Advance life support (ALS)	D = Drugs, E = ECG, F = Fibrillation
Phase 3: Prolonged life support	Postresuscitation care

- *Circulation:* The brain cannot survive for more than 3 minutes without circulation. Hence, start chest compressions immediately for a patient without central pulsations.
  - *Chest compressions (cardiac massage):*
    - Place the patient on a hard surface (wooden board)
    - The palm of one hand is placed in the concavity of the lower half of the sternum two fingers above the xiphoid process (avoid xiphisternal junction → fracture and injury). The other hand is placed over the hand on the sternum.
    - *Shoulders* should be positioned directly over the hands with the *elbows* locked straight and arms extended. Use your upper body weight to compress.
    - Sternum must be depressed *at least 5 cm* in adults, and *2–4 cm* in children, and *1–2 cm* in infants.
    - *Push hard and push fast.* Must be performed at a rate of 100–120/min.
    - During CPR, the ratio of chest compressions to ventilation should be: single rescuer = 30:2 and in the presence of 2 rescuers, *chest compressions must not be interrupted for ventilation*.
    - Chest compressions must be continued for 2 minutes before reassessment of cardiac rhythm (2 minutes = equivalent to 5 cycles 30:2).
  - *Assessment of the adequacy of chest compressions:* Systolic BP = 60–80 mm Hg, diastolic BP (>40 mm Hg), and COP = 30% of normal.
  - *Complications of chest compressions:* Fractures of rib/sternum, rib separation, pneumothorax, hemothorax, contusions of lung, lacerations of liver, and fat emboli
- *Airway:* Loss of consciousness usually produces obstruction of airway due to loss of the muscle tone in the airway and falling back of the tongue. Hence, *clear the airway. Basic techniques for airway patency:*
  - *Head tilt, chin lift:* Place one hand on the forehead and the other on the chin. The head is tilted upward to displace the tongue anteriorly.
  - *Jaw thrust method:* In this, angles of mandible are grasped with both hands and the mandible is lifted forward.
  - *Finger sweep:* Sweep out foreign body in the mouth by index finger in unconscious patients and *not in a conscious or convulsing patient.*
  - *Heimlich maneuver:* It is useful to remove the foreign body in a conscious patient. It is done while the patient is standing up or lying down. In this, subdiaphragmatic abdominal thrust elevates the diaphragm and expels a blast of air from the lungs that displaces the foreign body. In infants, this is performed by a series of blows on the back and chest thrusts.
- *Breathing:* Rescue breathing can be mouth-to-mouth breathing or mouth-to-nose breathing (if there is serious injury of the mouth or it cannot be opened). With the airway open (using the head-tilt, chin-lift maneuver),

pinch the nostrils shut for mouth-to-mouth breathing and cover the person's mouth with rescuer making a seal.
- *Mouth-to-mouth breathing*: With the airway held open, pinch the nostrils closed, take a deep breath and seal your lips over the patient's mouth. Blow steadily into the patient's mouth watching the chest rise as if the patient was taking a deep breath. Volume of each rescue breath should produce visible chest rise.
- *Mouth-to-nose breathing:* Seal the mouth shut and breathe steadily through the nose.
- *Mouth-to-mouth and nose:* It is used in infants and small children.
- *Assessment of restoration of breathing and circulation*: Contraction of pupil, improved color of the skin, free movement of the chest wall, swallowing attempts, and struggling movements
- *Indications for termination of BLS:* Pulse and respiration returns, emergency medical help arrives, physician declared patient is deceased, in a non-health setting, another indication to stop BLS would be that the rescuer was exhausted and physically unable to continue to perform BLS.
- **Advanced life support (ALS):** The purpose is to restore normal cardiac rhythm by defibrillation when the cause is tachyarrhythmia, or to restore cardiac output by correcting other reversible causes of cardiac arrest. It includes:
  - Circulation by cardiac massage
  - Airway management by equipment
  - Breathing by advanced techniques.
  - Defibrillation by manual defibrillator.
  - Drugs

Advanced techniques for airway patency: (1) face mask, (2) oropharyngeal airway, (3) nasopharyngeal airway, (4) laryngeal mask airway, (5) endotracheal intubation, (6) combitube, (7) cricothyrotomy, and (8) tracheostomy

Advanced breathing: Expired air contains $16\% \, O_2$ so supplemental $100\% \, O_2$ should be used as soon as possible. Successful breathing is achieved by delivery of a tidal volume of *800–1,200 mL* in adults at a rate of *10–12 breaths/min* in adults. Advanced techniques include:
1. *Self-inflating resuscitation bag* (Ambu bag)
2. *Mechanical ventilator or in ICU*

Advanced circulation
- It consists of continuation of chest compression and establishing an intravenous access, attaching a cardiac monitor/defibrillator, assessing the rhythm, defibrillation, and administering appropriate drugs for rhythm as well as the condition
- Continuous chest compression is performed at the rate of 100/minute and ventilation is provided at 8–10 breaths/minute (1 breath/6–8 seconds).

Rhythm in cardiac arrest
It may be—(1) shockable rhythm (ventricular tachycardia/ventricular fibrillation) and (2) nonshockable rhythm (asystole and pulseless electrical activity).

- Rhythm checks should be performed done only after 2 minutes of CPR and not immediately following a defibrillation attempt.

Shockable rhythms: Ventricular fibrillation or pulseless ventricular tachycardia (VT)

Defibrillation: Completely depolarize all myocardial cells so SA node can re-establish as pacemaker. Voltage of electricity discharge is high from 150 to 360 J (biphasic) and 360 J (monophasic). Continue CPR for 2 minutes and briefly check the monitor for rhythm. If VT/VF persists, give second shock and immediately resume CPR and continue for 2 minutes, and repeat this cycle.

Drugs
- **Adrenaline:** Given as a *vasopressor* α-1 effect (not as an inotrope). *Dose is 1 mg (0.01 mg/kg) IV every 4 minutes* (alternating cycles) while continuing CPR.
  - Given: (1) Immediately in nonshockable rhythm (non-VT/VF), (2) In VF or VT, given after the 3rd shock.
  - *Repeated* in alternate cycles (every 4 minutes)
  - Once adrenaline always adrenaline.
- **Amiodarone:** Given in shockable rhythm *after the 3rd shock*. If unavailable, give *lidocaine* 100 mg IV (1–1.5 mg/kg). *Dose is 300 mg IV* bolus (5 mg/kg).
- **Vasopressin (ADH):** 40 IU single dose once.
- **Magnesium:** *Given* (1) VF/VT with hypomagnesemia, (2) Torsade de pointes, and (3) digoxin toxicity. *Dose is 2 g IV.*
- **Calcium:** *Dose is 10 mL of 10%* calcium chloride IV.
  - *Indications:* PEA caused by hyperkalemia, hypocalcemia, hypermagnesemia, and overdose of calcium channel blockers.
  - Calcium solutions and $NaHCO_3$ should not be given simultaneously by the same route.
- **Thrombolytics:** Fibrinolytic therapy is considered when cardiac arrest is caused by proven or suspected *acute pulmonary embolism*. If a fibrinolytic drug is used in these circumstances, consider performing CPR for at least 60–90 minutes before termination of resuscitation attempts. Examples are alteplase and tenecteplase (old generation: streptokinase).
- **Sodium bicarbonate:** Used in—(1) severe metabolic acidosis (pH < 7.1), (2) life-threatening hyperkalemia, and (3) tricyclic antidepressant overdose
  - *Dose*: (Half correction) 1/2 base deficit × 1/3 body weight
  - *Adverse drug reactions*: (1) Increases CO_2 load, (2) inhibits release of O_2 to tissues, (3) impairs myocardial contractility, and (4) causes hypernatremia.
- **Atropine:** Its routine use in *pulseless electrical activity* (PEA) and asystole is not useful. It is *indicated* in sinus bradycardia or AV block causing hemodynamic instability. *Dose is 0.5 mg IV*. It is repeated up to a maximum of 3 mg (*full atropinization*).

Nonshockable rhythms: Pulseless electrical activity (PEA) and asystole:
- PEA is characterized by cardiac electrical activity in the absence of any palpable pulse. They usually have some very weak mechanical myocardial contractions and do not produce a detectable pulse.

- Start CPR. Begin with chest compressions, and continue for 2 minutes before the rhythm check is repeated.
- Give 1 mg adrenaline IV immediately and re-check rhythm after 2 minutes of CPR.
- If PEA or asystole persists, continue CPR and re-check rhythm every 2 minutes. Administer adrenaline every 3–5 minutes. Do not give atropine.
- Check rhythm. If it shows change, check for pulse. If pulse appears, start post-resuscitation care. If there is still no pulse, continue CPR with rhythm check every 2 minutes and adrenaline every 3–5 minutes. If the rhythm develops into VF/VT, defibrillate the patient.

IV fluids: Infuse fluids rapidly, if hypovolemia is suspected. Use *normal saline* (0.9% NaCl) or *Ringer's* solution. *Avoid dextrose*, which is redistributed away from the intravascular space rapidly and causes hyperglycemia, which may worsen neurological outcome after cardiac arrest. Dextrose is indicated only if there is *documented hypoglycemia.*

Postresuscitation care:
- Maintain adequate airway and support breathing.
- Continue cardiac monitoring.
- Vasoactive medications (norepinephrine, dobutamine, and epinephrine) and IV fluids to support circulation.
- Avoid hyperthermia, hyperglycemia (maintain blood sugar <200 mg/dL).
- Treating the precipitating cause of cardiac arrest.

SYNCOPE

Definition
Syncope is defined as a transient loss of consciousness due to inadequate cerebral blood flow with loss of postural tone.
- It is associated with loss of postural tone, with spontaneous return to baseline neurologic function without any resuscitative efforts.
- **Presyncope** is the term used for lightheadedness in which the individual thinks he/she may black out.
- **Classical vasovagal syncope:** Syncope triggered by emotional or orthostatic stress, such as venipuncture (experienced or witnessed), painful or noxious stimuli, fear of bodily injury, prolonged standing, heat exposure, or exertion.

Mechanism: Global hypoperfusion of cerebral cortices or focal hypoperfusion of the reticular activating system—
- About 1/3 of individuals may develop a syncopal episode during their lifetime.
- Its incidence increases with age (sharp rise at age 70 years).
- Cardiac syncope has a high incidence (about 24%) of subsequent cardiac arrest.

Causes of Syncope
Causes of syncope are described in **Box 9.17.**

Box 9.17: Causes of syncope.

Cardiac causes:
- **Cardiac arrhythmias:** Ventricular tachycardia, paroxysmal supraventricular tachycardia, long QT syndrome, Brugada syndrome, and bradycardia (Mobitz type II or 3rd degree heart block)
- **Structural cardiac or cardiopulmonary disease:** Cardiac valvular disease (AS, MS, and PS), obstructive cardiomyopathy, atrial myxoma, acute aortic dissection, pericardial disease/tamponade, pulmonary embolus/pulmonary hypertension, and acute myocardial infarction/ischemia

Noncardiac causes:
- **Neurocardiogenic syncope "vasovagal or vasodepressor syncope":** Classical vasovagal syncope, situational syncope, carotid sinus syncope, glossopharyngeal neuralgia, and micturition syncope
- **Orthostatic hypotension:** Autonomic failure, which may be primary (e.g., pure autonomic failure, multiple system atrophy, and Parkinson's disease with autonomic failure) or secondary (e.g., diabetic neuropathy)
- **Neurovascular syncope:** Vascular steal syndromes

(AS: aortic stenosis; MS: mitral stenosis; PS: pulmonary stenosis)

INVESTIGATIONS
- **Electrocardiogram (ECG):** Factors that suggest arrhythmia-induced syncope are prolonged intervals (QRS and QTc), severe bradycardia, pre-excitation, and evidence of myocardial infarction.
- Holter monitoring
- Echocardiography
- **Neurological:** CT brain and MRI, electroencephalography (EEG)
- **Laboratory evaluation:** Full blood count (FBC) and hematocrit, RBS, electrolytes, and pregnancy test
- Head up tilt table test.

COR PULMONALE
- Cor pulmonale is a Latin word means "pulmonary heart" and is defined as *symptoms and signs of fluid overload secondary to lung disease.*
- Cor pulmonale is a disease of the right ventricle characterized by its hypertrophy and dilation with or without failure secondary to diseases directly affecting the lung parenchyma, pulmonary vasculature, and chest bellows or central. This excludes pulmonary alterations produced due to diseases that primarily affect the left side of the heart (e.g., congenital heart diseases).

Etiology
Etiology of cor pulmonale is described in **Box 9.18.**

Clinical Features
Usually, the signs and symptoms are minimal except in the advanced stage. Mostly, the clinicians focus on the disease producing cor pulmonale rather than on cor pulmonale itself.

> **Box 9.18: Causes of cor pulmonale.**
>
> **Diseases of lung:** *Chronic obstructive pulmonary disease (COPD, e.g., chronic bronchitis and emphysema), pulmonary tuberculosis, interstitial lung disease, high altitude dwelling, cystic fibrosis, and pleural fibrosis*
> **Diseases of pulmonary circulation:** *Recurrent pulmonary thromboembolism, primary pulmonary hypertension, collagen vascular diseases, and chronic liver disease*
> **Diseases of thorax:** *Kyphoscoliosis, neuromuscular diseases, sleep apnea syndrome, and obesity*
> **Diseases of respiratory control:** *Brainstem lesions, central sleep apnea—Ondine's curse.*

Symptoms

Similar to those of right side heart failure: Fatigability, dyspnea on exertion, syncope, chest pain, palpitation, abdominal distension, edema of the lower extremity, exercise-induced peripheral cyanosis, and excessive daytime somnolence.

Signs

- Pedal edema
- Accentuated A wave of the jugular venous pulsations and prominent jugular V wave, indicating the presence of tricuspid regurgitation.
- Palpable left parasternal lift
- Accentuated pulmonic component of the second heart sound, right-sided S_4 heart sound, and ejection systolic murmur in the pulmonary area. In addition, there may be pansystolic murmur of tricuspid regurgitation or early-diastolic murmur of pulmonary regurgitation.
- **Overt right side heart failure:** A patient with chronic cor pulmonale reveals following signs:
  - Increasing peripheral edema
  - *Jugular venous pressure*: Raised and hepatojugular reflux positive
  - Tender hepatomegaly and enlargement of heart
  - Right ventricular third heart sound and a gallop rhythm, and right-sided fourth heart sound.

Management of Chronic Cor Pulmonale

These include—(1) general measures, (2) additional measures in cor pulmonale due to COPD, and (3) surgical treatment.

- **General measures:**
  - *Nonpharmacological treatment:*
    - Oxygen therapy
    - Phlebotomy
    - Noninvasive positive pressure ventilation (NIPPV)
  - *Pharmacological treatment:*
    - Diuretics.
    - Anticoagulation
    - Vasodilators
- **Treatment to decrease pulmonary hypertension:**
  - Treatment of underlying disease
  - Oxygen therapy is the most important treatment for reducing pulmonary hypertension. The long-term oxygen therapy retards its progression of pulmonary hypertension and oxygen therapy should be started, if the arterial oxygen tension is 55 mm Hg or less.
- **Treatment of right heart failure:**
  - Restriction of salt intake
  - *Digoxin*: Role not clear
  - Diuretics
- **Chronic anticoagulation** with Warfarin may benefit patients with cor pulmonale due to thrombo-occlusive pulmonary disease.
- **Surgical treatment:**
  - *Pulmonary embolectomy*: If pulmonary emboli are not resolved.
  - *Heart lung transplantation*: For primary pulmonary hypertension.

CIRCULATORY FAILURE: SHOCK

Definition

- Shock (acute circulatory failure, low-output state) is defined as a state with impaired cardiac pump, circulatory system, and/or volume that can lead to compromised blood flow to tissues.
- **Kumar and Parrillo (1995):** Shock is a state in which profound and widespread reduction of effective tissue perfusion leads first to reversible, and then if prolonged, to irreversible cellular injury.

Classification and Causes

Classification and causes of shock are described in **Table 9.42**.

Stages of Shock

Stages of shock are described in **Table 9.43**.

Pathogenesis of Various Types of Shock (Flowchart 9.5)

Types of Shock

- **Neurogenic shock:**
  - Neurogenic is the rarest form of shock. It is caused by the loss of sympathetic control of resistance vessels resulting in massive dilatation of arterioles and venules.
  - A type of distributive shock that results from the loss or suppression of sympathetic tone.
  - Causes massive vasodilatation in the venous vasculature—venous return to heart—cardiac output.
  - Most common cause is spinal cord injury above T6.

Clinical Features

Clinical features of various types of shock are described in **Table 9.44**.

- **Sepsis syndrome:** SIRS with confirmed infectious process associated with organ failure or hypotension
- **Two phases:**
  1. *"Warm" shock early*: Hyperdynamic response and vasodilation
  2. *"Cold" shock*: Late phase—hypodynamic response
- Decompensated state

Chapter 9: Cardiology

Table 9.42: Classification and causes of shock.

Type of shock and insult	Causes	Physiologic effect	Compensation
Cardiogenic: Heart fails to pump blood out	Myocardial infarction (MI), arrhythmia, aortic stenosis, mitral regurgitation, myocarditis, rupture of papillary muscle, and right ventricular infarction with excessive diuretic therapy	Decreased cardiac output	Baroreceptor mechanism. Increased systemic vascular resistance. Increased heart rate and contractility
Obstructive: Heart pumps well, but the outflow is obstructed	Extracardiac obstructive causes, such as pericardial effusion, tension pneumothorax, tamponade, and acute massive pulmonary embolism		
Hypovolemic: Heart pumps well, but *not enough blood volume* to pump	Hemorrhage, fluid loss (vomiting, diarrhea, and burns)		
Distributive: Heart pumps well, but there is *peripheral vasodilation*	Septic, anaphylactic, and neurogenic shock Pancreatitis, burns, and multi-trauma via activation of the inflammatory response	Reduced systemic vascular resistance	Increased cardiac output. Increased heart rate and contractility No change in neurogenic shock

Table 9.43: Stages of shock.

Stage	Pathophysiology	Clinical findings
Insult (initial stage)	*Example*: Splenic rupture with blood loss	
Preshock (compensatory stage)	Hemostatic compensation Mean arterial blood pressure (MAP) = Reduced Decreased cardiac output is compensated by increase in heart rate and systemic vascular resistance	MAP is maintained Heart rate will be increased Extremities will be cool due to vasoconstriction
Shock (progressive stage)	Compensatory mechanisms fail	MAP is reduced. Tachycardia, dyspnea, and restlessness
End organ dysfunction (refractory stage)	Cell death and organ failure	Decreased renal function, liver failure, disseminated intravascular coagulopathy, and death

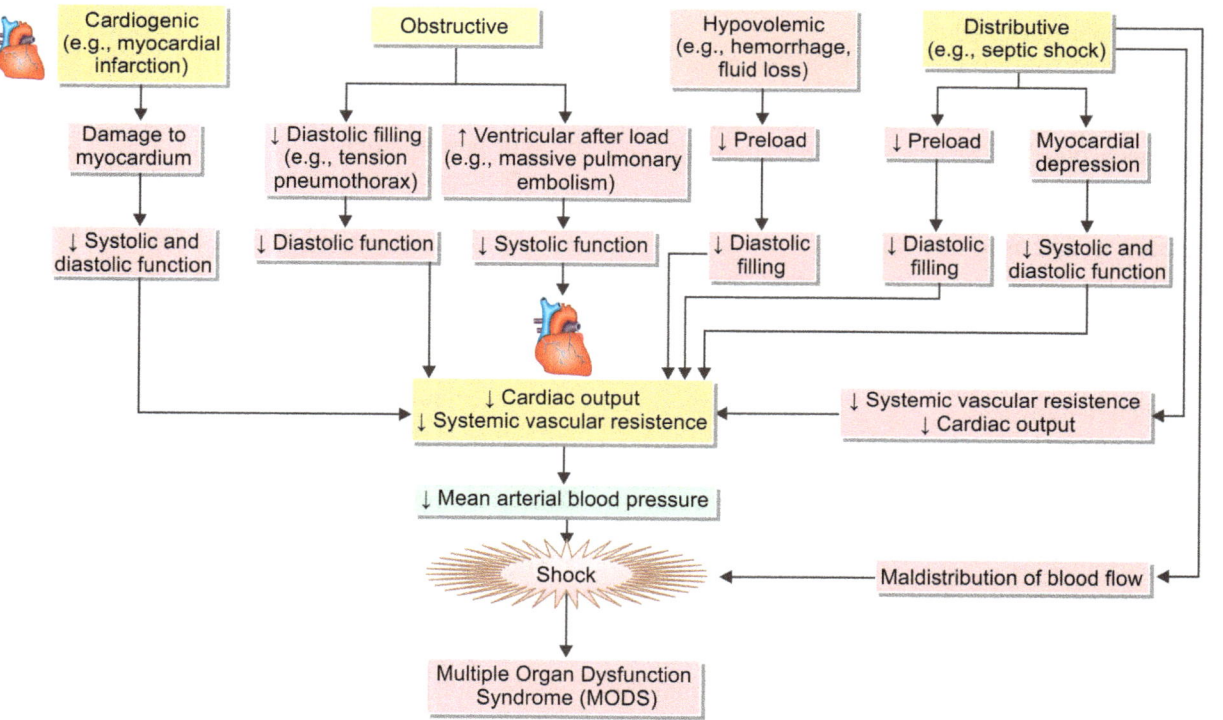

Flowchart 9.5: Pathogenesis of various types of shock.

Table 9.44: Clinical features of various types of shock.

	Hypovolemic shock	Distributive shock	Cardiogenic shock	Obstructive shock
Heart rate	Increased	Increased (normal in neurogenic shock)	Increased or decreased	Increased
Jugular venous pressure (JVP)	Low	Low	High	High
Blood pressure	Low	Low	Low	Low
Skin	Cold	Warm (cold in severe shock)	Cold	Cold
Capillary refill	Slow	Slow	Slow	Slow

- **Anaphylactic shock:**
  - A type of distributive shock that results from widespread systemic allergic reaction to an antigen.
  - This hypersensitivity reaction is *life threatening*.
- **Cardiogenic shock:**
  - The impaired ability of the heart to pump blood. Pump failure of the right or left ventricle.
  - Most common cause is left ventricular myocardial infarction (anterior). It occurs when > 40% of ventricular mass damage.
  - Mortality rate is 80% or more.

Management of Shock

Goals of management arem(1) treat reversible causes, (2) protect ischemic myocardium, and (3) improve tissue perfusion.

Patient Monitoring

- Initial assessment (ABC)
- **Airway:**
  - Does patient have mental status to protect airway?
  - Glasgow Coma Scale (GCS) less than "eight" means "intubate"
  - Airway is compromised in anaphylaxis.
- **Breathing:** If patient is conversing with you, airway (A) and breathing (B) are fine, place patient on oxygen.
- **Circulation:** Vitals (heart rate and blood pressure), two large-bore IV, start fluids (careful if cardiogenic shock), and put on continuous monitor.
  - In a trauma, perform ABCDE, not just ABC.
- **Deficit or disability:**
  - Assess for obvious neurologic deficit.
  - Moving all four extremities—yes/no pupils-reaction
  - Glasgow Coma Scale (M6, V5, and E4).
- **Exposure:** Remove all clothing on trauma patients.

General Measures

- **Optimize oxygen content:**
  - *Hemoglobin*: Check, if appears pale or anemic, check coagulation status.
  - *Oxygen saturation (SaO_2)*: Just a pulse oximeter tells you the SpO_2. Check SaO_2 on ABG.
- **Optimize cardiac output:**
  - Cardiac output (CO) = Stroke volume (SV) ×Heart rate (HR)
  - Stroke volume depends on preload, contractility, and afterload:
    - *Preload*: Look at response to fluid bolus.
      - If improves, BP could be suggestive of decreased preload (volume) and a reasonable contractility.
      - If no improvement or worsening, BP could be suggestive of a contractility problem or excess preload (volume) situation
      - Look at CVP
    - *Contractility:*
      - Check any history suggestive of ischemic disease or congestive cardiac failure (CCF)
      - Check ECHO and ECG
      - A high systolic pressure could be suggestive of good contractility.
    - *Afterload:*
      - Check ECHO, if suggestive of any obstructive features.
      - If peripheries cold could indicate increased vascular resistance
      - If peripheries warm could indicate vasodilation and decreased vascular resistance
      - A low diastolic blood pressure could indicate low vascular resistance.
      - A high-diastolic blood pressure could indicate increased vascular resistance.
- **Heart rate:**
  - If low, two possible interventions namely electric pacing or pharmacological intervention.
  - If high, two possible interventions namely electric cardioversion/defibrillation or pharmacological intervention.

Optimize Blood Pressure

- **Vasopressors and inotropes (sympathomimetic amines and vasopressin) (Table 9.45):**
  - Dobutamine alone is useful to augment cardiac output, if arterial pressure is near-normal. Otherwise, a combination of dopamine and dobutamine is preferred initial sympathomimetic agents.
  - *Vasopressin:*
    - Vasopressin constricts vascular smooth muscle directly via V1 receptors, and also increases responsiveness of the vasculature to catecholamines.
    - Vasopressin may also increase blood pressure by inhibition of vascular smooth muscle nitric oxide production.
  - *Milrinone* can be used to increase cardiac contractility
  - *Steroids* can be used in specific types as septic shock

Table 9.45: Common sympathomimetic amines used in shock.

Sympathomimetic amine (receptor activated) and dose	Actions
Dopamine (Dopaminergic + α + β_1) • 0.2–1 mg/min	Vasodilation of renal, mesenteric, cerebral, and coronary vessels Increase myocardial contraction, heart rate, and cardiac output. Rise in systolic blood pressure
Dobutamine (β_1) • 2–8 µg/kg/minute	Marked increase in myocardial contraction, minimal increase in heart rate, and minimal peripheral vessels vasodilatation
Noradrenaline (α + β_1) • 2–8 µg/minute	Increased myocardial contraction, heart rate, cardiac output, and rise in blood pressure Vasoconstriction in skin, muscle, and splanchnic beds. Coronary vasodilation
Adrenaline (α + β_1 + β_2) • 1–8 µg/kg/minute	Increased myocardial contraction, heart rate, and cardiac output. Rise in mean blood pressure. Vasoconstriction in most except skeletal muscles and coronary arteries. Vasodilatation in skeletal muscles and coronary arteries
Isoproterenol (β_1 + β_2) • 5–10 µg/min	Increased myocardial contraction, heart rate cardiac output, and rise in systolic blood pressure. Vasodilatation mainly in skeletal muscles
Phenylephrine (α_1) • 30–60 µg/min	Vasoconstriction

Treatment of Underlying Cause

- **Hypovolemic shock:**
  - Rapid replacement of blood, colloid, or crystalloid
  - Identify source of blood or fluid loss and treat it. Endoscopy/colonoscopy or angiography
- **Cardiogenic shock (Box 9.19)**
  Extra-cardiac obstructive shock:
  - *Pericardial tamponade*: Pericardiocentesis and surgical drainage (if needed)
  - *Pulmonary embolism*:
    - Heparin
    - Ventilation/perfusion lung scan
    - Pulmonary angiography
    - *Consider*: Thrombolytic therapy and embolectomy at surgery
- **Septic shock:**
  - Identify site of infection and drain, if possible
  - Antimicrobial agents (key rules)
  - ICU monitoring and support with fluids, vasopressors, and inotropic agents

Management of Neurogenic Shock

Hypovolemia: Treat with careful fluid replacement for BP<90 mm Hg, UO <30 cc/h:
- Observe closely for fluid overload
- Vasopressors may be needed
- **Hypothermia:** Warming. Avoid large swings in patient's body temperature
- Treat hypoxia

Box 9.19: Cardiogenic shock.

Left ventricular infarction:
- Intra-aortic balloon pump (IABP)
- Cardiac angiography
- Revascularization: Angioplasty and coronary bypass

Right ventricular infarction: Fluid and inotropes with PA catheter monitoring

Mechanical abnormality:
- Echocardiography
- Corrective surgery

- Maintain ventilatory support
- Alpha agonist to augment tone, if perfusion still inadequate:
  - Dopamine (>10 mg/kg per min)
  - Ephedrine (12.5–25 mg IV every 3-4 hour)
- Treat bradycardia with atropine 0.5–1 mg doses to maximum 3 mg, may need transcutaneous or transvenous pacing temporarily.

DEEP VENOUS THROMBOSIS

Common Sites of Venous Thrombosis

- **Deep venous system of lower extremities** (95% of pulmonary emboli arise from here):
  - Other systemic veins, especially pelvic veins
  - Right atrium, especially in patients with atrial fibrillation and cardiac failure
  - Right ventricle

Risk Factors

Risk factors of deep venous thrombosis (DVT) and embolism are mentioned in **Box 9.20**.

Box 9.20: Risk factors (predisposing factors) for venous thrombosis and embolism.

Primary (genetic)
- **Deficiency of antithrombotic (anticoagulant) factors** (e.g., Antithrombin III deficiency, protein C and S deficiency)
- **Increased prothrombotic factors** (e.g., activated protein C (APC) resistance (factor V mutation/ factor Va/ factor V Leiden).

Secondary (acquired)
- **Surgery:** Major abdominal/pelvic, hip/knee surgery, postoperative intensive care
- **Obstetrics:** Pregnancy, postpartum
- **Cardiorespiratory disease:** COPD, congestive cardiac failure
- **Lower limb conditions:** Fracture, varicose veins
- **Malignancy:** Abdominal/pelvic, advanced/disseminated cancers, concurrent chemotherapy
- **Antiphospholipid antibody syndrome**
- **Miscellaneous:** Increasing age, prolonged bed rest, prolonged immobilization, trauma

Clinical Features of Deep Venous Thrombosis

- Clinical detection is difficult, as DVT is silent in 50% of cases.
- Low-grade fever
- Pain, tenderness, warmth, and swelling of calf muscles
- "Homan's sign" is pain in the calf on forceful dorsiflexion of foot
- Later, there is cyanosis, edema, and venous gangrene of the affected limb

Wells probability score: It quantifies pretest probability of DVT.

Investigations

- D-dimer is elevated (>500 ng/mL) in most patients but is not specific.
- Doppler (duplex) ultrasonography is useful, but highly operator dependent.

Treatment of Deep Venous Thrombosis

- Bed rest with legs elevated to 15°
- Physiotherapy to legs
- Graduated elastic stockings (compression stockings) should be used routinely to prevent post-thrombotic syndrome
- Start treatment with heparin (as in pulmonary embolism) as well as warfarin and continue with warfarin
- Anticoagulation with warfarin should be maintained for 3–6 months
- Low molecular weight heparins (LMWHs)

PULMONARY EMBOLISM

Types

- Acute massive pulmonary embolism where the embolus lodges in the main pulmonary artery (may result in death)
- Pulmonary infarction from embolism to smaller pulmonary artery
- Recurrent silent pulmonary embolism resulting in chronic pulmonary hypertension and chronic right heart failure

Causes and Risk Factors

- Pulmonary embolism usually results from dislodgement of venous thrombi of the deep veins of lower limb and pelvis
- Causes of pulmonary embolism are the same as that for venous thrombosis
- "Economy class syndrome" (or traveler's thrombosis) is a rare condition
- The incidence through various studies appears to be in the range of 0.25/100,000 passengers in flights longer than 8 hours.

Clinical features of Pulmonary Embolism and Pulmonary Infarction

- Sudden onset of unexplained breathlessness is the most common symptom
- Retrosternal discomfort from right ventricular ischemia
- Syncope
- Pleuritic chest pain and hemoptysis in pulmonary infarction
- Supraventricular tachyarrhythmias
- Sudden onset or worsening of congestive heart failure
- Sudden deterioration in a patient with chronic obstructive lung disease.

Physical Findings

- A low-grade fever may occur with infarction
- Central cyanosis in massive pulmonary infarction
- Pleural friction rub and a small pleural effusion
- Tachycardia is the most consistent and most important physical sign
- Clinical evidence of DVT may be present

Wells Scoring System

To determine probability of pulmonary embolism, Wells scoring system is used.

Diagnosis

Electrocardiogram may show tachycardia, changes of acute pulmonary hypertension, and right ventricular enlargement with strain.

Other abnormalities include atrial fibrillation or flutter; an S wave in lead I, a Q in Lead III and an inverted T in lead III ($S_1 Q_3 T_3$ pattern).

Arterial blood gas studies may reveal hypoxemia, hypocapnia, and respiratory alkalosis.

The best screening test is a measurement of the D-dimer levels in the blood, spiral CT pulmonary angiography (CT-PA), perfusion scanning of the lungs, and pulmonary angiography.

A V/Q scan uses less radiation and contrast.

Management

Anticoagulation

- Unfractionated heparin is given at an initial dose of 5,000–10,000 units intravenously, followed by maintenance.
- Along with heparin, oral warfarin should be started with the intention of keeping the INT at 2.5–3.0, this may take 4–5 days after which heparin is stopped.
- Anticoagulation is maintained for at least 6 months.

Thrombolytic Therapy

- It is used in patients with major embolism with hypotension.
- **Agents currently used for thrombolysis are:**
  - Streptokinase
  - Urokinase
  - Tissue plasminogen activator (tPA)

Surgical Therapy

- Inferior vena caval filters to prevent recurrent emboli
- Pulmonary embolectomy

HYPERLIPIDEMIA

Hyperlipidemia is characterized by an abnormality in the lipid profile, consisting of a variety of disorders with raised total cholesterol, low-density lipoprotein (LDL), or triglyceride (TG), or conversely, lower levels of high-density lipoprotein (HDL).

Classification and Causes

- **Primary hyperlipidemia:** It is a genetic disorder of lipid metabolism (e.g., familial hypercholesterolemia). It is characterized by a genetic mutation, which causes impaired clearance of LDL from the circulation due to absence of LDL receptors.
- **Secondary hyperlipidemia:** These are characterized by hyperlipidemia secondary to a disease/disorder other than the genetic defect **(Table 9.46)**.
- Therapeutic drug classes, their effect on lipid profile and side effects are presented in **Table 9.47**.

Ezetimibe inhibits the absorption of cholesterol from the diet.
Omega-3 fatty acid is useful to reduce TG levels. Dose is 1–2 g/day.

Newer agents
- **Torcetrapib** is a cholesteryl ester transfer protein (CETP) inhibitors.
- **Proprotein convertase subtilisin/kexin type-9 (PCSK9) inhibitors:** Two PCSK9 inhibitors are approved.

Evolocumab is dosed at 140 mg subcutaneously every 2 weeks or 420 mg SC every 4 weeks. *Alirocumab* is dosed at 75 or 150 mg every 2 weeks or 300 mg every 4 weeks.

Management

- Therapeutic lifestyle changes
- **Patients with normal-weight, dyslipidemia (BMI 18.5–24.9 kg/m^2):** Focus on healthy eating and regular exercise.
- **Overweight and obese patients (BMI ≥25 kg/m^2):** Reduce caloric intake from fats, simple carbohydrate, and ≥30 minutes physical activity most days.
- Intake of soluble fiber to be increased (10–25 g/day).
- Diet (rich fruits, vegetables, nuts, whole grains, monounsaturated oils; low red meat, animal fat) reduces LDL 5–15% (ATP III TLC diet).
- **Aerobic exercise:** Running, walking, cycling, and swimming enhance weight reduction and facilitate achieving optimum lipid levels.

Table 9.46: Causes of secondary hyperlipidemia.

Increased LDL cholesterol level	Increased triglyceride level	Decreased HDL cholesterol level
Diabetes mellitus, hypothyroidism, nephrotic syndrome, and obstructive liver disease *Drugs:* • Anabolic steroids • Progestins • β-adrenergic blockers (without intrinsic sympathomimetic action) • Thiazides	Alcoholism, diabetes mellitus, hypothyroidism, obesity, and renal insufficiency *Drugs:* • β-adrenergic blockers (without intrinsic sympathomimetic action) • Bile acid binding resins • Estrogens • Ticlopidine	• Cigarette smoking, diabetes mellitus, hypertriglyceridemia, menopause, obesity, and uremia • Anabolic steroids • Beta-adrenergic blockers (without intrinsic sympathomimetic action) • Progestins

(LDL: low-density lipoprotein; HDL: high-density lipoprotein)

Table 9.47: Drug classes, their effect on lipid profile, and side effects.

Drug class	Total cholesterol levels	LDL levels	HDL levels	Triglycerides	Side effects
Bile acid binding resins	20%	10–20%	3–5%	Neutral	Unpalatability, bloating, constipation, and heartburn
Nicotinic acid	25%	10–25%	15–35%	20–50%	Flushing, nausea, glucose intolerance, and abnormal liver function test
Fibric acid analogs	15%	5–15%	14–20%	20–50%	Nausea and skin rash
HMG-CoA reductase inhibitors	15–30%	20–60%	5–15%	10–40%	Myositis, myalgia, and elevated hepatic transaminases

(LDL: low-density lipoprotein; HDL: high-density lipoprotein; HMG-CoA: β-hydroxy β-methylglutaryl-CoA)

OBJECTIVE-BASED SELF-EVALUATION

LONG QUESTIONS

1. Define angina. How do you differentiate it from non-cardiac chest pain? Discuss the management of stable angina pectoris.
2. Define and classify acute coronary syndrome. Discuss the management of acute inferior wall myocardial infarction.
3. List the indications and contraindication of thrombolysis in acute myocardial infarction. List the complications of acute myocardial infarction.
4. Classify hypertension as per JNC 8. List the causes of hypertension. Enumerate the complications of hypertension.
5. List antihypertensive agents with examples for each class. Enumerate hypertensive emergencies.
6. Discuss the pathogenesis, diagnostic criteria, and management of acute rheumatic fever.
7. Discuss the symptoms, signs, complications, and management of mitral stenosis.
8. Discuss the symptoms, signs, complications, and management of mitral regurgitation.

9. Discuss the symptoms, signs, complications, and management of aortic stenosis.
10. Discuss the symptoms, signs, complications, and management of aortic regurgitation
11. Discuss the etiology, clinical features, and management of subacute bacterial endocarditis.
12. Classify heart failure. List the causes of heart failure. Discuss the clinical features and management of acute left ventricular failure.
13. Discuss the etiology, clinical features, and management of ventricular tachycardia.
14. Discuss the etiology, clinical features, and management of atrial fibrillation.
15. Describe the steps in cardiopulmonary resuscitation.
16. Define and classify circulatory shock. Discuss the management of cardiogenic shock.
17. Discuss pulmonary thromboembolism under the following headings—risk factors, clinical features and management.

SHORT ANSWER QUESTIONS

1. Pathogenesis of atherosclerosis
2. Cardiac enzymes in ACS
3. Complications of acute myocardial infarction
4. Antianginal agents
5. Antiplatelet drugs
6. Prinzmetal angina
7. Modified Jones criteria
8. Secondary hypertension
9. Acute rheumatic carditis
10. Rheumatic chorea
11. Peripheral signs of aortic regurgitation
12. Differences between acute and subacute endocarditis
13. Culture-negative endocarditis
14. Modified Duke criteria
15. Bacterial endocarditis prophylaxis
16. Management of acute pulmonary edema
17. Classify cardiomyopathies
18. Classify congenital heart diseases with examples
19. Causes of syncope
20. Tetralogy of Fallot
21. Lipid lowering agents
22. Causes of secondary hyperlipidemia
23. Cor pulmonale
24. Causes of cardiac arrest
25. Eisenmenger's syndrome

MULTIPLE CHOICE QUESTIONS

1. Angina pectoris and syncope are most likely to be associated with:
    a. Mitral stenosis
    b. Aortic stenosis
    c. Mitral regurgitation
    d. Tricuspid stenosis

2. Which of the following is recommended for blood culture sampling in infective endocarditis?
    a. 2 culture sets separated by at least 1 hour over 24 hours
    b. 2 culture sets separated by at least 2 hours over 24 hours
    c. 3 cultures sets separated by at least 1 hour over 24 hours
    d. 3 culture sets separated by at least 2 hours over 24 hours

3. Antibiotic prophylaxis for dental procedure in infective endocarditis is indicated in all, *except*:
    a. Prosthetic valves
    b. Mitral valve prolapse without regurgitation
    c. Previous infective endocarditis
    d. Repaired congenital heart disease

4. Assays of which of the following biomarkers is most commonly used in the diagnosis of heart failure or ventricular myocyte damage?
    a. Brain natriuretic peptide (BNP)
    b. Atrial natriuretic peptide (ANP)
    c. Endothelin-1 (ET-1)
    d. Adrenomedullin

5. A patient comes with sudden respiratory distress. On examination, bilateral basal crepitations are present over chest suggestive of pulmonary edema. Further evaluation revealed normal alveolar wedge pressure. The likely cause is:
    a. Narcotic overdose
    b. Congestive heart failure
    c. Myocardial infarction
    d. Cardiogenic shock

6. Drug of choice for management of acute pulmonary edema is:
    a. Furosemide
    b. Hydrochlorothiazide
    c. Spironolactone
    d. Triamterene

7. An elderly patient presents with hypertension and diabetes, proteinuria without renal failure. Antihypertensive of choice is:
    a. Furosemide
    b. Methyldopa
    c. Enalapril
    d. Propranolol

8. A 40-year-old male patient presents to the emergency department with central chest pain for 2 hours. The ECG shows ST segment depression and cardiac troponins are elevated. He is administered aspirin, clopidogrel, nitrates and LMWH, in the emergency department and shifted to the coronary unit. The best recommended course of further action should include:
    a. Immediate revascularization with thrombolytics
    b. Early revascularization with PCI
    c. Continue conservative management and monitoring of cardiac enzymes and ECG
    d. Continue conservation management and plan for delayed revascularization procedure after patient is discharged

9. The most common source of pulmonary embolism is:
   a. Amniotic fluid embolism
   b. Calf vein thrombi
   c. Thrombi from large veins of leg
   d. Cardiothoracic surgery
10. A patient with acute inferior wall myocardial infarction has developed shock. Which of the following is the most likely cause of shock?
    a. Cardiac rupture
    b. Interventricular septal perforation
    c. Papillary muscle rupture
    d. Right ventricular infarction

=== ANSWERS ===

| 1. b | 2. c | 3. b | 4. a | 5. a |
| 6. a | 7. c | 8. b | 9. c | 10. d |

Renal System

CHAPTER OUTLINE

- Functions of Kidney
- Terminologies
- Nephritic Syndrome
- Nephrotic Syndrome
- Acute Kidney Injury
- Chronic Kidney Disease
- Urinary Tract Infection

FUNCTIONS OF KIDNEY

- *Excretion* of many metabolic breakdown products (including ammonia, urea and creatinine from protein, and uric acid from nucleic acids), drugs, and toxins
- Regulation of *water and electrolyte balance*
- Maintenance of *acid–base balance*
- *Reabsorption* of essential substances
- Secretion of hormones, such as *erythropoietin and renin*
- Metabolism of *vitamin D*
- Regulation of blood pressure

TERMINOLOGIES

Azotemia

- **Definition:** It is a *biochemical abnormality* characterized by an *elevation of the blood urea nitrogen (BUN) and creatinine* levels. It is mainly due to a decreased glomerular filtration rate (GFR).
- **Causes:** Azotemia can be divided into prerenal, renal, and postrenal.

Glomerular Filtration Rate

- Measurement of the GFR is required to know the exact level of renal function. It is necessary to calculate GFR when the serum (plasma) urea or creatinine is within the normal range.
- GFR for an average adult is about 125 mL/min. Formula for calculation of GFR is presented in **Table 10.1**.

Urine Volume

A healthy adult excretes about 600–2,000 mL of urine in 24 hours. Volume is measured by collecting 24-hour urine samples in a measuring cylinder.

Oliguria

Oliguria is decreased production of *urine usually <400 mL of urine per day or <17 mL per hour*. On an average diet, about 300–500 mL urine/day is required to excrete the solute load at maximum concentration.

Causes of oliguria: Causes are mentioned in **Table 10.2**.

Anuria

Anuria is defined as urine output that is <100 mL/24 h or 0 mL/12 h. Anuria more commonly suggests reduced production of urine or obstruction to urine flow from both

Table 10.1: Formulas used to estimate estimated glomerular filtration rate (eGFR)/creatinine clearance (CrCl).

MDRD	GFR in mL/min per 1.73 m² = 175 × Serum $Cr^{-1.154}$ × $age^{-0.203}$ × 1.212 (if patient is black) × 0.742 (if female)	
Cockroft–Gault	CrCl = [(140 – age) × TBW] / (S.cr × 72) (× 0.85 for females)	
The Schwartz equation: It is a simple bedside formula to estimate glomerular filtration rate (GFR) in children: $$\text{GFR (mL/min/1.73 m}^2\text{)} = \frac{\text{Height (cm)} \times 0.55}{\text{Serum creatinine (mg/dL)}}$$		
CKD-EPI	Male	141 × min (serum Cr/0.9,1) – 0.411 × maximum (serum Cr/0.9,1) × 1.209 × 0.993 Age × {1.159 if black}
	Female	141 × min (serum Cr/0.7,1) -0.329 × maximum (serum Cr/0.7,1) – 1.209 × 0.993 Age × {1.159 if black} × 1.018

(CKD-EPI: chronic kidney disease epidemiology collaboration; Cr: creatinine; MDRD: modification of diet in renal disease)

Table 10.2: Causes of oliguria.

Nonrenal conditions	Renal diseases
• Excess loss of fluid • Hypovolemia • Shock • Congestive heart failure • Cirrhosis • Pancreatitis and sepsis • Peritonitis	• Acute glomerulonephritis • Acute tubular necrosis (ATN) • Acute interstitial nephritis • Obstructive nephropathy

> **Box 10.1:** Causes of anuria.
>
> ❖ **Obstruction:**
>   - Bilateral ureteric obstruction
>   - Prostatic or urethral obstruction
> ❖ Renal stones
> ❖ Tumors
> ❖ **Renal ischemia:** Bilateral renal arterial or venous occlusion
>
> All causes of oliguria can lead to anuria.

kidneys (until proved otherwise). Bladder outflow obstruction must always be considered first.

Causes of anuria are mentioned in **Box 10.1**.

Polyuria

Polyuria is defined as *persistent large increase in urine volume of >3 L/day and 2 L/m² in children*. This term should exclude normal individuals who take large amount of fluid and, therefore, form large volumes of urine. Polyuria may be either due to—(1) increased urinary solute excretion (osmotic/solute diuresis) or (2) pure water diuresis.

Causes of polyuria are mentioned in **Box 10.2**.

Proteinuria

- Healthy adults may daily excrete <150 mg of total proteins and <30 mg/d of albumin.
- Proteinuria is defined as the *urinary excretion of >150 mg of protein/day*. It is one of the most common signs of renal disease. Pyrexia, exercise, and adoption of the upright posture (*postural proteinuria*) may also increase urinary protein output. Types of proteinuria and causes are mentioned in **Table 10.3**.
- **Amount of pathological proteinuria:** It may be "mild" (<1.0 g/day), "moderate" (1.0–3.5 g/day), or "massive"/"heavy" (>3.5 g/day).

Albumin: creatinine ratio:

Measurement of 24-hour urinary excretion rates provides the most precise measure of microalbuminuria. However, it is often difficult to obtain 24-hour urine, it is more convenient to measure urinary albumin:creatinine ratio in a random urine sample and generally *albumin:creatinine ratio (ACR)* of 2.5–20 corresponds to albuminuria of 30–300 mg daily respectively **(Table 10.4)**. The adequacy of the collection can be estimated by quantifying the 24-hour urine creatinine and comparing this value to the expected urine creatinine.

> **Box 10.2:** Causes of polyuria.
>
> 1. **Pathological polyuria:**
>   - *Increased excretion of solute (osmotic diuresis):* Glycosuria–hyperglycemia, administration of mannitol, and hypercalcemia. Urea diuresis and sodium diuresis.
>   - *Defective renal concentrating ability:* Diabetes insipidus, papillary necrosis, and diuretic phase of ATN
>   - *Failure of production of ADH:* Idiopathic (50%), mass lesion, trauma, and infection
>   - *Drugs/toxins:* Diuretics, lithium, and alcohol
> 2. **Primary (or psychogenic) polydipsia:** Excess fluid intake
>
> (ADH: antidiuretic hormone; ATN: acute tubular necrosis)

Table 10.3: Types of proteinuria and their causes.

Types of proteinuria	Causes
Transient proteinuria	Fever, heavy exercise, noradrenaline/albumin infusion
Orthostatic proteinuria	Usually in 2–5% of adolescents, rare above age of 30
Overflow proteinuria	Myeloma, hemoglobinuria, and myoglobinuria
Glomerular proteinuria	Primary glomerular diseases, secondary glomerular diseases, diabetic nephropathy, and hypertensive nephrosclerosis
Tubulointerstitial proteinuria	Heavy metal intoxications, autoimmune or allergic interstitial inflammation, and drug-induced interstitial injury
Postrenal proteinuria	Urinary tract infections, nephrolithiasis, and tumor

Table 10.4: Classification of proteinuria.

	Dipstick (not accurate)	Albumin–creatinine ratio (in mg/g)	Protein–creatinine ratio (in mg/g)
Normal to mildly increased KDIGO A1	Negative to trace	<30	<150
Moderately increased KDIGO A2 (previously microalbuminuria)	Trace to +	30–300	150–500
Severely increased KDIGO A3 (previously macroalbuminuria)	+ or greater	>300	>500
Nephrotic range proteinuria	+++ or ++++	>2,200	>3,500

Microalbuminuria

- Normal urine contains <30 mg of albumin/day (<20 µg of albumin per minute).
- **Definition:** Microalbuminuria is the *presence of albumin (small amounts) in urine about >30 to <300 mg/day*. It is defined as the persistent elevation of the urinary albumin excretion of 30–200 mg/L (or 20–200 µg/min) in an early morning urine sample. It indicates early and possibly reversible glomerular damage.
- It is so named because conventional dipsticks cannot detect albumin levels of 30–300 mg/day (if urine volume is normal). An increase in albumin excretion between these two levels is so-called microalbuminuria.
- **Significance:** The presence of albumin in the urine is a sign of glomerular abnormality.
  - **Diabetes mellitus:**
    - Microalbuminuria is an *early indicator of diabetic glomerular disease*. It is widely used as a predictor of the development of nephropathy in diabetics (raised fractional excretion of magnesium is a more sensitive

marker than microalbuminuria in detecting early diabetic nephropathy).
- In diabetic patients, presence of microalbuminuria is associated with *increased cardiovascular mortality*.
- **Essential hypertension:** In hypertensive patients, microalbuminuria predicts cardiovascular morbidity and mortality.
- **Normotensive individuals:**
  - *Risk marker for the presence of cardiovascular disease predicts progression of nephropathy* when it increases to frank albuminuria (>300 mg/day).
  - *Atherosclerosis:* Persistent microalbuminuria is also associated with an increased risk of atherosclerosis and cardiovascular mortality.

> **Treatment**
> ❖ Microalbuminuria can be reduced, and its progress to overt proteinuria can be prevented or retarded by *aggressive reduction of blood pressure (especially with ACE inhibitors or angiotensin receptor blockers) and control of diabetes mellitus*.
> ❖ Blood pressure should be maintained at or below 130/80 mm Hg in patients with diabetes or kidney disease.

Hematuria

Hematuria may be visible on gross examination and reported by the patient as bloody urine (*macroscopic/overt hematuria*), or invisible and detected on dipstick/chemical testing of urine (*microscopic hematuria*—three or more red blood cells per high-power field).

Sites and causes of hematuria are described in **Figure 10.1** and **Table 10.5**.

Glycosuria

❑ Blood glucose level varies between 70 and 120 mg/dL. This may increase to 120–160 mg/dL after a meal. Normally, all the glucose in the blood is filtered through the glomerulus and reabsorbed at the proximal tubules.

Table 10.5: Probable site of bleeding and its features.

Probable sites of bleeding	Suggestive features
Urethra	Blood is seen at the start of voiding and then the urine becomes clear
Urinary bladder or above	Blood diffusely presents throughout the urine
Glomerular origin	• Cola-colored urine • Red-cell casts (glomerulonephritis) • Dysmorphic erythrocytes (irregular outer cell membrane) • Acanthocytes (erythrocytes with one or more membrane protrusions of variable size and shape)
Renal pelvis and lower urinary tract	Pink- or red-colored urine
Prostate or bladder base	Blood only at the end of micturition
Lower urinary tract origin	• Isomorphic erythrocytes in urine • Microscopic clots of clumped erythrocytes in urine

❑ If the renal threshold (the lowest blood glucose level that will result in glycosuria) is exceeded (usually >180–200 mg/dL), the excess glucose will not be reabsorbed into the blood and will be eliminated in the urine as in cases of diabetes mellitus. The presence of detectable amounts of *glucose in urine* is termed *glycosuria*.

GLOMERULAR DISEASES

GLOMERULONEPHRITIS (GN)

Inflammation of glomeruli and *most are* due to an *immunologically mediated injury*.

Causes of GN are mentioned in **Box 10.3**.

> **Box 10.3:** Causes of glomerular diseases.
>
> ❖ **Primary glomerulonephritis/glomerulopathies:**
>   ❑ *Acute proliferative glomerulonephritis*: Postinfectious and others
>   ❑ Rapidly progressive (crescentic) glomerulonephritis
>   ❑ Minimal-change disease
>   ❑ Membranous glomerulopathy
>   ❑ Membranoproliferative glomerulonephritis
>   ❑ Focal segmental glomerulosclerosis
>   ❑ IgA nephropathy
>   ❑ Chronic glomerulonephritis
> ❖ **Systemic diseases with glomerular involvement:**
>   ❑ *Systemic immunological diseases*: Systemic lupus erythematosus
>   ❑ *Metabolic diseases*: Diabetes mellitus
>   ❑ *Vasculitis*: Microscopic polyarteritis/polyangiitis, Wegener granulomatosis, Henoch–Schonlein purpura
>   ❑ Amyloidosis
>   ❑ Goodpasture syndrome
>   ❑ Bacterial endocarditis
> ❖ **Hereditary disorders:**
>   ❑ Alport syndrome
>   ❑ Thin basement membrane disease
>   ❑ Fabry disease

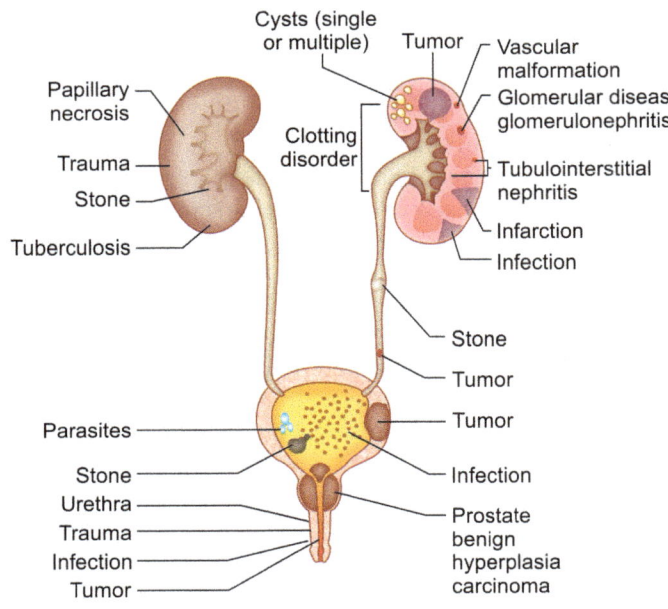

Fig. 10.1: Sites and common causes of bleeding from the urinary tract.

Pathogenesis

The main mechanism is antibody-mediated glomerular injury.

- **Immune complex mediated:**
  - Glomerular injury develops due to deposition of *circulating antigen–antibody complexes* (immune complexes) in the glomerulus. There is trapping of circulating antigen–antibody complexes within glomeruli, which results in glomerular damage. The antibodies are not against any of glomerular constituents, and the immune complexes localize within the glomeruli.
  - The antigen may be exogenous (e.g., bacteria as in post-streptococcal glomerulonephritis (PSGN) or endogenous (e.g., antibodies to host DNA in patients with SLE).
- **Antiglomerular basement membrane (GBM) antibody-induced GN:** It develops due to injury by antibodies to the insoluble *fixed (intrinsic) glomerular basement antigens*. Anti-GBM antibody-induced GN is responsible for <5% of cases of GN. This type of injury is caused due to antibodies, which are produced against intrinsic fixed antigens (that are normal components) of the GBM proper.

Characteristics of acute nephritic syndrome are presented in **Box 10.4**.

> **Terms used in glomerular diseases:**
> - **Focal:** Some glomeruli, but not all show the lesion
> - **Diffuse (global):** Most of the glomeruli (>75%) show the lesion
> - **Segmental:** Only a part of the glomerulus is affected (most focal lesions are also segmental, e.g., focal segmental glomerulosclerosis).
> - **Proliferative:** Increase in cell numbers due to hyperplasia of one or more of the resident glomerular cells with or without inflammation.
> - **Membranous:** Capillary wall thickening due to deposition of immune deposits or alterations in basement membrane.
> - **Crescent formation:** Proliferation of parietal epithelial cell with mononuclear cell infiltration in Bowman's space.

POST-STREPTOCOCCAL (POSTINFECTIOUS) GLOMERULONEPHRITIS

Post-streptococcal glomerulonephritis (PSGN) is specific subtype of postinfectious GN. It is common in developing countries and one of the common causes of *acute nephritic syndrome*.

Age group: Most frequently seen in *children between 6 and 10 years* of age, but may be developed in adults.

> **Box 10.4: Characteristics of acute nephritic syndrome.**
> - *Hematuria* (gross or microscopic)
> - *Red cell casts in the urine*
> - *Azotemia* (temporary)
> - *Temporary oliguria* (due to decreased glomerular filtration rate)
> - *Hypertension*
> - *Proteinuria**
> - *Edema**(periorbital, leg, or sacral)

*Not as severe as in nephrotic syndrome.

Etiology and Pathogenesis

- The *primary Streptococcal infection* usually involves the *pharynx* (pharyngitis) or the *skin* (impetigo/pyoderma). Skin infections are usually associated with overcrowding and poor hygiene.
- Only certain strains of *Group A β-hemolytic streptococci* are nephritogenic. More than 90% are due to *types 12, 4, and 1*.
- It is commonly associated with poor personal hygiene, overcrowding, and skin diseases, such as scabies.
- *It is an immunologically-mediated disease* and *evidences to support* this are:
  - *Latent period:* It manifests usually after a latent period of *1–4 weeks* following primary streptococcal infection. Cutaneous infections are associated with longer latent period. This latent period is compatible with the time required for the production of antibodies and the immune complex formation.
  - *Antibodies against streptococcal antigens:* Majority of patients show increased titers of antibodies against one or more streptococcal antigens. These antibodies include—antistreptolysin O, antideoxyribonuclease B (anti-DNase B), antistreptokinase, antihyaluronidase, and antinicotinyl adenine dinucleotidase.
  - *Hypocomplementemia:* Immune complexes activate and utilize complement components and more than 90% of patients reveal decreased complement (C3 and C4) levels in the blood (hypocomplementemia).
  - *Immune-complex deposits:* Electron microscopy shows glomeruli with electron-dense deposits of immune complexes.
  - Immunofluorescence shows granular fluorescence to the immune deposits.
  - *Streptococcal antigens in the glomeruli:* Many *cationic antigens* unique to nephritogenic strains of streptococci can be demonstrated in the glomeruli. Examples are nephritis-associated streptococcal plasmin receptor (NAPlr), streptococcal pyrogenic exotoxin B (SpeB), and its zymogen precursor (zSpeB).

Clinical Features

- Onset is often abrupt.
- Usually, the affected child suddenly develops *malaise, fever, nausea, oliguria, and hematuria* (characteristically, urine appears *smoky or red or cola-colored urine*) 1–4 weeks after recovery from a sore throat.
- *Periorbital edema* (causes puffiness of face) and *mild-to-moderate hypertension* are usually observed. Edema initially appears in areas of low tissue pressure (periorbital areas), followed by involvement of dependent portions of the body, and may be associated with ascites and/or pleural effusion.
- In adults, clinical features are atypical. They may present with the sudden appearance of *hypertension or edema, and elevation of blood urea nitrogen (BUN)*.

Investigations

Investigations are described in **Table 10.6**.

Table 10.6: Various laboratory findings in acute post-streptococcal (postinfectious) glomerulonephritis (PSGN).

Blood findings	Urinary findings

• Raised *antistreptococcal antibody*, titers, e.g., antistreptolysin O (ASO) titer
• Significant *reduction in serum concentration of complement* (C3) components
• *Urea and creatinine*: May be elevated and indicates renal impairment
	• Oliguria
	• Mild (variable degree) *proteinuria* (usually <1 g/day)
	• *Hematuria* (smoky or cola-colored urine)
	• Urine microscopy:
	  ▪ Red cells (particularly dysmorphic, i.e., distorted and fragmented red cells)
	  ▪ Red cell casts

Renal biopsy: Diffuse acute inflammation in the glomerulus with neutrophils and deposition of immunoglobulin (IgG) and complement. Electron microscopy shows electron-dense deposits in the subepithelial aspects of the capillary walls.

Management/treatment:
- *Supportive treatment during acute PSGN:* These include *rest, salt restriction, diuretics, and antihypertensives*
- *Dialysis* is necessary when there is severe oliguria, fluid overload, and hyperkalemia.
- *Steroids and cytotoxic drugs are of no value.* However, if recovery is slow or if RPGN develops, corticosteroids (methylprednisolone) may be of some help.

Complications
1. Rapidly progressive glomerulonephritis (RPGN)
2. Pulmonary edema
3. Hypertensive encephalopathy
4. Renal failure

Prognosis
Majority of patients with the epidemic form of PSGN have an *excellent prognosis*.
- **Children:** *Prognosis is good* and more than 95% totally recover. Minority may develop a rapidly progressive glomerulonephritis.
- **Adults:** *Less benign.* They may recover promptly or develop rapidly progressive GN or progress to chronic GN (hypertension and/or renal impairment).

Prevention
Pharyngitis caused by *Streptococci* should be treated promptly by antibiotics, which protects against development of GN.

Rapidly Progressive Glomerulonephritis/Crescentic Glomerulonephritis
Rapidly progressive glomerulonephritis is a *syndrome*, characterized by *rapid and progressive loss of renal function* (usually a 50% reduction in the GFR within 3 months) associated with *severe oliguria and signs of nephritic syndrome*. If not treated, death occurs due to renal failure within weeks to months. Histologically, it is characterized by *extensive crescents* (usually >50%).

NEPHROTIC SYNDROME
Features of nephrotic syndrome are mentioned in **Box 10.5**.

Box 10.5: Characteristics of nephrotic syndrome.
- Massive/heavy proteinuria (>3.5 g of protein/24 hours)
- Hypoalbuminemia
- Generalized edema
- Hyperlipidemia and lipiduria

Causes of Nephrotic Syndrome (Box 10.6)

☐ **Minimal change disease:**
- Minimal change disease (MCD) is named so because the *glomerular changes* are *absent or minimal and glomeruli appear normal under light microscopy*. But under electron microscopy, it shows *diffuse effacement (loss) of foot processes* of visceral epithelial cells (podocytes).
- MCD is the *major cause of nephrotic syndrome in children (80%), but it is less common in adults (20%)*.

☐ **Age:** Peak incidence between 2 and 6 years of age.

☐ **Focal and segmental glomerulosclerosis (FSGS):**
- FSGS is characterized by the *sclerosis* that *involves only part of the capillary tuft* (i.e., segmental) *of some glomeruli* (i.e., focal).
- It accounts for about *one-third of cases of nephrotic syndrome in adults*.
- It usually manifests as nephrotic syndrome or heavy proteinuria, hypertension, renal insufficiency, and occasionally hematuria.

☐ **Membranous nephropathy:**
- It is characterized by *uniform diffuse thickening of the glomerular capillary wall*. This is due to the accumulation of *electron-dense deposits along the subepithelial side* of the glomerular basement membrane.

Box 10.6: Causes of nephrotic syndrome.

A. **Primary (idiopathic) glomerular disease:**
  ☐ Membranous glomerulopathy (~30% in adults)
  ☐ Minimal change disease (~65% in children)
  ☐ Focal segmental glomerulosclerosis (~35% in adults)
  ☐ Membranoproliferative glomerulonephritis
  ☐ IgA nephropathy
  ☐ Mesangial proliferative

B. **Infection related:**
  ☐ Malaria (quartan malaria)
  ☐ Infective endocarditis
  ☐ Hepatitis B and C
  ☐ HIV
  ☐ Syphilis

C. **Systemic diseases:**
  ☐ Diabetes mellitus
  ☐ Amyloidosis
  ☐ Systemic lupus erythematosus
  ☐ Polyarteritis nodosa
  ☐ Wegener's granulomatosis

D. **Drug and toxins:** Penicillamine, gold, street heroin, and captopril

E. **Malignancy:**
  ☐ Carcinoma
  ☐ Melanoma
  ☐ Hodgkin's disease, chronic lymphatic leukemia

F. **Others:** Bee-sting allergy and hereditary nephritis

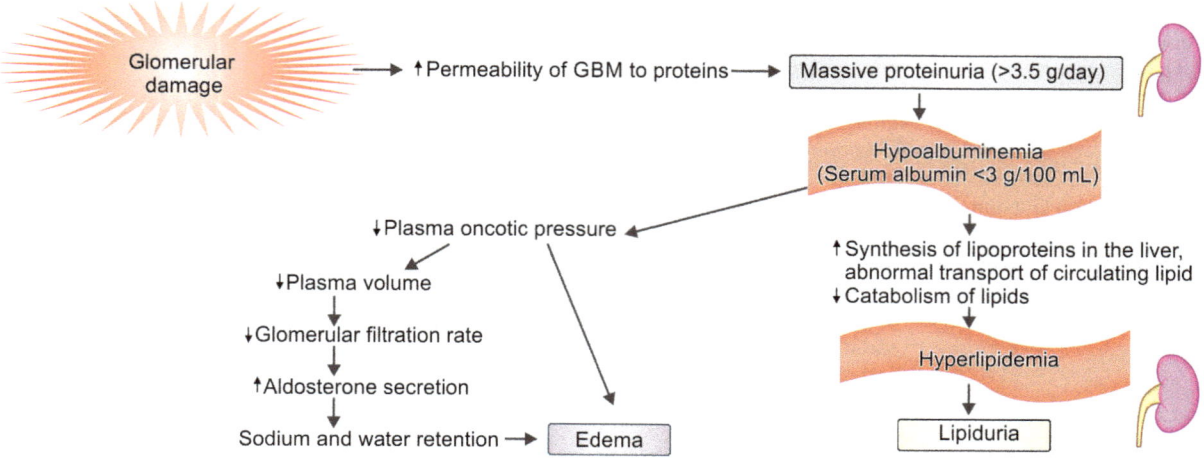

Fig. 10.2: Various characteristic features of nephrotic syndrome and its mechanism.
(GBM: glomerular basement membrane)

- It is a common cause (~30%) of the nephrotic syndrome in adults.
- *Gender and age:* Male predominance and high incidence between 30 and 50 years of age.

Pathophysiology (Fig. 10.2)

☐ *Massive proteinuria* is characterized by *daily loss of 3.5 g or more of protein* (less in children) in the *urine*.
  - Normally, the glomerular capillary wall acts as a size and charge-dependent barrier for the plasma filtrate.
  - Proteinuria in nephrotic syndrome is due to *increased permeability of glomerular capillary wall to plasma proteins*. This increased permeability is due to glomerular inflammation, change in the surface electrical charge, and an alteration in the pore size.

Table 10.7: Consequences of protein loss.

Nature of protein loss	Consequences
Hypoalbuminemia	• Edema and may also produce pleural effusion and ascites. Subungual edema may manifest as parallel white lines in the fingernail beds • Increased susceptibility to infections
Urinary losses of plasma proteins, such as thyroxin-binding globulin	Abnormalities in thyroid function tests, hypothyroidism
Deficiency of antithrombin III (due to urine loss)	Hypercoagulable state (consequences include DVT, pulmonary embolism, myocardial infarction, and stroke) and renal vein thrombosis
Loss of globulins in urine	Severe IgG deficiency leading to infections, such as spontaneous bacterial peritonitis
Loss of cholecalciferol-binding protein	Vitamin D deficiency state
Loss of transferrin	Microcytic, hypochromic anemia
Loss of metal-binding proteins	Metal deficiency, e.g., zinc and copper
Loss of drug-binding proteins	Altered drug pharmacokinetics

- The *major proportion of protein* lost in the urine is *albumin*, and rarely globulins. Consequences of protein loss are listed in **Table 10.7**.

☐ **Hypoalbuminemia:**
  - Massive proteinuria decreases the serum albumin levels (hypoalbuminemia).
  - *Hypoalbuminemia decreases the colloid osmotic pressure* of the blood resulting in a disturbance in the starling forces acting across peripheral capillaries.
  - The *hypovolemia also triggers the renin–angiotensin–aldosterone* system. This causes *increased reabsorption of sodium and water* by the kidney, resulting in edema.

☐ **Generalized edema:**
  - Soft and pitting
  - *Most marked in the periorbital regions* (**Fig. 10.3**) and dependent portions of the body.
  - Associated with pleural effusions and ascites.

☐ **Hyperlipidemia and lipiduria:**
  - *Hyperlipidemia:* Most patients with nephrotic syndrome have raised blood levels of cholesterol, triglyceride,

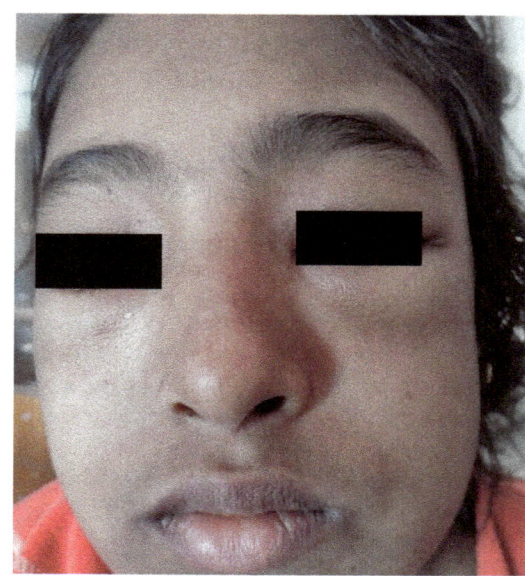

Fig. 10.3: Facial and periorbital puffiness in nephrotic syndrome.

very-low-density lipoprotein, low-density lipoprotein, lipoprotein a, and apoprotein. It *increases risk of atherosclerosis* and *cardiovascular disease*.
- *Causes of hyperlipidemia:* Increased *synthesis* of lipoproteins in the liver due to low-plasma colloid oncotic pressure.
- *Abnormal transport* of circulating lipid and *decreased catabolism* of lipids

☐ **Lipiduria:** Hyperlipidemia is followed by leakage of lipoproteins across the glomerular capillary wall → leaked lipoprotein is reabsorbed by tubular epithelial cells → then shed along with the degenerated cells → *appears in urine either as free fat or as oval fat bodies*.

Investigations in Nephrotic Syndrome

☐ **Urine examination:**
- *Proteinuria:* 24-hour urinary protein estimation.
- *Microscopy:* Red cells and red cell casts and waxy casts may be present. However, in minimal change disease, RBCs and red cell casts are not seen. It shows lipiduria.

☐ **Serum albumin:** *Reduced*
☐ **Serum cholesterol:** *Raised*
☐ **Renal biopsy:** *May be necessary* for histological diagnosis
☐ **Other investigations:** Depending on the suspected secondary causes, appropriate investigations are to be performed.

Management

General measures:
Measures to reduce proteinuria: These measures are necessary, if immunosuppressive drugs and other specific measures against the underlying cause do not benefit.
❖ *Angiotensin-converting enzyme (ACE) inhibitors and/or angiotensin II receptor antagonists*: They *reduce proteinuria* in all types of GN and also slow *the rate of progression of renal failure* by lowering glomerular capillary filtration pressure. Blood pressure and renal function should be monitored regularly during their administration.

Measures to control complications:
❖ *Treatment of edema:*
  ☐ Initially, it is treated by *dietary salt (sodium) restriction, rest and a thiazide diuretic* (e.g., chlorthalidone, bendroflumethiazide). The weight loss should not be more than 1 kg/day. Aggressive diuretic therapy may precipitate acute renal failure (ARF) due to reduction in intravascular volume.
  ☐ *If not responsive, furosemide 40–120 mg daily* with the *addition of amiloride* (5 mg daily) and serum potassium concentration should be monitored.
  ☐ *Gut mucosal edema* in nephrotic syndrome may *cause malabsorption of diuretics* (as well as other drugs). Thus, if there is *resistance to oral diuretic treatment, parenteral administration is required*.
  ☐ In diuretic-resistant patients and those with oliguria and uremia in the absence of severe glomerular damage (e.g., in minimal change nephropathy), edema may be treated by *infusion of salt-poor albumin as a temporary measure combined with diuretic therapy*. However, most of infused albumin will be excreted by the kidneys within 1–2 days.
  ☐ *Dietary proteins:* It is advisable to *take normal protein and should be about 0.8–1.0 g/kg*. A high-protein diet (approximately 80–90 g protein daily) increases proteinuria and may be harmful in the long term. However, malnutrition should be prevented.
❖ *Hypercoagulable state:* It develops due to loss of coagulation factors (e.g., antithrombin) in the urine and an increase in production of fibrinogen by liver. It *predisposes to venous thrombosis and thromboembolism*. Therefore, *avoid prolonged bed rest*. Long-term *prophylactic anticoagulant therapy* is desirable and it is indicated in patients who have already developed deep venous thrombosis or arterial thrombosis.
❖ *Lipid abnormalities:* They *increase in the risk of myocardial infarction or peripheral vascular disease*. Hypercholesterolemia is treated with an HMG-CoA reductase inhibitor and dietary restrictions of lipids.
❖ *Vitamin D supplementation:* To be given, if there is biochemical evidence of vitamin D deficiency.
❖ *Sepsis:* It is a *major cause of death* in nephrotic syndrome. The increased susceptibility to infection is partly due to loss of immunoglobulin in the urine. They are particularly *susceptible to pneumococcal infections* and pneumococcal vaccine should be given to these patients. Early detection and aggressive treatment of infections should be done. Vaccinations prophylactically are advisable.

Treatment of underlying cause:
Minimal change disease:
❖ *In children:*
  ☐ *Initial treatment* by *high-dose corticosteroid* therapy with **prednisolone** 60 mg/m^2 daily (up to a maximum of 80 mg/day) for a maximum of 4–6 weeks.
  ☐ Followed by alternate day, prednisolone at a dose of 40 mg/m^2 (1 mg/kg in adults) for further 4–6 weeks
  ☐ *More than 95% of children respond* to the above therapy. Children who respond within the first 4 weeks of corticosteroid therapy are termed as "steroid responsive". Those who relapse on withdrawal of corticosteroid therapy are termed as "steroid dependent".
  ☐ *Relapse:*
    – One-third of patients relapse on steroid withdrawal, and remission is once more induced with *steroid therapy*.
    – In patients who have frequent relapses or develop unacceptable corticosteroid side effects, long-term remission can be achieved by a course of *cyclophosphamide* 1.5–2.0 mg/kg daily is given for 8–12 weeks *with concomitant prednisolone* 7.5–15 mg/day. Steroid unresponsive patients may also benefit by cyclophosphamide. Not more than two courses of cyclophosphamide should be given because of the risk of side effects (e.g., azoospermia).
    – An alternative to cyclophosphamide is *cyclosporin* 3–5 mg/kg/day, (cyclosporin is potentially nephrotoxic).

- *Adults*: *Response rates are significantly lower* and response may occur late (12 weeks with daily steroid therapy and 12 weeks of maintenance with alternate-day therapy).
- *Prognosis*: *Excellent*, although it may show remission and relapses.

Focal and segmental glomerulosclerosis:
- *Steroids*: It is *beneficial in only 20–30% patients* and usually prednisolone is given in the dose of 0.5–2 mg/kg/day.
- *Cyclosporin* may be effective in reducing or stopping urinary protein excretion.
- *Cyclophosphamide, chlorambucil, or azathioprine* may be used *as second-line therapy in adults*.
- About *50% progress to end-stage renal failure*.

Membranous glomerulonephritis:
- *Oral high-dose corticosteroids are not useful for* producing either a sustained remission of nephrotic syndrome or preserving renal function.
- *Alkylating agents*: Cyclophosphamide and chlorambucil are effective. However, because of long-term toxicity, these drugs should be reserved for patients who have severe or prolonged nephrosis (i.e., proteinuria >6 g/day for >6 months), renal insufficiency, and hypertension. *Cyclophosphamide, cyclosporine, and chlorambucil* in combination with steroids may be helpful.
- *Anti-B lymphocyte therapy is more effective* against T lymphocytes than broad-spectrum immunosuppressive agents. Anti-CD20 antibodies (rituximab, which ablates B-lymphocytes) improve renal function, reduce proteinuria, and increase the serum albumin.
- *Prognosis*: Spontaneous remission may occur in 40%, 3–40% may develop repeated remissions and relapses, and 10–20% patients may develop progressive renal failure.

IgA Nephropathy (Berger's Disease)

It is characterized by *focal and segmental proliferative GN with predominant IgA deposition in the glomerular mesangium*.
- It occurs in *children and young males*.
- It presents with *asymptomatic/painless microscopic hematuria or recurrent macroscopic hematuria* generally within *1–2 days after an upper respiratory or gastrointestinal viral infection*.
- Proteinuria occurs and in 5%, it can be in the nephrotic range.
- Occasionally, it may present as acute renal failure (ARF) or nephritic syndrome.

Hereditary Nephritis or Alport Syndrome

- It is most common familial nephropathy, characterized by familial occurrence of *progressive hematuria, nephritis, and sensorineural loss of hearing*.
- It is common in females. Male patients develop severe renal disease with progressive renal failure occurring before the fourth decade. Most females have a normal lifespan.

ACUTE KIDNEY INJURY (ACUTE RENAL FAILURE)

Definition

Acute kidney injury (AKI) is a clinical syndrome, defined as an *abrupt, deterioration of kidney function*, which is usually, but not invariably, reversible over a period of days or rarely over a few weeks. The deterioration in renal function is sufficiently severe to result in retention of nitrogenous wastes in the body (uremia) and other waste products are normally cleared by the kidneys. The other term used for this is azotemia.

It is *usually* but not invariably accompanied by *oliguria*.

Acute kidney injury is a medical emergency. It may produce sudden, life-threatening biochemical disturbances. *AKI includes an increase in serum creatinine by ≥0.3 mg/dL (27 µmol/L) within 48 hours or an increase to ≥1.5 times the presumed baseline value that is known or presumed to have occurred within the prior 7 days, or a decrease in urine volume to <3 mL/kg over 6 hours [Kidney Disease: Improving Global Outcomes (KDIGO)-AKI]*.

Classification of AKI

RIFLE Criteria (Table 10.8)

- The distinction between acute and CKD or acute or chronic kidney disease cannot easily be done in case of uremia. Acute Dialysis Quality Initiative group proposed the *RIFLE* (*R*isk, *I*njury, *F*ailure, *L*oss, *E*nd-stage renal disease) *criteria* to classify AKI.
- These criteria indicate that an increasing degree of renal damage is of predictive value for mortality.

Acute Kidney Injury Network (AKIN) Classification (Fig. 10.4)

Acute kidney injury network has proposed a modification of the RIFLE criteria. It includes less severe AKI, a time constraint of 48 hours, and gives a correction for volume status before

Table 10.8: RIFLE criteria for classification of acute kidney injury.

Grade	GFR criteria	Urine output criteria
Risk (Stage 1)	Increased serum creatinine × 1.5 times within 48 hours	Urine output <0.5 mL/kg/h × 6 hours
Injury (Stage 2)	Increased serum creatinine × 2–3 times	Urine output <0.5 mL/kg/h × 12 hours
Failure (Stage 3)	Increased serum creatinine × 3 times or serum creatinine (acute rise of = 0.5 mg/dL)	Urine output <0.3 mL/kg/h × 24 hours OR Anuria for 12 hours OR Initiation of renal replacement therapy
Loss	Persistent AKI = Complete loss of renal function >4 weeks	
End-stage kidney disease	Persistent renal failure >3 months	

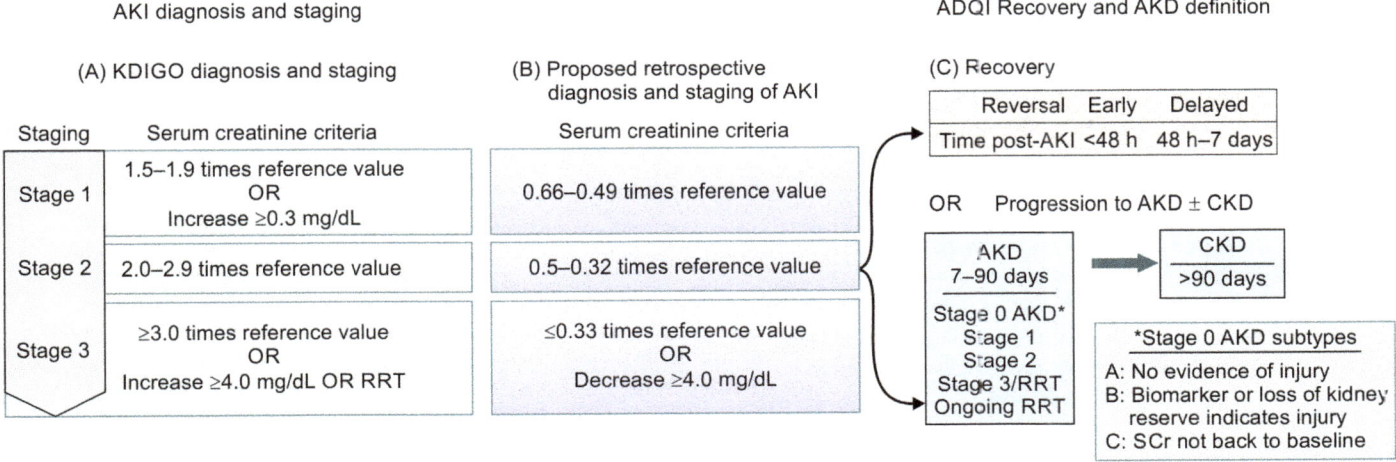

Fig. 10.4: Acute kidney injury network (AKIN) classification.

classification. According to this, AKI is classified into *three stages*.
- *Stage 1* is same as risk category of RIFLE with *addition of increase in serum creatinine by 0.3 mg/dL* within 48 hours.
- *Stages 2 and 3 are same as* injury and failure categories of RIFLE.

Causes

The etiology of AKI is diverse.
Classification and causes of acute kidney injury is discussed in **Figure 10.5 and Table 10.9**.

Clinical Features (Table 10.10)

General Symptoms
- Irrespective of the cause, ARF presents with symptoms related to uremia. These include *anorexia, nausea, vomiting, intellectual clouding, drowsiness, fits, coma, pruritus, hemorrhagic episodes* (e.g., epistaxis and gastrointestinal hemorrhage), and *dyspnea* due to fluid overload.
- *Physical findings* include asterixis, myoclonus, pericardial rub, and evidence of fluid overload in the form of edema, elevated jugular venous pressure (JVP), and crepitation.

Investigations

Serum creatinine and urea:
- The rate of rise in serum creatinine and urea is determined by the rate of protein catabolism (tissue breakdown).
- Raised serum creatinine and urea levels are the most consistent findings. In ARF, due to prerenal causes, there is a disproportionate elevation of serum urea in relation to serum creatinine.
  - *More than 50% loss of renal function must be lost before serum creatinine rises.*
  - *Serum creatinine does not reflect true GFR.* This is because several hours to days must elapse before a new equilibrium between presumably steady state production and decreased excretion of creatinine is established.

Other Investigations
- *Other biochemical findings* include *hyperkalemia, hypocalcemia, hyperphosphatemia, and hyperuricemia*.
- *Urine analysis:*
  - *In glomerulonephritis:* Proteinuria, red cells, and red cell casts
  - *RBCs/RBC casts:* Glomerulonephritis, vasculitis, malignant hypertension, and thrombotic microangiopathy
  - *WBCs/WBC casts:* Interstitial nephritis, GN, pyelonephritis, allograft rejection, and malignant infiltration of kidney
  - *Renal tubular epithelial (RTE) cells/RTE casts/pigmented casts:* Acute tubular necrosis (ATN), tubulointerstitial nephritis, acute cellular allograft rejection, myoglobinuria, and hemoglobinuria
  - *Granular casts:* ATN, GN, tubulointerstitial nephritis, and vasculitis
  - *Eosinophiluria:* Allergic interstitial nephritis, atheroembolic disease, pyelonephritis, cystitis, and GN

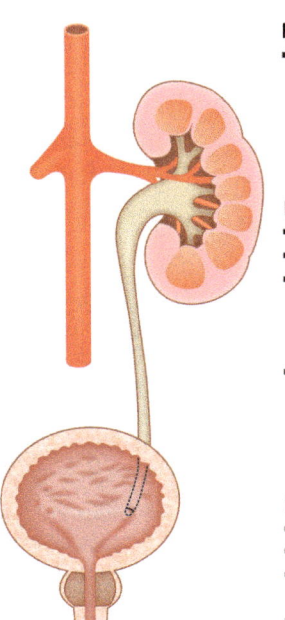

Prerenal
- Impaired perfusion:
  - Cardiac failure
  - Sepsis
  - Blood loss
  - Dehydration
  - Vascular occlusion

Renal
- Glomerulonephritis
- Small-vessel vasculitis
- Acute tubular necrosis
  - Drugs
  - Toxins
  - Prolonged hypotension
- Intestitial nephritis
  - Drugs
  - Toxins
  - Inflammatory disease
  - Infection

Postrenal
- Urinary calculi
- Retroperitoneal fibrosis
- Benign prostatic enlargement
- Prostate cancer
- Cervical cancer
- Urethral stricture/valves
- Meatal stenosis/phimosis

Fig. 10.5: Causes of acute kidney injury.

Table 10.9: Classification and causes of acute kidney injury.

Category	Abnormality	Possible causes
Prerenal	Hypovolemia	• Hemorrhage • Volume depletion • Renal fluid loss (over-diuresis) • Third space (burns, peritonitis, and muscle trauma)
	Impaired cardiac function	• Congestive heart failure • Acute myocardial infarction • Massive pulmonary embolism
	Systemic vasodilatation	• Antihypertensive medications • Gram negative bacteremia • Cirrhosis • Anaphylaxis
	Increased vascular resistance	• Anesthesia • Surgery • Hepatorenal syndrome • NSAID medications • Drugs that cause renal vasoconstriction (i.e., cyclosporine)
Intrinsic	Tubular	• Renal ischemia (*shock, complications of surgery, hemorrhage, trauma, bacteremia, pancreatitis, and pregnancy*) • Nephrotoxic drugs (*antibiotics, antineoplastic drugs, contrast media, organic solvents, anesthetic drugs, heavy metals*) • Endogenous toxins (*myoglobin, hemoglobin, and uric acid*)
	Glomerular	• Acute postinfectious glomerulonephritis • Lupus nephritis • IgA glomerulonephritis • Infective endocarditis • Goodpasture syndrome • Wegener disease
	Interstitium	• Infections (*bacterial and viral*) • Medications (*antibiotics, diuretics, NSAIDs, and many more drugs*)
	Vascular	• Large vessels (*bilateral renal artery stenosis and bilateral renal vein thrombosis*) • Small vessels (*vasculitis, malignant hypertension, atherosclerotic or thrombotic emboli, hemolytic uremic syndrome, and thrombotic thrombocytopenic purpura*)
Postrenal	Extrarenal obstruction	• Benign prostate hypertrophy • Improperly placed catheter • Bladder, prostate, or cervical cancer • Retroperitoneal fibrosis
	Intrarenal obstruction	• Nephrolithiasis • Blood clots • Papillary necrosis

(NSAIDs: nonsteroidal anti-inflammatory drugs; IgA: immunoglobulin A)

Table 10.10: Clinical features of acute kidney injury.

Type of acute kidney injury	History findings	Physical examination findings
Prerenal	• Volume loss (e.g., history of vomiting, diarrhea, diuretic overuse, hemorrhage, burns) • Reduced fluid intake • Cardiac disease • Liver disease	• Orthostatic hypotension and tachycardia • Cardiac disease • Poor skin turgor • Dilated neck veins, S3 heart sound, pulmonary rales, and peripheral edema • Ascites, caput medusae, and spider angiomas
Intrinsic renal:		
Acute tubular necrosis	History of receiving nephrotoxic medications (including over-the-counter, illicit, and herbal), hypotension, trauma or myalgias suggesting rhabdomyolysis, recent exposure to radiographic contrast agents	Muscle tenderness, compartment syndrome, and assessment of volume status
Glomerular	Lupus, systemic sclerosis, rash, arthritis, uveitis, weight loss, fatigue, hepatitis C virus infection, human immunodeficiency virus infection, hematuria, foamy urine, cough, sinusitis, and hemoptysis	Periorbital, sacral, and lower-extremity edema, rash, oral/nasal ulcers, and hypertension
Interstitial	Medication use (e.g., antibiotics, proton pump inhibitors), rash, arthralgias, fever, and infectious illness	Fever, drug-related rash (skin), and eosinophilia
Vascular	Nephrotic syndrome, trauma, flank pain, anticoagulation (atheroembolic disease), vessel catheterization, or vascular surgery	Skin changes, livedo reticularis, fundoscopic examination (showing malignant hypertension), abdominal bruits
Postrenal	Urinary urgency or hesitancy, gross hematuria, polyuria, stones, medications, and cancer	Bladder distention, pelvic mass, and prostate enlargement

- *Crystalluria*: Acute uric acid nephropathy, calcium oxalate (ethylene glycol intoxication), and drugs/toxins (acyclovir, indinavir, sulfadiazine, amoxicillin)
☐ **Proteinuria:**
- *Mild*—<1 g/day—ischemia or nephrotoxin-associated AKI
- *Moderate*—multiple myeloma and atheroembolism
- *Severe (nephrotic range) > 3.5 g/day*—glomerulonephritis, vasculitis, and toxins that affect both glomerulus and tubulointerstitium such as nonsteroidal anti-inflammatory drugs (NSAIDs), and minimal change disease
☐ **Electrocardiogram:** It may show features of hyperkalemia.
☐ **Chest radiograph:** It may show pulmonary edema and pleural effusion.
☐ **Others:**
- *In RPGN*: Systemic causes (e.g., Wegener's granulomatosis) must be excluded by appropriate investigations (e.g., cANCA). *A kidney biopsy may be necessary.*
- *In postrenal ARF*: Renal imaging by plain abdominal X-ray and ultrasonography may be useful.

- *Kidney injury molecule 1 (KIM 1):* Ischemia or nephrotoxin-associated AKI
- *Neutrophil gelatinase-associated lipocalin (NGAL)*: Cardiopulmonary bypass-associated AKI
- *Insulin-like growth factor-binding protein 7 (IGFBP7)*: Marker of development of severe AKI
- *Tissue inhibitor of metalloproteinase-2 (TIMP-2)*: Marker of development of severe AKI

Fractional Excretion of Sodium (FENa)

The ratio of sodium clearance to creatinine clearance increases the reliability of this index. However, it may remain low in some renal diseases. Fraction of filtered sodium load that is reabsorbed by the tubules—measure of kidney's ability to reabsorb sodium as well as endogenously and exogenously administered factors that affect tubular reabsorption.

It helps in differentiating between prerenal azotemia and ATN, but has limited role.

Complications of Acute Kidney Injury

Complications of acute kidney injury are discussed in **Box 10.7**.

Management
General measures and management of complications:
- **Fluid balance:** Advisable to *restrict fluid intake*—
  ☐ Amount of fluid to be given *depends upon* the *degree of edema, and fluid loss* through urine, gastrointestinal tract, and skin.
  ☐ Usually intake restricted to about *400 mL/day* in addition to the above-mentioned fluid losses.
- **Sodium balance:** *Sodium is restricted* to avoid volume expansion and overhydration—
  ☐ *Hyponatremia* is common and is usually *due to excessive fluid administration.*
  ☐ Hypernatremia may occur occasionally, due to excessive administration of sodium bicarbonate for correction of acidosis.
- **Potassium balance:** *Hyperkalemia is the leading cause of death* in ARF. Has to be treated with calcium gluconate, insulin-dextrose, nebulization with salbutamol, hemodialysis.
- **Acid–base balance:** In most patients, *acidosis* is of moderate degree and does not require treatment. However, in *advanced cases, intravenous sodium bicarbonate* may be necessary. Acidosis if accompanied by severe hyperkalemia and fluid overload is best treated with dialysis.
- **Calcium-phosphorus balance:** Both *hypocalcemia and hypercalcemia* are observed *in the maintenance phase* of ARF and are not serious clinical problems. *Phosphate retention* occurs in patients can be *controlled with aluminum hydroxide lanthanum carbonate, sevelamer, calcium acetate, or calcium carbonate* (bind phosphate within the GIT and eliminated in stool).
- **Diet:**
  ☐ Restrict dietary proteins to about 40 g/day. Suppress endogenous protein catabolism to a minimum level by giving as much energy as possible in the form of carbohydrates and fats. Patients treated by blood purification techniques are given 70 g or more protein/day.
  ☐ Hypercatabolic patients may *need higher nitrogen intake* to prevent negative nitrogen balance.
  ☐ Restrict the salt intake.
  ☐ *Vitamin supplements* are usually necessary.
- **Systemic complications of ARF:** *Infections* and *gastrointestinal bleeding* are two important complications—
  1. *Infectious complications* [very high (80%)] include pulmonary, urinary, and wound infections (in post-traumatic and postoperative patients). Infections should be treated promptly by *appropriate antibiotics.*
  2. *Gastrointestinal bleeding* (in 40% of patients) may prove fatal and treated by proton pump inhibitors and gastroprotective agents. Qualitative platelet dysfunction, which results in a hemorrhagic diathesis.
- **Use of drugs:** Great care is necessary in the use of drugs and nephrotoxic drugs should be avoided.

Treatment of the underlying cause of the AKI:
Identify the cause (by simple initial investigations such as ultrasound or may require additional investigations, including renal biopsy) and correct it, if possible.

Specific therapy:
- No specific treatment for ATN, other than restoring renal perfusion.
- *Intrinsic kidney disease may require specific therapy* (e.g., immunosuppressive drugs, such as corticosteroids and cyclophosphamide in some causes of *rapidly progressive glomerulonephritis*).
- "Postrenal" obstruction requires *urgent relief of obstruction*. Once the blood chemistry returns to normal, the underlying cause should be treated whenever possible.
- *Drug-induced* acute tubule-interstitial nephritis usually recovers after stopping the offending drug, but sometimes, short course of steroids may be helpful.
- *If conservative measures fail, dialysis and hemofiltration* may be necessary. These techniques purify blood and/or remove excess fluid. Main indications of dialysis and hemofiltration in ARF are listed in **Table 10.11**.

Box 10.7: Complications of acute kidney injury.

- *Metabolic*: Hyperkalemia, hypocalcemia, hyperphosphatemia, hypermagnesemia, hyperuricemia, and metabolic acidosis (increased anion gap)
- *Cardiovascular*: Cardiac arrhythmias, pulmonary edema, pericarditis/pericardial effusion
- *Gastrointestinal*: Gastrointestinal hemorrhage
- *Neurologic*: Encephalopathy, neuropathy, and seizures
- *Hematologic*: Anemia, bleeding—platelet dysfunction
- *Miscellaneous*: Infections (pneumonia, urinary tract infection, and septicemia)

Cause of death: Most common causes of death in ARF (in the absence of dialysis) are hyperkalemia and pulmonary edema, followed by infection and uremia.

Table 10.11: Indications of dialysis or hemofiltration in acute renal failure (ARF).

- Fluid overload refractory to diuretics and refractory pulmonary edema*
- Severe metabolic acidosis (pH <7.1)*
- Resistant hyperkalemia*
- Complications of uremia (e.g., pericarditis and encephalopathy, neuropathy)*
- Increased plasma urea (>180 mg/dL) and creatinine (>6.8 mg/dL)
- ESRD (end-stage renal disease)
- Severe biochemical derangement in the absence of symptoms (especially in an oliguric and hypercatabolic patients)
- Removal of drugs causing the acute renal failure (e.g., gentamicin, lithium, and severe aspirin overdose)
- Severe hyperphosphatemia (defined as >12 mg/dL)
- Tumor lysis syndrome
- Anuria for >12 hours

*Absolute indications

CHRONIC KIDNEY DISEASE

Chronic kidney disease (CKD) is previously termed chronic renal failure (CRF) or insufficiency.

Chronic kidney disease (CKD) refers to a spectrum of *long-standing* (more than 3 months), usually *progressive* processes associated with *irreversible worsening of renal function* and decline in glomerular filtration rate (GFR). *CKD spectrum ranges from abnormalities detectable only by laboratory testing to uremia.*

Revised chronic kidney disease classification based upon glomerular filtration rate and albuminuria KDIGO, 2013 is presented in **Figure 10.6**.

Causes of CKD

See **Table 10.12**.

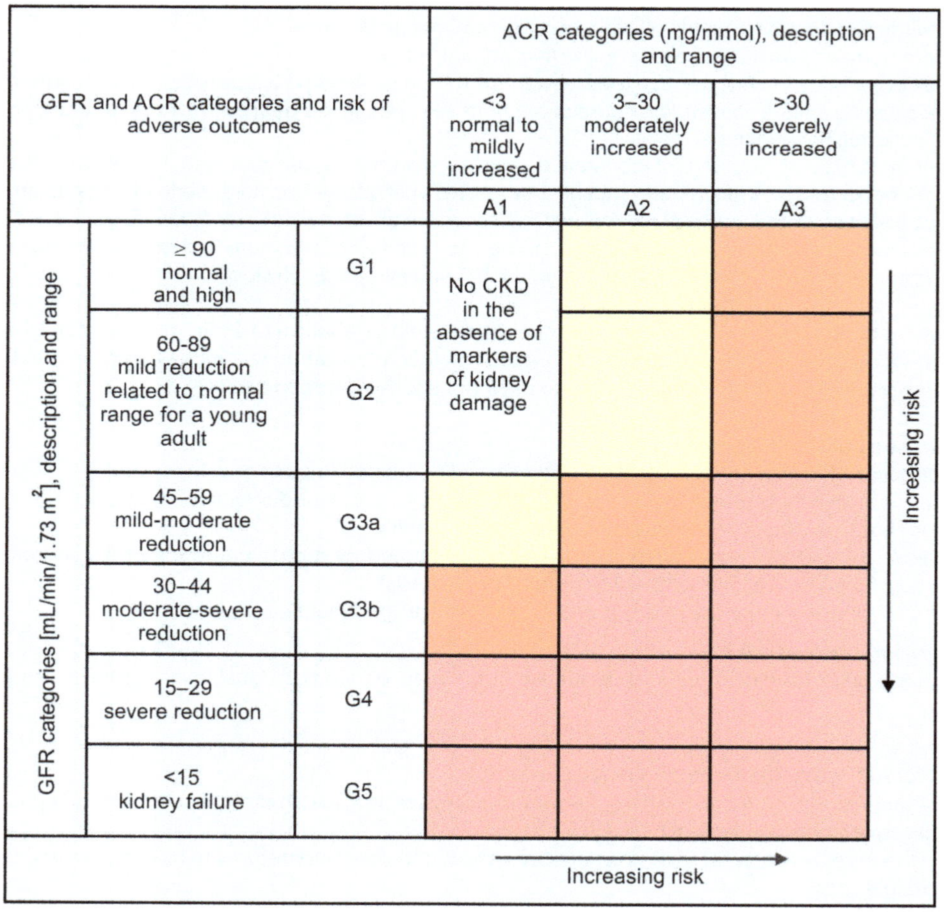

ACR categories (mg/mmol), description and range
GFR and ACR categories and risk of adverse outcomes
<3 normal to mildly increased
3–30 moderately increased
>30 severely increased
A1
A2
A3
GFR categories [mL/min/1.73 m2], description and range
≥ 90 normal and high
G1
60-89 mild reduction related to normal range for a young adult
G2
45–59 mild-moderate reduction
G3a
30–44 moderate-severe reduction
G3b
15–29 severe reduction
G4
<15 kidney failure
G5
No CKD in the absence of markers of kidney damage
Increasing risk
Increasing risk

Fig. 10.6: Revised chronic kidney disease classification based upon glomerular filtration rate (GFR) and albuminuria (KDIGO).

Table 10.12: Important causes of chronic kidney disease.

I. Glomerulopathies (GN)*:	IV. Obstructive*:
▪ Proliferative GN ▪ Crescentic GN ▪ Membranoproliferative GN ▪ Mesangiocapillary GN	▪ Calculus Tumors ▪ Retroperitoneal fibrosis Prostatic enlargement
II. Systemic and metabolic diseases: ▪ Diabetes* ▪ Systemic lupus erythematosus (SLE) ▪ Polyarteritis nodosa (PAN) ▪ Amyloidosis ▪ Gout	V. Vascular: ▪ Essential hypertension (accelerated)* ▪ Renovascular vasculitis (SLE, PAN, and scleroderma)
III. Interstitial: ▪ Chronic interstitial nephritis* ▪ Chronic pyelonephritis* ▪ Analgesic ▪ Tuberculosis ▪ Nephrocalcinosis	VI. Congenital: ▪ Polycystic kidney* ▪ Medullary cystic disease ▪ Alport syndrome

*Common causes of chronic renal failure

Clinical Features (Table 10.13 and Fig. 10.7)

Anemia: Various causes of anemia in CRF are listed in **Box 10.8**.

Metabolic bone disease: renal osteodystrophy:
The term "renal osteodystrophy" (bone mineral disorder) constitutes various forms of bone disease that may develop alone or in combination in chronic renal failure. It includes—(1) hyperparathyroid bone disease (osteitis fibrosa cystica), (2) osteomalacia, (3) osteoporosis, (4) osteosclerosis, and (5) adynamic bone disease.

Pathogenesis of bone disease (**Fig. 10.8**):
☐ Phosphate retention owing to reduced excretion by the kidneys release of fibroblast growth factor-23 (FGF-23) and other phosphaturic agents by osteoblasts as a compensatory mechanism. Actions of FGF-23 are:
  • Causes phosphaturia to normalize the plasma phosphate level.
  • It downregulates 1α-hydroxylase to reduce intestinal absorption of phosphate.
☐ Decreased production of the 1α-hydroxylase enzyme by the kidney results in reduced conversion of $25\text{-}(OH)_2D_3$ (25-hydroxyvitamin D) to the more metabolically active $1,25\text{-}(OH)_2D_3$ (1,25-dihydroxycholecalciferol). Its consequences are:
  • Decreased activation of vitamin D receptors (VDR) in the parathyroid glands leads to increased release of parathyroid hormone (PTH) causing secondary hyperparathyroidism.
  • Decreased intestinal absorption of calcium causes hypocalcemia, which leads in turn to increased PTH production by the parathyroid glands.
  • Phosphate retention also indirectly lowers ionized calcium and these together result in an increase in PTH synthesis and release. The raised serum phosphate combines with calcium in the extracellular space, causing ectopic calcification in blood vessels and other tissues.
  • PTH causes reabsorption of calcium from bone and increased reabsorption of calcium from proximal renal tubules.

Table 10.13: Clinical features of chronic kidney disease (CKD).

System	Clinical feature	Cause
Renal	Nocturia and polyuria	Impaired concentrating ability of kidney
Muscle	Generalized myopathy	Combination of poor nutrition, hyperparathyroidism, and vitamin D deficiency
Gastrointestinal	Malaise, loss of appetite (anorexia), nausea, vomiting, and diarrhea	Nitrogenous waste products
Metabolic	Paresthesia and tetany	Hypocalcemia
Endocrine	Loss of libido in both sexes • *Women*: Amenorrhea and menorrhagia • *Males*: Erectile dysfunction and oligospermia	Hypothalamic-pituitary axis dysfunction
Skeletal	Bone pain	Metabolic bone disease
Respiratory	Pleural effusion, interstitial lung disease, and calcification	Salt and water retention
Hematologic	*Symptoms due to anemia*: Fatigue and lassitude	Anemia is normochromic and normocytic type. Various causes mentioned in **Box 10.8**
Skin	Pruritus/itching, rash, and metastatic calcification	Retention of nitrogenous waste products of protein catabolism, hyperparathyroidism, and calcium-phosphate deposition
Immune system	Infections	Leukocyte functional defects and reduced cellular immunity
Cardiovascular	Atherosclerosis, heart failure, and hypertension	Hypertension, homocysteinemia, and calcification of heart valves
Neurologic	Peripheral neuropathy, mental slowing, clouding of consciousness and seizures, myoclonic twitching, coma, restless leg syndrome, or sensory deficits	Uremic toxins
Serosal inflammation	Pericardial or pleural pain and fluid, peritoneal fluid	Water retention

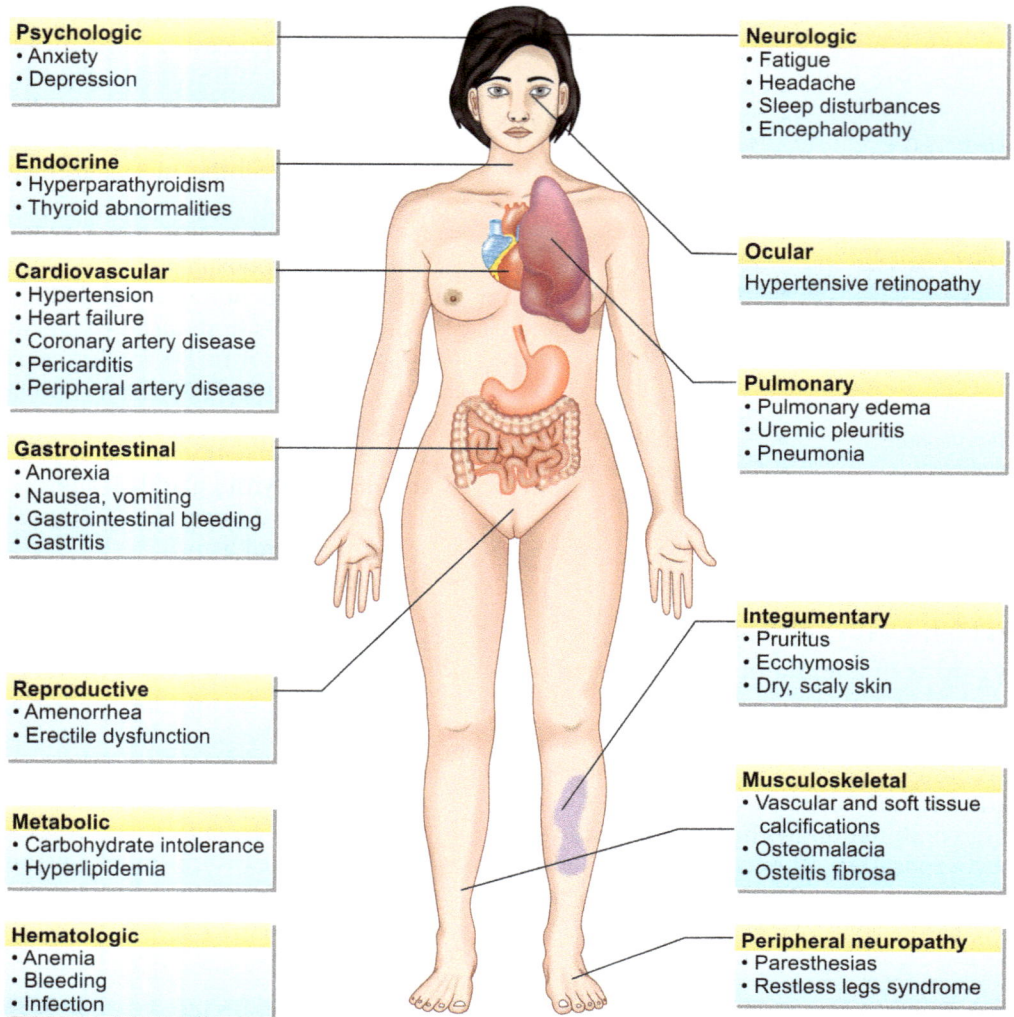

Fig. 10.7: Various clinical manifestations of chronic kidney disease (CKD).

Box 10.8: Causes of anemia in CRF.

- Deficiency of erythropoietin (most important)
- Toxic effects of uremia on bone marrow precursor cells
- Bone marrow fibrosis secondary to hyperparathyroidism
- **Deficiency of hematinic:** Iron, vitamin B_{12}, and folate because of reduced dietary intake due to anorexia. Intestinal absorption of iron is also impaired.
- **Increased red cell destruction:** Abnormal red cell membranes
- **Increased blood loss:**
  - Occult gastrointestinal bleeding
  - Blood sampling
  - Blood loss during hemodialysis
  - Capillary fragility
  - Due to platelet dysfunction and capillary fragility

(CRF: chronic renal failure)

- This prevents hypocalcemia induced by $1,25\text{-}(OH)_2D_3$ deficiency and phosphate retention.
- *Secondary hyperparathyroidism* causes increased osteoclastic activity, cyst formation, and bone marrow fibrosis (osteitis fibrosa cystica).
- Long-standing secondary hyperparathyroidism finally causes hyperplasia of the glands with autonomous or *"tertiary" hyperparathyroidism.*
- **Osteomalacia:** It is due to impaired mineralization of osteoid caused by deficiency $1,25\text{-}(OH)_2D_3$ and hypocalcemia.
- **Osteosclerosis:** Literally means "hardening of bone" characterized by increased bone density and is due to the direct result of long-standing parathyroid hormone excess. Alternating bands of sclerotic and porotic bone in the spine give rise to a characteristic *"rugger jersey"* appearance on X-ray.
- *Osteoporosis* is probably related to malnutrition and is commonly found in CRF, often after transplantation and the use of corticosteroids.
- *Adynamic bone disease* is the condition in which both bone formation and resorption are depressed.

Gastrointestinal complications: (1) Reduced gastric emptying and increased risk of reflux esophagitis, (2) increased risk of peptic ulceration and acute pancreatitis, and (3) constipation [especially in patients on continuous ambulatory peritoneal dialysis (CAPD)], and (4) gastrointestinal bleed.

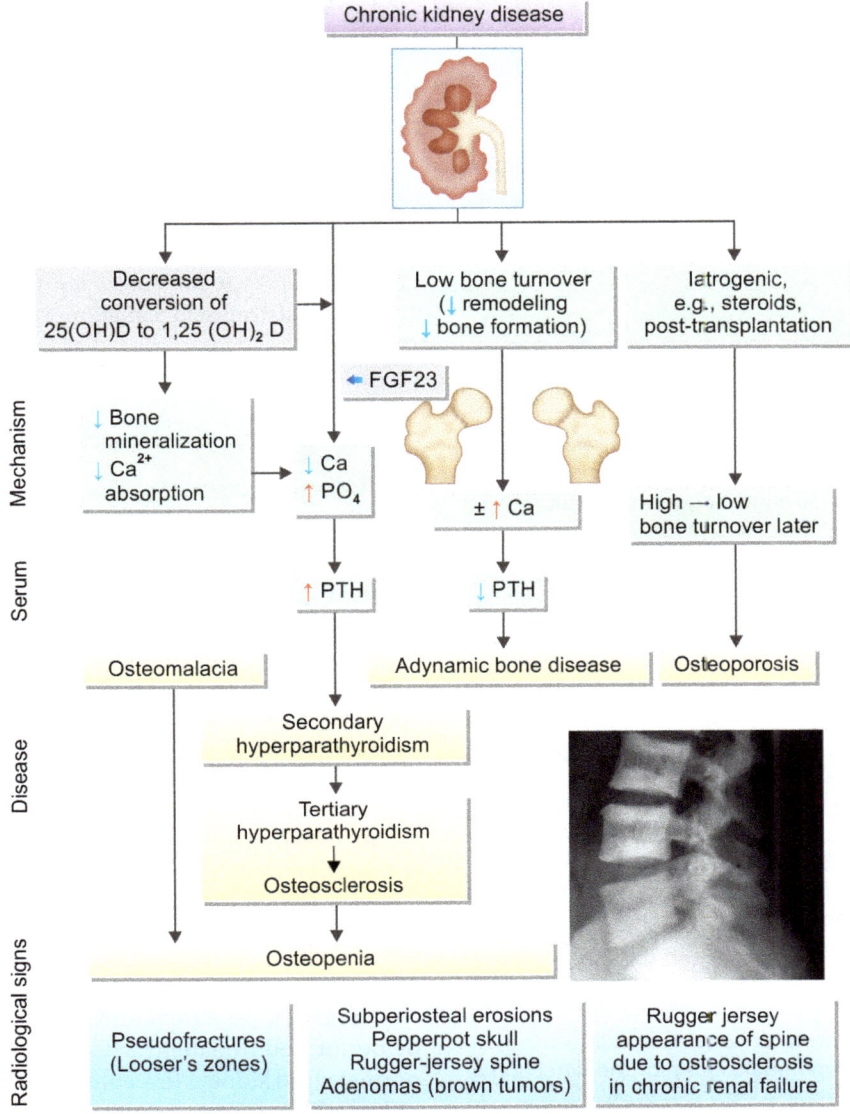

Fig. 10.8: Lateral spine X-ray showing rugger jersey appearance of spine.

[25-(OH)D$_3$: 25-hydroxyvitamin D; 1,25-(OH)$_2$D$_3$: 1,25-dihydroxycholecalciferol; FGF23: fibroblast growth factor 23; Ca: calcium; PO$_4$: phosphate; PTH: parathormone]

Metabolic abnormalities:
- **Gout:** Urate retention is a common in CRF.
- **Insulin requirement and resistance:** Insulin is catabolized by and to some extent excreted via the kidneys. Thus, insulin requirements in diabetic patients reduce as renal failure progresses. By contrast, end-organ resistance to insulin is observed in advanced renal impairment.
- **Lipid metabolism abnormalities:** These include— (1) impaired clearance of triglyceride-rich particles and (2) hypercholesterolemia.
- **Endocrine abnormalities:** These include—(1) hyperprolactinemia, (2) increased luteinizing hormone (LH) levels in both sex, (3) decreased serum testosterone levels, (4) absence of normal cyclical changes in female sex hormones, resulting in oligomenorrhea or amenorrhea, (5) abnormalities of growth hormone secretion and action, and (6) abnormal thyroid hormone levels.
- *Muscle dysfunction proximal myopathy.*

- **Nervous system:**
  - *Central nervous system:*
    - Unusual combination of depressed cerebral function and decreased seizure threshold.
    - *Dialysis disequilibrium* develops, if rapid correction of severe uremia is done by hemodialysis owing to osmotic cerebral swelling.
    - *Dialysis dementia* is a syndrome characterized by progressive intellectual deterioration, speech disturbance, myoclonus, and fits.
  - *Autonomic nervous system*: (1) Increased circulating catecholamine level, (2) impaired baroreceptor sensitivity, and (3) impaired efferent vagal function.
  - *Peripheral nervous system:* (1) Median nerve compression in the carpal tunnel due to β$_2$-microglobulin-related amyloidosis, (2) restless legs syndrome, and (3) polyneuropathy, and (4) psychiatric problems (anxiety, depression, phobias, and psychoses).

- **Cardiovascular disease:** *Increased (16-fold) incidence of cardiovascular disease*, particularly myocardial infarction, cardiac failure, sudden cardiac death and stroke, uremic pericarditis, or dialysis pericarditis. Hypertension develops in about 80% of patients with CRF.
- **Malignancy:** *Raised* incidence of malignancy. Malignant change can occur in polycystic kidney disease. Lymphomas, primary liver cancer, and thyroid cancers can also develop.

Investigations

Urinalysis

- **Physical examination:** Fixed specific gravity around 1.010 (isosthenuria) is seen in CRF.
- **Chemical examination:**
  - Hematuria may indicate glomerulonephritis.
  - Proteinuria, if heavy, is strongly suggestive of glomerular disease.
  - Glycosuria with normal blood glucose level is common in CRF.
- **Urine microscopy:**
  - White cells in the urine usually indicate *bacterial urinary infection*, sterile pyuria suggests papillary necrosis or renal tuberculosis.
  - *Eosinophils* indicate *allergic tubulointerstitial nephritis* or cholesterol embolization.
  - *Red cells* source may be from anywhere in the urinary tract between the glomerulus and the urethral meatus.
  - *Red-cell casts* are suggestive of *glomerulonephritis*.
  - *Granular casts* indicate *active renal disease*.
  - *Broad casts* are seen in CRF.
- Urine culture should be performed. Early-morning urine samples should be cultured for tuberculosis.

Urine biochemistry:
- *24-hour creatinine clearance* is useful to know the severity of renal failure.
- *Urine osmolality* is a measure of concentrating ability.
- *Urine electrophoresis* and immunofixation for the detection of light chains in myeloma.

Serum Biochemistry

- *Serum urea and creatinine*: The most consistent abnormalities in CRF are *elevated* levels of urea and creatinine. The level of serum creatinine correlates with the degree of renal damage.
- Electrophoresis and immunofixation for myeloma
- Extreme elevations of creatine kinase and a disproportionate elevation in serum creatinine and potassium compared to urea suggestive of rhabdomyolysis.
- Other biochemical abnormalities include hypocalcemia, hyperphosphatemia, hyperuricemia, and hyperkalemia.

Hematology

- Anemia
- *Eosinophilia* suggestive of allergic tubulointerstitial nephritis, vasculitis, or cholesterol embolism.
- *Peripheral smear* with *fragmented red cells (Burr cells) and/or thrombocytopenia* suggestive of *intravascular hemolysis* due to accelerated hypertension, hemolytic uremic syndrome, or thrombotic thrombocytopenic purpura.
- *Markedly raised erythrocyte sedimentation rate (ESR)* is suggestive of *myeloma*.

Immunology

- *Low complement components* may be seen in *active glomerular disease* (e.g., SLE, poststreptococcal glomerulonephritis).
- *Autoantibody screening* is helpful in autoimmune diseases (e.g., SLE).
- *Antibodies to streptococcal antigens* (ASOT and anti-DNase B), if poststreptococcal glomerulonephritis is suspected.
- *Antibodies to hepatitis B and C*
- *Antibodies to HIV* when HIV-associated renal disease is suspected
- *Malaria* can cause glomerular disease in the tropics

Radiological Investigation

- **Ultrasound:** Ultrasonography is done to assess the renal size and to exclude hydronephrosis. Renal ultrasound usually shows shrunken kidneys in CRF. *In diabetic glomerulosclerosis, amyloidosis, polycystic kidney diseases, HIV nephropathy bilateral hydronephrosis, and myeloma, the kidneys may be of normal size.*
- *Plain abdominal radiography and CT* (without contrast) is done to exclude low-density renal stones or nephrocalcinosis. CT may also useful for the diagnosis of retroperitoneal fibrosis and useful in some patients with suspected obstructive nephropathy.
- *Magnetic resonance angiography (MRI)* is useful in renovascular disease.

Renal Biopsy

Aim: To establish the nature and extent of renal disease, which help in treatment and predicting prognosis. It should be performed in patient with unexplained renal failure and normal-sized kidneys (exception diabetic glomerulosclerosis), unless there are strong contraindications.

Management of Chronic Renal Failure

Management of CRF can be divided into three parts:
1. Establishing the diagnosis and etiology of CKD and to detect any reversible factors
2. Measures to prevent/slow down the further damage to the kidney (progression of CKD)
3. Supportive measures (e.g., dialysis or transplantation) when necessary

Treatments aimed at specific causes of CKD: Optimization glucose control in diabetes mellitus, immunomodulatory agents for glomerulonephritis, and emerging specific therapies to retard cytogenesis in polycystic kidney disease. Any reversible factors should be detected and treated (**Box 10.9**).

Measures to reduce the symptoms and progression of CRF:
Following measures may stabilize or slow the decline of renal function.

- *Control of hypertension and proteinuria*: Goals of treatment include (1) blood pressure should be reduced <130/80 and proteinuria <0.3 g/24 hours. If creatinine is below 3 mg/dL, ACE inhibitors and angiotensin receptor blockers (ARBs) (inhibit the angiotensin-induced vasoconstriction of the efferent arterioles of the glomerular microcirculation) are the drugs of choice.

- **Diet:**
  - *Protein restriction* to 0.60 and 0.75 g/kg per day, i.e., about 40 g/day (with higher amount of essential amino acids). It reduces symptoms associated with uremia and may also slow the rate of renal decline at earlier stages of renal disease.
  - *Avoid foods with high potassium.*
  - *Salt restriction* is necessary in most of the patients. However, patients with salt-losing nephropathy (tubulointerstitial disease) require a high-salt intake.
- *Slowing progression of diabetic renal disease* by control of blood glucose and maintaining HbA_1c in the range of 7.0–7.5.
- **Use of lipid-lowering agents:** Hypercholesterolemia is common in patients with significant proteinuria, and in patients with CKD. Lipid lowering reduces vascular events in non-dialysis CKD.
- Cessation of smoking
- Exercise and weight reduction
- Avoid nephrotoxic medications

> **Box 10.9: Reversible factors in chronic kidney disease.**
>
> - **Hypovolemia:** Vomiting, diarrhea, excessive diuresis, and congestive heart failure
> - **Urinary tract obstruction:** Nephrolithiasis, papillary necrosis, and bladder outlet obstruction
> - Infection
> - Uncontrolled or accelerated hypertension
> - **Nephrotoxic drugs:** Aminoglycosides, cephalosporins, tetracycline, amphotericin, radio-contrast agents, NSAIDs, and diuretics
> - **Electrolyte and metabolic disorders:** Hyperphosphatasemia, hyperuricemia, acidosis
> - **Vasculitis:** Systemic lupus erythematosus, Wegener's granulomatosis, and microscopic polyarteritis
> - **Pregnancy:** Eclampsia

Treatment of anemia in chronic renal failure (Table 10.14): The anemia of erythropoietin (EPO) deficiency is treated with recombinant (synthetic) human EPO (erythropoietin-alpha or -beta, or the longer-acting darbepoetin-alpha). Administration of erythropoietin-alpha through subcutaneous route is contraindicated in CRF and the intravenous route is used, initially 50 U/kg of epoetin-alpha over 1–5 min three times/week. EPO is less effective in the presence of iron deficiency, active inflammation, or malignancy, and in patients with aluminum overload (found in dialysis).

Table 10.14: Drugs used in treatment of anemia in chronic renal failure.

	Initiation dose in CKD—nondialysis dependent	Initiation dose in dialysis-dependent CKD
• Erythropoietin	• 20–50 U/kg 3 times/week (if given IV, IV dose is 20–30% higher than SC dose)	
• Darbepoetin-alpha	0.45 µg/kg every 4 weeks (SC or IV)	0.45 µg/kg once weekly (SC or IV) Or 0.75 µg/kg every 2 weeks (SC or IV)
• Epoetin-β	• 0.6 µg every 2 weeks (SC or IV)	

- Blood pressure, hemoglobin concentration, and reticulocyte count are measured every 2 weeks and the dose adjusted to maintain a target hemoglobin level of 10–12 g/dL.
- Hemoglobin >13 g/dL has been associated with increased incidence of cardiovascular mortality.

- Some newer agents tried in management of anemia in CKD:
  - *Prolyl hydroxylase inhibitors:* Roxadustat and vadadustat
  - *Erythropoietin-mimicking peptide:* Peginesatide
- **Treatment of hypocalcemia and hyperphosphatemia:** Both should be treated aggressively.
  - *Hypocalcemia:* It is treated with calcitriol or alphacalcidol (1-α-hydroxyvitamin D_3) or paricalcitol (19-nor-1,25-dihydroxyvitamin D_3) and calcium supplementation.

Serum calcium level should be monitored to avoid hypercalcemia. Oral calcium carbonate also decreases the bioavailability of dietary phosphates.

- **Hyperphosphatemia:** It is treated with phosphate binders. Previously, aluminum hydroxide was used to bind phosphate in the gut and was producing aluminum toxicity. Others include:
  - Calcium carbonate and calcium acetate (serum calcium should be monitored).
  - Polymer sevelamer carbonate (an anion-exchange resin).
  - Lanthanum carbonate (a nonaluminum, noncalcium phosphate-binding agent) has higher incidence of side effects.

Treatment of hyperparathyroidism: By the use of—
- Calcium carbonate or acetate
- Vitamin D analogs
- Calcimimetics activate the calcium-sensing receptor in the parathyroid gland, thereby inhibiting PTH secretion. Cinacalcet is used in patients who are on dialysis.

Maintenance fluid and electrolyte balance:
- **Fluid retention:** If there is evidence of fluid retention, intake of dietary sodium is restricted and loop diuretics may be necessary.
- **Hyperkalemia:** Usually responds to dietary restriction of potassium intake. Occasionally, ion-exchange resins may be necessary to remove potassium in the gastrointestinal tract. If hyperkalemia occurs during diuretic therapy, reduce or stop potassium-sparing diuretics, ACE inhibitors, and ARBs.
- **Acidosis:** Sodium bicarbonate may be effective, but can cause edema and hypertension owing to extracellular fluid expansion. Calcium carbonate, also used as a calcium supplement and phosphate binder, is useful in treating acidosis.

Table 10.15 lists the differences between acute kidney injury (AKI) and chronic kidney disease (CKD).

URINARY TRACT INFECTIONS

A urinary tract infection (UTI) is associated with multiplication of organisms in the urinary tract and is defined as

Table 10.15: Differences between acute kidney injury (AKI) and chronic kidney disease (CKD).

	AKI	CKD
Previous history of kidney disease	Absent	Present
Previous elevated creatinine >3 months	Absent	Present
Anemia	Absent	Present
Hypertension	±	++
Kidney size (ultrasound)	Not contracted	Contracted
Complications: Hyperphosphatemia, hypocalcemia, neuropathy, osteodystrophy, and band keratopathy	Absent	Present

the presence of more than 10^5 organisms/mL in the midstream sample of urine (MSU).

Classification of Urinary Tract Infections (Table 10.16)
- **Lower urinary tract infections:** These include cystitis (bladder), prostatitis, and urethritis.
- **Upper urinary tract infections:** These include infection of kidneys and their collecting systems (pyelonephritis) and perinephric abscess.

Etiology
Causative organisms: *Majority* (~85%) of urinary tract infection are the caused by *gram-negative bacilli*, which are normal inhabitants of the intestinal tract (enteric origin).
- *Most common pathogens*: *Escherichia coli* (80% cases), *Proteus, Klebsiella, Enterobacter,* and *Pseudomonas.*
- *Less common*: *Streptococcus faecalis*, staphylococci, and fungi.

Table 10.16: Clinical spectrum of urinary tract infection.

Asymptomatic bacteriuria (ABU)	Symptomatic (disease)

Presence of bacteriuria (>10^5/mL or two occasions in females and on one occasion in males) indicating UTI but without symptoms.
• Common in pregnancy
• Occurs in the absence of symptoms
• Does not usually require treatment
	• Includes:
	  ▪ Acute urethritis
	  ▪ Acute cystitis
	  ▪ Acute prostatitis
	  ▪ Acute pyelonephritis
	  ▪ Renal abscess
	  ▪ Septicemia with septic shock
	• Requires antimicrobial therapy

- *In immunocompromised patients*: Viruses (polyoma virus, cytomegalovirus, and adenovirus).

Pathogenesis
Pathogenesis is shown in **Figure 10.9**.

Clinical Features
Clinical features are described in **Table 10.17**.

Uncomplicated versus complicated infection **(Table 10.18):**

Investigations
Urine Examination
- **Dipstick tests:** Most gram-negative organisms reduce nitrates to nitrites, and dipstick tests (nitrite test) are used to detect nitrite in urine. Dipsticks that detect significant pyuria depend on the release of esterases from leukocyte (leukocyte esterase test). Positive dipstick tests for both nitrite and leukocyte esterase are highly predictive of acute infection.
- **Microscopic examination:** For leukocytes, leukocyte casts, and red cells
- **Culture and sensitivity** of a freshly voided clean-catch midstream specimen of urine

Table 10.17: Symptoms and signs of UTI.

Constitutional:	
• Malaise • Listlessness • Fever • Chills • Nausea and vomiting	
Upper tract—symptoms: • Flank pain • Backache • Heaviness in the flank	**Upper tract—signs:** • Flank/CVA tenderness • Flank mass • Scoliosis • Psoas spasm
Lower tract—symptoms: • Frequency • Scalding urination • Urgency • Strangury • Hematuria • Turbid urine (pyuria) • Foul-smelling urine • Pneumaturia/fecaluria	**Lower tract—signs:** • Suprapubic tenderness • Bladder distension (bladder outlet obstruction) • Urethral discharge • Urethral tenderness
Genital—female—symptoms: • Leukorrhea • Dyspareunia • Pruritus vulvae	**Genital—female—signs:** • Vaginal discharge • Pelvic organ prolapse • Atrophic vaginitis
Genital—male—symptoms: • Pain in the urethra • Deep perineal pain • Orchialgia	**Genital—male—signs:** • Phimosis, balanoposthitis • Urethral tenderness • Periurethral abscess • Perineal tenderness (Cowperitis) • Signs of epididymo-orchitis • Prostatic enlargement on DRE

(CVA: cerebrovascular accident; DRE: digital rectal examination; UTI: urinary tract infection)

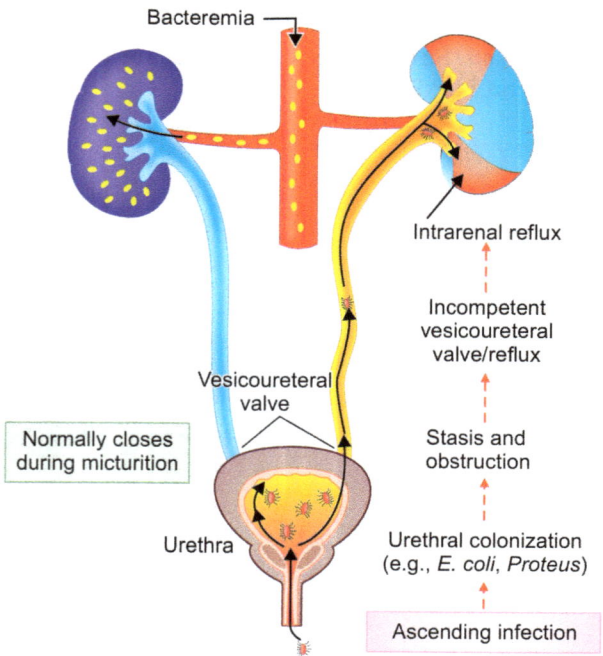

Fig. 10.9: Pathogenesis of acute pyelonephritis. More common mode is ascending infection. Hematogenous infection results from bacteremic spread.

Table 10.18: Differences between uncomplicated versus complicated UT infection.

Features	Uncomplicated urinary tract infection	Complicated urinary tract infection
Characteristics	UTI occurring in patients with functionally normal urinary tracts	UTI occurring in patients with abnormal urinary tracts (e.g., with stones, or associated diseases, such as diabetes mellitus) or infection that extends beyond the bladder
Lesions	Includes cystitis or urethritis due to bacterial colonization of the bladder or urethra	Infection of renal parenchyma and renal pelvis (pyelonephritis) or prostate (prostatitis)
Sex affected	Much more in females than in males	Infection in men is often considered complicated
Predisposing factors	May not be obvious	Usually occurs in presence of obstructive lesions or following instrumentation on urinary tract
Clinical features	Burning on urination and frequent urination without fever or flank pain	Accompanied by fever or flank pain • Costovertebral angle tenderness • Pelvic or perineal pain in men (prostatitis)
Prognosis	Responds well to treatment and persistent or recurrent infection seldom results in serious kidney damage	May be difficult to treat and relapses after treatment are common
Sequelae	Rare	Common such as sepsis, metastatic abscesses, and renal failure

Special Investigations

- **Prostatitis:**
  - Per rectal examination of the prostate
  - Prostatic massage followed by urine culture
- **Cystitis:** Cystoscopy
- **Renal ultrasonography computed tomography of kidneys, ureters, and bladder (CT-KUB), MR urogram:** To identify obstruction, cysts, and calculi
- **Intravenous urography (IVU), including a post-void film of bladder:** To identify physiological and/anatomical abnormalities of urinary tract.
- **Dimercaptosuccinic acid (DMSA) renal scan:** For pyelonephritis
- **Micturating cystourethrogram** *(MCU)* to identify vesicoureteric reflux and disturbed bladder emptying
- In females with recurrent UTI, *pelvic examination* to exclude cystocele, rectocele, and uterine prolapse

Treatment

- **Antibiotic therapy:** The choice of antibiotic depends on the result of urine culture and sensitivity of urine.
  - The commonly employed antibiotics include cotrimoxazole (trimethoprim and sulfamethoxazole 1 double-strength tablet two times daily), ampicillin (250 mg three times daily), amoxicillin (250 mg 250 mg 8-hourly three times daily), oral cephalosporin, nitrofurantoin (50 mg three times daily), and quinolones. Treatment is over 3–5 days in uncomplicated infections (nitrofurantoin for 7 days) and for 7–10 days in complicated infections.
- **Hospitalized patients:**
  - No risk factors for infection with a multidrug-resistant organism ceftriaxone (1 g IV once daily) or piperacillin-tazobactam (3.375 g IV every 6 hours)
  - At least one risk factor for infection with a multidrug-resistant organism, antipseudomonal carbapenem (imipenem 500 mg IV every 6 hours, meropenem 1 g IV every 8 hours, or doripenem 500 mg IV every 8 hours)
  - If *Enterococcus* species or methicillin-resistant *Staphylococcus aureus* (MRSA) is suspected, add vancomycin, daptomycin, or linezolid.
  - "Single-shot" treatment with 3 g of amoxicillin or 1.92 g of cotrimoxazole can be used in patients with bladder symptoms of <36 hours duration and without any previous history of UTI.
  - If patient has calculi, catheter, or other obstructions, no antibiotic is necessary unless symptomatic.
- **Fluid intake:** A high (2 L daily) fluid intake during treatment and for some subsequent weeks to initiate water diuresis, so as to maintain a high rate of urine flow.
- **Other measures:**
  - Regular complete emptying of urinary bladder at 2- to 3-hour intervals
  - Alkalinization of urine
  - Urinary analgesics (e.g., phenazopyridine) and antispasmodics (e.g., hyoscyamine) to be given for detrusor spasm
  - If patients presents for the first time with high fever, loin pain, and tenderness, urgent renal ultrasound examination is performed to exclude an obstructed pyonephrosis. If this is present, percutaneous nephrostomy is performed to drain it.
  - Cranberry juice inhibits adherence of uropathogens to uroepithelial cells, hence advisable to prevent recurrent UTI.
  - *In females*: The incidence of UTIs can be reduced by—(1) adequate perineal hygiene, (2) emptying the bladder before bedtime and before and after intercourse, and (3) application of 0.5% cetrimide cream to periurethral area before intercourse. Atrophic vaginitis should be identified and treated in postmenopausal women.
  - Avoidance of constipation (may impair bladder emptying).

Asymptomatic bacteriuria: It requires treatment—(1) if a patient is pregnant, (2) in case of renal transplantation, or (3) before planning for a urologic surgery. Treatment of asymptomatic bacteriuria in pregnant women decreases the occurrence of pyelonephritis.

Acute Pyelonephritis

Acute pyelonephritis is an acute suppurative inflammation of upper urinary tract affecting the tubules, interstitium, and renal pelvis. There is often coincident cystitis.

Clinical Features

- **Classic triad:** The classic triad is—(1) Loin pain, (2) fever, and (3) tenderness over the kidneys. Presence of this

triad and significant bacteriuria usually indicates acute pyelonephritis.
- Sudden onset of pain in one or both loins (costovertebral/renal angle), radiating to the iliac fossa and suprapubic area
- Fever with chills and rigors, and malaise
- Tenderness and guarding in the renal angle
- Dysuria, frequency, and urgency. Frequent passage of small amount of urine accompanied by scalding. Cloudy urine
- Acute pyelonephritis caused by the presence of obstruction (e.g., stone, tumor, bladder neck obstruction, and enlarged prostate) can be very severe and may progress to renal abscess.
- Rarely, acute pyelonephritis may be associated with necrotizing papillitis/papillary necrosis. Causes include diabetes mellitus, chronic urinary obstruction, analgesic nephropathy, and sickle-cell disease.

Management
Intravenous antibiotics: Intravenous ampicillin, amoxicillin plus aminoglycosides (e.g., tobramycin), cephalosporin (e.g., cefuroxime), quinolone (e.g., ciprofloxacin) or a combination β-lactam/β-lactamase inhibitor (piperacillin–tazobactam) or carbapenem (meropenem)

OBJECTIVE-BASED SELF-EVALUATION

LONG QUESTIONS
1. Discuss the pathogenesis, clinical features, and management of poststreptococcal glomerulonephritis.
2. List the etiology of nephrotic syndrome. Discuss the clinical features and complications of minimal change disease.
3. Define acute kidney injury. List the causes and complications of acute kidney injury.
4. List the causes of chronic kidney disease. Describe the staging system of CKD.
5. Discuss the clinical features of chronic kidney disease.
6. Classify urinary tract infections. Discuss the clinical differences between complicated and uncomplicated UTI.

SHORT ANSWER QUESTIONS
1. List the differences between nephritic and nephrotic syndrome
2. List the etiology of acute kidney injury
3. Microalbuminuria
4. List the complications of chronic kidney disease
5. Glomerular filtration rate
6. Indications for hemodialysis
7. RIFLE criteria
8. Complications of nephrotic syndrome
9. IgA nephropathy
10. Acute pyelonephritis
11. Hematuria
12. List the causes of acute glomerulonephritis

MULTIPLE CHOICE QUESTIONS
1. Oliguria is defined as reduction in urine output:
   a. <400 mL/24 hr
   b. <300 mL/24 hr
   c. <200 mL/24 hr
   d. <100 mL/24 hr
2. A 22-year-old obese man presents with mild ankle edema and urinalysis shows protein +++ with no blood. A diagnosis of nephrotic syndrome proteinuria of 8 g/24 hours. What is the most likely diagnosis?
   a. Focal segmental glomerulosclerosis
   b. Membranoproliferative glomerulonephritis
   c. Membranous nephropathy
   d. Minimal change disease
3. Hypercoagulation as a complication in nephrotic syndrome is caused by:
   a. Loss of antithrombin ill
   b. Decreased fibrinogen
   c. Increase in protein C
   d. Loss of globulin
4. In stage 5 chronic kidney disease the glomerular filtration rate is below:
   a. 25 mL/min per 1.73 m^2
   b. 15 mL/min per 1.73 m^2
   c. 5 mL/min per 1.73 m^2
   d. 0 mL/min per 1.73 m^2 (anuria)
5. Leukocyte esterase dipstick test in urine is done for:
   a. Bacteriuria
   b. Pyuria
   c. Hematuria
   d. Proteinuria
6. Most common cause of CKD in adults is:
   a. Hypertension
   b. SLE
   c. Diabetes mellitus
   d. Drug induced
7. All are true of nephrotic syndrome, *except*:
   a. RBC casts in urine
   b. Hypoproteinemia
   c. Edema
   d. Hyperlipidemia
8. Following are features of acute glomerulonephritis, *except*:
   a. Polyuria
   b. Hematuria
   c. Hypertension
   d. Oliguria
9. A 16-year-old female patient presents with upper respiratory tract infection. After 15 days, she develops hematuria. Probable diagnosis is:
   a. IgA nephropathy
   b. Wegener's granulomatosis
   c. Henoch Schönlein purpura
   d. Post-streptococcal glomerulonephritis
10. RIFLE criteria is used for diagnosis of:
    a. Acute kidney injury
    b. Acute splenic injury
    c. Acute liver injury
    d. Acute bowel injury

11. Most common cause for prerenal azotaemia is:
    a. Hypovolemia
    b. Glomerulonephritis
    c. Pyelonephritis
    d. Renal artery stenosis
12. Most common organism producing urinary tract infection is:
    a. *Streptococcus faecalis*
    b. *Escherichia coli*
    c. *Klebsiella*
    d. *Pseudomonas*
13. Microalbuminuria is the presence of albumin in urine about:
    a. >30 to <300 mg/day
    b. <30 mg/day
    c. >30 to <300 g/day
    d. <30 g/day
14. Cockroft–Gault formula is used to calculate:
    a. Sodium deficit
    b. Bilirubin degradation
    c. Glomerular filtration rate
    d. Core body temperature
15. What is the leading cause of death in the patients with CKD?
    a. Cardiovascular
    b. Hyperkalemia
    c. Infection
    d. Uremia

ANSWERS

1. a	2. d	3. a	4. b	5. b
6. c	7. a	8. a	9. d	10. a
11. a	12. b	13. a	14. c	15. a

Neurology

CHAPTER OUTLINE

- Symptomatology
- Migraine
- Cluster Headache
- Tension-Type Headache
- Stroke and Cerebrovascular Disease
- Seizures and Epilepsy
- Meningitis
- Neurosyphilis
- Encephalitis
- Trigeminal Neuralgia
- Bell's Palsy
- Intracranial Pressure
- Coma
- Brain Death

SYMPTOMATOLOGY

Weakness and Paralysis

Categories

- **Upper motor neurons:** These consist of corticospinal interneurons, which arise from the motor cortex and descend to the spinal cord where they activate the lower motor neurons (anterior horn cells) through synapses.
- **Lower motor neurons:** The term "motor neuron" is usually used only to the efferent neurons that actually innervate muscles (the lower motor neurons). A motor neuron consists of nerve cell (neuron), which is located in the anterior horn cell of the spinal cord and its fibers (axon) projects outside the spinal cord to directly or indirectly control effector organs, mainly muscles and glands. Motor neuron axons are efferent nerve fibers and carry signals from the spinal cord to the effectors to produce effects.
- **Figure 11.1** shows the structure of nervous system.

Signs of Upper and Lower Motor Neuron Disease

Signs of upper and lower motor neuron disease are described in **Table 11.1**.

Ataxia

Ataxia is a disorder characterized unsteadiness and impaired coordination of regulating body posture and the rate, range, force, and direction of movement. Usually seen in cerebellar diseases (stroke, tumors) or involvement of posterior column of spinal cord—Sensory ataxia (Vitamin B_{12} deficiency, syphilis).

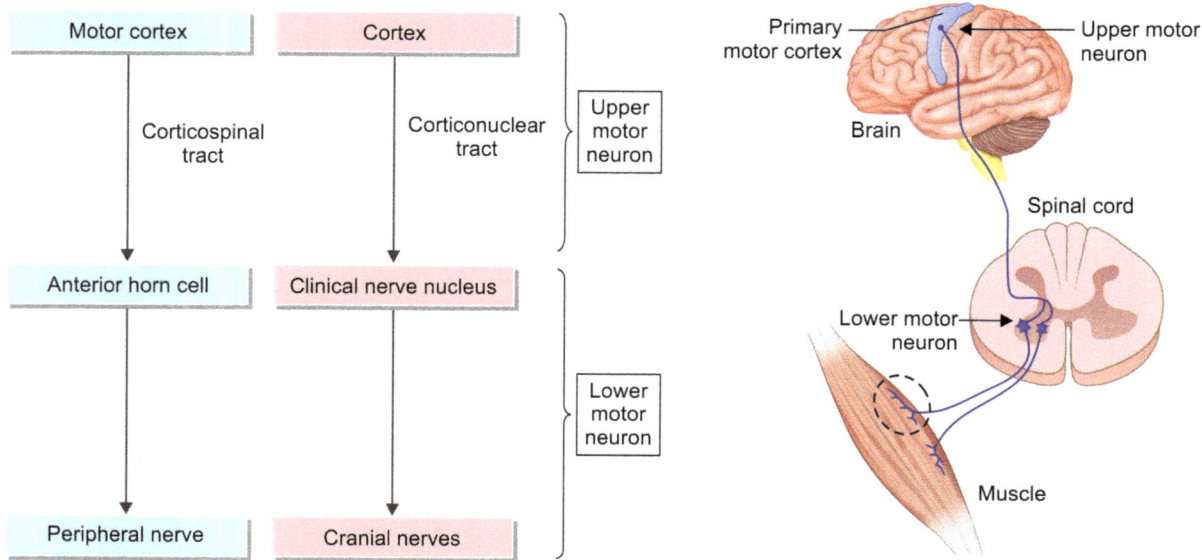

Fig. 11.1: Structure of nervous system.

Table 11.1: Signs of upper and lower motor neuron disease.

Sign	Upper motor neuron	Lower motor neuron
Atrophy	None (rarely disuse atrophy)	Severe wasting
Muscles affected	Group of muscles	Single
Fasciculations	None	Common
Tone	Hypertonia-rigidity/spasticity	Decreased (hypotonia)
Distribution of weakness	Distal predominant/regional	Predominantly proximal (except neuropathy)/segmental
Tendon reflexes	Exaggerated/hyperactive	Hypoactive/lost
Babinski sign	Present	Absent
Flexor spasms, clonus	Present	Absent

Vertigo

- **Definition:** Vertigo is defined as an abnormal perception (hallucination/illusion) of movement (a sensation of rotation or tipping) of either the environment or self (body or part of it). The individual feels that the surroundings are spinning or moving.
- The most common cause is benign paroxysmal positional vertigo (BPPV). Other causes include Meniere's disease, vertebral artery ischemia, vestibulitis, and drugs.
- The perceived movement may be falling down, or rotating or there is a sensation of spinning of the outside world. It is often accompanied by nausea or vomiting.

Aphasias

- Aphasia is loss or defective language content of speech resulting from damage to the speech centers within the dominant (usually left in 97%) hemisphere. A language disturbance occurring after a right hemisphere lesion in a right hander is known as crossed aphasia.
- It includes defect in or loss of the power of expression by speech, writing or gestures or a defect in or loss of the ability to comprehend spoken or written language or to interpret gestures.
- Aphasia may be categorized according to whether the speech output is fluent or nonfluent.
  - **Fluent aphasias** (receptive aphasias) are impairments mostly due to the input or reception of language, with difficulties either in auditory verbal comprehension or in the repetition of words, phrases, or sentences spoken by others. For example, Wernicke's aphasia.
  - **Nonfluent aphasias** (expressive aphasias) are difficulties in articulating, with relatively good auditory, verbal comprehension. For example, Broca's aphasia.

DYSARTHRIAS

Dysarthria involves the abnormal articulation of sounds or phonemes. Could be due to facial, tongue, or palatal paralysis. Scanning and staccato speech is seen in cerebellar disease.

Apraxia

Apraxia is impaired ability (inability) to carry out (perform) skilled, complex, organized motor activities in the presence of normal basic motor, sensory, and cerebellar function. Examples of complex motor activities: dressing, using cutlery, and geographical orientation.

Agnosia

Agnosia is failure to recognize objects (e.g., places, clothing, persons, sounds, shapes or smells), despite the presence of intact sensory system.

Functions of Cerebral Hemispheres

Cerebral dominance aligns limb dominance with language function. Right-handed individuals almost always (>95%) have the dominant left hemisphere, and about 7% of left handers have a dominant right hemisphere (**Fig. 11.2**).

HEADACHE

Headache is among the most common reasons patients seek medical attention.

Classification of Headache (Table 11.2 and Fig. 11.3)

- **Primary headaches:** Benign, recurrent, no organic disease as their cause. It affects the quality of life of the patient.
- **Secondary headaches:** Underlying organic disease.

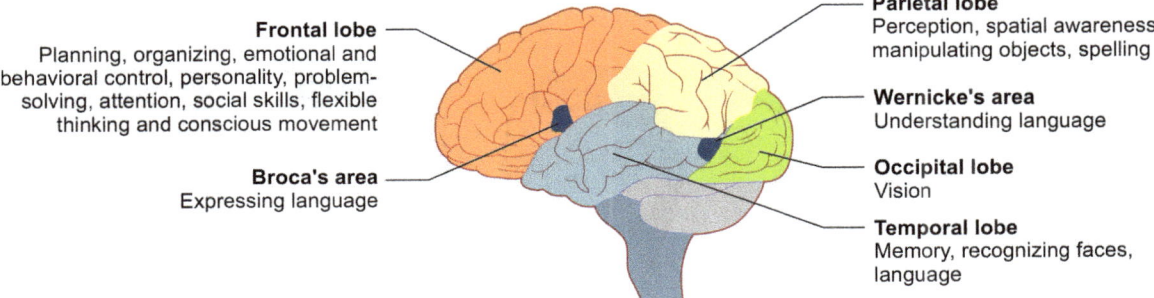

Fig. 11.2: Functions of various lobes of cerebral hemispheres.

Table 11.2: Classification of headache.

Primary headache		Secondary headache
Type	**%**	1. Head or neck trauma
• Tension-type	69	2. Cranial or cervical vascular disorder. Arterial dissection, Cerebral venous thrombosis
• Migraine	16	3. Noninfectious inflammatory disease
• Idiopathic stabbing	2	▪ Intracranial neoplasm
• Exertional	1	▪ High and low-cerebrospinal fluid pressure headache
• Cluster	0.1	4. Substance use or its withdrawal
• Other primary headache: ▪ Paroxysmal hemicrania ▪ SUNCT (Short-lasting unilateral neuralgiform headache attacks with conjunctival injection and tearing) ▪ SUNA (Short-lasting unilateral neuralgiform headache attacks with cranial autonomic symptoms)		5. Disorder of homeostasis—Hypoxia, hypercarbia, hypoglycemia 6. Psychiatric disorder—Somatization 7. Cranial neuralgia 8. Infection— meningitis 9. Disorder of cranium, neck, face, eyes, ears, nose, sinus, teeth, mouth, or other facial structure

MIGRAINE

Migraine is a **neurovascular disease** caused by neurogenic inflammation and characterized by **severe, recurring headaches.**

- It is the second most common cause of headache. It usually characterized by an episodic severe pain on one side of the head (headache) and usually associated with certain features such as sensitivity to light, sound, or movement; nausea and vomiting often accompany the headache.
- **Gender:** F:M ratio is 5:1.

Classification

- **Migraine without aura or common migraine:** Does not give any warning signs before the onset of headache. It occurs in about 70–80% of migraine patients.
- **Migraine with aura or classical migraine:** Gives some warning signs called "aura" before the actual headache begins. About 20–30% migraine patients experience aura. The most common aura is visual and may include both positive and negative (visual field defects) features.
- **Retinal migraine:** It involves attacks of monocular scotoma or even blindness of one eye for less than an hour and associated with headache.
- **Childhood periodic syndromes:** It involve cyclical vomiting (occasional intense periods of vomiting), abdominal migraine (abdominal pain, usually accompanied by nausea), and benign paroxysmal vertigo of childhood (occasional attacks of vertigo). They may be precursors or associated with migraine.
- **Complicated migraine:** Describes migraine headaches and/or auras that are unusually long or unusually frequent, or associated with a seizure or brain lesion.
- **Basilar migraine:** Occipital headache, preceded by vertigo, diplopia, and dysarthria, visual and sensory symptoms (brainstem symptoms).
- **Hemiplegic migraine:** Rare autosomal dominant disorder characterized by prolonged headache lasting hours or days, followed by hemiparesis and/or coma that recovers slowly over days.
- **Ophthalmoplegic migraine:** Migraine associated with transient 3rd nerve palsy with/without involvement of pupil; sometimes also affect 4th and 6th nerve.
- **Vestibular migraine** (also called migrainous vertigo) associated vertigo.
- **Catamenial migraine:** Migraine associated with menstruation-associated migraine.

Pathogenesis

- **Genetic factors:** Play a role in causing the neuronal hyperexcitability. Migraine is usually polygenic. Rarely, familial migraine is associated with mutations in the α1 subunit of the P/Q type voltage-gated calcium channel or neuronal sodium channel (SCN1A), and **a dominant** loss of function mutation in a potassium channel gene (TRESK). Migraine is frequently associated with positive family history, and similar phenomena occur in disorders such as CADASIL.
  - Genes for **familial hemiplegic migraine**
  - *FHM1—CACNA1A*—Neuronal p/q calcium channel-Increases neurotransmitter release.
- **Hormonal influences:** Female preponderance and the frequency of migraine attacks at certain points in the menstrual cycle due to hormonal fluctuations. Estrogen-containing oral contraception can exacerbate migraine in few patients.

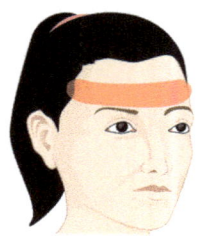
Tension

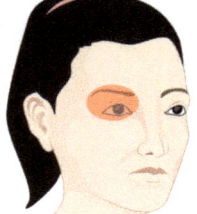
Cluster

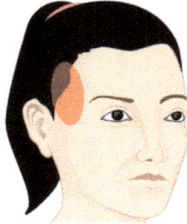
Giant cell arteritis

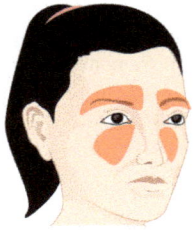
Sinus

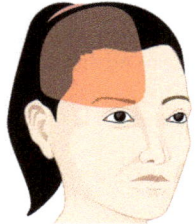
Migraine

Fig. 11.3: Headache types.

- **Right-to-left cardiac shunt:** Migraine with aura has been associated with patent foramen ovale (PFO), atrial septal defect (ASD) and pulmonary arteriovenous malformations (AVMs) in hereditary hemorrhagic telangiectasia (Osler-Weber-Rendu syndrome).
- **Several theories** have been proposed for the pathogenesis of migraine.

Vascular theory: Constriction of intracerebral blood vessel produces aura. Vasodilatation of intracranial/extracranial blood vessel produces headache phase.

Serotonin theory: Decreased serotonin levels linked with migraine and specific serotonin receptors found in blood vessels of brain.

- **Neurogenic theory:** The aura (see clinical features later) is thought to be due to spreading cortical depression wave of neuronal depolarization followed by depressed activity spreading slowly anteriorly across the cerebral cortex from the occipital region. This spreading process occurs at a rate of about 3 mm/minute. Dysfunction of activation of cells in the trigeminal nucleus releases vasoactive neuropeptides [e.g., calcitonin gene-related peptide (CGRP), substance P and other vasoactive peptides including 5HT] by activated trigeminovascular neurons. They produce painful meningeal inflammation and vasodilation.
- Dopamine plays a role and most migraine symptoms can be induced by dopaminergic stimulation. There is dopamine receptor hypersensitivity in patients with migraine.

Cortical Spreading Depression (CSD)

- Wave of activation followed by reduced activity that spreads across the surface of the brain
- Initial dilation conducted with intrinsic velocity ahead of CSD, Subsequent constriction and eventual dilation.

Astrocyte Calcium Waves

- Slowly propagated waves evoked by wide variety of stimuli
- Associated with active release of ATP, glutamate, K+, lactate, prostanoids, and interleukins

Precipitating factors

Anything can initiate or precipitate or amplify an attack. Common triggers are: excess stress, glare, exposure to bright light, loud noises/sounds, smoke or strong scents, menstruation, lack or excess of sleep, cheese, caffeine, alcohol, chocolate, citrus fruit, food additives such as monosodium glutamate, vasodilators, hunger, physical exertion, stormy weather, or barometric pressure changes and contraceptive pills, etc.

Clinical Features

Headache is usually hemicranial, throbbing, and associated with nausea and vomiting.

- **Migraine without aura** (previously called "common" migraine).
  - About 70–80% of patients with migraine have characteristic headache but without aura.
  - Typically attacks are episodic and start at puberty and prevalence increases in 4th decade. May show variable degree of spontaneous remissions.
  - The scalp may be tender to touch during episodes (allodynia is production of pain from normally nonpainful stimuli) and the patient prefer to be still in a dark and quiet environment.
  - Other symptoms associated with migraine headache include photophobia, phonophobia, vertigo, scalp tenderness, and cutaneous allodynia.
- **Migraine with aura** (previously known as classical migraine) **(Fig. 11.4)**
  - *Migraine aura:* About 20–30% of patient with migraine experience malaise, irritability, behavioral change, or focal neurological symptoms for some hours or days immediately preceding the headache phase.

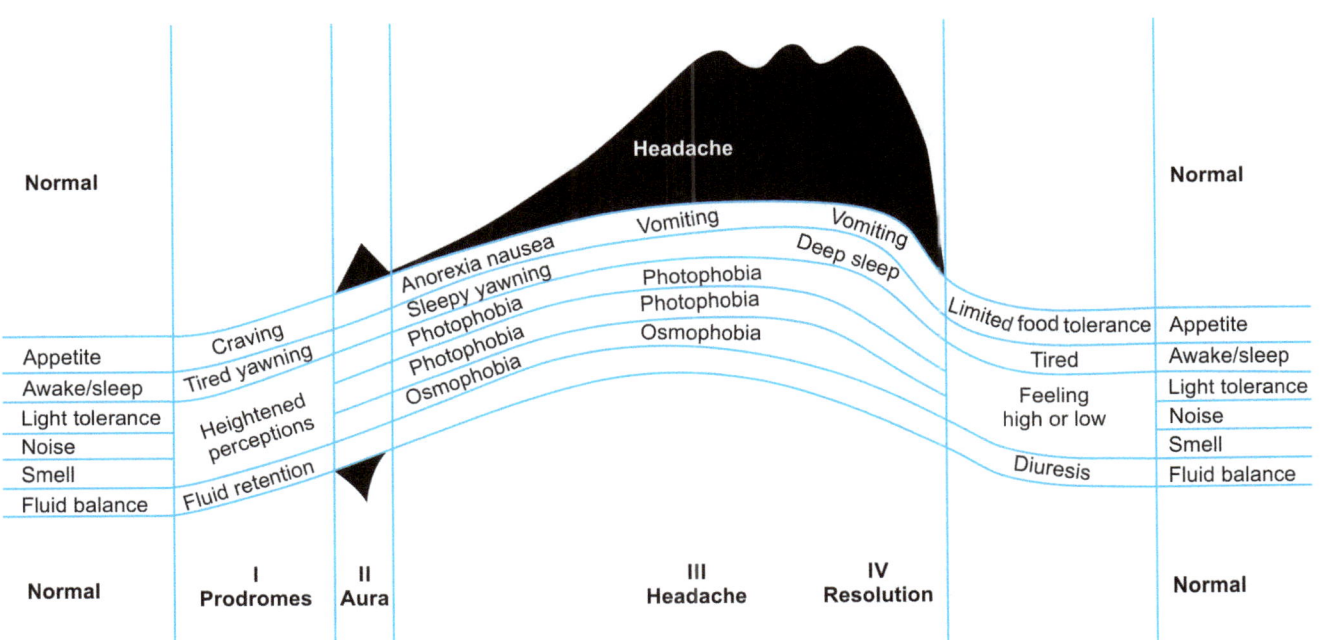

Fig. 11.4: Migraine phases.

- *Types of aura:*
  1. *Visual aura:* It is most common type characterized by positive visual symptoms such as shimmering, teichopsia (silvery zigzag lines also called **fortification spectra**) flashing lights or fragmentation of the image (like looking through a pane of broken glass) or scintillating spots across the visual fields for up to 40 minutes. Sometimes there may be temporary patchy visual field loss which may move across the visual field (scotomas) and even evolve into hemianopia or tunnel vision.
  2. *Sensory aura:* It consists of positive sensory symptoms such as tingling followed by numbness, spreading over 20–30 minutes, from one part of the body to another.
  3. *Language aura:* Dominant hemisphere involvement may cause transient speech disturbance.
  4. *Motor aura:* Transient weakness.
- **Duration of aura:** Usually evolves over 5–20 minutes with symptoms changing as the wave of spreading neuronal depression moves across the surface of the cortex. It rarely lasts for more than 60 minutes and is followed immediately by the headache phase.

Diagnostic Criteria (Table 11.3)

Strongest Predictors of Migraine

- *Are you nauseated or sick to your stomach when you have a headache?*
- *Has a headache limited your activities for a day or more in the last 3 months?*
- *Does light bother you when you have a headache?*
  Patients who answer positively to 2 out of 3 have a 93% chance of having migraines.

  Always rule out other causes of headache—*RED* flags of headache **(Table 11.4)**

Complications of Migraine

- **Status migrainosus** is a debilitating migraine attack lasting for more than 72 hours.
- **Persistent aura without infarction** is defined by aura symptoms persisting for 1 week or more with no evidence of infarction on neuroimaging.

Table 11.3: Simplified diagnostic criteria for migraine.

Repeated attacks of headache lasting 4–72 hours (untreated) with	
At least two of the following features:	Plus at least one of the following features:
• Unilateral pain	• Nausea/vomiting
• Throbbing pain	• Photophobia and phonophobia
• Motion sensitivity (headache aggravated with head movement or physical activity)	• Normal physical examination, no other reasonable cause for the headache
• Moderate or severe intensity	

Table 11.4: RED flags of headache.

	Mnemonic SNNOOP10
• "Worst" headache ever • First severe headache • Subacute worsening over days or weeks • Altered level of sensorium/consciousness • Abnormal neurologic examination • Fever or unexplained systemic signs • Significant weight loss • Vomiting that precedes headache • Pain induced by bending, lifting, cough, Worsens with Valsalva maneuvers • Pain which disturbs sleep or presents immediately upon awakening • Known systemic illness, history of trauma, cancer or HIV • New onset headache in a patient >50 years of age • Focal neurologic deficits, jaw claudication • Morning headache associated with nausea and vomiting • Pain associated with local tenderness (e.g., region of temporal artery)	• **S**ystemic symptoms including fever • **N**eoplasm history • **N**eurologic deficit (including decreased consciousness) • **O**nset is sudden or abrupt • **O**lder age (onset after age 50 years) **P10** • **P**attern change or recent onset of new headache • **P**ositional headache • **P**recipitated by sneezing, coughing, or exercise • **P**apilledema • **P**rogressive headache and atypical presentations • **P**regnancy or puerperium • **P**ainful eye with autonomic features • **P**ost-traumatic onset of headache • **P**athology of the immune system such as HIV • **P**ainkiller (analgesic) overuse (e.g., medication overuse headache) or new drug at onset of headache

- **Migrainosus infarction:** Migraine attack, occurring in a patient with migraine with aura, in which one or more aura symptoms persist for more than 1 hour and neuroimaging, shows an infarction in a relevant brain area.
- **Migraine aura-triggered seizure** is a seizure triggered by an attack of migraine with aura.

Management (Flowchart 11.1)

Nonpharmacological Treatment (General Measures)

- Explanation that migraine has no grave prognosis.
- Identification of triggers and avoidance of identified triggers or exacerbating factors to prevent attacks. Women with aura should avoid estrogen treatment (oral contraception or hormone replacement). Lifestyle modification wherever possible.
- **Other measures:** Meditation, relax techniques, and psychotherapy.

Pharmacological Treatment

- **Abortive treatment:** Treatment of acute attack.
- **Preventive treatment:** Drug prophylaxis.

Treatment of an acute attack

- **Analgesic:** Simple analgesia such as aspirin, paracetamol, or nonsteroidal anti-inflammatory agents.
- Nausea may be treated by an antiemetic (metoclopramide or domperidone).

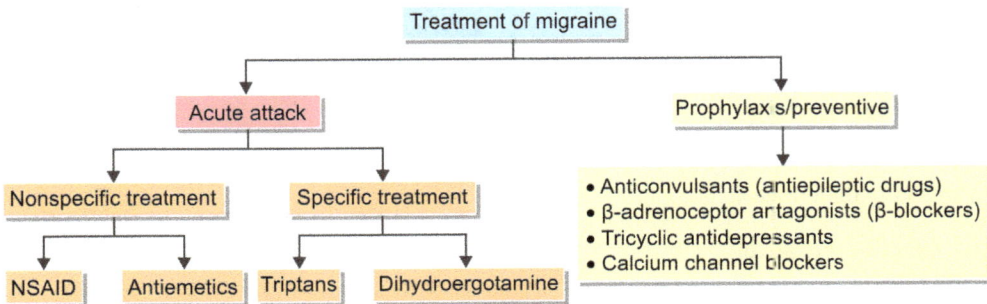

Flowchart 11.1: Treatment of migraine.

- **Severe attacks:** If there is previously no relief with an NSAID, use "triptans".
    - *Triptans:* (e.g., sumatriptan, almotriptan, eletriptan, frovatriptan, naratriptan, rizatriptan, and zolmitriptan).
        - Sumatriptan: 50–100 mg tablet/5–20 mg nasal spray/ 6 mg S/C
        - Rizatriptan: 5–10 mg tablet
        - Frovatriptan: 2.5 mg oral
        - Almotriptan: 12.5 mg
        - Eletriptan: 40–80 mg
        - Zolmitriptan: 2.5 mg oral/5 mg intranasal spray
    - *Mode of action:* Potent 5HT1B/1D agonists, inhibit release of CGRP and substance P, inhibit activation of the trigeminal nerve and inhibit vasodilation in the meninges.
    - *Administration triptans* are available as oral preparations, nasal spray, and subcutaneous injections.
    - *Contraindications:* Ischemic heart disease or stroke, high-risk for coronary artery disease, pregnancy, hemiplegic, or basilar migraine and use with ergots.
- CGRP antagonists (e.g., **erenumab, fremanezumab, galcanezumab**) are very effective for acute treatment of migraine.
- **Lasmiditan,** a selective serotonin 1F receptor agonist has been tried.
- Single-pulse **transcranial magnetic stimulation** (TMS).

Drug prophylaxis
- Indications for drug prophylaxis in migraine are listed in **Box 11.1**.
- Various drugs can be used and the most frequently used are:
    - Anticonvulsants (antiepileptic drugs): **Valproate** (800 mg) or **topiramate** (100–200 mg daily) are the most effective options.
    - β-adrenoceptor antagonists (β-blockers), e.g., **propranolol** slow release 80–160 mg daily.
    - Tricyclic antidepressants, e.g., **amitriptyline** 10 mg increasing weekly in 10 mg steps to 50–60 mg or Dosulepin (10–200 mg at night).
    - Methysergide 1–2 mg TID in resistant cases (prolonged use may produce retroperitoneal and mediastinal fibrosis).
    - Botulinum toxin has been tried as a treatment for chronic migraine.
    - Vasoactive drugs and calcium channel blockers: These include **flunarizine** (5–10 mg OD at bed time), verapamil (80–160 mg three times a day), and methysergide are used in refractory cases. Pizotifen is rarely used.
    - **Memantine** MDA receptor antagonist, blocks glutamate
    - Nonprescription medications: Riboflavin (B_2) 400 mg daily, Magnesium Oxide 400 mg daily, Coenzyme Q10 150 mg daily, Feverfew 10–30 mg daily, Butterbur (Petadolex) 50–75 mg BID, and Melatonin.

CLUSTER HEADACHE

- Cluster headache (migrainous neuralgia) is distinct from migraine and is less common than migraine.
- **Age and gender:** Usually occurs in young adult in the third decade (20 and 40 years) with male predominance (M: F = 5:1).

Clinical Features

- Cluster headache is **periodic with recurrent bouts** of identical headaches beginning at the **same hour for weeks at a time** (the eponymous "cluster"). Patients may develop either one or several attacks within a 24-hour period.
- Cluster headache causes **severe (excruciating)** and **worst, stabbing/boring, unilateral periorbital/retro-orbital pain with parasympathetic autonomic features** in the same eye (e.g., unilateral lacrimation, nasal congestion, and conjunctival redness/injection or even a transient Horner's syndrome). The pain is so severe that they may commit suicide.
- **Circadian periodicity:** Usually cluster period lasts for few weeks and followed by remission for months to years. They typically recur a year or more later often at the same time of year.

Diagnostic Criteria for Cluster Headache

Diagnostic criteria for cluster headache are shown in **Box 11.2**.

Box 11.1: Indications for drug prophylaxis in migraine.

- Patients who have very frequent headaches (more than 2–3 week)
- Attack duration >48 hours
- Migraine-related disability ≥3 days/month
- Headache extremely severe
- Migraine accompanied by severe aura
- Contraindication to acute treatment
- Unacceptable adverse effects with acute migraine treatment
- Patient's preference

> **Box 11.2: Diagnostic criteria for cluster headache.**
>
> At least five attacks fulfilling following:
> - Severe or very severe unilateral orbital, supraorbital, and/or temporal pain lasting 15–180 minutes, if untreated.
> - Headache is accompanied by at least one of the following.
>   - Autonomic features: Unilateral
>   - Conjunctival redness/injection and/or lacrimation or
>   - Nasal congestion and/or rhinorrhea or
>   - Edema of eyelid
>   - Sweating on the forehead and face or
>   - Miosis and/or ptosis or
>   - Restlessness or agitation.
> - Frequency of attacks: From one every other day to eight/day

Management of Cluster Headache

- **Acute attacks:** Analgesics are not useful and acute attacks are usually halted by:
  - **Subcutaneous injection of sumatriptan** (6 mg) is the drug of choice for acute treatment. It works quickly and usually shortens an attack to 10-15 minutes. There is no evidence of tachyphylaxis. Oral sumatriptan is not effective. Sumatriptan (20 mg) and zolmitriptan (5 mg) nasal sprays are also effective or
  - **Inhalation of 100% oxygen** at 10-12 L/min for 15-20 minutes. Many respond very well.
  - The brevity of the attack probably prevents other migraine therapies from being effective. **Octreotide** is effective in the treatment of acute cluster headaches.
- **Most prophylactic migraine drugs are often ineffective.** Attacks can be prevented in some patients by sodium valproate, lithium, verapamil, methysergide and/or a short course of **oral corticosteroids.**

TENSION-TYPE HEADACHE

Most common type of headache.

Pathophysiology is incompletely understood, and few consider this as a milder version of migraine.

Clinical Features

Characteristic features of headache are:
- Pain is "dull" "tight", or like a "pressure", and it may be accompanied by a sensation of a band round the head or pressure at the vertex.
- It is of constant character and generalized, but often radiates forward from the occipital region. It may be episodic or persistent.
- Severity may vary, and is not associated vomiting or photophobia. The pain often progresses throughout the day.
- Tenderness may be present over the skull vault or in the occiput.

Management

- Carefully assess, followed by discussion of likely precipitants and reassurance that the prognosis is good.
- Physiotherapy (with muscle relaxation and stress management) may be helpful.

Table 11.5: Comparison of most common primary headaches.

Characteristic	Migraine	Tension	Cluster
Age of onset	25–55 years	30–50 years	20–40 years
Location	60–70% unilateral	Bilateral	Unilateral, orbital, supraorbital, temporal
Duration of episode	4–72 hours	30 min–7 days	15–180 minutes
Severity	Moderate to severe	Mild to moderate	Extremely severe
Type	Pulsating, throbbing	Pressing, tightening but not pulsating	Boring, searing
Pattern	1–2 attacks per month	<180 attacks per year (or <15 attacks per month)	1–8 attacks per day separated by pain-free periods
Associated symptoms	Nausea, vomiting, photophobia, phonophobia (2 of these)	Either photophobia or phonophobia, but not both, no nausea or vomiting	Conjunctival injection, lacrimation forehead/facial swelling, nasal congestion, rhinorrhea, ptosis, miosis, eyelid edema

- Low-dose amitriptyline may be beneficial. Investigation is rarely required.

Differences between most common primary headaches are presented in **Table 11.5**.

STROKE AND CEREBROVASCULAR DISEASE

Stroke

- **A stroke (cerebrovascular accident is a vague** term which should be avoided) is defined as a syndrome of rapid **(abrupt) onset of a neurologic deficit** that is attributable to a focal vascular cause.
- **World Health Organization (WHO) definition:** Stroke is a defined as, a clinical syndrome consisting of **"rapidly developing clinical signs of focal (or global) disturbance of cerebral function,** with **symptoms lasting for 24 hours or longer or leading to death,** with **no apparent cause other than of vascular origin".**
- **Progressing stroke (or stroke in evolution):** It is a stroke in which the focal neurological deficit worsens after the patient first presents. It may be due to increasing volume of infarction, secondary hemorrhage in the infarcted area or increasing cerebral edema.
- **Complete stroke:** Rapid onset with persistent focal neurological deficit which does not progress beyond 96 hours.
- **Evolving stroke:** Gradual stepwise development of neurological deficits.

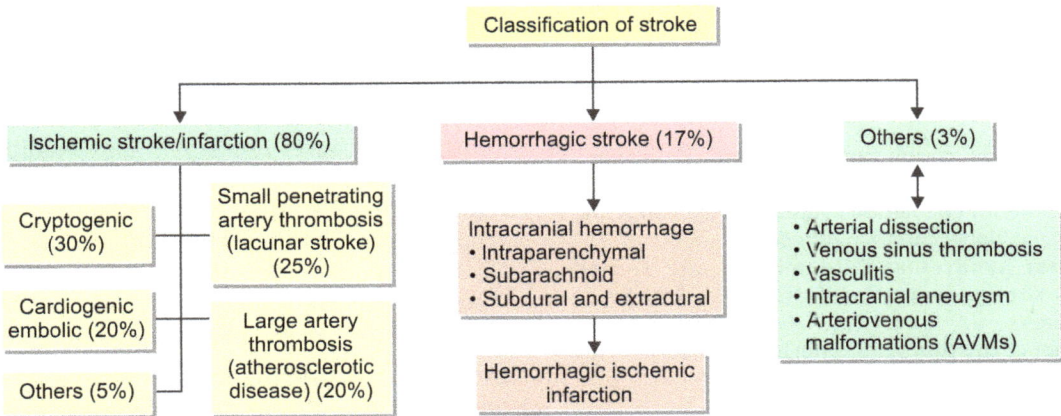

Flowchart 11.2: Classification of stroke.

- Focal cerebral deficits that develop slowly (over weeks to months) are unlikely to be due to stroke and are more suggestive of tumor or inflammatory or degenerative disease.
- **Transient ischemic attack (TIA):**
  - *Reversible ischemic neurological deficit (RIND):* In some cases, deficits last for longer than 24 hours but resolve completely or almost completely within a few days.
  - *Stuttering hemiplegia:* Internal carotid lesions are characterized by repeated episodes of TIA followed by fully evolved stroke.

Types of Stroke (Flowchart 11.2)

About 80% of patients develop **cerebral infarction** due to inadequate blood flow to part of the brain, and most of the remainder develops an **intracerebral hemorrhage (ICH).**

- **Ischemic stroke: Cerebral infarction** is **most commonly caused by thromboembolic disease** secondary to atherosclerosis in the major extracranial arteries (carotid artery and aortic arch). About 20% of infarctions are caused by emboli from the heart, and about 20% are caused by thrombosis in situ caused by intrinsic disease of small perforating vessels (lenticulostriate arteries), producing lacunar infarctions.
- **Hemorrhagic stroke: Intracranial hemorrhage** is caused by bleeding directly into or around the brain. Neurological symptoms are produced by compression, toxic effects, or raised intracranial pressure.
- **Hemorrhagic conversion of ischemic stroke**
  - This may occur after thrombolytic drugs (alteplase) are administered to patients with an ischemic stroke or where a patient has a large cerebral clot, which tends to be more common with cardioembolic strokes
  - The major adverse effect of thrombolysis is symptomatic ICH, observed in around 6–7% of cases.
  - The risk of symptomatic ICH increases with age, high blood pressure, very severe neurological deficits, severe hyperglycemia, and with early ischemic changes on computed tomography (CT) scans
- **Cerebrovascular anomalies** such as intracranial aneurysm and AVMs.

Risk (Predisposing) Factors for Stroke

Risk factor for stroke are described in **Table 11.6**.

Small Vessel (Lacunar) Stroke

- Small penetrating arterial branches of 200–800 μm in diameter, supply the deep brain parenchyma. Each of these small branches can be occluded either by atherothrombotic disease at its origin or by the development of occlusive vasculopathy—lipohyalinotic thickening (consequence of hypertension).

Table 11.6: Risk factors for stroke in patients of all age groups.

High-risk	
• Hypertension (including isolated systolic) • Smoking • Diabetes mellitus • Atrial fibrillation • Drugs: Cocaine, amphetamine • Dilated cardiomyopathy • Endocarditis	• High cholesterol • Obesity • Vasculitis: Systemic vasculities [e.g., polyarteritis nodosa (PAN), granulomatosis with polyangiitis (Wegener's) etc.], primary CNS vasculitis, meningitis (syphilis, tuberculosis, fungal, bacterial, zoster)
Low-risk	
• Migraine • Oral contraceptives or alcohol • Patent foramen ovale	• Recent myocardial infarction • Prosthetic valve • Sleep apnea
Additional risk factors that are more common in young patients	
Hypercoagulable disorders	
• Protein C and S deficiencies • Antithrombin III deficiency • Antiphospholipid syndrome • Factor V Leiden mutation • Prothrombin G20210A heterozygous mutation	• Sickle-cell anemia • Hyperhomocysteinemia • Thrombotic thrombocytopenic purpura • Arterial dissection • Infections (e.g., syphilis, HIV) • Systemic malignancy

- Thrombosis of these vessels causes small infarcts that are referred to as lacunes. These infarcts range in size from **0.2 to 15 mm** in diameter.

Oxford shire Community Stroke Project (OCSP)—Bamford classification

- **TACS Total anterior circulation syndrome:** Hemianopia, hemiparesis, and higher cortical dysfunction
- **PACS Partial anterior circulation syndrome:** Any two of TACS criteria or isolated higher cortical dysfunction
- **LACS Lacunar syndrome:** Pure motor, pure sensory, sensorimotor strokes, clumsy hand-dysarthria syndrome or ataxic hemiparesis
- **POCS Posterior circulation syndrome:** Isolated hemianopia or brainstem or cerebellar signs

Treatment of Ischemic Stroke—"Time is brain"

Treatments designed to reverse or lessen the amount of tissue infarction and improve clinical outcome fall into six categories: (1) IV thrombolysis, (2) endovascular techniques, (3) antithrombotic treatment, (4) medical support, (5) neuroprotection, and (6) stroke centers and rehabilitation.

Intravenous thrombolysis
- Intravenous administration for recombinant t-PA within 3 hours of the onset of symptoms reduces disability and mortality from ischemic stroke.
- Indications and contraindications for r-tPA **(Table 11.7)**
- **Administration:** Administer at the rate of 0.9 mg/kg intravenously (maximum 90 mg) as 10% of total dose as an intravenous bolus and remainder of dose as a continuous intravenous infusion over 60 minutes.

Endovascular mechanical thrombectomy
It is an alternative or adjunctive treatment of acute stroke in patients who are ineligible for, or have contraindications to, thrombolytics or in those who have failed to have vascular recanalization with IV thrombolytics.

Antiplatelet therapy
- **Platelet inhibition:** Aspirin 150 mg PLUS clopidogrel 75 mg daily. **Note:** Glycoprotein IIb/IIIa receptor inhibitor abciximab causes excess ICH and should be avoided in acute stroke.
- Randomized studies of unfractionated heparin, low-molecular-weight heparins, or heparinoids have shown no proven benefits in the reduction of stroke-related mortality, stroke-related morbidity, early stroke recurrence, or stroke prognosis except in the case of cerebral venous thrombosis.

Anticoagulation for acute ischemic stroke
Routine use of anticoagulation for acute ischemic stroke is not recommended. Only indications for anticoagulants are:
- Conditions with potential high risk of early cardiogenic re-embolization (e.g., atrial fibrillation)
- Symptomatic arteriosclerotic stenosis with crescendo TIAs
- Known hypercoagulable states
- Cerebral venous sinus thrombosis.

Medical support
- **Prevention of the common complications of bedridden patients:**
  - *Infections (pneumonia, urinary, and skin):* Prophylactic antibiotic.
  - *Deep venous thrombosis (DVT) with pulmonary embolism:* Subcutaneous heparin and pneumatic compression stockings to prevent DVT.
  - *Others:* Catheterization, Ryle's tube (RT) feeding, maintenance of hygiene, etc.
- **Maintenance of blood pressure:** Collateral blood flow within the ischemic brain is dependent on the blood pressure; hence it is to be maintained.
  - Treat if BP >220/120 mm Hg
  - BP goals in the first 24–48 hours post stroke:
    - No IV tPA: <220/120 mm Hg
    - IV tPA: <185/110 mm Hg
  - First-line agent: labetalol, nicardipine and clevidipine, second-line: nitroprusside (if DBP >120 mm Hg)
  - *Avoid excessive lowering of BP just to give t-PA—"Do not kill the penumbra to save the penumbra"*
  - Do not use antihypertensive drug except left ventricular failure, aortic dissection, acute myocardial infarction, acute renal failure and hypertensive encephalopathy
- **Fever:** It is detrimental and should be treated with antipyretics and surface cooling.
- **Serum glucose** should be monitored and kept at <6.1 mmol/L (110 mg/dL) using an insulin infusion, if necessary.
- **Decreasing intracranial tension (ICT):** By water restriction and IV mannitol, oral glycerol, head end elevation.
- **Hemicraniectomy** (craniotomy and temporary removal of part of the skull) markedly reduces mortality.
  - People with middle cerebral artery (MCA) infarction who meet all of the criteria below should be considered for **decompressive hemicraniectomy.**

Table 11.7: Indications and contraindications for r-tPA.

Indications for r-tPA	Contraindications for r-tPA
• Clinical diagnosis of stroke • Onset of symptom to time of drug administration ≤3 hours (time window: 3–4.5 hours) • Age ≥18 years • CT scan showing no hemorrhage or infarct size >1/3rd of the middle cerebral artery (MCA) territory • Consent by patient or surrogate	• Sustained BP >185/110 mm of Hg despite treatment • Platelets <100,000/μL • Hematocrit <25% • Glucose <50 or >400 mg% • Use of heparin/warfarin within 48 hours and prolonged activated partial thromboplastin time (aPTT) or international normalized ratio (INR) • Prior intracranial hemorrhage • Prior stroke or head injury within 3 months • Major surgery in preceding 14 days • Minor stroke symptoms • GI bleed in preceding 21 days • Recent myocardial infarction (within 3 months) • Coma or stupor • Pregnancy • Age >80 years

Endovascular treatment approaches
- EKOS (ultrasound enhanced thrombolysis)
- NeuroFlo (perfusion augmentation)
- **Mechanical endovascular thrombectomy.**

Statins
Atorvastatin, rosuvastatin (10–20 mg).

Neuroprotection
Drugs that block the excitatory amino acid pathways (nimodipine, **magnesium lubeluzole**, basic fibroblast growth factor, and citicoline) protect neurons and glia in animals, but they have not yet been proven to be beneficial in humans.

Rehabilitation
- Proper rehabilitation of the stroke patient includes **early physical, occupational, and speech therapy.** It is directed toward educating the patient and family about the patients' neurologic deficit, preventing the complications of immobility (e.g., pneumonia, DVT and pulmonary embolism, pressure sores of the skin, and muscle contractures), and providing encouragement and instructions in overcoming the deficit.
- *Goal of rehabilitation:* It is to **return the patient to home and to maximize recovery.** The use of **restrain therapy** (immobilizing the unaffected side) has been shown to improve hemiparesis following stroke, even years following the stroke.

SUBARACHNOID HEMORRHAGE

- Subarachnoid hemorrhage (SAH) is a pathologic condition in which the **blood enters the subarachnoid space.**
- SAH is less common than ischemic stroke or ICH. It accounts for about 5% of strokes.
- **Most common cause** of SAH **is trauma.**
- **Most common cause of spontaneous SAH** is an **aneurysmal** (saccular or "berry aneurysms") **bleed (65–80%).**
- SAH causes intense reductions in cerebral blood flow (CBF), reduced cerebral autoregulation, and acute cerebral ischemia.
- The overall case fatality varied from 32 to 67%.
- Risk factors for SAH **(Table 11.8).**

Clinical Features of Subarachnoid Hemorrhage (SAH)

- **Headache:** Most common symptom (97%). Usually severe (the worst headache of my life) and sudden **(thunderclap)** in onset. Few patients may have milder warning headaches (sentinel headaches) in 2–8 weeks preceding the major hemorrhage. Headache may pulsate toward the occiput and sometimes may be felt as neck pain. Occipital and posterior cervical pain may signal a posterior inferior cerebellar artery (PICA) or anterior inferior cerebellar artery aneurysm. If there is expanding middle cerebral artery aneurysm, pain may be observed in or behind the eye and in the low temple. Headache commonly occurs on physical exertion, straining, and sexual excitement.
- **Vomiting** may be present.
- **Other symptoms:** Decreased consciousness and alertness, seizure (10%), and stiff neck, etc.
- **Rerupture/rebleed:** The rerupture of an untreated aneurysm in the first month following SAH is approximately 30%, with the peak in the first 7 days.

Physical Examination
- Patient is usually distressed and irritable, with photophobia.
- Neck stiffness (and a positive Kernig's sign) due to subarachnoid blood may be present but this may take few hours to develop. Focal hemisphere signs, e.g., intracerebral hematoma may cause hemiparesis or aphasia.
- Rarely, third nerve palsy may be developing due to local pressure from an aneurysm of the posterior communicating artery.
- **Fundoscopy:** May show **subhyaloid hemorrhage,** which is canoe-shaped (**SAH plus subhyaloid hemorrhage = *Tersen syndrome*),** produced due to tracking of blood along the subarachnoid space around the optic nerve.

Investigations
- **CT scan:** It shows blood in the subarachnoid space (if performed in the first few days), intracerebral hematoma, hydrocephalus, associated brain ischemia, and occasionally aneurysmal location.
- **Lumbar puncture:** It should be performed when clinical suspicion of SAH is high, CT scan does not reveal subarachnoid blood, and there is no mass effect. In the initial few hours cerebrospinal fluid (CSF) will be uniformly blood stained.

Management
- Immediate treatment is absolute **bed rest** (for 4 weeks) and **supportive measures.** These include protecting the airway, managing blood pressure and raised ICP, pain management, and sedation. It should be discussed urgently with a neurosurgical team. Patient is advised to gradually resumption of physical activities after recovery.
- *Control of hypertension:* In conscious patients without raised ICP, active treatment of hypertension is necessary. A target mean arterial pressure of 130 mm Hg is recommended. Drugs include labetalol, esmolol, or nicardipine. Sodium nitroprusside should be avoided because may cause increase of ICP.
- **Avoid strictly:** *Hypovolemia, hypotension, hyperthermia, hyperglycemia and hyponatremia* are important to prevent delayed cerebral ischemia.

Table 11.8: Risk factors for subarachnoid hemorrhage.

• Hypertension	• Slight increased risk with advancing age
• Cigarette smoking	• Alcohol consumption (debatable)
• Oral contraceptives	• Following cocaine abuse
• Diurnal variations in blood pressure	• Increased incidence of polycystic kidneys, fibromuscular dysplasia of extracranial arteries, Ehler-Danlos syndrome, moyamoya, AV malformations and coarctation of aorta
• Pregnancy and parturition	
• Slight increased risk during lumbar puncture and/or cerebral angiography in patient with cerebral aneurysm	

- **Calcium channel blocker:** Nimodipine (30–60 mg IV for 5–14 days, followed by 360 mg orally for a further 7 days) provides a modest but significant improvement in outcome by reducing cerebral arterial vasospasm. It is given for 3 weeks to prevent delayed ischemia in the acute phase and decreases mortality.
- **Prophylactic anticonvulsants**
- **Interventional management:** Early aneurysm repair prevents rerupture/rebleeding and improve blood flow. An aneurysm can be "clipped" by a neurosurgeon or "coiled" by an endovascular surgeon.

SEIZURES AND EPILEPSY

- *Seizure:* It is a **paroxysmal event due to abnormal, excessive, hypersynchronous discharges from** an aggregate of **central nervous system** (CNS) **neurons.**
- *Epilepsy:* It is a condition in which an individual has **recurrent seizures due to a chronic, underlying process.**
- An individual with a single seizure or recurrent seizures due to correctable or avoidable circumstances does not necessarily have epilepsy.

Classification of Seizures (Tables 11.9 and 11.10)

Focal Seizures

Focal seizures without dyscognitive features
- In this type, **consciousness is fully preserved during the seizure** and the clinical manifestation is relatively simple.
- Focal seizures can cause motor, sensory, autonomic, or psychic symptoms without an obvious alteration in consciousness.
- A focal motor seizure arising from the right primary motor cortex near the area controlling hand movement will note the onset of involuntary movements of the contralateral, left hand.
- Three additional features of these seizures are:
  1. *Jacksonian march:* Representing the **spread of seizure activity over a progressively larger region of motor cortex.** In Jacksonian seizures, march of symptoms occur where if it is motor, clonic jerking starts at a point. For example, it may start at face and spreads to upper limb, then to lower limb and then on to opposite side to become a generalized fit. This denotes the path of spread of the epileptic activity and is called Jacksonian spread/march.

Table 11.9: New classification of seizures.

Focal seizures: It can be further described as having motor, sensory, autonomic, cognitive, or other features	
Generalized seizures	
• Absence (typical/atypical)	• Atonic
• Tonic-clonic (in any combination)	• Myoclonic
• Clonic	• May be focal, generalized, or unclear
• Tonic	
Unknown: Epileptic spasms	

Table 11.10: International League against Epilepsy (ILAE) classification of seizure types 2017.

Generalized onset seizures	
• Tonic-clonic	• Typical
• Clonic	• Atypical
• Tonic	• Myoclonic
• Myoclonic	• Eyelid myoclonia
• Myoclonic-tonic-clonic	
• Myoclonic-atonic	
• Atonic	
• Epileptic spasms	
Focal onset seizures	
Motor onset	**Nonmotor onset**
• Aware	• Aware
• Impaired awareness	• Impaired awareness
• Unknown awareness	• Unknown awareness
• Automatisms	• Autonomic
• Atonic	• Behavior arrest
• Clonic	• Cognitive
• Epileptic spasms	• Emotional
• Hyperkinetic	• Sensory
• Myoclonic	
• Tonic	
• Focal to bilateral tonic-clonic	• Focal to bilateral tonic-clonic
Unknown onset seizures	
Motor	**Nonmotor**
• Tonic-clonic	• Behavior arrest
• Epileptic spasms	
Unclassified seizures	

  2. *Todd's paralysis or the localized paresis:* It is a condition characterized by brief, temporary paralysis that follows a seizure. It may occur **for minutes to hours in the involved region following** the seizure.
  3. *Epilepsia partialis continua:* Analogous to partial status epilepticus. It is often quite refractory to medical therapy.
- **Other manifestations:** Changes in somatic sensation (e.g., paresthesia), vision (flashing lights or formed hallucinations), equilibrium (sensation of ailing or vertigo), and autonomic function (flushing, sweating, and piloerection).

Focal seizures with dyscognitive features
- Focal seizure activity may be accompanied by a transient impairment of the patient's ability to maintain normal contact with the environment.
- Patient is **unable to respond to visual or verbal commands** during the seizure and has impaired recollection or awareness of the ictal phase.
- The seizures **frequently begin with an aura** (i.e., focal seizures without dyscognitive features) that is stereotypic for the patient.

- The start of the ictal phase is often a **sudden behavioral arrest or motionless stare,** and this marks the onset of the event for which the patient will be amnesic.
- The behavioral arrest is usually accompanied by oromandibular or hand automatisms, which are involuntary, automatic behaviors that have a wide range of manifestations.
- **Automatisms** may consist of very basic behaviors such as chewing, lip smacking, swallowing or picking movements of the hands or more elaborate behaviors such as a display of emotion or running.

Complex partial seizures (temporal lobe seizures)
Focal seizures arising from the temporal or frontal cortex may also cause alterations in hearing, olfaction, or higher cortical function (psychic symptoms like to sensation of unusual intense odors (e.g., burning rubber or kerosene) or sounds (crude or highly complex sounds) or illusions that objects are growing (metamorphopsia) smaller (micropsia) or larger (macropsia). When such symptoms precede focal seizures with dyscognitive features or secondarily generalized seizure, these seizures serve as a warning, or aura.

Absence Seizures (Petit Mal)
- Sudden, brief lapses of **consciousness without loss of postural control.**
- **It lasts for only a few seconds and consciousness returns rapidly** and there is no postictal confusion.
- Usually accompanied by subtle, bilateral motor signs such as rapid blinking of the eyelids, chewing movements, or small-amplitude, clonic movements of the hands. Absence seizures can be typical or atypical.
- Onset usually in childhood (ages 4–8 years) or early adolescence and are the main seizure type in 15–20% of children with epilepsy.
- May occur hundreds of times in a day without the knowledge of parents or the child.
- First clue may be often unexplained "daydreaming" and a decline in school performance recognized by a teacher.
- **EEG:** Generalized, symmetric, 3-Hz spike-and-wave discharge that begins and ends suddenly, superimposed on a normal EEG background which can be provoked by hyperventilation.

Generalized, Tonic-Clonic Seizures (GTCS) (Grand Mal)
- Main type of seizure in 10% of all individuals with epilepsy.
- Usually **begins abruptly without warning.** Some may develop vague premonitory symptoms which are distinct from the stereotypic auras associated with focal seizures that generalize.
- **Initially,** there is **tonic contraction of muscles throughout the body** leading to **loud moan or ictal cry, cyanosis,** biting of the tongue, etc.
- Marked enhancement of sympathetic tone leads to increase in heart rate, blood pressure, and pupillary size.
- **After 10–20 seconds, clonic phase starts** with **superimposed relaxation** which progressively increases until the end of ictal period.
- **Postictal phase** is characterized by **unresponsiveness, muscular flaccidity, and excessive salivation, bladder or bowel incontinence.**
- Patients **gradually regain consciousness** over **minutes to hours** with accompanying postictal confusion, headache and muscle ache.
- **EEG:** Generalized high-amplitude, polyspike discharges in tonic phases, which in the clonic phase typically interrupted by slow waves to create a spike-and-wave pattern.
- **Other variants** include pure tonic and pure clonic type.

Atonic seizures
- Characterized by **sudden loss of postural muscle tone** lasting **1–2 seconds.**
- **Consciousness is briefly impaired,** but there is usually **no postictal confusion.**
- May cause only a quick head drop or nodding movement, while a longer seizure will cause the patient to collapse.
- They **are rarely seen in isolation** and are usually seen in association with known epileptic syndromes.
- **EEG:** Brief, generalized spike-and-wave discharges followed immediately by diffuse slow waves that correlate with the loss of muscle tone.

Myoclonic seizures
- **Sudden, brief jerky muscle contraction** that may involve **one part of the body or the entire body.**
- Normal, common physiologic forms of myoclonus are the sudden jerking movement observed while falling asleep and hiccups.
- Most pathologic myoclonus commonly seen in association with metabolic disorders, degenerative CNS diseases, or anoxic brain injury.
- Myoclonic seizures are the predominant feature of juvenile myoclonic epilepsy.
- **EEG:** May show bilaterally synchronous spike-and-wave discharges synchronized with the myoclonus.

Epilepsy Syndromes
Epilepsy syndromes are disorders in which **epilepsy is a predominant feature,** and there is sufficient evidence to suggest a common underlying mechanism.

Juvenile myoclonic epilepsy
- Juvenile myoclonic epilepsy (JME) is a **generalized seizure** disorder of **unknown cause** that appears in **early adolescence** and is usually characterized by **bilateral myoclonic jerks** that may be single or repetitive.
- The myoclonic seizures are **most frequent in the morning** after awakening and can be provoked by sleep deprivation.
- Lifelong treatment is necessary and **sodium valproate** is the drug of choice.

Lennox-Gastaut syndrome
- Lennox-Gastaut syndrome is seen in children between the age of 1 and 8 years and is characterized by the following triad:
  - **Multiple seizure types** (usually including generalized tonic-clonic, atonic, and atypical absence seizures).
  - **EEG:** Shows **slow (<3 Hz) spike-and-wave discharges** and a variety of other abnormalities.
  - **Impaired cognitive function** in most but not all patients.

- Lennox-Gastaut syndrome is an epileptic encephalopathy **associated with CNS disease or dysfunction** from a variety of causes, including developmental abnormalities, perinatal hypoxia/ischemia, trauma, infection, and other acquired lesions.
- A similar syndrome in infancy that often evolves into Lennox-Gastaut syndrome is **West syndrome**, characterized by infantile spasms, Salaam attacks, other findings of cerebral dysfunction, and abnormal EEG pattern (Hypsarrhythmia).

Mesial temporal lobe epilepsy syndrome
- Mesial temporal lobe epilepsy (MTLE) is the **most common syndrome** associated with complex partial seizures and is an example of symptomatic, partial epilepsy.
- Characteristic **hippocampal sclerosis** on MRI is an essential element in the pathophysiology of MTLE for many patients.
- Recognition of this syndrome is especially important because it tends to be **refractory to treatment with anticonvulsants but responds extremely well to surgical intervention.**

Febrile Seizure
- Usually occur between **3 months and 5 years of age** and have a peak incidence between 18 and 24 months.
- It **is generalized, tonic-clonic seizure** in child **during a febrile illness** in the setting of a common childhood infections.
- The seizure is likely to occur during the rising phase of the temperature curve (i.e., during the first day)
- A **simple febrile seizure** is a **single, isolated** event, brief, and symmetric in appearance. **Complex febrile seizures** are characterized **by repeated seizure activity,** duration >15 minutes, or by focal features.
- Simple febrile seizures are not associated with an increase in the risk of developing epilepsy; while complex febrile seizures have a risk of 2–5%. Other risk factors include the presence of pre-existing neurologic deficits and a family history of nonfebrile seizures.

Causes of Seizures According to Age

For causes of seizures according to age, *see* **Box 11.3.**

Laboratory Studies
- **Routine investigations:** These include serum glucose, calcium, electrolytes, renal and hepatic functions.
- **Lumbar puncture:** If indicated.
- **EEG:** May help establish the diagnosis of epilepsy, classify the seizure type, and provide evidence for the existence of a particular epilepsy syndrome.
  - The presence of electrographic seizure activity, i.e., of abnormal, repetitive, rhythmic activity having an abrupt onset and termination, clearly establishes the diagnosis.
  - The EEG findings may also be helpful in the interictal period by showing certain abnormalities that are strongly supportive of epilepsy. Such epileptiform activity consists of bursts of abnormal discharges containing spikes or sharp waves.
  - EEG is normal in 40% of epileptic patients.
- Neuroimaging studies (MRI preferred over CT).

Box 11.3: Causes of seizures according to age.

Neonates (<1 month)
- Perinatal hypoxia and ischemia
- Intracranial hemorrhage and trauma
- CNS infections
- Metabolic

Infants and children (>1 month and <12 years)
- Febrile seizures
- Genetic disorders (metabolic, degenerative, primary epilepsy syndromes)
- CNS infections

Adolescents (12–18 years)
- Trauma
- Genetic disorders
- Infection

Young adults (18–35 years)
- Trauma
- Alcohol withdrawal

Older adults (>35 years)
- Cerebrovascular disease
- Trauma (including subdural hematoma)
- Brain tumor
- Alcohol withdrawal
- Degenerative diseases

Seizures and Syncope

Differences between seizures and syncope are listed in **Table 11.11.**

Table 11.11: Differences between seizures and syncope.

Features	Seizures	Syncope
Immediate precipitating factor	Usually none	Emotional stress, Valsalva, orthostatic hypotension, cardiac etiologies
Premonitory symptoms	None or aura (e.g., odd odor)	Tiredness, nausea, diaphoresis, tunneling of vision
Posture at onset	Variable	Usually erect
Transition to unconsciousness	Often immediate	Gradual over seconds
Duration of unconsciousness	Minutes	Seconds
Duration of tonic or clonic movements	30–60 seconds	Never more than 15 seconds
Facial appearance during event	Cyanosis, frothing at mouth	Pallor
Disorientation and sleepiness after event	Many minutes to hours	<5 minutes
Headache, muscle pain, tongue bite incontinence	Often, tongue bite—lateral	Rarely, tongue bite—tip

Treatment

Indications to Initiate Antiepileptic Drug Therapy
- Antiepileptic drug therapy should be **started in any patient with recurrent seizures of unknown etiology** or a **known cause that cannot be reversed within short time.**
- Selection of antiepileptic drugs **(Table 11.12)**. Certain AEDs such as phenytoin and carbamazepine can worsen myoclonic seizure. Hence, proper AED for proper seizure must be given.

Treatment Modification
- If a treatment is modified recently, one should wait for at least four half-lives of the drug before further modifying dosage.
- If one drug is unable to control seizures then another drug should be considered when either maximum dose of the first drug is reached or the patient starts showing intolerable side effects.
- Whenever a new drug is added, the first drug is continued till the second drug controls seizures. Only after achieving adequate seizure control the first drug should be gradually withdrawn.

Indications for Discontinue Therapy
- Complete medical control of seizures for 1–5 years.
- Single seizure type, either focal or generalized.
- Normal neurologic examination (including intelligence)
- Normal EEG

Treatment of Refractory Epilepsy
- Therapy combines first line drugs, i.e., carbamazepine, phenytoin, valproic acid and lamotrigine.
- If these drugs are unsuccessful, then the addition of a newer drug such as levetiracetam and topiramate is indicated.

Table 11.12: Selection of antileptic drugs in seizures.

Seizure types	1st choice	2nd choice
Monotherapy for generalized-onset tonic-clonic seizures	Valproate, topiramate	Zonisamide, levetiracetam, lamotrigine phenytoin, carbamazepine
Absence seizure	Ethosuximide, valproate	Zonisamide, levetiracetam, topiramate, felbamate, clonazepam
Monotherapy for partial seizures	Carbamazepine, oxcarbazepine, phenytoin, topiramate	Lamotrigine, gabapentin, levetiracetam
Myoclonic	Valproate, levetiracetam, clonazepam	Zonisamide, topiramate
Status epilepticus	Diazepam, lorazepam	Phenytoin IV, phosphenytoin IV
Febrile convulsions	Diazepam rectal 0.5 mg/kg	
Infantile spasms	Corticotropin Corticosteroids Zonisamide	Clonazepam, nitrazepam, vigabatrin, phenobarbital

- Patients with myoclonic seizures resistant to valproic acid may respond to a combination of valproic acid and ethosuximide.

Surgical Treatment of Refractory Epilepsy
- About 20–30% of patients with epilepsy are resistant to medical therapy. **Ketogenic diet**—has been advised to decrease seizure recurrence. Low carbohydrate, adequate protein, high fat has been advised.
- **Anteromedial temporal lobe** (temporal lobectomy) or a **more limited removal of the underlying hippocampus** and **amygdala** (amygdalohippocampectomy).
- Focal seizures arising from extratemporal regions may be abolished by a focal neocortical resection with precise removal of an identified lesion (lesionectomy).
- **Others:** Hemispherectomy, corpus callosotomy, etc.
- **Vagus nerve stimulation** (VNS) may be used; some of these cases, although the benefit for most patients seem to very limited.

Antiepileptic Drugs for Chronic Use
For Antiepileptic drugs for chronic use and antiepileptic drugs and their adverse reactions and uses, see **Tables 11.13 and 11.14.**

Table 11.13: Antiepileptic drugs for chronic use.

Type of drug		Examples
Na^+ channel blockers		Phenytoin, carbamazepine, oxcarbazepine, primidone, valproic acid, lamotrigine, topiramate, zonisamide, phenobarbital, gabapentin, felbamate
Ca^{2+} channel blockers		Ethosuximide, phenobarbital, zonisamide
Drugs that potentiate GABA	Increase opening time of channel	Phenobarbital
	Increase frequency of openings of channel	Diazepam, lorazepam, clonazepam
	Increase GABA in synapse	Valproic acid
	Increase GABA metabolism	Gabapentin
	Increase GABA release	Gabapentin
	Block GABA transaminase	Vigabatrin
	Block GABA transporter (GAT-1)	Valproic acid, tiagabine
	Facilitate GAD (Glutamic acid decarboxylase) Increase GABA synthesis	Valproic acid
	Synaptic vesicle protein 2A binding	Levetiracetam (inhibits presynaptic calcium channels)
	AMPA agonist	Perampanel

Table 11.14: Antiepileptic drugs and their adverse reactions and uses.

Drug	Adverse reactions	Uses
Phenytoin	Ataxia and nystagmus, cognitive impairment, hirsutism, gingival hyperplasia, coarsening of facial features, dose-dependent zero order kinetics, exacerbates absence seizures, 'Fetal hydantoin syndrome'	Partial seizure, generalized (including tonic-clonic) seizures, contraindicated in absence seizures. **Nonseizure indications** include trigeminal neuralgia, manic-depressive disorders
Carbamazepine	Auto induction of metabolism, nausea and visual disturbances, granulocyte suppression, aplastic anemia, exacerbates absence seizures	Partial seizure (including tonic-clonic). **Contraindicated in absence seizures. Nonseizure indications** include trigeminal neuralgia, manic-depressive disorders
Oxcarbazepine	Hyponatremia, less hypersensitivity and induction of hepatic enzymes than with carbamazepine	
Phenobarbital	Sedation, cognitive impairment, behavioral changes, induction of liver enzymes, may worsen absence and atonic seizures	Useful for partial, generalized tonic-clonic seizures, and febrile seizures
Primidone	Same as phenobarbital Sedation occurs early Gastrointestinal disturbances	Effective against partial and generalized tonic-clonic seizures
Valproate	Elevated liver enzymes, nausea and vomiting, abdominal pain, heartburn, tremor, hair loss, syncratic, hepatotoxicity, teratogen (spina bifida)	A broad spectrum anti-seizure drug to the most partial and generalized seizures, including myoclonic and absence seizures). **Nonseizure indications include:** Migraine (prophylaxis), bipolar disorder
Ethosuximide	Gastric distress, including, pain, nausea and vomiting, lethargy and fatigue, headache, hiccups, euphoria, skin rashes	Drug of choice for absence seizures
Clonazepam	Sedation is prominent. Ataxia, behavior disorders	Long-acting drug with efficacy for absence seizures. Also effective in some cases of myoclonic seizures. Has been tried in infantile spasms
Lamotrigine	Dizziness, headache, diplopia, nausea, somnolence, rash	Presently use as add-on therapy with valproic acid. Also effective in generalized and myoclonic seizures in childhood and absence seizures preferred in elderly
Topiramate	Somnolence, fatigue, dizziness, cognitive slowing, paresthesia, nervousness, confusion, urolithiasis	Myoclonic seizures, migraine
Zonisamide	Drowsiness, cognitive impairment, high incidence of renal stones	Effective against partial and generalized tonic-clonic seizures
Felbamate	Aplastic anemia, severe hepatitis	Third-line drug used only for refractory partial seizure cases
Vigabatrin	Drowsiness, dizziness, weight gain, agitation, confusion, psychosis	Use for infantile spasms, partial seizures and contraindicated if pre-existing mental illness is present
Tiagabine	Dizziness, nervousness, tremor, difficulty concentrating, depression, asthenia, emotional liability, psychosis, skin rash	Effective against partial and generalized tonic-clonic seizures
Gabapentin	Somnolence, dizziness, ataxia, headache, tremor	Used as an adjunct in partial and generalized tonic-clonic seizures. Neuropathy
Levetiracetam	Somnolence, incoordination, irritability, mood swings, psychosis	Effective for GTCS, JME. Preferred in elderly

STATUS EPILEPTICUS

Status epilepticus (SE) refers to **continuous seizures or repetitive, discrete seizures with impaired consciousness** in the interictal period.

Status epilepticus is an epileptic seizure of greater than 5 minutes or more than one seizure within a 5-minute period without the patient returning to normal between them. Previous definitions used a 30-minute time limit.

Subtypes

- **Generalized convulsive status epilepticus** (GCSE), e.g., persistent, generalized electrographic seizures, coma, and tonic-clonic movements.
- **Nonconvulsive status epilepticus,** e.g., persistent absence seizures or focal seizures, confusion or partially impaired consciousness, and minimal motor abnormalities.

Etiology of Status Epilepticus

For etiology of status epilepticus, *see* **Table 11.15**.

Table 11.15: Etiology of status epilepticus.

• Stroke, including hemorrhagic	• Remote brain injury/ congenital malformations
• Low AED levels	• Infections
• Alcohol withdrawal	• Brain neoplasms
• Anoxic brain injury	• Idiopathic
• Metabolic disturbances	

Clinical Features

☐ Self-perpetuating, generalized tonic-clonic seizure, or
☐ Series of generalized tonic-clonic seizures
☐ Without return to consciousness in between seizures.

Phases

☐ **Initial compensatory phase:** Sympathetic overdrive, increased CO, increased BP.
☐ **Decompensation** → homeostatic failure
☐ Reduced → CO/sugar/lactate/O_2 levels leading to:
  • Cardiorespiratory collapse
  • Electrolyte imbalance
  • Rhabdomyolysis and delayed tubular necrosis
  • Hyperthermia
  • Multiorgan failure (MOF)
  • Raised ICP and cerebral edema.

Complications

These include aspiration, hypotension, cardiac arrhythmias, and renal or hepatic failure.

Diagnosis

☐ **Diagnosis of nonconvulsive status epilepticus in critically ill patients.**
☐ Correlate with poorer outcome.
☐ EEG patterns are difficult to interpret (equivocal patterns)—criteria are **not** validated.
☐ A trial of rapidly acting IV AED is used to observe improvement in both clinical → EEG by several hours.

Management of Status Epilepticus

For management of status epilepticus, *see* **Table 11.16**.

MENINGITIS

Classifications of Meningitis

For classifications of meningitis, *see* **Table 11.17**.

Acute Bacterial (Pyogenic/Purulent) Meningitis

Relative frequency of various bacterial species causing meningitis varies with age.
☐ **Neonatal period:** Major causative agents include gram-negative bacilli (principally *Escherichia coli*), *Listeria monocytogenes*, and group B streptococci.
☐ **Infants and children:** Major causes in children beyond 1 month of age are *Haemophilus influenzae* and *Neisseria meningitidis*.

Table 11.16: Management of status epilepticus.

First 5 minutes
- Check emergency ABC's
- Give O_2
- Obtain IV access
- Begin ECG monitoring
- Check fingerstick glucose
- Draw blood for serum electrolytes, RFT, magnesium, calcium, phosphate, CBC, LFTs, AED levels, ABG, troponin
- Toxicology screen (urine and blood)

6–10 minutes
- Thiamine 100 mg IV; 50 mL of D50 IV unless adequate glucose known
- Lorazepam 4 mg IV over 2 minutes; if still seizing, repeat × 1 in 5 minutes
- If no rapid IV access give diazepam 20 mg PR or midazolam 10 mg intranasally, buccally or IM

10–20 minutes
- If seizures persist, begin fosphenytoin 20 mg/kg IV at 150 mg/min, with blood pressure and ECG monitoring. OR
- Phenytoin 15–20 mg/kg at 30–50 mg/min

Reasonable to bypass this step, or perform subsequent step simultaneous with fosphenytoin loading

10–60 minutes: One (or more) of the following 4 options (intubation usually necessary except for valproate):
1. Continuous IV midazolam: Load: 0.2 mg/kg; repeat 0.2–0.4 mg/kg boluses every 5 minutes until seizures stop, up to a maximum total loading dose of 2 mg/kg. Initial rate: 0.1 mg/kg/hour. Continuous IV dose range: 0.05–2.9 mg/kg/hour. OR
2. Continuous IV propofol: Load: 1 mg/kg; repeat 1–2 mg/kg boluses every 3–5 minutes until seizures stop, up to maximum total loading dose of 10 mg/kg. Initial continuous IV rate: 2 mg/kg/h. Continuous IV dose range: 1–15 mg/kg/hour. Avoid >48 hours of >5 mg/kg/hour (increased risk of propofol infusion syndrome). OR
3. IV valproate: 40 mg/kg over ~10 minutes. If still seizing, additional 20 mg/kg over ~5 minutes. OR
4. IV phenobarbital: 20 mg/kg IV at 50–100 mg/min.

60 minutes
- Continuous IV pentobarbital. Load: 5 mg/kg at up to 50 mg/min; repeat 5 mg/kg boluses until seizures stop. Initial continuous IV rate: 1 mg/kg/hr. Continuous IV-dose range: 0.5–10 mg/kg/hour; traditionally titrated to suppression-burst on EEG.

Perform neuroimaging when convulsive activity is controlled:
- Begin continuous EEG, if patient does not awaken rapidly or if continuous IV Rx is used.
- Treat metabolic abnormalities and hypothermia.
- Lumbar puncture and antibiotics can be considered if infection is suspected.

SE not controlled even with anesthetic agents is called super refractory SE, for which IV Ig/pulse steroid can be tried as last resort.

☐ **Adolescents and in young adults**: Meningococcus (*Neisseria meningitides*) is the most common pathogen.
☐ **Extremes of life:** *Streptococcus pneumoniae* and *Listeria monocytogenes*.

Table 11.17: Classifications of meningitis.

Infective	

1. **Bacterial meningitis**
  ▪ Common organisms: *Streptococcus pneumonia, Neisseria meningitidis, Haemophilus influenzae*
  ▪ Uncommon organisms: *Staphylococcus aureus, Staphylococcus epidermidis,* Group B streptococci, *E. coli, Klebsiella, Proteus* spp., *Listeria monocytogenes.*
  ▪ Rare organisms: *Salmonella, Shigella, Clostridium perfringens, Neisseria gonorrhoeae*
	3. **Viral meningitis (aseptic meningitis)**
	  ▪ Enteroviruses (Coxsackie, poliovirus)
	  ▪ Mumps virus
	  ▪ Arboviruses
	  ▪ HIV
	  ▪ Herpes simplex-2

2. **Tuberculous meningitis (TBM):** *Mycobacterium tuberculosis*	4. **Spirochetal:** Leptospirosis, Lyme disease, syphilis 5. **Rickettsial:** Typhus fever 6. **Protozoal:** Cysticerci, amoeba, *Naegleria* 7. **Fungal:** *Cryptococcus neoformans, Candida, Histoplasma, Blastomyces, Coccidioides, Sporothrix*
Noninfective (sterile)	

1. **Malignant disease**
  ▪ Breast cancer
  ▪ Bronchial cancer
  ▪ Leukemia (leukemic meningitis)
  ▪ Lymphoma
2. **Subarachnoid hemorrhage (SAH)** (causes meningismus)
	3. **Inflammatory disease (may be recurrent)**
	  ▪ Sarcoidosis
	  ▪ Systemic lupus erythematosus, rheumatoid arthritis
	  ▪ Behçet's disease
	  ▪ Vasculitis

Predisposing conditions
- **For pneumococci:** Other pneumococcal infections (pneumonia, sinusitis, otitis media), splenectomy, hypogammaglobulinemia, complement deficiency.
- **For Neisseria meningitides:** Complement deficiency (including properdin), B-serotype (not protected by vaccine is responsible for one-third of cases). Usually associated with petechial or purpuric skin lesions.
- **Listeria monocytogenes:** Important cause in neonates (<1 month), pregnant women, >60 years and immunocompromized persons.

Clinical manifestations
- **Classic triad:** (1) Fever, (2) headache, and (3) nuchal rigidity.
- **Consciousness:** Vary from lethargy to coma (>75%).
- Nausea, vomiting and photophobia are common
- **Seizure/convulsions** (especially in children) may be initial presentation or present during course (20–40%).
  - *Focal:* Due to arterial ischemia, infarction, cortical venous thrombosis, or focal edema.
  - *Generalized or status:* Due to hyponatremia, cerebral anoxia, or toxic effects of antimicrobial drugs.
- **Classic signs of meningitis:**
  - *Cervical rigidity/neck stiffness*
  - *Kernig sign:* Knee pain with hip flexion
  - *Brudzinski sign:* Knee/hip flexion when the neck is flexed.
- **Occasionally cranial nerve palsies,** with focal neurologic deficits such as visual field defects, dysphasia, and hemiparesis may occur.
- **Raised ICP:** One of the complications of bacterial meningitis and CSF pressure may be raised to 180–400 mm H_2O. Disastrous complication of ICP is cerebral herniation.
  - *Other signs:* Reduced level of consciousness, papilledema, dilated poorly reactive pupil, VIth cranial nerve palsy, decerebrate posture, Cushing reflex (bradycardia, hypertension, and irregular respiration).

Complications of bacterial meningitis
- Obstructive hydrocephalus
- Thrombophlebitis of leptomeningeal veins may lead to venous thrombosis, cerebral infarction, focal infection of the underlying brain parenchyma
- Chronic adhesive arachnoiditis
- Cerebral abscess
- Subdural empyema
- Focal neurologic deficits (e.g., cranial nerve palsy, hemiparesis)
- Sensorineural hearing loss
- Vasculitis of cranial vessel
- Epilepsy
- **Waterhouse-Friderichsen syndrome:** It results from meningitis-associated septicemia with hemorrhagic infarction of the adrenal glands and cutaneous petechiae. It occurs most often with meningococcal and pneumococcal meningitis.

Diagnosis
- **By examination of the CSF:** It is usually obtained by lumbar puncture. Lumbar puncture should be postponed, if there is papilledema and or focal neurologic findings suggestive of an intracranial mass lesion. It can be done only after ruling out the same by CT or MRI.
- **Blood culture:** If meningitis seems likely, blood should be sent for culture and sensitivity and empirical antimicrobial therapy should be started while the neuroimaging study is being carried out.
- CSF findings in bacterial meningitis and other meningitis **(Table 11.18)**.

Treatment
Antibiotics used in empirical therapy of bacterial meningitis and focal CNS infections.

A. Empirical therapy
S. pneumoniae and *Neisseria meningitides* are common organisms. Due to emergence of penicillin and cephalosporin resistant of *S. pneumoniae* a combination therapy of 3rd or 4th generation cephalosporin (ceftriaxone, cefotaxime, cefepime) and vancomycin, plus acyclovir (HSV is a differential diagnosis) and doxycycline (tick infection) is given as empirical therapy.

B. Specific antimicrobial therapy
- *Neisseria meningitides*
  - **Penicillin sensitive:** Penicillin G-250,000–300,000 U/kg/day in divided doses, Ampicillin (3 g intravenous TID/QID)

Table 11.18: CSF findings in meningitis.

	Normal	Acute pyogenic	Acute viral (aseptic)	Tuberculous
Physical examination	Clear and colorless	Turbid and forms coagulum	Clear	Clear and colorless, forms cobweb on standing due to coagulation of fibrinogen
CSF pressure	60–150 mm of H_2O	Raised above 180 mm of H_2O	Raised above 250 mm of H_2O	Raised above 300 mm of H_2O
Total protein	20–40 mg/100 mL (<0.45 g/L)	>50–200 mg/100 mL	>40 mg/100 mL	50–150 mg/100 mL
Glucose	45–80 mg/100 mL (>50–60% of blood level)	0–20 mg/l00 mL (Usually <40 mg/dL)	Normal	Decreased: May be <45 mg/100 mL
Chlorides	720–750 mg/100 mL	600–700 mg/100 mL	Normal	450–600 mg/100 mL
Cells				
Polymorphs	Usually absent	1,000–5,000/mL	Absent	0–5 cells/µL
Lymphocytes	0–5 cells/µL	5–50 cells/µL	10–2000 cells/µL	50–5000 cells/µL
Gram stain/ZN stain	-	Bacteria +	-	AFB + (Ziehl-Neelsen/auramine stain) or tuberculosis culture positive

- *Penicillin resistant:* Ceftriaxone 2 g intravenous BID/Cefotaxime 2 g intravenous BID
- 7 days IV dose are adequate.
- All close contacts should be given chemoprophylaxis with rifampicin for 2 days or azithromycin (500 mg once) or one IM ceftriaxone (250 mg).
- ☐ *Streptococcus pneumonia*
  - Should be tested for penicillin and cephalosporin sensitivity
  - *Penicillin sensitive:* Penicillin G
  - *Penicillin-intermediate:* Ceftriaxone/cefotaxime/cefepime
  - *Penicillin-resistant:* Ceftriaxone/cefotaxime/cefepime+vancomycin
  - 2 weeks IV is adequate.
  - Lumbar puncture is to be repeated 24–36 hours after initiation to see the response
  - Intraventricular vancomycin may be more effective than IV or intrathecal.
- ☐ **Gram-negative bacilli (except *Pseudomonas*):** Ceftriaxone/cefotaxime for 3 weeks
- ☐ *Pseudomonas aeruginosa*: Ceftazidime/cefepime/meropenem
- ☐ *Staphylococci spp*:
  - *Methicillin sensitive:* Nafcillin
  - *Methicillin resistant:* Vancomycin (1 g intravenous TID) (IV or intraventricular)
- ☐ *Listeria monocytogenes*: Ampicillin for 3 weeks. Gentamicin may be added in critical ill cases. Trimethoprim and sulfamethoxazole is alternative
- ☐ *H. influenzae*-**intermediate:** Ceftriaxone/cefotaxime/cefepime
- ☐ *Streptococcus agalactiae*: Penicillin G/ampicillin
- ☐ *Bacteroides fragilis:* Metronidazole
- ☐ *Fusobacterium spp:* Metronidazole.

C. Adjunctive therapy
- ☐ **Dexamethasone** inhibits synthesis of IL-1β and TNF-α, decrease CSF out flow resistance, and stabilize blood-brain barrier (BBB).
- ☐ It is to be given 20 minutes before antimicrobial therapy. It is less effective if given 6 hours after antibiotic therapy.

D. Treatment of raised ICP
- ☐ Elevation of head end of the bed to 30–45 degrees, hyperventilation, and administration of mannitol.
- ☐ Duration of therapy: 7 days for *N. meningitides,* 7–10 days for *H. influenzae,* 10–14 days for *S. pneumoniae,* and 3 weeks for gram-negative bacilli.

Tubercular Meningitis

In India, tubercular meningitis (TBM) remains the most common form of meningitis.

Risk factors
- ☐ Previous history of exposure to tuberculosis or illness.
- ☐ Immunocompromised state of AIDS
- ☐ Young children.

Pathology
- ☐ Main neuropathologic finding is **basal meningeal exudates** containing mainly mononuclear cells.
- ☐ **Tubercles may** be seen on the meninges and on the surfaces of the brain.
- ☐ The **ventricles may be dilated** as a result of hydrocephalus, and the ependymal surface may be covered by **exudates.**
- ☐ **Hydrocephalus** is common in children and most develop symptoms in 2–3 weeks.
  - **Communicating type:** Common, due to blockage of basal cistern by exudates in acute phase or adhesive leptomeningitis in chronic phase.
  - **Obstructive type:** Less common, due to narrowing or occlusion of aqueduct by ependymal inflammation, tuberculomas, or obstruction of outlet of IV ventricle.
- ☐ Arteritis can cause cerebral infarction, and basal inflammation; and fibrosis can compress cranial nerves.

Clinical features
- ☐ **Onset:** Usually subacute/chronic. Acute: children—50%, adult—14%.
- ☐ **Past history of TB:** Children—50%, adult—10%.
- ☐ **Prodromal symptoms:** 2–3 weeks, vague ill health, apathy, irritability, anorexia, changes in behavior.

- **Features of meningitis:** Headache, vomiting, fever, and focal neurological deficit.
- **Features of raised intracranial pressure (ICP)**
  - *Convulsions* (focal/generalized—20-30%).
  - *Cranial nerve palsy:* 20-30% (6th cranial nerve).
  - *Loss of vision:* Partial/complete. Due to optochiasmatic exudate and arteritis.
- **Other presentation:** Hemiplegia, facial nerve palsy, optic atrophy, abnormal movement, oculomotor palsy, choroid tubercle, etc.
- **In untreated cases:** Consciousness deteriorates, pupillary abnormality, pyramidal signs due to hydrocephalus and tentorial herniation.

Investigations
- **CSF study**
  - Discussed earlier
  - **Adenosine deaminase** (ADA) produced by T-lymphocytes elevated in CSF (60-100%).

Complications of tubercular meningitis
- Raised intracranial pressure (ICP), cerebral edema
- Basal meningitis with cranial nerve palsy—II, III, IV, VI, and VII
- Focal neurologic deficit and seizure
- Hydrocephalus
- Tuberculoma
- Opticochiasmatic pachymeningitis: Visual loss
- **Endocrine abnormality:** Growth hormone and gonadotropin
- **Hypothalamic disorder:** Loss of control of blood pressure and temperature, delayed or precocious sexual development
- Diabetes insipidus, syndrome of inappropriate ADH secretion (SIADH).

Management
- Antituberculous treatment (ATT) for one and a half year in uncomplicated cases is usually sufficient.
- **Steroids:** It is recommended to give steroids during initial 6 weeks to decrease the possibility of adhesion formation. Steroids prevent complications. There is no definite duration for which treatment might be continued, but should be judged on the basis of neuroimaging findings.
- **Surgical intervention:** If hydrocephalus, tuberculoma, or abscess develops. Tubercular abscess needs drainage.

Viral Meningitis/Aseptic Meningitis
- Viral infections of the meninges (meningitis) or brain parenchyma (encephalitis) often present as acute confusional states.
- Children and young adults are frequently affected.

Etiology
Common viruses include:
- **Enteroviruses** (most common, i.e., coxsackie viruses, echoviruses, and human enteroviruses): At least **two-thirds** of the cases of CSF culture-negative aseptic meningitis are due to enteroviruses.
- **Herpes simplex virus-2 (HSV-2) meningitis:** It may occur during the initial episode of genital herpes. Most cases of benign recurrent lymphocytic meningitis (previously called as Mollaret's meningitis) appear to be due to HSV
- **Arthropod-borne viruses:** These are transmitted through infected insect vectors.
- **HIV: Aseptic meningitis** is a common manifestation of primary exposure to **HIV. Cranial nerve palsies,** most commonly involving cranial nerves V, VII and VIII are more common in HIV meningitis than in other viral infections.
- **Mumps** can also cause meningitis.

Clinical manifestations
Fever, headache, and meningeal irritation. Other features include malaise, myalgia, anorexia, nausea and vomiting, abdominal pain, and/or diarrhea.

Laboratory diagnosis
- **CSF examination:** Discussed earlier
- **Polymerase chain reaction (PCR):** Amplification of viral-specific DNA or RNA from CSF by PCR important method for the diagnosis of CNS viral infection.

Treatment
- **Symptomatic** and hospitalization is not required.
- **Oral or intravenous acyclovir** may be of benefit in patients with meningitis caused by **HSV-1 or 2** and in cases of severe **EBV or VZV infection.**
- Patients with **HIV** should receive highly **active retroviral therapy.**

■ NEUROSYPHILIS

- *Treponema pallidum* invades nervous system within 3 to 18 months (may take years to develop) after primary infection.
- **Neurosyphilis** may be asymptomatic or symptomatic. Initial event is usually in the form of asymptomatic meningitis. Later it may produce more damage. All forms of neurosyphilis have meningitis of variable severity. Secondary to meningitis, the blood vessels show endarteritis obliterans.

Asymptomatic Neurosyphilis
- Asymptomatic invasion of CNS by treponema is common and occur within few months of primary infection by *Treponema pallidum.*
- Neurosyphilis may develop in 25% cases of latent syphilis. Many of them may develop symptomatic neurosyphilis.
- CSF shows lymphocytosis with increased protein and low glucose. Antibodies in the CSF, is the most specific test for neurosyphilis. Venereal disease research laboratory test is positive.
- **Treatment:** Penicillin.

Symptomatic Neurosyphilis
- It takes one of several forms, although mixed features are common
- Major categories of symptomatic neurosyphilis.
  - Meningeal syphilis
  - Chronic meningovascular disease
  - Parenchymatous syphilis
    - General paresis of insane
    - Tabes dorsalis

Meningeal Syphilis
- Symptoms of meningitis may develop at any time after infection, but usually occur within 2 years after primary infection.
- Symptoms:
  - These include headache, neck stiffness, seizures, altered sensorium and cranial nerve palsies. It may show skin rash on palms and soles.
  - Papilledema with symptoms of increased intracranial pressure (ICP) may develop.
  - Patient is afebrile and CSF is abnormal.

Meningovascular Syphilis
- Chronic meningitis involves base of the brain, cerebral convexities, and spinal leptomeninges.
- Usually presents 6–7 years after primary infection. However, it can develop as early as 6 months and as late as 10–12 years.
- It should be suspected when a young patient develops stroke (generally subacute), which results in hemiparesis, aphasia, visual loss, etc. Other features include headache, vertigo, insomnia, and psychological abnormalities.

CSF Findings
Gold standard test for diagnosis is VDRL from CSF. This is highly specific but only 30–70% sensitive for neurosyphilis. CSF FTA-ABS is more sensitive but not specific because false positives are common.

General Paralysis of Insane
- It develops about 20 years after primary infection.
- Shows generalized/diffuse brain parenchymal disease with **dementia;** hence called as general paresis of insane.
- Clinical manifestation includes personality changes, illusions, delusions, hallucinations, dementia (reduced memory), hyperactive reflexes, and Argyll Robertson pupils.

Tabes Dorsalis
- Tabes dorsalis is the parenchymal form of neurosyphilis characterized by **demyelination of posterior column, dorsal root and dorsal root ganglia** in the spinal cord.
- Usually develops 20–25 years after primary infection.
- **Symptoms:** Severe lightening pains in trunk and extremities, ataxia and urinary incontinence.
- **Signs:** Patchy tactile sensory loss and severe impairment of proprioception with sensory ataxia. Muscular strength is normal and tendon jerks are absent. Complications include trophic lesions such as perforating ulcers of feet and Charcot joints. Argyll Robertson pupils may also be observed in tabes dorsalis.
- **Visceral crisis:** It consists of sudden epigastric pain with vomiting that Abadie's sign (Pinching of, or the application of firm pressure to, the Achilles tendon does not result in pain) lasts for hours. Barium studies show pylorospasm (gastric crisis). Other crisis includes intestinal crisis with diarrhea, rectal crisis with tenesmus, genitourinary crisis with strangury and pharyngeal-laryngeal crisis with gulping movements and dyspnea.

Treatment
- **Penicillin:** Drug of choice and given in the dose of 18–24 million units/day for 15–20 days.
- If patient is sensitive to penicillin: Erythromycin and tetracycline 0.5 g 6 hourly for 20–30 days.

Follow-up
- Re-examine the patient every 3 months and CSF examination at 6 months interval.
- If CSF is normal and VDRL titers are reduced, no further treatment is necessary. However, if CSF remains abnormal, patient should be treated by another full course of penicillin.

ENCEPHALITIS

Viral Encephalitis
- In meningitis, the infectious process and associated inflammatory response is limited largely to the meninges, whereas in encephalitis, the brain parenchyma is also involved.
- Encephalitis is characterized by nonsuppurative inflammation of brain by an inflammatory process.

Etiology
Viruses causing encephalitis
- Epidemics of encephalitis are caused by arboviruses
- Herpesvirus
  - Herpes simplex virus I (MC)
  - Varicella zoster virus
  - Epstein-Barr virus
- Arthropod-borne viruses
- West Nile virus
- Japanese encephalitis
- Colorado tick fever
- Others: Rabies, enteroviruses, mumps, cytomegalovirus

Clinical Manifestations
- Acute febrile illness with evidence of meningitis and encephalitis.
- Altered level of consciousness (ranging from mild lethargy to coma), an abnormal mental state, and evidence of either focal or diffuse neurologic signs or symptoms.
- It may have hallucinations, agitation, personality change, behavioral disorders and at times a frankly psychotic state.
- Focal or generalized seizures occur in many patients with encephalitis.
- Most common focal neurological findings: Aphasia, ataxia, upper or lower motor neuron patterns of weakness, involuntary movements (e.g., myoclonic jerks, tremor), and cranial nerve deficits (e.g., ocular palsies, facial weakness).
- Involvement of the hypothalamic pituitary axis may result in temperature dysregulation, diabetes insipidus, or the development of the syndrome of inappropriate secretion of antidiuretic hormone (SIADH).

Laboratory Diagnosis
CSF
- **CSF examination:** Indistinguishable from that of viral meningitis and typically consists of lymphocytic

pleocytosis, a mildly elevated protein concentration, and a normal glucose concentration.
- **CSF PCR:** Primary diagnostic test for CNS infections caused by CMV, EBV, HHV-6 and enteroviruses.
- **CSF culture:** Limited utility.

Serologic studies and antigen defection
Demonstration of antibodies or antigens.

Brain biopsy
Reserved for patients in whom CSF PCR studies fail to lead to a specific diagnosis, who have focal abnormalities on MRI, and who continue to show progressive clinical deterioration despite treatment with acyclovir and supportive therapy.

MRI, CT, and EEG Management
- **General measures:** Care of the unconscious patient. Anticonvulsants may be needed. Brain edema is managed with dexamethasone 4 mg 6 hourly.
- Acyclovir is given for herpes encephalitis

DISEASES OF CRANIAL NERVES

Vth Cranial Nerve: Trigeminal Nerve

Trigeminal Neuralgia (Tic Douloureux)
- Trigeminal neuralgia is also known as **prosopalgia or Fothergill's disease.** Tic Douloureux means painful jerking.
- It is a neuropathic disorder. It is defined as sudden, episodes of usually unilateral, severe, brief, stabbing, intense, lancinating, recurring pain in the distribution of one or more branches of the Vth cranial nerve (trigeminal nerve).
- Middle age and later. Usually start in the 6th and 7th decades and major risk factor is hypertension.

Etiology
Usually produced due to compression of the trigeminal nerve at or near the pons by an ecstatic vascular loop. Pain like trigeminal neuralgia can be seen in other conditions

Causes of trigeminal neuralgia
- Usually idiopathic
- Demyelination
- Multiple sclerosis
- Petrous ridge compression
- Post-traumatic neuralgia
- Intracranial tumors
- Intracranial vascular abnormalities
- Viral etiology

Clinical features
Pain
- **Characteristics of pain:** Sudden, unilateral, intermittent (paroxysmal), sharp, shooting/knifelike/lancinating/electric shock like. Pain rarely crosses the midline. In extreme cases, the patient will have a motionless face known as the "frozen or mask-like face". In 10–12% of cases it is bilateral and usually due to intrinsic brainstem pathology (e.g., multiple sclerosis) or expanding cranial tumor (acoustic schwannomas, meningiomas, epidermoid).
- **Duration of pain:** Pain is of short duration (lasting seconds), but may recur with variable frequency (may be many times a day). Attacks do not occur during sleep.
- Pain occurs along the cutaneous distribution of the fifth nerve (Full or branches). Pain usually commences in the mandibular division but may spread to involve the maxillary and occasionally the ophthalmic divisions.
- Pain is precipitated by minor trauma to the trigger zones (e.g., slight touch, chewing, shaving, rinsing mouth, exposure to cold wind). Common trigger zones can be external/cutaneous (around the ala of nose, corners of lips, and cheek) or internal/intraoral (teeth, gingivae, tongue). Trigger area on the face are so sensitive that touching or even air currents can trigger an episode.
- Neither objective signs of sensory loss nor signs of V nerve dysfunction can be demonstrated on examination.
- **Differential diagnosis:** Reactivation of the varicella zoster virus is seen in older people and has predilection for ophthalmic division of the trigeminal nerve.
- **Treatment:**
  - **First line of treatment: Carbamazepine** (anticonvulsant) to be started with a dose of 100–200 mg/day, increase in 2–3 weeks to 200–400 mg TID.
  - **Second line of treatment:** Baclofen, lamotrigine, oxcarbazepine, phenytoin, gabapentin, pregabalin, and sodium valproate.
  - **Long-acting anesthetic agents:** Localized pain is managed by injecting any of the following into the particular branch of the nerve.
    - Alcohol injection
    - Peripheral glycerol injection.
- **Surgery:** Indicated if drug fails or not tolerated.
  - Peripheral neurectomy (nerve avulsion)
  - Open procedures (intracranial procedures)
  - Microvascular decompression
  - Percutaneous rhizotomies
  - *Gamma knife radiosurgery:* Using stereotactic imaging of the trigeminal nerve root entry zone, radiation to delivered to trigeminal nerve.

VIIth Cranial Nerve: Facial Nerve

Causes of Facial Nerve Palsy
See **Table 11.19 and Figure 11.5.**

Table 11.19: Causes of facial nerve palsy.

Unilateral	Bilateral
Upper motor neuron (UMN)	**Upper motor neuron (UMN)**
• Vascular (stroke)	• Vascular (multi-infarct dementia)
• Tumor	
• Multiple sclerosis	• Motor neuron disease
Lower motor neuron (LMN)	**Lower motor neuron (LMN)**
• **Bell's palsy**	• Guillain-Barré syndrome
• Ramsay Hunt syndrome	• Sarcoidosis (Uveoparotid fever)
• Parotid tumor	• Leprosy
• Head injury	• Lyme's disease
• Skull base tumor	• Leukemia
• Basal meningitis	• Lymphoma
• Diabetes mellitus	• Moebius syndrome
• Hypertension	• Melkersson Rosenthal syndrome
• Chronic suppurative otitis media	• Toxin: Thalidomide
	• Bilateral Bell's palsy

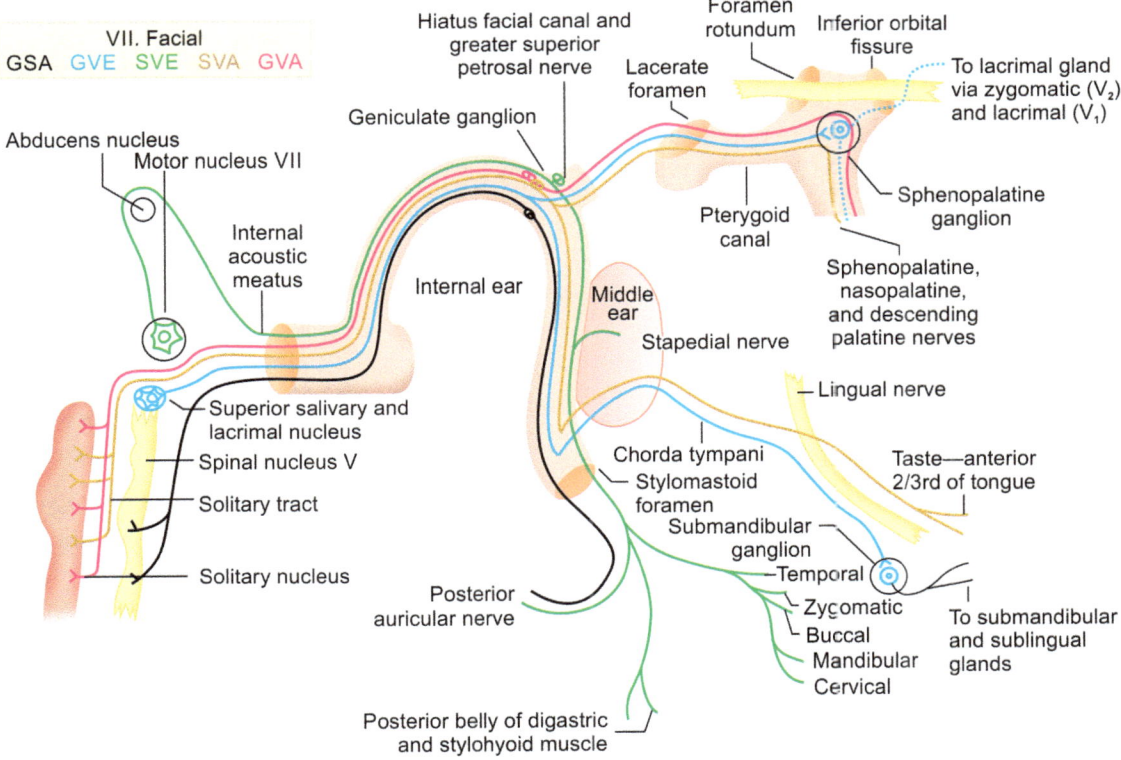

Fig. 11.5: Facial nerve anatomy.

BELL'S PALSY

Most common form of unilateral isolated lower motor neuron (LMN) type of facial paralysis is Bell's palsy.

Pathophysiology

- Main cause of Bell's palsy is thought to be latent herpes viruses (herpes simplex virus type 1 and herpes zoster virus), which are reactivated from cranial nerve ganglia. It causes **swelling of nerve within** the tight petrous bone **facial canal.**
- Herpes zoster virus shows more aggressive biological behavior than herpes simplex virus type 1.
- PCR techniques have isolated herpes virus DNA from the facial nerve during acute palsy.
- Inflammation of the nerve initially results in a reversible neuropraxia.

Clinical Manifestations

- **Race:** Slightly higher in persons of Japanese descent. Familial incidence 4.1%.
- **Age and gender:** Highest in persons aged 15–45 years. It is rare below the age of 15 years and above the age of 60 years. No gender difference exists.
- **Onset is fairly abrupt,** with **pain around the ear** preceding the unilateral facial weakness (maximal weakness by 48 hours). Patients often describe the face as "numb" and sometimes give the history of exposure to cold.
- **Associated symptoms:** Hyperacusis, decreased production of tears and saliva, and altered taste, otalgia or aural fullness and facial or retroauricular pain.
- Less common in pregnancy but prognosis is significantly worse in pregnant women.
- **Examination:** Shows features of isolated lower motor neuron facial paralysis. On the affected side **following features are observed.** These include:
  - **Paralysis of all the muscles of facial expression (Fig. 11.6A).**
  - Dropping of corner of mouth, effacement of creases and skin fold.
  - Involvement of frontalis makes frowning difficult. Eye closure is weak because of involvement of orbicularis oculi

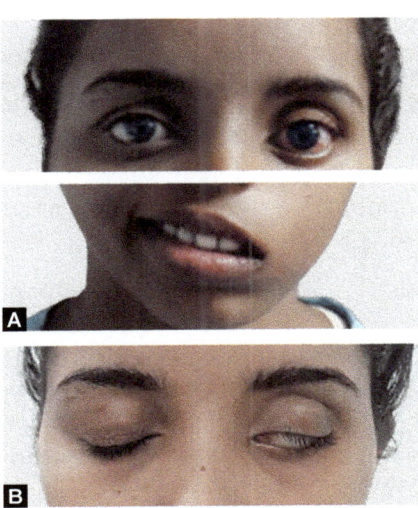

Figs. 11.6A and B: (A) Bell's palsy; (B) Bell's phenomenon.

- Drooling of saliva from angle of mouth.
- Action of the levator anguli oris on the normal side makes the angle of mouth to deviate to the opposite side of the lesion, when the patient shows his teeth.
- When the closure of the eyelid is attempted, the eye on the paralyzed side rolls upward (Bell's phenomenon) **(Fig. 11.6B)**.
- Due to exposure of the cornea, patient may develop exposure keratitis and corneal ulceration.

Investigation

- No specific confirmatory diagnostic test.
- CSF may show mild lymphocytosis.
- MRI may reveal swelling and uniform enhancement of the geniculate ganglion and facial nerve and in some cases, entrapment of the swollen nerve in the temporal bone.

Differences between Upper Motor and Lower Motor Neuron Facial Palsy

For differences between upper motor and lower motor neuron facial palsy, see **Table 11.20**.

Differences between Bilateral Upper Motor and Bilateral Lower Motor Neuron Facial Palsy

For differences between bilateral upper motor and bilateral lower motor neuron facial palsy, see **Table 11.21**.

Sequelae of Bell's Palsy

- **Incomplete recovery:** Facial asymmetry persists; eye cannot be closed resulting in epiphora. A weak oral sphincter causes drooling and difficulty in taking food.
- **Exposure keratitis:** Eye cannot be closed, tear film from the cornea evaporates causing dryness, exposure keratitis and corneal ulcer.
- **Synkinesis (mass movement):** When the patient wishes to close eye corner of mouth also twitches or vice versa.

Table 11.20: Differences between upper motor and lower motor neuron facial palsy.

UMN (upper motor neuron) facial palsy	LMN (lower motor neuron) facial palsy
Lower part of the face is involved	Both lower and upper part of the face is involved
No Bell's phenomenon	Bell's phenomenon is seen
Taste is not affected	Taste is affected
No hyperacusis	Hyperacusis may be present if nerve to stapedius is involved
Usually associated with hemiplegia	Usually not associated unless any pontine lesion is present causing crossed hemiplegia
Site of the lesion is above facial nucleus usually in the internal capsule	Usually in the nucleus or distal to the nucleus
No wasting or atrophy	Wasting or atrophy may be present

Table 11.21: Differences between bilateral upper motor and bilateral lower motor neuron facial palsy.

Bilateral UMN palsy	Bilateral LMN palsy
Emotional fibers-spared	Bell's phenomenon present
Emotional incontinence present	Emotional fibers—affected
Associated with bilateral long tract signs	Long tract signs—absent
Jaw jerk—exaggerated	Jaw jerk—normal
Corneal reflex—present	Corneal reflex—absent
Taste sensation—spared	Taste sensation—absent
Gag reflex—exaggerated	Gag reflex- Normal

- **Tics and spasm:** Result of faulty regeneration of fibers. Involuntary movements are seen on the affected side of face.
- **Contractures:** Results from fibrosis of atrophied or fixed contraction of a group of muscles.
- **Crocodile tears (gustatory lacrimation):** Unilateral lacrimation with mastication. Due to faulty regeneration of parasympathetic fibers which now supply lacrimal gland instead of the salivary glands.
- **Frey' syndrome (gustatory sweating):** Sweating and flushing of skin over the parotid during mastication. It results from parotid surgery.
- Anomalous regeneration of the seventh nerve fibers. Originally connected with the orbicularis oculi come to innervate the orbicularis oris, closure of the lids may cause a retraction of the mouth. Jaw opening causing closure of the eyelids on the side of the facial palsy is termed **Marcus-Gunn jaw-winking phenomenon.**

Treatment

- Severe facial weakness may produce inability to blink and lead to **exposure keratitis.** Use of **lubricating eye drops** may be needed, and **paper tape** to close the eye during sleep.
- Massage of weekend muscles.

Medical Treatment of Bell's Palsy

- Steroids (Prednisolone) 1 mg/kg/day for 5–7 days and then tapered over the next one week.
- Antiviral agents: for 5–7 days.
  - Famciclovir 500 mg BD.
  - Valacyclovir 500 mg BD.
  - Acyclovir 800 mg five times a day.
- **Surgical decompression**—only if no resolution of symptoms after 2 weeks.

INTRACRANIAL PRESSURE

Raised Intracranial Pressure

- Normal intracranial pressure in adults is less than 10–15 mm Hg. There are normal regular waves due to pulse and respiration.

- With increased pressure "pressure waves" appear. With continued rise of ICP, the perfusion pressure (PP) falls. When PP falls CBF is reduced. Electrical cortical activity fails, if CBF is 20 mL/100 g/min.
- When intracranial pressure reaches mean arterial pressure circulation to the brain stops.
- Raised intracranial pressure (RIP) may be caused by mass lesions, cerebral edema, obstruction to CSF circulation causing hydrocephalus, impaired CSF absorption, and cerebral venous obstruction.

Common Causes of Raised ICP

For common causes of intracranial pressure, see **Table 11.22**.

Clinical Features

- Signs and symptoms of underlying cause.
- **Features of raised ICP (Table 11.23).**

Table 11.22: Common causes of raised intracranial pressure.

Primary or intracranial causes	
Mass lesions • **Intracranial hemorrhage** (traumatic or spontaneous): Extradural or subdural hematoma, intracerebral hemorrhage • **Brain tumor:** Posterior fossa tumor or high-grade gliomas • **Infective:** Cerebral abscess, tuberculomas, cysticercosis, hydatid cyst • **Colloid cyst** (in ventricles)	**Disturbance of CSF circulation** • **Obstructive (noncommunicating) hydrocephalus:** Obstruction within ventricular system • **Communicating hydrocephalus:** Obstruction outside ventricular system • Obstruction to venous sinuses • Cerebral venous thrombosis • Trauma (fractures overlying sinuses)
Diffuse brain edema or swelling • Meningoencephalitis • Trauma (diffuse head injury, near-drowning) • Subarachnoid hemorrhage • Metabolic (e.g., water intoxication) • Idiopathic intracranial hypertension • Postneurosurgery	
Secondary or extracranial causes	
• Hypoxia or hypercarbia (hypoventilation) • Hyperpyrexia • Drug and toxins (e.g., valproate sodium, lead intoxication)	• Hepatic failure • Seizure • Reye's syndrome • High-altitude cerebral edema

Table 11.23: Features of raised intracranial pressure (ICP).

- Diffuse anterior headache worse on lying/straining
- Vomiting
- Diplopia (6th nerve involvement)
- Papilledema
- Bradycardia, raised blood pressure
- Impaired conscious level: Drowsiness and mental deterioration
- Seizures

COMA

Definitions

Consciousness

- It means the state of patient's awareness of self and environment and his responsiveness to external stimulation and inner need.
- Consciousness is maintained by two separate anatomical and physiological systems:
  - Ascending reticular activating system (ARAS) projecting from brainstem to thalamus determines arousal (the level of consciousness).
  - Cerebral cortex determines the content of consciousness.

Confusion

- Traditionally referred as **"clouding of sensorium"**!
- It denotes inability to think with customary speed, clarity, and coherence, accompanied by some degree of inattentiveness and disorientation.
- Confusion results most often from process that influences the brain globally, such as toxic or metabolic disturbance or a dementia.

Drowsiness

- The inability to sustain a wakeful state without application of stimuli externally is called drowsiness.
- Slow arousal is elicited by speaking to the patient or applying a tactile stimulus.

Stupor

- A state in which the person can be aroused only by repeated vigorous stimuli is called as stupor.
- There is either absence or slow and inadequate response to spoken commands.
- It is common to find restless or stereotyped motor activity. In these patients there is a reduction in the natural shifting of positions.
- When left unstimulated, these patients quickly return to a sleep-like state.

Lethargic/Drowsiness

- Patient can usually be aroused or awakened and may then appear to be in complete possession of her senses, but promptly falls asleep when left alone. It resembles normal sleepiness.
- For example, high brainstem disturbances.

Obtundation

Refers to moderate reduction in the patient's level of awareness such that stimuli of mild to moderate intensity fail to arouse; when arousal does occur, the patient is slow to respond.

Coma

Coma is a condition characterized by a deep sleep-like stage from which the patient cannot be aroused even with vigorous, continuous stimulation. The patient does not make any localized responses. However, the patient may grimace or show withdrawal responses to painful stimuli.

Classification of Coma

For classification of coma, see **Table 11.24**.

Table 11.24: Classification of coma.

Coma without focal signs or meningism
- **Exogenous intoxicants:** Alcohol, barbiturate, opiates
- **Endogenous metabolic disturbances:** Anoxia, hypoglycemia, diabetic ketoacidosis (DKA), hyperosmolar non-ketotic state (HONK), uremia, hepatic failure, hyponatremia or hypernatremia, Addisonian crisis, carbon monoxide poisoning, myxedema
- **Severe systemic infections:** Septicemia, typhoid fever, cerebral malaria, pneumonia, peritonitis, Waterhouse Friderichsen syndrome
- **Circulatory collapse** (shock) from any cause
- **Postseizure states**
- Hypertensive encephalopathy
- Hyperthermia and hypothermia
- Concussion
- Acute hydrocephalus

Coma with meningism
- Subarachnoid hemorrhage (SAH)
- Acute bacterial meningitis
- Viral meningoencephalitis
- Neoplastic meningitis
- Parasitic meningitis
- Pituitary apoplexy

Coma with focal signs
- Hemispheral hemorrhage or massive cerebral infarction
- Brainstem infarction
- Brain abscess, subdural empyema, herpes encephalitis
- Epidural and subdural hemorrhage, brain contusion
- Brain tumor
- Miscellaneous: TTP, fat embolism, ADEM, cortical vein thrombosis, focal infarction caused by bacterial endocarditis

Assessment of Coma

Assessment of coma is done by Glasgow coma scale (GCS) (Table 11.25).

Table 11.25: Glasgow coma scale (GCS).

Eye opening		Best verbal response		Best motor response	
				Obeys commands	6
		Oriented and converses	5	Localizes pain	5
Open spontaneously	4	Converses, but disoriented, confused	4	Exhibits flexion withdrawal	4
Open only to verbal stimuli	3	Uses inappropriate words	3	Decorticate rigidity	3
Open only to pain	2	Makes incomprehensible sounds	2	Decerebrate rigidity	2
Never open	1	No verbal response	1	No motor response	1

Maximum score = **15**
Minimum score = **3**
Coma is equal to GCS of less than **8 or less**.

BRAIN DEATH

Brain death occurs from irreversible brain injury, which is sufficient to permanently eliminate all cortical and brainstem function (i.e., loss of all functions of the brain, including the brainstem).
- Because the vital centers in the brainstem maintain cardiovascular and respiratory functions, brain death is incompatible with survival despite mechanical ventilation and cardiovascular and nutritional supportive measures.
- Significance of brain death:
  - It permits the withdrawal of costly life-saving equipment and drugs.
  - Family can be offered the opportunity for organ donation.

Diagnosis of Brain Death

Brain death is a **clinical diagnosis**. No other tests are necessary and complete clinical examination including independent brain death determinations by two licensed physicians is conclusive.

Clinical Evaluation (Prerequisites)
- Establish known irreversible cause of coma.
- The first and foremost critical step in establishing the diagnosis of brain death is to **establish an irreversible, untreatable cause of the brain injury** (e.g., global ischemia due to cardiac arrest, intracranial bleed, and severe head injury).
- **Exclude** potentially **reversible conditions** such as hypothermia, drug intoxication, poisoning, metabolic disorders (e.g., hypoglycemia, acidosis, electrolyte imbalance). Hypothermia should also be excluded—rectal temperature must exceed 35°C.
- Achieve body temperature >36°C.
- Achieve normal systolic BP (>100 mm Hg).

Clinical Evaluation (Neuroassessment)
- **Establish coma**
- **Establish absence of brainstem reflexes**
  - Pupillary reflex (absent)
  - Eye movements
    - *Occulocephalic:* Absent (dolls-eye movements)
    - *Occulovestibular:* Absent (cold caloric test)
  - Facial sensation and motor response: No corneal reflex, no jaw reflex, no grimacing to deep pressure on nail bed, supraorbital ridge or temporomandibular joint
  - Pharyngeal (gag) reflex absent
  - Tracheal (cough) reflex absent.
- **Establish Apnea by Apnea Test**
  - **Prerequisites for apnea test:** Body temperature >36°C, systolic blood pressure >100 mm Hg, normal electrolytes profile, normal $PaCO_2$ (35–45 mm Hg).
  - **Procedure of apnea test**
    - Connect a pulse oximeter and disconnect the ventilator.
    - Deliver 100% O_2 by catheter through endotracheal tube at 6 L/minute.
    - Observe for respiratory movement at least for 8–10 minutes.
    - Discontinue testing: If BP drops to <90 mm Hg and PaO_2 decreases to 85% by pulse oximetry for 30 seconds.

- **If respiratory drive/movement** is observed after 8 minutes. Take next blood sample for blood gas studies. This indicates apnea test result is negative.
- **Absence of respiration drive:** If respiratory **movements are absent** and arterial $PaCO_2$ is 60 mm Hg or 20 mm Hg increase over a baseline normal $PaCO_2$ indicates apnea **test** result is **positive** and **supports the clinical diagnosis of brain death.**

Ancillary Tests/Confirmatory Testing
- Electroencephalography (EEG): Electrocerebral silence absence of electrical activity during at least 30 minutes.
- Cerebral angiography: Absence of intracranial blood flow.
- PET: Glucose metabolism studies/dynamic nuclear brain scan: "Hollow-skull" sign of brain death.

Documentation
Time of death is the time the arterial $PaCO_2$ reached the target value OR when ancillary test is officially interpreted.

OBJECTIVE-BASED SELF-EVALUATION

LONG QUESTIONS
1. List the common types of headache. Discuss the types, clinical features, and management of migraine.
2. Discuss the clinical features, complications, and management of Bells palsy.
3. List the types of epilepsy. Discuss the management of status epilepticus.
4. Discuss the clinical features, investigations, and management of tuberculous meningitis.
5. Discuss the clinical features, investigations, and management of trigeminal neuralgia.
6. Discuss the risk factors, clinical features, and management of subarachnoid hemorrhage.

SHORT ANSWER QUESTIONS
1. Glasgow coma scale
2. Differences between seizure and syncope
3. Risk factors for stroke
4. Causes for facial nerve palsy
5. Causes of coma
6. CSF findings in bacterial meningitis
7. Prophylaxis of migraine
8. Clinical features of neurosyphilis
9. Clinical features of migraine
10. Types of migraine
11. Classification of stroke
12. Absence seizures
13. List the common organisms causing encephalitis

MULTIPLE CHOICE QUESTIONS
1. A 46-year-old woman is seen or complaints of very sharp pain lasting about 1 minute over her right cheek and lips. These pain episodes occur in clusters with intense pain during the episode. When an episode occurs, it is present both day and night and can recur over a period of about a week. Paroxysms of pain can be elicited by washing her ace. On physical examination, there is no sensory or motor loss in the right ace:
   a. Initiate treatment with carbamazepine 100 mg with a goal dose of 200 mg qid
   b. Perform an MRI/magnetic resonance angiography (MRA) of the brain
   c. Refer patient or electromyography and nerve conduction study
   d. Refer patient or microvascular decompression surgery
2. Migraine is associated with release of:
   a. Neurotensin
   b. Substance P
   c. Calcitonin gene related peptide (CGRP)
   d. Cholecystokinin
3. Which of the following is a feature of acute Wernicke's disease?
   a. Global confusion
   b. Impairment of eye movements
   c. Gait ataxia
   d. All the above
4. A patient with a head injury who has eye opening to speech, no verbal responses and withdrawal motor responses would have a Glasgow coma scale score of:
   a. 5 b. 6
   c. 7 d. 8
5. Tic Douloureux affects which cranial nerve?
   a. Optic b. Trigeminal
   c. Facial d. Olfactory
6. A state in which the person can be aroused only by repeated vigorous stimuli is called:
   a. Coma b. Stupor
   c. Obtundation d. Confusion
7. Argyll-Robertson pupils is classically caused by:
   a. Herpes b. Tuberculosis
   c. Syphilis d. HIV
8. Gingival hyperplasia, ataxia and nystagmus, cognitive impairment, hirsutism are side effects of:
   a. Phenytoin b. Valproate
   c. Zonisamide d. Carbamazepine
9. Lymphocytic meningitis with cob web formation is classical of:
   a. Tuberculous meningitis b. Aseptic meningitis
   c. Fungal meningitis d. Cryptococcal meningitis
10. Medical treatment of Bell's palsy includes:
    a. Acyclovir and steroids
    b. Carbamazepine
    c. Aspirin and atorvastatin
    d. Azithromycin and hydroxychloroquine

ANSWERS
1. a 2. c 3. d 4. d 5. b
6. b 7. c 8. a 9. a 10. a

Hematology

CHAPTER OUTLINE

- Anemia
- Platelet Disorders
- Clotting Disorders
- Thrombosis
- Leukemia
- Myeloproliferative Diseases
- Plasma Cell Dyscrasias
- Lymphoma
- Stem-cell Therapy
- Bone Marrow Transplantation

DISORDERS OF RED BLOOD CELL

Hemoglobin Structure

A hemoglobin molecule is a conjugated protein composed of iron-containing pigment called *heme* and protein *globin*. About 65–70% of hemoglobin is synthesized in normoblasts and 30–35% is synthesized at the reticulocyte stage.

- Each molecule of *heme* consists of protoporphyrin with an iron in ferrous state (Fe^{++}). Heme synthesis occurs mainly in the mitochondria of normoblasts.
- Each *globin* chain is made up of *two pairs of distinct polypeptide* chains (composed of a number of amino acids) bound to a heme molecule.
  - *Hemoglobin A (HbA)* is composed of two α and two β globin chains $\alpha_2\beta_2$ and normally represents more than 95% of the hemoglobin in adult red blood cell (RBCs). Fetal hemoglobin is replaced by adult hemoglobin during the 1st year of life (hemoglobin switching).
  - *Fetal hemoglobin (HbF)* contains two α- and two γ-globin chains (α_2 and γ_2). It is the major hemoglobin (70–90%) during fetal development and is normally found in low levels in adults.
  - *Hemoglobin A2* (α2 and δ2) is normally found at low levels in adults (2%).
  - Normal hemoglobins in the adult are Hb-A (α_2 and β_2) and Hb-A_2 (α_2 and δ_2)
  - Normal hemoglobins in the fetus are Hb-F (α_2 and γ_2) and Hb-Bart's (γ_4)

ANEMIA

- It is defined as *decrease* of *hemoglobin concentration (Hb)/RBC count/hematocrit (PCV)* below normal for the patient's age, sex, and altitude of residence
- **Normal adult hemoglobin:**
  - *Males:* 13–17 g/dL
  - *Females:* 12.0–15.0 g/dL

Classification

Classification of anemia is given in **Table 12.1**.

Clinical Features (Fig. 12.1; Tables 12.2 and 12.3)

- **Pallor:** Skin, palms, oral mucous membrane, nail beds, and palpebral conjunctiva
- **Pulse:** Tachycardia and wide-pulse pressure
- **Cardiovascular system:** Cervical venous hum, hyperdynamic precordium, ejection systolic murmur (best heard over the pulmonary area), cardiac dilatation, and later signs of cardiac failure
- **Edema**

Iron Metabolism (Fig. 12.2)

Iron is required for synthesis of normal heme of hemoglobin. Its deficiency leads to decreased erythropoiesis and anemia.

Distribution of Iron

Iron is an essential metal present in the human body. The total body iron content (3–4 g) is divided into functional and storage compartments (**Table 12.4**). Iron in the body is extensively recycled between the functional and storage pools.

- **Functional:** Approximately, 80% (2.5 g) of the functional iron is present in hemoglobin. The remaining functional iron is found in myoglobin and iron-containing enzymes (catalase, cytochromes, and peroxidases).
- **Storage:** The storage pool contains 15–20% (0.5–1.5 g) of total body iron. Free iron is highly toxic because it can result in tissue damage due to its capacity to form free radicals. Therefore, iron is bound to protein and stored in the body in two forms namely—"*ferritin*" and "*hemosiderin.*" The storage iron can be readily mobilized whenever there is increase in the requirements of iron, as may occur after blood loss. Two-thirds of the iron is stored as ferritin and one-third as hemosiderin.
  - *Ferritin* (Fe^{3+}) is a protein–iron complex (apoferritin + iron) found in all tissues but particularly in liver, spleen,

Table 12.1: Classification of anemia.

Morphological classification:		
Normocytic normochromic	Microcytic hypochromic	Macrocytic
Etiological classification:		
Blood loss:		
Acute		**Chronic**
• Loss of large volume over a short period • *Trauma*, postpartum bleeding		• Small volume over a long period • Peptic ulcer, hemorrhoids, carcinoma colon, hookworms, and excessive menstrual loss
Impaired red cell production:		
Disturbed proliferation and maturation		**Marrow replacement**
Defective DNA synthesis: • Megaloblastic anemias: Deficiency or impaired utilization of vitamin B_{12} and folic acid • Anemia of renal failure: Deficiency of erythropoietin • Anemia of chronic disease: Iron sequestration and relative erythropoietin deficiency • Anemias of endocrine disorders *Defective hemoglobin synthesis*: • Defective heme synthesis: Iron deficiency and sideroblastic anemia • Defective globin synthesis: Thalassemia		*Primary hematopoietic neoplasms:* • Acute leukemia • Myelodysplastic syndromes *Marrow infiltration (myelophthisic anemia)* Metastatic neoplasms *Disturbed proliferation and differentiation of stem cells* • Aplastic anemia • Pure red cell aplasia
Increased red cell destruction (hemolytic anemias):		
Intrinsic (intracorpuscular)		**Extrinsic (extracorpuscular)**

Hereditary:
• Abnormal membrane: Spherocytosis and elliptocytosis
• Enzyme deficiencies: Glucose-6-phosphate dehydrogenase and pyruvate kinase
• Disorders of hemoglobin synthesis:
  ▪ *Deficient globin synthesis:* Thalassemia
  ▪ *Hemoglobinopathies:* Sickle cell anemia
Acquired:
Membrane defects: Paroxysmal nocturnal hemoglobinuria
		Antibody-mediated:
		• Isohemagglutinins: Transfusion reactions, Rh disease of the newborn
		• Autoantibodies: Idiopathic, primary, drug-associated, and systemic lupus erythematosus
		Mechanical trauma to RBCs:
		• Microangiopathic hemolytic anemia: Disseminated intravascular coagulation
		Infections: Malaria

(RBC: red blood cell)

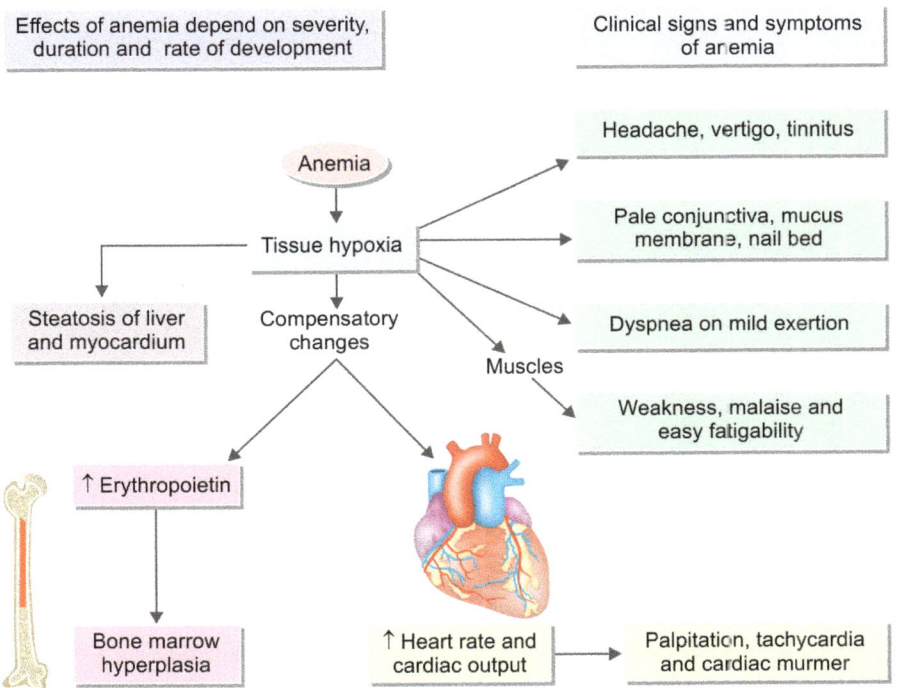

Fig. 12.1: Clinical signs and symptoms of anemia.

Table 12.2: Various signs of anemia suggesting the probable etiology.

Sign	Probable etiology
Angular cheilitis, blue sclera, and koilonychia	Iron deficiency anemia
Glossitis	Iron, vitamin B_{12}, and folate deficiency anemia
Neurological changes (neuropathy, dementia, and ataxia), knuckle pigmentation	Vitamin B_{12} deficiency
Jaundice	Hemolytic anemia and megaloblastic anemia
Splenomegaly	Malaria, chronic hemolytic anemia, acute infection, leukemia, lymphoma, portal hypertension, megaloblastic anemia, and iron deficiency anemia (rare)
Frontal bossing, dental malocclusion, and skin ulcers	Chronic hemolytic anemia (e.g., β-thalassemia and sickle cell anemia)
Leg ulcers	Sickle cell disease

Table 12.3: History suggesting the possible etiology of anemia.

Signs and symptoms	Possible etiology of anemia
Known normal complete blood cell count in the past	Probably not a hereditary/congenital disorder
Anemia known since childhood	Inherited/congenital hemolytic anemia
Splenectomy, gallstones, and/or jaundice	Chronic hemolytic anemia and liver disease
Family history of splenectomy, gallstones, and/or jaundice	Hereditary hemolytic anemia (RBC enzyme or membrane disorder, thalassemia, or hemoglobinopathy)
Poor or unconventional diet, malnutrition, or severe alcoholism	Bone marrow hypoplasia and folate deficiency
Paresthesias, foot numbness, loss of balance, or altered mental status	Cobalamin (vitamin B_{12}) deficiency
Gastrectomy, surgical removal of the ileum, and chronic malabsorption disorder	Cobalamin (vitamin B_{12}) deficiency
Chronic gastritis, peptic ulcer disease, chronic use of ASA or NSAIDs, recurrent epistaxis or rectal bleeding, melena, menorrhagia, metrorrhagia, multiple pregnancies, duodenal surgery, or gastrectomy	Iron deficiency
Chronic rheumatologic, immunologic, infectious, or neoplastic disease	Anemia of inflammation and autoimmune hemolytic anemia
Decreased urine output	Anemia secondary to renal insufficiency
Dark urine	Hemolytic anemia (intravascular hemolysis)
Recent onset of infections, mucosal and skin bleeding, easy bruising, or oral ulcerations	Bone marrow aplasia/hypoplasia, acute leukemia, myelodysplasia, and myelophthisis
Occupational/environmental toxin exposure (benzene, ionizing radiation, and lead)	Bone marrow aplasia/hypoplasia, acute leukemia, myelodysplasia, and lead poisoning
Drug/medication exposure:	
• Penicillin, cephalosporin, procainamide, quinidine, quinine, and sulfonamide	Drug-induced immune hemolytic anemia
• Fava beans, dapsone, and naphthalene	Oxidant-induced hemolysis (G6PD deficient)
• Cancer chemotherapeutic drugs (recent use)	Bone marrow aplasia/hypoplasia, oxidant damage, fluid retention/dilutional anemia, and megaloblastic anemia
• Cancer chemotherapeutic drugs (past use)	Bone marrow hypoplasia, myelodysplasia, and acute myeloid leukemia
• Chloramphenicol, gold salts, sulfonamides, and anti-inflammatory drugs	Bone marrow aplasia/hypoplasia
• Ethanol and chloramphenicol	Acute reversible bone marrow toxicity
• Methotrexate, azathioprine, pyrimethamine, trimethoprim, zidovudine, sulfa drugs, hydroxyurea, and antimetabolites	Bone marrow aplasia/hypoplasia and megaloblastic anemia

(G6PD: glucose-6-phosphate dehydrogenase)

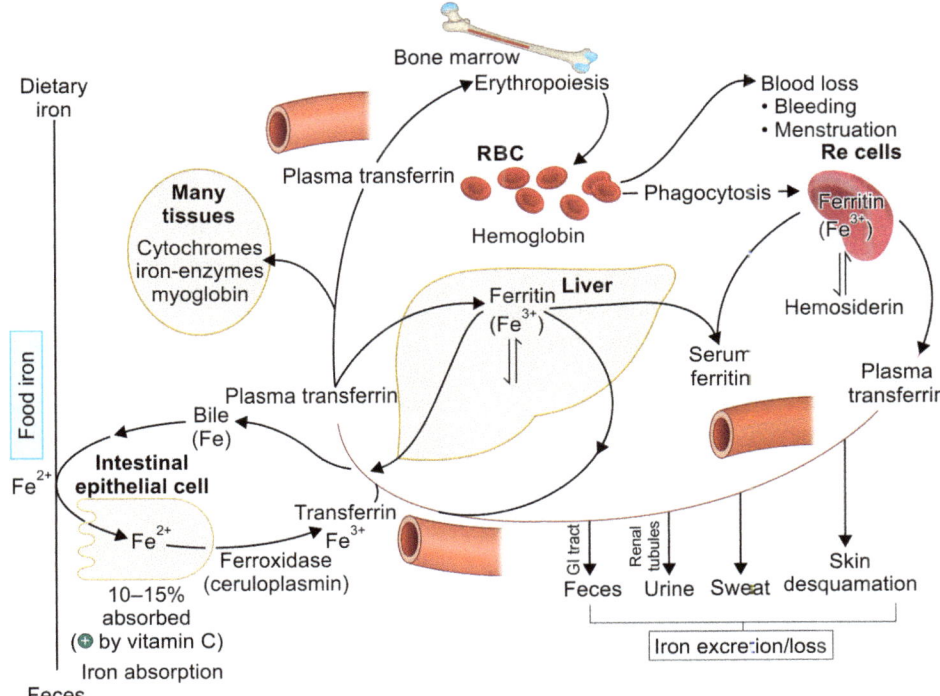

Fig. 12.2: Iron metabolism.

Table 12.4: Iron distribution in healthy young adults.

Pool	Grams	%
Functional:		
Hemoglobin	2.5	68
Myoglobin	0.15	4
Transferrin (iron-binding blood plasma glycoprotein)	0.003	0.1
Iron-containing enzymes	0.02	0.6
Storage:		
Ferritin and hemosiderin in tissue	1.0	27
Ferritin and serum	0.0001	0.004

bone marrow, and skeletal muscles. Very small amounts of ferritin circulate in the serum, the value normally being 15–300 µg/L. *Serum ferritin levels reflect the iron stores* and is a sensitive indicator of the amount of iron in the body. Serum ferritin level is usually below 12 µg/L in iron deficiency and it is very high (as high as 5,000 µg/L may be observed) in conditions associated with iron overload. Ferritin is water-soluble and not visible by light microscopy.

- *Hemosiderin* is an aggregate of iron and protein, which is found in the reticuloendothelial cells of bone marrow, spleen, and liver. It is formed when iron is in excess (amorphous iron deposition).

Daily requirements: Recommended dietary allowance is 10–15 mg. The daily requirement in adult males is 5–10 mg/day and in females 20 mg/day.

Dietary sources: The diet contains iron either in the form of heme contained in animal products and/or non-heme iron in vegetables. Of 10–50 mg in the diet, only 10–15% is normally absorbed.

Iron Absorption

Site of absorption: Iron is absorbed from the *duodenum* and *proximal jejunum*. Iron balance is maintained mainly by regulating the dietary absorption of iron (by the synthesis of apoferritin within mucosal cells).

Transport of Iron

- **Transferrin:** Iron is transported in plasma by the iron transport protein *transferrin*, which is synthesized in the liver. The major function of plasma transferrin is to deliver iron to erythroid precursors for the synthesis of hemoglobin. In normal individuals, transferrin is about 33% saturated with iron, with an average serum iron levels of 120 µg/dL in men and 100 µg/dL in women. Thus, the total iron-binding capacity of serum is in the range of 310–340 µg/dL. Unsaturated transferrin protects against infections (iron overload and infection).
- **Lactoferrin:** It binds iron in milk. It has antimicrobial effect (protects newborns from gastrointestinal infections).
- **Haptoglobin:** It binds hemoglobin in the plasma.

Iron Excretion/Loss

Iron metabolism is unique, as it is very efficiently utilized and reutilized by the body. There is no physiological regulated mechanism for iron excretion and 1–2 mg/day is lost by shedding of epithelial cells of gastrointestinal (GI) tract, skin epithelial cells (by sweat), and renal tubules; and by menstruation, pregnancy, multiple births, lactation, and bleeding.

Regulation of Iron Balance

Iron is essential for cellular metabolism; at the same time, excess of it is highly toxic. Therefore, the total body iron stores must be properly regulated. Iron balance is mainly achieved by regulating the absorption of iron in the diet. As body stores decrease, the absorption of iron rises and vice-versa.

Hepcidin:

It is synthesized in the liver and is the *central* (key) *regulator of iron homeostasis* and it *controls* intestinal iron *absorption* of plasma iron concentrations, tissue iron distribution, and *storage*.

- **Ferroportin is the cellular iron exporter, which exports iron into plasma:**
  - From absorptive enterocytes
  - From macrophages that recycle the iron of senescent erythrocytes
  - From hepatocytes that store iron
- The major mechanism of hepcidin is the regulation of transmembrane iron transport. Hepcidin binds to ferroportin and forms hepcidin–ferroportin complex. This complex is degraded in the lysosomes and thus degrades its receptor ferroportin. By this mechanism, hepcidin reduces resorption of iron in the intestine and inhibits iron transfer from the enterocyte to plasma (thereby reduces concentration of iron in plasma).
- When hepcidin levels rise, it lowers iron absorption in the intestine; iron gets stored (locked) within enterocytes forming mucosal ferritin and is shed with the cells. It also lowers iron release from hepatocytes and macrophages (through degradation of ferroportin) leading to decreased serum iron.

Significance of hepcidin:
- Increased hepcidin concentration is seen in inflammation (chronic disease anemia).
- Reduced hepcidin production → hereditary hemochromatosis

Functions of Iron

- **Heme iron:** Hemoglobin, myoglobin, cytochrome c oxidase, and catalase
- **Non-heme iron:** Fe-S complexes (xanthine oxidase) and DNA synthesis (ribonucleotide reductase)

Iron Deficiency Anemia

Causes of iron deficiency anemia are described in **Table 12.5**.

Clinical Features

- Usual symptoms and signs of anemia
- **Advanced iron deficiency:**
  - Cheilosis/angular stomatitis
  - Glossitis
  - Brittle fingernails, platynychia, and *koilonychia* (spooning of the fingernails)
  - Blue-tinged sclerae
  - *Pica:*
    - Unusual craving for substances with no nutritional value like clay or chalk
    - Craving for ice (pagophagia) specific to iron deficiency or for clay (geophagia) or starch (amylophagia)

Table 12.5: Causes of iron deficiency anemia.

Decreased iron intake:	Increased demand/requirement for iron:
• Milk-fed infants • Elderly with improper diet, poor dentition • Low socioeconomical sections • Vegetarians (poorly absorbable inorganic iron)	• Rapid growth in infancy or adolescents • Pregnancy and lactation
Decreased absorption of iron:	**Increased iron loss:**
• Total/partial gastrectomy • Intestinal absorption is impaired in sprue, other causes of intestinal steatorrhea, and chronic diarrhea • Specific items in the diet, such as phytates of cereals, tannates, carbonates, oxalates, phosphates, and drugs, can impair iron absorption	• Chronic blood loss due to bleeding from the gastrointestinal tract (peptic ulcers, gastric or colonic carcinoma, hemorrhoids, hookworm infestation, schistosomiasis, or NSAID) • Urinary tract (renal or bladder tumors) • Genital tract (menorrhagia and uterine cancer)

- *Plummer-Vinson syndrome/Patterson-Kelly-Brown/Sideropenic dysphagia:* Esophageal/postcricoid webs result in dysphagia for solids than liquids.

Stages of Iron Deficiency (Fig. 12.3)

- **Stage 1:** *Negative iron balance* is characterized by decreased bone marrow iron stores.
- **Stage 2:** *Iron-deficient erythropoiesis*—erythropoiesis is impaired when serum iron falls to <50 µg/dL (<9 µmol/L) and transferrin saturation to <16%.
- **Stage 3:** *Iron deficiency anemia*—microcytosis and then hypochromia develop. Eventually, iron deficiency affects tissues, resulting in symptoms and signs.

Laboratory Investigations

Laboratory investigations for iron deficiency anemia are described in **Table 12.6**.

Serum iron profile in iron deficiency anemia is described in **Table 12.7**.

Differential diagnosis for microcytic hypochromic anemia is given in Table 12.8.

Management

- Identify and treat the underlying cause for deficiency.
- **Oral iron therapy:** Most patients can be treated with oral iron preparations. Ferrous sulfate (200 mg three times daily, a total of 180 mg ferrous iron), ferrous gluconate (300 mg twice daily, only 70 mg ferrous iron), ferrous fumarate (325 mg two or three times daily), and others.
- **Parenteral iron therapy:**
  - *Indications:*
    - Intolerant to oral iron preparation
    - Severe malabsorption
    - Primary blood loss is uncontrollable
    - Chronic GI tract disease (e.g., inflammatory bowel disease), which may worsen with oral iron
  - Iron dose in mg = Body weight (kg) × 2.3 × (normal Hb-patient's hemoglobin, g/dL) + 500 or 1,000 mg (to provide body iron stores)

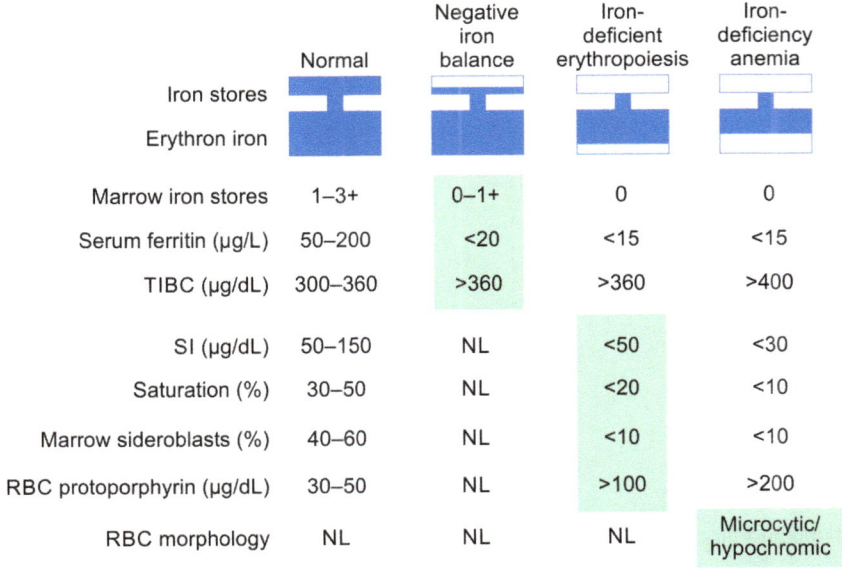

Fig. 12.3: Staging of iron deficiency anemia.
(RBC: red blood cell; SI: serum iron; TIBC: total iron binding capacity)

Table 12.6: Laboratory investigations for iron deficiency anemia.

To confirm iron deficiency	Investigation of the cause of iron deficiency
Hemoglobin and hematocrit (PCV): Decreased	**Stool:** Examine for occult blood and hookworm infestation
Red cell indices: MCV: <80 fL; MCH: <25 pg; MCHC: <27g/dL. RDW: Increased, >15%. Earliest sign of iron deficiency	
Peripheral smear: Microcytic hypochromic RBCs (**Fig. 12.4**). Severe anemia: ring/pessary, pencil/cigar-shaped cells with moderate anisocytosis and poikilocytosis	**Endoscopy:** This includes upper gastrointestinal endoscopy, sigmoidoscopy, and colonoscopy
Reticulocyte count: Low for degree of anemia	
Bone marrow: Moderate erythroid hyperplasia and micro-normoblastic maturation	**Urine:** Examine for parasites, such as schistosomiasis
Absence of bone marrow iron: "Gold standard" test, demonstrated by negative Prussian blue reaction	
Hepcidin: Decreased Hepcidin regulates iron concentrations and tissue iron distribution	Investigations for malabsorption

(MCH: mean corpuscular hemoglobin; MCHC: mean corpuscular hemoglobin concentration; MCV: mean corpuscular volume; PCV: packed cell volume)

Table 12.7: Serum iron profile in iron deficiency anemia (IDA).

	Normal range	Value in IDA	Observation
Serum ferritin	15–300 µg/L	<15 µg/L	Low
Serum iron	50–150 µg/dL	10–15 µg/dL	Low
Serum transferrin saturation	30–40%	<15%	Reduced
Total plasma iron-binding capacity (TIBC)	310–340 µg/dL	350–450 µg/dL	Increased
Serum transferrin receptor (TFR)	0.57–2.8 µg/L	3.5–7.1 µg/L	Increased
Red cell protoporphyrin	30–50 µg/dL	>200 µg/dL	Increased

Table 12.8: Differential diagnosis for microcytic hypochromic anemia.

Iron deficiency	Anemia of chronic disease
Thalassemia	Sideroblastic anemia
Lead poisoning	

- *Preparations*: Iron-sorbitol, iron-dextran (imferon), iron sucrose, or sodium ferric gluconate, ferric carboxymaltose, and iron isomaltoside
- ☐ **Red cell transfusion:**
  - *Indication:* It is reserved for patients who have symptoms of anemia, cardiovascular instability, continued and

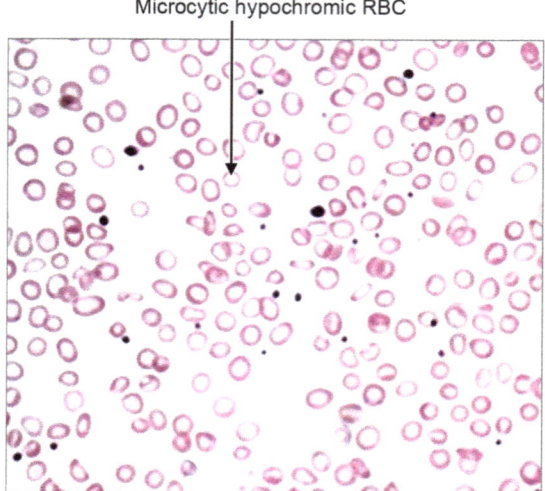

Fig. 12.4: Microcytic hypochromic red blood cell (RBC).

excessive loss of blood loss from any site, and require immediate intervention.
- Transfusions correct the anemia acutely as well as transfused red cells provide a source of iron for reutilization.

Macrocytic Anemia

Vitamin B_{12} and folic acid are closely related and both are essential for normal DNA synthesis and nuclear maturation.

Vitamin B_{12} Metabolism

- Vitamin B_{12} is present only in animal proteins and dairy products and not present in vegetables. Therefore, strict vegetarians do not get an adequate quantity of vitamin B_{12}.
- A balanced diet (not rigid vegetarian!) contains significantly large amounts of vitamin B_{12}, which accumulate in the body (liver) and are enough for several (about 3) years. Hence, if there is any dietary deficiency or malabsorption of vitamin B_{12}, its clinical manifestations appear only after about 2–4 years.
- Normal daily requirement is about 2–3 μg.

Absorption, transport, and storage (Fig. 12.5):

- Vitamin B_{12} in food is usually in coenzyme form (as deoxyadenosylcobalamin and methylcobalamin) and bound to binding proteins in the diet.
- In the stomach, peptic digestion at low pH is required for release of vitamin B_{12} from binding protein in the food. The released vitamin B_{12} binds with salivary protein called *haptocorrin*, which is secreted in salivary juice.
- These haptocorrin-B_{12} complexes leave stomach along with unbound special protein called *intrinsic factor* (IF), which is produced by gastric (fundus and cardia) parietal (oxyntic) cells.
- As haptocorrin-B_{12} complexes pass into the second part of the duodenum, pancreatic proteases release vitamin B_{12} from haptocorrin. Vitamin B_{12} then associates with the intrinsic factor and forms IF-B_{12} complex.
- This stable IF-vitamin B_{12} complex is transported to the ileum, where it is endocytosed by ileal enterocytes. These

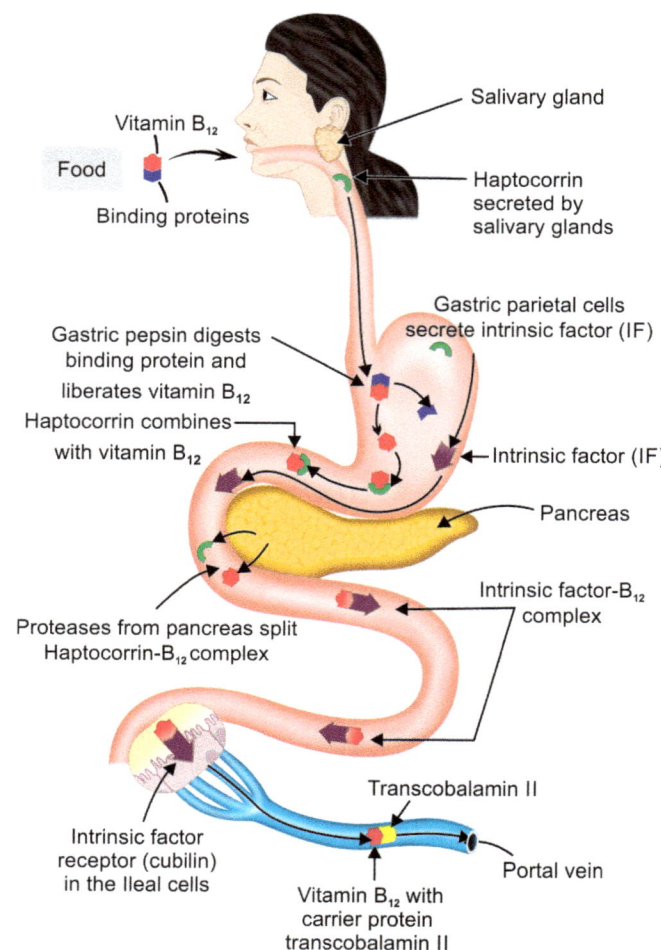

Fig. 12.5: Mechanism of vitamin B_{12} absorption.

ileal enterocytes express a receptor on their surfaces for the intrinsic factor. These receptors are called *cubilin*.
- In the ileal epithelium, vitamin B_{12} combines with a major carrier protein, transcobalamin II, and is actively transported into the mucosal cells and then into the blood.
- Transcobalamin II-vitamin B_{12} complex delivers vitamin B_{12} to the liver and other cells of the body, particularly rapidly proliferating cells in the bone marrow and mucosal lining of the gastrointestinal tract.

Role of vitamin B_{12}:
Vitamin B_{12} is essential for:
- Normal hemopoiesis
- Maintenance of normal integrity of the nervous system

Vitamin B_{12} is indirectly required for DNA synthesis in various metabolic steps and its deficiency impairs DNA synthesis. There are two biologically active forms of cobalamin in the body, both act as coenzymes, namely—(1) methylcobalamin and (2) adenosylcobalamin.
- Methylcobalamin is the main form of vitamin B_{12} in plasma, and is an essential coenzyme for conversion of homocysteine to methionine and formation of tetrahydrofolate (THF) from methyl THF **(Fig. 12.6)**. During the former reaction, vitamin B_{12} loses its methyl group and this is replaced from methyl THF, the principal form of folic acid in plasma. Tetrahydrofolate is essential

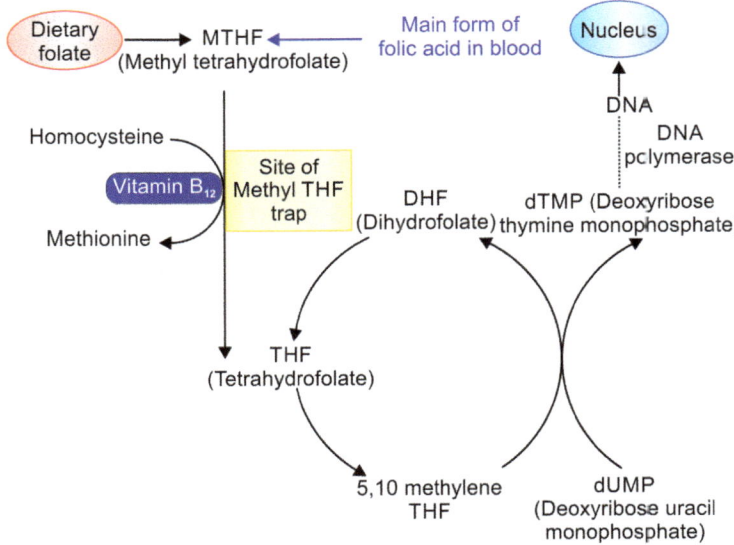

Fig. 12.6: Inter-relation and role of vitamin B_{12} and folate in DNA synthesis.

for the generation of a precursor of DNA known as deoxythymidine monophosphate (dTMP).

In vitamin B_{12} deficiency, main cause of impaired DNA synthesis is that methyl THF is not converted into THF. Methyl THF accumulates in the cell and is known as "*Methyl THF trap.*" Lack of folic acid is the next cause of anemia in vitamin B_{12} deficiency, as the anemia invariably improves with folic acid administration.

- Deoxyadenosylcobalamin form of vitamin B_{12} is a coenzyme required for conversion of methylmalonyl coenzyme A (CoA) to succinyl malonyl CoA (**Fig. 12.7**). Deficiency of vitamin B_{12} causes increased levels of methylmalonic acid in plasma and urine. This results in the formation of abnormal fatty acids, which get incorporated into neuronal lipids. Consequently, this predisposes to myelin breakdown and is probably responsible for neurologic complications of vitamin B_{12} deficiency.

Folic Acid Metabolism

- **Daily requirement:** 50–200 mg
- **Source:** Green vegetables, yeast, legumes, fruits, and animal proteins are the richest sources. The folic acid in these foods is largely in the form of polyglutamates. Polyglutamates are sensitive to heat (thermolabile); boiling, steaming, or frying, and which destroys most of the folic acid (destroyed by cooking). Intestinal conjugates split the polyglutamates into monoglutamates.

- **Site of absorption:** Proximal jejunum. During intestinal absorption, they are modified to 5-methyltetrahydrofolate, the normal transport form of folic acid (FA).
- **Storage:** Folate is mainly stored in the liver and is enough for about 3 months and hence the manifestations of folate deficiency appear after about 3 months.

Role of folic acid:

Active form of folic acid is tetrahydrofolate (THF), which is the biologic "middleman" involved in metabolic processes, which synthesize DNA. The various reactions in which folic acid plays a main role are:

- Purine (required for DNA and RNA) synthesis
- Conversion of homocysteine to methionine, a reaction also requiring vitamin B_{12}
- *Deoxythymidylate monophosphate synthesis*: 5,10-methylene THF polyglutamate is required for conversion of dUMP to dTMP and DNA, a rate-limiting step in pyrimidine synthesis.

Folic acid is associated with metabolism of histidine: Histidine is metabolized to formiminoglutamic acid (FIGLU), which combines with THF to form glutamic acid (**Fig. 12.8**). In FA deficiency, this reaction cannot take place and therefore FIGLU accumulates and is excreted as such in urine. This is used as a test to measure folic acid deficiency.

Megaloblastic Anemia

Megaloblastic anemia is described in **Table 12.9**.

Pernicious anemia (PA):

Chronic autoimmune disorder characterized by atrophic gastritis with loss of parietal cells in the gastric mucosa, which causes failure of production of intrinsic factor.

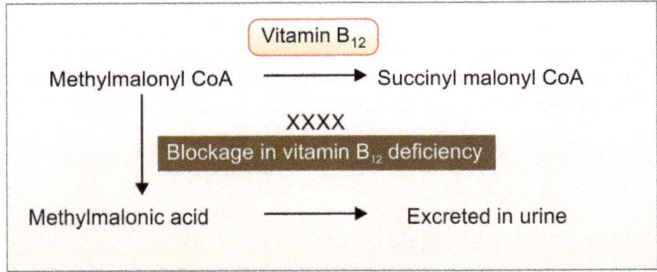

Fig. 12.7: Role of vitamin B_{12} in methylmalonyl coenzyme A (CoA) metabolism.

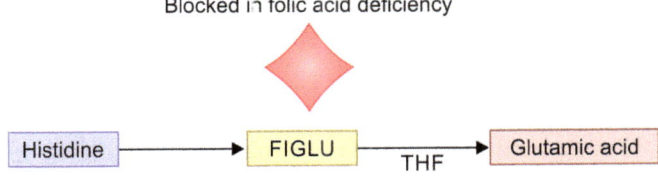

Fig. 12.8: Role of folic acid in metabolism of histidine.
(FIGLU: formiminoglutamic acid; THF: tetrahydrofolate)

Table 12.9: Megaloblastic anemia.

Vitamin B$_{12}$ deficiency	Folic acid deficiency
Decreased intake: Inadequate diet—"pure vegetarians"	**Decreased intake:** Inadequate diet—alcoholism, malnutrition
Increased demand: Pregnancy, hyperthyroidism, and disseminated cancer	**Increased loss:** Hemodialysis

Impaired absorption:
• *Gastric*: Deficiency of gastric acid or pepsin or intrinsic factor
  ▪ Pernicious anemia
  ▪ Postgastrectomy
  ▪ *Drugs*: Prolonged use of H2-receptor blockers and proton-pump inhibitors
• *Intestinal*:
  ▪ Loss of absorptive surface:
   – Malabsorption syndromes
   – *Diffuse intestinal disease*: Lymphoma and systemic sclerosis
   – Ileal resection and Crohn disease
  ▪ Competition for vitamin B$_{12}$: Bacterial overgrowth in blind loops and diverticula of bowel, *Diphyllobothrium latum*
	Impaired absorption:
	• *Malabsorption states*: Nontropical and tropical sprue, celiac disease
	• Diffuse infiltrative diseases of the small intestine (e.g., lymphoma)
	• *Drugs*: Anticonvulsant phenytoin, oral contraceptives, metformin, and cholestyramine
	
	Increased demand: Pregnancy, lactation, infancy, disseminated cancer, markedly increased hematopoiesis (hemolytic anemias), chronic exfoliative skin disease, chronic inflammatory, and infective diseases

Abnormal cobalamin transport: Transcobalamin II deficiency	**Impaired utilization:** Folic acid antagonists (antifolate drugs), such as methotrexate, trimethoprim, pyrimethamine, pentamidine, 5-fluorouracil, and hydroxyurea
Others: Antifolate drugs, e.g., methotrexate; independent of either cobalamin or folate deficiency	

There is presence of autoantibodies in most of the patients. *Two major types* of autoantibodies are found:
- **Anti-intrinsic factor (IF) antibody:**
  - *Type I (blocking) antibody*: It blocks binding of vitamin B$_{12}$ to IF, presents in 50–75% of the cases, and is detected in both plasma and gastric juice.
  - *Type II (binding) antibody* attaches to IF–vitamin B$_{12}$ complex and prevents its binding to receptors in the ileal mucosa, and presents in about 40% of patients.
- **Parietal cell (type III) antibody:** It is directed against α and β subunits of gastric proton pump (H$^+$, K$^+$-ATPase) in parietal cells but is neither specific for PA nor other autoimmune disorders, found in 90% of patients with PA as well as in older patients with chronic nonspecific gastritis. Diagnosis/laboratory findings of megaloblastic anemia are given in **Table 12.10**.

Clinical features (Fig. 12.11):
Vitamin B$_{12}$ deficiency:
- **Classic triad:** Weakness, sore throat, and paresthesia
- Painful red "beefy" tongue due to glossitis and atrophy of papillae. Loss of taste and appetite

Table 12.10: Diagnosis/laboratory findings of megaloblastic anemia.

Peripheral blood:	
Hemoglobin, hematocrit	Reduced
Red cell indices	MCV raised above 100 fL
Peripheral smear (Fig. 12.9)	Pancytopenia
RBCs	Macrocytic and oval (egg-shaped macro-ovalocytes) Most macrocytes lack the central pallor. Marked variation in the size and shape of red cells (anisopoikilocytosis) *Dyserythropoiesis*: Basophilic stippling, Cabot ring, and Howell–Jolly bodies
WBCs	Decreased WBC count (leukopenia) *Hypersegmented neutrophils (more than five nuclear lobes)*: First and specific morphological sign of megaloblastic anemia. These neutrophils are also larger than normal
Platelets	Decreased
Reticulocyte count	Normal-low. *Reticulocytosis*: Response to small doses of parenteral vitamin B$_{12}$
Bone marrow: • Markedly hypercellular • Megaloblastic type of erythropoiesis • *Granulocytic precursors*: Nuclear-cytoplasmic asynchrony as giant metamyelocytes and band forms • *Megakaryopoiesis*: Normal or increased in number	
Bone marrow iron	Moderately increased
Diagnostic/specific tests for vitamin B$_{12}$ deficiency	
Serum vitamin B$_{12}$ levels: Reduced and levels are very low (<200 pg/μL) *Serum methyl malonic acid (MMA) and homocysteine levels*: Raised *Urinary excretion of methylmalonic acid*: Raised **Schilling test** for vitamin B$_{12}$ absorption, discontinued in 2003, once provided invaluable information on the locus and mechanism of cobalamin malabsorption **(Fig. 12.10)**	
Diagnostic/specific tests for folic acid deficiency: • *Serum folic acid levels*: Reduced • *FIGLU in urine*: Excessively excreted	

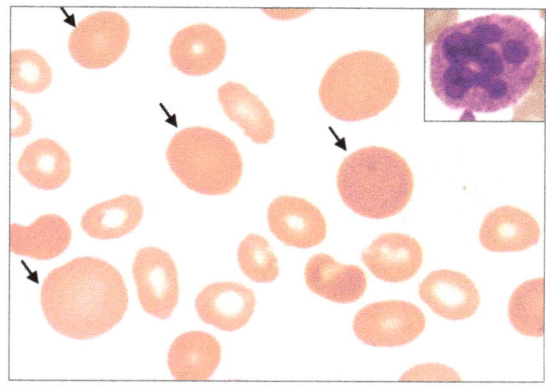

Fig. 12.9: Peripheral blood smear showing macro-ovalocytes (short arrows) and hypersegmented neutrophil (inset).

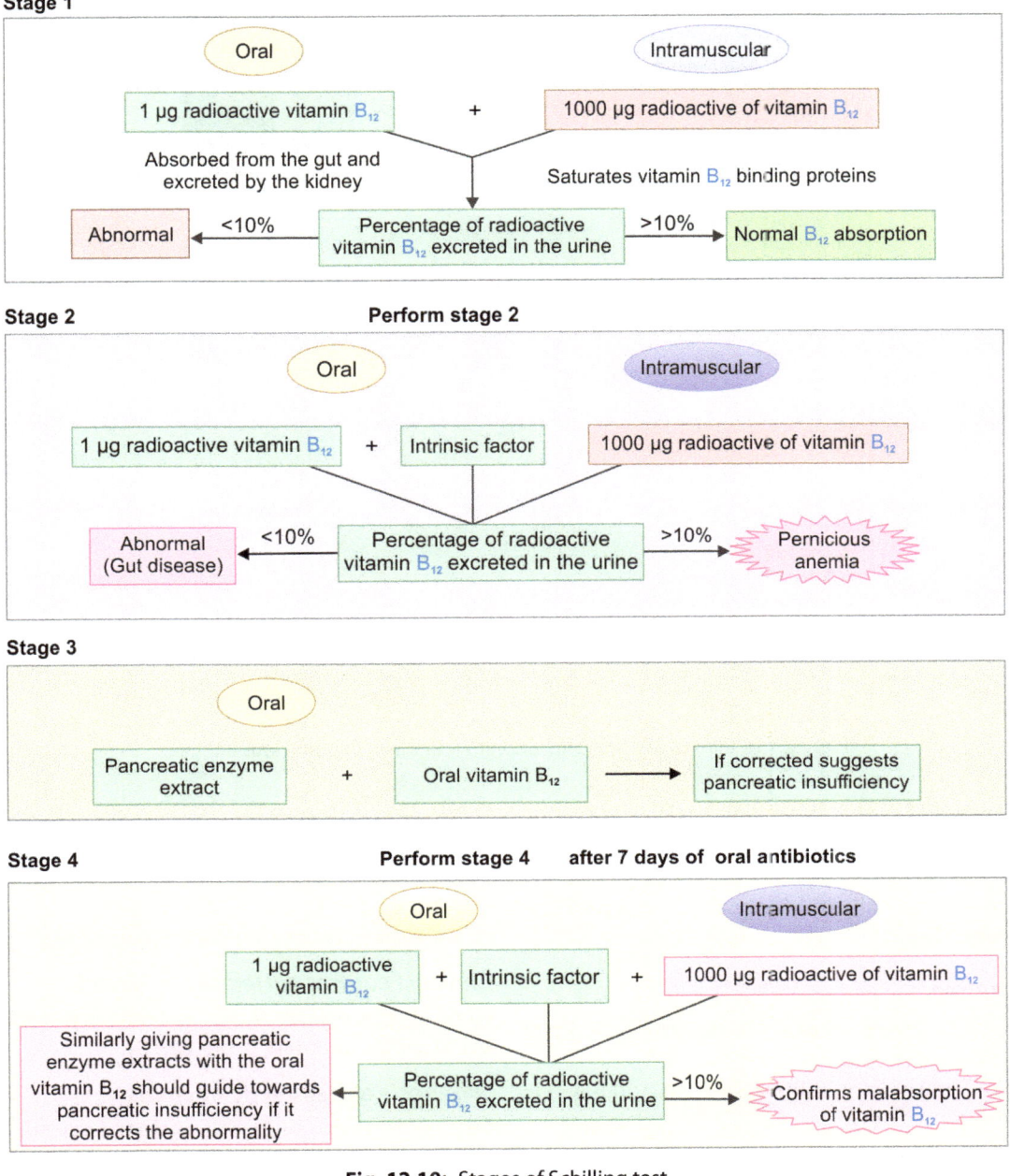

Fig. 12.10: Stages of Schilling test.

- **Lemon-yellow color:** Pallor and mild jaundice caused by excess breakdown of hemoglobin
- **Neurological features:**
  - *Peripheral nerves*—peripheral neuropathy: Glove and sock distribution of paresthesia. Tingling begins in tips of toes and progresses proximally—bilateral and symmetric. Loss of ankle reflexes
  - *Spinal cord*: Subacute combined degeneration of the cord—
    - *Posterior columns*: Impaired/diminished vibration and position sensation
    - *Corticospinal tracts*: Upper motor neuron signs—ataxic and uncoordinated gait
  - *Cerebrum:* Depression and loss of memory (dementia) and optic atrophy
- Positive Romberg sign and Lhermitte's sign may be elicited.

Folate deficiency: Similar to vitamin B_{12} deficiency without neurological features.

Management:
Treat the underlying cause, whenever possible.
Vitamin B_{12}/cobalamin: Vitamin B_{12} therapy—cyanocobalamin, hydroxocobalamin, and methylcobalamin
- *Dosage:*
  - *Initial dose:* Six intramuscular injections of hydroxocobalamin 1,000 μg at 3–7-day intervals.
  - *Maintenance dose:* 1,000 μg to be given intramuscularly every 3 months for rest of the patient's life. Methylcobalamin, metabolically active form of vitamin B_{12}, can also be used.

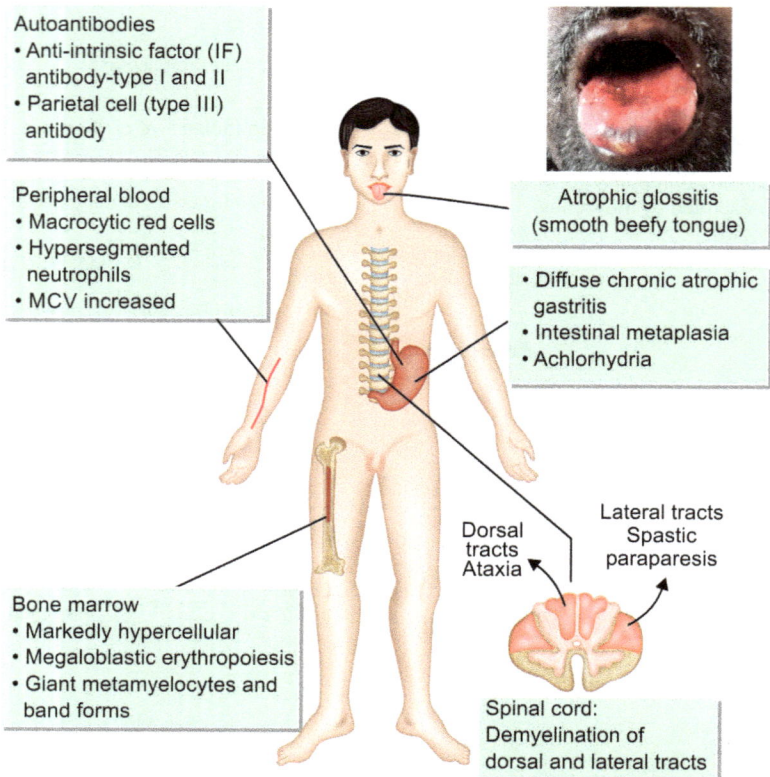

Fig. 12.11: Clinical features and laboratory findings in pernicious anemia.

Folate deficiency: Oral dose of 5 mg folate (folic acid) daily for 3 weeks will treat acute deficiency and 5 mg once weekly is adequate maintenance therapy.

Causes of nonmegaloblastic macrocytic anemia are described in **Table 12.11**.

Hemolytic Anemia

Anemia that results due to increase in the rate of red cell destruction is known as hemolytic anemia.

Lifespan of red cells (normal lifespan is 90–120 days) is shortened.

Classification of Hemolytic Anemias

The hemolytic anemias are classified in a variety of ways:
- **Location of hemolysis:** Intravascular and extravascular hemolytic disorders **(Fig. 12.12)**
- **Source of defect:** Intracorpuscular defect or extracorpuscular mechanism
- **Mode of onset:** Hereditary and acquired disorders **(Table 12.12)**.
- **Clinical point of view:** Acute or chronic

Clinical Features of Hemolytic Anemia

Clinical features depend on the severity, duration, and type of hemolytic anemia **(Table 12.13)**.

Diagnosis of Hemolytic Anemias

Diagnosis of extravascular and intravascular hemolysis is described in **Table 12.14**.

Features of increased RBC production: Compensatory mechanism to hemolysis, there is increased production of red cells.
- **Bone marrow:** Compensatory erythroid hyperplasia
- **Peripheral smear:** Reticulocytosis. Other findings vary depending on the cause—
  - Nucleated red cells and polychromasia
  - Macrocytosis (due to increased reticulocyte count and folate deficiency)
  - Spherocytes (hereditary spherocytosis and autoimmune hemolytic anemia)
  - Marked anisopoikilocytosis, hypochromic red cells, and target cells in thalassemias
  - Fragmented red cells (microangiopathic anemia and prosthetic cardiac valve)
- **Radiological changes:** Hair on end appearance in skull radiograph (thalassemia and sickle cell anemia)

Table 12.11: Causes of nonmegaloblastic macrocytic anemia.

Physiological causes	
Pregnancy	Newborn
Pathological causes:	
Alcohol excess	Reticulocytosis
Chronic liver disease	Hypothyroidism
Postsplenectomy	Myeloproliferative disorders
Hematological disorders: • Aplastic anemia • Sideroblastic anemia • Pure red cell aplasia	**Drugs:** • Azathioprine • Hydroxycarbamide

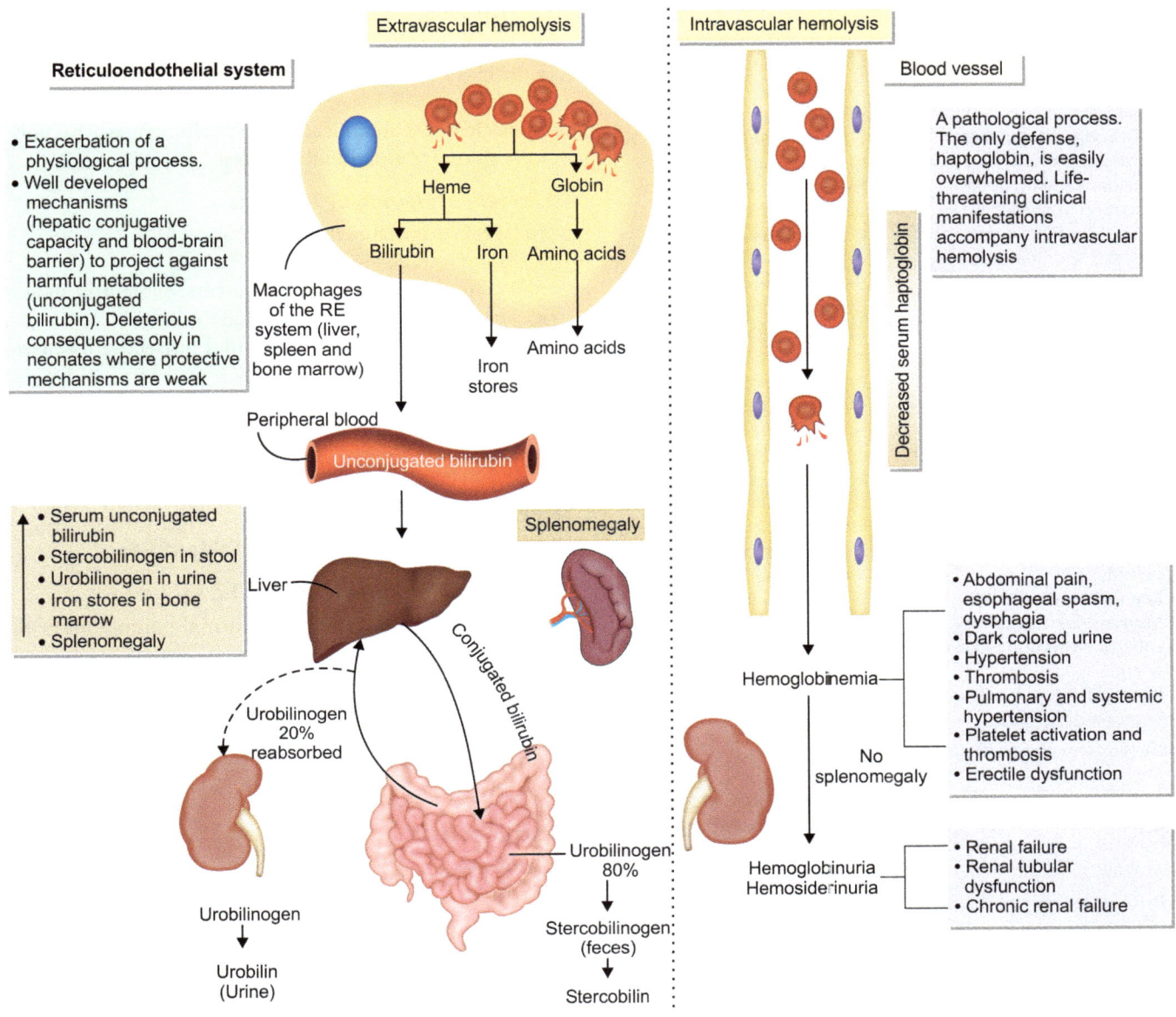

Fig. 12.12: Mechanism and consequences of extravascular and intravascular hemolysis.

Table 12.12: Hereditary and acquired hemolytic anemia.

Hereditary	Acquired
Defects in red cell membrane	**Immunohemolytic anemias**

• Hereditary spherocytosis
• Hereditary elliptocytosis
• Stomatocytosis
• Abetalipoproteinemia (acanthocytosis)
	Autoimmune hemolytic anemias:
	• *Due to warm antibodies:* • *Due to cold antibodies:*
	  ▪ Idiopathic ▪ Cold agglutinin disease
	  ▪ Secondary ▪ Paroxysmal cold hemoglobinuria
	• Hemolytic disease of the newborn

Red cell enzyme deficiencies	**Fragmentation syndromes**
• Pyruvate kinase deficiency • Hexokinase deficiency • Glucose-6-phosphate dehydrogenase deficiency (G6PD)	• Hemolytic uremic syndrome • Thrombotic thrombocytopenic purpura • Disseminated intravascular coagulation • Prosthetic cardiac valves
Defects in globin synthesis—hemoglobinopathies:	**Miscellaneous**
• Thalassemia—quantitative • Sickle cell syndromes—qualitative • Alpha thalassemia • Unstable hemoglobin disease	• *Drugs:* Oxidant drugs (primaquine and dapsone) • *Chemical* (naphthalene, nitrites and nitrates, and oxidizing chemicals) • *Thermal injury:* Burns *Paroxysmal nocturnal hemoglobinuria*

Table 12.13: Clinical features of hemolytic anemia.

Symptoms/history	Physical findings/signs
• Mild jaundice • Symptoms due to anemia • **Urine color:** It appears normal (acholuric) and turns dark on standing due to oxidation of urobilinogen to urobilin. Black urine (hemoglobinuria) is seen in intravascular hemolysis (malaria, mismatched blood transfusion, and G6PD deficiency) • Infections • **Splenic pain:** Enlargement or infraction of spleen • **Acute crisis:** Due to sudden fall in hemoglobin—fever, joint pains, and abdominal pain • **Pigment gallstones:** Chronic hemolysis • **Leg ulcers manifest in adult males:** Hereditary spherocytosis and sickle cell anemia • **Family history:** Congenital hemolytic anemias	• Anemia • Mild jaundice • **Splenomegaly:** Some cases of hemolytic anemia—thalassemia and hereditary spherocytosis • **Chronic leg ulcers:** Sickle cell anemia • **Skeletal abnormalities:** Expansion of bone marrow in some congenital hemolytic anemias due to increased erythropoiesis, manifests as enlargement of maxillary bones and frontal bossing and malocclusion of the teeth due to overgrowth of upper jaw (thalassemic facies). • Signs of systemic disease—predisposing to hemolysis. • **Signs of cholelithiasis:** Cholecystitis

(G6PD: glucose-6-phosphate dehydrogenase)

Table 12.14: Diagnosis of extravascular and intravascular hemolysis.

Extravascular hemolysis	Intravascular hemolysis
• Anemia	
• Unconjugated hyperbilirubinemia (jaundice)	
• Increased urobilinogen in urine leading to high-colored urine	
• Shortened red cell life span (demonstrated by ^{51}Cr-labeled red blood cells)	
• Decreased plasma haptoglobin and hemopexin	
Splenomegaly	Increased plasma LDH, hemoglobinemia, hemoglobinuria, hemosiderinuria (demonstrated by Prussian blue reaction) and methemoglobinemia (in some)

(LDH: lactate dehydrogenase)

Tests for Cause of Hemolysis

☐ **Common tests:**
  • *Peripheral smear examination*: Red cell morphology—
    ▪ Spherocyte (hereditary spherocytosis and autoimmune hemolytic anemia)
    ▪ Sickle cell (sickle cell anemia)
    ▪ Target cell (thalassemia)
    ▪ Acanthocyte
    ▪ Schistocyte (intravascular hemolysis—fragmented red cells, helmet cells, and triangular cells)
    ▪ Malarial parasite
  • *Coombs' test*
  • *Osmotic fragility, sucrose lysis, and Ham's test*
  • *Heinz body preparation*
  • *Hemoglobin electrophoresis*
  • *High-performance liquid chromatography (HPLC)*
  • *Measurement of enzyme activity*
☐ **Specific tests:** Identification of specific cause of hemolysis is dealt under individual diseases.

Treatment of Hemolytic Anemias

☐ **General supportive therapy:**
  • Blood transfusions
  • Treatment of infections, leg ulcers, cholelithiasis, etc.
  • *Splenectomy*: In some selected diseases
☐ **Specific therapy:** Dealt with under respective diseases.

Hemoglobinopathies

Table 12.15 discusses about different types of hemoglobinopathies.

Sickle-Cell Anemia

Sickle-cell anemia is described in **Table 12.16**.

Etiology and Pathogenesis (Fig. 12.13)

It is caused by production of abnormal hemoglobin called sickle hemoglobin (HbS).

In HbS, there is an adenine (A) to thymidine (T) substitution (GAG → GTG) in codon 6 of the β-globin gene. This point mutation results in *replacement of the normal glutamic acid residue by a valine* and alters the solubility or stability of the hemoglobin.

Clinical Features

In children:

☐ Infant till 3 months may be asymptomatic, because of the protective role of HbF. Since, HbF disappears after 3rd

Table 12.15: Different types of hemoglobinopathies.

Qualitative defect in (structurally abnormal) hemoglobins:	Combined qualitative and quantitative defects in hemoglobins:
• Hemoglobin S • Hemoglobin C • Hemoglobin D Punjab	• Hemoglobin E • Sickle-cell β-thalassemia
Quantitative defect in hemoglobins: Thalassemias (α, β-thalassemia)	**Acquired hemoglobinopathies:** • Methemoglobinemia due to toxic exposures • Carboxyhemoglobinemia

Table 12.16: Sickle-cell anemia.

Sickle-cell anemia (SS)	Homozygous state in which both β-globin chains are abnormal
Sickle-cell trait (AS)	Heterozygous state in which one gene is defective for HbS (abnormal) and other gene is for HbA (normal)
Compound heterozygous	Both β-globin chains having different abnormalities (HbSC and HbS-β-thalassemia)

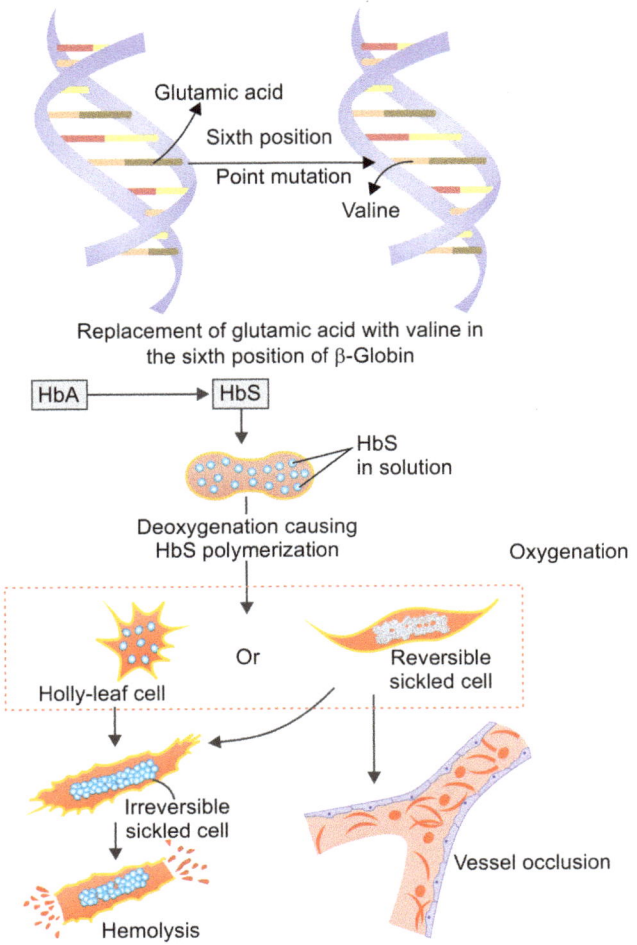

Fig. 12.13: Pathogenesis of sickle cell anemia.

- **Changes in spleen:** Splenomegaly is observed during early childhood. Repeated episodes of splenic infarct result in atrophy of the spleen (*autosplenectomy*).
- **Acute chest syndrome** can develop in both children and adults. It is due to infection or infarction in the lung and presents with pain in the chest, fever, respiratory distress, and hypoxemia.
- **Others** include acute coronary syndrome and stroke. Chronic hypoxia in children is responsible for generalized impairment of growth and development.

In adults (Fig. 12.14):
- **Anemia:** Patients develop severe hemolytic anemia, which is exacerbated by secondary folate deficiency. Chronic anemia presents with fatigue, frequent infections, cardiomegaly, and systolic murmurs. Chronic hemolytic anemia causes increased levels of unconjugated (indirect) bilirubin, which predisposes to development of pigmented bilirubin gallstones. Cholelithiasis may lead to cholecystitis.
- **Crises:** Irreversibly sickled cells have a shortened survival and plug vessels in the microcirculation. Any new syndrome or episode that develops rapidly in sickle cell anemia is termed crises. The protracted course of sickle cell anemia is frequently exacerbated by a variety of crises. Four types of crises are encountered. These are:
  - **Infarction (sickling) crisis (vaso-occlusive crisis):** Blockage of microcirculation by sickled red cells causes hypoxic injury and infarction.

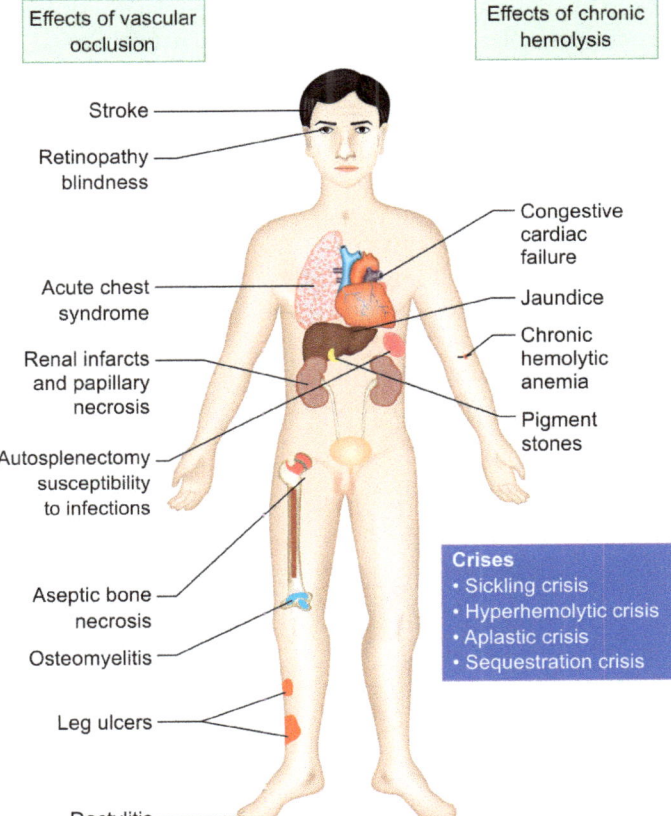

Fig. 12.14: Various effects of vascular occlusion and hemolysis in sickle cell anemia.

month, majority of cases present after 3 months and before 1st year of life.
- **Prone to infections:** Children are susceptible to acute infections with encapsulated organisms. Common infections are pneumococcal pneumonia, meningitis due to *S. pneumonia* and osteomyelitis due to *Salmonella*. Increased susceptibility to infections is because of hypofunction of spleen and defects in the alternative complement pathway, which impair opsonization of encapsulated bacteria, such as *pneumococci* and *Haemophilus influenzae*. Septicemia and meningitis are the most common causes of death in children. Increased frequency of *osteomyelitis* is because of repeated bone infarcts, which act as nidus for infection.
- In children, *bone involvement* may resemble acute osteomyelitis. They manifest as the *hand-foot syndrome, dactylitis* of the bones of the hands or feet or both. It is due to microinfarcts in the carpal and tarsal bones.
- **Sequestration crisis:** It usually occurs in children with chronically enlarged but normal functioning spleen. Sudden trapping of blood in spleen or liver causes rapid enlargement of the organ with resultant drop in hematocrit and hypovolemic shock. This may require blood transfusions.

- It is most common and the hallmark of sickle cell disease.
- It clinically presents with acute, severe pain in the affected region. It commonly involves bones, lungs, liver, and spleen.
  - *Bone*: Sudden attacks of bone pain are due to ischemia and infarction. Avascular necrosis of the head of femur is also common.
  - *Lung*: Involvement presents with fever, cough, chest pain, and pulmonary infarcts and known as *acute chest syndrome (dangerous)*. These are sometimes initiated by a simple lung infection.
  - *Spleen*: Acute abdominal pain caused by infarcts of spleen and leads to autosplenectomy.
  - *Other sites of infarction*: Mesenteric infarction results in acute abdominal pain, cerebral infarctions result in hemiplegia, infarction of renal papillae results in hematuria, and retinal microinfarcts result in loss of vision.
- *Aplastic crisis:* Temporary suppression of bone marrow erythropoiesis may develop due to an acute infection of erythroid progenitor cells by parvovirus B19.
- *Hemolytic crisis* is characterized by episodes of increased sequestration and destruction of red cells. It presents with marked increase in hemolysis with a sudden lowering of hemoglobin, rapid enlargement of liver and spleen, and reticulocytosis.
- *Sequestration crisis* (described above)
- Other crisis encountered rarely is hypoplastic crisis and megaloblastic crisis (due to inadequate folate).

Investigations
- **Evidences of hemolysis (see above)**
- **Blood count:** Hb is in the range 6–8 g/dL with a high reticulocyte count (10–20%).
- **Peripheral smear:** *Sickle cell*—long, curved cells with pointed ends (**Fig. 12.15**)
- **Hyposplenism:** Howell–Jolly bodies (small nuclear remnants), *target cells* (due to red cell dehydration), *and ovalocytes*
- **Erythrocyte sedimentation rate (ESR)** is low because sickle cells do not form rouleaux.
- **Sickling test:** Sickling is induced by adding a reducing agent, such as 2% sodium metabisulfite or sodium dithionite to blood sample.
- **Sickle solubility test:** A mixture of HbS in a reducing solution (e.g., sodium dithionite) gives a turbid appearance because of precipitation of HbS, whereas normal Hb gives a clear solution.
- **Hemoglobin electrophoresis:** No Hb-A, 80–95% Hb-SS, and 2–20% HbF. HbS—slow moving hemoglobin compared to HbA and HbF. In sickle cell trait (heterozygous state), HbS is 20–40% and the rest is HbA.

Management
Anemia:
- **Blood transfusion** is required to increase the oxygen-carrying capacity, to replace sickle-shaped RBCs with normal cells, and to restore blood flow. Acute transfusions—life-saving, chronic transfusions—reduce the incidence and severity of most complications.
  - Heart failure, transient ischemic attacks (TIAs), strokes, acute chest syndrome, and severe anemia due to aplastic crises and acute splenic sequestration
  - *Repeated transfusions* reduce the proportion of circulating HbS to less than 20% to prevent sickling, before elective procedures and pregnancy. Chronic RBC transfusion reduces the chance of recurrent ischemic stroke.
  - *Exchange transfusions*: These may be necessary in patients with severe or recurrent crises, or before emergency surgery. Whether exchange transfusion is preferable to simple transfusion in the acute chest syndrome, stroke, or other acute complications has not been established by clinical trials.
  - Infarction crises are managed with hydration, oxygen, analgesics, and transfusion with RBC concentrate in selected cases.

Iron overload: It develops due to repeated transfusions, can result in heart and liver failure and other complications. It is treated by using iron chelators (deferoxamine or deferasirox).

Hydroxycarbamide (hydroxyurea): It is therapy for patients with severe symptoms. 10–30 mg/kg/day increases HbF and

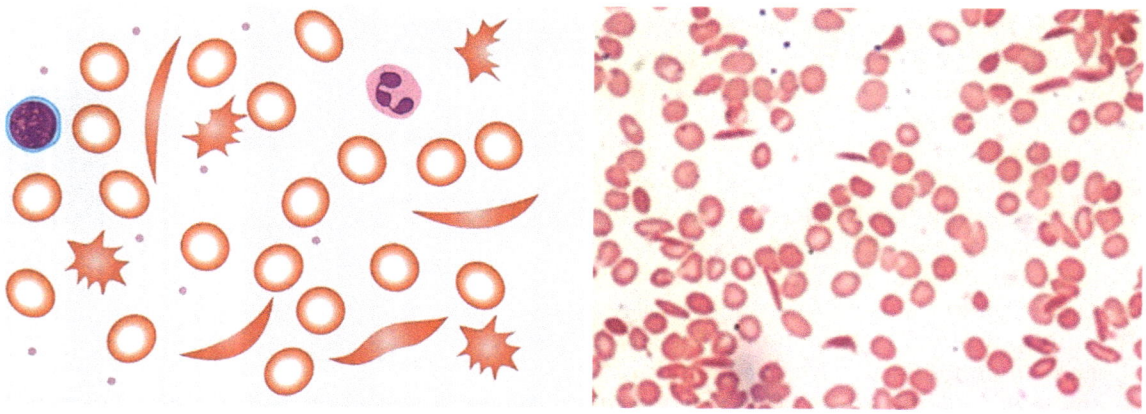

Fig. 12.15: Peripheral smear with sickle cells.

suppress neutrophil and reticulocyte counts (sickle cell crisis). It reduces episodes of pain, the acute chest syndrome, and need for blood transfusions.

Acute painful crisis:
- Supportive therapy with intravenous fluids, oxygen, antimicrobial agents, and adequate analgesia
- **Acute severe pain:** Narcotic, analgesia (morphine); milder pain—codeine, paracetamol, and NSAIDs
- **Inhaled nitric oxide** inhibits platelet function, reduces vascular adhesion of red cells, and is also a vasodilator. It provides short-term pain relief and reduces opiate requirements in acute painful episodes. Avoid hypoxia and respiratory depression. Nasal oxygen should be employed as appropriate to protect arterial saturation.

Acute chest syndrome is treated with antibiotics, maintenance of arterial oxygenation, pain relief, bronchodilators, and if required, exchange transfusion.

Curative:
- **Bone marrow/stem cell transplantation:** In children and adolescents younger than 16 years of age with who have severe complications (strokes, recurrent chest syndrome, or refractory pain) can provide definitive cure.
- **Gene therapy:** It is intensively pursued, but no safe measures are currently available.

Hereditary Spherocytosis

- It is most common inherited hemolytic anemia in adults.
- **Autosomal dominant** inheritance is observed in more than 75% cases.
- Defect in the RBC membrane is due to cytoskeleton protein (e.g., *ankyrin, band 3, spectrin, or band protein 4.2*) deficiency.
- This results in red cells losing part of the cell membrane, as they pass through the spleen and assume spheroidal shape (spherocytes) that are less deformable (rigid) and more susceptible to osmotic lysis.

Clinical Features

- It is present during or anytime from the neonatal period to adulthood.
- **Family history:** 75% HS is inherited as autosomal dominant trait with strong family history of anemia, jaundice, splenomegaly, and cholelithiasis.
- **Anemia:** Anemia is usually mild to moderate.
- **Jaundice:** Intermittent attacks of jaundice
- **Splenomegaly:** Moderate splenic enlargement is characteristic, constant (500–1,000 g) feature

Complications

- Cholelithiasis (pigment gallstones)
- Chronic leg ulcers
- Aplastic crises due to parvovirus B_{19} infection
- Hemolytic crises (rare)

Investigations

- **Anemia:** Usually mild, but occasionally can be severe.
- **Peripheral blood film** shows *spherocytes* and reticulocytes (Fig. 12.16).

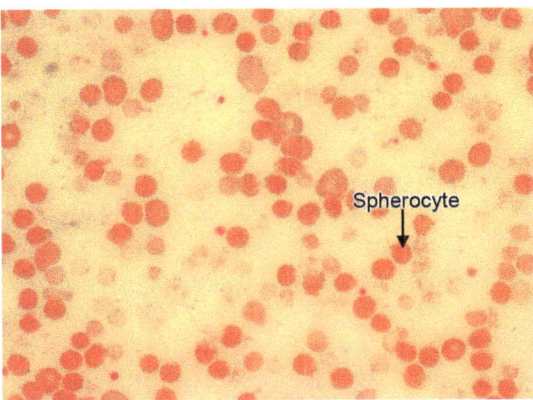

Fig. 12.16: Peripheral blood smear with numerous spherocytes (arrow) in hereditary spherocytosis.

- **Demonstration of a hemolytic state:** Raised serum bilirubin and urinary urobilinogen
- **Increased osmotic fragility:** It may be absent in mild cases and may be positive in autoimmune hemolytic anemia.

Treatment

- **Splenectomy:** It is treatment of choice and not to be done before 6 years. It corrects anemia and its complications, increases infection risk. It should be preceded by pneumococcal and *Haemophilus influenzae* immunization and followed by lifelong penicillin prophylaxis.
- **Folic acid supplementation:** In patients without splenectomy
- Regular blood transfusions are required in few patients with severe disease

Thalassemias

β-thalassemia syndromes are described in **Table 12.17.**

β-Thalassemia Major

β-thalassemia major (Mediterranean or Cooley's anemia) is the homozygous form of β-thalassemia characterized by absent or reduced synthesis of β-chain.
- It is most common in Mediterranean countries, parts of Africa, and Southeast Asia. In India, it is common among certain communities (e.g., Sindhi, Punjabi, Gujarati, and Parsee) in North India and less common in South India.
- **Anemia** is produced due to diminished synthesis of HbA, ineffective erythropoiesis, and extravascular hemolysis.
- **Consequences of ineffective erythropoiesis:**
  - *Marked erythroid hyperplasia:* Severe hemolytic anemia stimulates erythropoietin (EPO) production by kidney leading to marrow erythroid hyperplasia.
  - *Changes in the bone:* Thalassemic facies and hair on end appearance of skull X-ray
  - Extramedullary hematopoiesis

Pathogenesis and clinical features (Fig. 12.17)

- **Severe anemia:** Infants with thalassemia major are well at birth but develop moderate-to-severe anemia 6–9 months after birth, when hemoglobin synthesis switches from HbF to HbA.

Table 12.17: β-thalassemia syndromes: Based on the genetic defect (β⁺ or β⁰).

β-thalassemia major	β-thalassemia intermedia	β-thalassemia minor
Homozygous disorder. Most severe form Either no production of β-chains (β⁰) or it is markedly reduced (β⁺) *Anemia*: Severe, transfusion dependent High level of HbF in the blood	Double heterozygous state *Anemia*: Moderately severe, not transfusion dependent	Also called β-*thalassemia trait* Heterozygous state Asymptomatic with mild anemia

α-thalassemia syndromes:

Each cell has four genes coding for α-globin, two on each chromosome. Each gene contributes to 25% of the total α-globin chains. Severity depends on the number of genes deleted or affected. Deleted genes may vary from 1 to 4

1 gene affected	2 genes affected	3 genes affected	4 genes affected
Silent carrier state	α-thalassemia trait	HbH disease	*Hb Bart's*: Hydrops fetalis *Incompatible with life*: Stillbirths or die shortly after birth Pale, edematous, and hepatosplenomegaly

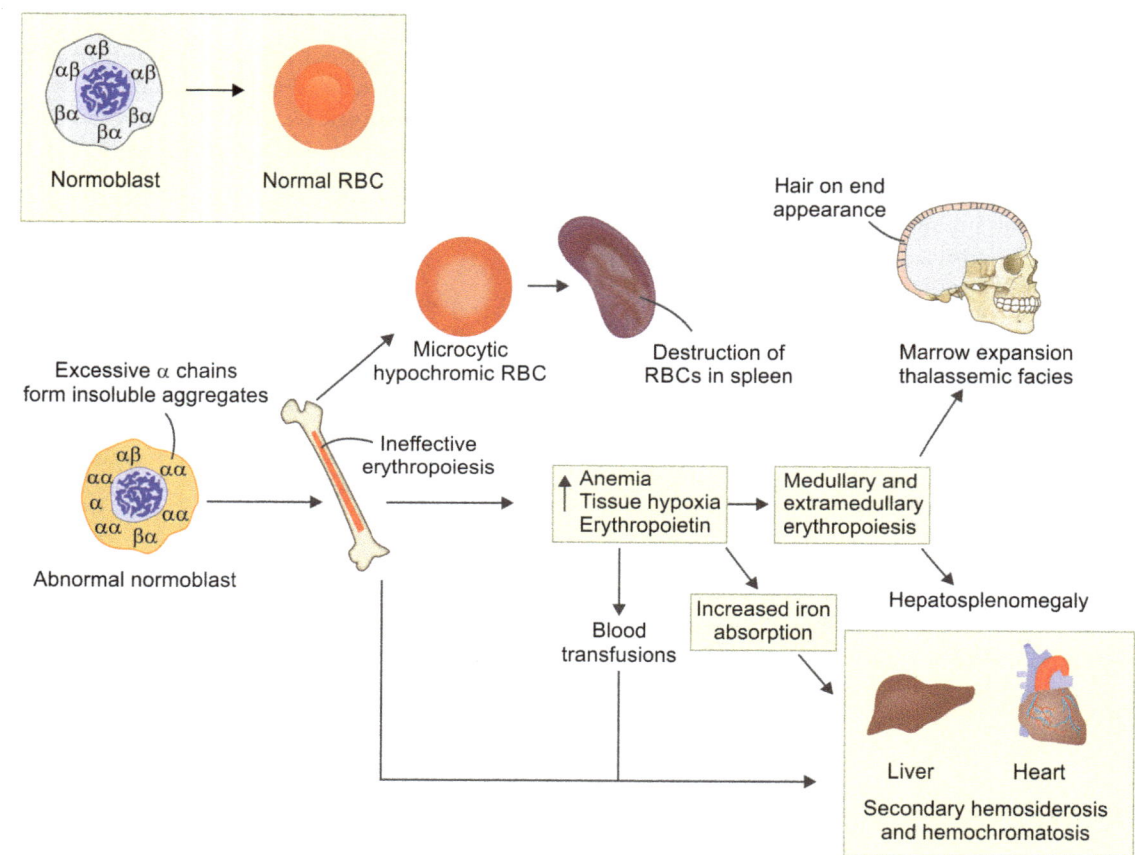

Fig. 12.17: Pathogenesis of β-thalassemia major and its consequences.

- **Retardation of growth and development:** Untreated/untransfused children *fail to thrive* (growth retardation) and die early within 4–5 years of age from the effects of anemia. They are *susceptible to recurrent bacterial infections.*
- **Changes in bone:** In those who survive longer, bone marrow hyperplasia causes expansion and widening of marrow and gives the *classical X-ray changes.*
  - *Thalassemic (Chipmunk) facies* **(Fig. 12.18A):** Due to enlargement and distortion of craniofacial bones (frontal bossing of the skull, prominent malar eminence, depression of bridge of nose, and hypertrophy of the maxillae, which tend to expose the upper teeth)
  - *Hair on end ("crew-cut") appearance* **(Fig. 12.18B):** In the skull X-ray due to new bone formation
- **Splenomegaly** may be massive and enlarges up to 1,500 g due to hyperplasia and extramedullary hematopoiesis.
- **Liver** (hepatomegaly) and lymph nodes also may show extramedullary hematopoiesis.
- **Hemosiderosis:** Although blood transfusions improve the anemia but iron overload will lead to hemosiderosis and secondary hemochromatosis. This may be due to increased gastrointestinal absorption of iron. It damages organs like heart, liver, and pancreas.
  - Cardiac hemosiderosis results in arrhythmias, heart blocks, and congestive heart failure.

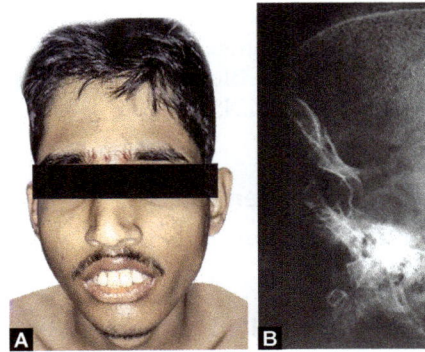
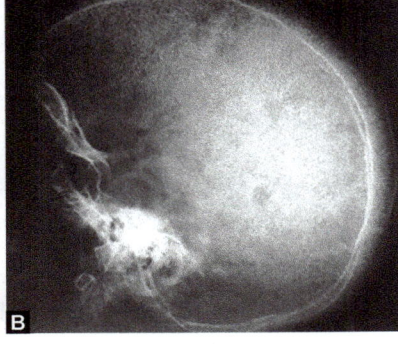

Figs. 12.18A and B: (A) Chipmunk facies in thalassemia; (B) Skull X-ray showing crew-cut appearance due to new bone formation.

- Hepatic hemosiderosis results in cirrhosis.
- Pancreatic hemosiderosis results in diabetes.
- *Pituitary:* It leads to hypogonadotropic hypogonadism
☐ Treated patients can survive beyond 40 years of age.

Investigations:
☐ **Peripheral smear (Figs. 12.19A and B):** Marked *microcytic hypochromic anemia*, moderate-marked anisopoikilocytosis. Target cells nucleated red cells
☐ **HbF level is increased** (30–92%)
☐ **Markedly reduced or absent hemoglobin A** (HbA)
☐ Osmotic fragility test shows increased resistance to hemolysis
☐ Skull radiograph shows a *"hair-on-end" appearance*
☐ Evidence of thalassemia minor in both parents
☐ **Red cell distribution width (RDW):** Within normal limits (in contrast to iron deficiency anemia)

Management:
☐ **Maintenance of Hb:** Long-term folate supplementation and blood transfusions to keep Hb >10 g/dL.
☐ **Iron overload:** Chelating agent, desferrioxamine (parenterally), is indicated if serum ferritin >1,500 μg/L. Ascorbic acid 200 mg daily along with desferrioxamine increases the urinary excretion of iron in response to desferrioxamine. Deferiprone and deferasirox are oral iron chelators.
☐ **Splenectomy** is indicated in children with massive symptomatic splenomegaly and those with progressively increasing requirement of blood transfusion.

☐ **Bone marrow transplantation:** In young patients
☐ **Management of associated complications**, e.g., congestive heart failure and endocrinopathies

Glucose-6-phosphate Dehydrogenase Deficiency

It is an X-linked disorder and is the most common enzyme deficiency. RBCs deficient in glucose-6-phosphate dehydrogenase (G6PD) deficiency cannot keep glutathione in reduced state. RBCs are susceptible to injury by both exogenous and endogenous oxidants.

Clinical Features
☐ Most are clinically asymptomatic; however, all of them have an increased risk of developing acute hemolytic anemia (AHA), neonatal jaundice (NNJ), and rarely, chronic nonspherocytic hemolytic anemia (CNSHA).
☐ **Acute hemolytic anemia:** Due to intravascular hemolysis, it is the most dramatic clinical presentation of G6PD deficiency. It develops after exposure to an oxidative stress and the triggers include:
- *Drugs:* Antimalarials (primaquine, quinine, and chloroquine), sulfonamides (sulfamethoxazole), antibacterial/antibiotics (cotrimoxazole, nitrofurantoin), antipyretics/analgesics (acetanilide phenazopyridine) dapsone, quinidine, methylene blue, nitrofurantoin, etc.
- *Fava beans* (favism)
- *Infections:* Viral and bacterial
☐ **Neonatal jaundice** is a feature of Mediterranean type. Hemolytic anemia is very rarely severe. Jaundice may be due to decreased hepatic elimination of bilirubin. Severe neonatal jaundice, if not adequately treated with phototherapy, may result in kernicterus or even death.
☐ **Chronic nonspherocytic hemolytic anemia (CNSHA):** It develops in very small minority of patients. It is seen in males and patients usually have a history of severe neonatal jaundice and chronic anemia. The degree of chronic anemia is variable, and some patients have may require intermittent transfusions. They have reticulocytosis, gallstones, and splenomegaly. Hemolysis is mainly extravascular.

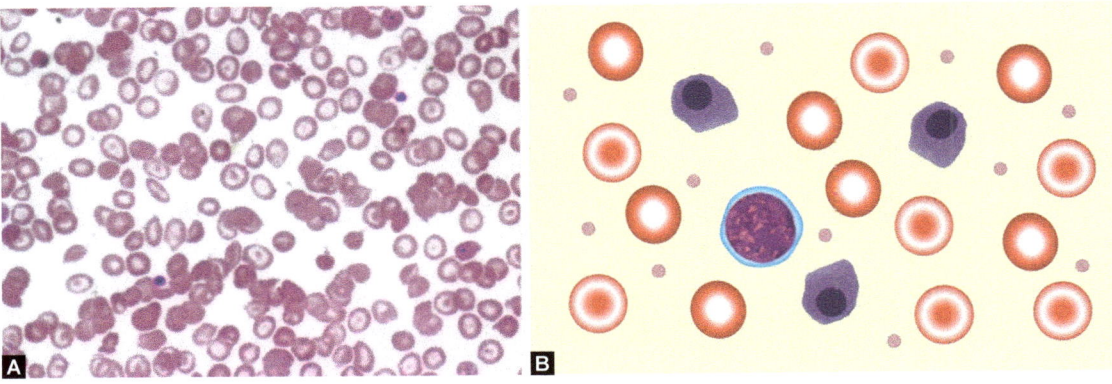

Figs. 12.19A and B: Peripheral blood smear in β-thalassemia showing target cells and nucleated red cells.

The G6PD deficiency (African variety) has a protective effect against *Plasmodium falciparum*.

Laboratory Findings/Investigations

- **Intravascular hemolysis:** Raised unconjugated bilirubin, hemoglobinemia, hemoglobinuria, high lactate dehydrogenase (LDH), and low or absent plasma haptoglobin.
- **Anemia:** Moderate-extremely severe. Both intravascular and extravascular hemolysis.
- **Peripheral blood film:** Normocytic and normochromic with anisopoikilocytosis, reticulocytosis, and spherocytes, bite (blister) cells, and Heinz bodies **(Fig. 12.20)**.
- **Confirmation of diagnosis:** Estimating G6PD activity of the red cell. This should be estimated several days after the acute hemolytic episode. This is because if done during or immediately after acute hemolysis, it may give a falsely normal value, as the young red cells and reticulocytes have near normal G6PD levels.

Treatment/Management of G6PD Deficiency

- **Removal of triggering agent** and avoiding further exposure to triggering factors in previously screened patients. Once cause is recognized, in most cases, no specific treatment is required.
- Management of neonatal jaundice is similar to any other cause of neonatal hyperbilirubinemia.
- **Supportive therapy for anemia:** Blood transfusion and regular folic acid supplements in CNSHA
- Treatment of infection

Normocytic, Normochromic Anemia

Normocytic, normochromic anemia is described in **Table 12.18**.

Differentiating Hypochromic Microcytic Anemias

Differentiation of hypochromic microcytic anemias is described in **Table 12.19**.

Pancytopenia

Pancytopenia is described in **Table 12.20**.

Sideroblastic Anemias

These are rare inherited or acquired disorders of refractory anemia characterized by presence of ring sideroblasts, excess storage iron in the bone marrow, and increased serum iron concentration **(Table 12.21)**.

Diagnostic feature is the presence of ring sideroblasts in the bone marrow.

Treatment

- Withdrawal of causative agent
- Occasional cases may respond to pyridoxine or folic acid
- Supportive treatment with transfusions
- Erythropoietin

Paroxysmal Nocturnal Hemoglobinuria

- In paroxysmal nocturnal hemoglobinuria (PNH), the red cells are abnormally sensitive to complement-mediated intravascular hemolysis.
- **Intravascular hemolysis:** Urine voided at night (nocturnal) and morning on waking is dark in color. Hemolysis is due to reduced pH of blood during sleep, which enhances the activity of complement. Hemoglobin in acidic urine is converted into acid hematin, which colors the urine dark brown. Urinary iron loss may be sufficient to cause iron deficiency.
- Mild jaundice and mild hepatosplenomegaly are often present.

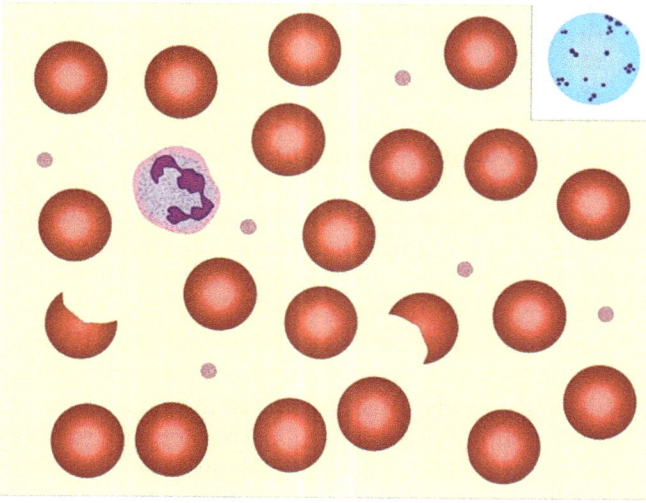

Fig. 12.20: Peripheral blood smear in G6PD deficiency with "bite cells".
[Inset: Heinz bodies (supravital stain)]

Table 12.18: Normocytic, normochromic anemia.

Decreased red cell production	Increased red cell loss or destruction
Anemia of chronic disease Chronic renal failure Chronic liver disease *Endocrine disorders*: Hypopituitarism, hypothyroidism, and hypoadrenalism **Hematological disorders:** • Marrow hypoplasia or aplasia • Myeloproliferative neoplasms • Myelofibrosis • Sideroblastic anemia	Acute blood loss Hypersplenism **Hematological disorders:** • Hemoglobinopathies (sickle cell disease) • Hereditary spherocytosis • Glucose-6-phosphate dehydrogenase (G6PD) deficiency • Microangiopathic anemias (disseminated intravascular coagulation, thrombotic thrombocytopenic purpura, and hemolytic uremic syndromes) • Autoimmune hemolytic anemia • Paroxysmal nocturnal hemoglobinuria
Expansion of plasma volume: Pregnancy	

Table 12.19: Differentiation of hypochromic microcytic anemias.

	Iron deficiency anemia	Thalassemia trait	Anemia of chronic disease	Sideroblastic anemia
MCV	Reduced	Very low for degree of anemia	Low normal or normal	Inherited—low Acquired—high
Serum iron: (normal 60–170 µg/dL)	Reduced	Normal to high	Reduced	Raised
Serum total iron-binding capacity (normal 300–350 µg/dL)	Raised	Normal	Reduced	Normal
Serum ferritin (normal 15–300 µg/dL)	Reduced	Normal	Normal or raised	Raised
Serum-soluble transferrin receptors	Increased	Normal or raised	Normal	Normal or raised
Iron in marrow	Absent	Present	Present	Present
Iron in erythroblasts	Absent	Present	Absent or reduced	Ring forms
Hemoglobin A_2 (normal <3%)	Reduced	Increased	Normal	Reduced

(MCV: mean corpuscular volume)

Table 12.20: Pancytopenia.

Decreased bone marrow function:	
Aplastic anemia: Idiopathic, secondary, and inherited **Myelodysplastic syndromes (MDS):** *Bone marrow infiltration with:* • Leukemia (e.g., hairy cell leukemia) • Lymphoma and myeloma • Tumors (carcinoma) • Granulomatous diseases (e.g., TB and sarcoidosis)	• *Nutritional deficiencies*: Megaloblastic anemia • Paroxysmal nocturnal hemoglobinuria • Myelofibrosis (rare) • Hemophagocytic syndrome
Increased peripheral destruction: Hypersplenism	

Table 12.21: Different types of sideroblastic anemias.

Inherited sideroblastic anemia: X-linked disease—transmitted by females	
Acquired sideroblastic anemia: *Primary:* Myelodysplasia *Secondary:* Drugs, e.g., isoniazid, cycloserine, chloramphenicol, busulfan, and D-penicillamine Alcohol abuse Lead toxicity	Myeloproliferative neoplasms Myeloid leukemia Primary pyridoxine deficiency Others (e.g., rheumatoid arthritis and carcinoma)

- *Thrombosis*: Very common—Budd-Chiari syndrome. Portal or cerebral vein thrombosis is often the cause of death.
- It may begin or progress to aplastic anemia.

Diagnosis
- Ham's test and sucrose lysis test
- Flow cytometry—detects red cells that are deficient in GPI-linked proteins (CD55 and CD59).

Treatment
- **Supportive measures:** Blood transfusions (severe anemia) and control of infections

- **Eculizumab:** Humanized monoclonal antibody prevents cleavage of C5 and membrane attack complex, reducing intravascular hemolysis, hemoglobinuria, and transfusion requirements.
- Long-term anticoagulants may be necessary for patients with recurrent thrombotic episodes.

Methemoglobinemia
Causes and treatment of methemoglobinemia are described in **Table 12.22**.

Autoimmune Hemolytic Anemia
Classification of autoimmune hemolytic anemia (AIHA) is described in **Box 12.1**.

Investigations
- Evidence of hemolytic anemia
- Spherocytosis (due to red cell damage) and macrocytes in peripheral blood
- Direct antiglobulin (Coombs') test is positive
- Autoantibodies may have specificity for the Rh blood group system (e.g., for the e antigen).
- **Autoimmune thrombocytopenia** and/or neutropenia may also be present (Evans' syndrome)

Treatment
- **Corticosteroids (e.g., prednisolone in doses of 1 mg/kg daily):** These are effective in about 80% of patients. Initially,

Table 12.22: Causes and treatment of methemoglobinemia.

Causes of methemoglobinemia:	
Hereditary: Deficiency of methemoglobin reductase	*Acquired*: drugs and toxins (nitrites, nitrates, primaquine, dapsone, phenacetin, phenazopyridine, metoclopramide, and nitroglycerin)
Treatment:	
Methemoglobin reductase deficiency: Oral methylene blue or ascorbic acid **Severe methemoglobinemia:** Intravenous methylene blue	

> **Box 12.1:** Classification of autoimmune hemolytic anemia (AIHA).
>
> **Based on antibody type:**
> *Warm antibody type (IgG antibodies active at 37°C):*
> ❖ Primary (idiopathic)
> ❖ Secondary:
>   □ Autoimmune disorders (systemic lupus erythematosus and others)
>   □ Drugs (e.g., methyldopa, penicillins, and quinidine)
>   □ *Lymphomas*: Hodgkin's lymphoma and chronic lymphatic leukemia
> *Cold agglutinin type (IgM antibodies active at 4–18°C):*
> ❖ Acute:
>   □ Mycoplasma infection
>   □ Infectious mononucleosis
> ❖ Chronic:
>   □ Idiopathic
>   □ Lymphomas
> *Cold hemolysin type (Donath–Landsteiner antibodies):* Rare; seen mainly in children; usually postviral
> **Based on etiology:**
> ❖ Idiopathic (50%)
> ❖ Secondary (50%):
>   □ Drugs, e.g., methyldopa, penicillins, and quinidine
>   □ Mycoplasma infection
>   □ Infectious mononucleosis
>   □ Autoimmune disorders (systemic lupus erythematosus and others)
>   □ Lymphomas

for first 2–4 weeks, prednisolone 60 mg daily, followed by gradual tapering of the dose
- **Avoid blood transfusion** (autoantibodies may cause difficulty in cross-matching)
- **Danazol with prednisone** as first-line therapy
- **Splenectomy**
- **Intravenous immunoglobulin:** Temporary treatment before splenectomy for those refractory to steroids
- **Rituximab:** Monoclonal antibody directed against CD20 antigen expressed on B-lymphocytes.

Anemia of Chronic Disease

Causes

It occurs in a wide variety of chronic diseases.
- **Chronic infections:** Infective endocarditis, tuberculosis, and osteomyelitis
- **Chronic immune disorders:** Crohn's disease, rheumatoid arthritis, and systemic lupus erythematosus
- **Associated with malignant tumors** (e.g., carcinoma of lung and breast)

Investigations

- **Peripheral smear:** Normocytic normochromic red cells
- **Increased storage iron** in the marrow (Prussian blue staining)
- **Raised serum ferritin** because of the inflammatory process
- *Reduced total iron-binding capacity* (TIBC) and *reduced serum iron*
- Reduced transferrin levels and normal serum-soluble transferrin receptor level

Management

Treat the underlying disorder. Recombinant erythropoietin therapy may be tried, if the anemia is not corrected after treatment of the underlying disorder.

Aplastic Anemia

It is characterized by pancytopenia (anemia, neutropenia, and thrombocytopenia) with hypocellular bone marrow (less than 30% cellularity), and no leukemic, or other abnormal cells in the peripheral blood or bone marrow.

Causes of Aplastic Anemia

Causes of aplastic anemia are discussed in **Table 12.23**.

Treatment/Management

- **Removal of the causative factor**/agent wherever possible (refer causes of aplastic anemia)
- **Providing supportive care** while awaiting bone marrow recovery:
  - Prevention and treatment of infections
  - Treatment of hemorrhage
  - Treatment of anemia by red cell transfusion
- **Severe aplastic anemia:**
  - *Stem cell transplantation:* It is treatment of choice for patients under 40 years who have an HLA-identical sibling donor. In patients over the age of 40, there is high risk of graft-versus-host disease.
  - *Immunosuppressive therapy:* Patients without HLA-matched siblings and >40 years of age—
    - Antilymphocyte globulin (ALG) and cyclosporine combination produces hematological response rate of 60–80% (destroy activated suppressor cells)
    - Androgens (e.g., oxymetholone) are sometimes useful in patients not responding to immunosuppression and those with moderately severe aplastic anemia.

Table 12.23: Causes of aplastic anemia.

Inherited:
• Fanconi anemia
• Diamond–Blackfan anemia
• Telomerase defects
Acquired
Idiopathic:
• Acquired defects in stem cell
• Immune mediated
Secondary:

• **Chemical agents:** ▪ *Dose related:* Cytotoxic drugs (alkylating agents, antimetabolites), Benzene, inorganic arsenicals, and chloramphenicol ▪ *Idiosyncratic:* Chloramphenicol, phenylbutazone, penicillamine, carbamazepine, gold salts, organic arsenicals, and methylphenylethylhydantoin	• **Physical agents:** Whole-body irradiation • **Viral infections:** ▪ Hepatitis (unknown type) ▪ Epstein–Barr virus infections ▪ Cytomegalovirus infections ▪ Herpes zoster (varicella zoster) ▪ HIV

- *Steroids* have little role in severe aplastic anemia and are useful for serum sickness induced by ALG. Steroids are used in children with congenital pure red cell aplasia (Diamond–Blackfan syndrome) and in some adults with pure red cell aplasia associated with a thymoma.

PLATELET DISORDERS

Patterns of bleeding in platelet and coagulation disorders are described in **Table 12.24**.

Laboratory Investigations

The different laboratory investigations for platelet disorders are described in **Table 12.25**.

Thrombocytopenia

Table 12.26 describes the thrombocytopenia.

General Clinical Manifestations (Table 12.27)
- **Skin:** Purpura, petechiae, and ecchymoses
- **Mucous membranes:** Epistaxis, hemorrhagic bullae in oral mucosa, genitourinary, and gastrointestinal (GI) bleeding
- Severe thrombocytopenia produces fundal hemorrhage and intracranial bleeding

Laboratory Investigations
- **Platelet count:** Reduced and manifestations roughly correlate with the platelet count.
- **Hess test (capillary fragility test/tourniquet test) may be positive:**
  - *Principle:* Measures the ability of capillaries to withstand the increased stress.
  - *Procedure:* Sphygmomanometer cuff is tied to the upper arm and the cuff is inflated to 80 mm for 5 minutes.
    - Release the pressure after 5 minutes and the number of petechiae present in a circle of 5-cm diameter on the flexor aspect of forearm (below the bend of the elbow) is noted.
    - *Normal:* 0–5 petechiae

Table 12.24: Distinguishing patterns of bleeding in platelet and coagulation disorders.

Characteristics	Platelet/vascular disorders	Coagulation disorders
Onset	Spontaneous and develops immediately after trauma/surgery	Delayed bleeding after trauma/surgery
Type of lesion	Petechiae and ecchymoses	Hematomas
Sites	Skin and mucous membrane	Deep tissues
Mucous membrane	Common from nose, mouth, gastrointestinal and genitourinary tracts	Uncommon except from gastrointestinal or genitourinary tract
Into the joint	Absent	Common in severe factor deficiencies
Into the muscle	Following trauma	Spontaneous
Local pressure	Effective	Ineffective

Table 12.25: Laboratory investigations for platelet disorders.

Name of the test	Evaluation
Blood count and film	Number, morphology, and blood disorder—leukemia or lymphoma
Platelet count (150–350 × 10^3/mm^3)	Platelets
Bleeding time (<9 minutes)	Platelet function, von Willebrand factor
Prothrombin time (12–14 seconds)	Extrinsic pathway—factors V, VII, and X; factor II, X, and XII; and factor II
Activated partial thromboplastin time (33–45 seconds)	Intrinsic pathway—factors I and II
Thrombin time (3–5 seconds > control)	Common pathway—factors I and II
Clot retraction	Platelets
Fibrinogen concentration	Fibrinogen
Fibrin degradation products (FDPs)	Lysis of fibrin

Table 12.26: Thrombocytopenia.

Increased platelet destruction	Decreased production of platelets

Immune mediated
• Primary: Idiopathic thrombocytopenic purpura—acute and chronic
• Secondary:
  ▪ Autoimmune: Systemic lupus erythematosus
  ▪ Alloimmune: Post-transfusion or during pregnancy
  ▪ Drugs: Quinidine, heparin, and sulfa compounds
  ▪ Infections: HIV, infectious mononucleosis, and CMV
Nonimmune mediated:
• Disseminated intravascular coagulation
• Thrombotic thrombocytopenic purpura
• Hemolytic uremic syndrome
• Mechanical destruction
• Microangiopathic hemolytic anemias
	Generalized diseases of bone marrow
	• Aplastic anemia: Congenital and acquired
	• Marrow infiltration: Leukemia and disseminated cancer
	• Selective impairment of platelet production:
	  ▪ Drugs: Alcohol, thiazides, cytotoxic drugs, and alcohol
	  ▪ Infections: Measles and HIV
	• Ineffective megakaryopoiesis:
	  ▪ Megaloblastic anemia
	  ▪ Myelodysplastic syndromes

Sequestration: Hypersplenism: Portal hypertension, lymphomas, and myeloproliferative disorders	Dilutional

(CMV: cytomegalovirus; HIV: human immunodeficiency virus)

Table 12.27: Clinical features associated with decreased platelet count.

Platelet count/μL	Clinical features
30,000–50,000	Post-traumatic bleeding
<30,000	Spontaneous bleeding
<10,000	Intracranial bleeding

- *Interpretation:* Positive test—more than 10 petechiae and is observed in vascular purpura, defective platelet function, thrombocytopenia, and scurvy
- **Bleeding time (BT):** Prolonged, and it bears a close relationship to platelet count.
- **Bone marrow:**
  - Normal or increased number of megakaryocytes indicates increased platelet destruction, hypersplenism, or ineffective platelet production.
  - Decreased number of megakaryocytes indicates reduced production of platelets

Management
Treatment of underlying cause: Severe, life-threatening bleeding (fundal hemorrhages and intracranial hemorrhage) can be temporarily treated by platelet transfusions.

Qualitative Platelets Defects
These are characterized by prolonged bleeding time and normal platelet count.

These produce defects in the formation of hemostatic plug and thus result in bleeding **(Table 12.28)**.

Immune (Idiopathic) Thrombocytopenic Purpura (Fig. 12.21)
Autoimmune disorder is characterized by increased destruction of platelets by autoantibodies directed against platelet membrane GPIIb/III and GPIb/IX.

Pathogenesis
- Antiplatelet antibodies demonstrated in approximately 80% of patients and are of the IgG type.
- Antibody-bound platelets are removed and prematurely destroyed by the spleen causing thrombocytopenia.

Table 12.28: Classification of platelet function disorders.

Hereditary	Acquired
Disorders of adhesion: Bernard–Soulier syndrome	*Drugs:* Aspirin, non-steroidal anti-inflammatory drugs (NSAID), dipyridamole, and sulfinpyrazone
Disorders of secretion: Storage pool deficiency	*Renal failure* (uremia)
Disorders of aggregation: Glanzmann thrombasthenia	*Hematologic malignancies:* Myeloproliferative and myelodysplastic disorders

- *Spleen:* It is site of destruction of platelets and important site of autoantibody synthesis. Splenectomy shows improvement in about 75–80% of patients.
- Although destruction of sensitized platelets is the major mechanism responsible for thrombocytopenia, the autoantibodies probably also affect production of platelets by megakaryocytes and also impair platelet function.

Clinical Features (Tables 12.29 and 12.30)
- No physical signs other than those due to bleeding and anemia (menorrhagia and epistaxis)
- May be associated with hemolysis (Evan's syndrome)

Investigations and Diagnosis
- **Platelet count:**
  - Thrombocytopenia (below 80×10^9/L)
  - Should be repeated using sodium citrate to exclude pseudothrombocytopenia caused by platelet aggregation and clumping in EDTA tubes
- **Tourniquet test (Hess test):** Positive
- **Bleeding time (BT):** Prolonged
- **Bone marrow:**
  - Moderate increase in number of immature and mature forms of megakaryocytes

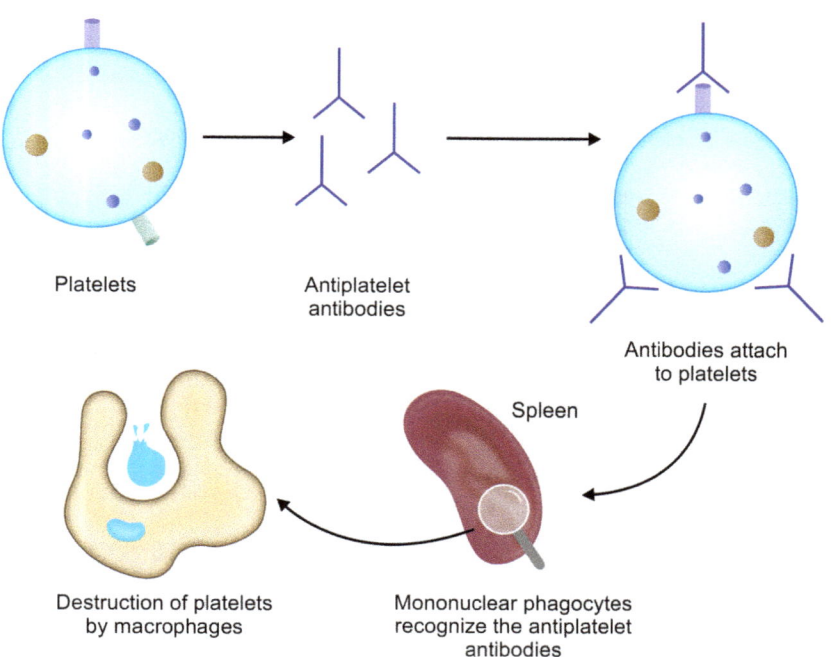

Fig. 12.21: Immune (idiopathic) thrombocytopenic purpura.

Table 12.29: Clinical features.

Primary	Secondary

Most cases are primary
• Subtypes:
  ▪ *Acute*: More common in children
  ▪ *Chronic*: Persistence of thrombocytopenia for >6 months, more common in adults
	Observed in several diseases such as systemic lupus erythematosus, acquired immunodeficiency syndrome (AIDS), and hepatitis C, following viral infections and as a complication of drug therapy

Table 12.30: Differences between acute and chronic immune (idiopathic) thrombocytopenic purpura (ITP).

	Children	Adults
Occurrence:		
Peak age (years)	2–4	15–40
Sex (F:M)	Equal	1.2–1.7
Presentation:		
Onset	Acute (<1 week)	Insidious (>2 months)
Symptoms	Purpura (<10% with severe bleeding)	Purpura (typically bleeding not severe)
Platelet count	Most <20,000/L	Most <20,000/L
Antecedent infection	Usually follows an antecedent upper respiratory viral infection	Usually no preceding history of viral infection
Course:		
Spontaneous remission	83%	2%
Chronic disease	24%	43%
Response to splenectomy	71%	66%
Eventual complete recovery	89%	64%
Morbidity and mortality:		
Cerebral hemorrhage	<1%	3%
Hemorrhagic death	<1%	4%
Mortality of chronic refractory disease	2%	5%

- Usually not performed in acute ITP, unless treatment is necessary on clinical grounds
- Important in chronic ITP to rule out thrombocytopenia resulting from bone marrow failure
- Decrease in number of megakaryocytes argues against the diagnosis of immune (idiopathic) thrombocytopenic purpura (ITP).

☐ **Antiplatelet antibodies:** Not widely available but may be demonstrated in blood. Negative test does not exclude ITP.

Treatment (Box 12.2)

☐ **Children:** Mild acute ITP usually does not require treatment.
☐ **Adults:** Platelet counts >30 × 10⁹/L usually do not require treatment. Even lower platelet counts may require treatment, if they have spontaneous bruising or bleeding.

Box 12.2: Treatment of immune (idiopathic) thrombocytopenic purpura (ITP).

- High-dose corticosteroids
- Splenectomy
- Intravenous immunoglobulin (i.e., IgG)
- Rho (D) immunoglobulin (anti-D)
- *Immunosuppressive therapy:* Vinca alkaloids (vincristine and vinblastine), azathioprine, cyclophosphamide, cyclosporine combination chemotherapy, and mycophenolate mofetil
- *Plasmapheresis:* Emergency measure to remove antibodies from the plasma
- *TPO mimetic drugs:* Eltrombopag or romiplostim
- *Specific immunomodulatory monoclonal antibodies:* Rituximab

Other therapies:
- *Danazol:* Androgen with low virilizing activity has been tried in ITP
- *Dapsone*

Platelet transfusions: Reserved for intracranial or extreme hemorrhages, where emergency splenectomy may be justified

Emergency treatment: It is necessary in case of life-threatening bleeding. It consists of intravenous administration of methylprednisolone (30 mg/kg, maximum dose 1 g) over 20 to 30 minutes along with platelet transfusion. This is followed by intravenous immunoglobulin.

Table 12.31: Causes of thrombocytosis.

Primary (autonomous production)	Secondary (reactive thrombocytosis)
Myeloproliferative neoplasms: • Essential thrombocytosis • Polycythemia vera • Chronic myeloid leukemia *Myelodysplastic syndrome*	• Iron deficiency • Malignancy (paraneoplastic feature) • Post-hemorrhage: Acute or chronic • Following splenectomy • Following major surgery • *Inflammatory disorders*: Rheumatoid arthritis and inflammatory bowel disease

☐ **Indications for treatment:**
- Overt hemorrhage (treated with platelet concentrates)
- Platelet counts below 20,000/mm³
- Organ- or life-threatening bleeding irrespective of the circulating platelet count

Thrombocytosis (Table 12.31)

Platelet count more than 450,000/mm³ is known as thrombocytosis.

CLOTTING DISORDERS

Hemophilia A (Factor VIII Deficiency)

It is a most common hereditary X-linked recessive disease with a reduction in the amount or activity of factor VIII (antihemophilic factor). About 30% have no family history and may be due to acquired mutations.

Antihemophilic factor is secreted by the liver and has a half-life of 12 hours. In the blood, it is carried bound to the von Willebrand factor (vWF).

Factor VIII serves as a cofactor for factor IX in the activation of factor X in the coagulation cascade. Reduced amount or activity of factor VIII is associated with life-threatening bleeding.

Bleeding is due to both inadequate coagulation and inappropriate clot removal (fibrinolysis).

Inheritance

- X-linked recessive disorder. Males are affected and females are carriers. Incidence: 1 in 10,000 males
- Females can be hemophilic, if:
- She is born to an affected father and a carrier mother (25% risk)
- Inactivation of the X chromosome such as Turner's syndrome (45 × O)
- Inactivation of normal X-chromosome due to unfavorable lyonization (rare)
- A hemophiliac male's daughters will be carriers, while sons will be normal.
- A hemophilia female carrier can have—a hemophiliac boy, a carrier girl, and two normal children.
- Gene can be traced within families by using gene probes.
- Degree of deficiency of factor VIII and severity of bleeding tend to be similar in all the affected members of the same family.

Molecular genetics have detected a variety of defects in hemophilia. The mutations include deletions, inversions, point mutations, and insertions.

Normal level of factor VIII in the blood is 0.50–1.50 IU/mL. Hemophilia A may be classified based on the factor VIII activity in blood (**Table 12.32**).

Clinical Features

Clinical severity depends on the level of factor VIII activity and is presented in the **Table 12.33**:
- **Excessive bleeding:** Hemophilia A is characterized by excessive bleeding but is unusual until the child is about 6-month old.
- **Post-traumatic bleeding:** Bleeding following trauma is characteristically "delayed"
- **Severity of bleeding:** Range from mild to severe
- Petechiae observed in platelet and vascular disorders are not seen in hemophilia

Laboratory Investigations

- **Bleeding time**—normal
- **Clotting time**—prolonged

Table 12.32: Factor VIII level and clinical severity in hemophilia A.

Classification	Factor VIII Level	Clinical features
Severe	≤1% of normal (≤0.01 U/mL)	• Spontaneous hemorrhage from early infancy • Frequent spontaneous hemarthroses and hemorrhages, requiring factor replacement
Moderate	1–5% of normal (0.01–0.05 U/mL)	• Hemorrhage secondary to trauma or surgery • Occasional spontaneous hemarthroses
Mild	6–30% of normal (0.06–0.3U/mL)	• Hemorrhage secondary to trauma or surgery • Rare spontaneous hemorrhage

- **Platelet count**—normal
- **Prothrombin time**—normal
- **Activated partial thromboplastin time (aPTT)**—increased (normal 35–45 seconds) to 50 seconds—few minutes
- **Factor VIII assay**—confirmation of diagnosis, to assess factor VIII levels and severity of disease

Management

- **Replacement therapy:**
  - Factor VIII concentrate is available as plasma-derived and recombinant products
  - *Indications of replacement therapy:*
    - Early treatment of spontaneous bleeding
    - Severe or prolonged wound and tissue bleeding
    - Control of bleeding during and after surgery and trauma
    - *Prophylaxis*: In all patients with severe hemophilia so as to prevent recurrent bleeding into joints and subsequent joint damage (arthropathy)
- **Nontransfusion therapy in hemophilia:**
  - *DDAVP (1-amino-8-D-arginine vasopressin)*
  - *Antifibrinolytic drugs*

Complications: About 15% of the patients receiving factor VIII therapy develop inhibitory antibodies that bind and inhibit factor VIII.

- **Treatment for patients with factor VIII inhibitors:** Immune tolerance induction (ITI) is the most effective strategy of eradication of inhibitor with steroids or other immunosuppressants.

Table 12.33: Clinical features of hemophilia A (factor VIII deficiency).

Hemarthroses	Bleeding into muscles	Others
Frequent and spontaneous hemorrhage into large joints—knee, elbow, ankle, wrist, and hip **Spontaneous or follows minor trauma** • *Acute stage*: Affected joint is swollen, hot, and tender; movements severely restricted—gradually subside over a period of days • *Consequences*: Recurrent bleeding into joints will lead to crippling deformities and disuse atrophy of muscles around the joint	*Commonly*—calf and psoas muscles **Consequences:** • *Psoas hematomas*: Femoral nerve compression resulting in sensory disturbances over thigh and weakness of quadriceps • *Calf hematomas*: Contraction and shortening of the Achilles tendon	• Easy bruising • Massive bleeding following trauma or procedures (dental extraction) • Cerebral hemorrhage • Hematuria and ureteric colic due to passage of blood clots

- Antibodies to antihemophilic globulin (AHG) may occur de novo in nonhemophiliacs as part of an immunological disorder such as systemic lupus erythematosus.

Hemophilia B (Christmas Disease)

It is a deficiency of factor IX.
- **Mode of inheritance:** X-linked disorder
- **Clinical features:** Similar to hemophilia A. Patients with severe disease present with muscle hematomas and hemarthroses, which progresses to crippling joint deformities.
- **Diagnosis:** Factor IX assay shows deficiency of factor.
- **Management:** Similar to hemophilia A—
  - *Replacement therapy:*
    - Fresh frozen plasma to treat mild-to-moderate bleeding
    - Recombinant factor IX—to treat moderate-to-severe bleeding
  - *Gene therapy:* It may be effective in managing severe disease.
  - Desmopressin is ineffective.

Von Willebrand Disease

It is characterized by defective platelet function and factor VIII deficiency, due to a deficiency or dysfunction von Willebrand factor (vWF).

Major categories: *vWF* gene—chromosome 12 and numerous mutations of the gene produce vWD.
- **Quantitative deficiency in vWF:**
  - *Type 1*: Autosomal dominant, relatively mild disorder
  - *Type 3*: Autosomal recessive disorder and is a severe disorder
- **Qualitative defects (dysfunction) in vWF:** Type 2 accounts for 25% of all cases and is usually an autosomal dominant disorder. There are several subtypes—
  - Type 2a is most common characterized by defective assembly of multimers.
  - Type 2b is caused by synthesis of an abnormal vWF with increased affinity for platelets, which results in thrombocytopenia.

Von Willebrand factor (vWF): Protein synthesized by endothelial cells and megakaryocytes—
- **Main functions (Fig. 12.22):**
  - Von Willebrand factor acts as a *carrier protein*, which binds to *factor VIII* and forms plasma factor VIII–vWF complex. vWF protects factor VIII and is important for its stability. It has no role in the coagulation cascade, but deficiency of vWF causes a secondary reduction of factor VIII causing coagulation defect.
  - vWF is the most important co-factor for adhesion of platelets to the exposed subendothelial collagen matrix by GpIb/IX. Hence, the deficiency of vWF results in a defect of platelet function.

Clinical Features
- Von Willebrand disease is variable and ranges from mild asymptomatic conditions to a severe hemorrhagic disorder.

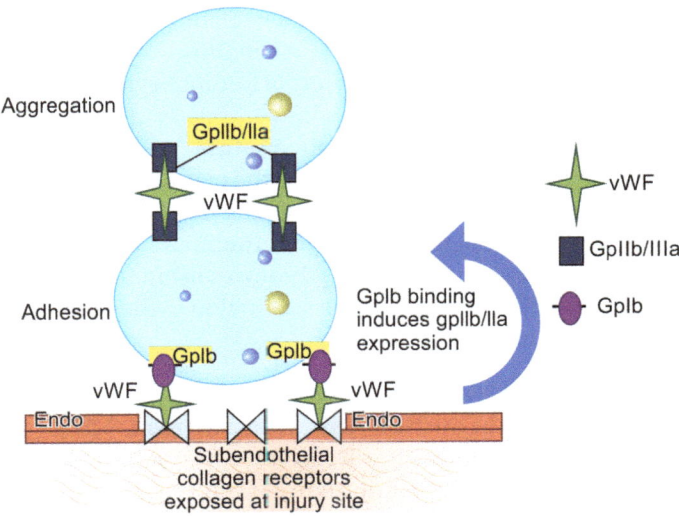

Fig. 12.22: Functions of von Willebrand factor (vWF).

- The symptoms are spontaneous bleeding from mucous membranes (e.g., epistaxis), excessive bleeding from wounds, or menorrhagia. In severe cases, manifestations may be similar to hemophilia A.

Laboratory Findings
- *Platelet count is normal*
- **Bleeding time** is *prolonged* despite a normal platelet count because of defect in platelet function
- **Tourniquet test (Hess test):** *Positive* due to defect in platelet adhesion
- **APTT:** *Prolonged* because vWF stabilizes factor VIII by binding to it. A deficiency of vWF gives rise to a secondary decrease in factor VIII levels.
- **vWF assay:** Plasma level of active vWF is *decreased*.

Management
- **Mild bleeding:** Desmopressin
- **Severe bleeding:** Intravenous cryoprecipitate or plasma-derived concentrates containing vWF and factor VIII. Recombinant activated factor VII (rFVIIa) has also been successfully used in vWD patients with severe hemorrhage refractory to vWF replacement therapy

Vitamin K Deficiency

It clinically manifests as ecchymoses, bleeding from injection sites, bruises, gum bleeding, hematemesis, melena, or hematuria

Prothrombin time and activated partial thromboplastin time are prolonged.

Administration of vitamin K in a dose of 5–10 mg stops bleeding within 1–2 days.

If blood loss is severe or response to vitamin K is inadequate, transfusion of fresh blood or fresh frozen plasma is indicated.

THROMBOSIS

Microangiopathic Hemolytic States

This syndrome consists of two closely related entities— *thrombotic thrombocytopenic purpura (TTP) and hemolytic uremic syndrome (HUS)*. The underlying basic defects are:

- Formation of microthrombi, initiated and perpetuated by platelet adhesion and aggregation in the microcirculation of vital organs and consequently of thrombocytopenia and organ dysfunction
- Microangiopathic hemolytic anemia, resulting from damage to erythrocytes traversing the platelet thrombi and adhesion to endothelium of the affected vessels. Hallmark of microangiopathic hemolytic anemia is presence of fragmented and damaged erythrocytes in circulation.
- Unlike in DIC, there is no gross alteration in the process of coagulation and fibrinolysis.

Thrombotic Thrombocytopenia Purpura

Thrombotic thrombocytopenia purpura (TTP) is severe microangiopathic hemolytic anemia (MAHA), characterized by systemic platelet aggregation, organ ischemia, profound thrombocytopenia (with increased marrow megakaryocytes), fragmentation of erythrocytes, fever, and renal failure.

Etiology and pathogenesis (Fig. 12.23):

- Normally, endothelial cells and megakaryocytes secrete normal vWF multimers into the plasma. These multimers spontaneously develop into unusually large multimers, which are effective in platelet adhesion.
- **Plasma protease enzyme:** ADAMTS-13 (vWF metalloprotease) regulates activity of vWF by cleaving hemostatically active unusually large multimers into normal multimers. ADAMTS-13 regulates size of vWF multimers and prevents platelet adhesion.
- **TTP:** Inherited or acquired deficiency of ADAMTS-13. Deficiency leads to accumulation of unusually large multimers of vWF in plasma.
- These large multimers promote platelet adhesion or promote intravascular platelet aggregation and cause spontaneous activation of the coagulation cascade.
- This results in hyaline thrombi throughout the microcirculation, leading to tissue ischemia and infarction that are characteristic of TTP.
- **Secondary causes:** These include pregnancy, oral contraceptives, SLE, infection, and drugs (ticlopidine and clopidogrel). They may or may not have associated antibodies to ADAMTS-13.

Clinical features:

The classic five symptoms of TTP are—(1) microangiopathic hemolytic anemia (MAHA) with schistocytosis (at least 3 cells per 100), (2) severe thrombocytopenia, (3) transient neurologic symptoms secondary to central nervous system ischemia, (4) fever, and (5) renal abnormalities including hematuria and/or proteinuria.

Laboratory findings:

- **Platelet count:** Markedly reduced often below 20,000/μL (thrombocytopenia)
- Peripheral blood smear shows fragmented red cells (called *schistocytes*) and numerous reticulocytes.
- **Prothrombin time (PT), partial thromboplastin time (PTT), and fibrinogen concentration:** Normal, because the coagulation system is not activated
- **Urine**—shows moderate proteinuria and both gross and microscopic hematuria.
- **Serum LDH**—raised due to release from ischemic tissues.
- **ADAMTS-13 activity**—reduced below 5–10% of normal.

Diagnosis: Schistocytes and elevated serum LDH (out of proportion to the degree of hemolysis) suggest the diagnosis of TTP.

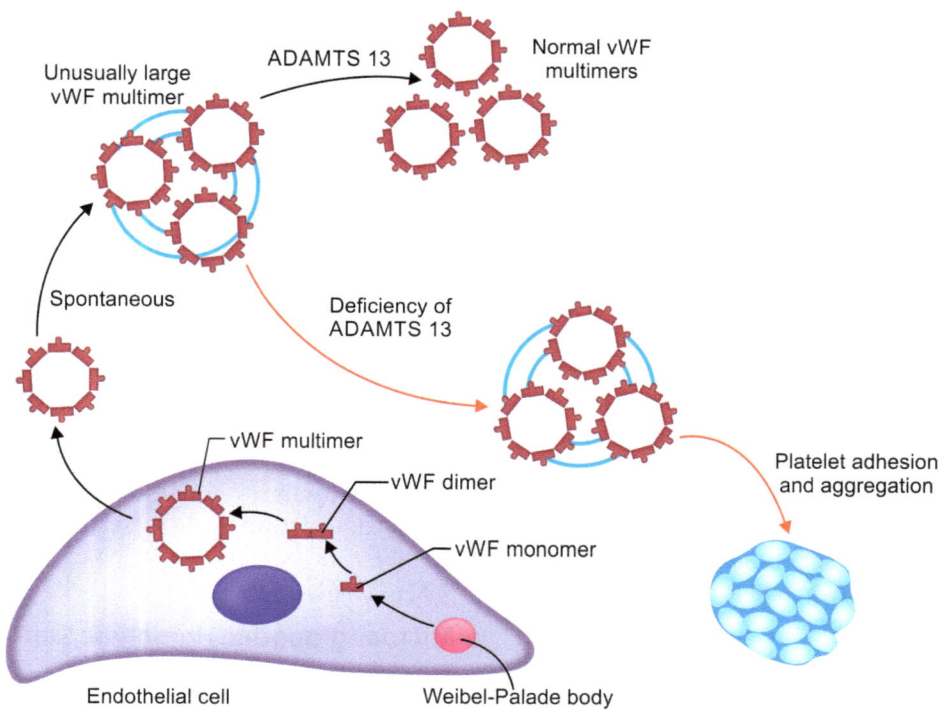

Fig. 12.23: Pathogenesis of thrombotic thrombocytopenia purpura (TTP).

Treatment:
- **Plasma exchange**
- **Corticosteroids:** Pulsed intravenous methylprednisolone is given acutely and is generally added to plasma exchange to suppress formation of antibody.
- **Rituximab:** It is a monoclonal antibody against CD20, suppresses antibody-producing cells. It is used in those patients who are refractory to plasma exchange and corticosteroids.
- **Splenectomy:** It is performed in resistant cases, which removes antibody-producing cells.
- **Platelet concentrates are contraindicated**.

Prognosis: Untreated cases have a mortality of up to 90% but with modern management, it has been reduced to about 10%.

Hemolytic–Uremic Syndrome

Hemolytic–uremic syndrome (HUS) is distinguished from TTP by the absence of fever and neurologic symptoms, the prominence of acute renal failure (uremia), frequent affection of children, and different pathogenesis.

Etiology and pathogenesis (Fig. 12.24):
- Develops following damage to the endothelium by toxins, drugs, or radiation
- A main cause of HUS in children and elderly is infectious gastroenteritis caused by *Escherichia coli* strain 0157:H7. *E. coli* produces a Shiga-like toxin, which is absorbed from the inflamed gastrointestinal mucosa, which enters circulation and damages endothelial cells of microvasculature, mainly in the renal glomerular capillaries and initiates platelet activation and thrombi formation.
- Red cells get trapped in the formed thrombi and undergo fragmentation resulting in schistocytes
- Splenic trapping of the fragmented red cells causes extravascular hemolysis.

Clinical features:
- **Age:** It is most common in children between 1 and 5 years of age few days after a bloody diarrhea. It also develops in adults following certain drugs and radiation therapy that damage endothelial cells.
- **Classical presentation:** It is triad of microangiopathic hemolytic anemia, thrombocytopenia, and renal failure (oliguria). Hematuria and hypertension are also common. Despite thrombocytopenia, bleeding manifestations are rare.
- **Complications:** Fluid overload may result in pulmonary edema and hypertensive encephalopathy.

Investigations:
- **Hemoglobin levels:** Decreased (anemia)
- **Platelet count:** Markedly reduced often below 20,000/μL (thrombocytopenia)

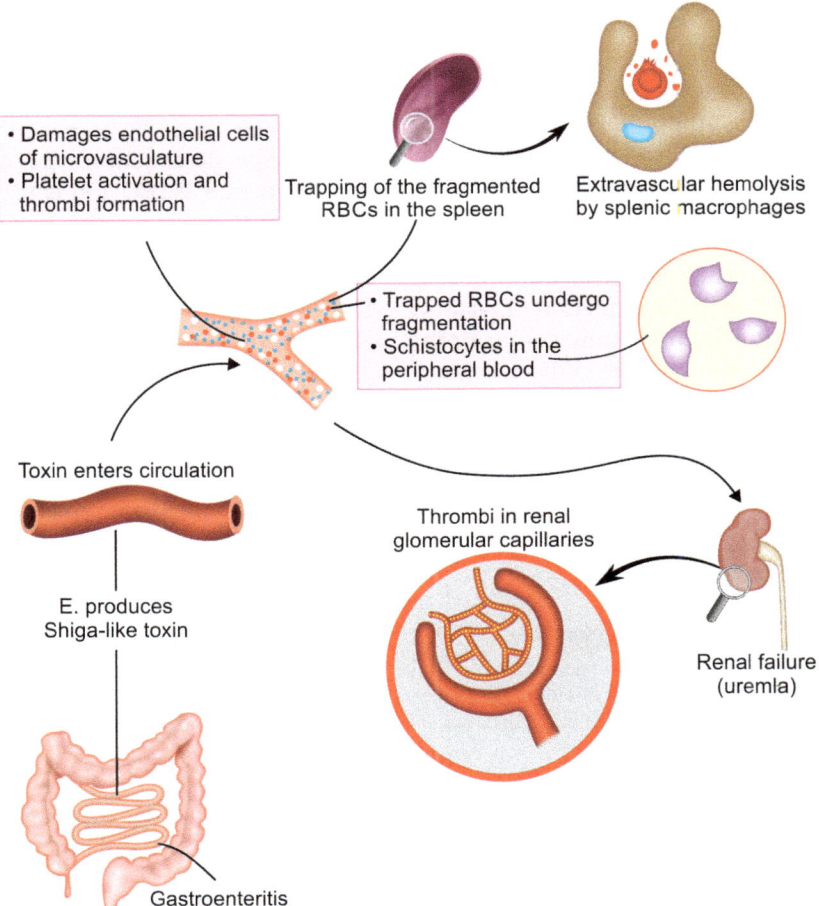

Fig. 12.24: Pathogenesis of hemolytic–uremic syndrome.

- **Peripheral blood smear:** Fragmented red cells (schistocytes) and numerous reticulocytes
- **LDH:** Elevated
- **Blood urea and creatinine:** Elevated
- **Urine:** May show proteinuria and red blood cells
- **PT and aPTT:** Normal
- **Stool:** Culture for enterohemorrhagic *E. coli*-positive; Shiga toxin-positive

Treatment:
- **Supportive care**—for the renal and hematological complications
- **Antibiotics**—if shigellosis is suspected/detected
- **Experimental**—eculizumab and monoclonal antibody to C5

Prognosis: With appropriate supportive care, they usually recover completely, but in more severe cases, renal damage may result in death.

Disseminated Intravascular Coagulation

Disseminated intravascular coagulation (DIC) is a widespread acute or chronic thrombohemorrhagic disorder in which a *combination of thrombosis and hemorrhage* develops as a secondary complication of wide variety of disorders **(Table 12.34)**.

Pathogenesis
Pathogenesis of DIC is shown in **Figure 12.25**.

Clinical Features
- Disseminated intravascular coagulation is serious, often fatal, and important clinical condition, which needs an immediate diagnosis and management. The symptoms of DIC depend on the nature, intensity, and duration of the underlying disorder.
- Signs and symptoms are related to the tissue hypoxia and infarction caused by the microvascular thrombosis; or with bleeding diathesis due to the depletion of factors and the activation of fibrinolytic mechanisms; or both **(Table 12.35)**. *Bleeding* is most common clinical feature

Table 12.34: Major disorders associated with disseminated intravascular coagulation.

Infections:	Massive tissue injury:
• Gram-negative bacterial sepsis • Meningococcemia and other bacteria • Fungi, viruses, Rocky Mountain spotted fever, and malaria	• Trauma and burns • Fat embolism • Surgery
Neoplasms:	**Vascular disorders:**
• Carcinomas of pancreas, prostate, lung, and stomach • Acute promyelocytic leukemia	Aortic aneurysm, giant hemangioma, and vasculitis
Obstetric complications:	**Miscellaneous:**
• Retained dead fetus • Septic abortion • Abruptio placentae • Amniotic fluid embolism • Toxemia and preeclampsia	• Snakebite • Liver disease • Acute intravascular hemolysis • Shock and heat stroke • Hypersensitivity

in acute *DIC*—ecchymoses, petechiae, or bleeding from mucous membranes or at the sites of venipuncture.
- **Microvascular thrombi**—ischemic necrosis of the organ with resultant dysfunction of the involved organ and occur most often with chronic underlying diseases. Organ dysfunction may manifest as hepatic, renal, cardiac or respiratory failure, or neurological disturbances. It may also result in gangrene of extremities and hemorrhagic necrosis of the skin.
- **Waterhouse–Friderichsen syndrome:** Occult thrombosis of adrenal vein thrombosis resulting in adrenal hemorrhage
- **Trousseau sign:** Migratory venous thrombosis in cancers
- **Multiorgan dysfunction syndrome (MODS):** It is frequent consequence of DIC and is usually due to bleeding into organs or thrombotic alteration in various organs (hepatic, cardiac, central nervous, renal, and pulmonary systems).

Laboratory Findings (Investigations) in DIC (Table 12.36)
- **Erythrocyte sedimentation rate (ESR):** Low
- **Peripheral smear:** Presence of schistocytes

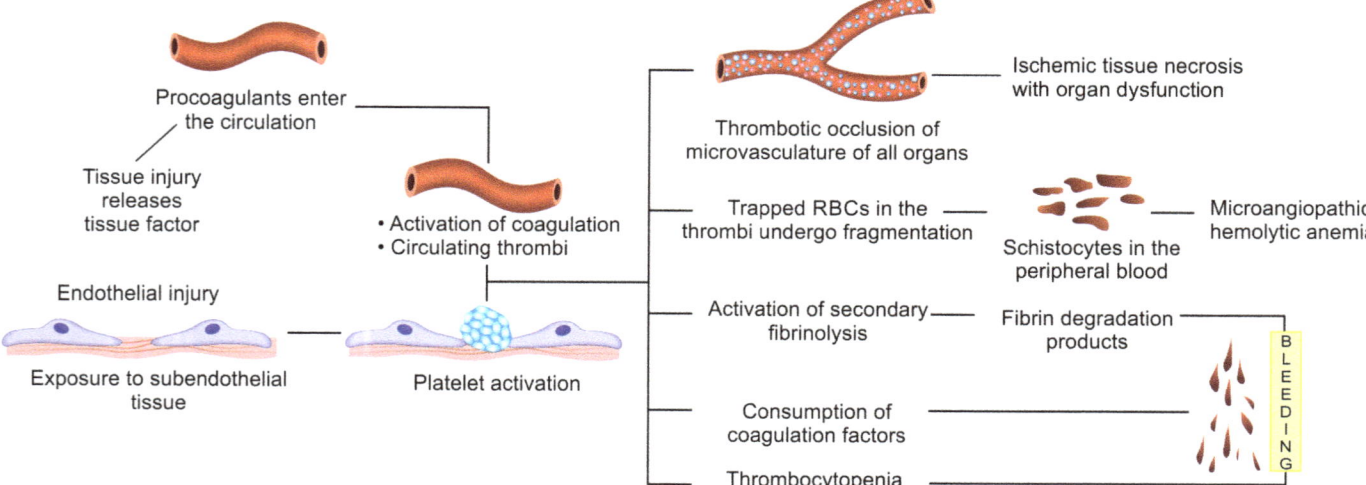

Fig. 12.25: Pathogenesis of disseminated intravascular coagulation (DIC).

Table 12.35: Effects and signs of disseminated intravascular coagulation (DIC).

Organ/site	Due to thrombi in microvasculature	Due to hemorrhagic diathesis
Central nervous system	Multifocal, delirium, and coma	Intracerebral bleeding
Renal system	Cortical necrosis—oliguria and azotemia	Hematuria
Skin	Focal ischemic necrosis and gangrene	Petechiae, ecchymoses, and bleeding at the sites of venipuncture
Gastrointestinal tract	Acute ulceration	Massive bleeding
Respiratory tract	Acute respiratory distress syndrome	
Mucous membranes		Epistaxis and gingival bleeding
Peripheral circulation	Fragmentation of trapped RBCs—microangiopathic hemolytic anemia	

Table 12.36: Routine laboratory value abnormalities in disseminated intravascular coagulation (DIC).

Test	Abnormality
Platelet count	Decreased
Prothrombin time	Prolonged
aPTT	Prolonged
Fibrin degradation products	Elevated
Protease inhibitors (e.g., protein C, AT, and protein S)	Decreased

(aPTT: activated partial thromboplastin time)

- **Screening assays**
- **Platelet count**—decreased because of utilization of platelets in microthrombi
- **Prothrombin time—increased**
- **aPTT—increased** because of consumption and inhibition of the function of clotting factors
- **Thrombin time (TT)**—increased because of decreased fibrinogen
- **Plasma fibrinogen**—decreased
- Presence of schistocytes (fragmented RBCs) in the peripheral smear
- **Confirmatory tests:**
  - *FDP (fibrin degradation/split products):* Secondary fibrinolysis results in generation of FDPs, which can be measured by latex agglutination.
  - *D-dimer test:* D-dimer is formed during fibrinolysis as a result of degradation of cross-linked fibrin by plasmin. D-dimmer levels are elevated and are specific for diagnosing DIC.

Management

- Control or elimination of the underlying cause, e.g., removal of a dead fetus, placenta, etc.
- Correction of precipitating factors, e.g., acidosis, dehydration, and hypoxia
- **Management of hemorrhagic symptoms:** It is necessary to maintain blood volume and tissue perfusion. Hemorrhagic symptoms are managed by transfusions of platelet concentrates, fresh frozen plasma (FFP), cryoprecipitate, and red cell concentrates.
  - *Platelet concentrates:* 1–2 units/10 kg
  - *Fresh frozen plasma:* 15–20 mL/kg
  - *Cryoprecipitate:* 1 unit/10 kg
- Replacement of coagulation or fibrinolysis inhibitors
- Drugs to control coagulation such as heparin or antifibrinolytic drugs have been tried in DIC.
  - *Heparin:* Low doses of continuous infusion heparin (5–10 U/kg per h) are often used in patients with thrombotic manifestations. It should be given after the correction of bleeding. Major indications for heparin therapy are:
    - Purpura fulminans during the surgical resection of giant hemangiomas and during removal of a dead fetus
    - Acute promyelocytic leukemia
  - Antifibrinolytic drugs, e.g., epsilon-aminocaproic acid (EACA) or tranexamic acid, prevent fibrin degradation by plasmin and may reduce bleeding episodes. However, they increase the risk of thrombosis and concomitant use of heparin is indicated.

LEUKEMIA

Classification

Traditional classification: Microscopic appearance of the cell and the speed of evolution **(Table 12.37)**.

Revised French–American–British (FAB) classification of acute and chronic leukemias (Tables 12.38 and 12.39):
- According to FAB, the marrow should show a blast count of 30% or more.

Table 12.37: Classification of leukemia.

Acute	Chronic
• Acute myeloblastic/myelocytic leukemia (AML)	• Chronic myeloid leukemia (CML)
• Acute lymphoblastic/lymphocytic leukemia (ALL)	• Chronic lymphocytic leukemia (CLL)

Table 12.38: Revised French–American–British (FAB) classification of acute myeloid leukemia (AML).

Type of AML	Type of ALL
M0: Minimally differentiated AML	L1
M1: AML without differentiation	L2
M2: AML with maturation	L3
M3: Acute promyelocytic leukemia	
M4: Acute myelomonocytic leukemia	
M5: Acute monocytic leukemia	
M6: Acute erythroleukemia (DiGugliemo's disease)	
M7: Acute megakaryocytic leukemia	

(ALL: acute lymphocytic leukemia)

Table 12.39: Chronic lymphocytic and myelocytic leukemia.

Chronic lymphocytic	Chronic myelocytic (myeloid)
• **B-cell CLL:** Common • T-cell CLL (rare), e.g., cell granular lymphocytic leukemia • Hairy cell leukemia • B-cell prolymphocytic leukemia (PLL)	• Ph^x positive • Ph^x negative, BCR^{xx} positive • Ph^x negative, BCR^{xx} negative • Eosinophilic leukemia

(Ph^x: Philadelphia chromosome; BCR^{xx}: breakpoint cluster)

☐ It includes parameters that affect namely—morphology, cytochemistry, immunophenotyping, cytogenetics, and molecular genetics.

World Health Organization (WHO) classification (2001) of acute myeloid and lymphoid leukemia incorporates parameters namely morphology, cytochemistry, cytogenetic, molecular genetics (which are related to prognosis), and clinical features **(Table 12.40)**. The number of blasts necessary for the diagnosis is more than 20% in bone marrow when compared to 30% in FAB classification.

Etiology of Leukemia

Risk Factors

In the majority of acute leukemia, the cause is not known. Numerous risk factors may cause mutations in the genes involved in regulating cell proliferation and differentiation. These genes include oncogenes and tumor suppressor genes. Sophisticated molecular techniques such as fluorescent in situ hybridization (FISH) and gene array technology have led to the understanding of leukemia at molecular level.

Environmental Factors

☐ **Ionizing radiation:** Ionizing radiation and X-rays are associated with increased risk of leukemia. The evidence for this association are:
  • *Atomic bombing:* Survivors of atomic bomb explosions in Hiroshima and Nagasaki, who had high incidence of AML and CML (chronic myeloid leukemia)
  • *Therapeutic radiation:* Increased risk of AML (secondary leukemia) in patients with malignancies/neoplasms treated by radiation
  • *X-ray fetus during pregnancy*

☐ **Drugs:** Drugs can cause secondary hematopoietic neoplasms.
  • Leukemia develops in patients who have been administered alkylating agents for neoplasms such as Hodgkin lymphoma. The various drugs include nitrogen mustard, chlorambucil, etc.
  • AML in myeloma patients treated with melphalan
  • Leukemia follows chemotherapy of lung and ovarian cancer. Some anticancer drugs induce myelodysplastic changes with certain chromosomal abnormalities and subsequently develop AML.

☐ **Chemicals:**
  • Benzene is used in paint industry, plastic glues, etc. It causes chromosomal abnormalities resulting in higher incidence of acute leukemia, myelodysplastic syndrome, and aplastic anemia.

☐ **Viruses:** Leukemia are often associated with human T-cell lymphotropic virus type 1 (HTLV-1)

☐ **Immunological:** Immune deficiency states

Genetic Disorders

A few genetic disorders may be associated with acute leukemia, e.g., Down's syndrome (ALL or AML), Fanconi anemia (AML), ataxia telangiectasia (ALL and NHL), and Klinefelter syndrome

Acquired Disorders

☐ Acquired stem cell disorders, such as PNH and aplastic anemia may transform into acute leukemia.
☐ **Myelodysplastic syndromes (MDS):** AML may develop de novo or secondary to MDS.

Acute Leukemia

Leukemia is defined as a group of malignant stem cell neoplasms characterized by failure of cell maturation,

Table 12.40: World Health Organization (WHO) classification showing major subtypes of AML.

Acute myeloid leukemia (AML):	
I. AML with genetic aberrations: ▪ AML with t (8;21) (q22; q22); *CBFα/ETO* fusion gene ▪ AML with inv (16) (p13; q22); *CBFβ/MYH*11 fusion gene ▪ AML with t (15;17) (q22;11-12); *RARα/PML* fusion gene ▪ AML with t (11q23; v); diverse *MLL* fusion genes ▪ AML with normal cytogenetics and mutated *NPM* **II. AML with MDS-like features:** ▪ With prior MDS ▪ AML with multilineage dysplasia ▪ AML with MDS-like cytogenetic aberrations: 5q-, 7q-, and 20q-	**III. AML—therapy-related** **IV. AML not otherwise specified:** ▪ AML minimally differentiated ▪ AML without maturation ▪ AML with myelocytic maturation ▪ AML with myelomonocytic maturation ▪ AML with monocytic maturation ▪ AML with erythroid maturation ▪ AML with megakaryocytic maturation
Acute lymphoid leukemia: *Precursor T-cell acute lymphoblastic leukemia* *Burkitt-cell leukemia*	**Precursor B-cell acute lymphoblastic leukemia:** • t (9;22) (q34; q11); BCR/ABC fusion gene • t (4;11) (q21; q23); MLL-AF4 fusion gene • t (1;19) (q23; p13.3); E2A/PBX1 fusion gene • t (12;21) (p13; q22); TEL/AML1

(MDS: myelodysplastic syndrome)

proliferating of leukocyte precursors (blast/immature cells), which fill the bone marrow and abnormal numbers and forms of immature white blood cells ultimately spill over into the peripheral blood.

Clinical Features

Though ALL and AML are distinct (immunophenotypically and genotypically), they usually have similar clinical features. Patient usually presents with nonspecific "flu-like" symptoms.

- **Bone marrow failure:** Replacement of normal marrow hematopoietic cells by leukemic blast cells—
  - *Anemia*—causes shortness of breath on effort, excessive tiredness/fatigue, and weakness.
  - *Neutropenia* results in life-threatening infections by bacteria or opportunistic fungi, *Pseudomonas*, and commensals. Fever develops due to septicemia. The infection may develop in the oral cavity, skin, lungs, kidneys, urinary bladder, and colon. The common presentations include respiratory infections (pneumonia), cellulitis, or sepsis.
  - *Thrombocytopenia* presents as bleeding manifestations in the form of petechiae, atraumatic ecchymosis, gum bleeding, epistaxis, urinary tract, and fundal hemorrhages. Intracranial bleeding is a serious and fatal complication, usually associated with headache, fundal hemorrhages, and focal neurological deficits.
  - Marrow expansion and infiltration of the subperiosteum cause bone pain (more common in ALL) and sternal tenderness.
- **Leukostasis:** Stasis of blood flow may develop when the blast count is above 50,000/mm³:
  - Cerebral leukostasis may cause headache, confusion, and visual disturbances.
  - Pulmonary leukostasis can cause dyspnea at rest, tachypnea, chest pain, pulmonary infarction, and acute respiratory distress syndrome.
- **Coagulopathy:** Both disseminated intravascular coagulation (DIC) and primary fibrinolysis may lead to hemorrhagic diathesis. DIC is observed in AML-M_3 (promyelocytic leukemia).
- **Extramedullary leukemic infiltration:**
  - Gingival hypertrophy and infiltration of skin (leukemia cutis)
  - Hepatosplenomegaly
  - Generalized lymphadenopathy
  - Leukemic meningitis is rare. It presents as headache and nausea. As the disease progresses, papilledema, cranial nerve palsies, seizures, and altered consciousness develop. Cerebrospinal fluid (CSF) characteristically shows leukemic blast cells, elevated proteins, and reduced glucose levels.
  - *Chloromas* are localized, solid, soft tissue tumor masses known as myeloblastomas, granulocytic sarcomas, or chloromas.
- **Metabolic abnormalities:** Hyperuricemia, elevated serum liver transaminases, and serum LDH are found in patients with acute leukemia.

Investigations

- **Confirmation of diagnosis:**
  - *Blood count:*
    - Hb—low
    - *Total leukocyte count*: Markedly raised, but usually less than 100×10^9/L (range—1×10^9/L to 500×10^9/L). Leukopenia is common in AML.
    - *Platelet count*: Markedly decreased
  - *Peripheral blood smear:*
    - It shows numerous blast cells and types of blasts can be identified morphologically and confirmed with immunophenotyping.
    - Auer rods are seen as rod-shaped red inclusion in the cytoplasm of myeloblast.
    - Severe normochromic anemia
  - *Bone marrow aspirate*—hypercellular with reduced erythropoiesis and reduced megakaryocytes. Blast cells > 20% (often approaching 100%)) and type of blast are confirmed by immunophenotyping (FISH), cytogenetic, and molecular genetics.
  - *Chest X-ray:* Mediastinal widening is often seen in T lymphoblastic leukemia.
  - *CSF examination*—to rule out occult central nervous system (CNS) involvement
- **For planning therapy:**
  - *Biochemical parameters:*
    - Serum urate
    - Liver function tests
    - Renal function tests
    - Coagulation studies
    - Plasma LDH
  - *Cardiac function:* ECG and direct tests of left ventricular function (echocardiogram or MUGA scan)

Management

At initial presentation, acute leukemia may be:
- Probably curable (childhood acute lymphoblastic leukemia)
- Possibly curable (de novo low-risk AML)
- Probably incurable (AML with adverse cytogenetic features in the elderly, secondary AML, and recurrent acute leukemia)

1. **Palliative therapy**—both chemotherapy and irradiation in addition to blood product support
2. **Curative therapy**—implies that cure is possible and does not mean that cure is guaranteed or even expected. The failure rate may be high.
   - *Active therapy:* The first and major decision to be taken is whether to give specific therapy or supportive therapy.
   - *Supportive care/therapy*—forms the basis of treatment for both curative and palliative therapy:
     - Treatment of anemia with repeated transfusion of packed red cells to avoid symptoms of anemia (hemoglobin >10 g/dL)
     - Prevention or control of bleeding due to thrombocytopenia with platelet transfusions

- *Treatment of infection*:
  - *Prophylactically:* Education about handwashing and isolation facilities. Use of selected antibiotics and antifungal agents
  - *Therapeutically:* Management of fever by identifying the microorganism and giving appropriate antimicrobial treatment in bacterial, fungal, protozoal, and viral infections.
- Barrier nursing
- Continuous monitoring of liver, kidney, and hemostatic functions
- *Maintenance of fluid and electrolyte balance*: In patients receiving chemotherapy, rapid lysis of leukemic cells may produce tumor lysis syndrome characterized by hyperuricemia, hypokalemia, and hyperphosphatemia. It can be prevented by close attention to hydration, urine alkalinization, and prophylactic allopurinol before starting chemotherapy.
- *Treatment of hyperleukocytosis*: Reduction in leukocyte counts can be achieved by using chemotherapy or hydroxyurea, and leukapheresis (removal of circulating cells and reinfusion of leukocyte-poor plasma)
- Psychological support

Bone marrow transplantation has to be considered in following condition:
- Acute myeloblastic leukemia in first remission in patients below 40 years of age
- Acute lymphoblastic leukemia (ALL) in first, second, or subsequent remission

Specific therapy
The specific therapy is intended to return the peripheral blood and bone marrow to normal (complete remission—CR).

Acute Lymphocytic Leukemia (Flowchart 12.1)
Specific therapy involves:
- **Remission induction** with combination chemotherapy:
  - Goal of induction therapy—to induce morphologic remission and to restore normal hematopoiesis in the bone marrow with less than 5% blasts.
  - Remission induction consists of combination chemotherapy including vincristine, prednisolone (dexamethasone), asparaginase (crisantaspase), and usually an anthracycline antibiotic, e.g., doxorubicin. It induces complete morphologic response within 4–6 weeks.
- **Consolidation phase**—includes administration of high-dose systemic therapy and CNS-directed treatment.
  - *Aim*: To eliminate disease in the central nervous system (CNS) and to reduce systemic minimal residual leukemic burden.
  - CNS-directed therapy consists of weekly or biweekly intrathecal therapy along with high-dose systemic therapy with methotrexate and 6-mercaptoputine. Cyclophosphamide and cytarabine (cytosine arabinoside) may also be used in consolidation phase.
- **Re-induction or re-intensification** (similar to induction phase) reduces chances of relapse.
- **Remission maintenance** to prevent relapse and affect cure. It involves administering drugs for 2 years or more and consists of daily 6-mercaptopurine and weekly methotrexate.

Acute Myeloid Leukemia (Flowchart 12.2)
Initial therapeutic goal is to quickly induce complete remission (CR) and further therapy to prolong survival and achieve cure. Curative therapy is given to the majority of adults below the age of 60 years (without any significant comorbidity).

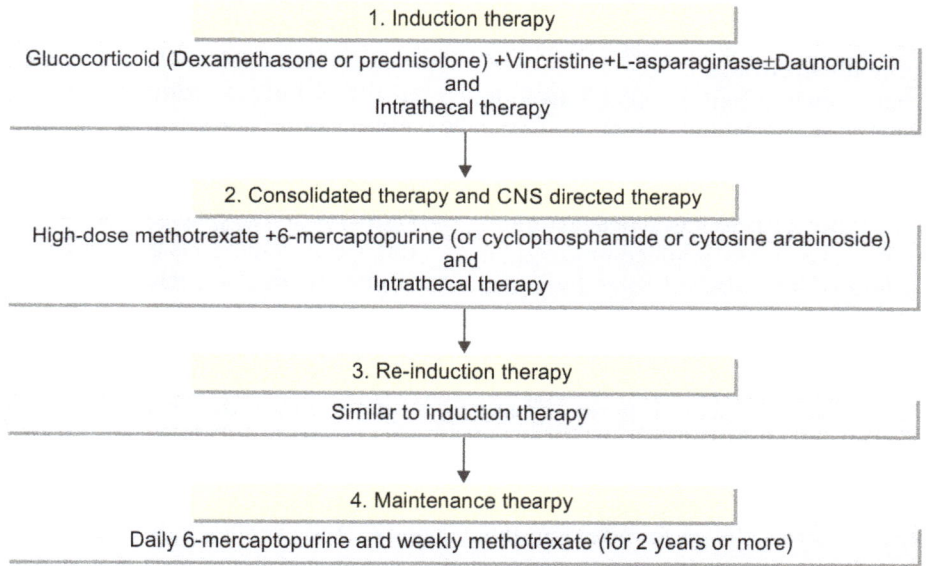

Flowchart 12.1: Treatment strategy of acute lymphocytic leukemia.

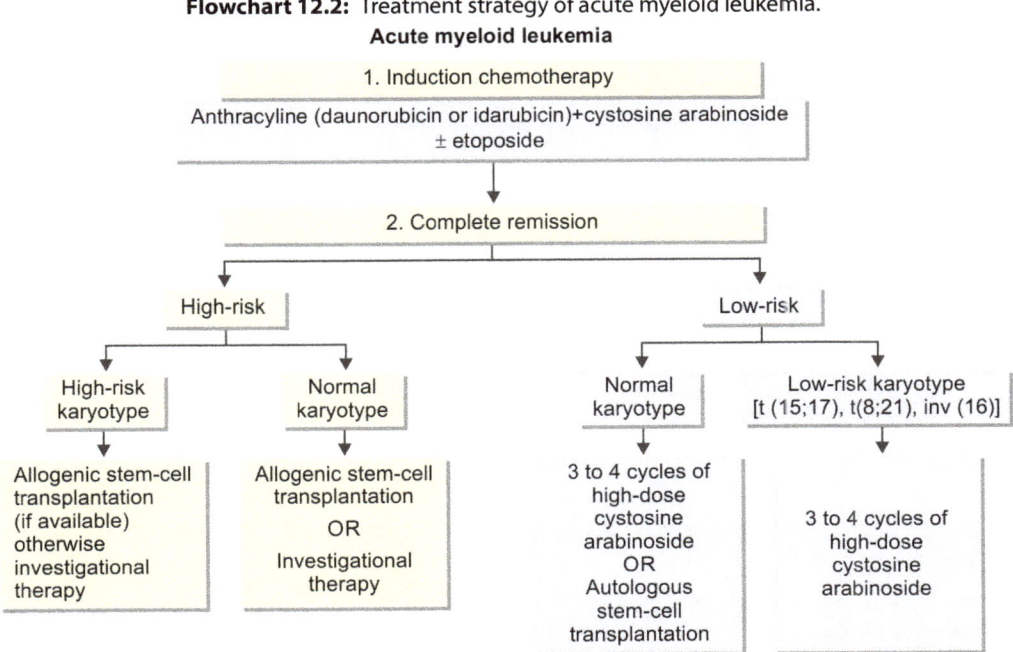

Flowchart 12.2: Treatment strategy of acute myeloid leukemia.

Specific therapy of the newly diagnosed patient with AML is usually divided into two phases—(1) induction and (2) maintenance (postremission) therapy.
- **Induction chemotherapy:** Moderately intensive combination chemotherapy that includes an anthracycline (e.g., daunorubicin or idarubicin) and cytosine arabinoside (cytarabine) ± etoposide. "High-risk" patients (include patients <70 years with high-risk karyotype) may only be treated with curative intent, if an HLA-identified sibling is available for stem cell transplantation.
- **Maintenance or postremission therapy**—for patients achieving remission with induction therapy in young patients (<60 years) consists of 3–4 cycles of high-dose cytosine arabinoside.
  - Low-risk patients in AML, patients with t (15;17) t (8;17) or inv (16) (i.e., low-risk karyotype) do not benefit from allogeneic stem cell transplantation during their first complete remission.
  - Patients with high-risk karyotypes should have stem cell transplantation because they respond poorly to conventional chemotherapy.

Acute Promyelocytic Leukemia (M3)

It is uncommon variant of AML associated with severe coagulation complications.

It has favorable prognosis. It responds well to combination of induction therapy plus all-*trans*-retinoic acid (ATRA). Alternatively, daunorubicin and cytarabine or idarubicin can be given.

Allogeneic transplantation is necessary, if the leukemia is not eliminated at the molecular level or following a second remission after recurrence.

In relapsed cases, arsenic trioxide (induces apoptosis via activation of the caspase cascade) has been also found to be effective.

Alternative chemotherapy: It is used to curb excessive leukocyte proliferation and not for achieving remission.

Hydroxyurea up to 4 g daily and mercaptopurine up to 150 mg daily are used to reduce leukocyte count without inducing bone marrow failure.

Poor prognostic factors in AML and ALL are given in **Table 12.41**.

Clinical features of acute lymphoblastic leukemia and acute myelogenous leukemia are discussed in **Table 12.42**.

Hairy Cell Leukemia

It is uncommon chronic malignant disorder of mature B cells with characteristic fine cytoplasmic projections.

Table 12.41: Poor prognostic factors in acute myeloid leukemia (AML) and acute lymphocytic leukemia (ALL).

Features	AML	ALL
Age	>60 years	<1 year or >9 years
TLC	>1,00,000/mm³	>50,000/mm³
French–American–British (FAB) type	M_0, M_5, M_6, and M_7	L_3 type
Chromosomal abnormality	High-risk karyotype [t (6;9), inv (3)]	Hypodiploidy (<45 chromosomes)
Other features	Secondary cause present Presence of DIC Auer rod absent Fibrosis on bone marrow examination Following myelodysplastic syndrome (MDS) Relapsed disease Secondary leukemia Extramedullary disease	Male gender Pro-B or T-cell ALL Mediastinal mass CNS involvement

(CNS: central nervous system; DIC: disseminated intravascular coagulation)

Table 12.42: Clinical features of acute lymphoblastic leukemia and acute myelogenous leukemia.

	Acute lymphoblastic leukemia	Acute myelogenous leukemia
Clinical features:		
Age	Predominantly children	Predominantly adults
Coagulopathy (DIC)	Absent	Seen in M3
Gingival hypertrophy and dermal infiltrate	Absent	Seen in M4 and M5
Hepatosplenomegaly	In majority (50–75%)	Frequent
Lymphadenopathy	More common	Less common
Leukemic meningitis	More common	Less common
Testicular involvement	In 10–20%	—
Eye involvement	More common	Less common
Investigations:		
Leukemic blasts	Lymphoblasts (10–15 μm) are smaller than myeloblasts, with a thin rim of agranular cytoplasm and round or convoluted nucleus	Myeloblasts (12–20 μm) are larger than lymphoblasts, with discrete nuclear chromatin and multiple nucleoli
Cytoplasmic Auer rods	Absent	Present in 10–20% (diagnostic)
Nuclear enzyme, terminal deoxynucleotidyl transferase (Tdt) in leukemic blasts	In more than 90%	Rarely present
Cytochemical staining:		
Myeloperoxidase	Negative	Positive
Sudan black B	Negative	Positive
Nonspecific esterase	Negative	Positive in M4 and M5
Periodic acid Schiff (PAS)	Positive >50% of cells (block positivity)	Negative

The term *hairy cell leukemia* is derived from the appearance of fine hair like cell membrane projections on the leukemic cells, under the phase-contrast microscope.

It affects middle-aged to elderly men, with a male-to-female ratio of 5:1.

Clinical Features

Hairy cell leukemia is mainly due to leukemic infiltration of bone marrow, liver, and spleen.
- **Massive splenomegaly** is common finding, hepatomegaly is less common, and lymphadenopathy is rare.
- **Pancytopenia**—marrow failure and splenic sequestration, and is found in more than 50% of cases.
- **Infections:** About one-third of patients present with infections especially with atypical mycobacteria, which may be due to monocytopenia. Infections are the most common cause of death.
- **Risk of secondary malignancies:** Hodgkin's lymphoma, non-Hodgkin's lymphoma, and thyroid cancer
- **Chemotherapy:** The purine analogs 2-chloroadenosine acetate (2-CDA) (cladribine) and pentostatin are highly effective with just one cycle of treatment. Rituximab is used in patients who do not respond to the above drugs.
- **Contraindicated drugs:** Corticosteroids and myelotoxic drugs

Prognosis

It follows an indolent course and prognosis is excellent.

Chronic Leukemia

Chronic Myeloid Leukemia

It is *myeloproliferative neoplasms* (MPN) of *pluripotent hematopoietic stem cell* characterized by *overproduction* of cells of the *myeloid series* (results in marked splenomegaly and leukocytosis) and the presence of the Philadelphia chromosome.

Balanced reciprocal translocation between long arm of chromosome 9 and chromosome 22 resulting in shortened chromosome 22 is known as Philadelphia chromosome (Fig. 12.26).

Molecular pathogenesis:

Philadelphia (Ph) Chromosome: It is acquired chromosomal abnormality of *hematopoietic stem cells. Balanced reciprocal translocation between the long arms of chromosomes 9 and 22 (t9;22)* increases the length of chromosome 9 and shortening of 22. The *shortened chromosome 22* is known as Philadelphia chromosome *(Ph).*

Natural course of CML: It has three phases:
- **Chronic stable phase:** Most of the CML are diagnosed in this phase and it lasts for about 3–5 years.
- **Accelerated phase:** It is more aggressive and lasts for few months.
- **Blast crisis phase:** It resembles acute (myeloid or lymphoid) leukemia and has poor prognosis.

Symptoms:
- **Age:** *Usually occurs between 40 and 60 years* of age.
- **Onset:** *Insidious*

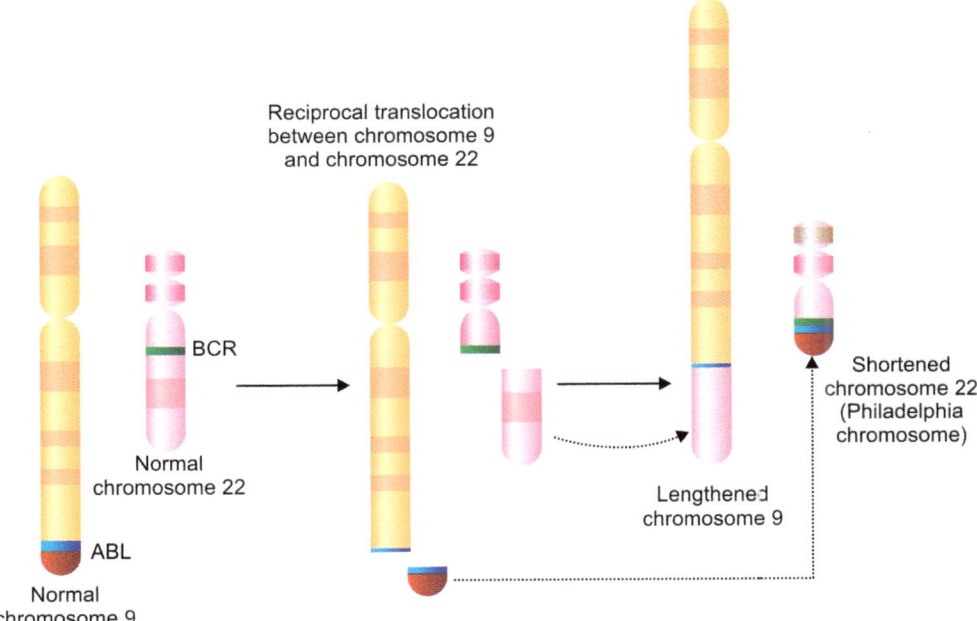

Fig. 12.26: Philadelphia (Ph) chromosome.

- **Symptoms:** Many patients are asymptomatic during early stage of CML and may be diagnosed during routine peripheral blood examination.
    - *Nonspecific symptoms:* Fatigue, weakness, weight loss, and anorexia
    - *Symptoms due to massive splenomegaly: Fullness of abdomen* (abdominal distension and postprandial fullness), reflux esophagitis, dyspnea, and dragging discomfort in the left hypochondrium due to splenomegaly (caused by leukemic infiltration and extramedullary hematopoiesis). Splenomegaly is moderate to severe and is characteristic feature in majority (80–90%) of patients.
    - *Symptoms of hypermetabolic state*: It is due to rapid turnover of cells and may result in symptoms such as fatigue, weakness, fever, sweating, heat intolerance, weight loss, and anorexia.
    - *Priapism*: Painful penile erection due to leukostasis (associated with marked leukocytosis or thrombocytosis).
    - Bleeding tendencies occur late in the disease.
- **Signs:**
    - *Pallor*—due to anemia
    - *Splenomegaly:* It is moderate-to-massive, nontender splenomegaly. It is due to leukemia infiltration and extramedullary hematopoiesis. Presence of tender spleen and splenic friction rub indicate splenic infarction.
    - Mild *hepatomegaly* as a result of leukemic infiltration may develop in 60–70% of cases.
    - *Sternal tenderness and bone pain:* It is due to hypercellularity of marrow and irritation of periosteum.

Investigations:
- **Hemoglobin** is usually less than 11 g/dL.
- **Total leukocyte count** is markedly raising, almost always more than 20,000/μL, often exceeding 100,000/μL. In untreated patients, the leukocyte count progressively increases.
- **Peripheral smear (Fig. 12.27):**
    - *RBC* shows moderate degree of *normocytic normochromic anemia*.
    - *WBC*:
        - *Shift to left (shift to immaturity)* with granulocytes at all stages of development (neutrophils, metamyelocytes, myelocytes, promyelocytes, and occasional myeloblasts). *Predominant cells* are *neutrophils and myelocytes* in an untreated patient. *Blasts* are usually *less than 10%* of the circulating white blood cells.
        - Increase in basophils (<20%) and eosinophils
    - *Platelets:* Count may be normal, increased, or decreased. Automated analyzers may give falsely elevated platelet counts due to disruption of granulocytes.
- **Bone marrow study:**
    - Markedly hypercellular due to marked hyperplasia of all granulocytic elements
    - About 20–30% of the patients may develop bone marrow fibrosis in late stages.
- **Philadelphia chromosome (Ph)** is positive in more than 95% of cases, in all three phases. In Ph-negative cases, evidence of translocation can be demonstrated by cytogenetics, reverse transcription–polymerase chain reaction (RT-PCR), and fluorescence in situ hybridization (FISH).
- **BCR-ABL fusion gene** can be demonstrated in peripheral blood or bone marrow.
- **Decreased neutrophil alkaline phosphatase (NAP)/ leukocyte alkaline phosphatase (LAP) score** and is usually below 20 (normal score range from 40–100) in majority of patients. This is helpful in differentiating CML from leukemoid reaction.

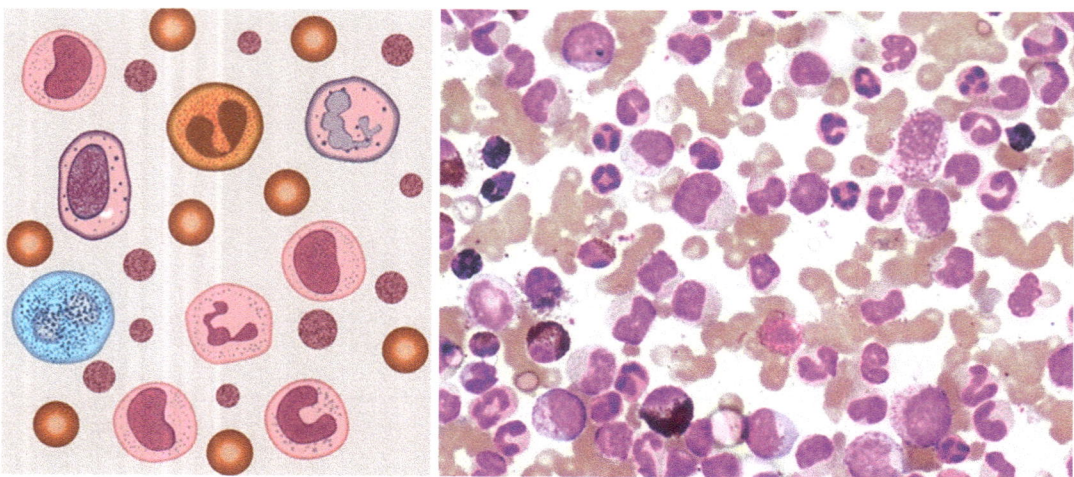

Fig. 12.27: Peripheral blood picture in chronic stable phase of chronic myeloid leukemia.

- **Biochemical findings:**
  - Serum LDH and uric acid are increased.
  - Serum alkaline phosphatase is increased.
  - Serum vitamin B_{12} is markedly elevated due to production of binding protein (transcobalamin) by the granulocyte series.
  - Marked thrombocytosis may raise serum potassium spuriously as platelets release potassium during clotting.
  - Blood sugar may be falsely decreased due to glucose uptake and metabolism by leucocytes.

Treatment:
- **Goal of therapy in CML**—complete molecular remission and cure:
  - Achieve prolonged, durable, nonneoplastic, and nonclonal hematopoiesis
  - Eradication of any residual cells containing the *BCR-ABL1* transcript
- **Chemotherapy:**
  - First-line treatment for the chronic phase of CML
  - If there is failure of response or progress on imatinib, options include—(1) second-generation tyrosine kinase inhibitors (such as dasatinib or nilotinib), (2) allogeneic bone marrow transplantation, or (3) classical cytotoxic drugs, such as hydroxycarbamide (hydroxyurea) or interferon-α or melphalan, and busulfan **(Table 12.43)**.
  - Hydroxyurea was widely used for initial control of disease and is still useful as palliative therapy. It does not decrease the frequency of the Ph chromosome or affect the onset of blast cell transformation but is used only to reduce leukocyte count. Chemotherapy is started with an induction dose, followed by a maintenance dose for a few months. The drug is reintroduced when the leukocyte counts rise.
- **Splenectomy:** It is indicated to relieve the symptoms due to massive splenomegaly and in repeated splenic infarctions.
- **Stem cell transplantation (SCT)**

Chronic Lymphocytic Leukemia

It is tumor of immature small round lymphocytes characterized by the accumulation of neoplastic mature looking lymphocytes in the peripheral blood, bone marrow, and lymphoid organs (spleen and lymph nodes).

Types:
- **B-cell origin:** More than 95% of the cases of CLL express the pan-B cell markers CD19 and CD20. And also, aberrant expression of T-cell antigen CD5 (found only in a small subset of normal B cells).
- **T-cell origin**—constitutes less than 5%.

Clinical features:
- It is the most common form of chronic leukemia.
- **Age:** Most of the patients at the time of diagnosis are over 50 years of age.
- **Sex:** More common in males than in females with a ratio of 2:1
- **Asymptomatic**—in about 25% of patients and is detected either because of nonspecific symptoms or routine blood examination for some other disease.
- **Nonspecific symptoms:** These include fatigue, loss of weight, and anorexia.
- **Painless generalized lymphadenopathy:** Initially, the cervical lymph nodes are enlarged and in later stages, there may be generalized lymphadenopathy. Involved nodes are rubbery, discrete, non-tender, small, and mobile.
- **Splenomegaly and hepatomegaly:** Mild degree is observed in very few cases.
- Transformation to diffuse large B-cell lymphoma (Richter syndrome)

Investigations:
- **Hemoglobin:** Usually below 13 g/dL, as the disease progresses, it may decrease below 10 g/dL. This is due to

Table 12.43: Drugs used and their dosage for induction and maintenance in chronic stable phase of chronic myeloid leukemia (CML).

Drug	Induction dose	Maintenance dose
Imatinib mesylate	300–400 mg/day	300–400 mg/day
Hydroxyurea (hydroxycarbamide)	0.5–2.0 g/day	0.5–2.0 g/day
Melphalan	4–12 mg/day	2–4 mg/day
Busulfan	4 mg/day	2–4 mg/day

marrow failure, but associated autoimmune hemolysis may also be contributory, when present.
- **Blood counts:** Total leukocyte count is increased and varies from $20 \times 10^9/L$ to $50 \times 10^9/L$. Platelet count may be normal or low.
- **Peripheral blood smear:**
  - Mild-to-moderate normocytic normochromic anemia
  - Lymphocytosis is the characteristic feature, which constitutes more than 50% of the white cells and absolute lymphocyte count should be more than $5000 \times 10^9/L$.
  - Lymphocytes are of mature type in majority of the cases.
  - Smudge cells or basket cells are disintegrated lymphocytes and is due to the rupture of neoplastic lymphocytes while making the peripheral smear due to its fragile nature.
  - *Platelets*: Normal or reduced in number (autoimmune thrombocytopenia)
- **Bone marrow:** It is involved in all cases of chronic lymphocytic leukemia (CLL) and its infiltration by mature lymphocytes results in hypercellular marrow.
- **Direct Coombs' test:** About 15–20% of patients manifest autoimmune hemolytic anemia and have positive direct Coombs' test.
- **Lymph node** biopsy shows well-differentiated, small, and non-cleaved lymphocytes.
- **Immunoglobulins:** Low or normal
- Serum folic acid levels are low.

Diagnostic criteria:
Diagnostic criteria of chronic lymphocytic leukemia are described in **Table 12.44**.

Clinical staging:
Clinical staging of chronic lymphocytic leukemia is discussed in **Tables 12.45 and 12.46**.

Lymphoid enlargement includes cervical, axillary, and inguinal lymph nodes.

Table 12.44: Diagnostic criteria of chronic lymphocytic leukemia.

Lymphocytosis	Immunophenotype
Absolute lymphocyte count should be more than $5000 \times 10^9/L$	Positive for B-cell surface antigens (CD19, CD20, and CD23)
Lymphocytosis for >2 months	Aberrant expression of T-cell antigen CD5
Lymphoid cells ≤55% atypical immature	Weak expression of monoclonal surface immunoglobulin with κ or λ light chains

Table 12.45: Binet staging.

Stage	Features	Survival
A	No anemia or thrombocytopenia Less than three lymphoid areas of enlarged	>10 years
B	No anemia or thrombocytopenia Three or more lymphoid areas enlarged	7 years
C	Anemia (Hb ≤10 g/dL) and or thrombocytopenia (<10,000/mm³) present, regardless of the number of areas of lymphoid enlargement	2 years

Table 12.46: Rai staging.

Stage	Features	Survival
0	Lymphocytosis only in blood (>5,000/mm³) and bone marrow	>10 years
I	Lymphocytosis with lymphadenopathy	9 years
II	Lymphocytosis with splenomegaly or lymphadenopathy or both	7 years
III	Lymphocytosis with anemia (hemoglobin <11 g/dL) and organomegaly	5 years
IV	Lymphocytosis with anemia, thrombocytopenia, and organomegaly	5 years

Table 12.47: Treatment options based on Binet staging.

Binet staging	Treatment
Stage A	No specific therapy required
Stage B	• No specific treatment, if asymptomatic • Medically unfit elderly patients with symptoms: Chlorambucil (oral) • Young patients: Fludarabine (IV) • Local radiotherapy to troublesome lymph nodes
Stage C	• Young patients: Fludarabine (IV) • Refractory cases: Combination chemotherapy with cyclophosphamide, doxorubicin, vincristine, and prednisolone (CHOP) • Rituximab in combination with fludarabine • Packed red cell transfusion (for anemia) with fludarabine • Prednisolone for patients with hemolytic anemia and thrombocytopenia • Splenectomy for symptomatic splenomegaly • Palliative total body irradiation

Treatment (Table 12.47):
Absolute indications for treatment—when any of the following features is present:
- Anemia (due to hemolysis) and increasing anemia or thrombocytopenia due to bone marrow failure
- Recurrent infection and fever without evidence of infection, extreme fatigue, night sweats, and weight loss
- Bulky or progressive lymphadenopathy; massive or progressive splenomegaly with discomfort
- Autoimmune cytopenias, not responsive to corticosteroids
- Progressive disease manifested by doubling of the lymphocyte count in 6 months.

MYELOPROLIFERATIVE DISEASES

These are clonal hematopoietic stem cell disorders, which are characterized by proliferation of one or more of the myeloid lineages (erythroid, granulocytic, megakaryocytic, and mast cells).

These are seen in adults with a peak in the 5th to 7th decade. Splenomegaly and hepatomegaly occur commonly due to sequestration of excess hematopoietic cells or proliferation of abnormal hematopoietic cells.

Classification of Myeloid Neoplasms (Table 12.48)

Classification includes five major entitles:
1. Acute myeloid leukemia (AML)
2. Myelodysplastic syndromes (MDS)
3. Myeloproliferative neoplasms (MPN)
4. Myelodysplastic/myeloproliferative neoplasms (MDS/MPN) overlap
5. Myeloid neoplasms associated with eosinophilia and specific molecular abnormalities

Polycythemia/Erythrocytosis

It is increase in the number of RBCs above normal in the circulating blood, usually with a corresponding increase in hemoglobin and packed cell volume (PCV) level. PCV is a more reliable indicator of polycythemia than is hemoglobin. The increase in red cells can be absolute or relative.

Relative polycythemia is characterized by decreased plasma volume with a normal red cell mass. They may result from dehydration following prolonged vomiting, diarrhea, or excessive use of diuretics.

Absolute polycythemia is characterized by a true increase in total red cell mass and can be subclassified as primary and secondary.

- **Primary polycythemia or polycythemia vera (PV)**—results from an intrinsic abnormality of the hematopoietic stem cells. It is an autonomous, erythropoietin (EPO) independent proliferation of erythroid cells due to an acquired, clonal hematopoietic stem cell disorder. PV is considered as one of the several neoplasms originating from myeloid stem cells (chronic myeloproliferative neoplasm).
- **Secondary polycythemia**—results as a compensatory response of red cell progenitors to an increase in EPO secretion. The erythropoietin secretion may be physiological as a response to general chronic tissue hypoxia or it may be pathological like in paraneoplastic syndromes.

Pathophysiologic classification of polycythemia is described in Box 12.3.

Clinical Features

- Usually appears insidiously, in late middle age (median age at onset—60 years)
- Most symptoms are due to the increased red cell mass and hematocrit.
- Plethora (excessive fullness of blood) and cyanosis due to stagnation and deoxygenation of blood in peripheral

Table 12.48: World Health Organization (WHO) classification (2008) of myeloproliferative neoplasm (MPN).

• Chronic myelogenous leukemia, *BCR-ABL1* positive	• Chronic eosinophilic leukemia not otherwise specified
• Chronic neutrophilic leukemia	• Mastocytosis
• Polycythemia vera (PV)	• Myeloproliferative neoplasm, unclassifiable
• Essential thrombocythemia (ET)	
• Primary myelofibrosis (PMF)	

Box 12.3: Pathophysiologic classification of polycythemia.

Relative:
- Reduced plasma volume with normal red cell mass (hemoconcentration) due to dehydration—low fluid intake, vomiting, diarrhea, sweating, and acidosis
- Gaisböck syndrome (spurious polycythemia)

Absolute (increased red cell mass)
Primary (low erythropoietin level)
Polycythemia vera (erythremia)
Secondary (high erythropoietin level)—erythrocytosis
Compensatory:
- Lung disease (e.g., COPD—chronic obstructive pulmonary disease)
- Living in high altitude
- Cyanotic congenital heart disease (tetralogy of Fallot and Eisenmenger's complex)
- Chronic carbon monoxide poisoning
- Sleep apnea syndrome
- Smokers

As a consequence of local hypoxia: Renal artery stenosis, end-stage renal disease, hydronephrosis, renal cysts (Polycystic kidney disease), and postrenal transplant erythrocytosis
Paraneoplastic: Erythropoietin-secreting tumors—renal cell carcinoma, hepatocellular carcinoma, cerebellar hemangioblastoma, uterine leiomyoma, and pheochromocytoma

---

vessels are early findings. Headache, dizziness, and visual problems result from vascular disturbances in the brain and retina.
- Increased incidence of thrombotic episodes and bleeding
- Secondary polycythemia, in addition, shows manifestations of the underlying disease.

Polycythemia Vera

- It is *acquired myeloproliferative neoplasm* arising from malignant transformation of *hematopoietic stem cell*.
- *Trilineage* (erythroid, granulocytic, and megakaryocytic) *hyperplasia* in the bone marrow
- It leads to *uncontrolled production of red cells, granulocytes, and platelets* (panmyelosis), *erythrocytosis* (polycythemia), and/or granulocytosis and thrombocytosis. PV is generally dominated by an elevated hemoglobin concentration and polycythemia is responsible for most of the clinical symptoms.
- It is one of the chronic myeloproliferative neoplasms.

Etiology

Etiology is not known. PV is partly due to a failure of apoptosis as a result of deregulation of the *Bcl-x* gene (anti-apoptotic gene); in addition, a mutation in the *in-tyrosine* kinase *JAK2 V617F* has been found; this stimulates low-grade erythropoiesis.

Clinical Features

- Onset is insidious.
- **Age and gender:** Late middle age (median age at onset is 60 years) and more common in males
- **Features due to increased viscosity and/or decreased cerebral perfusion:**

- Plethora (excessive fullness of blood) and deep dusky cyanosis due to stagnation and deoxygenation of blood in peripheral vessels are early findings.
- Headache, dizziness, vertigo, a sense of fullness in the head, rushing in the ears, visual problems, tinnitus, tiredness, syncope, and even chorea result from vascular disturbances in the brain and retina.
☐ Severe itching (pruritus) after a hot bath or when patient is warm is frequent and may be disabling.
☐ Thrombotic episodes, e.g., deep venous thrombosis, myocardial infarction, and thrombosis of hepatic veins (producing Budd–Chiari syndrome)
☐ **Bleeding manifestations** include epistaxis, bleeding from peptic ulcer, bruising, and intramuscular hemorrhages.
☐ Peptic ulcer is seen in few patients and is five times more frequent than general population.
☐ **Hyperuricemia**—may result in urate stones, gout, and uric acid nephropathy.
☐ **Physical findings:**
  - Injection of the conjunctivae, deep red palate, dusky red hands, and retinal venous engorgement
  - Splenomegaly is very common (~70%) and is useful in distinguishing PV from secondary polycythemia.
  - Hepatomegaly occurs in ~50%.

Diagnosis (Table 12.49)
☐ *Hemoglobin is increased ranging from* 14 to 28 g/dL
☐ *PCV (hematocrit)* is increased to about 60%. However, in many patients, the plasma volume is also increased giving rise to near-normal hematocrit. Hence, it is important to determine the red cell mass.
☐ *Red cell count is increased and usually about 6 million/mm³ (6 × 10¹²/L)*
☐ **Increased red cell volume and blood viscosity:** Red cell volume is determined by isotope dilution using the patient's ^{51}Cr-tagged red cells (>36 mL/kg in males and 32 mL/kg in females).
☐ Total white cell count (~70%) and platelet count (~50%) are usually increased.
☐ **Absolute basophil count** is increased to >100/µL in majority of patients
☐ **Arterial oxygen saturation** (PO$_2$) is normal and is useful for differentiating it from secondary polycythemia.
☐ **Erythropoietin (EPO) levels are decreased** in urine and serum, in contrast to secondary polycythemia.
☐ **Bone marrow**—shows either erythroid hyperplasia or hyperplasia of all elements (trilineage hyperplasia) and depletion of iron stores.
☐ *Leukocyte alkaline phosphatase (LAP)* is increased in majority of patients.
☐ *Serum vitamin B$_{12}$ and vitamin B$_{12}$-binding protein transcobalamin I (TC I) levels* are increased (not routinely measured).
☐ **Serum uric acid** is increased indicating increased cell turnover.
☐ Abnormal liver function tests
☐ **Janus kinase 2 (JAK2) mutations (JAK2V617F mutation):**
  - In ~95% patients with polycythemia vera and in ~50% of essential thrombocytosis and primary myelofibrosis
  - Janus kinases belong to tyrosine kinase family located on chromosome 9
  - JAK2 is used by the EPO; thrombopoietin and granulocyte colony-stimulating factor (G-CSF) receptors to transmit signals are involved in hematopoiesis.
  - JAK2 inhibitors are used for managing these patients.

The clinical course tends to proceed as a series of phases:
☐ **Proliferative phase:** Erythroid proliferation with increased red cell mass
☐ **Spent phase:** Excessive proliferation of erythroid cells ceases, resulting in stable or decreased erythrocyte mass
☐ Progression to myelofibrosis
☐ Acute myelogenous leukemia in 2–5% of cases

Complications
Complications are described in **Table 12.50**.

Treatment
Polycythemia vera (PV) generally has a very slow course.
☐ **Aim:** To maintain a normal blood count, PCV below 0.45 L/L, and the platelet count below 400 × 10⁹/L and to prevent the complications (mainly thromboses and hemorrhage)

Table 12.49: World Health Organization (WHO) diagnostic criteria for polycythemia vera (PV).

Major criteria	Minor criteria
Hb >18.5 g/dL (men), >16.5 g/dL (women) Or Hb or PCV >99th percentile of reference range Or Hb >17 g/dL (men) or >15 g/dL (women), if associated with a documented and sustained increase of ≥2 g/dL from baseline that cannot explained otherwise Or Elevated red cell mass >25% above mean normal predicted value	BM showing hypercellularity with trilineage (panmyelosis) myeloproliferation
	Subnormal serum EPO level
Presence of *JAF2V617F* (a mutation in *JAK2*) or similar mutation	Endogenous erythroid colony (EECs) growth
Diagnostic criteria for PV Either both major criteria + 1 minor criterion or first major criterion + 2 minor criteria	

(EPO: erythropoietin)

Table 12.50: Complications of polycythemia vera.

• Thrombotic and bleeding episodes	• Myelofibrosis and myeloid metaplasia
• Peptic ulcer due to *Helicobacter pylori*	• Erythromelalgia (thrombocytosis, involving the lower extremities with erythema, warmth, and pain, and occasionally digital infarction)
• Hyperuricemia (gout)	
• Sudden increase in splenic size	
• Acute nonlymphocytic leukemia	

- **Venesection:** Repeated venesection (phlebotomy) is the treatment of choice and relieves many of the symptoms of PV.
- **Chemotherapy:**
  - It is indicated, if patient is intolerant to venesection, or thrombocytosis occurs, or symptomatic or progressive splenomegaly develops
  - Continuous or intermittent treatment with *hydroxycarbamide (hydroxyurea)* is the treatment of choice in patients above 40 years. It controls thrombocytosis and is generally safer than alkylating agents (e.g., busulfan) and ^{32}P (phosphorus), which carry an increased risk of acute leukemia.
  - In younger patients, interferon-α is used.
- **Radioactive ^{32}P:** One dose may control for up to 1½ years but carries an increased risk to acute leukemia. In elderly patients, ^{32}P or low-dose intermittent busulfan may be more convenient.
- **Other measures:**
  - *Low-dose aspirin* may be used to reduce thrombotic episodes.
  - *Anagrelide (inhibits platelet aggregation)*—may be used, if thrombotic features develop despite above treatment.
  - Itching should be treated with antihistamines. If do not relive, hydroxyurea, interferon-α, and psoralens with UV light in "A" range (PUVA) may be helpful.
  - Asymptomatic hyperuricemia does not require treatment.

Primary Myelofibrosis

It is a clonal MPN characterized by increased fibrosis within the marrow, which replaces hematopoietic cells leading to cytopenias, splenomegaly, and extensive extramedullary hematopoiesis. The extramedullary hematopoiesis is seen in the spleen, liver, and, at times, in lymph nodes, kidneys, and adrenals.

It can arise from polycythemia vera (PV) or essential thrombocytosis (ET). **Table 12.51** shows the differences between polycythemia vera and secondary olycythemia.

Table 12.51: Differences between polycythemia vera and secondary polycythemia.

Feature	Polycythemia vera	Secondary polycythemia
Oxygen saturation	Normal	Low
EPO (erythropoietin) levels	Decreased	Increased
Blood counts:		
Total white cell count	Increased	Normal
Absolute basophil count	Increased	Normal
Platelet count	Increased	Normal
Leukocyte alkaline phosphatase (LAP)	Raised	Normal
Vitamin B_{12} levels	Increased	Normal
Bone marrow	Trilineage (panhyperplasia)	Erythroid hyperplasia
Splenomegaly	Present	Absent

Clinical Features
- Usually found above 60 years of age
- A significant number of cases develop acute myeloid leukemia.

Symptoms
- **Due to progressive anemia**—fatigue, weakness, and anorexia
- **Due to massive splenomegaly**—abdominal distension, postprandial fullness, reflux esophagitis, dyspnea, and dragging discomfort in the left hypochondrium
- **Hypermetabolic state**—fever, fatigue, weight loss, night sweats, and heat intolerance
- Bleeding tendencies due to thrombocytopenia develop at late stages.
- Death usually occurs due to portal hypertension and infections. Median survival is about 5 years.

Signs
- Massive splenomegaly and hepatomegaly
- Anemia, lymphadenopathy, bleeding manifestations, ascites, cardiac failure, and jaundice
- Hyperuricemia and secondary gout due to a high rate of cell turnover
- **Extramedullary hematopoiesis**—may produce paraspinal masses with spinal cord compression, ascites, and effusions (pleural and pericardial).

Investigations
- **Hemoglobin level** is normal in the early stages, but markedly reduced in the late stages.
- **Total leukocyte count** is normal/increased (early stages)/decreased (late stages).
- **Platelet count** is increased in early stages and decreased in the late stages.
- **Peripheral smear:** Moderate to severe degree of normochromic normocytic anemia accompanied by leukoerythroblastic blood picture (precursors of granulocytes and nucleated RBCs being present simultaneously). *Many tear drop-shaped red cells* (dacrocytes) are probably due to damage in the fibrotic marrow. *Basophilic stippling. Giant platelets* with vacuoles
- **Bone marrow:** The peripheral smear findings are not specific and bone marrow biopsy is diagnostic.
  - *Cellularity:* In early stages ("cellular phase"), it is often hypercellular and in later stages ("hypocellular phase"), it becomes hypocellular and diffusely fibrotic.
  - Megakaryocytes are large, dysplastic, and abnormally clustered.
- **LAP score** is raised
- **Philadelphia chromosome** is negative.
- ***JAK2-V617F*** mutation occurs in ~50% patients
- **Serum vitamin B_{12}**—moderately increased
- **Radiological examination**—shows increased bone density of vertebrate and proximal ends of long bones.

Treatment
No specific therapy exists for primary IMF.

- **Treatment of anemia:**
  - Correct other causes of anemia, such as gastrointestinal blood loss and folic acid deficiency (folic acid 5 mg daily)
  - Packed red cell transfusions
  - Neither recombinant erythropoietin nor androgens (such as Danazol) is consistently effective in controlling anemia but can be tried in some patients
  - Glucocorticoids (prednisolone) may control constitutional symptoms and autoimmune complications
  - Combination with low-dose thalidomide (50–100 mg/day) with prednisolone can control anemia and splenomegaly in a significant number of patients.
- **Treatment of splenomegaly:**
  - *Patients with cellular bone marrow and marked leukocytosis*: Busulfan 2 mg daily
  - Indications for splenectomy in selected cases:
    - With hypersplenism
    - If splenomegaly impairs alimentation and should be performed before cachexia sets in
  - *Splenic irradiation*—to reduce splenic size is reserved for patients, who cannot undergo splenectomy. Patients often develop severe cytopenias.
  - Hydroxyurea is useful to control splenomegaly but can produce myelosuppression that may exacerbate underlying anemia.
- **Treatment of extramedullary hematopoiesis**—by low-dose irradiation
- **Curative treatment:** *Allogenic bone marrow transplantation* is the only curative treatment. It should be performed in younger patients as most patients in IMF are above 60 years of age.
- **Others:**
  - Allopurinol can control hyperuricemia.
  - Etanercept (TNF-α antagonist) is used in patients with severe constitutional features.
  - JAK2 inhibitors are under trial.

Prognosis
Median survival varies from 27 to 135 months and depends on prognostic factors **(Table 12.52)**.

Myelodysplastic Syndrome

Clinical Features
- Myelodysplastic syndrome is usually found in patients above 60 years and slightly more common in males.
- It is detected incidentally on routine blood examination in about 50% of patients.
- Symptoms are due to cytopenias, which may be single lineage cytopenia, bicytopenia, or pancytopenia. Symptoms include weakness (anemia), infections (leukopenia), and hemorrhage (thrombocytopenia).
- Extramedullary hematopoiesis may occur leading to hepatomegaly and splenomegaly but is uncommon.
- About 10–40% progresses to AML. MDS was referred to as preleukemic syndrome.

Diagnosis
- **Minimal morphologic criterion for the diagnosis of an MDS:** Dysplasia in at least 10% of cells of any one of the myeloid lineages
- **Complete blood count**—may give clues to this diagnosis
- **Peripheral smear:**
  - Mild-to-moderate degree of macrocytic or dimorphic anemia with evidence of dyspoiesis
  - *WBC count*: Normal or low. Neutropenia with few blasts; the number of blasts determines type of MDS. The cytoplasm of neutrophils is hypogranular or agranular. The nuclei may show hyposegmentation with only two nuclear lobes (Pseudo-Pelger-Hüet cells), hypersegmentation, or ringed neutrophils.
  - Variable thrombocytopenia and presence of large hypogranular or giant platelets are seen.
  - *NAP score* is moderately or severely decreased
- **Bone marrow:** Varying degree of dyspoietic (disordered) differentiation affecting all non-lymphoid lineages (erythroid, granulocytic, monocytic, and megakaryocytic) associated with cytopenias.
- **Cytogenic study of the marrow** is most important for establishing the diagnosis.

Treatment
- **Therapy is supportive:**
  - Packed red cell transfusion for anemia
  - Platelet transfusions for bleeding due to thrombocytopenia
  - Antibiotic therapy for infections
  - Iron chelators to reduce iron overload from multiple transfusions
- EPO and G-CSF may be useful in some patients, to ameliorate symptoms.
- **Others:** Use of thalidomide, lenalidomide (a derivative of thalidomide), 5-azacytidine, and decitabine. 5-azacytdine and decitabine (hypomethylating agents) may reduce requirements of blood transfusion and is used to retard the progression of MDS to AML. Lenalidomide is found useful in the 5q-syndrome.
- Allogenic hematopoietic stem cell transplantation—curative. However, it may be performed in less than 5–10% of patients because MDS is most common during seventh or eighth decade of life.

PLASMA CELL DYSCRASIAS

Multiple Myeloma

Clinical Features (Table 12.53)
Insidious in onset. Peak incidence is seen during 6th to 7th decade, and males are more affected than females.

Table 12.52: Poor prognostic factors.

Age> 65 years	Hemoglobin level <10g/dL	Total WBC count >25,000/mm³
Presence of blasts in peripheral blood	Presence of constitutional symptoms	

Table 12.53: Clinical features of multiple myeloma.

Involved system	Features
Bone	• Localized bony swellings over vertebrae, skull, sternum, ribs, and clavicle • Bone pain due to pathological fractures • *Neurological symptoms*: Sensory and/or motor loss due to lesion in the vertebra compressing the spinal cord nerve root
Bone marrow	Anemia, leukopenia, and thrombocytopenia
Immune system	Humoral immune deficiency leading to increased susceptibility to infections, particularly of the respiratory system and urinary tract
Renal damage—multifactorial	• Bence Jones proteinuria, hypercalcemia, and immune deficiency • Nephrocalcinosis, amyloidosis, renal insufficiency, infections, or nephrotic syndrome
Bleeding tendency	Purpura, epistaxis, and gastrointestinal bleeding
Cryoglobulinemia Hyperviscosity syndrome	• *CNS:* Confusion headache, vertigo, nystagmus, postural hypotension and dizziness • *Retina*: Producing blurred vision, retinal venous congestion, and papilledema • *CVS*: Congestive cardiac failure
Neurological manifestations	Amyloid peripheral neuropathy, carpal tunnel syndrome, and compressive myelopathy

(CNS: central nervous system; CVS: cardiovascular system)

Osteosclerotic Myeloma (Poems Syndrome)

This syndrome is characterized by polyneuropathy, organomegaly, endocrinopathy, M protein, and skin changes (POEMS).

The major clinical features are a chronic inflammatory-demyelinating polyneuropathy with predominantly motor disability and sclerotic skeletal lesions.

Treatment

- **Autologous stem cell transplantation:** In young patients (<65 years) without renal failure, standard treatment is first-line high-dose chemotherapy for myeloablation (melphalan 20 mg/m² intravenously) to maximum response and then an autologous stem-cell transplantation.
- **Chemotherapy:** *Older patients—*
  - Thalidomide and alkylating agent (melphalan, cyclophosphamide, and chlorambucil) and prednisolone. Thalidomide is teratogenic. Recent studies have suggested that combination with thalidomide results in improved response rates and overall survival, albeit with increased toxicity.
  - Bortezomib—proteasome inhibitor is used in relapses, combined with doxorubicin and dexamethasone.
  - Lenalidomide in combination with steroids has been tried.

Younger patients (<65–70 years):
- Orally active cyclophosphamide, thalidomide, and dexamethasone-based induction (CTD), followed by a high-dose melphalan autograft
- **Radiotherapy:** It is effective for local problems such as severe bone pain, pathological fractures, and tumorous lesions. It is used as an emergency treatment of spinal cord compression complicating extradural plasmacytomas.

LYMPHOMA

Hodgkin Lymphoma

Hodgkin lymphoma (HL) is a malignant lymphoma characterized by a heterogeneous cellularity of specific *neoplastic cells* (Hodgkin cells and Reed–Sternberg cells) (1–3%) in a background of reactive non-neoplastic cells of various types.

- **Cell of origin:** Neoplastic Reed–Sternberg cells derived from germinal-center or immediate postgerminal-center B-cells indicating that most HLs are unusual tumors of B-cell origin.
- **Age:** Bimodal incidence, one peak in young adults (15–35 years) and the other in older adults (45–75 years)
- *Reed–Sternberg (RS) cell*
- *Reed–Sternberg cells* and its variants are *pathognomonic* and differentiate HL from NHL.
- Histological diagnosis of HL should not be made in their absence. They are necessary but not sufficient for diagnosis of classical Hodgkin lymphoma, and should be found in cellular background for the specific subtype.
- **Appearance of diagnostic Reed–Sternberg cells:** Giant cells with two large nuclei and nucleoli in each nucleus (owl's eye appearance)
- **Variants of RS cell:**
  - *Mononuclear variant:* Single, large, and round nucleus with a large eosinophilic inclusion-like nucleolus, also called as Hodgkin cells.
  - Lacunar cell variant
  - Mummified cell (necrobiotic) variant
  - Anaplastic/pleomorphic variant
  - Lymphohistiocytic variant (L and H cells/popcorn cell)—specific to lymphocyte predominance subtype
- **Immunophenotype:** Classical forms of HL are CD15⁺ and CD30⁺. Lymphocyte-predominant HL cells are CD15⁻ and CD30⁻.

Etiology

- **Epstein–Barr virus (EBV):** Young adults who have had previous infectious mononucleosis have an increased risk of develop and EBV genome is frequently identified in the Reed–Sternberg cells.
- **Genetic factors:** HLA-B18 is higher in patients with HL.
- **Immune status:** More in immunocompromised or with autoimmune diseases

Classification of Hodgkin Lymphoma (Fig. 12.28)

Rye's classification: The prognosis depends on the histological type (**Table 12.54**). Nodular sclerosing type is most common.

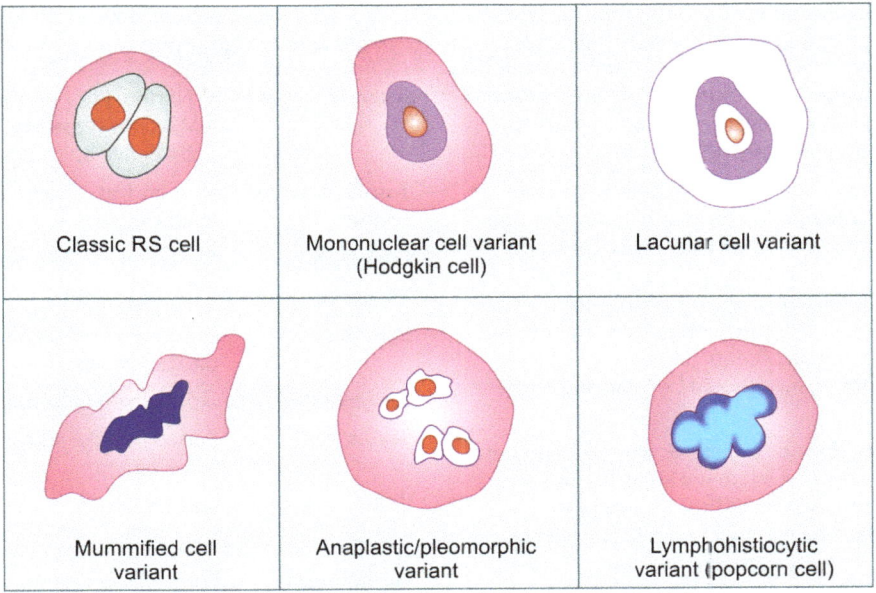

Fig. 12.28: Classification of Hodgkin lymphoma.

Table 12.54: Rye's classification of Hodgkin lymphoma.

Histological type	Prognosis
Lymphocyte predominant	Very good
Nodular sclerosing	Good
Mixed cellularity	Fair
Lymphocyte depleted	Poor

Table 12.55: World Health Organization (WHO) classification of Hodgkin lymphoma (HL).

Classical HL (>95%):	Nodular lymphocyte predominance (LP) Hodgkin's lymphoma (<5%)
• Nodular sclerosis (NS) classic HL • Mixed cellularity (MC) classic HL (most common type in India) • Lymphocyte-rich (LR) classic HL • Lymphocyte depletion (LD) classic HL	

The WHO classification of Hodgkin lymphoma is described in **Table 12.55**.

Clinical Manifestations

- **Most common presentation:** Painless enlargement of one lymph node group (unifocal) usually cervical, which spreads in a predictable manner (contiguous spread)
- **Other presentation:**
  - *Localized disease of mediastinum* (young women—cough due to mediastinal lymphadenopathy or axillary nodes, rarely in the abdominal, pelvic, or inguinal nodes).
  - *Generalized disease:* Hepatosplenomegaly and constitutional "B" symptoms are uncommon in the beginning but may become prominent as the disease advances.
  - *Rare sites:* Waldeyer's ring, mesenteric epitrochlear and popliteal nodes
- *Involvement of extralymphatic organs:* Not common, may occur in the later stages
- **Classical Pel–Ebstein fever:** Cyclical pattern, characterized by several days or weeks of fever alternating with afebrile periods. Rarely seen
- **Common symptoms:** Alcohol-induced pain at site of lymphadenopathy. Pruritus can be troubling.
- **Nephrotic syndrome:** Immune complex deposition, associated with depressed cell-mediated immunity, and increases risk of infections, such as herpes zoster, tuberculosis (TB), cryptococcus, *Cytomegalovirus (CMV)*, and candida.
- **Compression** by lymph node masses or *infiltration* of various organs may develop with mediastinal involvement—dysphagia, dyspnea, Horner's syndrome, hoarseness of voice, superior vena caval syndrome, and inferior vena caval obstruction.
- On examination, lymph nodes are discrete, non-tender, and have a "rubbery" consistency.

Clinical Staging

Cotswold's modification of the Ann Arbor classification is given in **Table 12.56**.

Investigations

Investigations done in Hodgkin lymphoma are described in **Table 12.57**.

Management (Tables 12.58 and 12.59)

- **Aim:** Curative intent with expectation of success
- Patients with localized disease receive a brief course of chemotherapy followed by radiotherapy to sites of node involvement and cured HD in >90% of cases.
- Presently, all stages of HL are treated initially with chemotherapy.
- Those with more extensive disease or with B symptoms receive a complete course of chemotherapy.

Table 12.56: Cotswold's modification of the Ann Arbor classification.

Stage	Definition
I	Involvement of a single lymph node region or lymphoid structure (e.g., spleen, Waldeyer's ring, and thymus) or involvement of a single extralymphatic site
II	• Involvement of two or more lymph node groups on same side of diaphragm (mediastinum is a single site; hilar nodes, when involved on both sides, constitute stage II disease) • Localized contiguous involvement of only one extranodal organ or site and lymph-node region(s) on the same side of the diaphragm (IIE). • Number of anatomic sites should be indicated by suffix (e.g., II$_3$)
III	Involvement of lymph node regions or structures on both sides of the diaphragm, which may also be accompanied by involvement of the spleen (IIIS) or by localized involvement of only one extranodal organ site (IIIE) or both (IIISE)
III$_1$	With/without splenic, hilar, celiac, or portal nodes
III$_2$	With para-aortic, iliac, or mesenteric nodes
IV	Diffuse or disseminated involvement of one or more extra nodal organs or tissues, with or without associated lymph-node involvement

E: Involvement of a single extranodal site, or contiguous or proximal to known nodal site of disease
A: No "B" symptoms
B: Place the patient in the "B" category when at least one of the following is observed—
1. Unexplained weight loss >10% of bodyweight during 6 months before staging
2. Recurrent unexplained fever >38°C during the previous month
Recurrent heavy night sweats during the previous month
Lymphatic structures are lymph nodes, spleen, thymus, Waldeyer's rings, appendix, and Peyer's patches. Liver and bone marrow are excluded.
Each stage is further divided into A or B based on the absence or presence of systemic symptoms (B symptoms), respectively

- **Chemotherapy:** Combination chemotherapy has been shown to be highly effective.
- **Early stage—"low risk":** Moderate chemotherapy, consisting of 2–4 cycles of ABVD followed by involved field irradiation (20–30 Gy). It has a 90% cure rate.
- **Advanced disease (including locally advanced unfavorable early stage):**
  - Cyclical chemotherapy with 6–8 cycles of ABVD with involved field irradiation to sites, which were initially bulky.
  - *Stanford V for ABVD:* It consists of weekly chemotherapy regimen of doxorubicin, vinblastine, mechlorethamine, etoposide, vincristine, bleomycin, and prednisone administered for 12 weeks and includes radiation therapy.
  - Escalated BEACOPP (bleomycin, etoposide, doxorubicin, cyclophosphamide, vincristine, prednisone, and procarbazine)
- Autologous bone marrow transplantation is successful in about 40% cases even after the failure of chemotherapy.

Table 12.57: Investigations done in Hodgkin lymphoma (HL).

Peripheral blood:	
Anemia	• Normocytic normochromic anemia • *Advance stage:* Microcytic anemia due to defective utilization of iron
Total leukocyte count	Normal, but sometimes neutrophil leukocytosis
Eosinophilia	Observed in ~20% of patients
Thrombocytosis	In some patients
Lymphopenia	Lymphocyte depletion and associated with bad prognosis
Terminal stages: Leukopenia and thrombocytopenia	
Serum ALP	Raised usually indicates bone marrow or liver involvement
ESR	May be raised
Biopsy:	
Lymph node biopsy	Surgically or percutaneous needle biopsy under radiological guidance
Liver biopsy	Diagnosis in patients with hepatomegaly
PET scan	Staging management of Hodgkin lymphoma
Staging of HL:	

- It predicts prognosis and guides choice of therapy. It requires physical examination and investigations:
  - Chest radiographs
  - Liver function tests
  - Renal function tests
  - Abdominal ultrasound
  - Bone marrow trephine and aspirate (clinically advanced disease—stage III, IV, "B" symptoms, and HIV-positive)
  - CT scans of neck, chest, abdomen, and pelvis
  - *Staging laparotomy* is rarely required (stage IIA or less and in whom mantle radiation is planned)
- With current treatment protocols, tumor stage rather than histological type is the most important prognostic variable.
- The cure rate of patients with stages I and IIA is close to 90%.
- Even with advanced disease (IVA and IVB), 60–70% 5-year disease-free survival is obtained.

(ALP: alkaline phosphatase; ESR: erythrocyte sedimentation rate; PET: positron emission tomography)

Table 12.58: Popular chemotherapy regimens used in the treatment of Hodgkin lymphoma.

Regimen	Drugs used
ABVD	Doxorubicin (adriamycin), bleomycin, vinblastine, and dacarbazine
MOPP	Mechlorethamine (mustine hydrochloride), vincristine, procarbazine, and prednisone
ABVD/MOPP	Alternating cycles of MOPP and ABVD
BEACOPP escalated	Bleomycin, etoposide, adriamycin, cyclophosphamide, vincristine, procarbazine, and prednisone in escalated dose

Late complications: Due to high-cure rates achieved with modern treatment.

- **Second malignancies:** Acute leukemia and solid organ cancers:

Table 12.59: Treatment plan for adults with Hodgkin lymphoma.

Stage of Hodgkin lymphoma	Prognostic category	Choice of treatment
IA or IIA, no bulky disease*		ABVD × 4, if complete remission after two cycles or ABVD × 2 + involved-region radiation therapy (IRRT)
IB, IIB, or any stage III or IV or bulky disease, any stage	≤3 adverse factors**	ABVD until two cycles past complete remission (minimum 6 and maximum 8)
	≥4 adverse factors**	BEACOPP escalated

*Bulky: Largest diameter of any single mass equal to or greater than 10 cm.
**Adverse factors: Male sex, older than 45 years of age, stage IV, hemoglobin less than 10.5 g/dL, WBC count greater than 15,000/mL, lymphocyte count less than 600/mL or less than 8% of the white cell count, or serum albumin less than 4 g/dL.

- *Acute leukemia:* Within 10 years of use of alkylating agents in combination with radiotherapy. The risk is higher with MOPP as compared to ABVD.
- Solid organ cancers usually develop after 10 years of radiotherapy.
- **Cardiac failure and accelerated coronary artery disease**—following radiotherapy
- Pulmonary fibrosis
- Hypothyroidism

Non-Hodgkin Lymphoma

- Lymphoma represents solid tumors of the immune system.
- It can be divided into Non-Hodgkin lymphoma (NHL) and Hodgkin lymphoma.
- About 80% of non-Hodgkin lymphomas (NHLs) are of B-cell origin and 20% of T-cell origin

Etiology (Table 12.60)

Etiology is not known in most of the cases. Genetic, environmental, and infectious agents are implicated.

Immune disorders occur in congenital or acquired immunodeficiency states.

- **Genetic factors/congenital immunodeficiency:** Increased risk of lymphoma in—
  - Family history: Siblings, first-degree relatives with lymphoma, or hematologic malignancies
  - Certain inherited syndromes, e.g., ataxia–telangiectasia and Wiskott–Aldrich syndrome
- **Acquired immune disorders:** Immune suppression, immunosuppressant drugs, used for solid organ transplantation, and HIV infection are associated with an increased incidence of lymphoma.

Pathology and Classification

Grading of NHL (Table 12.61):

- Size of the lymphoid cells is a guide to prognosis. Small lymphoid cells (mature lymphocytes) are low-grade and those with large lymphoid cells (immature lymphoid cells) show high-grade disease.
- **Follicular lymphomas** are low grade with good prognosis. Most diffuse lymphomas are high grade with poor prognosis

Table 12.60: Various factors associated with the development of non-Hodgkin lymphoma.

Genetic factors/inherited immune disorders:	Acquired immune disorders:
• Wiskott–Aldrich syndrome • Ataxia–telangiectasia	• Solid organ transplantation • Acquired immunodeficiency syndrome (AIDS) • Rheumatoid arthritis, SLE • Sjogren's syndrome • Hashimoto thyroiditis
Infectious agents:	**Occupational and environmental exposure:**
• *Human T-lymphotropic virus type 1* with adult T-cell leukemia/lymphoma • *Human herpesvirus 8* (Kaposi's sarcoma) associated with primary effusion lymphoma • *Hepatitis C virus*: Lymphoplasmacytic lymphoma and splenic marginal zone lymphoma • *Helicobacter pylori* is associated with gastric lymphoma of extranodal marginal zone/mucosa • *Epstein–Barr virus* is associated with Burkitt lymphoma and Hodgkin lymphoma, and mucosa-associated lymphoid tissue (MALT)	• Ionizing radiation • Herbicides • Organic solvents • Hair dyes • Ultraviolet light • High-fat diets and nitrates in drinking water • Heavy smoking associated with follicular lymphoma

Table 12.61: Grading of non-Hodgkin lymphoma (NHL).

Indolent or low grade	Highly aggressive/high grade	Aggressive/intermediate grade
• Small lymphocytic • Follicular, predominantly small cleaved cells • Follicular, mixed, small cleaved, and large cleaved cells	• Large cell, immunoblastic (B- or T-cell type) • Lymphoblastic • Small non-cleaved cell (Burkitt's and non-Burkitt's)	• Follicular, predominantly large cell, cleaved, and/or non-cleaved • Diffuse, small cleaved cell • Diffuse, large cell, cleaved, or noncleaved

- **WHO classification of lymphoid neoplasm:** It requires immunophenotyping, cytogenetics, fluorescent in situ hybridization (FISH), and antigen receptor gene rearrangement studies (**Table 12.62**).

Clinical Features

- **Age:** NHL can occur at any age, but the peak incidence is around 60 years.
- **Most common presentation:**
  - Painless firm, lymph node enlargement, or symptoms due to lymph node mass
  - *Extranodal involvement*: T-cell lymphoma involves bone marrow, gut, thyroid, lung, skin, testis, brain, and, more rarely, bone.

Table 12.62: World Health Organization (WHO) classification of lymphoid neoplasm.

Precursor B-cell neoplasms (immature B cells)	Precursor T-cell neoplasms (immature T cells)
Precursor B-lymphoblastic leukemia/lymphoma	Precursor T-lymphoblastic leukemia/lymphoma
Peripheral B-cell neoplasms (mature B cells)	*Peripheral T-cell and NK-cell neoplasms* (mature T cells and natural killer cells)
Chronic lymphocytic leukemia	T-cell prolymphocytic leukemia
B-cell prolymphocytic leukemia	Large granular lymphocytic leukemia
Lymphoplasmacytic lymphoma	Mycosis fungoides/Sezary syndrome
Mantle cell lymphoma	Peripheral T-cell lymphoma, unspecified
Follicular lymphoma	Anaplastic large cell lymphoma
Marginal zone lymphoma	Angioimmunoblastic T-cell lymphoma
Hairy cell leukemia	Adult T-cell leukemia/lymphoma
Plasmacytoma/plasma cell myeloma	Extranodal NK/T-cell lymphoma
Diffuse large B-cell lymphoma	
Burkitt lymphoma	

- *Bone marrow involvement* is more common in low-grade (50–60%) than high-grade (10%) and can produce cytopenias.
- Primary extranodal lymphomas present with soft tissue masses and symptoms relevant to the site. Waldeyer's ring and epitrochlear lymph nodes are frequently involved.
- *Pressure effects*: Due to NHL, include gut obstruction, ascites, superior vena caval obstruction, and spinal cord compression
- Involvement of liver and spleen results in hepatosplenomegaly.
- Patients with lymphoblastic lymphoma often present with an anterior mediastinal mass.
- Typically disseminates to the bone marrow and meninges and involves extranodal sites
□ NHL may be associated with "B" or systemic symptoms—weight loss, sweats, fever, and itching.
□ NHL is multicentric and spreads rapidly to non-contiguous areas, widespread at the time of diagnosis.
□ **Immunologic abnormalities:** Autoimmune hemolytic anemia and immune thrombocytopenia
□ **Paraneoplastic complications:** Neurological—demyelinating neuropathy, Guillain–Barré syndrome, autonomic dysfunction, peripheral neuropathy, skin—pemphigus, kidney—glomerulonephritis, and other systems—vasculitis, dermatomyositis, and cholestatic jaundice

Clinical Staging (Ann Arbor Classification)
Same staging system (**Table 12.56**) is used for both HL and NHL.

Investigations
Investigations required for staging disease are the same as that for Hodgkin lymphoma. Laparotomy is rarely required, only when retroperitoneal nodes are involved.
□ **Peripheral blood:**
  - *Anemia*: Moderate anemia may be observed when there is significant bone marrow involvement.
  - *Blood counts*: Usually normal, but few patients may show lymphocytosis.
  - Splenomegaly with hypersplenism or autoimmune hemolytic anemia may lead to reduced hemoglobin level, reticulocytosis, and positive Coombs' test.
□ **Bone marrow aspiration and trephine biopsy:** Marrow involvement is common with NHL.
□ **Other investigations:**
  - *Immunophenotyping*: It distinguishes T and B cell tumors, is done on blood, marrow, or lymph node material by flow cytometry and/or immunohistochemistry utilizing a minimal antibody panel (CD45, CD20, and CD3) to identify B, T, or NK subtypes.
  - *Immunoglobulin determination* is associated with IgG or IgM paraproteins.
  - *Measurement of uric acid levels:* Few very aggressive high-grade NHLs are associated with very high urate levels that can precipitate renal failure when treatment is started.
  - HIV testing
  - Serum levels of LDH, β_2-macroglobulin, and serum protein electrophoresis are often needed
  - *Diagnostic spinal tap* is required when a prophylactic instillation of cytarabine and methotrexate is indicated in high-risk patients (involvement of CNS, orbit, bone marrow, testis, spine, or skull base). It is indicated in HIV-associated lymphoma and highly aggressive lymphoma.

Management
Management of NHL is discussed in **Tables 12.63**.

CHOP-R	CVP-R	FCR
• Cyclophosphamide • Doxorubicin • Vincristine • Prednisone • Fixed dose rituximab	• Cyclophosphamide • Vincristine • Prednisone • Fixed dose rituximab	• Fludarabine • Cyclophosphamide • Rituximab

Difference between Hodgkin and non-Hodgkin lymphoma is described in **Table 12.64**.

Burkitt Lymphoma/Leukemia
It is highly aggressive, often extranodal B-cell lymphoma.

It is most common childhood malignancy worldwide and majority in children but can occur in all ages.

Male : female ratio is 3:1.

It often presents with extranodal involvement or as leukemia.

Three categories of Burkitt lymphoma are described in **Table 12.65**.

Table 12.63: Management of low- and high-grade non-Hodgkin lymphoma (NHL).

Low-grade NHL	High-grade NHL
Radiotherapy:	
Localized stage I disease	In few stages I patients without bulky disease Residual localized bulk disease after chemotherapy Spinal cord and other compression syndromes
Chemotherapy:	
• Oral therapy—chlorambucil (not curative) • Intensive IV chemotherapy in younger patients—better quality of life without any survival benefit	>90% of patients—IV combination chemotherapy—CHOP regimen (cyclophosphamide, doxorubicin, vincristine, and prednisolone)
Humanized monoclonal antibody therapy:	
• Rituximab, 131I-Tositumomab, and 90Y-Ibritumomab • Anti-CD20 antibody rituximab(R) alone or with chemotherapy, i.e., R-CVP recommended as first-line therapy	Combination with CHOP chemotherapy, rituximab (R) improves overall survival. R-CHOP: First-line therapy for those with stage II or greater diffuse large-cell lymphoma
Autologous bone marrow transplantation:	
	In relapsed chemosensitive disease

About 80% of cases are associated with a chromosomal translocation involving *myc* oncogene from chromosome 8 to the immunoglobulin (Ig) heavy chain region on chromosome 14 [t (8;14)].

Clinical Features

☐ **Endemic form**—presents as a rapidly growing jaw tumor in a young child (4-7 years). Mandibular and maxillary involvement leads to deformity, loosening of teeth, and extrusion of eye with loss of vision.
☐ **Sporadic form**—presents as an abdominal mass.
☐ **Immunodeficiency-associated (HIV) form** usually occurs with CD4 counts above 200/mm^3. It presents with abdominal involvement.
☐ **Abdominal involvement:** Mass due to bilateral involvement of kidneys, adrenals, ovaries, bowel, and lymph nodes.
☐ **Other sites:** CNS (adults), long bones, salivary glands, thyroid, testes, heart, breast, and bone marrow

Investigations

☐ **Histological examination:**
  • Distinctive, involved tissues are effaced by diffuse monotonous infiltrate of medium-sized lymphoid cells with round nuclei with clumped chromatin and multiple, centrally located nucleoli.
  • *Mitoses*—numerous, almost 100% of cells being in cell cycle.

Table 12.64: Difference between Hodgkin and non-Hodgkin lymphoma.

Characteristics	Hodgkin lymphoma	Non-Hodgkin lymphoma
Age	Bimodal peak incidence, 15–35 years and 45–70 years	Peak incidence around 60 years
"B" symptoms	More common	Less common
Alcohol-induced discomfort in lymph nodal region	Common	Not observed
Disease at the time of diagnosis	Usually well localized	Usually widespread
Site of involvement	Unifocal origin and arises in a single node or chain of nodes (cervical, mediastinal, and para-aortic)	Mostly involves multiple peripheral nodes (multicentric origin)
Pattern of spread	Orderly spread by contiguity, predictable	Noncontiguous spread, unpredictable
Epitrochlear node involvement	Rare	Common
Mediastinal involvement	Common	Uncommon
Mesenteric nodes, Waldeyer's ring	Rarely involved	Commonly involved
Bone marrow involvement	Late	Early
Extranodal involvement	Uncommon	Common
Neoplastic cells	Neoplastic cells—Hodgkin or Reed–Sternberg cells (1–5%)	Neoplastic cells form major tumor mass
Number of neoplastic cells	Few neoplastic cells (RS cells)	Majority of the cells are neoplastic

Table 12.65: Three categories of Burkitt lymphoma.

Endemic (African)	Sporadic (nonendemic)	Immunodeficiency associated
• Affects children and adolescents • Associated with EBV infection, corresponds malaria distribution • Involves extranodal sites, particularly the jaw, gastrointestinal tract, and gonads	Burkitt lymphoma	(HIV) lymphomas

(EBV: Epstein–Barr virus)

  • Plenty of *apoptotic* tumor cells. Nuclear remnants of the apoptotic cells are phagocytosed by benign macrophages, which are evenly, diffusely distributed

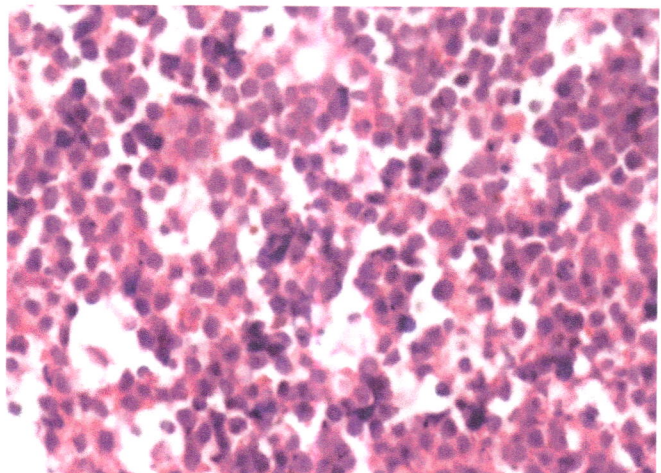

Fig. 12.29: Burkitt lymphoma composed of medium-sized lymphoid cells admixed with benign macrophages giving a "starry sky" appearance.

among the tightly packed basophilic tumor cells, creating a *"starry sky" pattern* (**Fig. 12.29**).
- **Chromosome analysis (Fig. 12.30):** The most common translocation results in movement of MYC-containing segment of chromosome 8 to chromosome 14q32, placing it close to *IGH* gene. Genetic notation for translocation is t(8:14)(q24; q32). As a result, MYC protein is overexpressed resulting in cell proliferation and stimulates apoptosis.
- Antibodies to EB viral capsid antigen may be detected (most—endemic type, many with sporadic and HIV-associated tumors).

Treatment
- Initiated urgently with curative intent whenever feasible
- Adequate hydration prior to the initiation of therapy to prevent the risk of tumor lysis syndrome
- Standard treatment comprises high-intensity, brief-duration cyclical combination chemotherapy
- Regimens include:
  - CHOP (cyclophosphamide, hydroxydaunorubicin or doxorubicin, vincristine, and prednisolone)
  - Rituximab plus EPOCH (etoposide, prednisolone, vincristine, cyclophosphamide, and doxorubicin)
  - CODOX-M/IVAC regimen (cyclophosphamide, vincristine, doxorubicin, methotrexate/ifosfamide, etoposide or VP-16, and cytarabine).
- Prophylactic central nervous system therapy is essential; intrathecal methotrexate or cytosine arabinoside is given in addition to high-dose systemic administration.
- Cure rates are high as 70–80%.

BLOOD TRANSFUSION

Red Cell Concentrates (Packed Red Cells)
General indications for RBC transfusion are described in **Table 12.66**.

Platelet Concentrate
Indications and contraindications of platelet transfusion are described in **Table 12.67**.

Granulocyte Concentrates
Granulocyte concentrates are prepared from single donors using cell separators.
Indications are severe neutropenia with definite evidence of bacterial infection.

Table 12.66: General indications for red blood cell (RBC) transfusion.

Replace acute blood loss due to hemorrhage or during surgery to relieve clinical features caused by insufficient oxygen delivery	• *Symptomatic anemia* • β-thalassemia major • Sickle cell anemia • Aplastic anemia • Severe anemia of any cause

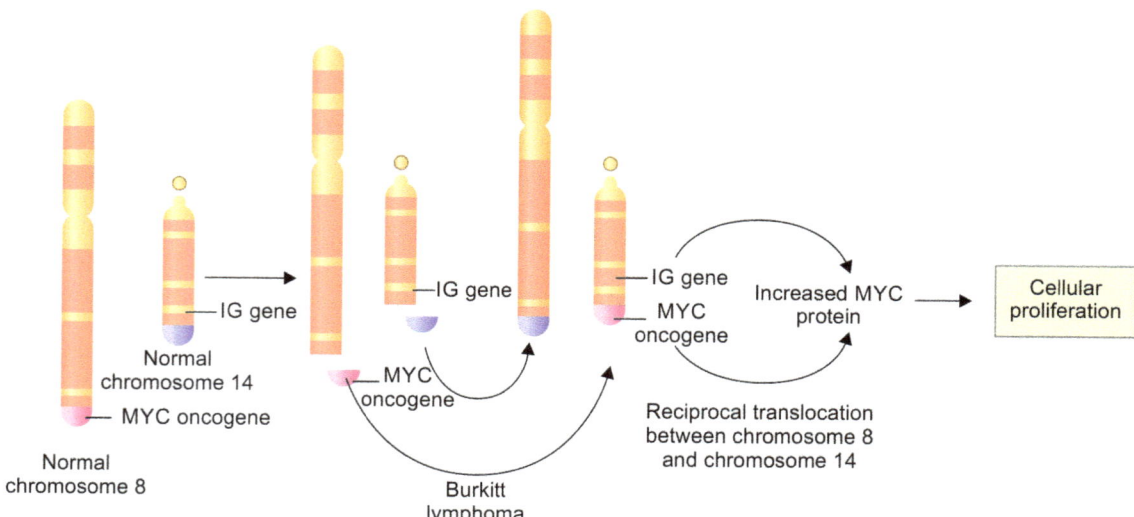

Fig. 12.30: Chromosomal translocation and activated mica oncogene in Burkitt lymphoma.

Table 12.67: Indications and contraindications of platelet transfusion.

Indications	Contraindication

Bleeding due to: Severe thrombocytopenia (when platelet count is less than 20,000/mm³)
• *Immune mediated:* Autoimmune thrombocytopenia—reserved for life-threatening bleeding
• *Secondary to bone marrow failure:*
  ▪ Chemotherapy induced
  ▪ Due to leukemia
  ▪ Dilutional
• Abnormal platelet function
• Disseminated intravascular coagulation (DIC)
Surgical or invasive procedures in thrombocytopenic patients
	• Thrombotic thrombocytopenic purpura (TTP)
	• Heparin induced thrombocytopenia (HIT)
	
	Relative contraindication: Idiopathic thrombocytopenic purpura (ITP) or post-transfusion purpura (PTP) because the survival of transfused platelets is very brief

Fresh Frozen Plasma

Indications: For replacement of coagulation factors in acquired coagulation factor deficiencies—
- Patients on anticoagulant drug therapy (Coumarin)
- Antithrombin deficiency
- Coagulopathy of liver diseases
- Vitamin K deficiency
- **Microangiopathic hemolytic anemia:** TTP, hemolytic uremic syndrome, and HELLP syndrome
- DIC

Cryoprecipitate

Indications:
- DIC, other conditions where fibrinogen level is very low (hypofibrinogenemia)
- It was used for hemophilia, factor XIII deficiency, and von Willebrand disease. However, it is no longer used for these disorders because of the greater risk of virus transmission compared with virus-inactivated coagulation factor concentrates **(Table 12.68)**.

Factor VIII and IX Concentrates

Freeze-dried preparations of coagulation factors are prepared from large pools of plasma from many donors.

Indications: *Hemophilia and von Willebrand disease*—when recombinant coagulation factors are unavailable. However, recombinant coagulation factor concentrates are the treatment of choice for patients with inherited coagulation factor deficiencies.

Table 12.68: Various coagulations factors and their amount in one unit of cryoprecipitate.

Coagulation factor	Quantity per unit
Fibrinogen	150–250 mg
Factor VIII	80–150 units
Von Willebrand factor	100–150 units
Factor XIII	50–75 units

Saline-washed Red Blood Cells

Effective means of removing leukocytes and plasma (up to 99%). This product is largely restricted to patients with antibodies to IgA or IgE, and those requiring red cells with minimal plasma as in thalassemia and paroxysmal nocturnal hemoglobinuria.

Frozen Red Blood Cells

Red blood cells can be frozen and stored up to 3 years by addition of glycerol as an endocellular cryoprotective agent. This procedure is used for storage of rare blood groups. Frozen red cells may be indicated for patients with history of severe allergic reactions to plasma or leukocyte factors, e.g., patients sensitized to IgA.

Irradiated Blood Products

Cellular blood products (red cells, platelets, and granulocytes) can be irradiated to a dose of 1,500 rads before transfusion in order to minimize the risk of transfusion-acquired graft-versus-host disease in immunocompromised individuals.

Immunoglobulins-Rh Immune Globulin

Indications:
- **Known or suspected inoculation of Rh negative mother with unknown or Rh positive fetal red cells:** Abortion, threatened abortion, ectopic pregnancy, amniocentesis, abdominal trauma in 2nd or 3rd trimester, and postpartum, if newborn is Rh positive.
- Following transfusion of Rh positive cellular blood products (e.g., platelets) to a Rh negative female of childbearing age or younger.
- Acute ITP resistant to steroids

Complications of Blood Transfusions

Complications of blood transfusion are given in **Table 12.69**.

Massive Transfusion

Massive transfusion is transfusion of more than 10 units of red cells or replacement of blood volume in 24 hours. The use of

Table 12.69: Complications of blood transfusion.

Immunological complications	Nonimmunological complications
Immediate reactions:	
• Acute hemolytic transfusion reactions • Febrile nonhemolytic reaction • Allergic reaction—urticaria • Anaphylactic reactions	• Transfusion-related acute lung injury (TRALI) • Circulatory overload • Air embolism
Delayed reactions:	
• Alloimmunization • Delayed hemolytic reactions (asymptomatic) • Transfusion-associated graft-versus-host disease • Post-transfusion purpura	• **Iron overload:** Transfusion hemosiderosis • Thrombophlebitis • **Infections:** Hepatitis (HBV, HCV, and HDV), HIV, malaria, cytomegalovirus, and syphilis

(HBV: hepatitis B virus; HCV: hepatitis C virus; HDV: hepatitis D virus)

large quantities of stored blood may lead to complications such as dilutional coagulopathy, circulatory overload, hyperkalemia, hypoglycemia, hypothermia, and citrate-induced hypocalcemia.

STEM-CELL THERAPY

Clinical application of stem-cell therapy is described in **Table 12.70**.

Table 12.70: Clinical application of stem-cell therapy.

Genetic diseases	Marrow failure syndromes
Red cell disorders: Thalassemia major and sickle cell disease	*Allogeneic or syngeneic BMT*
Immunodeficiencies: Severe combined immunodeficiency and X-linked agammaglobulinemia	Severe aplastic anemia, Fanconi syndrome, and PNH
Enzyme deficiencies: Gaucher's disease, mucopolysaccharidoses, and leukodystrophies	*Malignant diseases*
Granulocyte disorders: Chediak–Higashi syndrome, chronic granulomatous disease, and Kostmann syndrome	*Autologous, syngeneic, or allogeneic BMT*
Platelet disorders: Wiskott–Aldrich syndrome and Glanzmann's thrombasthenia	Acute leukemia and chronic leukemia
Other: Osteopetrosis	Myelodysplastic syndromes, Hodgkin's disease, non-Hodgkin lymphomas, breast cancer, and other solid tumors

(BMT: bone marrow transplantation; PNH: paroxysmal nocturnal hemoglobinuria)

BONE MARROW TRANSPLANTATION

Bone marrow transplantation is a type of hematopoietic stem cell transplantation **(Table 12.71)**.

Table 12.71: Indications for bone marrow transplantation.

Red blood cell disorders	WBC disorders
• Severe aplastic anemia • Thalassemia major • Fanconi anemia • Sickle cell disease • Pure red cell aplasia	• *Leukemia*: Acute lymphoblastic leukemia and chronic myeloid leukemia • Myelodysplastic syndromes • Hodgkin and non-Hodgkin lymphoma • Multiple myeloma
Immunological disorders	**Solid tumors**
Autoimmune diseases: Scleroderma and SLE Immune deficiency syndromes	Carcinoma breast, ovarian cancer, germ cell tumors, and neuroblastoma

(SLE: systemic lupus erythematosus; WBC: white blood cell)

OBJECTIVE-BASED SELF-EVALUATION

LONG QUESTIONS

1. Classify anemia. Discuss the etiology and clinical features of iron deficiency anemia.
2. Discuss iron metabolism. List the investigations done in a case of iron deficiency anemia.
3. Discuss the etiology, clinical features, and management of megaloblastic anemia.
4. Classify hemolytic anemias. Discuss the clinical features of thalassemia.
5. List the types of hemoglobinopathies. Enumerate the clinical features and complications of sickle cell anemia.
6. Discuss the pathogenesis, clinical features, and management of immune (idiopathic) thrombocytopenic purpura.
7. Discuss the inheritance, clinical features, and management of hemophilia A.
8. Discuss the inheritance, clinical features, and management of Von Willebrand disease.
9. Discuss the pathogenesis, clinical features, and management of thrombotic thrombocytopenia purpura.
10. Discuss the etiopathogenesis, clinical features and management of hemolytic–uremic syndrome.
11. Discuss the etiopathogenesis, clinical features and management of disseminated intravascular coagulation.
12. Discuss Hodgkin's lymphoma under the following headings—pathological types, staging and treatment options available.
13. Discuss chronic myeloid leukemia under the following headings—clinical features, specific investigations, and treatment options available.

SHORT ANSWER QUESTIONS

1. Microcytic hypochromic anemia.
2. Schilling test.
3. G6PD deficiency.
4. Autoimmune hemolytic anemia.
5. Pancytopenia—causes.
6. Causes of aplastic anemia.
7. Distinguishing patterns of bleeding in platelet and coagulation disorders.
8. Differences between acute and chronic immune (idiopathic) thrombocytopenic purpura (ITP).
9. Differences between polycythemia vera and secondary polycythemia.
10. Clinical features of multiple myeloma.
11. Ann Arbor classification.
12. Difference between Hodgkin and non-Hodgkin lymphoma.
13. Indications and contraindications of platelet transfusion.
14. Complications of blood transfusions.

15. Indications for hematopoietic stem cell transplantation.
16. Clinical application of stem cell therapy.
17. Classify myeloproliferative disorders.

MULTIPLE CHOICE QUESTIONS

1. In R-CHOP regimen for lymphoma R stands for:
   a. Rituximab
   b. Recombinant
   c. Revival
   d. Regenerative
2. Ann Arbor classification is used in:
   a. CLL
   b. CML
   c. Hodgkin's disease
   d. ALL
3. Presence of JAF2V617F mutation is diagnostic of:
   a. Multiple myeloma
   b. Polycythaemia vera
   c. Megaloblastic anemia
   d. Aplastic anemia
4. Tyrosine kinase inhibitors like imatinib is used in treatment of:
   a. AML
   b. ALL
   c. CLL
   d. CML
5. Christmas disease is caused by deficiency of factor:
   a. 7
   b. 8
   c. 9
   d. 10
6. Activated partial thromboplastin time is a measure of:
   a. Platelet function
   b. Extrinsic coagulation pathway
   c. Intrinsic coagulation pathway
   d. Common coagulation pathway
7. Normocytic and normochromic anemia with anisopoikilocytosis, reticulocytosis, and spherocytes, bite (blister) cells, and Heinz bodies is seen in:
   a. Glucose-6-phosphate dehydrogenase deficiency
   b. Hereditary spherocytosis
   c. Aplastic anemia
   d. Sickle cell anemia
8. Most common inherited hemolytic anemia in adults is:
   a. Glucose-6-phosphate dehydrogenase deficiency
   b. Hereditary spherocytosis
   c. Thalassemia
   d. Sickle cell anemia
9. Vitamin B12 is absorbed in the:
   a. Stomach
   b. Duodenum
   c. Jejunum
   d. Ileum
10. All the following are differential diagnosis for microcytic hypochromic anemia, *except:*
    a. Iron deficiency
    b. Thalassemia
    c. Lead poisoning
    d. Folic acid deficiency

ANSWERS

| 1. a | 2. c | 3. b | 4. d | 5. c |
| 6. c | 7. a | 8. b | 9. d | 10. d |

Nutrition

CHAPTER OUTLINE

- Nutritional Assessment
- Vitamin A
- Vitamin B Complex
- Vitamin C
- Scurvy
- Vitamin D
- Vitamin E (Tocopherol)
- Vitamin K
- Calcium Homeostasis
- Hyperparathyroidism
- Hypercalcemia
- Hypoparathyroidism
- Tetany
- Trace Elements
- Protein-Energy Malnutrition
- Obesity

NUTRITIONAL ASSESSMENT

Nutritional Anthropometry

(Discussed in Chapter 2 under General Physical Examination)

- **Body weight and body mass index (BMI)**
- **Skin-fold measurements:** Subcutaneous fat tissues normally account for half of the entire body fat mass, and the measurement of skin-fold thickness (SFT) gives information on the energy stores of the body, mainly fat stores (i.e., triglycerides). Biceps, triceps, subscapular, and suprailiac SFT is measured.
- **Mid-upper-arm muscle circumference (MAMC)** reflects the muscle mass, while the mid-arm muscle area (MAMA) gives information about the muscle protein stores, as half of the body's proteins are stored in the skeletal muscles. The MAMA is calculated from the MAMC and the triceps SFT [MAMA = MAMC − (0.314 × SFT)].
- **Assessment of body composition:** Body composition describes the body compartments, such as fat mass, fat-free mass, muscle mass, and bone mineral mass. The methods used are bioelectrical independence analysis, creatinine height index, dual energy X-ray absorptiometry, MRI, CT, dilution method, and neutron activation.
- **Laboratory investigations:** Complete blood count, lipid profile, electrolytes, albumin, transferrin, prealbumin/transthyretin (TTR), retinol-binding protein (RBP), and insulin-like growth factor 1 (IGF-1).

Signs and Symptoms of Micronutrient Deficiencies

See **Table 13.1**.

Recommended Dietary Allowances (RDAs)/Adequate Intake of Vitamins and Minerals

See **Table 13.2**.

Table 13.1: Signs and symptoms of micronutrient deficiencies.

Vitamin deficiency	Manifestation
Fat-soluble vitamins	
Vitamin A, retinol	Night blindness, keratomalacia, Bitot spots
Vitamin D, ergo/cholecalciferol	• Rickets/osteomalacia • Bone pain, costochondral beading • Proximal myopathy
Vitamin E, tocopherol	Hemolysis, posterior column signs, ataxia, muscle wasting, retinitis pigmentosa-like changes, night blindness
Vitamin K, Phylloquinone and other Menaquinone	Bruising, purpura, nose, and gastrointestinal (GI) bleeds
Water-soluble vitamin (B-complex and vitamin C)	
B_1 (Thiamine)	• Wernicke encephalopathy • Korsakoff syndrome • Beriberi • Nystagmus, sixth cranial nerve palsy, ataxia, dementia, neuropathy • Cardiac failure • Anemia

Contd...

Contd...

Vitamin deficiency	Manifestation
B_2 (riboflavin)	• Ariboflavinosis • Angular stomatitis, glossitis, magenta tongue
B_3 (niacin)	Pellagra dermatitis of sun-exposed areas, dementia, poor appetite, difficulty sleeping, confusion, sore mouth
B_4 (Adenine)*	• Immune dysfunction • Aging
B_5 (pantothenic acid)	Nausea, abdominal pain, paresthesia, burning feet
B_6 (pyridoxine)	Poor appetite, lassitude, oxaluria
B_7 (biotin)	Dermatitis, depression, lassitude, muscle pains, blepharitis
B_8 (ionositol)*	Depression and other psychiatric manifestations
B_9 (folic acid)	Macrocytic anemia, thrombocytopenia, and megaloblastic bone marrow
B_{10} (PABA)*	• Free-radical damage • Sun burns and skin rashes
B_{11} (salicylic acid) *	Works in tandem with vitamin B_{12}
B_{12} (cobalamine)	Subacute combined degeneration, macrocytic anemia, icterus, knuckle pigmentation
Vitamin C (ascorbic acid)	• Scurvy • Poor wound healing, fatigue, limb pain, scorbutic rosary, difficulty sleeping, gingivitis, perifollicular purpura, hyperkeratosis

*Note: Vitamin B4, 8, 10, 11 are no longer labeled as vitamins, as they do not fit the official definition of vitamin.

Minerals	
Iron	Koilonychia, smooth tongue, anemia, esophageal web
Copper	Microcytic hypochromic anemia, neutropenia, scurvy-like bone lesions, osteoporosis
Zinc	• Acrodermatitis enteropathica • Peristomal/perinasal/perineal erythema, thin hair, diarrhea, apathy, anorexia, growth failure, hypoglycemia • Distorted or diminished taste (hypogeusia)
Chromium	Peripheral neuropathy, hyperglycemia
Selenium	Cardiomyopathy
Iodine	Goiter
Others	
Protein deficiency	• Pitting edema • Hair: thinning, easily pluckable with dyspigmentation or flag sign, and change in texture to silken, sparse hair. • Dermatosis with desquamation of the so-called flaky-paint type, with or without hyperpigmentation.

Table 13.2: Recommended dietary allowances.

Vitamin or mineral	Recommended Dietary Allowance (RDA) or Adequate Intake (AI) Nutrients with AIs are marked with an (*)	Upper Tolerable Limit (UL) The highest amount you can take without risk
Calcium	Age 19–50: 1,000 mg/day Women age 51+: 1,200 mg/day Men age 71+: 1,200 mg/day	Age 19–50: 2,500 mg/day Age 51 and up: 2,000 mg/day
Chloride	Age 19–50: 2,300 mg/day Age 50–70: 2,000 mg/day Age 70 and older: 1,800 mg/day	3,600 mg/day
Choline (vitamin B complex)	Women: 425 mg/day * Men: 550 mg/day *	3,500 mg/day
Copper	900 µg/day	10,000 µg/day
Fluoride	Men: 4 mg/day * Women: 3 mg/day *	10 mg/day

Contd...

Contd...

Vitamin or mineral	Recommended Dietary Allowance (RDA) or Adequate Intake (AI) Nutrients with AIs are marked with an (*)	Upper Tolerable Limit (UL) The highest amount you can take without risk
Folic acid (folate)	400 µg/day	1,000 µg/day This applies only to synthetic folic acid in supplements or fortified foods. There is no upper limit for folic acid from natural sources.
Iodine	150 µg/day	1,100 µg/day
Iron	*Men:* 8 mg/day *Women age 19–50:* 18 mg/day *Women age 51 and up:* 8 mg/day	45 mg/day
Magnesium	*Men age 19–30:* 400 mg/day *Men age 31 and up:* 420 mg/day *Women age 19–30:* 310 mg/day *Women age 31 and up:* 320 mg/day	350 mg/day This applies only to magnesium in supplements or fortified foods. There is no upper limit for magnesium in food and water.
Manganese	*Men:* 2.3 mg/day* *Women:* 1.8 mg/day*	11 mg/day
Molybdenum	45 µg/day	2,000 µg/day
Phosphorus	700 mg/day	Up to age 70: 4,000 mg/day Over age 70: 3,000 mg/day
Selenium	55 µg/day	400 µg/day
Sodium	*Age 19–50:* 1,500 mg/day * *Age 51–70:* 1,300 mg/day * *Age 71 and up:* 1,200 mg/day *	2,300 mg/day
Vitamin A	*Men:* 900 µg/day *Women:* 700 µg/day	3,000 µg/day
Vitamin B$_3$ (Niacin)	*Men:* 16 mg/day *Women:* 14 mg/day	35 mg/day This applies only to niacin in supplements or fortified foods. There is no upper limit for niacin in natural sources.
Vitamin B$_6$	*Men age 19–50:* 1.3 mg/day *Men age 51 up:* 1.7 mg/day *Women age 19–50:* 1.3 mg/day *Women age 51 up:* 1.5 mg/day	100 mg/day
Vitamin C	*Men:* 90 mg/day *Women:* 75 mg/day	2,000 mg/day
Vitamin D (calciferol)	*Age 1–70:* 15 µg/day (600 IU, or international units)* *Age 70 and older:* 20 µg/day (800 IU)*	100 µg/day (4,000 IU)
Vitamin E (alpha-tocopherol)	22.4 IU/day (15 mg/day)	1,500 IU/day (1,000 mg/day) This applies only to vitamin E in supplements or fortified foods. There is no upper limit for vitamin E from natural sources.
Zinc	*Men:* 11 mg/day *Women:* 8 mg/day	40 mg/day

VITAMIN A

Vitamin A is the name given to a group of fat-soluble vitamins and includes provitamin A carotenoids and preformed vitamin A retinoid and carotenoids.

- **Dietary source**:
  - Provitamin A carotenoids—found in plants. For example, beta-carotene, alpha-carotene, and beta-cryptoxanthin. Sources—dark green and deeply colored fruits and vegetables.
  - Preformed vitamin A (retinol, retinal, retinoic acid, and retinyl esters) is the most active form of vitamin A; it is mostly found in animal sources of food and is also the form supplied by most supplements. Sources—liver, fish, milk, eggs, butter, cheese.

- **Functions of vitamin A:** Vitamin A has several metabolic roles. The main functions of vitamin A in humans are as follows:
  - *Maintenance of normal vision:* Vitamin A is essential for **dark adaptation** and its deficiency causes **nyctalopia**. Mainly controlled by retinaldehyde.
  - *Host resistance to infections:* Vitamin A deficiency causes keratinization of mucous membranes and thereby

increases the risk of infections. RBP is a **negative "acute phase protein"**.
- *Immune function:* Vitamin A has the ability to stimulate the immune system. Retinoids are required for normal growth, fetal development, fertility, hematopoiesis, and immune function.
- *Control of cell growth and differentiation:* Vitamin A is needed for the maintenance of the surface linings of the eyes, growth, and repair of epithelial cells, and integrity of the epithelial cells of the respiratory, urinary, and intestinal tracts. In vitamin A deficiency, mucus-secreting cells are replaced by keratin-producing cells and this process is known as squamous metaplasia.
- *Regulation of lipid metabolism:* Fatty acid metabolism, including fatty acid oxidation in fat tissue and muscle, adipogenesis, and lipoprotein metabolism require vitamin A.
- *Antioxidant:* Retinoids, beta-carotene, and some related carotenoids act as photoprotective and act as antioxidants.
- *Other functions:* Vitamin A is involved in growth of bone, reproduction, embryonic development and the regulation of adult genes.
- *Tretinoin*, i.e., all-trans-retinoic acid (ATRA) is also used to treat acute promyelocytic leukemia (APL), **isotretinoin,** is used to treat psoriasis and 13-cis-retinoic acid is used in the treatment of acne.

Vitamin A Deficiency

Causes of vitamin a deficiency are described in **Table 13.3**.

Clinical Features/Manifestations
- **Eye changes:**
  - Xerophthalmia describes a spectrum of eye disease caused by vitamin A deficiency, which includes Bitot's spots, corneal xerosis, and keratomalacia.
    - **Bitot's spots (Fig. 13.1):** In young children with vitamin A deficiency, areas of abnormal squamous cell proliferation and keratinization of the conjunctiva known as Bitot's spots can be seen.
    - Corneal xerosis refers to dryness of cornea.
    - **Keratomalacia:** In advanced disease, the cornea becomes hazy and erosions can develop, finally leading to its destruction (keratomalacia).
  - **Night blindness** (nyctalopia) and retinopathy
- **Skin changes:**
  - Hyperkeratosis
  - Phrynoderma (follicular hyperkeratosis)
  - Xerosis (**Fig. 13.2**)

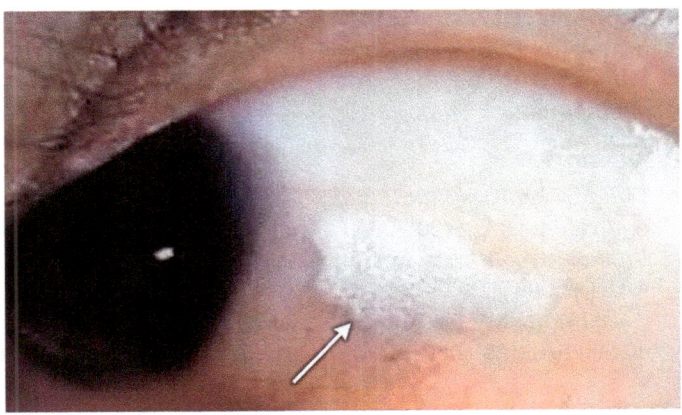

Fig. 13.1: Bitot's spot.

- **Impairment of humoral and cell-mediated immunity** causing increased susceptibility to infections.
- **Other features:**
  - Fatigue
  - Anemia
  - Diarrhea
  - Decreased growth rate
  - Decreased bone development
  - Infertility

Laboratory Investigations
- **Serum retinol level:** Normal range is 28–86 µg/dL (1–3 µmol/L). The level decreases in vitamin A deficiency.
- **Albumin levels** are indirect measures of vitamin A levels.
- **Complete blood count** (CBC) with differential count to be done, if there is a possibility of anemia, infection, or sepsis.

Diagnosis
- It is mainly on the basis of the **clinical features**. Response to replacement therapy is the best way for the diagnosis.
- Serum retinol levels less than 20 µg/dL suggest deficiency, or the ratio of retinol: RBP < 0.8 suggests deficiency.

Treatment
- Xerophthalmia (irrespective of stage) should be treated with 200,000 IU of vitamin A in oily solution, usually contained in a soft-gel capsule. Three doses: day 0, day 1, and day 14.
- If child is suffering from measles give two capsules of 200,000 IU for two consecutive days.

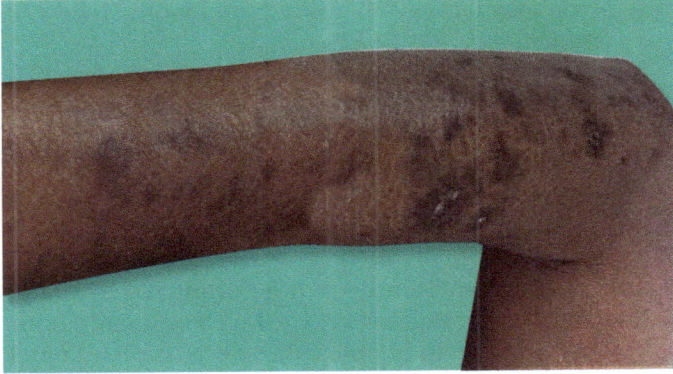

Fig. 13.2: Xerosis of skin in vitamin A deficiency.

Table 13.3: Causes of vitamin A deficiency.

Primary causes	Secondary causes
• Prolonged dietary deprivation • Vegetarians • Refugees • Chronic alcoholics • Toddlers • Preschool children	• Sprue • Cystic fibrosis • Pancreatic insufficiency • Duodenal bypass • Chronic diarrhea • Bile duct obstruction • Giardiasis and cirrhosis

- **Prophylactic vitamin A** at a dose of 200,000 IU every 6 months is to be given to all high-risk individuals. Patients with malabsorption syndrome need vitamin A supplements.

Prevention
- *Children between 1 and 5 years of age:* 60,000 retinol activity equivalent (RAE) (200,000 IU) per oral every 6 month
- *Infants <6 months:* It can be given a one-time dose of 15,000 RAE (50,000 IU).
- *6–12 months of age:* It can be given a one-time dose of 30,000 RAE (100,000 IU).

Vitamin A Toxicity
- **Types of toxicity:** Vitamin A toxicity can be **acute** (usually due to accidental ingestion by children) or **chronic**. Both types of toxicity cause **headache and increased intracranial pressure (pseudotumor cerebri).**
  - **Acute** toxicity also produces **nausea and vomiting, vertigo, diplopia, bulging fontanels, seizures, exfoliative dermatitis.** Single doses of 300 mg in adults or 100 mg in children can be harmful.
  - **Chronic** toxicity occurs with amounts higher than 10 times the recommended dietary allowances (RDA) causes changes in skin, hair (loss), and nails; liver and bone damage; double vision, ataxia, hyperlipidemia, and vomiting.
- **Retinol is teratogenic** and incidence of birth defects in infants is high with vitamin A intakes of >3 mg a day during pregnancy (**spontaneous abortions** and **fetal malformations**, including microcephaly and cardiac anomalies).
- **Carotenemia** is common among infants and toddlers who eat large amounts of carrots and green leafy vegetables. It can be confused with jaundice, but discoloration of skin spontaneously resolves once the intake of carotenoid rich food is reduced.

VITAMIN B COMPLEX

Thiamine (B_1)
- **Functions:** Thiamine is an important **water-soluble** vitamin.
  - Involved in **carbohydrate, fat, amino acid, glucose, and alcohol metabolism**.
  - Vitamin B_1 is **essential** for the **coenzyme**, thiamine pyrophosphate (TPP). It is required for the following reactions:
    - Decarboxylation of pyruvate (glycolytic pathway) to acetyl CoA (Krebs cycle)
    - Transketolase in the hexose monophosphate (HMP/pentose) shunt pathway
    - Decarboxylation of α-ketoglutarate to succinate (Krebs cycle)
  - Has an additional role in neuronal conduction.
- **Sources:** These vitamins can be produced by plants and some microorganisms. However, animals cannot synthesize them. In humans, the source is diet, though small amounts may be synthesized by intestinal bacteria.
- **Dietary sources:** Good dietary sources of thiamine are **whole wheat flour, unpolished rice, cereals, grains, beans, nuts, and yeast.** There is little or no thiamine in milled rice and grains. Thus, thiamine deficiency is more common in individuals who consume mainly a rice-based diet.
- It is also present in **liver, meat, and eggs**.
- **Requirement:** Up to 30 mg of thiamine can be stored in body tissues. Required daily allowance (RDA) is **0.5–0.9 mg daily for children, 1.2 mg daily for adult men, and 1.1 mg daily for nonpregnant adult women**.
- Causes of thiamine deficiency are listed in **Table 13.4**.

Thiamine Deficiency
Wet (Cardiovascular) Beriberi
- Wet beriberi is the term used for the **cardiovascular involvement** of thiamine deficiency.
- First effects are **vasodilatation, tachycardia**, a wide-pulse pressure, sweating, warm skin, and lactic acidosis. Later, **congestive heart failure** develops, causing orthopnea and pulmonary and peripheral edema. Marked cardiomegaly is present.
- **Infantile beriberi** occurs in infants (usually by age 3–4 weeks) who are breastfed by **thiamine-deficient mothers.** Heart failure can develop suddenly and presents with edema, aphonia, tachycardia, tachypnea, and absent deep tendon reflexes. If prompt treatment is not given, death occurs quickly.
- **Shoshin beriberi:** A more rapid form of wet beriberi is termed **acute fulminant cardiovascular beriberi.**

Dry Beriberi
- Dry beriberi usually manifests insidiously with **symmetrical peripheral neuropathy.**
- **Early symptoms:** There is bilateral and roughly symmetrical heaviness and stiffness of the legs.
- **Later symptoms:** These include weakness, numbness, and pins and needles (occurring in a stocking-glove distribution).

Table 13.4: Causes of thiamine deficiency.

Lack of thiamine intake	Decreased absorption
• Starvation state • Food items like milled rice, raw freshwater fish, raw shellfish, and ferns that have a high level of *thiaminase*. • Food high in *anti-thiamine factor*, such as tea, coffee, and betel nuts • Alcoholic state	• Chronic intestinal disease • Alcoholism • Malnutrition • Gastric bypass surgery • Malabsorption syndrome—celiac and tropical sprue
Increased consumption states	**Increased depletion**
• Diets high in carbohydrate or saturated fat intake • Pregnancy and lactation • Hyperthyroidism • Fever—severe infection Increased physical exercise	• Diarrhea • Peritoneal dialysis, hemodialysis, diuretic therapies • Hyperemesis gravidarum

- **Distribution of neuropathy:** They affect predominantly the lower limbs. They begin with paresthesias in the toes, burning in the feet (severe at night), muscle cramps in the calves, pains in the legs, and plantar dysesthesias.
- **Physical signs**: Calf muscle tenderness, difficulty rising from a squatting position, and decreased vibratory sensation in the toes. The ankle jerk reflexes are lost.
- Deficiency may also cause **degeneration of thalamus, mammillary bodies, and cerebellum.**

Biochemical Tests
- Measurement of thiamine, pyruvate, and lactate levels in blood or urine.
- Erythrocyte thiamine transketolase activity.

Management
- Complete bed rest
- 200 mg thiamine three times a day given till acute symptoms disappear, after that 10 mg/day till recovery
- Parenteral thiamine produces marked diuresis (in wet beriberi), resulting in dramatic improvement in the symptoms.

Wernicke's Encephalopathy (WE)
It is an acute neuropsychiatric condition. Initially, it is reversible biochemical brain lesion caused by depletion of vitamin B_1 (thiamine).
- **Clinical features:**
    - Wernicke's encephalopathy is a **triad of global confusion, ophthalmoplegia, and ataxia**, along with confusion. Impairment in the synthesis of one of the important enzymes of the **pentose phosphate pathway (erythrocyte transketolase)** may explain such a predisposition.
    - *Encephalopathy:* It is characterized by confusion, severe disorientation, indifference, and inattentiveness. There is also impaired memory and learning. If untreated patients will progress through stupor and coma to death.
    - *Oculomotor dysfunction:* Nystagmus, lateral rectus palsy, and lesions of the oculomotor, abducens, and vestibular nuclei resulting in conjugate gaze palsy.
    - *Gait ataxia:* Ataxia mainly involves stance and gait. It is probably due to a combination of polyneuropathy, cerebellar involvement, and vestibular dysfunction.
- **Diagnosis:** For confirmation of the diagnosis measure the circulating thiamine concentration or transketolase activity in red cells using fresh heparinized blood. MRI may show **periventricular lesions** surrounding third ventricle, aqueduct and fourth ventricle with **petechial hemorrhages** in acute cases and atrophy of mammillary bodies in chronic cases.
- **Management:**
    - Wernicke's disease is a medical emergency and requires immediate administration of thiamine.
    - **Dosage:** 500 mg of thiamine intravenously, infused over 30 minutes, three times daily for two consecutive days and 250 mg intravenously or intramuscularly once daily for an additional 5 days, in combination with other B vitamins.
    - Magnesium is often needed because it is a cofactor required for normal functioning of thiamine-dependent enzymes.
    - Wernicke encephalopathy may be precipitated by administration of intravenous glucose solutions to individuals with thiamine deficiency. In susceptible individuals, glucose administration should be preceded or accompanied by thiamine 100 mg IV.

Korsakoff's Psychosis/Syndrome
- Korsakoff's psychosis is caused by **deficiency of thiamine** with **involvement of central nervous system.**
- **Memory disturbances:** It is predominantly associated with **defect in retentive memory** (severe defect in storing new information and learning). Thus, there are **disturbances of short-term memory.** There are also marked deficits in anterograde and retrograde memory.
- Other features include apathy, an intact sensorium and relative preservation of long-term memory and other cognitive skills.
- **Confabulation:** It is a memory disturbance, characterized by the production of fabricated, distorted, or misinterpreted memories about oneself or the world, without the conscious intention to deceive. Attention and social behavior are relatively maintained. Affected individuals can perform conversation that may seem normal to an unsuspecting spectator.
- The syndrome is common in **chronic alcoholics**. It may also be seen with thiamine deficiency due to **gastric disorders** (e.g., carcinoma, chronic gastritis, or persistent vomiting).
- **Treatment:** Parenteral thiamine (100 mg IM daily for 7 days).

Vitamin B_2 (Riboflavin)
- **Source:** Milk and eggs, meats, fish, green vegetables, yeast, and enriched foods (fortified cereals and breads).
- **Actions:**
    - Essential component of coenzymes involved in multiple cellular metabolic pathways like tricarboxylic acid (TCA) cycle and beta-oxidation of fatty acids.
    - Flavoproteins are involved in multiple redox reactions and function as electron transporters.
- **Deficiency:**
    - *Causes:*
        - Anorexia nervosa
        - Malabsorptive syndromes
        - Glutaric acidemia type 1
        - Multiple acyl-coenzyme A (CoA) dehydrogenase deficiency (MADD)
        - Brown-Vialetto-Van Laere syndrome (defect in riboflavin transporter)
        - Long-term use of barbiturates can cause oxidation of riboflavin.

- Lactose intolerance because dairy products are a good source of riboflavin.
- *Features:*
  - Cheilitis
  - Stomatitis
  - Glossitis
  - Normochromic anemia
  - Seborrheic dermatitis
- Pure deficiency of riboflavin is rare.

Vitamin B$_3$ (Niacin)

- **Sources:**
  - Yeast, meats (especially liver), grains, legumes, corn used in tortilla, and seeds.
  - Tryptophan can be converted to a niacin derivative in the liver. However, it requires approximately 60 mg of tryptophan to produce 1 mg of niacin, and this process requires vitamin B$_6$ (pyridoxine).
- **Actions:** NAD/NADP are cofactors for many enzymatic redox reactions.
- **RDA:** Dosed as a "niacin equivalent" (NE), in which 1 NE is equal to 1 mg of niacin, or 60 mg of dietary tryptophan. RDA is 6–12 mg daily in children, 16 mg for adult males, and 14 mg daily for nonpregnant adult females.

Pellagra

- **Vitamin B$_3$ niacin (nicotinamide) deficiency** causes a metabolic encephalopathy called **pellagra.**
- It is found mostly in populations in which corn is the major source of energy in parts of China, Africa, and India. Pellagra means raw skin.

Causes:
- **Inadequate intake:** Maize or jowar (sorghum) diet, malnutrition, chronic alcoholism, anorexia nervosa.
- **Generalized malabsorption** (rare)
- **Drug-induced:**
  - Prolonged isoniazid therapy
  - Pyrazinamide
  - 6-mercaptopurine
  - 5-fluorouracil
  - Azathioprine
  - Ethionamide
  - Carbamazepine
  - Phenytoin
  - Phenobarbitone
- **Other disorders:**
  - *Hartnup's disease:* It is a rare genetic disorder, in which there is reduced absorption of basic amino acids including tryptophan by the gut.
  - *Carcinoid syndrome and pheochromocytoma:* In these conditions, tryptophan metabolism is diverted away from the formation of nicotinamide to form amines producing pellagra-like symptoms.

Clinical features:
Pellagra has been easily remembered a disease of four D's namely: (1) **dermatitis;** (2) **diarrhea;** (3) **dementia** (depression); and (4) **death**. However, these features are not always observed and the mental changes are not a true dementia.

1. **Skin manifestations:**
   - **Casal's necklace or collar rash:** Characteristic skin rash develops that is hyperpigmented and scaling that develops in skin areas exposed to sunlight. This rash forms a ring around the neck and is termed Casal's necklace (**Fig. 13.3**).
   - *Dermatitis:* Lesions of the skin may progress to vesiculation, cracking (ulceration), exudation, and secondary infection. Symmetrical chronic thickening, dryness and pigmentation may be seen on the dorsal surfaces of the hands.
2. **Gastrointestinal (GI) tract:**
   - *Diarrhea:* It may be in part due to proctitis and in part due to malabsorption. It is often a feature accompanied by anorexia, nausea, glossitis, and dysphagia indicating noninfective inflammation of the entire GI tract.
   - Other features include raw, painful, bright red tongue (glossitis), angular stomatitis, vaginitis, esophagitis, vertigo, and burning dysesthesia.
3. **Dementia:**
   - This occurs in chronic severe deficiency and may also develop hallucinations and acute psychosis.
   - Milder deficiency may present with depression, apathy and sometimes thought disorders.
   - Other neurologic symptoms include insomnia, anxiety, disorientation, tremor, delusions, dementia, and encephalopathy.

Diagnosis:
- Diagnosis in **endemic region** depends on the clinical features. Other vitamin deficiencies can also produce similar changes (e.g., angular stomatitis).
- **Dramatic improvement:** The response is usually rapid in the skin (within 24 hours), diarrhea and a striking improvement occurs in the patient's mental state **with nicotinamide** treatment.

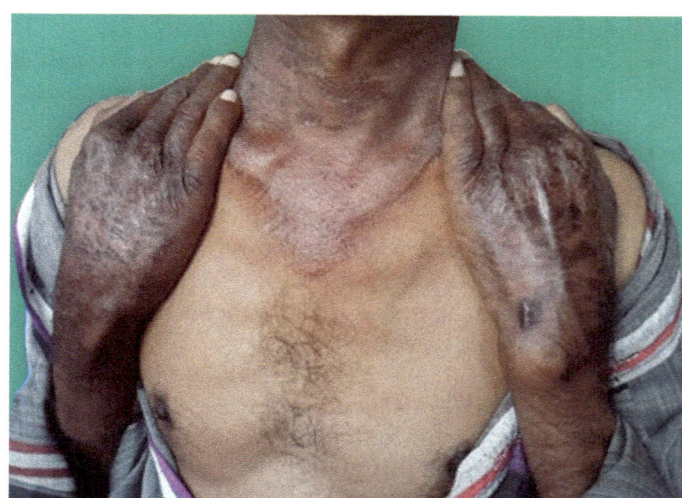

Fig. 13.3: Casal's necklace and dermatitis.

- Niacin status can be assessed by measuring urinary N-methylnicotinamide, 2-pyridonenicotinamide or by measuring the erythrocyte NAD: NADP (ratio).

Management/Treatment:
- **Nicotinamide:** 100–200 mg three times daily orally (approximately 300 mg daily) with a maintenance dose of 50 mg daily.
- **High-protein diet** with **adequate nutrients** and treatment of malnutrition.
- **Supplementation of other vitamin B** complex with **iron and folic acid** is also given, as other deficiencies are often likely to be present.
- In moderate-to-high doses (1–3 g a day) niacin is a well-established antihyperlipidemic agent.

Vitamin B_5 (Pantothenic Acid)

- **Sources:**
  - Egg yolk, liver, kidney, broccoli, and milk
  - Pantothenic acid is also produced by **bacteria in the colon**
  - Main dietary source of pantothenic acid is in the form of **coenzyme A.**
- **Actions:** CoA is involved in **metabolism** of vitamins A, D, cholesterol, steroids, heme A, fatty acids, carbohydrates, amino acids, and proteins.
- **RDA:**
  - The recommended intake for pantothenic acid is expressed as **adequate intake (AI)** rather than RDA.
  - The AI is 2–4 mg daily for children and 5 mg daily for adult men and women.
- **Deficiency:** Pantothenic acid deficiency is very rare in humans.
- **Clinical manifestations:**
  - Paresthesias and dysesthesias, referred to as "**burning feet syndrome**".
  - GI disturbance, depression, muscle cramps, hypoglycemia, ataxia, etc.
- **Diagnosis:**
  - Blood, plasma, serum, or urine pantothenic acid levels.
  - **Urine levels** are most reliable indicator of dietary intake.

Vitamin B_6 (Pyridoxine)

Vitamin B_6 consists of **pyridoxine, pyridoxamine, pyridoxal**, and the **phosphorylated derivatives** of each of these compounds.

- **Sources:**
  - Pyridoxine and pyridoxamine are predominantly found in plant foods.
  - Pyridoxal is most commonly derived from animal foods.
  - Meats, whole grains, vegetables, and nuts are the best sources.
- **Actions:**
  - Gluconeogenesis
  - Decarboxylation of amino acids
  - Conversion of tryptophan to niacin
  - Heme synthesis
  - Sphingolipid biosynthesis
  - Neurotransmitter synthesis
  - Steroid hormone modulation
  - Trans-sulfuration pathway by which homocysteine is converted into cystathionine and its subsequent conversion to cysteine.
- **RDA:**
  - 0.5–1 mg in children
  - 1.3 mg daily for young men and women
  - 1.7 mg daily for men older than 50 years
  - 1.5 mg daily for women older than 50 years
- **Deficiency:** Overt deficiency is rare.
- **Causes:**
  - *Drugs:* Isoniazid, penicillamine, hydralazine, and levodopa/carbidopa
  - Associated with—asthma, diabetes, alcoholism, heart disease, pregnancy, breast cancer, Hodgkin lymphoma, and sickle-cell anemia
- **Clinical manifestations:**
  - Nonspecific stomatitis, glossitis, cheilosis, irritability, confusion, and depression, and possibly peripheral neuropathy.
  - Severe deficiency is associated with **seborrheic dermatitis, microcytic anemia,** and **seizures**
  - A number of genetic syndromes affecting PLP-dependent enzymes, such as homocystinuria, cystathioninuria, and xanthurenic aciduria mimic vitamin B_6 deficiency.
  - An inborn error of pyridoxine metabolism is responsible for **pyridoxine-dependent epilepsy.**
  - Cystathionine synthase is a PLP-dependent enzyme, which produces cystathionine from serine and homocysteine. As a result, vitamin B_6 insufficiency can lead to elevations in plasma homocysteine concentrations, a risk factor for the development of atherosclerosis and venous thromboembolism.
- **Diagnosis:**
  - **PLP concentrations** >30 nmol/L (>7.4 ng/mL) are normal.
  - **Erythrocyte transaminase activity**, with and without PLP added.
  - Urinary 4-pyridoxic acid excretion >3.0 mmol/day
  - Urinary excretion of xanthurenic acid is normally <65 mmol/day following 2 g tryptophan loads. **Increased xanthurenic acid excretion** suggests vitamin B_6 deficiency due to abnormal tryptophan metabolism.
- **Treatment:**
  - 50 mg/day in regular deficiency
  - In case of deficiency secondary to certain drugs—higher doses of 100–200 mg/day are given.
- **Toxicity:** Peripheral neuropathy, dermatoses, photosensitivity, dizziness, and nausea have been reported with pyridoxine of over 250 mg/day.

Biotin

- **Sources:** Liver, egg yolk, soybean products, and yeast
- **Actions: Essential cofactor** for several carboxylase enzyme complexes involved in carbohydrate, amino acid, and lipid **metabolism.**
- **RDA:** The AI is 8–12 mcg daily for children and 30 mcg daily for adults

- **Deficiency:** Deficiency is rare.
- **Causes:**
  - Long-term **parenteral nutrition**
  - Consumption of **large amounts of raw egg whites** (which contain avidin, a substance that binds to biotin and prevents its absorption), can also lead to biotin deficiency.
  - Secondary biotin deficiency can occur due to **lack of a specific enzyme (biotinidase)**, which is required for release of protein-bound biotin to make it bioavailable
- **Clinical manifestations:**
  - **Dermatitis** around the eyes, nose, and mouth, conjunctivitis, alopecia
  - **Neurologic symptoms**, including changes in mental status, lethargy, hallucinations, and paresthesia
  - Myalgia, anorexia, and nausea.
  - Multiple carboxylase deficiency—inherited defects of biotin metabolism.
  - The **infantile form** is caused by a **deficiency of holocarboxylase synthetase** and presents in the first week of life with lethargy, poor muscle tone, and vomiting.
  - A **later-onset form** is caused by **biotinidase deficiency** and is associated with a slow but progressive loss of biotin in the urine, leading to organic aciduria; it is characterized by ataxia, ketoacidosis, dermatitis, seizures, myoclonus, and nystagmus.
- **Diagnosis:**
  - **Decreased urine biotin** concentrations
  - Increased urinary excretion of 3-hydroxyisovaleric acid after leucine challenge.
  - Decreased activity of biotin-dependent enzymes in lymphocytes.
- **Treatment:** Biotin in the dose of 10 mg/day

VITAMIN C

Vitamin C (ascorbic acid) is a **water-soluble** vitamin.
- **Sources:**
  - Citrus fruits, tomatoes, potatoes, Brussels sprouts, cauliflower, broccoli, strawberries, cabbage, and spinach.
  - Breast milk provides an adequate source of ascorbic acid for newborns and infants.
- **Metabolism:**
  - Ascorbic acid is absorbed in the **distal small intestine**.
  - Usual dietary doses of up to 100 mg/day are almost completely absorbed. As dietary concentrations increase, a smaller fraction is absorbed.
  - Pharmacologic dosing (>1,000 mg/day) can result in absorption rates of < 50%.
  - **Blood concentrations** of ascorbic acid are **regulated by renal excretion**. Excess amounts are filtered by renal glomeruli and reabsorbed via the tubules to a predetermined threshold.
  - **Dehydroascorbic acid** is the preferred form for **erythrocytes and leukocytes.**
  - The greatest concentrations of ascorbic acid are found in the **pituitary, adrenal, brain, leukocytes, and the eye.**
- **Functions:** These include:
  - **Formation of collagen** from procollagen. It is essential for **wound healing** and facilitates recovery from burns. It is needed for hydroxylation of proline to hydroxyproline (in protocollagen) and lysine to hydroxylysine (in mature collagen).
  - **Antioxidant properties:** Ascorbic acid is the **most active powerful reducing agent** controlling the redox potential within cells.
  - It is involved in intracellular electron transfer and supports **immune function**.
  - Promotes **absorption of nonheme iron**.
  - It is needed for the **formation of carnitine, hormones, neurotransmitters, and amino acids**.
  - Formation of **intercellular cement substances** in connective tissues, bones, and dentin, when defective, resulting in weakened capillaries with subsequent hemorrhage, and defects in bone and related structures.
- **RDA:**
  - 15–45 mg daily in children
  - 75 mg per day for adult women
  - 90 mg per day for men
  - Pregnant or lactating women and the elderly have requirements up to 120 mg/day

SCURVY

Scurvy is caused by deficiency of vitamin C.
- **Causes of vitamin C deficiency:**
  - Infants fed only on boiled cow's milk during the first year of life are at risk.
  - Individuals, who do not eat vegetables such as elderly, people who live alone (singly) and chronic alcoholics.
  - Pregnant and lactating women and those with thyrotoxicosis require more vitamin C because of increased utilization.
  - *Individuals at risk of deficiency:*
    - Anorexia nervosa or anorexia from other diseases, such as AIDS or cancer
    - Type 1 diabetes require increased vitamin C.
    - Patients undergoing peritoneal dialysis and hemodialysis
    - Diseases of small intestine, such as Crohn's, Whipple, and celiac disease.
- **Types of scurvy:** Adult scurvy and infantile scurvy.
  - *Adult scurvy:* Early symptoms may be nonspecific, with malaise, weakness, lethargy and muscle pain (myalgia may be due to reduced production of carnitine).
    - *Bone disease:* More common in growing children and manifests after 1–3 months. It is characterized by **deranged formation of osteoid matrix and bone pain. Fractures, dislocations**, and tenderness of bones are common in children.
    - *Hemorrhages:* Hemorrhaging is a **hallmark** feature of scurvy and can occur in any organ. Hair follicles

are one of the common sites of cutaneous bleeding. Marked tendency to bleed into the skin (easy **bruising, petechiae, ecchymosis, perifollicular hemorrhages**), bleeding into muscles, joints and underneath peritoneum. Bruising and hemorrhage may be spontaneous. Most commonly on the **legs and buttocks** where hydrostatic pressure is the greatest.
- *Delayed/poor wound healing* and breakdown of old scars.
- *Anemia:* It may cause high-output heart failure.
- *Gums:* Inflamed spongy gums (**gum swelling**) friability, bleeding, and infection with loosening of teeth; mucosal petechiae are common.
- *Skin changes:* Roughness, keratosis of hair follicles with "corkscrew" hair, perifollicular hemorrhages.
- *Nails:* Splinter hemorrhages.
- *Other features:* Emotional changes, shortness of breath.
- *Infantile scurvy (Barlow's disease):*
  - **Subperiosteal hemorrhage** into shafts of long bones.
  - **Scorbutic rosary** denotes enlargement of costochondral junctions, which are tender.
  - May be associated with **pectus excavatum**.
  - Retrobulbar, subarachnoid, and intracerebral **hemorrhages.**
  - Painful limbs giving rise to **"pseudoparalysis"**.
- ❏ Laboratory investigations and diagnosis
  - Diagnosis is usually made **clinically** in a patient who has skin or gingival signs and is at risk of vitamin C deficiency.
  - *Plasma and leukocyte vitamin C* levels can be measured.
    - Leukocyte vitamin C levels are more reliable as recent treatment will improve plasma levels but tissues will still be deficient in vitamin C.
    - **Plasma vitamin C level** of <11 μmol/L (0.2 mg/100 mL).
    - *Anemia:* It can be normochromic, normocytic (due to bleeding), megaloblastic (due to reduced erythropoiesis), or microcytic hypochromic anemia (due to impaired iron absorption and impaired heme synthesis).
    - *Hess' Capillary fragility* test can be checked by inflating a blood pressure cuff and looking for petechiae on the forearm.
    - **Bleeding time, clotting time, and prothrombin time:** To rule out other bleeding disorders.
  - *Imaging studies:* The findings include:
    - Loss of trabeculae results in a ground-glass appearance
    - Thinning of cortex
    - A line of calcified, irregular cartilage (**white line of Frankel**) may be visible at the metaphysis.
    - The epiphysis may be compressed and circular calcification surrounding epiphyseal center of ossification (**Wimberger ring sign**) (Fig. 13.4).
- ❏ Management/Treatment:

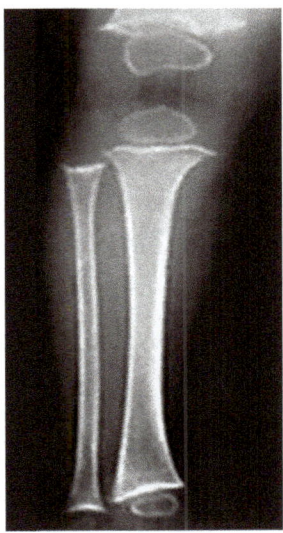

Fig. 13.4: X-ray of scurvy showing Frenkel line and Wimburger ring sign.

- *Ascorbic acid at 100 mg 3–5 times a day* until total of 4 g is reached, and then reduces the dose to 100 mg daily.
- *Encourage consumption of foods with high vitamin C:*
  - **Citrus fruits,** especially grapefruits and lemons.
  - **Vegetables** including broccoli, green peppers, tomatoes, potatoes, and cabbage.
  - The recommended dose for adults is 120 mg daily, although a dose of 60 mg daily is all that is required to prevent scurvy.
  - Diets high in vitamin C may lower the incidence of certain cancers, particularly esophageal and gastric cancers.
  - Vitamin C supplementation can be useful in upper respiratory tract infections, Chediak–Higashi syndrome and osteogenesis imperfecta.
  - There is inconclusive evidence of the protective role of vitamin C in the management of COVID-19 pneumonia.

VITAMIN D

Vitamin D is a **fat-soluble secosteroid** responsible for enhancing **intestinal absorption of calcium, iron, magnesium, phosphate, and zinc.**

- ❏ **Physiology (Fig. 13.5):**
  - *Vitamin D_3 (cholecalciferol):*
    - Produced in skin with direct sunlight, cod liver oil
    - Preferred form of supplementation
  - *Vitamin D_2 (ergocalciferol):*
    - Less effective as precursor to $1,25(OH)_2$-vitamin D
    - Hepatic conversion of vitamin D_3 to 25-OH-vitamin D (calcitriol)
    - Conversion of 25-OH-vitamin D to $1,25(OH)_2$-vitamin D (calcitriol)
- ❏ **Functions:** Vitamin D exists in two activated sterol forms. Its functions include:

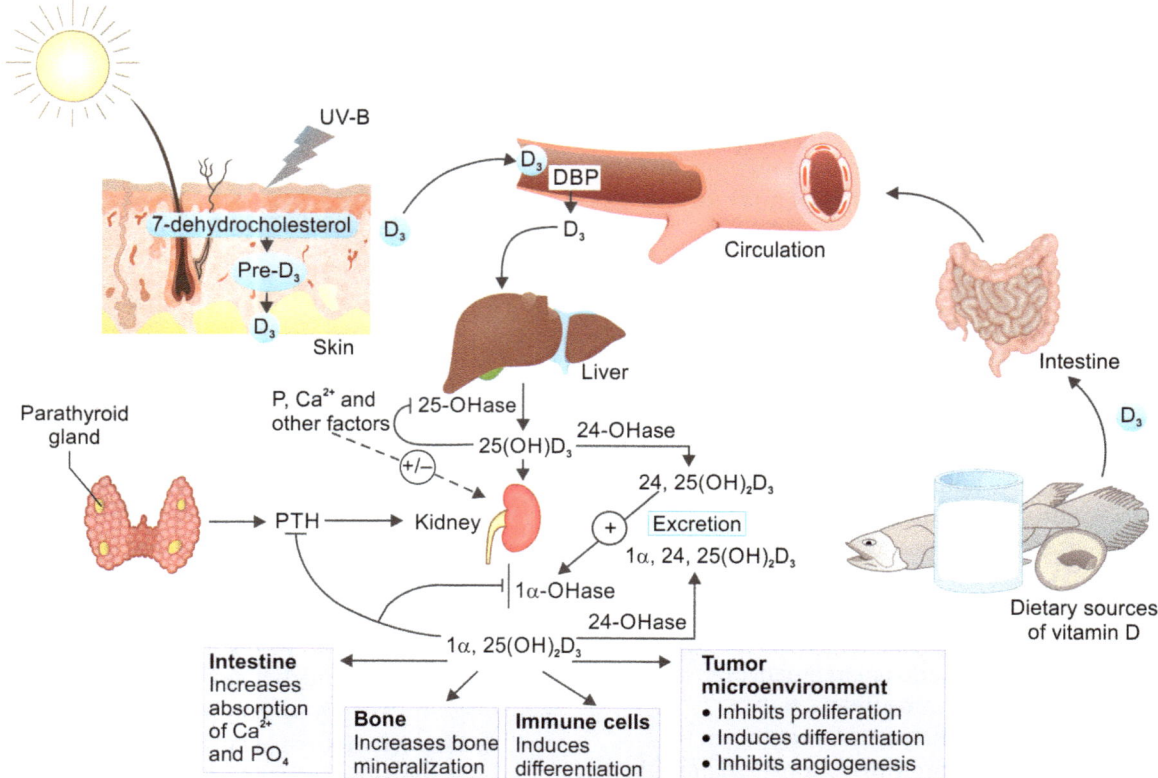

Fig. 13.5: Physiology of vitamin D.

- **Regulation of plasma levels of calcium and phosphorus:** The main functions of 1,25-dihydroxyvitamin D on calcium and phosphorus homeostasis are:
    - **Stimulates intestinal absorption of calcium:** 1,25-dihydroxyvitamin D stimulates intestinal absorption of calcium in the duodenum through the interaction of 1,25-dihydroxyvitamin D with nuclear vitamin D receptor (VDR).
    - **Stimulates calcium reabsorption in the kidney:** 1,25-dihydroxyvitamin D increases calcium influx in distal tubules of the kidney.
    - **Interaction with parathormone (PTH) in the regulation of blood calcium**
    - **Mineralization of bone:** Vitamin D plays a role in the **mineralization of osteoid matrix** and **epiphyseal cartilage** in both flat and long bones. Vitamin D stimulates osteoblasts to produce the calcium-binding protein osteocalcin, which is involved in the **deposition of calcium** during development of bone.
- **Antiproliferative effects:** The VDR is expressed in the parathyroid gland and 1,25(OH)$_2$ D has an antiproliferative effect on parathyroid cells and it suppresses the transcription of the parathyroid hormone gene.
- **Immunomodulatory:** Vitamin D is involved in the **innate and adaptive immune system**.

Vitamin D Deficiency

Diseases caused due to vitamin D deficiency are:

- **In children:** Deficiency of vitamin D in a growing child before the epiphyses has fused results in failure of growing bone to mineralize.
    - **Rickets:** Bone *softening* disease, deformity of *long bones* occurs.
- **In adults:**
    - *Osteomalacia:* Bone-thinning disorder, proximal muscle weakness, and bone fragility.
    - *Osteoporosis:* Decrease of bone mineralization and increased bone fragility.

Causes of Vitamin D Deficiency

- Impaired cutaneous production due to limited exposure to sunlight
- *Dietary absence*: Diets deficient in calcium and vitamin D
- Malabsorption
- Impaired hydroxylation by the liver to produce 25-hydroxyvitamin D
- Impaired hydroxylation by the kidneys to produce 1,25-dihydroxyvitamin D (vitamin D-dependent rickets type 1, chronic renal insufficiency)
- End-organ insensitivity to vitamin D metabolites [hereditary vitamin D-resistant rickets (HVDRR), vitamin D-dependent rickets type 2].

Rickets (Fig. 13.6)

- In children, before the closure of epiphyses, vitamin D deficiency causes retardation of growth associated with an expansion of the growth plate known as **rickets**.

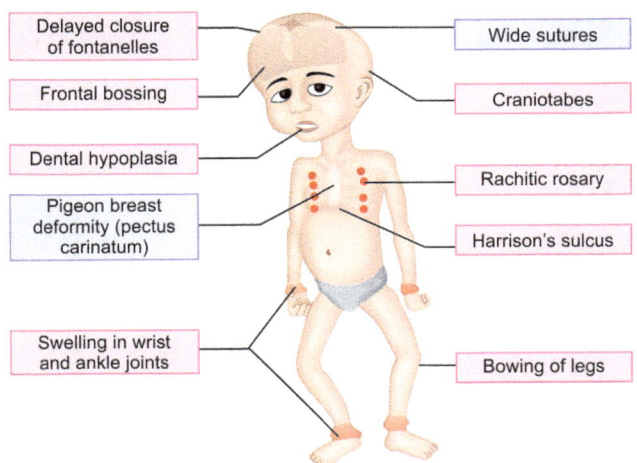

Fig. 13.6: Features of rickets.

- **Gross skeletal changes in rickets** depend on the severity and duration of the vitamin D deficiency and also the stresses to which individual bones are subjected.
- **During the nonambulatory stage of infancy**
  - *Head:*
    - **Craniotabes:** The skull appears square and box-like there is delayed closure of anterior fontanelle, frontal and parietal bossing.
    - **Frontal bossing:** Excess of osteoid produces frontal bossing and a squared appearance to the head.
    - Delayed eruption of primary teeth, enamel defects, and caries teeth.
  - *Chest:*
    - *Rachitic rosary:* Overgrowth of cartilage or osteoid tissue at the costochondral junction causes deformation of the chest producing the **"rachitic rosary".**
    - *Pigeon breast/chest deformity:* The weakened metaphyseal areas of the ribs are subject to the pull of the respiratory muscles and thus bend inward. This creates anterior protrusion of the sternum producing **pigeon-breast deformity** (pectus carinatum).
    - *Harrison's sulcus/groove:* It is due to the muscular pull of the diaphragmatic attachments to the lower ribs.
    - Respiratory infections and atelectasis.
- **During the ambulatory stage:**
  - This occurs when an ambulating child develops rickets. It is characterized by deformities affecting the spine, pelvis, and tibia. Scoliosis, kyphosis, and lumbar lordosis are characteristic.
  - *Bowing of the legs:* Due to affection of tibia, knock knees, anterior curving of legs.
- **Extraskeletal manifestations:**
  - *Seizures and tetany:* Secondary to hypocalcemia in vitamin D deficiency rickets.
  - *Hypotonia and delayed motor development:* In rickets developing during infancy.
  - *Protuberant abdomen, bone pain, waddling gait, and fatigue.*
  - *Asymptomatic:* Detected on radiological evaluation.
- **Investigations:**
  - *Wrist radiograph:* Findings include:
    - Lower ends of the shaft of radius and ulna become splayed
    - Epiphyseal surfaces—fuzzy and ill-defined
    - Unossified zone between shaft and radial epiphysis gets widened ("saucer" deformity).
    - **Figure 13.7** shows X-ray with splaying of epiphyses and bow legs.
  - *Blood:*
    - **Serum calcium:** Low
    - **Serum phosphate:** Low (due to associated secondary hyperparathyroidism).
    - **Serum alkaline phosphatase:** Increased due to increased osteoblast activity.
    - **Plasma 25-hydroxyvitamin D_3 level: Low** in most of the cases.
- **Treatment of rickets:**
  - Treat the underlying cause.
  - Supplementation diet with calcium and vitamin D.
  - **For nutritional deficiency** of vitamin D: Ergocalciferol, 1,50,000–6,00,000 IU orally or intramuscularly as a single dose. Or give Ergocalciferol in a dose of 2,000 IU every day.
- **Prevention:**
  - Adequate consumption of vitamin D (1,000–5,000 IU/day)
  - Adequate exposure to sunlight (from 30 minutes to 2 hours/week for infants).

Osteomalacia

- Vitamin D deficiency in **adults** is accompanied by hypocalcemia and hypophosphatemia which result in **impaired mineralization of bone matrix** proteins, a condition known as osteomalacia.
- Thus, it is a disorder of mineralization of the organic matrix of the skeleton in adults when the **epiphyseal growth plates have closed**. In contrast, in rickets, the growing skeleton is involved.

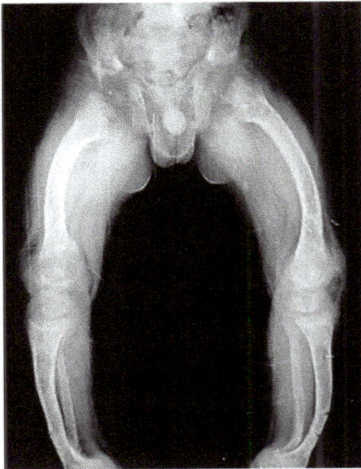 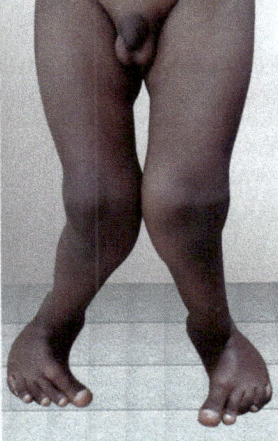

Fig. 13.7: X-ray of rickets showing splaying of epiphyses and bow legs.

Table 13.5: Causes of osteomalacia.

Causes	Features
Nutritional abnormalities	Dietary deficiency of vitamin D, parenteral nutrition
Malabsorption	Tropical sprue, celiac disease, hepatobiliary diseases, pancreatic insufficiency
Disorders of vitamin D metabolism	Vitamin D dependency type I and type II, anticonvulsants, chronic renal failure
Acidosis	Distal renal tubular acidosis (type I)
Phosphate depletion	Use of nonabsorbable antacids, tumor-associated osteomalacia
Others	Multiple myeloma, nephrotic syndrome, lead poisoning, inadequate sun exposure

Causes of osteomalacia:
Table 13.5 shows causes of osteomalacia.

Clinical features:
- **Bone pains, muscle weakness, fractures** of bones with minor trauma.
- Pain in the hip may cause **antalgic gait**.
- **Weakness of proximal muscle** results in waddling gait and may resemble primary muscle disease.
- **Collapse of vertebrae** causes local pain and deformity.
- Softening of skeleton may produce deformities, such as **kyphosis, coxa vara, pigeon chest,** and **triradiate pelvis** with a narrow pubic arch.

Laboratory investigations:
- Blood (same as for rickets as described earlier).
- **Urinary excretion of calcium:** Reduced.

Radiological findings:
- **Bone density:** Reduced (osteopenia).
- **Epiphyseal growth plate:** Increased in thickness, cupped and hazy at the metaphyseal border.
- **Cortical thinning:** Due to secondary hyperparathyroidism.
- **Other features:** Presence of nontraumatic fractures, radiolucent bands called pseudofractures (**Looser's zones**) (**Fig. 13.8**).

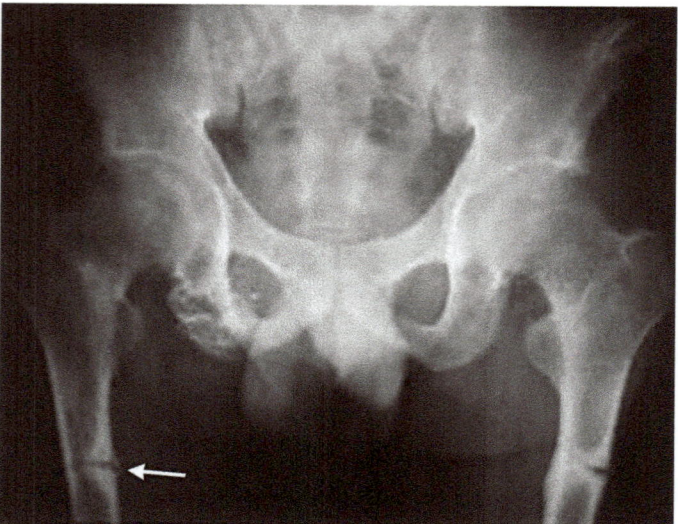

Fig. 13.8: X-ray shows looser zones (arrow) and osteopenia.

- **Bone scan** may be normal or show discrete foci of increased radionuclide uptake.
- **Bone mineral density** as assessed by dual-energy X-ray absorptiometry (DEXA) is reduced at spine, hip, and forearm, with the maximum deficits at the cortical-rich bone in the forearms.

Treatment:
- **Treat the underlying cause** wherever possible.
- **Dietary deficiency:** It is corrected by 1,000–4,000 IU of vitamin D_2 (ergocalciferol) or vitamin D_3 (cholecalciferol) for 3 months. This is followed by lower doses as maintenance. Vitamin D should be taken with fatty diet for maximum absorption.
- **Osteomalacia due to malabsorption:** Give 50,000–100,000 IU of vitamin D + calcium supplementation. Small doses of calcitriol (0.5–1.0 µg daily) also effective.
- **Chronic renal failure:** Calcitriol with weekly monitoring of calcium level.

Role of Vitamin D in Health and Disease
Role of vitamin D in health and disease is shown in **Table 13.6**.

Table 13.6: Role of vitamin D in health and disease.

Disease	Role
Parathyroid hormone	• Hypovitaminosis D causes secondary hyperparathyroidism which increases the risk of MI, HTN, and stroke
Malignancy	• Transcription of oncogenes involved in cell differentiation and proliferation is controlled: (c-myc, c-fos, c-sis) • There is an inverse relationship between sun exposure and cancer mortality. • 10 mg/mL rise in vitamin D level of associated with—17% reduction in cancer incidence, 29% reduction in all cancer mortality, and 45% reduction in GI cancer mortality
Nervous system function	• Vitamin D modulates neurotransmitter and neurological function • Has anticonvulsant and antidepressant effect. • 50% of multiple sclerosis patients are vitamin D deficient • Seizures are common with vitamin D deficiency
Anti-inflammatory function	• Suppresses and may prevent autoimmune diseases • Seems to reduce severity and frequency of childhood pneumonias

Contd...

Contd...

Disease	Role
Calcium homeostasis	• Calcium absorption increases as 25(OH) vitamin D blood levels increase
Cardiovascular function	• Risk of myocardial infarction doubles in patients with vitamin D deficiency • Heart failure patients have much lower vitamin D levels • HTN patients given UV light treatments three times/week for 6 weeks have shown mild decrease in BP
Diabetes type 1	• Infants and children who were supplemented with had decreased incidence of DM type 1 by 80%
Diabetes type 2	• Low vitamin D levels associated with insulin resistance and β-cell dysfunction • Postprandial glucose and insulin sensitivity are better in healthy adults with highest vitamin D levels • Highest vitamin D levels associated with 60% improvement in insulin sensitivity
Respiratory system	• Vitamin D supplementation provides significant protective effect against influenza • It is also associated with decrease in FEV_1 • Increased incidence of rhino-bronchial atopy
Osteoarthritis (OA)	• Vitamin D deficiency hastens the progression of OA hip and knee
Mood disorders	• Vitamin D supplementations improves general mood and hastens recovery in seasonal affective mood disorders
Polycystic ovary syndrome	• Deficiency exists in 60% of cases with normalization of menses and/or fertility within 3 months of supplementation
Pain	• Persistent, nonspecific musculoskeletal pain in 93% of patients had vitamin D deficiency • Low back pain patients (53%) have vitamin D deficiency
Autoimmune disease	• Vitamin D insufficiency in half of the patients with fibromyalgia + SLE, Graves' disease, ankylosing spondylitis and rheumatoid arthritis
Falls in the elderly	• Vitamin D deficiency reported to affect predominantly the weight-bearing antigravity muscles of the lower limb, which are necessary for postural balance and walking • Improvement in lower extremity muscle strength and balance with vitamin D supplementation thought to explain the reduced number of fall-related fractures

Hypervitaminosis D

- Hypervitaminosis D causes hypercalcemia, which manifest as:
  - Nausea and vomiting
  - Excessive thirst and polyuria
  - Severe itching
  - Joint and muscle pains
  - Disorientation and coma
  - Metastatic calcifications
- **Treatment of hypervitaminosis:** Hydration and treatment of hypercalcemia.

VITAMIN E (TOCOPHEROL)

- **Sources:** Almonds, vegetable oils, and cereals
- **Actions:**
  - Acts as free-radical scavenger and **antioxidant**
  - **Protects** LDL and PUFA in **membranes from oxidation**
  - **Inhibits prostaglandin synthesis**, activities of phospholipase A2, and protein kinase C.
- **Deficiency:**
  - *Causes:*
    - Pancreatic exocrine insufficiency
    - Cholestatic liver disease
    - Extensive resection or disease affecting small intestine
    - Ataxia with vitamin E deficiency, due to a mutation in the gene encoding hepatic alpha-tocopherol transfer protein (*TTPA*)
    - Abetalipoproteinemia, due to mutations in the microsomal triglyceride transfer protein.
- **Diagnosis:**
  - *Alpha-tocopherol levels* of <0.5 mg/dL (5 μg/mL or 11.5 μmol/L)—deficiency.
  - A normal result is > 0.8 mg.
- **Clinical manifestations:**
  - **Spinocerebellar syndrome**—ataxia, hyporeflexia, and loss of proprioceptive and vibratory sensation.
  - Ophthalmoplegia, skeletal myopathy, and pigmented retinopathy.
  - Brown bowel syndrome (**intestinal lipofuscinosis**) is a brown pigmentation of the bowel that occasionally presents with bowel dilatation and pseudo-obstruction (due to lipofuscin accumulation within the smooth muscle mitochondria).
  - Lifespan of red blood cells is shortened
  - In premature infants, vitamin E deficiency may cause a **hemolytic anemia**.
- **Treatment:**
  - *For infants and children:* 17–35 mg/kg/day of RRR-alpha-tocopherol.
  - *For adults:* 800–1,200 mg/day

VITAMIN K

- **Sources:**
  - Dietary vitamin K_1 (**phylloquinone**) is found in green vegetables like spinach and broccoli, and in some oils

- Vitamin K$_2$ (**menaquinone**) is found in bacterial flora, meat (especially liver), cheeses, fermented soybeans, and eggs.
- ❑ **Actions:**
  - **Coagulation:** Vitamin K is essential for activity of several carboxylase enzymes within hepatic cells, and therefore is necessary for the activation of coagulation factors **VII, IX, X, and prothrombin.**
  - Activation of proteins C and S
  - Reversal of coumarin-like anticoagulants
  - Bone formation
  - Coronary vascular calcification
- ❑ **Deficiency**
  - *Causes:*
    - Cystic fibrosis
    - Primary biliary cholangitis
    - Primary sclerosing cholangitis
    - Biliary atresia
    - Familial intrahepatic cholestasis and other inherited disorders associated with cholestasis
    - Malabsorption syndromes
    - Liver failure
    - Medications: 2nd, 3rd generation cephalosporins, orlistat (antiobesity drug)
    - Very high doses of vitamin E can cause vitamin K deficiency
  - *Clinical manifestations:*
    - Easy bruising
    - Mucosal bleeding
    - Splinter hemorrhages
    - Melena
    - Hematuria
    - Other manifestations of impaired coagulation.
  - *Diagnosis:*
    - Symptomatic patients with mild deficiency—only PT is elevated; in severe deficiency— both PT and aPTT are elevated.
    - Levels of PIVKA-II (**protein induced in vitamin K absence**), also known as des-gamma-carboxy prothrombin) are **more sensitive** than PT in detecting vitamin K deficiency. PIVKA-II is also elevated in the presence of vitamin K antagonists (VKA) drugs or certain tumors such as hepatocellular carcinoma.
    - Measuring **vitamin K-dependent factors** (i.e., prothrombin, factors VII, IX, X, or protein C). In patients who are vitamin K deficient, levels of these factors often are **less than 50%** of normal.
    - Phylloquinone levels also can be measured directly but are impractical for clinical use.
- ❑ **Treatment:**
  - Vitamin K can be administered in doses of **1–25 mg** (usually 10 mg) via oral, intramuscular, subcutaneous, or intravenous routes.
  - When vitamin K deficiency occurs in patients who are also receiving coumarin-like anticoagulants, doses of vitamin K should be minimized in order to prevent refractoriness to further anticoagulation.

CALCIUM HOMEOSTASIS

Distribution of Calcium

- ❑ Calcium weight is 400 mg/kg in infants and 950 mg/kg in adults.
- ❑ **Blood Ca^{++} level:** 8.5–10.2 mg/dL. Usually, 10 mg/100 mL (so 500 mg total in plasma = 0.5 g) **(Fig. 13.9)**.
- ❑ About 99% of total body calcium in the **bone**.
- ❑ Remaining 1% in **intracellular fluid (ICF), extracellular fluid (ECF), and cell membranes**.
- ❑ It can be divided in three components:
  1. 45% ionized
  2. 40% bound to albumin
  3. 15% complex with anions (citrate, phosphate)

Importance of Ionized Calcium

Ionized calcium (Ca^{++}) is physiologically important because it:
- ❑ Is one of the major intracellular messengers
- ❑ Precise levels are necessary for muscle contraction (cardiac, skeletal)
- ❑ Is responsible for exocytosis of secretory granules in neuronal synapses.
- ❑ Serves as second messenger in many cells.
- ❑ Is necessary for blood clotting.

Regulation of Calcium Levels

- ❑ It occurs in three different organs, namely
  1. *Small intestine:* Dietary Ca^{++} is absorbed in an active transcellular pathway in the duodenum and proximal jejunum. Paracellular calcium transport occurs throughout the length of the intestine.
  2. *Kidney:* Ionized Ca^{++} is filtered through the nephron, and can be excreted in the urine.
  3. *Bone:* Major storage site for Ca^{++}.
- ❑ **Calcium cycling in bone tissue:** Two processes that go on continuously and include bone formation and bone resorption.
  - Calcium phosphate crystals are called **"hydroxyapatite"**. The surfaces of crystals can exchange Ca^{++} and phosphate ions with extracellular fluid.
  - *Osteoblasts:* Synthesize a collagen matrix that holds calcium phosphate in crystallized form. Once surrounded by bone, osteoblast becomes osteocyte.
  - *Osteoclasts:* They break down bone (removes Ca^{++} from bone). Change local pH, causing Ca^{++} and phosphate to dissolve from crystals into extracellular fluids **(Table 13.7)**.

HYPERPARATHYROIDISM

Classification and Causes of Hyperparathyroidism

Causes and classification of hyperparathyroidism is described in **Table 13.8**.

Clinical Features of Hyperparathyroidism

- ❑ The most common clinical presentation of primary hyperparathyroidism (more than 70%) is asymptomatic hypercalcemia detected by routine biochemical screening.

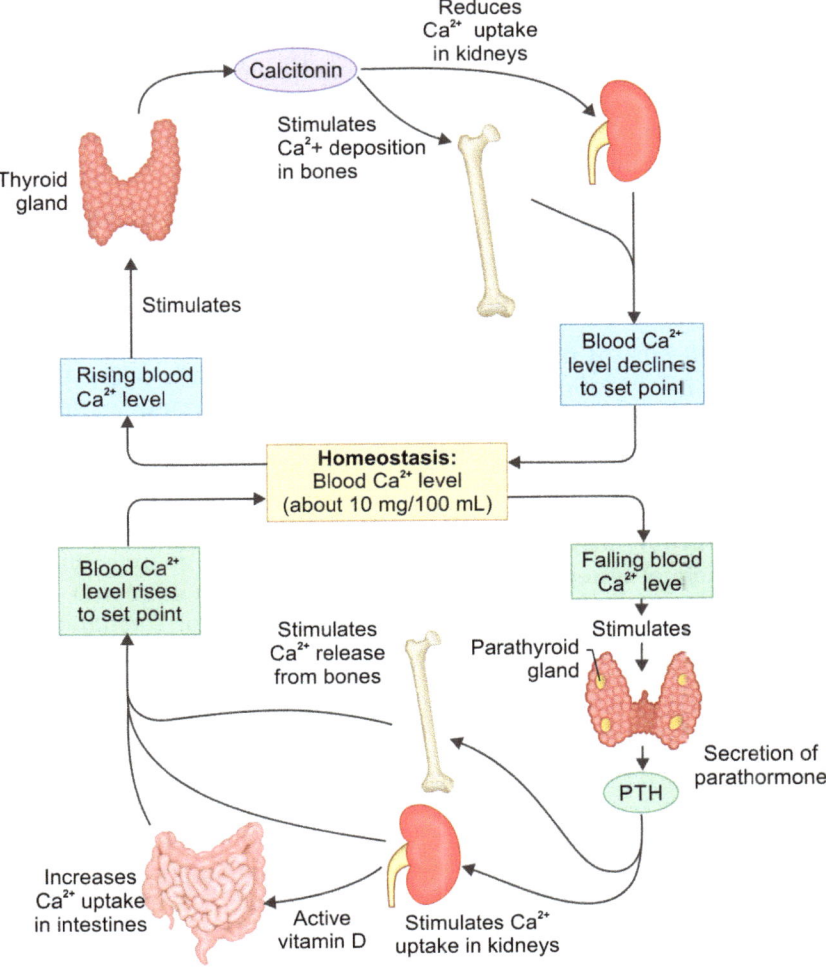

Fig. 13.9: Calcium metabolism.

Table 13.7: Hormonal regulators of calcium homeostasis.

Calcitonin (CT)	Parathormone (PTH)	Vitamin D (1, 25 vitamin D_3)

• Secreted from the parafollicular/C-cells in the thyroid gland.
• **Actions:**
  ■ Lowers Ca^{++} in blood.
  ■ Promotes deposition of Ca^{++} into bone.
  ■ It inhibits bone resorption by osteoclasts.
• **Control of secretion:** Increased plasma Ca^{++} stimulates C-cells to synthesize and release calcitonin.
	• Secreted from cells of the parathyroid glands (chief cells).
	• **Actions:**
	  ■ Increases Ca^{++} in the blood
	  ■ Increases Ca^{++} resorption from the bone
	  ■ Stimulates the osteoclasts
	  ■ Increases the number of osteoclasts
	  ■ Increases Ca^{++} resorption from the preurine filtrate in the nephron.
		• **Actions:** Vitamin D increases
		  ■ Calcium absorption from intestine.
		  ■ PO_4 absorption from intestine.
		  ■ Renal reabsorption of Ca and PO_4.
		  ■ Bone resorption from old bone and mineralize new bone (net resorption).
		• **Overall effect:** Increase serum Ca and PO_4.

Table 13.8: Classification and causes of hyperparathyroidism.

Type	Calcium	PTH	Causes
Primary: Autonomous secretion of PTH by parathyroid	Raised	Raised	Single adenoma (90%), multiple adenomata, nodular hyperplasia, and carcinoma of parathyroid
Secondary: Parathyroid hyperplasia with increased PTH secretion in an attempt to compensate for prolonged hypocalcemia	Low	Raised	Chronic renal failure, malabsorption, osteomalacia, and rickets
Tertiary: Adenoma formation and autonomous PTH secretion. Occurring in cases of secondary hyperparathyroidism	Raised	Raised	Chronic secondary hyperparathyroidism, post renal transplantation

- **Classical symptoms of primary hyperparathyroidism** are described by the adage *"moans, bones, stones, abdominal groans"*. However, nowadays only few patients present in this way.
  - *Moans:* Psychiatric manifestations—lethargy, fatigue, depression, memory loss, psychoses, neuroses, paranoia, confusion, stupor, and coma
  - *Bones:* Arthritis, osteomalacia, and osteitis
  - *Stones:* Renal stones, uremia, polydipsia, polyuria
  - *Groans:* Constipation, nausea, vomiting, peptic ulcers, indigestion, and pancreatitis
- **Nonspecific symptoms:** About 50% of patients are asymptomatic while others have nonspecific symptoms. These include: Anorexia, nausea, vomiting, constipation, weakness, fatigue, lassitude, tiredness, generalized aches, weight loss, pain, drowsiness, poor concentration, memory loss, and depression.
- **Manifestations of hyperparathyroidism:** Involve primarily the **kidneys** and the **skeletal system**.
  - *Renal manifestations:* Due either to deposition of calcium in the renal parenchyma or to recurrent nephrolithiasis.
    - **Recurrent renal calculi** (usually composed of either calcium oxalate or calcium phosphate).
    - **Nephrocalcinosis:** Deposition of calcium salts in the renal parenchyma.
    - Polyuria and polydipsia.
    - Loss of renal function with uremia, hypokalemia, hyperuricemia, hyperchloremic acidosis, and dilute urine.
  - *Skeletal manifestations:*
    - Bone pain, osteopenia, osteoporosis, fractures, and deformity due to osteitis fibrosa cystica (10–25% of patients)
    - Localized bone swelling/brown tumor (e.g., Mandible).
  - *Other manifestations:*
    - Hypertension is a common feature.
    - Calcification of cornea (observed by slit-lamp examination), arterial walls and soft tissues of hand.
    - Peptic ulcers
    - Myopathy
- A family history of hypercalcemia or primary hyperparathyroidism secondary to a parathyroid adenoma raises the possibility of multiple endocrine neoplasia (MEN) syndrome. Features of MEN syndromes are presented in **Table 13.9**.

Investigations

- **Biochemical investigations:** Estimation of several fasting serum calcium and phosphate samples should be done.
- **Hallmark of primary hyperparathyroidism:**
  - **Hypercalcemia** and **hypophosphatemia** with **detectable or elevated intact PTH levels** during hypercalcemia. When this combination is present in an asymptomatic patient then further investigation is usually unnecessary. Established hypercalcemia in more than one serum measurement accompanied by elevated immunoreactive PTH (iPTH) is characteristic.
  - Serum concentrations of 1,25 dihydroxy vitamin D may therefore be at upper limits of normal or elevated.
  - **Correction of serum calcium concentrations:** It should be corrected to the prevailing serum albumin concentration. Calcium level is corrected for low albumin levels by adding 0.8 mg/dL to the total serum calcium level for every 1.0 g/dL by which the serum albumin concentration is lower than 4 g/dL.
  - May be associated with **mild hyperchloremic acidosis**.
  - **Calcium/creatinine (Ca/Cr) clearance ratio:** (24-hour urine Ca × serum Cr) ÷ (serum Ca × 24-hour urine Cr)
- **Urine investigations:**
  - *Hypercalciuria (24-hours urinary calcium) (>200–300 mg/24 hours):* Observed in ~30% of patients.
  - *Increased markers of bone resorption:* These include urinary pyridinoline, deoxypyridinoline and N-telopeptide of collagen.
- **ECG findings:**
  - Shortened QT interval
  - Rarely cardiac arrhythmias
  - Rarely ST segment elevation
- **Radiological abnormalities:**
  - Most sensitive and specific radiologic finding of **osteitis fibrosa cystica** is **subperiosteal resorption of cortical bone**, best seen in high-resolution films of the phalanges.

Table 13.9: Features of multiple endocrine neoplasia syndromes.

MEN 1 (Wermer's syndrome)	MEN 2A (Sipple syndrome)	MEN 2B
• Parathyroid hyperplasia (very common) • Pancreatic tumors (benign or malignant) 　▪ Gastrinoma 　▪ Insulinoma 　▪ Glucagonoma 　▪ VIPoma • Pituitary tumor 　▪ Growth hormone-secreting 　▪ Prolactin-secreting 　▪ ACTH-secreting • **Other tumors:** Lipomas, carcinoids, adrenal, and thyroid adenomas	• Medullary carcinoma of the thyroid • Pheochromocytoma (benign or malignant) • Parathyroid hyperplasia	• Medullary carcinoma of the thyroid • Pheochromocytoma • Mucosal neuromas, ganglioneuromas • Marfanoid habitus • Hyperparathyroidism (very rare)

- A similar process in the **skull** leads to a **salt-and-pepper appearance**.
- Bone cysts or **brown tumors** may be evident as osteolytic lesions.
- The other important skeletal consequence of hyperparathyroidism is **osteoporosis**. Unlike other osteoporotic disorders, hyperparathyroidism often results in the preferential loss of cortical bone.
- Dental films may disclose loss of the lamina dura of the teeth, but this is a nonspecific finding also seen in periodontal disease.
- *Nephrocalcinosis:* Appear as scattered opacities within the renal outline.
- *Soft tissue calcification:* For example, calcification of arterial wall.
- *DEXA and CT scan:* Reveal reduced bone density.
- **Investigations for localization of the tumor:** Parathyroid imaging is generally indicated only for patients who have undergone previous parathyroid surgery. Investigations to localize the tumor include:
  - **High-resolution ultrasonography, CT scanning,** and **subtraction imaging** and **scintigraphy** with technetium 99 sestamibi.
  - **Selective neck vein catheterization** with PTH estimation.

Treatment

- **Primary hyperthyroidism:**
  - Patients with **symptomatic** primary hyperparathyroidism should undergo **parathyroid surgery,** which is the only definitive therapy.
  - Guidelines for surgery in asymptomatic primary hyperparathyroidism (2014): Any **one** of the following criteria.
    - Serum calcium: >1 mg/dL above the upper limit of normal.
    - BMD by DXA: T-score <-2.5 at lumbar spine, total hip, femoral neck, or distal 1/3 radius.
    - Vertebral fracture by radiograph, CT, MRI, or VFA.
    - Creatinine clearance <60 mL/min
    - 24-hour urine for calcium >400 mg/day and increased stone risk by biochemical stone risk analysis.
    - Presence of nephrolithiasis or nephron-calcinosis by radiograph, ultrasound, or CT.
    - Age < 50 years
  - For patients who are **unable to have surgery** and whose primary indication for surgery is symptomatic and/or severe hypercalcemia, **Cinacalcet** is preferred over bisphosphonates.
  - *Cinacalcet:* In primary hyperparathyroidism, initially: Oral, 30 mg twice daily; increase dose incrementally every 2-4 weeks (to 60 mg twice daily, 90 mg twice daily, and 90 mg 3 or 4 times daily) as necessary to normalize serum calcium levels.
- **Secondary hyperparathyroidism:**
  - Treatment of chronic kidney disease (CKD)
  - According to Kidney Disease Outcomes Quality Initiative (KDOQI) guidelines, in all dialysis patients, Serum phosphate should be maintained between 3.5 and 5.5 mg/dL, serum calcium should be maintained <9.5 mg/dL and PTH values should be maintained less than 2-9 times the upper limit for the PTH assay.
  - Treatment options for increased PTH include **calcimimetics, calcitriol, or synthetic vitamin D analogs**. In a recent update, oral calcitriol is comparable to IV Vitamin D analog for hemodialysis patients with secondary hyperparathyroidism.
  - **Cinacalcet**: In secondary hyperparathyroidism, initially orally: 30 mg once daily; increase dose incrementally every 2-4 weeks (to 60 mg once daily, 90 mg once daily, 120 mg once daily, and 180 mg once daily) as necessary to maintain iPTH level between 150 and 300 pg/mL. May be used alone or in combination with vitamin D and/or phosphate binders.
- **Tertiary hyperparathyroidism:** Parathyroidectomy.

HYPERCALCEMIA

- Normal serum calcium level is **8-10 mg/dL** (2.0-2.5 mmol/L)
- Normal ionized calcium levels are **4-5.6 mg/dL** (1-1.4 mmol/L).
- **Raised calcium level** is known as hypercalcemia.
- Hypercalcemia is considered as **mild,** if the total serum calcium level is between 10.5 and 12 mg/dL (2.6-3 mmol/L), **moderate** 12-14 mg/dL, and **severe** when the level is above 14 mg/dL.
- Hypercalcemia is one of the **most common biochemical abnormalities**. It is often detected incidentally during routine biochemical investigation in asymptomatic patients. However, it can present with chronic symptoms and occasionally as an acute emergency.
- In patients with hypoalbuminemia or hyperalbuminemia, the measured calcium concentration should be corrected in view of the albumin abnormality.

Causes of Hypercalcemia

Causes of hypercalcemia are described in **Table 13.10.**

Clinical Features

Refer clinical features of hyperparathyroidism earlier.

Management

Treatment of Acute Hypercalcemia

- **Adequate rehydration and volume expansion** are essential, usually at least 4-6 L of 0.9% saline on day 1, and 3-4 L for several days thereafter.
- Diuretics after correction of volume (not recommended in the present day due to potential complications and the availability of drugs that inhibit bone resorption, which is primarily responsible for the hypercalcemia.): For example, **furosemide** 40-160 mg/day or **ethacrynic acid** 50-200 mg/day. Forced diuresis with 4-6 L of intravenous fluid/day and furosemide 2 hourly.
- Sodium, potassium and magnesium should be supplemented. Saline decreases concomitant reabsorption of sodium and calcium in both the proximal and distal renal tubules, and enhances urinary excretion of calcium.

Table 13.10: Causes of hypercalcemia.

Parathyroid hormone related with normal or elevated PTH levels	Vitamin D related with Low PTH levels
• Primary hyperparathyroidism (most common) or tertiary hyperparathyroidism • MEN syndromes • Lithium therapy—induced hyperparathyroidism • Familial hypercalciuric hypercalcemia	• Vitamin D intoxication: Iatrogenic or self-administered excess • Granulomatous diseases (sarcoidosis, tuberculosis, and berylliosis) • Lymphoma • Idiopathic hypercalcemia of infancy
Malignancy related with Low PTH levels (second most common cause)	**High bone turnover**
• Multiple myeloma • PTH related protein secretion: Tumors of lung and kidney • Secondary deposits in bone: Breast carcinoma • Production of osteoclastic factors by tumors	• Long-term immobilization • Hyperthyroidism • Drugs, e.g., thiazide diuretics, etc. • Paget's disease with immobilization
Associated with renal failure	**Excessive calcium intake**
• Secondary hyperparathyroidism • Aluminum toxication	• Milk-alkali syndrome • Parenteral nutrition

- **Intravenous bisphosphonate** is the treatment of choice for hypercalcemia of malignancy or of undiagnosed cause. Concurrent administration of **zoledronic acid** 4 mg IV over 15 minutes or **pamidronate** 60–90 mg over 2 hours.
- **Calcitonin** (4 IU/kg IV 6-hourly), tachyphylaxis develops after 24–48 hours.
- **Prednisolone** (20–40 mg daily) is effective in few instances (e.g., in myeloma, lymphoma, sarcoidosis, and vitamin D excess).
- Oral phosphate (sodium cellulose phosphate) 5 g three times daily.
- **Denosumab**: For hypercalcemia refractory to ZA or in patients in whom bisphosphonates are contraindicated due to severe renal impairment. Starting dose 120 mg every 4 weeks.
- **Cinacalcet**: Reduces the serum calcium in patients with severe hypercalcemia due to parathyroid carcinoma and in hemodialysis patients with an elevated calcium-phosphorous product and secondary hyperparathyroidism.
- **Dialysis**: Treatment of last resort, HD with little or no calcium in the dialysis fluid.

HYPOPARATHYROIDISM

Deficient secretion of PTH which manifests itself biochemically by:
- Hypocalcemia
- Hyperphosphatemia
- Diminished or absent circulating iPTH
- Clinically, the symptoms of neuromuscular hyperactivity.

Causes of Hypoparathyroidism

- **Surgical hypoparathyroidism: Most** common. It may be due to the removal of the parathyroid glands or due to interruption of blood supply to the parathyroid glands. Postparathyroidectomy (**hungry-bone syndrome**)
- **Idiopathic hypoparathyroidism:** Occurs at an **early age** (genetic origin) with autosomal recessive mode of transmission "multiple endocrine deficiency-autoimmune-candidiasis" (**MEDAC**) syndrome.
  - "Juvenile familial endocrinopathy"— "Hypoparathyroidism—Addison's disease—mucocutaneous candidiasis (HAM) syndrome"
  - Circulating antibodies for the parathyroid glands and the adrenals are frequently present.
  - Other associated disease: Pernicious anemia, ovarian failure, autoimmune thyroiditis, and diabetes mellitus.
- **Infantile hypoparathyroidism**
- **Infiltrative diseases:** Granulomatous, iron overload, metastases
- **Radiation-induced destruction**
- **HIV**
- **Pseudohypoparathyroidism** (resistance to PTH)
- **Functional hypoparathyroidism:** In patients who has chronic hypomagnesemia of various causes. Magnesium is necessary for the PTH release from the glands and also for the peripheral action of the PTH.
- **DiGeorge syndrome** is a familial condition where the hypoparathyroidism is associated with intellectual impairment, cataracts and calcified basal ganglia, and occasionally with specific autoimmune disease.
- **Malabsorption syndrome:** Presumably secondary to decreased calcium level and may lead to steatorrhea with longstanding untreated disease.

Clinical Features

- **Acute:**
  - Neuromuscular irritability (**tetany**)
  - Paresthesia (peri oral and extremities)
  - Muscle twitching
  - Carpopedal spasm
  - Trousseau's sign
  - Chvostek's sign
  - Seizures
  - Laryngospasm
  - Bronchospasm
  - Prolonged QT interval
  - Hypotension, heart failure and arrhythmia
  - Papilledema

- **Chronic:**
  - Ectopic calcification (basal ganglia)
  - Extrapyramidal signs
  - Parkinsonism
  - Dementia
  - Subcapsular cataracts
  - Abnormal dentition
  - Dry skin

Treatment

- To effectively treat hypocalcemia in patients with magnesium deficiency, hypomagnesemia should be corrected first.
- **Acute cases:**
  - *Symptomatic:* **IV calcium** (initially, 10 mL ampule of 10% **calcium gluconate** in 50 mL of 5% dextrose infused over 10–20 minutes, followed by an intravenous infusion of calcium gluconate) with oral **calcitriol** (0.5 μg two times daily).
  - *Asymptomatic:* IV calcium if serum corrected calcium is ≤7.5 mg/dL. Oral calcium (1–4 g of **calcium carbonate** daily in divided doses) should be initiated as soon as the patient is able to take supplements orally.
- **Chronic cases:**
  - *Calcium:* **Calcium carbonate** or **calcium citrate** 1,000–2,000 mg daily in divided doses.
  - *Vitamin D:*
    - *Calcitriol (drug of choice), initial:* 0.25–0.5 μg daily and maintenance: 0.5–2 μg daily.
    - *Alfacacidol:* Initial 0.25 μg daily and Maintenance 0.5–1 μg daily
    - *Dihydrotachysterol:* 0.2–1.2 mg daily.
  - *Hydrochlorothiazide:* If needed for hypercalciuria, 12.5–50 mg daily
  - Second-line therapy by subcutaneous **recombinant human PTH**.

TETANY

It is characterized by **neuromuscular irritability** manifested clinically by **sensory, muscular dysfunction,** and **autonomic manifestations**.

Causes of Tetany (Table 13.11)

- Tetany is caused due to **hypocalcemia** or **alkalosis** or **hypomagnesemia**.
- Respiratory alkalosis alone (e.g., hyperventilation) can cause tetany, even in the absence of underlying hypocalcemia.
- Tetany is unusual among patients with chronic renal failure and hypocalcemia (occasionally severe) because of the protective effect of concurrent metabolic acidosis.
- Occurs when there is acute fall in **serum ionized calcium to <4.3 mg/dL** and **total calcium concentration to 7–7.5 mg/dL**.

Clinical Features

- Symptoms begin with **perioral and acral paresthesia** leading to hyperventilation—respiratory alkalosis—exacerbation of paresthesia.

Table 13.11: Causes of tetany.

Due to hypocalcemia	
Increased phosphate levels • Chronic renal failure (common) • Phosphate therapy	**Vitamin D deficiency** • Osteomalacia/rickets • Vitamin D resistance
Hypoparathyroidism • Surgical—after neck exploration (thyroidectomy, parathyroidectomy—common) • Congenital deficiency (DiGeorge syndrome) • Idiopathic hypoparathyroidism (rare) • Severe hypomagnesemia	**Others** • Acute pancreatitis (quite common) • Citrated blood in massive transfusion (not uncommon) • Low plasma albumin, e.g., malnutrition, chronic liver disease • Malabsorption, e.g., celiac disease
Resistance to PTH Pseudohypoparathyroidism	**Drugs** • Calcitonin • Bisphosphonates
Due to alkalosis	
• Repeated vomiting of gastric juice • Excessive intake of oral alkali	• Hyperventilation, e.g., hysteria • Primary hyperaldosteronism
Due to hypomagnesemia	

- **Motor symptoms:** Stiffness, clumsiness, myalgia, muscle spasms, cramps, carpal spasm, spasm of the respiratory muscles, and laryngismus stridulus.
- **Autonomic manifestations** are diaphoresis, bronchospasm, and biliary colic.
- The classic physical findings in patients with neuromuscular irritability due to latent tetany are:
  - *Chvostek's sign:* It is elicited by tapping the skin over the facial nerve in front of the external auditory meatus. It causes an **ipsilateral contraction of the facial muscles**, but up to 10% of normal population has a positive test.
  - *Trousseau's sign:* Inflate BP cuff on arm to 20 mm Hg > systolic BP for 3 minutes and watch for **carpopedal spasm** [flexion at the wrist, flexion at the metatarsophalangeal (MP) joints, extension of the interphalangeal (IP) joints adduction thumbs/fingers]. It may also be induced by voluntary hyperventilation for 1–2 minutes after release of the cuff.

Treatment

- **Control of tetany:**
  - *Calcium gluconate:* Slow intravenous (over 10 minutes) injection of 20 mL of 10% solution of calcium gluconate is rapidly effective in controlling the tetany.
  - *Magnesium:* If tetany is not relieved by above treatment, administration of magnesium may be necessary.
- **Correction of alkalosis:**
  - If alkalosis is due to persistent vomiting, treat with **intravenous isotonic saline and potassium**.
  - If alkalosis is due to alkali excess, it should be withdrawn. If needed, ammonium chloride 2 g 4 hourly orally will control tetany.
- **Hysterical hyperventilation:** It may be controlled by **rebreathing expired air from a suitable bag** or inhalation of 5% carbon dioxide in oxygen.

TRACE ELEMENTS

- The term "trace" is used for concentrations of elements **not exceeding 250 µg/g of extracellular matrix.**
- Trace elements are **naturally occurring, homogeneous, inorganic substances** required in humans in amounts less than 100 mg/day.
- Classification of trace elements is presented in **Table 13.12**.
- There are about 15 trace elements of which only **10 are essential** nutrients in humans.
- These include iron, zinc, copper, chromium, selenium, iodine, fluorine, manganese, molybdenum, and cobalt.

Iron

Deficiency state:
- Asymptomatic
- Anemia (discussed in Chapter 12: Hematology)

Fluorosis

- **Fluorine:** Fluorine's **ionic form** is known as fluoride.
- It is a component of **bone mineral** and alters its physical characteristics.
- Fluoride helps to **prevent dental caries**, because it increases the resistance of the enamel to acid attack.
- Requirement in adults is between 1.5 and 4 mg/day and 96% of fluorides in the body found in **bone and teeth.**
- **Deficiency:** Intake of < 0.1 mg/day in infants and < 0.5 mg/day in children predisposes to an increased incidence of dental caries.
- **Toxicity:** Results in **fluorosis.** This develops when fluoride content in the water is high (> 3–5 ppm).
  - *Acute* ingestion of >30 mg/kg body weight usually manifests with GI symptoms, such as diarrhea, vomiting leading to renal failure and may cause death.
  - *Dental fluorosis:* It is characterized by mottling of teeth where the enamel loses its luster; teeth appear chalky white with transverse yellow bands. It becomes rough, pigmented, pitted, and brittle (fluorite teeth).
  - *Skeletal fluorosis:* Its features are:
    - **Sclerosis of bones** (especially of spine, pelvis and limbs).
    - **Calcification** of ligaments, interosseous membrane (**Fig. 13.10**) and tendinous insertions.
    - **Osteoporosis with** brittle bones.

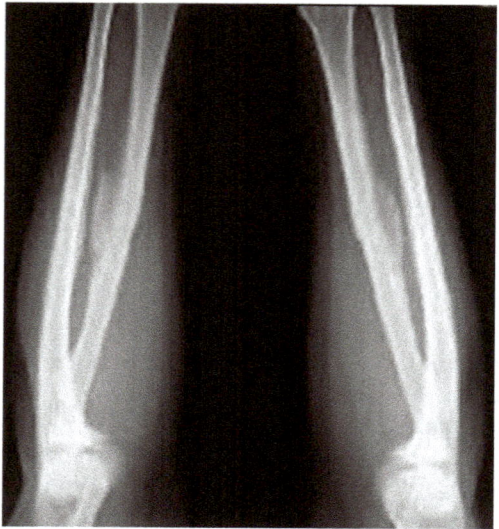

Fig. 13.10: X-ray of fluorosis showing calcification of interosseous membrane.

- **Severe pain and stiffness** in joints, stiffness in neck and backbone, bow legs. Other features are weakness, anemia, and weight loss.

PROTEIN-ENERGY MALNUTRITION

- Protein-energy malnutrition (PEM) is the deficiency of macronutrients or energy and protein in the diet.
- It is a nutritional disorder, which affects all the segments of population like children, women, and adult males particularly from the backward and downtrodden communities.

Different Types of PEM

- **Clinical forms:**
  - Kwashiorkor
  - Marasmus
  - Marasmic kwashiorkor
- **Subclinical forms:**
  - Underweight
  - Wasting
  - Stunting

Marasmus

- *Marasmus* is the childhood form of **starvation.**
- It develops **due to inadequate intake of protein and calories.**
- It is characterized by **emaciation** with apparent muscle wasting and loss of body fat.
- Marasmus is common in children below the age of 2 years.
- The marasmic children are so weak that they may not have even energy to cry, which most often is barely audible.
- The child is extremely wasted with very little subcutaneous fat with the skin hanging loosely particularly over the buttocks.
- Edema is absent and there are no skin and hair changes.
- However, frequent diarrheal episodes leading to dehydration and micronutrient deficiencies of vitamin A, iron, and B-complex are common.

Table 13.12: Classification of trace elements.

Essential trace elements	Trace elements that are probably essential	Potentially toxic elements with possible essential functions in low doses
• Iodine • Zinc • Selenium • Copper • Molybdenum • Chromium • Cobalt • Iron	• Manganese • Nickel • Silicon • Boron • Vanadium	• Fluoride • Lead • Cadmium • Mercury • Arsenic • Lithium • Tin • Aluminum

Signs and symptoms of marasmus:
- Extreme muscle wasting "skin and bones"
- Loose and hanging skin folds
- Old man's or monkey faces
- Absolute weakness

Kwashiorkor (Figs. 13.11A and B)
- Kwashiorkor develops due to an **inadequate protein intake with reasonable caloric** (energy) intake.
- Kwashiorkor is an African word, meaning a "disease of the displaced child", who is deprived of adequate nutrition.
- Mostly in children between the ages of **1** and **3** years, when they are completely weaned (taken off the breast).
- The three essential manifestations or signs of kwashiorkor are:
  1. Edema (swelling of feet)
  2. Growth failure
  3. Mental changes
- It may be **precipitated by infections** (e.g., measles, malaria, and diarrheal illnesses).
- Child appears **apathetic and lethargic with severe anorexia**.
- *Edema*: In kwashiorkor, marked protein deprivation causes **hypoalbuminemia** leading to **generalized or dependent edema.**
- *Skin lesions*: Children with kwashiorkor have characteristic *skin lesions*. This consists of alternating zones of hyperpigmentation, and hypopigmentation, producing **"flaky paint" appearance**.
- **Hair changes:** The hair is **dry and sparse**. There may be loss of color or alternating bands of pale and darker hair (**Flag sign**).
- **Moon face:** The cheeks may seem swollen with fluid or fatty tissue and often be slightly sagging.
- **Micronutrient deficiencies:** Almost all the children manifest anemia (due to iron deficiency) of some degree.
- Eye signs of vitamin A deficiency are also common.
- Manifestations of vitamin B complex deficiency are also noted in many cases.
- **Other features:** The other features that differentiate kwashiorkor from marasmus are:
  - Abdomen is distended due to **hepatomegaly** (presence of enlarged, fatty liver) and/or **ascites.**
  - Development of apathy, listlessness, and **loss of appetite**.
  - Defects in immunity and secondary **infections**.

Marasmic Kwashiorkor
- Sometimes, in areas where PEM is common, malnourished children exhibit the features of both kwashiorkor and marasmus. Such changes could occur during the transition from one form of severe PEM to another **(Table 13.13)**.
- These children will have extreme wasting of different degrees (representing marasmus) and also edema (a sign of kwashiorkor).
- **Signs and symptoms of marasmic kwashiorkor:**
  - Extreme muscle wasting—"skin and bones"
  - Loose and hanging skin folds
  - Old man's or monkey's face
  - Absolute weakness
  - Edema

Treatment of PEM
- **Diet:** Treatment of cases of kwashiorkor or marasmus involves mainly providing appropriate nutrition support. The child should receive a diet that provides adequate amounts of energy and protein. Both of these are required in larger quantities than normal.

Table 13.13: Biochemical signs specific to PEM.

Biochemical changes	Marasmus	Kwashiorkor
Serum albumin	Normal or slightly decreased	Low
Urinary urea per g of the creatinine	Normal or decreased	Low
Urinary hydroxyproline index	Low	Low
Serum free amino acid ratio	Normal	Elevated
Anemia	May be observed	Common iron and folate deficiency may be associated
Pancreatic secretions	Reduced enzymatic activity	Reduced enzymatic activity

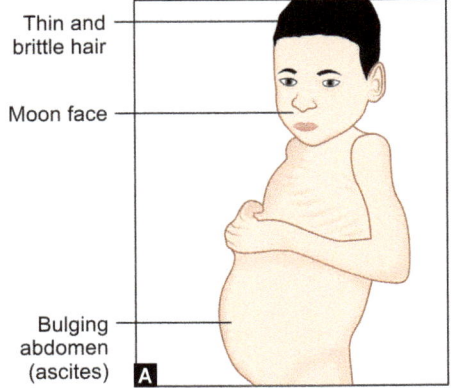 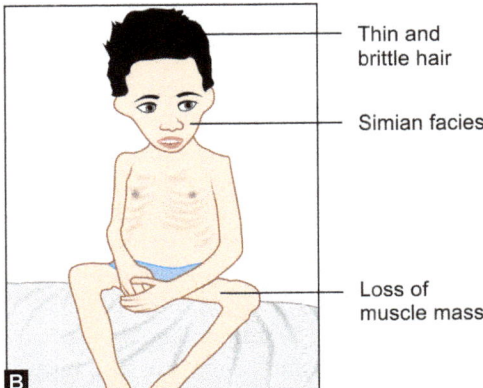

Figs. 13.11A and B: Types of malnutrition: (A) Kwashiorkor; (B) Marasmus.

- The child should be given the following concentrations:
  - Energy: 170–200 kcal per kg of body weight
  - Protein: 3–4 g/kg of body weight
- *Vitamin and mineral supplements:*
  - All cases of severe PEM require multivitamin preparation to meet the increased demands during recovery.
  - Iron (60 mg) and folic acid (100 mg) may be given daily to correct anemia.
- *Oral rehydration:*
  - Since diarrhea is very common in severe PEM, correction of dehydration is the first step in the treatment.
  - Home made (salt-sugar mixture) or commercial oral rehydration solution (ORS) can be administered to correct dehydration.
  - Intravenous fluids are required only in severe dehydration.
- *Control of infections and infestations:*
  - Appropriate antibiotics should be started immediately since infections are the immediate cause of death in many children.
  - Children with intestinal infestations like giardiasis and ascariasis should be treated.
- "Prevention is better than cure". So it becomes extremely important that we make sincere efforts to prevent and control PEM.

OBESITY

- **Definition:** Obesity is defined as an accumulation of **excess body fat (adipose tissue) that is of sufficient magnitude to impair health.** Latin word "obesus" meaning stout, fat, or plump.
- **Measurement of obesity:**
  - *BMI:* Weight/height^2 in kg/m^2
  - *Anthropometry:* Skin-fold thickness
  - *Densitometry:* Underwater weighing
  - CT/MRI imaging
  - Electrical impedance
- Classification of overweight and obesity by BMI **(Table 13.14)**
- **Types of obesity according to body fat distribution:** The distribution of the stored fat is important in obesity and accordingly obesity is divided into:
  - *Central ("abdominal", "visceral", "android", or "apple-shaped") obesity:*
    - This type of obesity shows **increased accumulation of fat in the trunk** and in the **abdominal cavity** (in the mesentery and around viscera).
    - It is associated with a **greater risk** for several diseases (e.g., type 2 diabetes, the metabolic syndrome, and cardiovascular disease) than generalized obesity.
    - *Increased waist:* **Hip ratio:** >0.9 in females, >1 in males is abnormal.
    - *Hypothesis:* intra-abdominal adipocytes are more lipolytically active than others—release free fatty acids into portal circulation—cause adverse metabolic reactions, especially on the liver.
  - *Generalized ("gynoid" or "pear-shaped") obesity:* This type is characterized by excess accumulation of **fat diffusely in the subcutaneous tissue**.

Etiology

Accumulation of fat in obesity can be considered by the result of **caloric imbalance** between the energy consumption (**intake** of calories) in the diet and **energy expenditure** through exercise and bodily functions.

Etiology and Risk Factors of Obesity

Etiology and risk factors of obesity are shown in **Table 13.15**.

Potentially Reversible Causes of Obesity and Weight Gain

Endocrine Factors
- Hypothyroidism
- Cushing's syndrome
- Insulinoma Stein–Leventhal syndrome
- Hypothalamic damage (e.g., due to trauma, tumor)

Drug-induced
- **Psychiatric and neurologic medications:** Atypical antipsychotics (e.g., olanzapine, pizotifen, sodium valproate, flunarizine)
- **Steroid hormones:** Progestational steroids, corticosteroids, hormonal contraceptives
- **Antidiabetic agents:** Insulin (most forms), sulfonylureas, thiazolidinediones
- **Antihypertensive agents:** α- and β-adrenergic receptor blockers

Pathologic Consequences of Obesity (Complications of Obesity)

Morbidity and mortality: Obesity is associated with an **increase** in mortality and morbidity. Obese individuals are at risk of early death, mainly from diabetes, coronary heart disease, and cerebrovascular disease.

Metabolic Complications of Obesity

- Central obesity or upper body fat distribution is associated with increased concentration of free-fatty

Table 13.14: Nutritional status based on the WHO and "Asian criteria" values.

Nutritional status	WHO criteria BMI cut-off	"Asian criteria" BMI cut-off
Underweight	<18.5	<18.5
Normal	18.5–24.9	18.5–22.9
Overweight	25–29.9	23–24.9
Preobese	–	25–29.9
Obese	>30	>30
Obese type-1 (obese)	30–40	30–40
Obese type-2 (morbid obese)	40.1–50	40.1–50
Obese type 3 (super obese)	>50	>50

Table 13.15: Etiology and risk factors of obesity.

Genetic aspects	Environmental factors
• Obesity is a **polygenic disorder**, with small contributions from a number of different genes. • Single-gene (**monogenic forms**) disorders are rare and produce severe childhood obesity—mutations in the leptin gene and leptin receptor gene, mutations of *POMC* (proopiomelanocortin), *Mc4R* (melanocortin-4 receptor) genes	• **Food:** Many environmental factors can influence food intake. • Increased consumption of energy-dense foods, larger food portion size, and increased variety of food, increased availability, reduced cost, and increased caloric beverages (soft drinks, juices) promote obesity
• A few **genetic condition in which obesity** is a feature including the Prader–Willi and Laurence–Moon–Biedl syndromes	• **Physical activity:** (1) exercise (fitness and sports-related activities); (2) work-related physical activity; and (3) nonexercise, nonemployment (spontaneous) activity • Increased sedentary behavior, reduced activities of daily living, and decreased physical activity promote obesity
Reversible causes of obesity and weight gain	
Minority of patients presenting with obesity have specific cause, which can be identified and treated (**Table 13.16**). Compared to idiopathic obesity, these patients have short history of marked weight gain	

acid (FFA), which can produce several metabolic complications of obesity.

☐ **Insulin resistance and type 2 diabetes mellitus:**
  • Insulin resistance is the decrease/failure of response of target (peripheral) tissues to insulin action.
  • Insulin resistance can develop in obesity and may produce type 2 diabetes mellitus.
  • **Central/upper body/visceral obesity** is found in more than 80% of patients with **type 2 diabetes.**

☐ **Causes of insulin resistance in obesity:**
  • **Obese individuals** have **excess** circulating **FFAs** and there is an **inverse correlation between fasting plasma FFAs and insulin sensitivity.** Central obesity is associated with **insulin resistance. Excess intracellular FFAs increases gluconeogenesis.**
  • **Adipokines: Adipose tissue** acts as a functional endocrine organ and **secrets variety of proteins** into the systemic circulation, which are **termed as adipokines** (or adipose cytokines). **In obesity, adiponectin (one of the adipokines) levels are reduced,** which contributes to insulin resistance.

☐ **Consequences of insulin resistance:**
  • *Muscle:* Hyperglycemia and diabetes mellitus
  • *Kidneys:* Salt retention and hypertension
  • *Ovaries:* Increase testosterone and polycystic ovary syndrome (PCOS)
  • *Heart:* Increase plasminogen activator inhibitor (PAI 1) and acute coronary syndrome
  • *Cancers:* Colon, prostrate, breast
  • *Sympathetic system:* Increased cytokines and blood pressure.

☐ **Dyslipidemia:**
  • Upper body obesity and type 2 diabetes mellitus are associated with an atherogenic lipid profile. Dyslipidemia includes **increased triglycerides, increased low-density lipoprotein (LDL) cholesterol with very low-density lipoprotein (VLDL) cholesterol**, decreased **high-density lipoprotein (HDL)** cholesterol, and decreased levels of the vascular protective adipokine adiponectin.
  • Dyslipidemia increases the risk of cardiovascular diseases (**atherosclerosis, cardiomyopathy**) in the metabolic syndrome.

Endocrine Manifestations of Obesity

Endocrine manifestations of obesity in men and women are shown in **Table 13.17.**

Mechanical Complications of Obesity

☐ **Osteoarthritis:** Extremity degenerative joint disease (osteoarthritis) and also gout.
☐ **Venous stasis/varicose veins**
☐ **Acanthosis nigricans:** Reflects the severity of underlying insulin resistance.

Table 13.16: Potentially reversible causes of obesity and weight gain.

Endocrine factors	
• Hypothyroidism • Cushing's syndrome • Insulinoma	• Stein–Leventhal syndrome • Hypothalamic damage (e.g., due to trauma, tumor)
Drug induced	
• **Psychiatric and neurologic medications:** Atypical antipsychotics (e.g., olanzapine) pizotifen, sodium valproate, flunarizine • **Steroid hormones:** Progestational steroids, corticosteroids, hormonal contraceptives	• **Antidiabetic agents:** Insulin (most forms), sulfonylureas, thiazolidinediones • **Antihypertensive agents:** α- and β-adrenergic receptor blockers

Table 13.17: Endocrine manifestations of obesity.

Men	Women
• Plasma testosterone and SHBG are reduced • Increase estrogen • Gynecomastia seen • Secondary sexual characters preserved	• Increased androgen • Decrease SHBG • PCOS • Not only fertility but their chances of IVF success reduces

- **Increased friability of skin:** It may be seen especially in skinfolds, thereby increasing the risk of fungal and yeast infections.
- **Urinary incontinence**
- **Pulmonary disease:**
  - These include reduced chest wall compliance, increased work of breathing, increased minute ventilation (due to increased metabolic rate), and decreased functional residual capacity (FRC) and expiratory reserve volume.
  - *Obstructive sleep apnea:* Sleep apnea is common in patients with severe obesity. Sleep apnea can be obstructive (most common), central, or mixed and is often associated with an increased risk of hypertension, right heart failure and sudden death. Obesity hypoventilation syndrome is also known as **Pickwickian syndrome**.
  - *Obesity and asthma:* Reduced total lung capacity (TLC), reduced residual volume (RV), and FRC.
  - *Obesity and cancer*

Males	Females
Esophagus	Gallbladder
Colon	Bile ducts
Rectum	Breasts
Pancreas	Endometrium
Liver	Cervix
Prostate	Ovaries

  - Obesity is the biggest preventable cause of cancer after smoking.
  - Accounts for 14% of cancer deaths in men and 20% in women.
- *Gastrointestinal disorders:* Following are more prevalent in obese patients:
  - *Gastroesophageal reflux disease*
  - *Gallstones:* Obesity is associated with increased secretion of cholesterol in the bile, supersaturation of bile, and a higher incidence of gallstones, especially cholesterol gallstones.
  - *Fatty liver (steatosis) and nonalcoholic steatohepatitis (NAFLD):* NAFLD can progress to hepatic cirrhosis and rarely to hepatocellular carcinoma.

Clinical Assessment, Investigations, and Diagnosis

Aims of assessing of obesity are to:
- **Evaluate and severity of obesity:** Severity of obesity can be quantified using the BMI
- **Exclude an underlying cause**
- **Identify complications**
- **Prepare a management plan**

Appearance of a patient with morbid obesity is shown in **Figure 13.12**.

Management

- **Goal:**
  - Initially to reduce weight by about 10% from baseline
  - Reduce weight of about 0.5–1 kg/week for 6 months.
- **Lifestyle modification diet:**
  - Low calorie diet, low in saturated fats, low density foods, normal protein intake, and increased fibers in diet.
  - 1,000 kcal deficits produce 1 kg weight loss per week. No matter what the calorie intake is the constituents remain in same proportion (i.e., carbohydrates 55%, fat 30%, and protein 15%).
  - **Total fasting: Not recommended.** There is diuresis, natriuresis, and all deficiencies.

Types of Diet in the Treatment of Obesity (Table 13.18)

- **Physical activity:** Regular physical activity enables to maintain loss of weight. Has to be done under supervision. Moderate exercise to be done for 30–45 minutes and 3–5 days/week.
- **Behavioral modification:** (1) Useful as adjunct to diet and physical exercise, (2) Patient often needs motivation to lose weight.
- **Drug therapy (pharmacotherapy):** Lifestyle modification should be considered before starting drug therapy.

Table 13.18: Types of diet in the treatment of obesity.

Fixed energy diet	Low calorie diet	Very low-calorie diet (VLCD)
• 1,200–1,800 kcal • Intake is limited by controlling portion sizes, menu choice and composition • Minimal self-monitoring • Lack of compliance to this rigid pattern	• 800–1,000 kcal • Applicable to most of the patients • Fewer restrictions than VLCD • Supplementation of vitamins and minerals • Reduction of 6–7 kg observed over a year	• 400–600 kcal • Even below one's basal metabolic rate • Used for period of 1–2 months under medical supervision • 45–70% protein, 30–50% carbohydrates and 2 g fat • Supplementation of vitamins, minerals and trace elements • Greater weight loss compared to restrictive diets

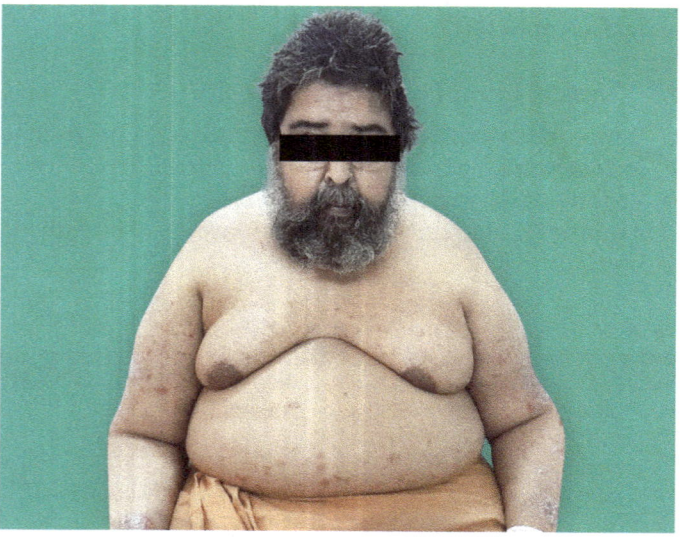

Fig. 13.12: Appearance of a patient with morbid obesity.

- *Centrally acting drugs*
  - *Sibutramine:*
    - *Mechanism of action:* Centrally acting, mono amine reuptake inhibitor (primarily serotonin and norepinephrine). By sympathetic stimulation, it prevents decrease in BMR. It reduces appetite.
  - *Rimonabant:*
    - *Mechanism of action:* Endocannabinoid (CB1) receptor blocker. It has both central and peripheral actions and reduces weight and weight-related metabolic factors.
    - *FDA approval:* BANNED
    - *Side effects:* Depression, anxiety, suicidal tendencies.
- *Peripherally acting drugs:*
  - *Orlistat:*
    - *Mechanism of action:* Nonsystemic reversible inhibitor of gastric and pancreatic lipases by forming a covalent bond with serine residue. It acts on stomach and intestine.
  - *Olestra:* Olestra is synthesized using a sucrose molecule, which can support from 6–8 fatty acid chains arranged radially like an octopus. Too large to move through the intestinal wall and be absorbed. Same taste and mouth feel as fat. Approval as a food additive up to 35% replacement of fats in home cooking and 75% in commercial uses.
- *Others:*
  - *Phentermine:* Amphetamine like drug, act centrally to reduce appetite. It has low addictive potential, modest efficacy and CVS side effects.
  - *Metformin:* Decreases appetite and thereby reduces weight. Since most DM II patients are obese, this is a good choice in DM II.
  - *Tesofensine (TE)* is a norepinephrine, dopamine, and serotonin reuptake inhibitor. Primarily used as an appetite suppressant.
  - *Betahistine:* Stimulates the histamine-1 receptor and reduce the craving not only for food in general but for fatty foods in particular. Not approved by FDA.
  - *Amylin (pramlintide):* Part of the endocrine pancreas and contributes to glycemic control. Functions as a synergistic partner to insulin.
  - *Liraglutide*, a GLP-1 agonist (1.8 or 3 mg daily), is an option for overweight or obese patients.
  - *Lorcaserin*, serotonin agonist approved by FDA
  - *Combination therapy:*
    - Phentermine-topiramate
    - Bupropion-naltrexone
- **Bariatric surgical techniques:**
  - *Indications:*
    - BMI ≥40 kg/m² without comorbid illness
    - BMI 35.0–39.9 kg/m² with at least one serious
    - Divided into three groups **(Figs. 13.13A to C)**
      1. *Malabsorptive procedures:* Induce decreased absorption of nutrients by shortening the functional length of the small intestine (e.g., biliopancreatic diversion and Roux-en-Y gastric

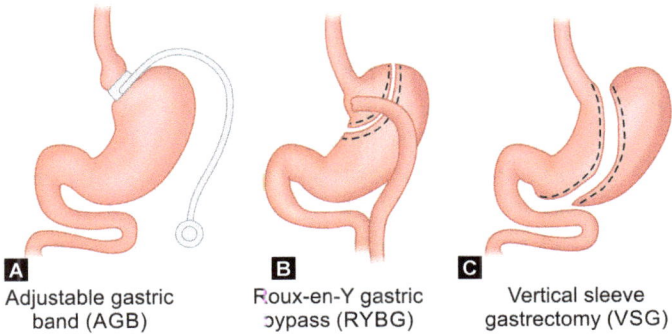

Figs. 13.13A to C: Various surgical options for the treatment of obesity.

  bypass). These procedures cause deficiency of nutrients, malnutrition and in some cases, anastomotic leaks and the dumping syndrome (e.g., with the duodenal switch).
      2. *Restrictive procedures:* Reduce the storage capacity of the stomach and as a result early satiety arises, leading to a decreased caloric intake (e.g., adjustable gastric banding, vertical banded gastroplasty, and sleeve gastroplasty).
      3. *Restrictive plus malabsorptive procedures* (e.g., duodenal switch, Roux-en-Y gastric bypass, intragastric balloon).
- **Liposuction:** It is the removal of large amounts of fat by suction (liposuction). It does not deal with the underlying cause and weight regain frequently occurs. There is no reduction in cardiovascular risk factors with the procedure.
- **Others:**
  - Electrical stimulation (vagal blockade) systems
  - *Hydrogels:* Hydrogels are orally administered products, taken twice daily before meals, which expand in the stomach and intestines to create a sensation of satiety. They are not systemically absorbed, and are eliminated through the feces.
  - *Dietary supplements:* Although over-the-counter dietary supplements are widely used by individuals attempting to lose weight-like ephedra, green tea, chromium, chitosan, and guar gum. These are not recommended and are inadequate and unsafe methods to lose weight.

OBJECTIVE-BASED SELF-EVALUATION

LONG QUESTIONS

1. What is the RDA of vitamin A? Discuss the clinical features of vitamin A deficiency and its management.
2. Briefly outline calcium metabolism. Discuss the clinical features and management of hyperparathyroidism.
3. How do you calculate body mass index? Classify nutritional status based on BMI. Add a note on the etiology of obesity.
4. Define obesity. Discuss the complications and management of obesity.
5. What are dietary sources of vitamin B_1? Discuss the clinical features and management of vitamin B_1 deficiency.

Chapter 13: Nutrition

6. What are the types of protein–energy malnutrition? Discuss the clinical features and management of the same.
7. Discuss the role of vitamin D in health and disease.
8. Discuss the clinical features and management of vitamin D deficiency in children and adults.
9. What are dietary sources of vitamin C? Discuss the clinical features and management of vitamin C deficiency.
10. What are dietary sources of vitamin B_3? Discuss the clinical features and management of vitamin B_3 deficiency.
11. What are dietary sources of vitamin B_{12}? Discuss the clinical features and management of vitamin B_{12} deficiency.

SHORT ANSWER QUESTIONS

1. Nutritional assessment
2. Tetany
3. Causes of hypercalcemia
4. Differences between marasmus and kwashiorkor
5. MEN syndromes
6. Pellagra
7. Beriberi
8. Scurvy
9. Rickets
10. Clinical signs of vitamin deficiency
11. Hypervitaminosis A
12. Management of obesity
13. Wernicke-Korsakoff syndrome
14. Vitamin K
15. Hypoparathyroidism

MULTIPLE CHOICE QUESTIONS

1. A 75-year-old male with liver disease and poor nutrition develops alopecia, dermatitis and paronychia. Which vitamin deficiency can lead to these symptoms?
   a. Calcium b. Selenium
   c. Zinc d. Magnesium
2. What food is a good source of vitamin D?
   a. Red meat
   b. Green leafy vegetables
   c. Herring
   d. Salmon
3. A 3-year-old child was born at term, with no congenital anomalies. She is now only 70% of normal body weight. On examination, she shows dependent edema of the lower extremities as well as an enlarged abdomen with palpable fluid wave. Her desquamating skin shows irregular areas of depigmentation, and hyperpigmentation. Which of the following nutritional problems is most likely present in this child?
   a. Marasmus b. Scurvy
   c. Niacin deficiency d. Kwashiorkor
4. 24-year-old man has a history of multiple and recurrent pulmonary infections since childhood. He also has noted foul smelling stools for the past 10 years. Laboratory studies show an elevated sweat chloride test. He has a quantitative stool fat of 10 g/day. A deficiency state involving which of the following nutrients is most likely to develop in this patient?
   a. Vitamin B_1 b. Vitamin D
   c. Iron d. Calcium
5. A 60-year-old woman has developed red, roughened skin in sun-exposed areas over the past 2 years. She also has a chronic, watery diarrhea. On physical examination she exhibits memory loss with confusion. These findings are most consistent with which of the following vitamin deficiencies?
   a. Vitamin A b. Thiamine
   c. Niacin d. Pyridoxine
6. A 6-year-old child has complained of pain in his legs for the past year. On physical examination, there is bowing deformity of his lower extremities. Plain film radiographs of his lower legs shows widened epiphyses and bowing of tibiae. Bone mineral density appears normal, consistent with failure of osteoid matrix formation. Which of the following vitamin deficiencies is this child most likely to have?
   a. D b. E
   c. C d. B_3
7. It is observed that pregnant women who do not get a diet that includes green, leafy vegetables develop a specific nutritional deficiency that affects their developing fetuses. Which of the following abnormalities is most likely to be found with increased frequency in these fetuses?
   a. Anencephaly
   b. Diaphragmatic hernia
   c. Low birth weight
   d. Congenital cytomegalovirus
8. A clinical study is performed involving dietary iron metabolism in adults. It is observed that intestinal absorption of iron can be enhanced in patients with iron deficiency anemia by supplementing their diet with another nutrient. Which of the following vitamins is most likely to have this effect?
   a. A b. B_1
   c. C d. D
9. A 50-year-old man chronic alcoholic has had increasing dyspnea for the past year. On physical examination, his temperature is 37°C, pulse 106/min, respiratory rate 20/min, and blood pressure 90/60 mm Hg. He has diffuse crackles at lung bases. A chest X-ray shows pulmonary edema and cardiomegaly. Echocardiography shows an ejection fraction of 40%. Laboratory studies show hemoglobin 14 g/dL, hematocrit 42%, and WBC count 8320/microliter. A deficiency in which of the following vitamins is most likely to produce these findings?
   a. A b. B_1
   c. B_2 d. K
10. A 50-year-old man has a 15-year history of chronic alcohol abuse. He has had worsening problems with ambulation for the past year. On physical examination, his gait is

ataxic. MR imaging of the brain shows diminished size of the mamillary bodies and of the cerebellar vermis. He is most likely to have a deficiency of which of the following vitamins?
   a. A
   b. B_1
   c. D
   d. E

11. A 30-year-old primigravida is in her 8th month of gestation. She is feeling increasingly tired and weak. Laboratory studies include a CBC which shows Hgb 9.7 g/dL, Hct 28.8%, MCV 71 fL, platelet count 289,000/microliter, and WBC count 5600/microliter. On the peripheral blood smear, the RBCs show increased variation in size and shape, with many that are hypochromic and microcytic. Which of the following dietary deficiencies is she most likely to have?
   a. Folic acid
   b. Vitamin B_{12}
   c. Iron
   d. Calcium

12. A 30-year-old man with a 10-year history of chronic alcohol abuse has noted during the past year that he has bruising with minimal trauma. On physical examination he has abdominal enlargement with a fluid wave. He has pitting edema to the knees. He has palmar erythema. Laboratory studies show he has a prothrombin time of 30 seconds (control 12). His hemoglobin is 13.8 g/dL, hematocrit 44.4%, MCV 94 fL, platelet count 229,000/microliter, and WBC count 6630/microliter. Which of the following nutrients is most likely to be of benefit in treating this man?
   a. Vitamin C
   b. Niacin
   c. Vitamin K
   d. Folic acid

13. It is observed that some commonly available foods have more vitamin A than others. Which of the following is most likely to provide the best source for vitamin A in the diet?
   a. Milk
   b. Meat
   c. Beer
   d. Carrots

14. A 14-year-old girl has been under a physician's care for the past year after diagnosis of anorexia nervosa. Her BMI is now 17.8. On physical examination, she has cheilosis. Laboratory studies show hemoglobin 13.7 g/dL, hematocrit 41.0%, MCV 88 fL, platelet count 191,055/microliter, and WBC count 4930/microliter. Her serum glucose is 66 mg/dL. Which of the following nutrient deficiencies is most likely to cause her findings?
   a. Riboflavin
   b. Ascorbic acid
   c. Folic acid
   d. Niacin

15. A 40-year-old woman goes to the health food store to buy dietary supplements that she is convinced will help her to be more healthy and live longer. Instead, a year later she has increasing headaches, joint pain, nausea, vomiting, and weight loss. On physical examination she is noted to have dryness of the oral mucosa, and a mild degree of papilledema is noted on funduscopic examination. An excessive intake of which of the following nutrients is most likely responsible for her findings?
   a. Calcium
   b. Fluoride
   c. Vitamin A
   d. Niacin

16. A 44-year-old woman has been on and off diets for the past 10 years trying to lose weight. She has had no major illnesses during this time. Her BMI has ranged from 25 to 31 over that time. Which of the following problems is her pattern of dieting most likely to cause?
   a. Vitamin deficiencies
   b. Increased risk for osteoporosis
   c. Decreased risk for atherosclerosis
   d. Greater weight gain

17. A 7-year-old child develops gradual loss of vision over the past 2 years resulting in blindness. On physical examination, there is bilateral keratomalacia and corneal scarring. This child's blindness is most likely to have been prevented by adequate dietary intake of which of the following vitamins?
   a. A
   b. B_1
   c. B_6
   d. K

18. An 11-month-old infant is only 60% of ideal body weight. The baby is proportionately small in size. Upon physical examination, the baby is listless and does not respond with vocalization when touched. A small purplish contusion is noted over the right lower extremity. Which of the following is the most likely diagnosis?
   a. Marasmus
   b. Hypocalcemia
   c. Premature birth
   d. Vitamin C deficiency

19. A 45-year-old woman has felt increasingly fatigued. On physical examination, she has decreased sensation to touch in her lower extremities bilaterally. Laboratory studies show hemoglobin 10.1 g/dL, hematocrit 31.2%, and MCV 126 fL. Microscopic examination of her peripheral blood smear shows red blood cells that have macrocytosis and neutrophils with hyper segmentation of nuclei. Laboratory testing for which of the following nutrients is most likely to show a deficiency state?
   a. Folate
   b. Iron
   c. Cobalamin
   d. Pyridoxine

20. A 32-year-old woman has been having particularly heavy menstrual periods for the past year. She is becoming progressively fatigued. She then becomes pregnant. She receives no prenatal care. She delivers a term baby. During the delivery, bleeding is excessive. Which of the following nutrient deficiencies is most likely to be present in both mother and baby postpartum?
   a. Niacin
   b. Magnesium
   c. Vitamin K
   d. Iron

ANSWERS

1. c
2. c
3. d
4. a
5. c
6. c
7. a
8. c
9. b
10. b
11. c
12. c
13. d
14. a
15. c
16. d
17. a
18. a
19. c
20. d

14 Endocrinology

CHAPTER OUTLINE

- Disorders of Pituitary and Hypothalamus
- Acromegaly
- Diabetes Insipidus
- Thyroid Disorders
- Thyroiditis
- Adrenal Gland Disorders
- Diabetes Mellitus
- Complications of Diabetes
- Metabolic Syndrome

DISORDERS OF PITUITARY AND HYPOTHALAMUS

Pituitary Hormones and their Principal Actions
See **Table 14.1**.

Hypopituitarism

Definition

- Hypopituitarism is defined as **combined deficiency (partial or complete) of any of the anterior pituitary hormones**.
- Panhypopituitarism is defined as **deficiency of all anterior pituitary hormones**.
- It may be due to selective or multiple deficiencies of pituitary hormones or disease of the hypothalamus.

Etiology

See **Box 14.1**.

Clinical Features (Table 14.2)

The presentation is highly variable and depends on the underlying cause/lesion. Symptoms and signs depend on the degree of hypothalamic and/or pituitary deficiencies. Mild deficiencies may be asymptomatic.

- **Hypopituitarism secondary to pituitary tumors:** Symptoms are due to mass effects (e.g., headache, visual impairment, electrolyte alterations, and disorders of the autonomic nervous system produced by hypothalamic involvement). As the lesions progress (e.g., nonfunctioning pituitary tumors), there is a sequential loss of hormone secretion.
- PRL deficiency is rare, except for complete destruction of pituitary or genetic syndromes.
- The order of diminished trophic hormone reserve function by pituitary compression usually follows the order **GH>FSH>LH>TSH >ACTH**.

Table 14.1: Pituitary hormones and their principal actions.

Hormone	Actions
Anterior pituitary hormones	
Thyroid stimulating hormone (TSH)	Synthesis and secretion of thyroxine (T4) and triiodothyronine (T3)
Growth hormone (GH)	Growth induction
Follicle stimulating hormone (FSH) and luteinizing hormone (LH)	Sex steroid production, follicle growth, germ cell maturation *Males:* • FSH and LH: Spermatogenesis • FSH: Stimulates sertoli cells to secrete androgen binding protein (ABP), transferrin, plasminogen activator and inhibin • LH: Stimulates Leydig cells to produce testosterone *Females:* • FSH and LH are necessary for the development of corpus luteum during the luteal phase of menstrual cycle • FSH promotes growth and development of ovarian follicles during the follicular phase of menstrual cycle • LH (LH surge) induces ovulation
Prolactin (PRL)	Controls milk production by breasts
Adrenocorticotrophic hormone (ACTH)	Controls cortisol release from adrenal cortex and skin pigmentation
Posterior pituitary hormones	
Arginine vasopressin (AVP)	Promotes reabsorption of water by renal tubules
Oxytocin	Promotes uterine contraction and expression of milk from the breasts

> **Box 14.1:** Various causes of hypopituitarism.
>
> A helpful mnemonic is the phrase "nine I's": **Invasive, Infarction, Infiltrative, Injury, Immunologic, Iatrogenic, Infectious, Idiopathic, and Isolated.**
> - Isolated hormone deficiencies
> - Invasive tumors: Pituitary adenomas, cysts, metastasis, hypothalamic tumors
> - Injury: Surgery, irradiation, stalk section
> - Infarction: Sheehan's syndrome (postpartum pituitary necrosis), diabetic antepartum necrosis, carotid aneurysm
> - Cerebrovascular accidents (CVA): Ischemic stroke, subarachnoid hemorrhage, and pituitary apoplexy
> - Inflammatory diseases: Granulomatous disease, autoimmune (lymphocytic) hypophysitis
> - Infiltrative diseases: Hemochromatosis, amyloidosis, sarcoidosis, Langerhans cell histiocytosis, and early stages of lymphocytic hypophysitis.
> - Injury: Head trauma
> - Immunologic: Lymphocytic hypophysitis
> - Infections: Meningitis, tuberculosis, syphilis, fungal infection (*Candida*), and Hanta virus.
> - Developmental defects (Kallmann syndrome) and genetic diseases.

- Long-standing panhypopituitarism produces a classic picture of **pallor with hairlessness ("alabaster skin")**.

Management

Replacement therapy for adult hypopituitarism:
- **Adrenocorticotropic hormone:** Hydrocortisone 15–25 mg daily in divided doses. Mineralocortcoid replacement not needed.
- **Follicle-stimulating hormone/luteinizing hormone**
  - Female patients (any one)
    - Conjugated estrogen 0.65 mg/day
    - Micronized estradiol 1 mg/day
    - Ethinyl estradiol 0.02–0.05 mg/day
    - Estradiol skin patch 4–8 mg twice weekly
  - Male patients (any one)
    - Testosterone enanthate 200 mg IM every 2–3 weeks
    - Testosterone skin patch 2.5–5.0 mg/day; can increase dose up to 7.5 mg/day
    - Testosterone gel 3–6 g daily
- **Growth hormone (GH)**
  - *Adults:* Recombinant human GH (rhGH) starting dose 2–5 µg/kg subcutaneously daily. This weight-based recommendation is for the starting dose only. The goal should be to start with low doses and increase gradually until the serum IGF-1 concentration is normal.
  - *Children:* Recombinant human GH is 0.16–0.24 mg/kg/week, divided into once daily injections. Further adjustments of GH dose based on growth response, serum insulin-like growth factor 1 (IGF-1) levels, and body weight
- **Thyroid-stimulating hormone:** L (levo)-thyroxine dose of 1.6 µg/kg daily and adjusting dose according to serum free T4 levels in upper half of reference range.
- **Vasopressin:**
  - Intranasal desmopressin-rhinal tube 5–20 µg twice daily
  - Oral DDAVP (Desmopressin) 300–600 µg daily, usually in divided doses
- **Prolactin:** Recombinant human prolactin (r-hPRL), although not commercially available, has been used experimentally.

Sheehan's Syndrome

Sheehan's syndrome is a potentially life-threatening complication due to **infarction of pituitary gland following postpartum hemorrhage**.

Mechanism

During pregnancy, the pituitary gland is enlarged and is more vulnerable to ischemia. Postpartum hemorrhage and consequent systemic hypotension can cause pituitary infarction.

Clinical Features

- Earliest symptom is **failure to lactate.**
- **Failure to regain menstruation after delivery**

Table 14.2: Clinical features due to deficiencies of various pituitary hormones.

Deficiency	Features
GH deficiency (GH often the earliest to be lost)	Decreased growth in children but may be clinically occult in adult patients. GH deficiency is associated with a decreased sense of well-being, lethargy, muscle weakness, and increased fat mass with a decrease in lean body mass
LH and FSH deficiency	• Hypogonadism may precede the clinical appearance of a hypothalamic-pituitary lesion • Leads to loss of libido and impotence in males, and oligomenorrhea or amenorrhea in females • In both sexes, infertility and osteoporosis occur, axillary and pubic hair becomes sparse, and the skin becomes fine and wrinkled • In males, there may be gynecomastia and decreased frequency of shaving
ACTH deficiency	• Weakness, nausea, vomiting, anorexia, decreased libido, weight loss, fever, tachycardia, and postural hypotension may occur. Severe forms of deficiency cause death due to vascular collapse • Normal plasma electrolytes (relative preservation of mineralocorticoid production) • In contrast to the hyperpigmentation that occurs during states of ACTH excess (Addison's disease, Nelson's syndrome), depigmentation, and diminished tanning may develop due to ACTH insufficiency
TSH deficiency	Secondary hypothyroidism is usually less severe than primary hypothyroidism, and goiter is absent. Cold intolerance, dry skin, mental dullness, bradycardia, delayed relaxation phase of the deep-tendon reflexes, constipation, weight gain, hoarseness, and anemia are seen
PRL deficiency	Failure of lactation (postpartum)

- **Other symptoms of hypopituitarism:** They appear over months or years. Few patients may present acutely (hypotension, hyponatremia, and hypothyroidism).
- Coma and death can occur in severe cases.

Treatment of Sheehan's Syndrome
- Control of hemorrhage and volume replacement.
- Administration of deficient hormones.

ACROMEGALY

Acromegaly results from persistent hypersecretion of GH. Excess GH stimulates hepatic secretion of IGF-1, which causes most of the clinical manifestations of acromegaly.
- Excess secretion of GH prior to closure of epiphyseal growth plates in long bone before onset of puberty causes **pituitary gigantism**.
- Excess secretion **after puberty** causes **acromegaly**.
- Males and females are equally affected.

Etiology of Acromegaly
Excess of GH (GH excess) after puberty may be due to:
- **Pituitary tumor (somatotrope pituitary adenoma)** is the **most common cause**. Acromegaly is caused by GH secretion usually from a macroadenoma of pituitary gland. Few adenomas secrete both GH as well as prolactin.
- **Other tumors:** In a few patients, acromegaly is caused by tumors of the **pancreas, lungs, and adrenal glands** (either because they produce GH themselves or, more frequently they produce GHRH, the hormone that stimulates the pituitary to make GH).

Clinical Features
See **Table 14.3 and Figures 14.1A to C**.

Investigations
1. Biochemical investigations
- **IGF-1 levels:** It is the single best test useful in diagnosis. IGF1 is almost always elevated in acromegaly.
- **GH levels:** Acromegaly can be confirmed by assessment of GH secretion. Basal fasting GH levels [normal, 1–5 ng/mL (46–232 pmol/L)] are >10 ng/mL (465 pmol/L) in more than 90% of patients and range from 5 ng/mL (232 pmol/L) to >500 ng/mL (23,000 pmol/L), with a mean of approximately 50 ng/mL (2,300 pmol/L).
- **Oral glucose tolerance test:** The criterion for the diagnosis of acromegaly is a GH concentration greater than 1 ng/mL
- **Serum IGFBP-3** concentrations are elevated in patients with acromegaly.
- **Thyrotropin-releasing hormone (TRH),** in a dose of 500 µg intravenously, raises serum GH concentrations by 50% or more in approximately one-half of patients with acromegaly, with peak values occurring at 20–30 minutes.
- **Postprandial plasma glucose may be elevated**, and serum insulin is increased in 70% of patients.
- **Prolactin:** Shows mild to moderate elevation in about 30% of patients due to cosecretion of prolactin from the tumor.
- **Others:** Elevated serum phosphorus.

2. Radiological investigations (Figs. 14.2A to C)
- **MRI of pituitary:** If the biochemical tests are abnormal and GH hypersecretion is confined, MRI will almost always reveal and localize the pituitary adenoma usually a somatotroph adenoma (most common cause of acromegaly). If the MRI is normal, abdominal, chest imaging or DOTATATE PET scan should be performed to look for an ectopic source of hormone secretion.

Table 14.3: Various systems involved in acromegaly and presenting features.

System/tissue involved	Features
Local tumor effects	Pituitary enlargement, visual-field defects, cranial nerve palsy, headache
Somatic systems	Acral enlargement including thickness of soft tissue of hands and feet
Musculoskeletal system and neurological	Gigantism, prognathism, jaw malocclusion, widely spaced teeth, arthralgia and arthritis, carpal tunnel syndrome, acroparesthesia, proximal myopathy, hypertrophy of frontal bones, and osteoporosis
Skin and integumental	Skin tags, acanthosis nigricans, increased sweat and sebum resulting in moist and oily skin, enlargement of lips, nose, and tongue, increased heel-pad thickness
Gastrointestinal system	Macroglossia, colonic polyps, visceromegaly, pancreatic cancer
Cardiovascular system	Left ventricular hypertrophy, asymmetric septal hypertrophy, cardiomyopathy, hypertension, congestive heart failure, coronary artery disease
Pulmonary system	Sleep disturbances, sleep apnea (central and obstructive), narcolepsy
Visceromegaly	Tongue, thyroid gland, salivary glands, liver, spleen, kidney, prostate
Reproduction	Menstrual abnormalities, galactorrhea, decreased libido, impotence, low levels of sex hormone-binding globulin, gynecomastia
Multiple endocrine neoplasia type 1	Hyperparathyroidism, pancreatic islet cell tumors
Carbohydrate metabolism	Impaired glucose tolerance, insulin resistance, and hyperinsulinemia, diabetes mellitus
Lipid	Hypertriglyceridemia
Mineral	Hypercalciuria, increased levels of 25-hydroxyvitamin D3, urinary hydroxyproline levels increased
Electrolyte	Low-renin levels, increased aldosterone levels
Thyroid	Low thyroxine binding globulin levels, goiter

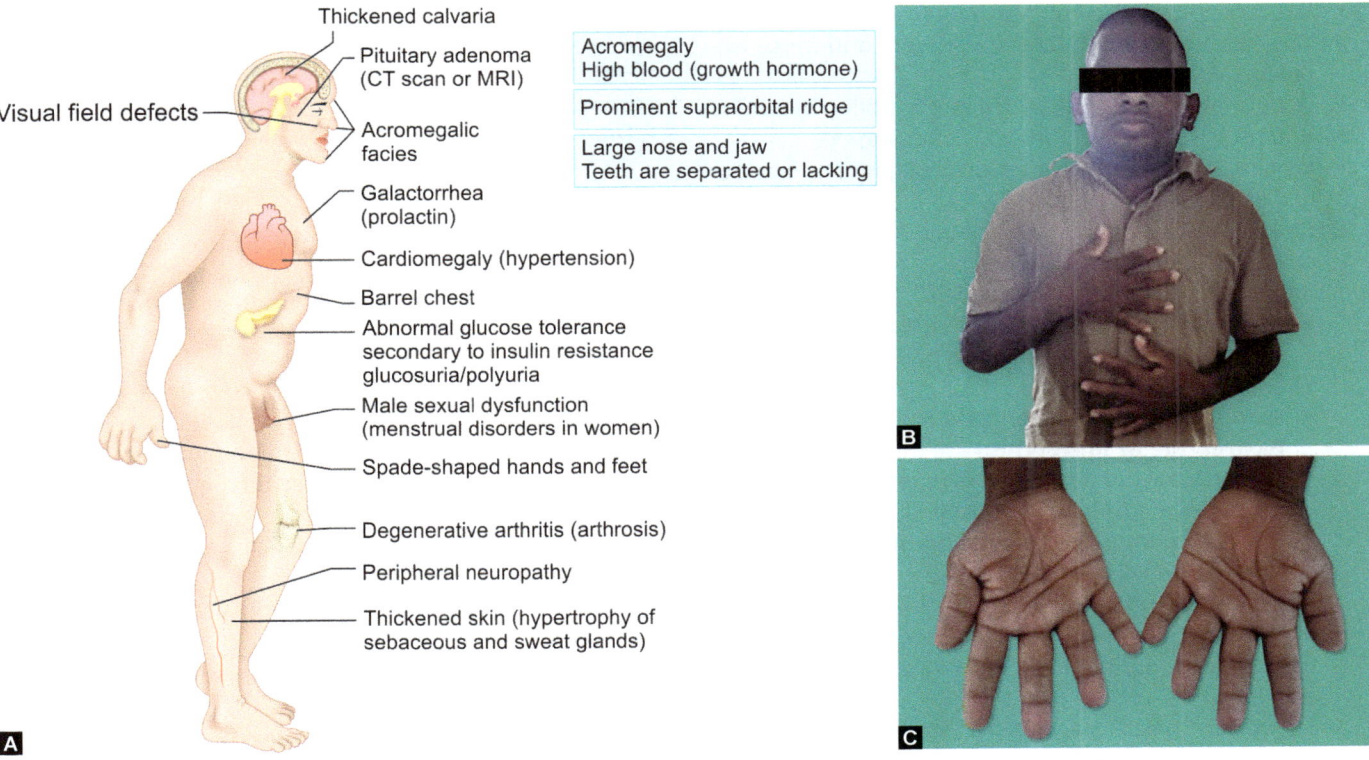

Figs. 14.1A to C: (A) Summary of various clinical features (diagrammatic); (B) Clinical features of acromegaly; (C) Acromegalic facies and thick and spade-shaped hands.

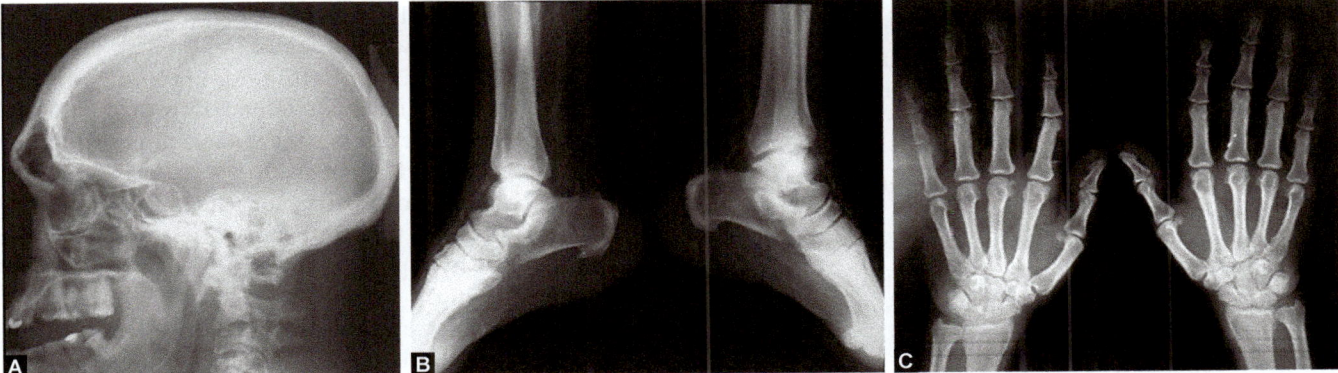

Figs. 14.2A to C: X-ray findings in acromegaly. (A) Lateral X-ray skull showing sellar enlargement, thickening of the calvarium, enlargement of the frontal and maxillary sinuses, and enlargement of the jaw; (B) X-ray ankle shows increased thickness of the heel pad in acromegaly; (C) X-ray of hand showing increased soft tissue bulk, "arrowhead" tufting of the distal phalanges.

- **X-ray**
  - *Plain films of skull:* Shows sellar enlargement in 90% of cases. Other findings may be thickening of the calvarium, enlargement of the frontal and maxillary sinuses, and enlargement of the jaw.
  - *Radiographs of the hand:* Shows increased soft tissue bulk, "arrowhead" tufting of the distal phalanges, increased width of intra-articular cartilages, and cystic changes of the carpal bones.
  - *Radiographs of the feet:* Shows similar changes to that of hand, and there is **increased thickness of the heel pad** (normal heel pad thickness <22 mm).
  - *X-ray of spine:* Scoliosis, calcification of spinal ligaments.

3. Pituitary function
Partial or complete anterior hypopituitarism is common

4. Visual field examination
Defects are common (e.g., bitemporal hemianopia).

Treatment of Acromegaly
Untreated acromegaly is associated with markedly reduced survival. Most deaths are due to **heart failure, coronary artery disease, and hypertension** related causes. Patients with acromegaly have an increase in neoplasia (i.e., carcinoma colon).

Treatment is indicated in all except the elderly or those with minimal abnormalities.

- **Surgery:** Trans-sphenoidal surgical removal of pituitary adenoma is the first-line therapy.
- **Medical therapy: Indication for primary treatment with drugs:** Patients

- Without risk of visual impairment from the tumor
- Who are not fit candidates for surgery and those who decline surgery
- With tumors that is unlikely to be controlled by surgery
- With persistence of acromegaly after surgery
- Who require the preservation of intact pituitary function (especially fertility).
□ **Drugs used:** There are three receptor targets for the treatment of acromegaly.
  1. *Somatostatin receptor ligands (SRL)*
     - About 90% GH-secreting adenomas express somatostatin receptor subtypes (SSTR), namely SSTR2 and SSTR5.
     - **Mode of action:** Somatostatin analogs (**octreotide, pasireotide or lanreotide**) are more effective than dopamine agonists and act on pituitary somatostatin receptors to produce inhibition of GH and IGF-I.
  2. *GH receptor antagonist:* **Pegvisomant** is a GH receptor antagonist, blocks peripheral IGF-1 action in almost all patients, and is indicated in patients who are inadequately controlled with other modalities or in patients experiencing clinically significant drug side effects.
  3. *Dopamine receptor agonists:* Act on D_2 receptors. **Bromocriptine or cabergoline** are dopamine receptor agonists and are useful in those with mildly elevated IGF-1.

Radiotherapy

□ **Indications:** It is usually employed as second-line treatment (1) if acromegaly persists after surgery, (2) in patients who are not fit candidates for surgical therapy, and (3) in whom medical therapy fails.
□ External radiotherapy or implantation of Yttrium into the gland.
□ Stereotactic radiosurgery (gamma knife, cyberknife).
□ **Others:** Treatment of associated conditions such as diabetes, hypertension, and hyperlipidemia.

PROLACTINOMA

□ **Prolactinoma** is a pituitary tumor that produces prolactin and is the most common functional pituitary tumor. Most of these tumors are microadenomas.
□ Elevated level of plasma prolactin is known as **hyperprolactinemia.**

Causes of Hyperprolactinemia
See **Box 14.2**.

Clinical Features
Hyperprolactinemia stimulates milk production in the breast and inhibits GnRH and gonadotropin secretion. It usually presents with:
□ **Hypogonadism, decreased libido, infertility,** and **galactorrhea** (spontaneous or expressible) in both sexes.
□ **In females: Amenorrhea, oligomenorrhea,** and **osteoporosis**

Box 14.2: Causes of hyperprolactinemia.

Physiological: Pregnancy, "stress", nursing, nipple stimulation
Pathological:
A. Drug-induced: Estrogens, opiates, dopamine-receptor antagonists (phenothiazines, butyrophenones, metoclopramide), dopamine-depleting agents (reserpine, methyldopa)
B. Disease states
  1. Pituitary adenomas (lactotroph, somatotroph-lactotroph, stalk compression by chromophobe tumors)
  2. Hypothalamic and stalk disease (craniopharyngiomas, irradiation, granulomas, stalk section/compression)
  3. Primary hypothyroidism
  4. Miscellaneous (cirrhosis, chronic renal failure, and seizures)

□ **In males: Hypogonadotropic hypogonadism** leading to loss of libido, impotence, infertility, gynecomastia, and rarely galactorrhea.
□ A sufficiently large macroadenoma usually produces visual field defects and headache.

Investigations
The investigation of prolactinomas is same as for the other pituitary tumors discussed earlier.
□ **Normal range for serum prolactin is approximately 5–20 µg/L.**
□ The diagnosis of hyperprolactinemia is made by a serum prolactin concentration that is well above the normal range >20 µg/L in men and postmenopausal women and >30 µg/L in premenopausal women.
□ Serum PRL over 150 µg/L in a nonpregnant woman is generally due to pituitary adenoma; a level of over 300 µg/L is almost diagnostic of tumor (even in a nursing mother).
□ **Visual fields** should be checked.
□ **Primary hypothyroidism** must be excluded.
□ **Anterior pituitary function** should be assessed, if there is evidence of hypopituitarism or radiological evidence of a pituitary tumor.
□ **MRI or contrast-enhanced CT scan of the pituitary:** It is needed if there are any clinical features suggestive of a pituitary tumor. It is desirable when prolactin is significantly elevated (above 1,000 mU/L). It can easily delineate macroprolactinoma (tumors above 10 mm diameter), but microprolactinoma (smaller ones) may be more difficult to delineate.

Treatment
□ Hyperprolactinemia is usually treated to prevent the long-term effects of estrogen deficiency or testosterone deficiency in the male.
□ **Medical treatment by dopamine agonists: Cabergoline** is the first choice with a dose of 0.25–0.5 mg twice a week. **Bromocriptine** (1.25–2.5 mg twice daily)
□ **Treatment of men with testosterone.**
□ Treatment of women with estradiol.
□ **Trans-sphenoidal removal:** It is indicated if dopamine agonists fails or in the presence of a large and invasive tumor.
□ **External radiotherapy:** Rarely necessary.

- **Asymptomatic patients** who do not require restoration of pregnancy give estrogens to prevent bone loss and should be regularly monitored.

DIABETES INSIPIDUS

Diabetes insipidus (DI) is a disorder in which polyuria due to decreased collecting tubule water reabsorption is induced by either decreased secretion of antidiuretic hormone [ADH; central DI (CDI)] or resistance to its renal effects [nephrogenic DI (NDI)].

It is characterized by the persistent passage of excessive **amounts of dilute urine** and thirst.

Types of Diabetes Insipidus

- **Primary deficiency** (neurogenic, pituitary, hypothalamic, cranial or CDI): It is due to agenesis or destruction of neurohypophysis.
- **Secondary deficiency:** It is due to inhibition of ADH secretion (primary polydipsia).
- **Deficient action of ADH** (NDI)
- Transient **DI of pregnancy** produced by accelerated metabolism of vasopressin by vasopressinases released from the placenta (gestagenic DI).

Causes of Diabetes Insipidus

See **Box 14.3**.

Clinical Features

- **Polyuria and polydipsia:** The urine output may range from 2 L/day with mild partial DI to over 10–15 L/day in patients with severe disease, nocturia, and compensatory excessive thirst (polydipsia) are the most marked symptoms.
- **Other features:** Change in mentation, insomnia, weight loss.
- Cool skin and mucous membranes
- If left untreated changes in loss of consciousness (LOC), tachycardia, tachypnea, hypotension (shock-like symptoms), but unlike hypovolemic shock, urine output is increased.
- Patients with NDI may also have manifestations related to underlying cause such as lithium toxicity, hypercalcemia, and hypokalemia.
- Can lead to **hypernatremia**, restlessness, agitation, diminished deep tendon reflexes, and seizures.

Complications

- Hypernatremia, dehydration and its neurological sequelae
- Growth retardation
- Hydronephrosis (due to excessive urine output).

Investigation and Diagnosis

- **Careful history, examination,** and document presence of **polyuria** (usually 2–15 L/24 hours).
- **Measurement of osmolality of plasma and urine:** It establishes the diagnosis.
  - Normally, plasma osmolality is <295 mOsmL/kg and urine osmolality (random specimen) is 50–1,200 mOsmL/kg.
  - In patients with DI and excess urine-free water, there is high or high-normal plasma osmolality (>295 mOsmL/kg) and low-urine osmolality (50–150 mOsmL/kg).
  - In primary polydipsia, plasma osmolality tends to be low and may be lower than urinary osmolality.
- Urine:
  - **High 24 hours urine volumes.** If the volume is <2 L, there is no need for further investigation.
  - **Clear and of low-specific gravity** of urine.
  - **Low-urine osmolality** and usually less than that of plasma osmolality.
- **Serum sodium is high or high normal** (hypernatremia) and indicates loss of water.
- **MRI of pituitary and hypothalamus** to identify hyperintensities in the posterior pituitary or thickening of the pituitary stalk can help determine the cause of CDI
- **Water deprivation test (Miller-Moses Test) (Fig. 14.3):**
  - *Indication*
    - Diagnosis or exclusion of DI.
    - To differentiate CDI and NDI
    - To differentiate diabetes insipidus from primary polydipsia.
  - *Procedure*
    - Should be done in the morning under observation with 8-hours fasting. No fluids (water deprivation) from 07:30 hours.
    - Measure plasma and urine osmolality, urine volume and weight hourly for up to 8 hours.
    - Abandon fluid deprivation, if weight loss is >5%.

Box 14.3: Causes of diabetes insipidus.

Central DI
- Idiopathic (30–50%)
- **Neoplastic or infiltrative lesions of hypothalamus** (pituitary tumors with suprasellar extension, metastases, leukemia, histiocytosis, craniopharyngioma, lymphoma, sarcoidosis, germinomas, pinealomas)
- Pituitary or hypothalamic surgery
- **Severe head injury,** usually associated with skull fracture
- Hypoxic encephalopathy
- Ruptured cerebral aneurysms
- Infections (e.g., encephalitis, TB, etc.)
- **Autoimmune:** Associated with thyroiditis
- Postsupraventricular tachycardia
- Anorexia nervosa

Familial: e-Wolfram syndrome (also known as **DIDMOAD** syndrome) characterized by DI, DM, optic atrophy, and deafness,

Nephrogenic DI
1. **Primary/congenital or familial:** X-linked recessive vasopressin receptor V2 mutation.
2. Autosomal dominant or autosomal recessive aquaporin-2 gene mutation.
3. **Acquired:** Chronic pyelonephritis, hypokalemia, hypercalcemia, sickle cell disease, protein-deprivation drug-induced (lithium, cidofovir, foscarnet, ifosfamide, ofloxacin, orlistat, demeclocycline, didanosine, amphotericin B, aminoglycosides, cisplatin, rifampicin, colchicine), amyloidosis, other renal diseases (chronic renal failure, obstructive uropathy, and polycystic disease), Sjögren's syndrome, postsurgery for craniophryngioma, and pregnancy.

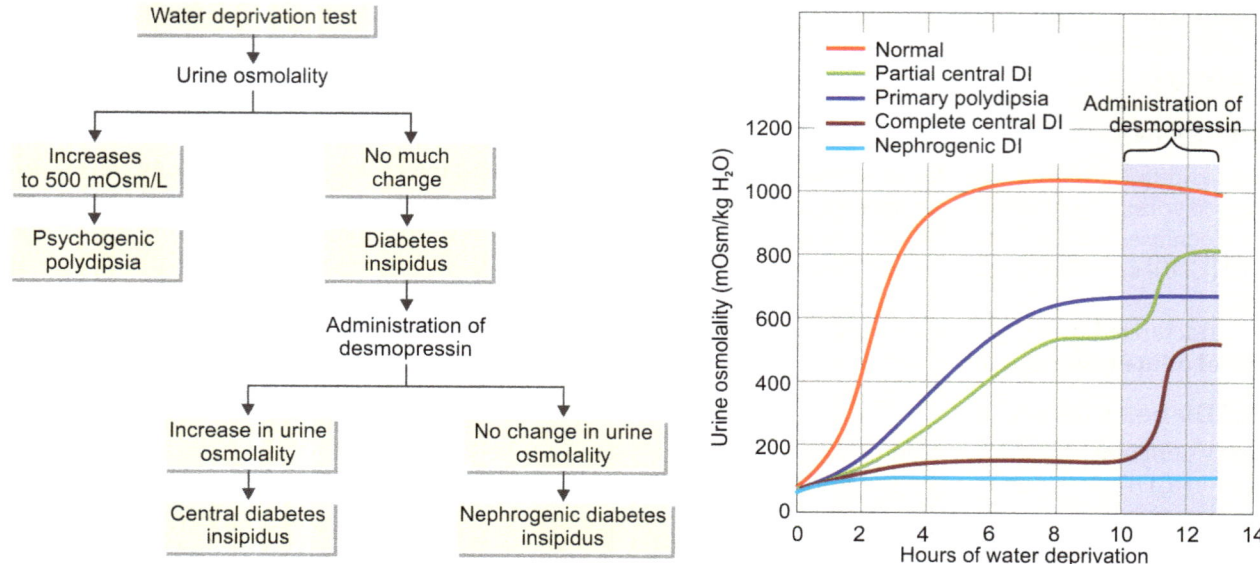

Fig. 14.3: Water deprivation test and its interpretation.

- If plasma osmolality >300 mOsm/kg and/or urine osmolality <600 mOsm/kg, ADH (vasopressin) is given in the dose of 2 μg IM at end of test. Allow free intake of fluids but measure urine osmolality for 2–4 hours.
- *Interpretation*
  - **Normal response:** With holding fluid in normal individuals, the plasma osmolality remains within normal range (275-295 mOsm/kg) while urine osmolality rises above 600 mOsm/kg (800-1,200 mOsm/kg).
    - Urine osmolality is greater than plasma osmolality after restriction of water.
    - Urine osmolality increase minimally (<10%) after exogenous ADH.
- *Primary polydipsia*
  - Patients with primary polydipsia start with low normal plasma osmolality (280 mOsm/kg).
  - Urine/plasma osmolality ratio rises to >2 after dehydration (water deprivation).
- *Central diabetes insipidus*
  - After water restriction in patients with DI, the plasma osmolality rises above normal (>300 mOsm/kg) without rise in urine osmolality (<600 mOsm/kg) or specific gravity of urine (normally urine osmolality rises to 1,000–1,200 mOsmL/kg after water restriction). Urine osmolality remain less than plasma osmolality and urine/plasma osmolality ratio remains <1.5.
  - After ADH is given, urine osmolality increases 100% in complete CDI and over 50% in partial CDI.
- *Nephrogenic diabetes insipidus*
  - Urine osmolality remain less than plasma osmolality.
  - After ADH, urine osmolality increases by <50%.
- Alternative to water deprivation test is by infusing hypertonic (5%) saline and measure ADH secretion in response to increasing plasma osmolality.

Treatment

Goals of Treatment
- **Balance fluid intake with output:** In acute cases, rapidly replace fluid and in chronic cases with slow replacement to prevent cerebral edema.
- Daily weights, accurate in/out, urine specific gravity, and osmolality.

Drugs
- **Desmopressin (DDAVP):** Drug of choice, an initial dose of 5 μg (rhinal tube) or 10 μg (metered spray) of the intranasal form is given at bedtime. This dose is titrated up in 5 μg increments as needed depending on the response of the nocturia and then additional daytime doses are added. The typical daily maintenance dose is 5–20 μg once or twice daily.
- **Chlorpropamide:** Increases the renal responsiveness to vasopressin. Hypoglycemia may develop.
- **Carbamazepine:** Is an alternate drug, which enhances ADH release and raises the sensitivity of the collecting duct toit.
- **Clofibrate:** Is a lipid lowering agent, which stimulates residual ADH production in the hypothalamus, therefore increasing ADH release from the posterior pituitary.
- **NSAIDs:** Work by inhibiting renal prostaglandin synthesis, which are ADH antagonists and also they decreasing the glomerular filtrationrate by prostaglandin-mediated effect of afferent arteriole dilation.

Treatment of Nephrogenic DI
- Provision of adequate fluids especially in cases of impaired thirst, calorie, and decreased dietary solute, such as low-sodium diet. Correct the underlying cause.
- **Thiazide diuretics** (e.g., hydrochlorothiazide 25 mg once or twice daily with a low-sodium diet) are the first-line therapy in NDI.

- **Amiloride (potassium sparing diuretic):** Additive effect with thiazide diuretic and may be particularly beneficial in patients with **reversible lithium nephrotoxicity** by possibly allowing lithium to be continued.
- **Exogenous ADH (DDAVP)**
- *NSAIDS:* Indomethacin

THYROID DISORDERS

Thyroid Function Tests

Various Thyroid Function Tests (Fig. 14.4)

1. Serum thyroid stimulating hormone/thyrotropin (TSH)
It is measured currently by TSH chemiluminometric assays. Normal range for serum TSH is approximately 0.4–5.0 mU/L.

Interpretation:
- **Thyroid diseases:** As a single test of thyroid function, TSH is the most sensitive index of thyroid function.
  - TSH levels can help in **differentiating hyperthyroidism, hypothyroidism, and euthyroidism** (normal thyroid gland function) in most cases.
  - Raised/elevated levels indicate primary hypothyroidism. Low/suppressed levels indicate primary thyrotoxicosis
- **Nonthyroid diseases:** Other conditions affecting TSH levels include:
  - TSH-secreting tumors of pituitary
  - Severe nonthyroidal illness (e.g., sick euthyroid syndrome)
  - Low TSH may be observed in first trimester of pregnancy, with high doses of corticosteroids, and patients ingesting Biotin supplements due to assay interference.
  - Secondary hypothyroidism due to hypothalamic-pituitary disease may produce low, normal or normal-high levels of TSH that are inappropriate for the very low-free T4 level.

2. Thyrotropin releasing hormone (TRH) stimulation test
It may be used in the investigation of hypothalamic pituitary dysfunction.
- Serum TSH is measured before and after the intravenous administration of TRH.
- **Use:** To differentiate secondary or tertiary hypothyroidism.
  - *Secondary hypothyroidism (pituitary disease):* TRH administration does not produce increase in TSH.
  - Tertiary hypothyroidism (hypothalamic disease): TRH administration produces delayed increase in TSH.
  - In primary hypothyroidism, TRH administration produces a prompt increase in TSH.

3. Serum-free T3 (Triiodothyronine fT3) and free T4 (Freethyroxine/fT4)
- Advantage of this test compared to the measurement of total T3 and T4 is that these are not influenced by changes in the thyroid hormone binding globulins (TBG), prealbumin, and albumin. Its level reflects secretory activity
- **Primary thyrotoxicosis:** fT3 and fT4 levels are elevated.
- **T3-thyrotoxicosis:** fT4 levels are normal and fT3 levels are elevated.
- **On T4 therapy:** fT4 levels are elevated and fT3 levels are normal.

4. Total serum thyroxine (tT4)
- Measured by automated competitive binding chemiluminometric assays.
- Its levels are altered by factors that affect the concentration of TBG.
- **Normal ranges are 4.6–11.2 µg/dL.**
- **Increased:** In hyperthyroidism, during pregnancy, estrogen therapy, tamoxifen use and as a congenital anomaly.
- **Decreased:** In hypothyroidism, nephritic syndrome, androgen therapy, liver failure, or drugs (e.g., salicylates, sulfonylureas and phenytoin).

5. Total serum triiodothyronine (tT3)
- Measured by automated competitive binding chemiluminometric assays. Its levels are subject to the same limitations as for tT4 in relation to TBG.
- **Normal range: 75–195 ng/dL.**

6. T3 resin uptake, free T4 index (FTI), effective T4 ratio
Nowadays, above three tests (4, 5, and 6) are not used.

7. Reverse T3 (rT3)
Reverse T3 (rT3) is mainly an inactive metabolite of T4 in peripheral tissues. It has extremely limited utility for assessing rare conditions such as consumptive hypothyroidism, MCT8 or SBP2 mutations, or possibly distinguishing central hypothyroidism from nonthyroidal illness in critically ill hospitalized patients.

8. Thyroglobulin (Tg)
It is synthesized by follicular cells, secreted into the lumen of the thyroid follicle, stored as a colloid, and is involved in iodination/synthesis of thyroid hormones.
- **Use:** To predict the outcome of therapy for hyperthyroidism.
  - *Increased:* Well-differentiated thyroid carcinoma, hyperthyroidism
  - *Decreased:* Total thyroidectomy or destruction of thyroid by radiation.

9. Uptake of radioactive iodine (RAIU) ortechnetium
- The iodine uptake activity of thyroid can be measured by administering orally a low/trace dose of radioactive iodine ^{131}I or ^{121}I and the radioactivity over the thyroid is measured after 4 hours, using a counter over the neck.
- Pregnancy and breastfeeding are **absolute contraindications** to radionuclide imaging. However, in the unusual

Basic thyroid evaluation

Free thyroxine or FT4	Thyroid-stimulating hormone (TSH)		
	Low	Normal	High
High	Primary hyperthyroid	NTI or patient on eltroxin	Secondary hyperthyroid
Normal	Subclinical hyperthyroid	Euthyroid	Subclinical hypothyroid
Low	Secondary hypothyroid	Nonthyroid illness (NTI)	Primary hypothyroid

Fig. 14.4: Basic thyroid evaluation.

instance where radioiodine uptake measurement is felt to be essential for a definitive diagnosis in a lactating woman, breast milk can be pumped and discarded for 5 days after ingestion of I^{123}, then breastfeeding may be resumed; breastfeeding should not be resumed, if the I^{131} isotope is used for determining the uptake.

- The amount of radioactivity that is taken up by the thyroid gland is known as radioactive iodine uptake (RAIU). Alternatively, thyroid uptake is measured by giving technetium-99m (^{99m}Tc) intravenously.
- **Uses of RAIU are:**
  - Evaluation of hyperthyroidism
  - Differentiate Graves from toxic goiter
  - Function of a thyroid nodule as hot or cold
- **Interpretation:** Normal uptake ranges from 10 to 35% in 24 hours.
  - *Uptake increased:* **Overactive** thyroid gland synthesizing excess T3 shows increased uptake of iodine. A very high RAIU is seen in hyperthyroidism (e.g., Graves' disease, toxic multinodular goiter, toxic adenoma, and early thyroiditis). Iodine/enzyme deficiency may show increased uptake even in the absence of thyrotoxicosis.
  - *Uptake decreased:* Low RAIU is seen in hypothyroidism, late thyroiditis. Excess iodine may show diminished uptake even in the presence or thyrotoxicosis. Acute autoimmune thyroiditis may manifest as low iodine uptake thyrotoxicosis.
- **Use:** To determine the functional activity and morphology of the thyroid gland.
  - **Very useful in determining the activity of a solitary thyroid nodule.** Functional nodule appears as a "hot" nodule, and a nonfunctional appears as a "cold" nodule.
  - **Useful in follow-up of patients with treated thyroid cancer.**
  - *Detection of ectopic thyroid tissue:* Confirmation a mass on the tongue as lingual thyroid, in the midline of the neck as thyroglossal duct, or in the mediastinum as substernal goiter.

10. Ultrasound of thyroid gland

Look for nodularity, vascularity, shape, microcalcifications, lymph nodes status, and for guided FNAC.

11. Thyroid auto antibody tests

The different types of thyroid autoantibodies responsible for the autoimmune thyroid disorders are:

- **Antimicrosomal antibody**
- **Antithyroid peroxidase (TPO) antibody (TPOAb):** They are involved in the tissue destructive process associated with hypothyroidism in Hashimoto and Atrophict hyroiditis.
- **Antithyroglobulin (Tg) antibody:** May be present in Hashimoto's thyroiditis and Graves' disease.
- **TSH receptor (TR) antibody (TRAb):** Classified as stimulating, blocking, or neutral. Stimulating antibodies (thyroid-stimulating immunoglobulins, TSI) cause Graves' disease. Thyroid receptor-blocking antibodies can cause hypothyroidism. Neutral antibodies bind the receptor but do not stimulate or block function.

12. Tests to determine etiology of thyroid disease

- **Calcitonin:** It is secreted by parafollicular C-cells and is increased in medullary carcinoma of thyroid.
- **Fine-needle aspiration cytology/excision biopsy:** It is helpful in diagnosis thyroid diseases.

THYROTOXICOSIS

Definition

Thyrotoxicosis is a state of circulating thyroid hormone excess (with hypermetabolic state) caused by exposure to **excessive levels of thyroid hormone** (free T3 and T4).

This increase in circulating hormone may be either from destruction of thyroid gland or from ectopic source.

Hyperthyroidism (thyroid overactivity): It is the **clinical consequence due to the excessive circulating thyroid hormone due to excessive thyroid function**/hyperfunction and is the **most common cause of thyrotoxicosis**. Its causes are listed in **Box 14.4**.

Few of the causes of hyperthyroidism/thyrotoxicosis are discussed below:

Graves' Disease

- Graves' disease is the most common form of thyrotoxicosis. It is characterized by one or more of the following features: **(1) thyrotoxicosis, (2) goiter, (3) orbitopathy (exophthalmos)**, and **(4) dermopathy (pretibial myxedema)**.
  Histology: Characterized by follicular hyperplasia, intracellular colloid droplets, cell scalloping, a reduction in follicular colloid, and a patchy (multifocal) lymphocytic infiltration.
- **Age, gender, and genetic susceptibility:**
  - It may occur at any age, with a peak incidence between **20 and 40 years** of age.
  - The diseases cluster in families and are **more common in women**.
  - The concordance rate in monozygotic twins is 20–40%.
  - Associated with certain alleles of CTLA-4

Box 14.4: Causes of hyperthyroidism.

Primary hyperthyroidism
Graves disease
❖ Toxic multinodular goiter
❖ Toxic adenoma (Plummer's disease)
❖ Iodine excess (Jod Basedow)
❖ Activating mutation of TSH receptor

Thyrotoxicosis without hyperthyroidism
❖ Subacute thyroiditis, hashitoxicosis
❖ Amiodarone induced
❖ Radiation induced
❖ Thyrotoxicosis factitia
❖ Struma ovarii
❖ Infarction of thyroid gland

Secondary hyperthyroidism
❖ TSH secreting pituitary adenoma
❖ Human chorionic gonadotropin-mediated hyperthyroidism (hyperemesis gravidarum, trophoblastic disease)
❖ Gestational thyrotoxicosis

- Associated with certain alleles of HLA on chromosome 6 namely, HLA-DRB1 08 and DRB3 0202.
- HLA- DRB1 07 is found to be protective.
- **Autoantibodies:** It is an autoimmune disorder with autoantibodies.
❑ **TSI or TSH-receptor antibodies of the stimulating type (TRAb):** IgG type of antibodies directed against the TSH receptors on the follicular cell of thyroid. They stimulate thyroid hormone production and enlargement of thyroid.
❑ **T cells:** Activated T cells release cytokines and increase the secretion of thyroid-specific autoantibodies from B cells. The current concept is that thyroid-specific T cells in Graves' disease primarily act as helper (CD4+ Th1) cells.
❑ **Ophthalmopathy and dermatopathy:** Observed in Graves' disease is due to immunologically mediated activation of fibroblasts in the extraocular muscles and skin. This along with accumulation of **glycosaminoglycans** and trapping of water causes edema initially. Later fibroblasts cause fibrosis.
❑ Genetic factors may be significant in a minority of cases (e.g., HLA-DR3-associated).
❑ **Hyperthyroidism may be triggered by viral or bacterial infections.** *E. coli* and *Yersenia enterocolitica* possess cell membrane TSH receptors. The antibodies produced against these microorganisms can cross-react with the TSH receptors (molecular mimicry).
❑ **Other mediating mechanisms:** Bystander activation and Thyroid cell HLA antigen expression.
❑ **Other precipitating causes:** Thyroid injury by radiation and drugs, stress, smoking, sex steroids, pregnancy, and fetal microchimerism, iodine and iodine containing drugs such as amiodarone.
Alemtuzumab, a monoclonal antibody against CD52, has been associated with a 10–15% incidence of new-onset Graves' disease.

Treatment-induced Hyperthyroidism
Drugs include iodine, amiodarone, iodine containing contrast media interferon-alpha, and rarely, lithium.
a. **Iodine-induced hyperthyroidism:** It develops following excess intake of iodine in diet or exposure to radiographic contrast media or iodine medication.
   - Usually develops in patients with autonomously functioning thyroid gland (e.g., nodular goiter/Graves' disease). It can also occur in endemic goiter and with iodine **(Jod-Basedow phenomenon)**.
   - It is characterized by suppressed serum TSH level with normal levels of circulating thyroid hormone.
   - Paradoxically, excess iodine uptake by the thyroid may inhibit the synthesis thyroid hormone **(Wolff-Chaikoff effect).** Thus, iodide toxicity can lead to iodine goiter, hypothyroidism or myxedema.
b. **Amiodarone-induced hyperthyroidism (AIT):** Amiodarone is a class III antiarrhythmic drug and 200 mg dose has 75 mg iodine. It can also induce hyperthyroidism which can be:
   - **Type I AIT:** It develops in patients with pre-existing multinodular goiter or latent Graves' disease. There is hyperthyroidism with increased synthesis of T4 and T3 and is triggered by the high iodine content of amiodarone. Jod-Basedow effect (refer above) occurs inpatients with underlying thyroid disease.
   - **Type II AIT:** It is not associated with previous thyroid disease. It is due to a direct cytotoxicity of the amiodrone on thyroid follicular cells leading to a destructive thyroid it is with release of T3 and T4. It produces a hyperthyroid phase which may last several weeks to months and may later progress to hypothyroid phase and eventual recovery in most but not all patients.

Thyrotoxicosis Factitia
❑ Exogenous hyperthyroidism is due to the surreptitious ingestion of thyroid hormone, it is termed thyrotoxicosis factitia.
❑ Patients are clinically thyrotoxic without eye signs of Graves.
❑ High doses of thyroxine lead to TSH suppression and causes shrinkage of the thyroid.
❑ Find cause or contamination and treat symptomatically.

Toxic Multinodular Goiter (Plummer's Disease)
❑ Result of diffuse hyperplasia of thyroid follicular cells whose functional capacity is independent of regulation by TSH.
❑ Goiter will be nodular.
❑ Constitutes 14% of thyrotoxicosis cases.
❑ Commonly occurs in elderly women (>50 years).
❑ T3 (greater), T4 raised, and TSH undetectable.

Toxic Solitary Adenoma/Nodule
❑ Constitutes <5% of all thyrotoxicosis (hyperthyroidism) cases and the solitary nodule is follicular adenoma.
❑ Usually occur in female >40 years of age.
❑ Suspected thyroid nodules merit close attention in the pediatric population because such nodules are much more likely to be malignant in children than they are in adults.

Clinical Features of Thyrotoxicosis (Table 14.4)
Classic symptoms include heat intolerance, tremor, palpitations, anxiety, weight loss, increased appetite increased frequency of bowel movements, and shortness of breath.
❑ **Elderly** patients present with anorexia, apathy, fatigue, weightloss, and dominant cardiovascular and myopathic features **(apathetic hyperthyroidism)**.
❑ **Younger** patients present predominantly with neurological manifestations.
❑ **Children** present with excessive height or excessive growth rate, or with behavioral problems (e.g., hyperactivity), and weight gain rather than loss.

Thyroid Orbitopathy (Eye Signs)
(Box 14.5 and Figs. 14.5A to D)
❑ An autoimmune disease of the retroocular tissues occurring in patients with Graves' disease. Although it has often been referred to as Graves' ophthalmopathy, or thyroid eye disease (TED), it is **primarily a disease of the orbit** and is better termed **Graves' orbitopathy**.

Chapter 14: Endocrinology

Table 14.4: Clinical features of thyrotoxicosis.

Organ/system involved	Symptoms
Thyroid	Diffuse or nodular enlargement, warmth and bruit (due to increased vascularity)
Gastrointestinal system	• **Weight loss**, **increased appetite**, vomiting, abdominal pain, increased gut motility, hyper defecation, malabsorption, diarrhea, steatorrhea, dysphagia due to goiter. • Celiac disease is also more prevalent in patients with Graves' disease.
Cardiovascular system	Tachycardia, exertional dyspnea, palpitations, hyperdynamic precordium, pulmonary hypertension, angina, **sinus tachycardia, atrial fibrillation,** wide pulse pressure, lowering of diastolic blood pressure cardiac failure, cardiomyopathy, "scratchy" midsystolic murmur (Means-Lerman scratch)
Neuropsychiatric system	• Nervousness, **irritability**, psychosis, emotional lability, fine **tremors**. Agitation and depression • Inability to concentrate, insomnia, hyperreflexia, cognitive impaiments, poor orientation and immediate recall, amnesia, constructional difficulty, proximal myopathy, bulbar myopathy, ill-sustained clonus
Respiratory system	Increased ventilation due to hypoxemia and hypercapnia, respiratory muscle weakness, decreased lung volume, large goiter causing tracheal obstruction, exacerbation of asthma and rise in pulmonary arterial systolic pressure.
Metabolic/endocrine	Increased bone resorption causing osteoporosis, periosteal new bone formation (**thyroid acropachy** seen in Graves' disease), dyslipidemia, hyperglycemia.
Hematologic	• Normocytic normochromic anemia. • Graves' hyperthyroidism may be associated with autoimmune hematologic disorders such as immune thrombocytopenia (ITP) and pernicious anemia. • Maybe prothrombotic, excess thyroid hormone was associated with a rise in prothrombotic factors, including factors VIII, IX, fibrinogen, von Willebrand factor, and plasminogen activator inhibitor-1.
Skin and integumentary system	• Soft, warm, moist, and smooth because of decrease in keratin layer. Increased sweating, pruritus, hives, onycholysis and softening of nails, palmar erythema, spider nevi, onycholysis, hyperpigmentation, vitiligo, and alopecia areata and clubbing. • Infiltrative dermopathy occurs only in patients with Graves' hyperthyroidism. The most common site is the skin overlying the shins, where it presents as raised, hyperpigmented, violaceous, orange-peel-textured papules (**pretibial myxedema**).
Genitourinary	• Urinary frequency and nocturia are common in hyperthyroidism. • In women, oligomenorrhea, amenorrhea and anovulatory infertility • In men, gynecomastia, reduced libido, and erectile dysfunction and abnormal/decreased spermatogenesis.
General	**Heat intolerance**, fatigue, gynecomastia, apathy, thirst, thymic enlargement in patients with Graves' disease.
Eyes	Stare, Lid lag, exophthalmos, proptosis, extraocular diplopia, exposure keratitis, lagophthalmos (classically seen in Graves' disease).

Note: Bold words indicate symptoms of greater discriminant value.

> **Box 14.5:** Eye signs of thyrotoxicosis.
>
> ❖ **Dalrymple sign:** Rim of sclera is seen all around the cornea, on looking straight forward.
> ❖ **Rosenbach's sign:** Fine tremor of the upper eyelids on slight closure of the eye.
> ❖ **Joffroy's sign:** Lack of wrinkling of the forehead when a patient looks upward.
> ❖ **Möbius sign:** Lack of convergence on looking to near object.
> ❖ **Von Graefe's sign (lid lag sign):** Lagging of the upper eyelid on looking downward without moving the head.
> ❖ **Stellwag's sign:** Staring look with in frequent blinking.
> ❖ **Vigouroux sign:** Eyelid fullness
> ❖ **Grove sign:** Resistance to pulling down the retracted upper lid)
> ❖ **Ballet sign:** Restriction of one or more extraocular muscles)
> ❖ **Kocher sign:** Staring look (upper sclera visible)
> ❖ **Naffziger's sign:** Standing behind, patient's neck is extended and examiner looks from behind along the superior orbital margin of the patient. Eyeball is seen beyond the superior orbital margin in exophthalmos.

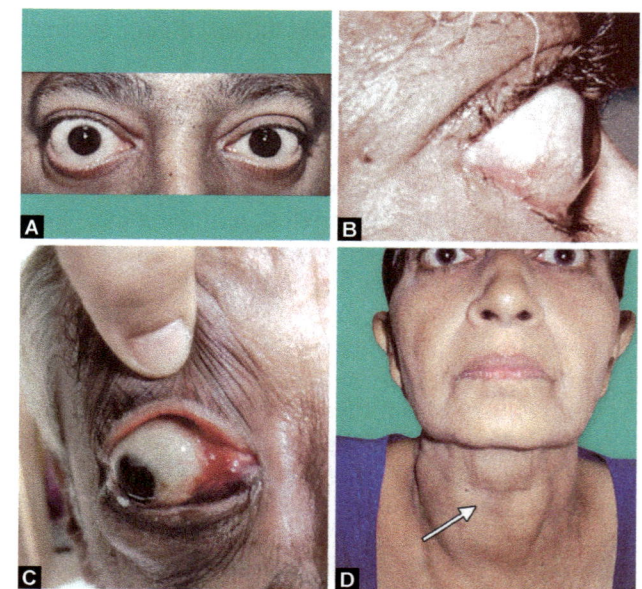

Figs. 14.5A to D: (A and B) Exophthalmos (front and side view); (C) Infiltration of extraocular muscles in hyperthyroidism; (D) Eye signs and enlarged nodular goiter (arrow).

- The ophthalmopathy causes **abnormal protrusion of the eyeball (exophthalmos)**. Sympathetic overactivity may produce a characteristic **wide, staring gaze, and lidlag**.
- It is observed in about 50% of the patients when first seen. It may precede Graves' disease by many years or may develop even after successful treatment of Graves' disease.
- The volume of both the extraocular muscles and retro-ocular connective tissue is increased, due to fibroblast proliferation, inflammation, and the accumulation of hydrophilic glycosaminoglycans (GAG), mostly hyaluronic acid.
- *Symptoms:* A gritty or foreign object sensation in the eyes, excessive tearing that is often made worse by exposure to cold air, wind, or bright lights, eye or retro-ocular discomfort or pain, blurring of vision, diplopia, color vision desaturation and loss of vision in severe cases.
- **Signs: Exophthalmos (proptosis) often asymmetric but can be symmetric, lid lag, lid retraction**, periorbital edema, corneal ulcers, chemosis, ophthalmoplegia, visual field defects and papilledema.

Pretibial Myxedema (Infiltrative Dermopathy)

- Formerly used to occur in 5% of patients with Graves' disease and 15% of patients with Graves' disease and ophthalmopathy. However, the incidence has declined due to early diagnosis and treatment of Graves' disease.
- Characterized by bilateral, asymmetric, nonpitting, scaly thickening, and induration of the skin.
- Lesion may be violaceous or slightly pigmented (yellow-brown) and often have an orange-peel appearance.
- The most frequent location is over the lower limbs, especially the pretibial areas or the dorsum of the foot. Rarely, the fingers and hands, elbows, arms, or face are affected (**Fig. 14.6**).
- Rarely, lesions progress to involve the legs, feet, or hands completely, resulting in a form reminiscent of elephantiasis.
- Occurs due to deposition of glycosaminoglycanse especially hyaluronic acid, secreted by fibroblasts under the stimulation of local cytokines arising from a lymphocytic infiltration.

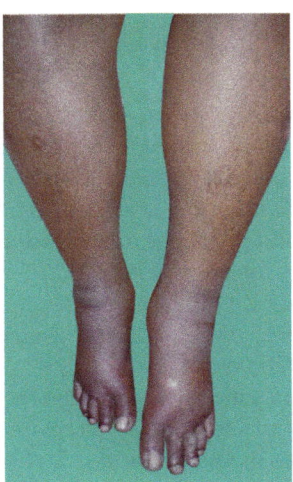

Fig. 14.6: Nonpitting pedal edema-myxedema.

Treatment of Pretibial Myxedema

Some patients do not seek treatment as they are asymptomatic. Indications for treatment are pruritus, local discomfort, the unsightly appearance of the lesions, or progression of lesions.

- **Nonpharmacologic** includes minimizing risk factors, such as avoiding tobacco, reducing weight, normalizing thyroid function and in severe cases, physiotherapy. Normalization of thyroid function does not necessarily improve pretibial myxedema.
- **Pharmacologic**
  - Topical 0.025% **fluocinolone acetonide** under plastic wrap.
  - Intralesional corticosteroids, if there is no improvement with topical treatment after 4–12 weeks, using **triamcinolone acetate** dose calculated according to 8 mg per 2 cm-diameter circle area at each session, but the total dose was not more than 100 mg at each session in a patient.
  - **Pentoxifylline** may be helpful in resistant cases.

Subclinical Hyperthyroidism
- **Clinical manifestations**
- **Laboratory findings:** Serum levels of free T4 and T3 are within normal limits. Serum TSH levels is subnormal (<0.5 mU/L).

Investigations of Graves' Disease
- **TSH levels: Very low or undetectable**. This is performed as the primary test, and normal level excludes thyrotoxicosis.
- **Serum T3 and T4 levels:** Raised in most cases. T3 thyrotoxicosis is associated with raised T3 levels and normal T4 level.
- **Absence of TSH response** following intravenous **TRH**.
- ^{131}I **uptake by the thyroid gland:** It may be increased, but not necessary to perform in most of the patients.
- **TSH receptor antibody (TRAb):** Present in most cases.
- Few patients may show minor LFT abnormalities, mild hypercalcemia, and glycosuria.

Other disorders associated with Graves' disease.
- **Autoimmune disorders**
  - *Endocrine:* Addison's disease, type 1 DM, Hashimoto's thyroiditis, primary gonadal failure, and hypophysitis.
  - *Nonendocrine:* Celiac disease, pernicious anemia, myasthenia gravis, immune thrombocytopenic purpura, rheumatoid arthritis, vitiligo, and alopecia areata.
- **Others:** Hypokalemic periodic paralysis and mitral valve prolapse.

Management of Hyperthyroidism of Graves' Disease

The therapeutic approach to Graves' hyperthyroidism consists of both rapid amelioration of symptoms with a beta blocker and measures aimed at decreasing thyroid hormone synthesis: the administration of a thionamide, radioiodine ablation, or surgery.

- **Symptom control:** Beta blocker, **propranolol** (drug of choice) in the dose of 20–40 mg 6 hourly or **atenolol** 25–50 mg/day to reduce symptoms for immediate relief due to sympathetic overactivity such as anxiety, palpitation, increased bowel activity, lid retraction, finger tremors.

❏ **Decrease thyroid hormone synthesis:** There are three treatment options for Graves' disease: **antithyroid drugs** (thionamides), **radioiodine**, or **surgery**. All three options are effective, but all three options have significant side effects. There is no consensus as to the "best" treatment.

❏ **Antithyroid drugs (ATD)** may be used initially to control hyperthyroidism (in addition to beta blockers) prior to definitive therapy with radioiodine or surgery; they may be prescribed for 1–2 years to attain a remission, or may be used long term.

Advantages

❏ No surgical risk, scar, or chances of injury to parathyroid or recurrent laryngeal nerve.
❏ Hypothyroidism, if induced, is reversible.
❏ Can be used even in children and young adults.

Disadvantages

❏ Prolonged (often lifelong) treatment is needed and relapse rate is high.
❏ Not practicable in uncooperative patient.

Indications: Primary therapy in **pregnancy**, in **children** and **adolescents** and **severe Graves' disease with eye changes**. The drugs include:

Thionamides: Methimazole, propylthiouracil, carbimazole

Mechanism of action: Inhibit the function of **TPO enzyme** and prevent binding of iodine to tyrosine (prevents iodination and organification).

❏ **Methimazole:** Primary drug to treat.
  - *Dose:*
    ■ Free T4 1 to 1.5 times the upper limit of normal, begin treatment with 5–10 mg once daily.
    ■ Free T4 1.5 to 2 times the upper limit of normal, begin treatment with 10–20 mg once daily.
    ■ Free T4 2 to 3 times the upper limit of normal, begin treatment on 20–40 mg daily in divided doses.
    ■ The dose is tapered to maintenance levels (5–10 mg/day) as the patient improves.
❏ **Propyl thiouracil:** Preferred during the first trimester of pregnancy.
  - *Dose:* 300 mg daily in 3 equally divided doses; 400 mg daily in patients with severe hyperthyroidism and/or very large goiters; usual maintenance: 100–150 mg daily in three divided doses.
❏ **Carbimazole:** It has additional immunosuppressive action.
  - *Dose:* Initially 20–60 mg daily given in 2–3 divided doses and maintenance 5–15 mg daily or alternatively 20–60 mg daily.
  - *Total duration of treatment:* 18–24 months.
  - *Adverse effects:* Rashes, urticaria, fever, arthralgia, blood dyscrasias **(agranulocytosis)**, hepatotoxicity, aplasia cutis in neonates.
❏ **Radioiodine ablation:** Preferred as definitive therapy of hyperthyroidism in nonpregnant patients except in patients with moderate or severe orbitopathy and chronic smokers.

Administered as a capsule I^{131}, induces extensive tissue damage by emitting gamma-radiation from within the follicles, resulting in ablation of the thyroid within 6–18 weeks.

- *Dose:* 185–555 MBq
- *Indications:* (i) Patients **above 40 years of age,** (ii) young patients with a short life-span due to some other reason, and (iii) young individuals who are sterilized.
- *Complication:* **Hypothyroidism**, infertility, secondary cancers.
- *Surgery:* **Subtotal thyroidectomy** is the **treatment of choice**.

  Surgical treatment is reserved for multinodular goiter (MNG) with following features:
  ■ Severe hyperthyroidism in children.
  ■ Pregnant women who cannot tolerate antithyroid drugs.
  ■ Large goiters with severe ophthalmopathy or with pressure symptoms.
  ■ Patients who require quick normalization of thyroid function
  ■ **Preparation for thyroidectomy:** It includes pretreatment with propranolol or atenolol, methimazole 5–40 mg depending on severity and potassium iodide (to decrease vascularity and make the gland firm) 8 mg iodide per drop, 5–7 drops three times daily for 2 weeks before surgery.
  ■ **Postoperative complications:** Hypothyroidism, hypoparathyroidism, hypocalcemia, and damage to recurrent laryngeal nerve.

❏ **Adjunctive therapies:** Oral radiocontrast agents' **sodium ipodate** and **iopanoic acid** are potent inhibitors of the peripheral conversion of T4 to T3.
  - *Dose:* of 500–1000 mg/day in combination with methimazole, can rapidly ameliorate severe hyperthyroidism and can also be used to prepare a hyperthyroid patient for early surgery.
  - Iodine elixirs, up to 10 drops of **saturated solution of potassium iodide** [SSKI, 50 mg iodide per drop (0.05 mL)] daily for 7–10 days is used perioperatively to reduce gland vascularity.
  - Glucocorticoids inhibit peripheral T4 to T3 conversion and, in patients with Graves' hyperthyroidism, reduce thyroid secretion.
  - **Cholestyramine**, given in a dose of 4 g four times daily with methimazole, lowers serum T4 and T3 concentrations more rapidly than methimazole alone.
  - *Potassium perchlorate:* It reduces uptake of iodine. It is more toxic and produces red cell aplasia. It is used only as temporary measure in iodine-induced thyrotoxicosis or when other therapy is not acceptable.
  - *Lithium:* Blocks thyroid hormone release, but its use has been limited by its toxicity.
  - *Rituximab:* May induce a sustained remission in patients with Graves' disease and low TSH-receptor antibodies (TRAb) levels, but its cost and side effects limit its utility.

❏ **Skeletal health:** Advised to ingest 1,200–1,500 mg elemental calcium daily through diet or supplements.

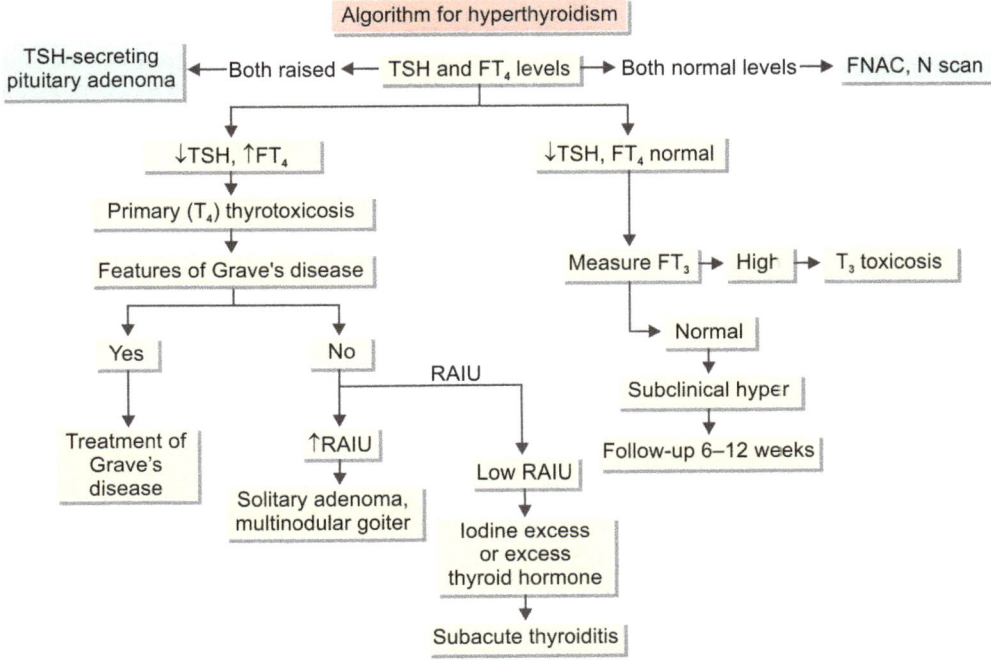

Flowchart 14.1: Approach to diagnosis in hyperthyroidism.

(FT$_4$: free tetrahydrothyronine; FT$_3$: free triiodothyronine; TSH: thyroid-stimulating hormone; RAIU: radioactive iodine uptake)

Approach for the hyperthyroidism is presented in **Flowchart 14.1**.

Hyperthyroid Crisis/Thyrotoxic Crisis/Thyroid Storm

It is a rare **life-threatening** medical emergency that develops as **complication of thyrotoxicosis** which is associated with a mortality of 10–30%.

Causes of Hyperthyroid Crisis

Thyroid storm can develop in patients with long standing untreated hyperthyroidism (Graves' disease, toxic multinodular goiter, solitary toxic adenoma). It is often precipitated by an acute event:

- **Severe infections** in a patient with previously undetected or inadequately treated hyperthyroidism/thyrotoxicosis.
- **Following surgery:** May develop **following subtotal thyroidectomy** in an ill-prepared patient or some other surgery in an undetected hyperthyroidism/thyrotoxicosis.
- **Following radiotherapy:** May occur with in a few days of ^{131}I therapy in an inadequately prepared patient. This is because of a transient rise in serum thyroid hormone levels caused due to acute damage by irradiation.
- **Other precipitating factors:** CVA, diabetic ketoacidosis, acute coronary syndrome, use of iodine contrast agent, acute iodine load, parturition, sudden withdrawal of antithyroid medications, stress, major trauma.

It is unclear why certain factors result in the development of thyroid storm. Hypotheses include a rapid rate of increase in serum thyroid hormone levels, increased responsiveness to catecholamines, or enhanced cellular responses to thyroid hormone. One study found that while the total T4 and T3 levels were similar to those seen in uncomplicated patients, the free T4 and free T3 concentrations were higher in patients with thyroid storm.

Clinical Features

- The clinical manifestations are due to marked hypermetabolism and excessive adrenergic response.
- Hyperpyrexia from 104 to 106°F is common and is associated with flushing and sweating.
- **Marked tachycardia** rates that can exceed 140 beats/min often with atrial fibrillation and high pulse pressure, hypotension, occasionally congestive heart failure occurs. A fatal outcome is associated with heart failure and shock.
- **Central nervous system symptoms** include marked **agitation, restlessness, delirium**, psychosis, stupor, and coma.
- **Gastrointestinal symptoms** include nausea, vomiting, diarrhea, abdominal pain, and hepatic failure with jaundice.
- **Physical examination** may reveal goiter, ophthalmopathy (in the presence of Graves' disease), lid lag, hand tremor, and warm and moist skin.

Laboratory findings: Low TSH and high free T4 and/or T3 concentrations. Nonspecific laboratory findings may include mild hyperglycemia secondary to a catecholamine-induced inhibition of insulin release and increased glycogenolysis, mild hypercalcemia due to hemoconcentration and enhanced bone resorption, abnormal liver function tests, leukocytosis, or leukopenia.

Treatment of Hyperthyroid Crisis

- Patients should be admitted in ICU, **rehydrated** and given **antibiotics,** if there is infection.
- **Control hyperthermia:** Aggressively by external cooling. **Acetaminophen should be used instead of aspirin** since the latter can increase serum free T4 and T3 concentrations by interfering with their protein binding.

- **Propranolol:** Either orally (60–80 mg every 4–6 hours) or intravenously (1–5 mg four times daily). It also blocks peripheral conversion of T4 to T3.

  The Japanese guidelines recommend **esmolol** over **propranolol** because of increased mortality in patients with congestive heart failure treated with propranolol.

  In patients with reactive airways disease, cardioselective beta blockers such as **metoprolol** or **atenolol** could be considered.
- **Propyl thiouracil** 200 mg orally every 4 hours (preferred as it decreases T4 to T3 conversion) or **methimazole** (20 mg orally every 4–6 hours) or **carbimazole** (inhibit the synthesis of new thyroid hormone) 15–30 mg stat followed by 15 mg TID. In an unconscious or uncooperative patient, carbimazole can be administered rectally with good effect.
- **Lugol's iodine:** 10 drops TID about 1 hour after the first dose of thionamide.
- **Sodium iopodate:** 500 mg/day orally will restore serum T3 levels to normal within 48–72 hours. This is a radiographic contrast medium which inhibits the release of thyroid hormones and also reduces the conversion of T4 to T3. Hence, more effective than potassium iodide or Lugol's solution.
- **Benzodiazepines:** For agitation.
- **Digoxin:** To control cardiac failure and atrial fibrillation (AF).
- **Plasmapheresis** has been tried when traditional therapy has not been successful; it removes cytokines, antibodies, and thyroid hormones from plasma.
- **Lithium** has also been given to acutely block the release of thyroid hormone. However, its renal and neurologic toxicity limit its utility.

HYPOTHYROIDISM

- Hypothyroidism is a **clinical syndrome resulting from a deficiency of thyroid hormones.** It results in a generalized slowing down of metabolic processes.
- **Infants and children:** Hypothyroidism results in marked **slowing of growth and development**, with serious permanent consequences, including mental retardation, when it occurs in infancy **(cretinism).**
- **Adults:** Hypothyroidism causes a **generalized decrease in metabolism**, with slowed heart rate, diminished oxygen consumption, and deposition of glycosaminoglycans in intracellular spaces, particularly in skin and muscle, producing in extreme cases the clinical picture of **myxedema.**

Classification and Etiology (Box 14.6)

- **Primary hypothyroidism:** Due intrinsic disorder of the thyroid gland. Accounts for over 95% of cases of hypothyroidism. There are **two** degrees of primary hypothyroidism:
- **Subclinical hypothyroidism**, defined as a high serum TSH concentration in the presence of normal serum free T4 and T3 concentrations.

> **Box 14.6:** Etiology of hypothyroidism.
>
> **Primary:**
> - Hashimoto's thyroiditis (chronic autoimmune thyroiditis)
> - Radioactive iodine therapy for Graves' disease
> - External neck irradiation
> - Subtotal thyroidectomy for Graves' disease, nodular goiter, or thyroid cancer
> - Excessive iodide intake (radiocontrast dyes)
> - Subacute thyroiditis (usually transient). Postpartum thyroiditis
> - Iodide deficiency
> - Drugs: Lithium, interferon-alpha, amiodarone, PTU, methimazole, ethionamide, ipilimumab, pembrolizumab, and nivolumab.
> - Environmental exposures: Polybrominated diphenyl ethers (fire retardant)
> - Infiltrative diseases: Fibrous thyroiditis (Riedel's thyroiditis), hemochromatosis, scleroderma, leukemia, cystinosis.
> - Dyshormonogenesis **(Pendred syndrome)**
>
> **Secondary:** Hypopituitarism due to pituitary adenoma, pituitary ablative therapy, or pituitary destruction, Sheehan syndrome, trauma, hypophysitis, nonpituitary tumors such as craniopharyngiomas, infiltrative diseases, and inactivating mutations in the gene for either TSH or the TSH receptor.
>
> **Tertiary:** Hypothalamic dysfunction (rare). It can also be caused by mutations in the gene for the TRH receptor. Hypothalamic damage results from tumors, trauma, radiation therapy, or infiltrative diseases.
> Rarely peripheral resistance to the action of thyroid hormone.

- **Overt hypothyroidism**, defined as a high-serum TSH concentration in the presence of a low serum-free T4 concentration.
- **Central hypothyroidism:** It is rare and is caused due to failure of TSH and TRH production due to disease of anterior pituitary (**secondary hypothyroidism**) or hypothalamus (**tertiary hypothyroidism**).

Hashimoto's Thyroiditis (Chronic Autoimmune Thyroiditis)

- **Most common cause** of primary hypothyroidism in iodine sufficient areas of the world.
- Organ-specific **autoimmuned is order** of thyroid characterized gradual thyroid failure with or without goiter formation by lymphoid infiltration of thyroid leading to apoptosis, fibrosis, and atrophy.
- The two major forms of Hashimoto's thyroiditis are **goitrous autoimmune thyroiditis** and **atrophic autoimmune thyroiditis** (often called **primary myxedema**), with the common pathologic feature being lymphocytic infiltration and follicular destruction.
- Patients have **TRAb** that block the effects of endogenous TSH, antibodies to TPO and thyroglobulin.
- The cause of Hashimoto's thyroiditis is thought to be a combination of genetic susceptibility and environmental factors.
- Several mechanisms have been proposed for the pathogenesis of Hashimoto's thyroiditis. These include molecular mimicry and bystander activation including the involvement of thyroid cell expression of HLAs and

activation of thyroid cell apoptosis by a Fas ligand-Fas interaction.
- It may be observed in **some patients of Graves' disease** treated with antithyroid drugs 10–20 years earlier.
- Patients have **high-risk of** developing **other autoimmune disorders** such as type 1 diabetes mellitus, pernicious anemia, and Addison's disease.

Clinical Features (Table 14.5)
- Depends on the duration and severity of the hypothyroidism.
- **Consequence of prolonged hypothyroidism:**
  - **Infiltration of many body tissues** by the mucopolysaccharides, hyaluronic acid and chondroitin sulfate.
  - **Infiltration of the dermis** produces nonpitting edema (myxedema). The term myxedema refers to the **accumulation of mucopolysaccharides in the subcutaneous tissues**. It is most marked in the skin of the hands, feet and eyelids.
  - *Myxedema facies:* It is a peculiar facial appearance characterized by striking **periorbital puffiness** (due to myxedema), scanty eyebrows, **facial pallor** (due to vasoconstriction and anemia), or a **lemon-yellow tint to the skin** (due to **carotenemia** produced by reduced conversion of carotene to vitamin A), purplish lips and malar flush.
- **Most cases** of hypothyroidism are **not clinically obvious** and should be kept in mind when individuals complain of nonspecific symptoms such as tiredness, weight gain, depression or carpal tunnel syndrome. Many cases are diagnosed on biochemical screening.

Investigations of Primary Hypothyroidism (Flowchart 14.2)
Majority of hypothyroidism results from an intrinsic disorder of the thyroid gland (primary hypothyroidism).
- **Serum TSH:** It is the investigation of choice. **High** TSH level **confirms primary hypothyroidism.**
- **Serum T4 levels: Low** level confirms the hypothyroid state.
- **Thyroid and other organ-specific antibodies** may be found.
- **Other abnormalities:**
  - **Increased serum aspartate transferase** from muscle and/or liver
  - *Increased serum lactate dehydrogenase (LDH) and creatine kinase (CK):* With associated myopathy
  - **Hypercholesterolemia and hypertriglyceridemia**
  - *Hyponatremia:* Due to an increase in ADH and impaired free-water clearance.
  - *Anemia:* Usually normochromic and normocytic
  - *Electrocardiogram (ECG):* Demonstrates sinus bradycardia, low voltage QRS complexes and ST segment and T wave abnormalities.
  - *Chest radiograph:* May reveal enlarged cardiac shadow.

Treatment of Hypothyroidism
- Hypothyroidism is treated with **T4**.
  - Replacement therapy with **levothyroxine sodium** is given for life, once daily dosage **(1.6 µg/kg/day).**
  - *Initial dose:* It depends upon the severity of the deficiency and on the age and fitness of the patient.
- **For young healthy patients:** 1.6 µg/kg/day.

Table 14.5: Clinical features of hypothyroidism.

Organ/system involved	Symptoms
General	Lethargy, somnolence, **weight gain, goiter (iodine deficiency and Hashimoto's thyroiditis)**, cold intolerance, hoarse voice, pallor, and cognitive dysfunction
Thyroid	Enlargement of the gland
Gastrointestinal	Reduced appetite, constipation, decreased taste, gastric atrophy, celiac disease, ileus, macroglossia, NAFLD, and ascites
Cardiorespiratory	Angina, **bradycardia, diastolic** hypertension, cardiac failure, **pericardial effusion,** pleural effusion, dyslipidemia, hyperhomocysteinemia, fatigue, shortness of breath on exertion, rhinitis, hypoventilation and reduced pulmonary responses to hypoxia and hypercapnia.
Neuromuscular	Aches and pains, muscle stiffness, delayed relaxation of tendon reflexes **(Woltman's sign)***, carpal tunnel syndrome, **depression,** psychosis, cerebellar **ataxia**, deafness, myotonia, proximal myopathy, pseudohypertrophy of muscles and Hashimoto encephalopathy
Skin	**Myxedema** (nonpitting edema of the skin of hands, feet and eyelids), dry flaky skin and hair, alopecia, brittle nails, vitiligo, purplish lips and malar flush, carotenemia, erythema ab igne, xanthelasmas, madarosis (thinning of lateral one-third of eyebrows)
Reproductive	**Pubertal delay, menorrhagia**, infertility, galactorrhea (hyper- prolactinemia), impotence
Hematological	Macrocytosis, normochromic, normocytic hypoproliferative anemia and hypothyroidism-associated hypocoagulable state.
Renal	Impaired GFR, renal dysfunction, raised creatinine.
Miscellaneous	**OSA** mostly due to macroglosia, **hyponatremia.**

Note: Bold words indicate symptoms of greater discriminant value.

*Woltman's sign (hung up ankle jerk) is due to decreased myosin ATPase activity and decreased rate of reaccumulation of calcium in the sarcoplasmic reticulum

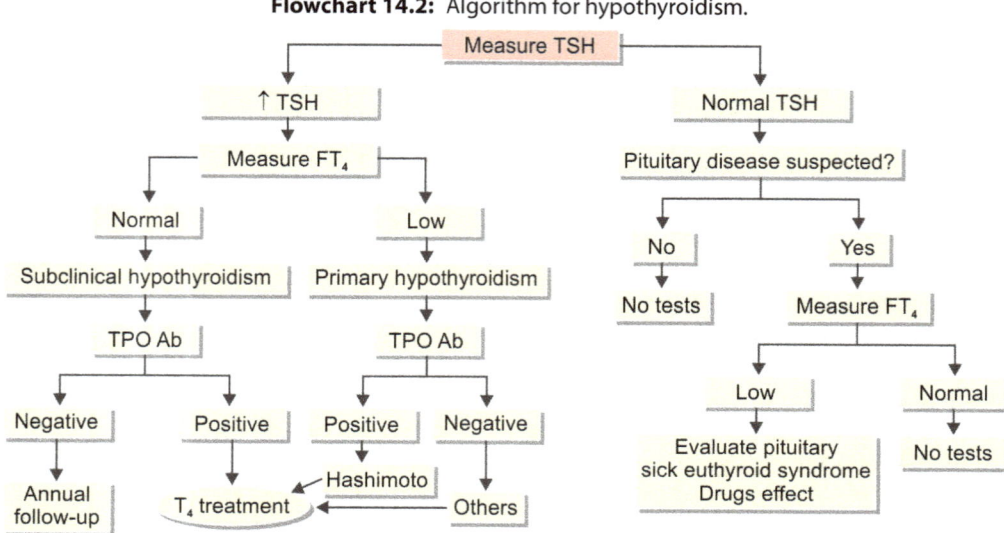

Flowchart 14.2: Algorithm for hypothyroidism.

(T4: free tetrahydrothyronine; TPOAb: thyroid peroxidase antibodies; TSH: thyroid-stimulating hormone)

- **For older patients or those with coronary heart disease:** 25–50 µg/day
  - *Timing:* Should be taken on an empty stomach with water, ideally an hour before breakfast.
  - The patient with symptomatic improvement should be re-evaluated and serum TSH measured in 4–6 weeks. If the TSH remains above the reference range, the dose of T4 can be **increased by 12–25 µg/day in older patients**, or it can be increased by a higher dose in younger patients. The patient will require a repeat TSH measurement in 6 weeks.
- **For patients with heart disease:** 12.5–25 µg/day and increase by 12.5–25 µg/day, if needed, at 6–8 weeks intervals. Few patients with ischemic heart disease may develop angina or worsen with therapy. They require β-blockers, vasodilators or CABG or angioplasty.

Dosage adjustments
- **Age:** In elderly start with half dose.
- **Severity and duration of hypothyroidism:** Increase the dose in severe cases
- **Weight:** 0.5 µg/kg/day increase up to 3.0 µg/kg/day
- **Malabsorption:** Requires increase dose
- **Concomitant drug therapy:** Thyroxine only to be taken on empty stomach
- **Pregnancy:** 25–50% increase in dose, safe in lactating mother
- **Presence of cardiac disease:** Start low dose or alternate day treatment.

Monitoring
- **Goal:** It is to **normalize TSH level** regardless of cause of hypothyroidism and to **restore T4 within the normal range**.
- **Adequacy of replacement: Assessed clinically** and by **thyroid function tests** after 6 weeks on a steady dose.

- Complete suppression of TSH should be avoided because it may cause atrial fibrillation and osteoporosis.
- Lifelong therapy is needed.

Myxedema Coma

Myxedema coma is a very rare, life-threatening medical emergency with a high-mortality rate that develops as a complication of severe hypothyroidism.

The **hallmarks** of myxedema coma are **decreased mentation** and **hypothermia.** Other features are bradycardia, hyponatremia, hypoglycemia, hypotension, puffiness of the hands and face, puffy nose, swollen lips, enlarged tongue, hypoventilation, and features of the precipitating cause/illness.

- **Epidemiology and precipitating factors:** It can occur as the culmination of severe long-standing hypothyroidism with older women being most affected.
- It can be precipitated by an acute event in a poorly controlled hypothyroid patient, such as infection, myocardial infarction, hypothermia, surgery, drugs (amiodarone, β-blockers, diuretics, anesthetic agents, barbiturates, lithium, narcotics, and phenothiazines), cardiac failure, hypoxia, hyponatremia and hypercapnia.
- **Warning signs:** Presence of cool pale skin (due to **hypothermia**—body temperature may be as low as 25°C), absence of mild diastolic hypertension and altered sensorium.
- **Laboratory findings:**
  - Serum **free T4 is low**, serum **TSH** is usually **high** but sometimes only slightly elevated.
  - Serum **cortisol**, may be low in patients with central hypothyroidism with associated hypopituitarism and secondary adrenal insufficiency.
  - **Serum creatine phosphokinase** mostly markedly raised.
  - **Hyponatremia**

Management of Myxedema
See **Table 14.6**.

Sick Euthyroid Syndrome/Nonthyroid Illness State
- Nonthyroidal illness influences thyroid hormone production and action at multiple levels, including H-P-T axis, thyroid hormone transport, and metabolism.
- Changes in thyroid function in the setting of systemic illness, surgery, or fasting not caused by primary thyroid or pituitary dysfunction are referred to as the nonthyroidal illness syndrome (also called "sick euthyroid syndrome"). Also called "low-T3 syndrome", due to the most common abnormality, a decreased level of serum total T3.
- Measurement of serum T4 concentration can be normal, low or elevated.
- Serum TSH is usually normal but can be influenced by nonthyroidal illness.
- Conditions associated with euthyroid sick syndrome include malnutrition, HIV, anorexia nervosa, trauma, myocardial infarction, chronic renal failure, diabetic ketoacidosis, cirrhosis and sepsis.
- Treatment with thyroxine is not recommended.

Subclinical Thyroid Diseases

Subclinical Hypothyroidism
- Subclinical hypothyroidism is defined as an increased serum TSH in the presence of a normal serum-free T4.
- Prevalent in women and elderly persons
- Common causes of subclinical hypothyroidism (**Box 14.7**)

Table 14.6: Management of myxedema coma. Treatment must be started before biochemical confirmation of the diagnosis.

Abnormality	Treatment
Hypothyroidism	Initial intravenous dose of 200–400 µg T4, followed by daily IV dose of 50–100 µg until oral dose is possible. Total serum T4 should increase by 2–4 µg/dL. IV T3, initially 5–20 µg, followed by 2.5–10 µg every 8 hours.
Hypocortisolemia	IV hydrocortisone 100 mg every 8 hours.
Hypoventilation	Intubation and mechanical ventilation
Hypothermia	Gentle warming of patient with blankets (passive rewarming), no active rewarming as it increases the risk for vasodilation and further hypotension.
Hyponatremia	Mild fluid restriction, 3% saline
Hypotension	Cautious volume expansion with crystalloid or whole blood and vasopressors.
Hypoglycemia	Glucose administration
Precipitating event	Identification and elimination by specific treatment (liberal use of empirical antibiotics)
Other measures	Monitor cardiac output and pressures whenever needed, cautious use of intravenous fluids, high-flow oxygen or assisted ventilation

Box 14.7: Common causes of subclinical hypothyroidism.
- Iatrogenic
- Hashimoto's thyroiditis
- Postpartumthyroiditis, painless thyroiditis
- Thyroid infiltration (amyloidosis, sarcoidosis, hemochromatosis, etc.)
- Medications: Amiodarone, lithium, interferon, sorafenib
  - Partial thyroidectomy
  - Head and neck radiation

Clinical Consequences
- Progression to overt hypothyroidism 4% yearly
- Risk of CV disease especially when TSH >10 mU/L: Diastolic dysfunction, diastolic hypertension, increase in LDL-C, increased hsCRP, alteration in coagulation parameters, endothelial dysfunction
- Decreased fertility
- NAFLD
- Neuropsychiatric manifestations and increased risk for Alzheimer disease.

Indication for treatment with levothyroxine
- Patients with serum TSH >10.0 mU/L
- Patients <65–70 years, asymptomatic with TSH ≥7 mU/L
- Patients <65–70 years, symptomatic with TSH from *upper limit of normal* to 6.9 mU/L.
- Patients who are infertile, ovulatory dysfunction, or planning for pregnancy.
- Symptoms or signs of hypothyroidism
- Goiter
- High serum anti-TPO antibodies.
- High-vascular risk including ischemic heart disease, diabetes, and dyslipidemia.

Subclinical Hyperthyroidism
- It is defined as **normal** serum-free T4 and T3 in the presence of **subnormal** TSH (<0.5 mU/L).
- Prevalence between 0.7 and 12.4 %
- Natural course: 40–60% normalize. About 0.5–8% progresses to overt hyperthyroidism.

Effects of subclinical hyperthyroidism
- **Cardiac effects** of subclinical hyperthyroidism: Resting tachycardia, coronary heart disease, heart failure, atrial fibrillation, LV hypertrophy
- **Noncardiac effects:** Osteoporosis, decreased bone mineral density, increased risk of fractures, muscle weakness, dementia, etc.

Causes of subclinical hyperthyroidism
See **Box 14.8**.

THYROIDITIS

Subacute Thyroiditis (De Quervain's Thyroiditis)
A spontaneously remitting, painful, and subacute inflammatory disease of thyroid characterized by transient inflammation of the thyroid gland.
- Most prevalent in the temperate zone.
- Strongly associated with HLA-B35

> **Box 14.8: Causes of subclinical hyperthyroidism.**
> - Iatrogenic (exogenous subclinical hyperthyroidism)
> - Autonomously functioning thyroid adenomas and multinodular goiters (endogenous subclinical hyperthyroidism)
> - Graves' disease (endogenous subclinical hyperthyroidism)
> - Thyroiditis
> - Euthyroid patients with Graves' orbitopathy
> - Early Graves'
> - Graves' disease in remission
> - High hCG

- **Gender and age:** Affect women more often than men (3–5:1). It is most common in young adults and middle age.

Clinical Features

- **Prodromal viral symptoms:** Often proceded by a viral infection (e.g., coxsackie, mumps, adenovirus, measles) of upper respiratory tract. Prodromal symptoms include fever, malaise, and pain in the neck with tachycardia and local thyroid tenderness.
- **Anterior neck pain** in the region of thyroid is the **presenting symptom** is majority of cases and occurs abruptly and may be sometimes unilateral.
  - It **may radiate to the ear, mandible, or occiput**. Pain may shift to the contralateral lobe (**creeping thyroiditis**).
  - Pain may be **aggravated** by **moving the head, swallowing, or coughing**.
- **Functional impairment: Initially** there is **hyperthyroidism** followed by **euthyroidism** and **later** followed by a period of **hypothyroidism**. Finally, **full recovery occurs in 4–6 months**. In about 5% of cases hypothyroidism may persist.
- **Signs: Enlarged diffusely or as symetrically** and **tender thyroid gland.**

Laboratory Findings

- **Mildly elevated** serum-free T4 and T3 and **low** serum TSH
- **Erythrocyte sedimentation rate (ESR):** Elevated (>50 mm/hours may exceed 100 mm/hours)
- **CRP** may be **elevated**
- **High** serum thyroglubulin
- **Mild** anemia
- **Leukocyte counts:** Normal or slightly elevated
- **Serum IL-6 and Tg concentrations:** Increased during the thyrotoxic phase.
- **Thyroid radionuclide uptake** is reduced or absent.
- **Thyroid antibodies** are **transiently detectable** at low titers in a minority of patients.

Treatment

- **Mild cases:** Salicylates (**aspirin** 2,600 mg daily) or NSAIDS (**naproxen** 500–1,000 mg daily in two divided doses or **ibuprofen** 1,200–3,200 mg daily in 3–4 divided doses) relieve pain and tenderness
- **Severe cases:** Corticosteroids (**prednisone** 40 mg/day) have a more dramatic and rapid effect.
- Symptoms of thyrotoxicosis should be managed with beta-adrenergic blocking agents (**propranolol** 40–120 mg, **propranolol LA** 80 mg daily, or 25–50 mg **atenolol** daily)
- If TSH >10 mU/L or associated with symptoms, 50–100 mg of **Levothyroxine** for 6–8 weeks.

Hashimoto's Thyroiditis

- Organ-specific **autoimmune is order** of thyroid characterized gradual thyroid failure with or without goiter formation by lymphoid infiltration of thyroid leading to apoptosis, fibrosis, and atrophy with high titers of circulating:
  a. **Antithyroid peroxidase (TPO) antibody (TPOAb)** in 95% patients.
  b. **Antithyroglobulin (Tg) antibody** in 60–80% patients.
- **Most common cause** of primary hypothyroidism in iodine sufficient areas of the world.
- The two major forms of Hashimoto's thyroiditis are **goitrous autoimmune thyroiditis** and **atrophic autoimmune thyroiditis** (often called **primary myxedema**),
- **Age and gender:** Most often diagnosed between 50 and 60 years of age, more frequent in women than in men with a sex ratio of approximately 7:1.
- **Association with other autoimmune diseases:** Often associated with ulcerative colitis or type 1 diabetes mellitus, pernicious anemia, and Addison's disease.

Pathology: Lymphocytic infiltration (lymphoid follicles with germinal center), fibrosis, follicular cell hyperplasia, and presence of **oxyphil cells** (Askanazy cells/Hürthle cells).

Clinical Features

- **Most** patients are **asymptomatic.** Some may have a feeling of tightness or fullness in the neck. Neck pain and tenderness are rare.
- **Hypothyroidism: Most common cause** of **goitrous hypothyroidism**. About 25% present with hypothyroidism and remaining are at a higher risk of developing in future years. Hashitoxicosis is seen in the acute phase.
- Chronic autoimmune thyroiditis is a **component of type 2 autoimmune polyglandular syndrome**
- **Physical examination:** Diffuse enlargement of thyroid with firm or rubbery consistency.

Investigations

- **Thyroid function tests:** Show features of **hypothyroidism**
- **TPOAb** in 95% patients
- **Antithyroglobulin (Tg) antibody** in 60–80% patients
- **Antinuclear factor (ANF)** may be found in patients below the age of 20 years
- **Ultrasound of thyroid:** Reduced echogenicity
- **Fine-needle aspiration cytology (FNAC) of thyroid.**

Complication

An increased risk for **thyroid lymphoma** (rare).

Treatment of Hashimoto's Thyroiditis

- **Levothyroxine** (150–200 µg/day) is indicated for the treatment of hypothyroidism and it may produce shrinkage of goiter. The dose of thyroxine should be sufficient enough to suppress serum TSH to low but detectable levels.

Riedel's Thyroiditis (Sclerosing Thyroiditis/Ligneous Thyroiditis/Invasive Fibrous Thyroiditis)

- Rare, chronic inflammatory disorder of unknown etiology.
- Characterized by dense fibrosis of the thyroid gland and adjacent perithyroidal tissues (parathyroid glands, the recurrent laryngeal nerve, and trachea), and extracervical areas (fibrous mediastinitis, retroperitoneal fibrosis, retro-orbital fibrosis, sclerosing cholangitis, and pancreatitis).
- Women are four times more likely than men to be affected, and it most commonly occurs between the ages of 30 and 50 years

Clinical Features

- Usually present with a long history of a painless, progressively increasing anterior neck mass. Most patients are euthyroid.
- **Pressure symptoms:** Dysphagia, cough, hoarseness, stridor, attacks of suffocation may be present. Local obstructive pneumonia and superior vena cava syndrome have been reported as presenting symptoms
- **Physical examination:** A **stony-hard or woody thyroid** mass, which varies in size from small to very large. It may involve one or both lobes and is **fixed to surrounding structures.**

Investigations

- **Thyroid function test:** 25–67% has subclinical or overt hypothyroidism.
- **Thyroid antibodies:** May be found in about 45% of patients.
- **Serum calcium:** May be low due to parathyroid invasion.
- **Imaging: Ultrasonography** shows heterogeneous hypoechoic lesions that may infiltrate the perithyroid muscles, and **Doppler** shows absence of vascular flow in the Riedel's regions. **CT/MRI** shows extent of fibrosis. Riedel's thyroiditis is hypermetabolic on **FDG-PET**.
- The differential diagnosis based on FNAC includes subacute thyroiditis, a fibrosing variant of Hashimoto's thyroiditis, radiation-induced thyroiditis, and malignancy, specifically a paucicellular variant of anaplastic cancer.
- Definitive diagnosis can be established pathologically only by open biopsy, since FNAC may be difficult to interpret due to insufficient thyroid epithelial cells but may reveal mononuclear cells and fibrous tissue.

Treatment

- If untreated, this condition may stabilize or regress.
- **Glucocorticoids** has reduced enlargement and induced softening of mass in a few patients, however, therapy is long term and it recurs when steroids are tapered.
- **Tamoxifen:** 10–20 mg twice daily
- **Rituximab** intravenous 375 mg/m² monthly for 3 months
- **Mycophenolate mofetil:** 1 g twice daily
- **Surgery:** Indicated to relieve tracheal and esophageal compression or to rule out malignancy. Surgery should be limited to relieve the obstruction and extensive resection is not indicated to avoid injury to adjacent adhering structures.
- **Radiation:** Low dose in cases refractory to other treatment.

ADRENAL GLAND DISORDERS

Hormones Secreted by the Adrenal Gland

See **Table 14.7**.

Table 14.7: Various hormones secreted by adrenal gland.

Site	Category	Hormone produced
Adrenal cortex		
Zona glomerulosa	Mineralocorticoid	Aldosterone
Zona fasciculata	Glucocorticoid	Cortisol
Zona reticularis	Androgens	• Dehydroepiandrosterone sulfate • Dehydroepiandrosterone • Androstenedione
Adrenal medulla	Catecholamines	• Adrenaline • Noradrenaline

CUSHING'S SYNDROME

Cushing's syndrome is the term used to describe the **clinical state of increased free circulating glucocorticoid.**

- It occurs *most often following the therapeutic administration of synthetic steroids* or ACTH.
- **Cushing's disease** results from corticosteroid excess due to **pituitary-dependent bilateral adrenal hyperplasia**. The pituitary tumors producing Cushing's disease are usually microadenomas (<10 mm in size), which usually do not cause symptoms by local mass effect. It usually develops sporadically but may be a component of multiple endocrine neoplasia type 1.

Causes of Cushing's Syndrome (Table 14.8)

A Cushingoid appearance can be caused by excess alcohol consumption (pseudo-Cushing's syndrome)—the pathophysiology is poorly understood.

Table 14.8: Causes of Cushing's syndrome.

ACTH-dependent causes	ACTH-independent causes
• ACTH-secreting pituitary tumor (**Cushing's disease**): 68% • Nonpituitary ACTH-secreting neoplasm (ectopic ACTH syndrome): 12% • Small cell carcinoma of the lung • Endocrine tumors of foregut origin • Pancreatic islet cell tumor • Medullary carcinoma thyroid • Bronchial carcinoid • Pheochromocytoma • Ovarian tumors • CRH-secreting neoplasm (ectopic CRP syndrome): <1%	• Adrenal adenoma: 10% • Adrenal carcinoma: 8% • Micronodular hyperplasia: <1% • Macronodular hyperplasia: <1% • McCune-Albright syndrome • Iatrogenic (use of corticosteroids)

Clinical Features (Figs. 14.7 and 14.8A to D, Table 14.9)

- Systemic fungal infections and tinea versicolor may develop in untreated patients.
- Higher risk of coronary artery disease and venous thrombosis.

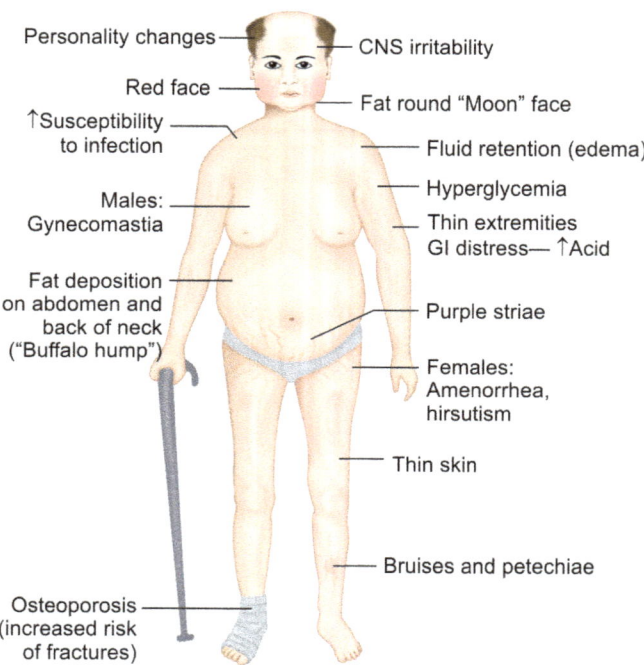

Fig. 14.7: Clinical features of Cushing's syndrome.

Table 14.9: Clinical features of Cushing's syndrome (% prevalence).

Clinical feature	Prevalence	Cause
General		
Weight gain/obesity	90%	Accumulation of fat and retention of fluid
Central obesity ("lemon on match-stick")		Centripetal distribution of fat
Buffalo hump		Fat accumulation at the lower part of neck
Moon face		Rounded plethoric appearance
Hypertension	85%	Increase in plasma volume and sodium retention
Skin		
Hirsutism	70–75%	Increased secretion of adrenal androgen
Plethoric appearance		Thinning of the skin
Purplish striae over abdomen, buttocks, and thighs		Thinning of the skin from collagen breakdown
Bruising		Thinning of blood vessels from collagen breakdown
Musculoskeletal		
Back pain	80%	Osteopenia, osteoporosis and vertebral compression fractures
Muscle weakness	65%	Proximal myopathy and **hypokalemia**. Loss of protein in muscle
Gonadal dysfunction		
Menstrual disorders (oligomenorrhea, amenorrhea),	70–85%	Gonadal dysfunction
Decreased libido and impotence		
Neuropsychiatric		
Emotional lability, depression, euphoria, psychosis, irritability	85%	
Metabolic		
Glucose intolerance	75%	Metabolic abnormalities
Diabetes	20%	
Hyperlipidemia	70%	
Polyuria	30%	
Kidney stones	15%	

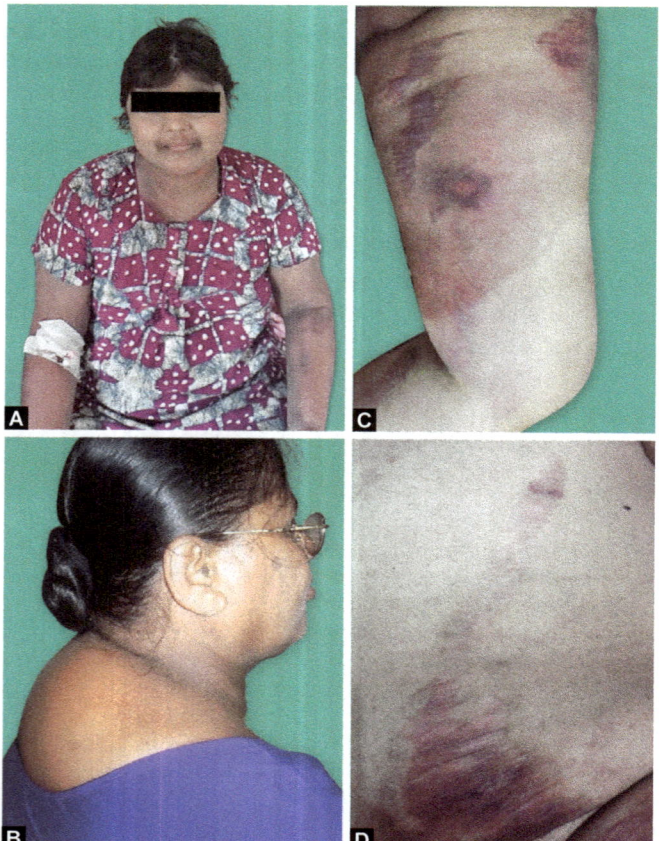

Figs. 14.8A to D: Features of Cushing's syndrome: (A) Cushing's habitus, obesity and moon facies; (B) Buffalo hump; (C and D) Pigmented striae.

- The predominant clinical features of Cushing's syndrome are those of glucocorticoid excess.
- Skin pigmentation occurs only with ACTH-dependent causes.
- Impaired glucose tolerance or frank diabetes is common, especially in the ectopic ACTH syndrome.
- Hypokalemia due to the mineralocorticoid activity of cortisol is common with ectopic ACTH secretion.

- Proximal muscle weakness, sleep apnea, osteoporosis, hypertension are common features of the disease.

Features of Cushing's Syndrome Due to Ectopic ACTH Secretion (Box 14.9)

- Impaired glucose tolerance due to gluconeogenesis.
- Hypokalemic alkalosis due to the mineralocorticoid activity of cortisol.
- Skin pigmentation.

Investigations in Cushing's Syndrome (Flowchart 14.3)

There are two phases of the investigation:
1. Confirmation of the presence or absence of Cushing's syndrome.
2. Differential diagnosis of its cause (e.g., pituitary, adrenal, or ectopic).
   - Most obese, hirsute, hypertensive patients do not have Cushing's syndrome
   - Some cases of mild Cushing's have relatively subtle clinical signs.
   - Confirmation rests on demonstrating inappropriate cortisol secretion, not suppressed by exogenous glucocorticoids
   - Random cortisol measurements are of no value.

Confirmatory tests to establish the presence of Cushing's syndrome (2008 Endocrine Society Clinical Guidelines)
- **48-hour low-dose dexamethasone test:** Normal individuals suppress plasma cortisol to <50 nmol/L. Patients with Cushing's syndrome fail to show complete suppression of plasma cortisol levels. This test is highly sensitive (>97%).
- **24-hour urinary-free cortisol measurements:** This is simple, but less reliable—repeatedly normal values (corrected for body mass) render the diagnosis most unlikely, but some patients with Cushing's have normal values on some collections (approximately 10%).
- **Plasma cortisol levels:** In normal individuals, measurement of plasma cortisol levels at 8 AM and 12 midnight will show the lowest levels at midnight. This circadian rhythm is lost in Cushing's syndrome and the cortisol levels remain the same throughout the day. A midnight level below 1.8 µg/dL is normal, and has a high sensitivity for excluding Cushing's syndrome. However, it has a low specificity.
- **Overnight 1 mg dexamethasone suppression test**
- **Low dose dexamethasone suppression test**
- **Late-night salivary cortisol (two measurements):** It may be used as a screening test for Cushing's syndrome. Concentration of cortisol in saliva is highly correlated with free plasma cortisol, irrespective of salivary flow rates and stable at room temperature for 1 week.

Tests that establish the cause of Cushing's syndrome
- The first step in the evaluation is to distinguish whether hypercortisolism is ACTH dependent or ACTH independent (primary adrenal disease) by measuring ACTH, best performed by **two-site immunoradiometric assay (IRMA)**
- **Plasma ACTH level at 8 AM (Table 14.10)**
- **Imaging for ACTH independent conditions (primary adrenal disease):** The next procedure after ruling out ACTH dependency is **CT** of the adrenal glands to look for adrenal mass.

Note: Bilateral hyperplasia or bilateral macronodular adrenal hyperplasia may be seen with ACTH-dependent disease)

- In patients with **ACTH dependent Cushing's**, the final stage of the diagnostic evaluation is to determine the source of ACTH by:
  - **High-dose dexamethasone suppression test** 8 mg dexamethasone given orally at 11pm, blood sample

> **Box 14.9:** Mnemonic for Cushing's syndrome.
>
> **C:** Central obesity, Collagen fiber weakness, Comedones (acne)
> **U:** Urinary free cortisol increased along with glucose
> **S:** Striae, Suppressed immunity
> **H:** Hypercortisolism, Hypertension, Hyperglycemia, Hypercholesterolemia
> **I:** Iatrogenic due to administration of corticosteroids
> **N:** Non-iatrogenic, Neoplasms
> **G:** Glucose intolerance, Growth retardation

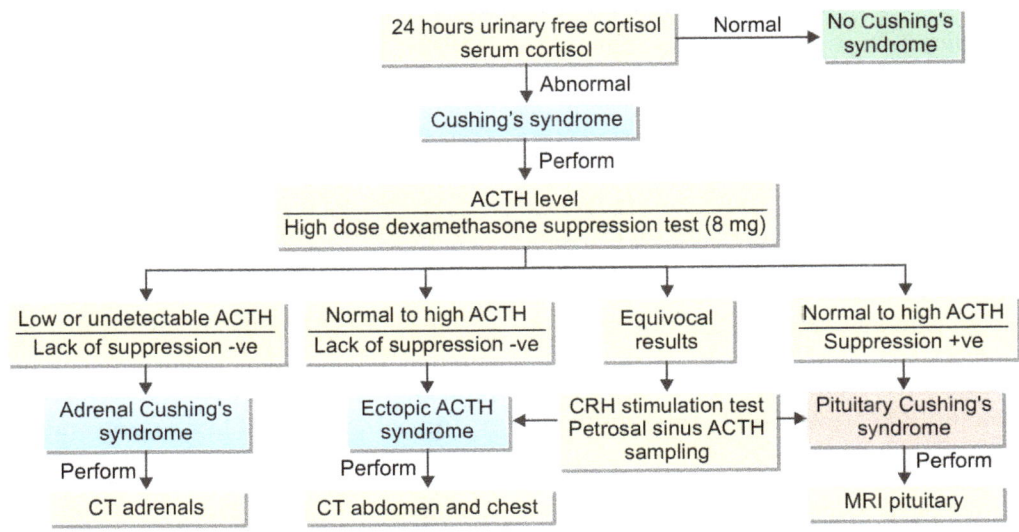

Flowchart 14.3: Algorithm of Cushing's syndrome.

Table 14.10: Interpretation of plasma ACTH level at 8 am.

Level of plasma ACTH	Probable source of ACTH as
Normal levels (20–80 ng/L)	Pituitary
Intermediate values (80–300 ng/L)	Pituitary dependent disease or ectopic ACTH syndrome
Very high levels (>300 ng/L)	Ectopic ACTH syndrome
Low ACTH (<10 ng/L)	Adrenal tumors, macronodular adrenal hyperplasia or exogenous steroid administration

drawn at 8 am the next day for serum cortisol, usually <5 µg/dL in most patients with Cushing's.
- **CRH stimulation test:** Patients with Cushing's have ACTH and cortisol increases within 45 minutes after the IV administration of CRH.
  - Increased in pituitary dependent disease
  - Unchanged in ectopic ACTH syndrome and tumors of adrenal gland.
- **Vasopressin stimulation test:** Stimulates ACTH in most patients with Cushing's disease.
- **Petrosal venous sinus catheterization:** ACTH is measured in petrosal and peripheral venous plasma before and within 10 minutes after administration of CRH.
- **Plasma potassium levels**
  - **Normal** in **pituitary-dependent disease** and tumors of adrenal gland.
  - **Low** (3.5 mmol/L) in **ectopic ACTH syndrome**.

Other investigations
- **Biochemical investigations:** Blood glucose, cholesterol, and LDL may be raised.
- **Radiological investigations**
  - **Plain radiograph** of the skull. Radiograph of chest to detect lung cancer.
  - **CT scan** of anterior mediastinum, upper abdomen and pancreas to rule out tumors.
  - **CT/MRI** head and MRI abdomen.

Management
1. **Exogenous Cushing's syndrome:** Taper and withdraw the glucocorticoid.
2. **Cushing's disease**
   - *Treatment of choice:* Trans-sphenoidal adenomectomy when there is clear circumscribed microadenoma. In the remaining patients subtotal (85–90%) resection of anterior pituitary.
   - *Radiotherapy and radiosurgery:* For recurrent or residual ACTH-secreting tumors. External pituitary irradiation alone is slow acting and useful in only 50-60% of cases.
   - *Medical therapy to reduce ACTH:* Needed when surgery is delayed, contraindicated or unsuccessful. "Block and replace strategy" with **ketoconazole** 200 mg TID and increased to 400 mg TID. If ketoconazole is unsuccessful in controlling cortisol secretion, it should be maintained at a total dose of 1,200 mg/day and **metyrapone** or **mitotane** (adrenolytic) should be added.
   - Pituitary targeted therapies have been tried. Only the somatostatin analog, **pasireotide**, and the dopamine agonist, **cabergoline** (and the combination of the two), have shown potential benefit
   - *Bilateral adrenalectomy:*
     - Bilateral total adrenalectomy with lifelong daily glucocorticoid and mineralocorticoid replacement therapy is the final definitive cure.
     - Done if the diagnosis is uncertain. Followed by pituitary irradiation with Yttrium-90 implantation to prevent the development of Nelson's syndrome.
     - Prednisolone and fludrocortisone should be given postoperatively for a variable length of time.
3. **Adrenal tumors**
   - *Surgical resection*
     - **Adrenal adenomas:** Surgical removal. Postoperatively, prednisolone is given as a replacement therapy till the contralateral adrenal, hypothalamus, and pituitary recovers.
     - **Adrenal carcinomas:** Surgical resection, irradiation of tumor bed, and administration of adrenolytic drug (mitotane).
     - **Medical adrenalectomy:** Medications that inhibit steroidogenesis include ketoconazole, metyrapone, mitotane, aminoglutethimide, and octreotide
4. **Ectopic ACTH syndrome**
   - Surgical excision of benign tumors (e.g., bronchial carcinoid).
   - Radiotherapy and chemotherapy: For malignant tumors.
   - Recurrent tumors may be treated with ketoconazole, metyrapone, or aminoglutethimide.

Nelson's Syndrome
- Nelson's syndrome is **increased pigmentation** (because of high levels of ACTH) associated with an enlarging pituitary tumor postbilateral adrenalectomy.
- It occurs in about 20% of cases after bilateral adrenalectomy for Cushing's disease.
- The syndrome is rare now that adrenalectomy is an uncommon primary treatment, and its incidence may be reduced by pituitary radiotherapy soon after adrenalectomy.
- **Treatment:** Nelson's adenoma may be treated by pituitary surgery and/or radiotherapy.

Hyperaldosteronism/Conn's Syndrome
Excessive production of the aldosterone hormone is called hyperaldosteronism.

Classification
- **Primary hyperaldosteronism:** Develops due to an abnormality in the zona glomerulosa of the adrenal gland.
- **Secondary hyperaldosteronism:** Develops due to the stimulation of aldosterone secretion by angiotensin II following activation of renin-angiotensin system.

Primary hyperaldosteronism
Etiology
- Adrenal adenoma (**Conn's syndrome**)
- Bilateral hyperplasia of zona glomerulosa/ bilateral adrenal hyperplasia
- Idiopathic

- **ACTH-dependent** (glucocorticoid-responsive or dexamethasone-suppressible): This is characterized by secretion of aldosterone under ACTH control. Therefore, treatment consists of **administration of glucocorticoids** to suppress release of ACTH.

Consequences: Excess secretion of aldosterone results in **sodium retention, potassium loss, and metabolic alkalosis.**

Clinical features
- **Hypertension:** Most important clinical consequence of hyperaldosteronism
- **Tetany** due to metabolic alkalosis
- **Muscle weakness** due to hypokalemia.
- **Polyuria and polydipsia** due to nephrogenic DI.

Investigations

Investigation for diagnosis:
- **Hypokalemia:** However, normal serum potassium does not exclude the diagnosis.
- **Urinary potassium loss:** Levels >30 mEq/day during hypokalemia are inappropriate
- **Plasma aldosterone concentration (PAC):** Elevated (>10 ng/dL) and is not suppressed with 0.9% saline infusion (2 L over 4 hours, 8 am to 12 pm, ideally when the patient is seated) or flurocortisone administration.
- **Suppressed plasma renin activity (PRA)** or immunoreactivity.
- **PAC: PRA ratio** *[Plasma aldosterone: renin ratio (ARR)]*: Used as the screening test for primary hyperaldosteronism. A level above 20 is abnormal when plasma aldosterone is measured in ng/dL and PRA is measured in ng/mL/min.
- **Confirmatory aldosterone suppression test**
- **Others**
  - *Oral salt loading test:* After controlling hypertension and hypokalemia, a high sodium diet (5,000 g sodium diet) should be given for 3 days. On the third day of this diet, a 24-hour urine specimen is collected for measurement of aldosterone, sodium, and creatinine. The 24-hour sodium excretion should be >4,600 mg to indicate proper sodium loading. Urine aldosterone excretion >12 µg/day indicates hyperaldosteronism.
  - *Oral captopril test:* In primary hyperaldosteronism, this test does not produce any significant decrease in PAC.

Investigation for differential diagnosis
- **CT/MRI scanning:** To detect adenoma and hyperplasia. Scanning of the adrenal with selenium-75 cholesterol to detect an adenoma.
- **Adrenal vein catheterization:** To detect hypersecretion of aldosterone.
  - Unilateral hypersecretion in adenoma.
  - Bilateral hypersecretion in hyperplasia.
- **Dexamethasone suppression**
  - Lowers plasma aldosterone transiently in adenoma.
  - Prolonged suppression in glucocorticoid sensitive hyperaldosteronism.
- **Measurement of 18-OH-cortisol levels.**
  - Very high levels observed in adenomas and glucocorticoid-responsive hyperplasia.
  - Slightly raised in idiopathic hyperplasia.

Management of primary hyperaldosteronism
- Potassium (K^+) supplementation
- Unilateral disease: Laparoscopic adrenalectomy, bilateral if multiple tumors are present. Surgery is the definitive treatment in unilateral disease.
- Patients with bilateral hyperaldosteronism, mineralocorticoid therapy are administered.
- **Aldosterone antagonists:** Spironolactone and eplerenone are useful in patients where surgery cannot be performed. High dose of spironolactone (up to 400 mg/day) may be required. A few patients may develop gynecomastia with spironolactone and the incidence is lower with eplerenone. Amiloride (10–40 mg/day) may also be tried.

Secondary hyperaldosteronism
Secondary hyperaldosteronism is secondary to an extra-adrenal cause. The aldosterone release occurs in response to activation of the renin-angiotensin system. It is characterized by *increased levels of plasma renin* that stimulates the zona glomerulosa.

Causes of secondary hyperaldosteronism
- **Physiological:**
  - Salt depletion from inadequate intake or excessive loss through kidney or gastrointestinal tract
  - Pregnancy (due to estrogen-induced increases in plasma reninsubstrate)
- **Pathological:**
  - Inadequate renal perfusion: Excessive diuretic therapy, nephrotic syndrome, liver failure, congestive cardiac failure, Bartter's syndrome accelerated or malignant phase of hypertension, severe renal artery stenosis
  - Renin-secreting renal tumor (very rare)

Adrenocortical Insufficiency

Adrenocortical insufficiency, or hypofunction, may be due to primary adrenal disease (primary hypoadrenalism) or decreased stimulation of the adrenals due to a deficiency of ACTH (secondary hypoadrenalism).

ADDISON'S DISEASE

Addison's disease or chronic adrenocortical insufficiency is an uncommon disorder resulting from progressive destruction of the entire adrenal cortex.

Causes of Adrenocortical Insufficiency

Primary Adrenocortical Insufficiency (Adrenal Causes)
- **Autoimmune adrenal insufficiency** (isolated adrenal insufficiency, polyglandular autoimmune syndrome type 1 and 2)
- **Metastatic malignancy** (lung, breast, stomach, colon carcinomas) or lymphoma
- **Adrenal hemorrhage**
  - Waterhouse-Friderichsen syndrome
  - Anticoagulation therapy
- **Infectious:** Tuberculosis, CMV, disseminated fungal infection (histoplasmosis, coccidioidomycosis), HIV, syphilis, and African trypanosomiasis.
  - Adrenal infarction: APLA, SLE
  - Adrenoleukodystrophy and adrenomyeloneuropathy.

- **Infiltrative disorders:** Amyloidosis, hemochromatosis, sarcoidosis
  - Bilateral adrenalectomy
  - Congenital adrenal hyperplasia
  - Familial glucocorticoid deficiency and hypoplasia
  - *Drugs:* Ketoconazole, fluconazole, metyrapone, aminoglutethimide, mitotane, etomidate, rifampin, cyproterone acetate
  - Kearns-Sayre syndrome

Secondary Adrenocortical Insufficiency (Inadequate Acth)

- Exogenous glucocorticoid therapy
- **Hypopituitarism:** Selective removal of pituitary
- Pituitary apoplexy
- Granulomatous disease of pituitary (tuberculosis, sarcoidosis, eosinophilic granuloma)
- Secondary tumor deposits in pituitary (breast, bronchus)
- Postpartum pituitary infarction (Sheehan's syndrome)
- Pituitary irradiation

Clinical Features of Addison's Disease (Table 14.11 and Figs. 14.9A and B)

- Clinical features are produced due to the deficiency of glucocorticoid, mineralocorticoid, and androgen as well as excess of ACTH.
- Fatigue and weight loss are the most prominent symptoms.
- Primary adrenal failure may present
  - Acute with hypotension and acute circulatory failure, with shock out of proportion to severity of current illness, dehydration, an "acute abdomen", unexplained hypoglycemia and unexplained fever (Addisonian crisis); or
  - Chronic with vague features of ill health, sometimes including gastrointestinal symptoms, features suggestive of postural hypotension, and salt craving.
- Skin pigmentation is nearly always present in primary adrenal insufficiency (but not in secondary).
- **Cardinal features of Addison's disease:** Hypotension, pigmentation, and previous history of acute adrenal crisis following stress, or slow recovery from illness.
- **Other autoimmune diseases associated with Addison's disease:** Hashimoto's thyroiditis, primary atrophic hypothyroidism, pernicious anemia, type 1 diabetes mellitus, primary ovarian failure and hypoparathyroidism.
- **Type II polyglandular autoimmune syndrome** is characterized by the association of two or more of the above endocrinopathies.
- **Type I polyglandular autoimmune syndrome** is the combination of adrenal insufficiency, hypoparathyroidism, and chronic mucocutaneous candidiasis.

Table 14.11: Clinical features of adrenocortical insufficiency.

Glucocorticoid deficiency	Mineralocorticoid deficiency	Adrenal androgen deficiency	ACTH excess
Fasting hypoglycemia	Hypotension	Decreased axillary hair in females	Pigmentation of exposed areas, pressure areas like elbows, knees and knuckles, palmar creases, mucous membranes, conjunctive and recently acquired scars, perineum, axillae and areolae of breasts [due to increased production of pro-opiomelanocortin (POMC), that is cleaved into adrenocorticotropic hormone (ACTH) and melanocyte-stimulating hormone (MSH)]
Increased insulin sensitivity	Dizziness	Decreased pubic hair in females	
Muscle weakness	Salt craving	Loss of libido in females	
Morning headache	Weight loss	Asymptomatic—during prepuberty	
Increased production of POMC—increased melanin	Anorexia		
Increased pigmentation—palmar creases, gingival border, axilla	Electrolyte anomalies (hyponatremia, hyperkalemia, metabolic acidosis)		
Fatigue, malaise, weakness, weight loss, anorexia, nausea, vomiting, diarrhea or constipation, postural hypotension			

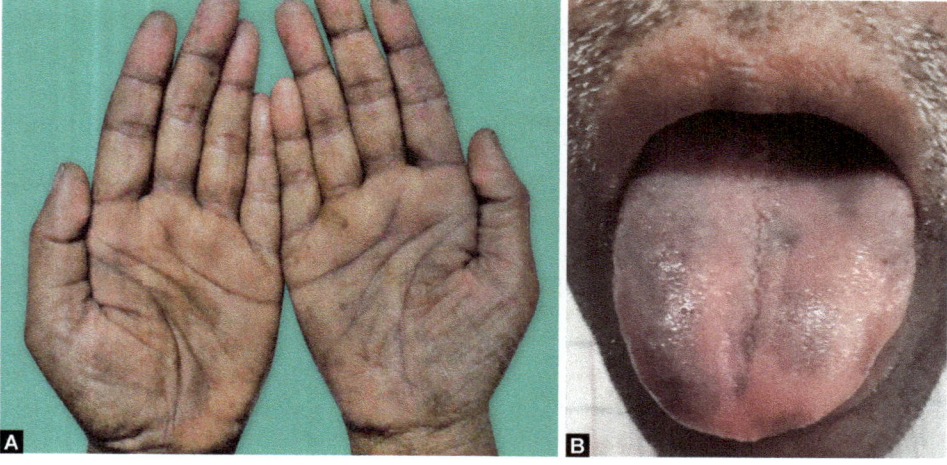

Figs. 14.9A and B: (A) Pigmentation of palms; (B) Oral pigmentation in Addison's disease.

- **Type II polyglandular autoimmune syndrome/Schmidt syndrome** is the association of Addison's disease and Hashimoto's thyroiditis.

Investigations

- **Early Morning (6 am) cortisol level**
  - Normally, levels are 10–20 μg/dL
  - Levels less than 3 μg/dL is suggestive of adrenal insufficiency.
  - Levels >11 μg/dL exclude AI
  - Random cortisol in ill patient → 20 μg/dL reassuring.
- **Morning salivary cortisol concentration**
  - Levels below 1.8 ng/mL are highly suggestive of adrenal insufficiency.
  - Levels above 5.8 ng/mL rules out adrenal insufficiency.
- **Plasma ACTH level:** Elevated in adrenal insufficiency.
- **ACTH stimulation test:** There is failure of rise in plasma cortisol level following the administration of 0.25 mg (standard high dose test) of synthetic ACTH (cosyntropin)
  - *Low dose test (1 mg)*
    - Baseline and 30-minute cortisol levels
    - More physiological ACTH level/stimulation
    - Useful in central AI
    - Useful for assessing recovery after chronic steroid treatment.
  - *High dose (250 mg) test*
    - Baseline, 30- and 60-minute levels
    - Stronger stimulation than 1 mg test.
- **Metyrapone test:** Useful to detect partial ACTH deficiency and partial secondary adrenal insufficiency.
- **Insulin-induced hypoglycemia test:** Insulin at a dose of 0.15 U/kg is administered to achieve hypoglycemia of 35 mg/dL or less. Cortisol levels are measured at 0, 30, and 45 minutes.
- **Corticotropin-releasing hormone test:** To differentiate between secondary and tertiary adrenal insufficiency.
- **Other investigations:**
  - PRA is high and plasma aldosterone levels are low or normal.
  - *Radiograph:*
    - Tuberculous adrenalitis: Chest radiograph may show evidences of pulmonary tuberculosis
    - Plain radiograph of abdomen, CT scan, and MRI scan may show calcification in the adrenal gland.
- **Adrenal autoantibodies:** Adrenal cortex antibody (ACA) and anti-21-OH-hydroxylase antibody
- Elevated blood urea, hyponatremia and hyperkalemia.
- **Blood sugar:** Low levels.
- **Peripheral blood:** Mild anemia, mild eosinophilia.
- **Central AI:** Evaluate for secretion of other pituitary hormones.

Management

- **Primary adrenal insufficiency:**
- **Acute treatment:**
  - Normal saline for volume resuscitation
  - Look for/treat hypoglycemia by 25%D
  - Steroids **(Table 14.12)**:

Table 14.12: Types of steroids.

Type of steroid	Anti-inflammatory action compared to hydrocortisone
Short acting	
Hydrocortisone	1
Cortisone acetate	0.8
Intermediate acting	
Prednisone	4
Prednisolone	4
Methylprednisolone	5
Triamcinolone	5
Long acting	
Dexamethasone	30
Betamethasone	30

  - Loading dose: 50–100 mg/m² **hydrocortisone** IV/IM
  - Continue hydrocortisone with 50–100 mg/m²/day, divided 6th or 8th hourly
  - Long-term treatment:
    - Daily glucocorticoid replacement (hydrocortisone): 10–15 mg/m²/day in divided doses.
    - Daily mineralocorticoid replacement: Fludrocortisone 0.05–0.2 mg daily
- **Stress conditions**
  - Primary goal is to avoid serious consequences of an adrenal crisis
  - *Illness:*
    - Minor stress (e.g., sore throat, rhinorrhea, T (temperature) <38°C) may not require increase in dose
    - Moderate stress (e.g., severe URTI) double the glucocorticoid (GC) replacement dose.
    - Major stress (e.g., T >38°C and/or vomiting), three to four times the GC replacement dose.
- **Surgery:**
  - During general anesthesia, +/– surgery, the GC requirements increases greatly
  - Dose equivalent to 100–150 mg hydrocortisone for major surgical procedures in divided doses.
  - Stress dosing is generally continued until the patient can tolerate oral intake, is afebrile, and is hemodynamically stable
- Tuberculous adrenalitis causing Addison's disease is treated with anti-tuberculous chemotherapy.

Acute Adrenal Crisis

Acute adrenal crisis is a state of acute adrenocortical insufficiency and occurs in patients with Addison's disease who are exposed to the stress of infection, trauma, surgery, or dehydration due to salt deprivation, vomiting, or diarrhea.

Other causes: Acute adrenal crisis can also develop after
- Bilateral adrenal infarction
- Bilateral adrenal hemorrhage: Adrenal hemorrhage and often death may occur following meningococcemia (**Waterhouse-Friderichsen syndrome**).

It is rare with secondary adrenal insufficiency.

Clinical Features

- **Major manifestations:**
  - Shock (out of proportion to severity of illness), but may present with nonspecific symptoms such as weakness, fatigue, lethargy, anorexia, nausea, vomiting, abdominal pain, confusion or coma.
  - Abdominal tenderness "acute abdomen" and unexplained fever.
- **Crisis in patients with long-standing adrenal insufficiency:** Show features of chronic adrenal insufficiency and may show hyperpigmentation (due to chronic ACTH hypersecretion) weight loss, serum electrolyte abnormalities.

Laboratory Findings

Laboratory findings that suggest the diagnosis of acute adrenal crisis: **hyponatremia, hyperkalemia, hypercalcemia, azotemia lymphocytosis, eosinophilia, and hypoglycemia.**

Management

- Establish IV access with a large bore needle.
- Withdraw blood for serum electrolytes, glucose, and routine plasma cortisol and ACTH. **Do not wait for results.**
- IV Infusion 2–3 L of normal saline bolus. Avoid iatrogenic fluid overload.
- IV **Hydrocortisone** 100 mg, followed by 50 mg IV every 6 hours OR 200 mg/day IV infusion.
- After initial stabilization, continue IV NS at a slower rate for next 24–48 hours.
- Search and manage possible precipitating cause.
- In case patient is not a known case of AI, do short ACTH stimulation test.
- Determine the type of AI
- Taper parenteral glucocorticoid over 1–3 days, to oral maintenance dose.
- Start mineralocorticoid replacement with **fludrocortisone** 0.1 mg by mouth daily when saline infusion is stopped.

STEROID THERAPY

Common indication and contraindications of steroids (Table 14.13)

Side Effects of Corticosteroids Therapy

See **Table 14.14**.

Waterhouse-Friderichsen Syndrome

- It is characterized by **acute hemorrhagic** infarction **(destruction) of both the adrenal glands** and is usually associated with fulminant **meningococcal septicemia**. It produces cutaneous petechiae, vasomotor collapse and shock.
- Can occur at any age but is more common in children.
- **Abrupt in onset** and profound prostration occurs within a few hours. It produces petichiae, purpuric lesion, and hemorrhage into the skin.
- **Prompt recognition and appropriate therapy:** Intravenous fluids, high dose antibiotics (penicillin, cephalosporins, sulfonamides), vasopressors, inotropes, plasma transfusion, steroids must be instituted immediately, or death follows within hours to a few days due to cardiac and/or respiratory failure.

Table 14.13: Common indication and contraindications of steroids.

Common indication of steroids	Common contraindications of steroids
- Bronchial asthma - Raised intracranial tension - Cerebral edema - Connective tissue diseases (e.g., rheumatoid arthritis, SLE) - Nephrotic syndrome - Adrenal insufficiency - Shock, septicemia - Leukemia, lymphoma, as an adjunct in chemotherapy for malignancies - Carditis - Demyelinating diseases - Tuberculosis of pericardium and tuberculous meningitis - Transplant rejection, graft-versus-host disease (GVH), bone marrow transplantation - Psoriasis, inflammatory bowel disease - **Eye conditions:** Scleritis, chorioretinitis	- Active tuberculosis - Peptic ulcer - Bleeding tendencies - Diabetes - Uncontrolled hypertension - Active infection

PHEOCHROMOCYTOMA

- Pheochromocytoma is a very rare tumor of the sympathetic nervous system composed of chromaffin cells that secretes catecholamines.
- Important because they are a rare cause of surgically correctable hypertension.
- **Rule of 10s for pheochromocytoma.**
  - 10% extraadrenal (closer to 15%)
  - 10% abdominal
  - 10% occur in children
  - 10% familial (now modified as closer to 25%)
  - 10% sporadic are bilateral or multiple (more if familial)
  - 10% not associated with hypertension
  - 10% malignant
  - 10% discovered incidentally
  - 10% recur (more if adrenal)

Clinical Features

- The classic triad of symptoms in patients with a pheochromocytoma consists of episodic headache, sweating, and tachycardia
- **Paroxysmal hypertension:**
  - Characterized by episodes of **pallor or flushing, headache sweating, palpitations, and anxiety** (fear of death).
  - Paroxysms last 10–60 minutes duration, daily to monthly
  - **Paroxysms are spontaneous or precipitated by:**
    - Diagnostic procedures, intra-arterial contrast
    - Drugs (opioids, unopposed beta-blockade, anesthesia induction, histamine, ACTH, glucagon, metoclopramide)

Table 14.14: Adverse effects of glucocorticoids.

Immune system	Bones
• Increased susceptibility to infections, re-activation of latent tuberculosis • Lymphopenia • Suppression of inflammation impaired wound healing • Suppression of delayed hypersensitivity reaction	• Osteoporosis • Avascular necrosis • Bone pains • Fracture
GIT • Gastric erosions, peptic ulceration, masked perforation, hemorrhage from stomach and duodenum. • Pancreatitis	**Muscles** • Myopathy
Cardiovascular • Hypertension • Fluid retention • Accelerated atherosclerosis • Ischemic heart disease (IHD)	**Metabolic** • Glucose intolerance or development of frank diabetes mellitus • Weight gain • Hyperlipidemia • Hypokalemia • Alkalosis • Fluid and salt retention • Negative nitrogen balance-muscle wasting
Masked perforation, hemorrhage from stomach and duodenum. **Psychiatric** • Depression • Insomnia • Euphoria • Steroid psychosis	**Endocrine** • Growth retardation • Menstrual irregularities • Hypothalamic-pituitary-adrenal axis suppression • Impotence • Acute adrenal insufficiency, Cushingoid features
Skin • Acne rubeosis steriodica • Hirsutism • Striae • Ecchymoses • Thin, fragile skin • Panniculitis (on withdrawal)	**Neurological** Pseudotumor cerebri **Eye** • Cataract • Glaucoma

- Strenuous exercise, movement that increases intra-abdominal pressure (lifting, straining)
- Micturition (bladder paraganglioma)
☐ **Sustained hypertension is more common than paroxysmal hypertension.**
☐ **Complications of hypertension:** Stroke, myocardial infarction, cardiomyopathy, and left ventricular failure.
☐ **Gastrointestinal symptoms:** Abdominal pain, vomiting, constipation, and weight loss.
☐ **Hypercalcemia:** Observed in associated MEN2 hyperparathyroidism
☐ **Mild glucose intolerance**
☐ **Lipolysis and weight-loss**

Investigations (Table 14.15)

Plasma metanephrine is the most sensitive test

Other investigations

☐ **Chromogranin A:** It is a major secretory protein present in the soluble matrix of chromaffin granules and is elevated.
☐ **Provocative** (glucagon provocative test) and adrenolytic (clonidine, phentolamine test) tests: Rarely necessary.
☐ **CT/MRI scan:** To localize tumor.
☐ **Scintigraphy:** Useful for localization of tumor and includes
- MIBG (^{123}I-labeled meta-iodo benzyl guanidine) scintigraphy.

Table 14.15: Laboratory findings in pheochromocytoma.

Investigation	Level	Sensitivity	Specificity
24-hour urine Vanillylmandelic acid (VMA)	Raised	63%	94%
24-hour urine metanephrines and normetanephrines	Raised	76%	94%
24-hour urine free catecholamines	Raised	83%	88%
24-hour urine free catecholamines + metanephrines	Raised	90%	98%
Plasma catecholamines	Raised	85%	80%
Plasma metanephrines	Raised	99%	89%

- Somatostatin receptor scintigraphy using ^{111}indium-labeled diethylene triamine pentaacetic acid octreotide scan.
- (^{18}F) fluoro dihydroxyphenylalanine (DOPA) PET scan.
☐ **Plasma noradrenaline:** Selective venous sampling and estimation of plasma noradrenaline level may be useful in localizing the tumor in difficult cases

Management

Excision of the tumor is the main treatment. Special care has to be taken preoperatively, intraoperatively and postoperatively.

Chapter 14: Endocrinology

Preoperative preparation regimens

☐ Combined α + β-blockade to be given at least 2 weeks preoperatively to control the hypertension. Antihypertensive agents used are: **phenoxybenzamine** (preferred drug for preoperative preparation) Initial dose is 10–20 mg in divided doses every 2–3 days as needed, final dose will be 20–100 mg/day. Other drugs used are selective α_1-blocker (prazosin, terazosin, or doxazosin).

☐ Beta blockers should never be started first. Drugs such as **propranolol** or **metoprolol** are used. Dose should be adjusted to control tachycardia. Typical maximum doses in this setting are 120 mg of propranolol or 200 mg of metoprolol.

☐ High sodium diet—patients are encouraged to start a diet high in sodium content (>5,000 mg daily) on the second or third day because of the catecholamine-induced volume contraction and the orthostasis associated with alpha-adrenergic blockade.

☐ If uncontrolled add
- Metyrosine
- *Calcium channel blockers:* **Nicardipine** and **amlodipine** are most commonly used in this setting; the starting dose of nicardipine is 30 mg twice daily of the sustained-release preparation and the starting dose of amlodipine is 2.5 or 5 mg administered once daily.
- Avoid diuretics as already ECF volume contracted
- Intraoperative blood pressure needs to carefully monitored and controlled.
- Postoperative hypotension can be avoided by adequate fluid replacement and hypoglycemia (10–15% of patients) due to removal of catecholamine suppression of insulin secretion by glucose infusion.

Short Stature

☐ Short stature is defined as a height that is below the 2.3th percentile OR two or more standard deviations below the mean for chronological age and gender for a given population.

☐ A growth velocity that is below the 5th percentile for age and gender is called growth deceleration (e.g., <5 cm/year after the age of 5 years).

☐ **Dwarfism** is defined as short stature for the age of the patient.

☐ Most common causes of dwarfism are familial short stature and constitutional delay of growth and puberty.

Causes of Short Stature

See **Table 14.16**.

Table 14.16: Causes of short stature.

Nonendocrine causes	Endocrine disorders
Constitutional short stature Familial short stature Genetic short stature Intrauterine growth retardation and SGA syndromes of short stature • Turner's syndrome and its variants • Noonan's syndrome • Prader–Willi syndrome • Laurence–Moon and Bardet-Biedl syndromes	GH deficiency and variants • Congenital GH deficiency • With midline defects • With other pituitary hormone deficiencies • Isolated GH deficiency • Pituitary agenesis • Acquired GH deficiency • Hypothalamic-pituitary tumors
Nonendocrine causes	**Endocrine disorders**
Chronic disease	• Hypothalamic-pituitary tumors
Cardiac disorders (left-to-right shunt, congestive heart failure)	• Histiocytosis X
Pulmonary disorders (cystic fibrosis, asthma)	• Central nervous systemic infections
Gastrointestinal disorders: Malabsorption (e.g., celiac disease)	• Head injuries
Hematologic disorders	• GH deficiency following cranial irradiation
• Sickle cell anemia	• Central nervous system vascular accidents
• Thalassemia	• Hydrocephalus
Renal disorders	• Empty Sella syndrome
• Renal tubular acidosis	• Abnormalities of GH action
• Chronic uremia	• GH insensitivity (Laron's dwarfism)
Immunologic disorders	• Pygmies
• Connective tissue disease	• Psychosocial dwarfism
• Juvenile rheumatoid arthritis	• Hypothyroidism
Chronic infection (TB)	• Glucocorticoid excess (Cushing's syndrome)
Malnutrition	• Pseudohypoparathyroidism
• Voluntary dieting	• Disorders of vitamin D metabolism
• Anorexia nervosa	• Diabetes mellitus, uncontrolled
• Cancer chemotherapy	• Diabetes insipidus, untreated

Tall Stature

Tall stature is defined as height above 97th percentile for chronological age and sex or more than 2 SD above the mean for a defined population.

Causes of Tall Stature
See **Table 14.17**.

DIABETES MELLITUS

Introduction

Definition
Diabetes mellitus is a metabolic cum vascular syndrome of multiple etiologies characterized by chronic hyperglycemia with disturbances of carbohydrate, fat, and protein metabolism resulting from defects in insulin secretion, insulin action, or both leading to changes in both small blood vessels (microangiopathy) and large blood vessels (macroangiopathy).

Classification and Etiology

Diabetes mellitus is classified according to etiopathogenesis that leads to hyperglycemia into different groups **(Box 14.10)** but **majority of cases fall into one of two** broad classes namely: **type 1** (not type I) and **type 2** (not type II).

- **Type 1 DM:** In this there is **absolute (complete or near total) deficiency of insulin.** It is subdivided into two subtypes namely **type 1 A,** which is due to **autoimmune** destruction of β-cells and **type 1 β** where the cause of β-cell destruction is **unknown.**
- **Type 2 DM:** It constitutes a **heterogeneous group** characterized by variable degrees of **insulin resistance, impaired insulin secretion, and increased glucose production.** It also develops due to several genetic and metabolic syndromes.
  - **Risk categories:** Type 2 DM is usually preceded by a period of abnormal glucose homeostasis classified as **impaired fasting glucose (IFG) or impaired glucose tolerance (IGT).**

Etiopathogenesis of Type 1 Diabetes Mellitus (T1DM)

Accounts for ~ **5–10%** of all cases
- **Age:** Most common in **childhood (younger than 20 years** of age). Since, it can develop at any age; the term "juvenile diabetes" should be avoided.

Table 14.17: Causes of tall stature.

Nonendocrine causes	Endocrine disorders
Constitutional tall stature, genetic tall stature	Pituitary gigantism
Cerebral gigantism, homocystinuria	Sexual precocity
Marfan's syndrome, Beckwith-Wiedemann syndrome, XYY and XYYY syndromes, Klinefelter's syndrome, syndromes of tall stature	Thyrotoxicosis
	Infants of diabetic mothers

Box 14.10: Classification of diabetes mellitus.

I. **Type 1 diabetes** (destruction of beta cell usually leading to absolute deficiency of insulin)
- Type 1 A: Immune-mediated
- Type 1 B: Idiopathic

II. **Type 2 diabetes** (may range from predominantly insulin resistance with relative insulin deficiency to a predominantly insulin secretory defect with insulin resistance)

III. **Other specific types of diabetes**
A. **Genetic defects of β-cell development or function characterized by mutations in:**
 - Hepatocyte nuclear transcription factor (HNF) 4 a (maturity-onset diabetes of the young 1 -MODY 1)
 - Glucokinase (MODY 2)
 - HNF-1 a (MODY 3)
   – Insulin promoter factor 1 (MODY 4)
   – Hepatocyte nuclear factor-1-beta (MODY 5)
   – Neurogenic differentiation factor-1 (MODY 6)
B. **Genetic defects in insulin action:** Type A insulin resistance, leprechaunism, Rabson-Mendenhall syndrome, lipodystrophy syndromes
C. **Exocrine pancreatic defects:** Pancreatitis, pancreatectomy, hemochromatosis, pancreatic neoplasm, cystic fibrosis, fibrocalculous pancreatopathy
D. **Endocrinopathies:** Acromegaly, Cushing syndrome, hyperthyroidism, pheochromocytoma, glucagonoma
E. **Infections:** Cytomegalovirus, coxsackie B virus, congenital rubella (Hepatitis C virus infection has been associated with an increased incidence of diabetes, but it is uncertain if there is a direct relationship)
F. **Drugs** or chemical induced: Glucocorticoids, pentamidine, nicotinic acid, thyroid hormone, diazoxide, β-adrenergic agonists, thiazides, phenytoin, α-interferon, asparaginase, tacrolimus
G. **Genetic** syndromes **sometimes associated with diabetes:** Down syndrome, Klinefelter syndrome, Turner syndrome, Wolfram's syndrome, DIDMOAD (diabetes insipidus, diabetes mellitus, optic atrophy, and deafness), Friedreich's ataxia, Huntington's disease, Laurence-Moon-Biedl syndrome, myotonic dystrophy, porphyria, Prader-Willi syndrome
H. Uncommon forms of immune-mediated diabetes: 'Stiff-man' syndrome, anti-insulin receptor antibodies

IV. **Gestational diabetes mellitus (GDM)**

V. **Latent autoimmune diabetes in adults (LADA)**

Etiology
- **Autoimmune disease** characterized by:
  - **Pancreatic β-cell destruction**
  - **Absolute deficiency of insulin.**
- **Idiopathic:** It is a rare form in which there is no evidence for autoimmunity.

Pathogenesis of Type 1 Diabetes Mellitus (Fig. 14.10)

- It is an **autoimmune disease** that involves interplay of both genetic susceptibility and environmental factors.
  - **Genetic susceptibility:** Incidence of type 1 diabetes is greater in twins of affected individuals than in the general population, and greater in monozygotic than in dizygotic twins.

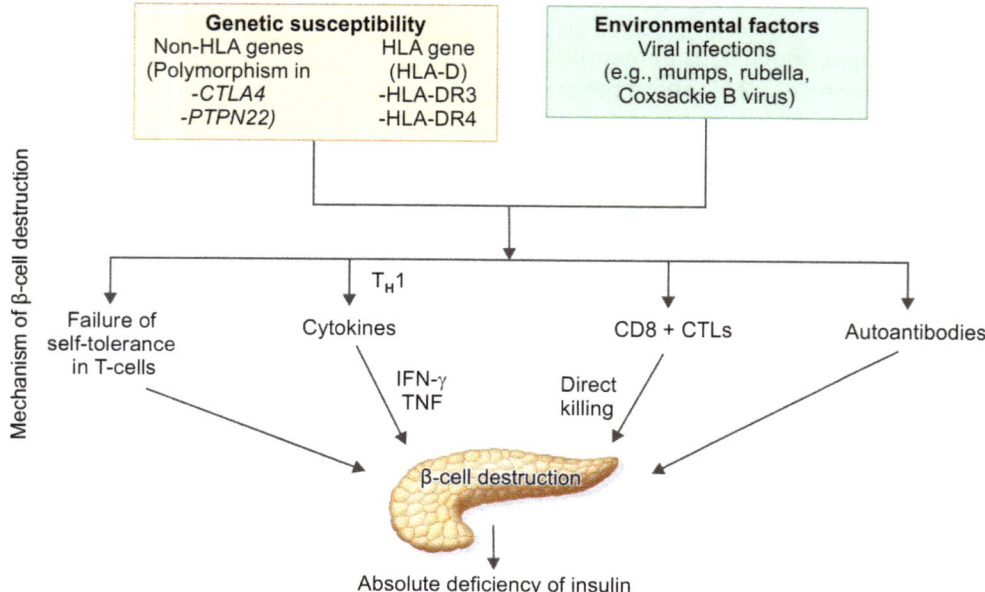

Fig. 14.10: Pathogenesis of type 1 diabetes mellitus.

- **HLA genes:** About 95% of patients with type 1 diabetes have either human leukocyte antigen **(HLA)-DR3 or HLA-DR4, or both,** compared with the general population.
  - **Environmental factors:** Viral infections may trigger islet cell destruction and associations have been found between type 1 diabetes and infection with *mumps, rubella, coxsackie B, or cytomegalovirus.* Environmental event initiates the process in genetically susceptible individuals. Relative deficiency of vitamin D may also be responsible.
  - **Mechanisms of β-cell destruction:** The autoimmune damage starts many years before the disease becomes clinically evident. An inflammatory response in the pancreas called **"insulitis"** develops and there is infiltration of the islets with activated T lymphocytes.
- **Phases in the development of diabetes mellitus:**
  - **Phase with normal glucose tolerance:** In most of the patients, islet cell autoantibodies appear much earlier than overt diabetes. Beta cell mass and insulin secretion progressively decreases however normal levels of blood glucose are maintained.
  - **Phase of impaired glucose intolerance:** Features of diabetes do not become evident even with destruction of 70–80% of beta cells. At this point, residual functional beta cells cannot maintain glucose tolerance and patient develops glucose intolerance.
  - **Phase of frank diabetes:** Stress, infection or puberty may be associated with increased insulin requirements and may trigger the *transition* from glucose intolerance to frank diabetes.
  - *Honeymoon phase:* After the initial clinical presentation of frank type 1 DM, a phase may occur during which time patient is euglycemic with modest doses of insulin or, rarely without insulin for some time. This is referred to as "honeymoon phase". This usually lasts for a few months after which the patient develops frank DM again.
    - **H**yperglycemia and ketosis occur after **more than 90% of the β cells have been destroyed** by an autoimmune process.
    - **Immunologic markers:** These include autoantibodies against islet cell, insulin, glutamic acid decarboxylase (GAD65), zinc transporter ZnT8 and tyrosine phosphatase IA-2 and IA-2p. One or more of these autoantibodies are detected in 85–90% of individuals when fasting hyperglycemia is initially detected.
- **Slow-burning variant of type 1DM:** It is characterized by slower progression to insulin deficiency and develops in later life and is sometimes called **latent autoimmune diabetes in adults (LADA).** LADA may be difficult to distinguish from type 2 DM.

Pathogenesis of Type 2 Diabetes Mellitus (Fig. 14.11)

Type 2 diabetes is a **multifactorial disease.** The four major factors are increasing **age, obesity, ethnicity, and family history.**

Type 2 diabetes is associated with central obesity, hypertension, hypertriglyceridemia, and decreased HDL cholesterol (metabolic syndrome).
- **Environmental factors** play a role and include:
  - **Sedentary lifestyle**
  - **Dietary habits and associated obesity.** Over-eating, obesity and under activity is associated with the development of type 2 DM.
- **Genetic factors:** It is much more significant in type 2 DM than in type 1 DM.
  - Type 2 diabetes has a **concordance rate of 35–60% in monozygotic twins compared with 17–30% in dizygotic twins.**

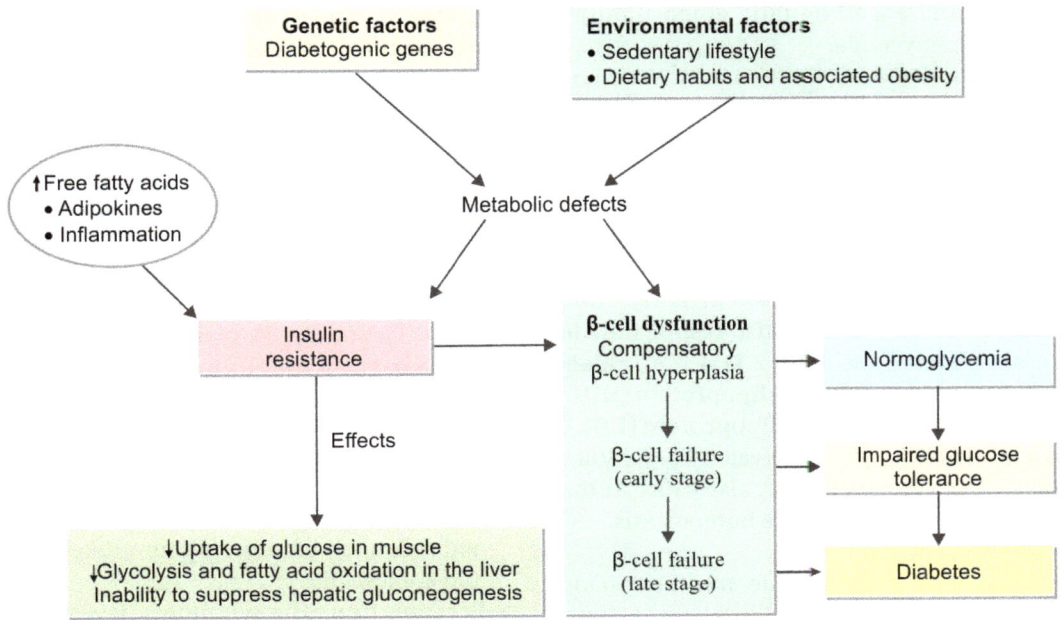

Fig. 14.11: Pathogenesis of type 2 diabetes. Insulin resistance associated with obesity is induced by free fatty acids, adipokines, and chronic inflammation in adipose tissue. Insulin resistance causes β cells of pancreas to undergo compensatory hyperplasia and the resulting hypersecretion of insulin maintains normoglycemia. However, at some point, β-cell compensation is followed by β-cell failure, and diabetes develops.

- Lifetime risk for type 2 diabetes in an offspring is more than double **if both parents** are **affected.**
- Diabetogenic genes have been found.
❑ In contrast to type 1 DM, in type 2 DM there is no HLA relationship and there is no evidence of an autoimmune basis. Pancreatic β-cell mass is intact in type 2 DM, in contrast to type 1 DM. The α-cell mass is increased.

Characteristics of Type 2 DM

These include: (1) insulin resistance, (2) abnormal/impaired insulin secretion/action, (3) increased hepatic production of glucose, and (4) abnormal fat metabolism.

Genome-wide association studies (GWASs) have linked aberrations in more than 40 different genes with an increased risk of T2DM. These genes are involved in the regulation of various biological processes, including cellular development, differentiation, and physiological functions.

Epigenetics and DNA methylation play an important role in the pathogenesis of T2DM, including insulin production, β cell secretion, and resistance. This regulation can either occur by affecting the DNA methylation of the insulin gene itself or by affecting the DNA methylation status of other genes that regulate insulin production, secretion, and sensing.

Insulin Resistance

❑ Insulin resistance is **the decrease/failure of target (peripheral) tissues to insulin action.**
❑ Main factors in the development of insulin resistance are combination of genetic susceptibility and **obesity.** The obesity accompanying type 2 DM is central obesity and central adipose tissue is more "lipolytic" than peripheral sites. Insulin resistance is induced by free fatty acids, adipokines, and chronic inflammation in adipose tissue.

❑ **Consequences of insulin resistance:**
  - **Decreased uptake of glucose in muscle** results in postprandial hyperglycemia. The defects in the uptake are due to defect in the receptors present in target tissues and usually at the postreceptor level.
  - **Reduced glycolysis** and **fatty acid oxidation** in the liver.
  - **Inability to suppress hepatic gluconeogenesis**
❑ Abnormalities of insulin secretion and action
❑ **β-cell dysfunction:** Abnormalities (abnormal/impaired) of insulin secretion develops early in the course of type 2 diabetes and is due to β-cell dysfunction. β-cell dysfunction is multifactorial in origin. In type 2 diabetes, β-cell dysfunction manifests as **inadequate insulin secretion by the pancreatic β cells (relative insulin deficiency)** in association with insulin resistance and hyperglycemia.
❑ **Compensatory β-cell hyperplasia:** Pancreatic β cells **initially respond** to long-term demands of peripheral insulin resistance **by undergoing compensatory hyperplasia leading to increased insulin secretion (hypersecretion).** Thus, the hyperinsulinemic state can compensate for peripheral resistance and maintain normal blood glucose for years.
  - *β-cell failure (early stage):* However, at some point, β cells exhaust their capacity to adapt. β-cell compensation cannot maintain normal blood sugar level. This stage, the patient develops impaired glucose tolerance.
  - *β-cell failure (late stage):* The early stage of cell failure is followed by decreased insulin secretion, hyperglycemia and frank diabetes develops.
❑ **Increased hepatic production of glucose:** Relative lack of insulin is associated with increased production of glucose from the liver (due to inadequate suppression of gluconeogenesis) and reduced glucose uptake by

peripheral tissues. Increased hepatic glucose output produces fasting hyperglycemia.

- **Abnormal fat metabolism:** Insulin resistance in adipose tissue causes lipolysis and increased production of free fatty acid from adipocytes. This leads to increased synthesis of lipid [very-low-density lipoprotein (VLDL) and triglyceride] in hepatocytes. Deposition of fat in the liver is a common association with central obesity and is increased by insulin resistance and/or deficiency. The deposition of fat/lipid or steatosis in the liver may result in nonalcoholic fatty liver disease (NAFLD). This is also responsible for the dyslipidemia observed in type 2 DM [i.e., **raised triglycerides, decreased high-density lipoprotein (HDL), and raised small dense low-density lipoprotein (LDL)**].

  Hyperglycemia (**glucotoxicity**) and elevated free fatty acid levels (**"lipotoxicity"**) and dietary fat may also cause further beta cell loss and deterioration of glucose homeostasis.

- **Phases of insulin resistance:**
  - *Phase 1:* Normal plasma glucose due to compensatory increase in insulin secretion.
  - *Phase 2:* Worsening of insulin resistance leading to post-prandial hyperglycemia despite elevated insulin secretion.
  - *Phase 3:* Insulin resistance remains constant, decline in beta cell function produces fasting hyperglycemia.

  Clinical findings in insulin resistance: Acanthosis nigricans, skin tags.

  Pathophysiology of type 2 diabetes mellitus—the ominous octet is presented in **Figure 14.12**.

Clinical Features of Diabetes Mellitus

Usually, the clinical features of type 1 and type 2 DM are distinctive.

Type 1 Diabetes Mellitus

- **Age:** Usually begins before the age of 30 years but can occur at any age.
- Weight is normal to lean (wasted).
- **Classical triad of diabetes:** The onset of symptoms may be abrupt, with **polyuria, polydipsia, polyphagia** to metabolic derangements. Weight loss may develop over days or weeks.
- DKA may be the initial presentation in approximately 25% of adults with newly diagnosed type 1 diabetes.
- **Insulin requirement:** In the initial 1 or 2 years, the exogenous insulin required may be minimal because of endogenous insulin secretion. But later, its requirement suddenly increases.
- Characteristically, the **plasma insulin is low** and **C peptide levels are low** and unmeasurable. *Glucagon levels are raised and suppressible with insulin.*

Type 2 Diabetes Mellitus

- **Age:** Usually begins in older **above the age of 40 years** and frequently in **obese individuals.** Due to increase in obesity and sedentary lifestyle, it is now detected also in children and adolescents.
- **Presentation:** The symptoms develop gradually, over a period of months to years. **Polyuria, polydipsia, nocturia, blurred vision, unexplained weakness or weight loss.**
- Polyuria occurs when the serum glucose concentration rises significantly above 180 mg/dL, exceeding the renal threshold for glucose reabsorption, which leads to increased urinary glucose excretion.
- Glycosuria causes osmotic diuresis (i.e., polyuria) and hypovolemia, which in turn can lead to polydipsia.
- In **asymptomatic individuals,** the **diagnosis is made after routine blood** (hyperglycemia) **or urine testing (glycosuria).**
- Patients may complain of symptoms like lack of energy, blurring of vision (due to glucose induced changes in refraction) or pruritus vulvae or balanitis caused by *Candida* infection.
- Many patients may present with one of the chronic complications of diabetes and are found to be diabetic on investigations. These include: Staphylococcal

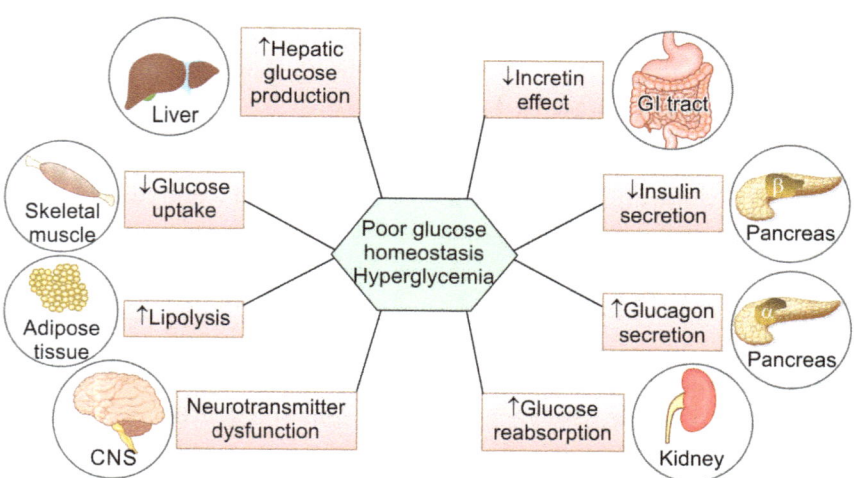

Fig. 14.12: Pathophysiology of type 2 diabetes mellitus—THE OMINOUS OCTET. Multiple drugs in combination may be needed to improve glucose homeostasis. The treatment should target the underlying pathophysiology.

skin infections, retinopathy, polyneuropathy, erectile dysfunction, and arterial disease (myocardial infarction or peripheral gangrene).
- Adults with type 2 diabetes can present with a hyperosmolar hyperglycemic state, characterized by marked hyperglycemia, severe dehydration, and obtundation, but without ketoacidosis. Diabetic ketoacidosis (DKA) as the presenting symptom of type 2 diabetes is also uncommon in adults.
- **Insulin levels in the plasma are normal to high.** Glucagon levels are raised, but resistant to insulin.

Latent Autoimmune Diabetes in Adults
- LADA is a form of **autoimmune type 1 diabetes,** which is diagnosed in individuals who are older than the usual age of onset of type 1 diabetes. Often, LADA is mistaken for **type 2 diabetes,** based on their age at the time of diagnosis.
- Alternate terms for "LADA" include late-onset autoimmune diabetes of adulthood, slow onset type 1 diabetes, and 'type 1.5:

Features of LADA
- **Age:** Usually less than or equal to 25 years age.
- **Clinical presentation:** Similar to non-obese type 2 diabetes.
- Initial control achieved with diet alone or diet plus oral antidiabetic drugs (OAD). Insulin dependency occurs within months (rarely can take years). LADA shares an increased frequency of risk for an HLA-DQB1 genotype than patients with type 1 diabetes and for a variant in the transcription factor 7-like 2 (TCF7L2) gene with patients with type 2 diabetes.
- **Other features of type 1 DM**
  - Low fasting and post glucagon stimulated C peptide levels
  - ICA and GAD65 positive.
- **Importance of diagnosis:** High-risk of progression to insulin dependency.
  - Avoid metformin treatment
  - Early introduction of insulin therapy.

Maturity Onset Diabetes of the Young
Maturity onset diabetes of the young (MODY) is a heterogeneous disorder characterized by noninsulin-dependent monogenic form of diabetes diagnosed at a young age (<25 years) with autosomal dominant transmission and lack of autoantibodies accounting for 2–5% of diabetes.
- **Mutations** in several **transcription factors** or in **glucokinase** result in insufficient insulin release from pancreatic β-cells, causing MODY. Almost 11 subtypes of MODY are identified based on the mutated gene.
- MODY **can occur at any age.** About 70% forms of MODY are MODY-3 (hepatic transcription factor-1 gene) and 10% MODY-2 (glucokinase gene).

Features of Maturity Onset Diabetes of the Young
- **Age:** Young onset of diabetes <25 years of age strong family history of early onset diabetes (2–3 generations affected)
- Evidence of macrovascular complications in earlier generation
- Sulfonylurea sensitivity. Non-insulin dependence (not requiring insulin even after 5 years of diagnosis).
- Absence of insulin resistance phenotype: normal blood pressure, triglycerides, HDL

Subtypes of MODY (Table 14.18)
Differences between type 1 DM, type 2 DM, and MODY are listed in **Table 14.19**.

Fibrocalculous Pancreatic Diabetes
- Pancreatogenic diabetes is classified by the American Diabetes Association and by the World Health Organization as **type 3c diabetes mellitus (T3cDM) (Box 14.11)**
- Prevalence of 5–10% among all patients with diabetes mellitus.
- Seen almost exclusively in developing countries, fibrocalculous pancreatic diabetes (FCPD) is characterized by a triad of abdominal pain, steatorrhea, and diabetes.
- Genes implicated are SPINK-1, Cathepsin B, CTFR genes.
- 70% are males in their second and third decades.

Table 14.18: Types of maturity onset diabetes of the young (MODY).

MODY type	Defective chromosome	Mutation in	Phenotypic features
1.	20 q	HNF-4α (hepatocyte nuclear factor)	Adolescent/early adult: Progressive in insulin secretory defect
2.	7 p	GCK (glucokinase gene)	Since birth: Stable mild fasting hyperglycemia
3.	12 q	HNF-1α	Adolescent/early adult: Progressive insulin secretory defect
4.	13 q	IPF-1 (insulin promoter factor)	Early adult: Very rare, mild diabetes
5.	17 q	HNF-1 β	Adolescent: Progressive diabetes
6.	2 q	Neuro D1	Early adult: Rare
7.	2 p	KLF-11	Early adult: Pancreatic atrophy
8.	9 q	CEL (carboxyl ester lipase)	Early adult: Rare
9.	7 q	Pax-4	Early adult: Rare
10.	11 p	INS	Rare
11.	8 p	BLK	Rare

Table 14.19: Differences between type 1 DM, type 2 DM, and MODY.

Features	Type 1 DM	Type 2 DM	MODY
Frequency	Common	Increasing	2–5% of type 2 DM
Genetics	Polygenic	Polygenic	Monogenic autosomal dominant
Family history	<15%	>50%	100%
Ethnicity	Different races	Different races	Asians, Polynesians, indigenous Australians
Age of onset	Throughout childhood	Post-puberty	<25 years
Severity of onset	Acute and severe	Mild	Mild/asymptomatic
Ketosis/diabetic ketoacidosis	Common	Uncommon	Rare
Obesity association	–	>90%	+/–
Acanthosis nigricans and metabolic syndrome	Absent	Common	Absent
Autoimmunity	Positive	Negative	Positive
Pathophysiology	β cell destruction	Insulin resistance and relative insulinopenia	β-cell dysfunction

> **Box 14.11:** Criteria for diagnosis of diabetes (American Diabetes Association, 2016).
>
> Typical symptoms of DM (polyuria, polydipsia, polyuria, weight loss) + random plasma glucose ≥**200 mg/dL** (symptoms of diabetes + random whole blood glucose >175 mg/dL)
>
> **or**
>
> Fasting plasma glucose ≥**126 mg/dL** (fasting whole blood glucose ≥110 mg/dL).
>
> **or**
>
> 2-hour plasma glucose ≥**200 mg/dL** during an oral glucose tolerance test (OGTT) (whole blood ≥175 mg/dL during an oral 75 g glucose tolerance test).
>
> **or**
>
> Glycated hemoglobin (HbA1c) ≥**6.5%**

- Classically, patients are malnourished with low BMI, but very high insulin requirements. While the presence of microvascular complications are similar as in other types of diabetes, the presence of macrovascular complications are rare, believed to be due to young age, lean body, and low lipid levels
- Risk of pancreatic cancer is very high in this population

Diagnosis of Diabetes Mellitus

- **Classical symptoms:** Diabetes may present with polyuria, polydipsia and polyphagia. There may significant weight loss despite polyphagia.
- **Symptoms due to depressed immune status:** Diabetes is associated with immune dysfunction. It may result in activation of pulmonary tuberculosis, non-healing of wounds, candidal pruritus vulvae or balanitis, recurrent styes and recurrent urinary tract infections.
- **End-organ involvement:** Some patients may present with symptoms of end-organ involvement such as retinopathy, nephropathy or neuropathy.
- **Risk factors of DM:** Some patients may have identifiable risk factors such as obesity, pregnancy and first-degree relatives of known diabetics.

Normal Glucose Levels

Normally the **blood glucose levels** are maintained in a very narrow range of **70–120 mg/dL.**

Glycemia can be classified into three categories: euglycemia (normal), prediabetes (impaired) and diabetes (**Table 14.20**).

Management of Diabetes Mellitus

Medical Nutrition Therapy

Medical nutrition therapy should optimally manage the "**ABC**s" of diabetes control: glycated hemoglobin (**A**1C), **b**lood pressure, and low-density lipoprotein (LDL) **c**holesterol.

Medical nutrition therapy for diabetes **has to be individualized,** with consideration given to eating habits and lifestyle factors. There must be flexibility in use of ordinary foods for patients and families. The best diet advised is the Mediterranean Diet.

Medical nutrition therapy can reduce the HbA1c levels by 0.6–1.4%, if strictly adhered to.

- A **regular pattern of meals** (and snacks) is important to maintain a constant daily intake of carbohydrate, and protects against hypoglycemia. Mild deviations in one or two meals do not matter. It is overall long-term dietary pattern that is important.

Table 14.20: WHO criteria: Levels of blood glucose in normal, prediabetes, and diabetes in glucose tolerance test.

	Euglycemic	Pre-diabetes (impaired glucose tolerance)	Diabetes
Fasting glucose level	<100 mg/dL	>100 mg/dL but less than 126 mg/dL	>126 mg/dL on more than one occasion
2-hour OGTT (75 g anhydrous glucose in water)	<140 mg/dL	>140 mg/dL but <200 mg/dL	>200 mg/dL

- Diet in the management of diabetes **varies with the type of disease.**
- In **insulin-dependent** patients and those on intensive insulin regimens, since adjustment of insulin can cover wide variations the composition of the **diet is not of critical importance.**
- In **noninsulin-dependent** patients who are not on exogenous insulin, **rigorous adherence to diet** is needed, as the endogenous insulin reserve is limited. The increased demand produced by excess calories or increased intake of rapidly absorbed carbohydrate cannot be met.
- **Caloric content of the diet:** It is first decision to be taken based on the need to gain, lose, or maintain current weight. **Two basic types of diet** used in the treatment of diabetes are: (i) **low calorie weight reducing diets** and (ii) **weight maintenance diets.** Dietary prescriptions, should be such that there is daily deficit of 500 kcal, provide a realistic diet and produce a weekly weight loss of around 0.5 kg. Calorie recommendations for adults carrying out "average" activity are 36 kcal/kg for men and 34 kcal/kg for women. Recommended diabetic diet should aim at achieving a BMI of 22. If weight loss cannot be achieved, weight maintenance (rather than gain) is an important goal.
- **Low glycemic index of pulses and pulse-incorporated cereal foods:** Including grams and pulses in rice or wheat-based starchy high GI diets reduces the glycemic index and brings satiety along with adequate supply of calories. Meals with mixed sources of cereals, pulses, and legumes contribute to regulation of insulin and glycemic responses.
- **Protein requirement:** Minimal protein requirement for good nutrition is about **0.9 g/kg of body weight/day** (acceptable range is 1.0–1.5 g/kg/day) and should constitute **10–15% of the total calorie intake.** Very low protein diets may retard the progression of diabetic nephropathy. Protein content should be limited to 0.8 g/kg/day, or about 10% of daily calories, once nephropathy develops.
- **Fat:** The calories required through carbohydrate and fat must be determined individually. **Restriction of fat** is necessary **if weight loss is desired,** because of the high energy value of fat compared to protein and carbohydrate. An **average recommendation** of fat for non-obese diabetic patients and those without hyperlipidemias **is 30% or less of total calories,** with 10% each as saturated, monounsaturated and polyunsaturated fats. Monounsaturated fats improve plasma lipid profile with reduction in total and LDL cholesterol without lowering HDL cholesterol in type 2 DM patients.
- **Carbohydrate:** After choosing the protein and fat content, the remaining calories are to be derived from carbohydrate. It should **constitute 50–55% of the daily caloric intake,** of which significant amount should be in the form of nonstarch polysaccharide, as dietary fiber. Foods with higher fiber content have a lower glycemic index. **Restrict mono and disaccharides** (fructose, sucrose, and glucose). The nonnutritive sweeteners saccharin, aspartame, sucramate and acesulfame K are used to reduce energy intake without loss of palatability.
- **Fiber and diabetes mellitus:** Increasing the intake of dietary fibers is known to have a favorable effect on the overall metabolic health. Fiber-rich foods contain complex carbohydrates that are resistant to digestion and thereby reduce glucose absorption and insulin secretion
- **Alcohol consumption:** It accounts for extra calories and has tendency to inhibit gluconeogenesis. Thus, it may potentiate the hypoglycemic action of sulfonylureas and insulin. In addition, alcohol predisposes towards the development of lactic acidosis in patients taking metformin. Hence, it should be avoided.

Recommended intake of various nutrients in diabetic patients is presented in **Table 14.21.**

Pattern of distribution of calories is presented in **Table 14.22.**

Exercise

Advantages: Exercise **improves insulin sensitivity, reduces fasting, and postprandial glucose,** and has **metabolic, cardiovascular and psychological benefits** in diabetic patients.

Based on all available evidence, the ADA and IDF recommend a total of at least 150 minutes of moderate-intensity physical activity per week that can be a combination of aerobic activities (such as walking or jogging) or resistance training

Aerobic exercise: Adults with diabetes are encouraged to decrease sedentary time and to perform 30–60 minutes of

Table 14.21: Recommended intake of various nutrients in diabetic patients.

Nutrient	Recommended intake
Carbohydrate	~50–60% of total calories
Protein	15–20% of total calories
Total fat	25–35% of total calories
Saturated fat	<10% of total calories (<7% in dyslipidemia)
Polyunsaturated fat	~10% of total calories
Monounsaturated fat	Up to 20% of total calories
Cholesterol	<300 mg/day (<200 mg/day in dyslipidemia)
Total calories	Adjust based on age, weight and height. • Sedentary individuals: 30 Kcal/kg/day • Moderately active individual: 35 Kcal/kg/day • Heavily active individuals: 40 Kcal/kg/day

Table 14.22: Pattern of distribution of calories.

Percentage of total calories	Provision for
20	Breakfast
35	Lunch
15	Late evening feed
30	Dinner

moderate-intensity aerobic activity on most days of the week. Shorter-duration, intensive exercise may be appropriate for physically fit individuals

Resistance training: In the absence of contraindications (e.g., moderate to severe proliferative retinopathy, severe coronary artery disease), people with type 2 diabetes should also be encouraged to perform resistance training (exercise with free weights or weight machines) at least twice per week.

Cardiovascular risk factor management

In addition to glycemic control, vigorous cardiac risk reduction (smoking cessation; blood pressure control; reduction in serum lipids with a statin; diet, exercise, and weight loss or maintenance; and antiplatelet therapy aspirin for those with established atherosclerotic cardiovascular disease) should be a top priority for all patients with type 2 diabetes.

Oral Hypoglycemic (Glucose-Lowering) Drugs

Agents used for treatment of type 1 and type 2 diabetes are listed in **Table 14.23**. Based on their mechanisms of action, oral hypoglycemic drugs are subdivided into agents that increase insulin secretagogues, reduce glucose production, increase insulin sensitivity, enhance GLP-1 action, or promote urinary excretion of glucose. Various categories of oral hypoglycemic drugs are listed in **Table 14.23**.

Biguanides: Metformin

- Activates cyclic AMP kinase, inhibits mitochondrial glycerol-3 phosphate dehydrogenase.
- It reduces both fasting level of blood glucose and the degree of postprandial hyperglycemia in patients with type 2 diabetes but has no effect on normal subjects. It is thought to act by inhibiting the hepatic gluconeogenesis.

Table 14.23: Agents used for treatment of type 1 and type 2 diabetes.

	Mechanism of action	Examples	HbA1c reduction (%)	Specific advantages	Specific disadvantages
Oral					
Biguanides	Hepatic glucose production	Metformin	1–2	Weight neutral/mild weight loss do not cause hypoglycemia, inexpensive	Diarrhea, nausea, lactic acidosis, vitamin B_{12} deficiency (0.5%).
Insulin secretagogues: Sulfonylureas	Insulin secretion	Glibenclamide (glyburide), glipizide, gliclazide, glimipiride	1–2	Inexpensive	Hypoglycemia, weight gain sulfonamide allergies
Insulin secretagogues: Non-sulfonylureas	Insulin secretion	Repaglinide, nateglinide, nitiglinide	1–2	Short onset of action, lower postprandial glucose	Hypoglycemia
Insulin secretagogues: Dipeptidyl peptidase IV inhibitors	Prolong endogenous GLP-1 action	Saxagliptin, sitagliptin, vildagliptin, linagliptin, teneligliptin, evogliptin	0.5–0.8	Do not cause hypoglycemia	Nasopharyngitis Meniscus lesions Headache Contact dermatitis Osteoarthritis Tremor
α-Glucosidase inhibitors	↓ GI glucose absorption	Acarbose, miglitol, voglibose	0.5–0.8	Reduce postprandial glycemia	GI flatulence, liver function abnormalities Contraindicated in kidney disease, inflammatory bowel disease
Thiazolidinediones *Contraindication: CHF, liver disease*	↓ Insulin resistance ↑ glucose utilization	Rosiglitazone, pioglitazone	0.5–1.4	Lower insulin requirements	Peripheral edema, CHF, weight gain, fractures, macular edema; rosiglitazone may increase cardiovascular risk
Sodium glucose cotransporter 2 (SGLT2) inhibitors	Help eliminate glucose in the urine	Canagliflozin, dapagliflozin, empagliflozin, remoglifozin	0.4–1.1	No hypoglycemia, weight loss	Genital and urinary infections
Bile acid sequestrants					
Bile acid sequestrants *Contraindications: Elevated plasma triglycerides*	Bind bile acids, mechanism of glucose lowering not known	Colesevelam	0.5		Constipation, dyspepsia, abdominal pain, nausea, triglycerides interfere with absorption of other drugs, intestinal obstruction

Contd...

Contd...

	Mechanism of action	Examples	HbA1c reduction (%)	Specific advantages	Specific disadvantages
Parenteral					
Insulin	↑ Glucose utilization, ↓ hepatic glucose production, and other anabolic actions	*Refer* Table 14.25	Not limited	Known safety profile	Injection, weight gain, hypoglycemia
GLP-1 receptor agonists *Contraindications: Renal disease, agents that also slow GI motility*	↑ Insulin, ↓ glucagon, slow gastric emptying satiety	Exenatide, liraglutide	0.5–10	Weight loss, do not cause hypoglycemia	Injection, nausea, risk of hypoglycemia with insulin secretagogues, pancreatitis, renal failure
Amylin agonists *Contraindication: Agents that also slow GI motility*	Slow gastric emptying, ↑ glucagon	Pramlintide	0.25–0.5	Reduce postprandial glycemia; weight loss	Injection, nausea, risk of hypoglycemia with insulin
Medical nutrition therapy and physical activity	↓ insulin resistance, ↑ insulin secretion	Low-calorie, low-fat diet, exercise	1–3	Other health benefits	Compliance difficult, long-term success low

- Reduces HbA1c 1.5–2 %
- It is particularly useful in obese patients or those patients who are not responding optimally to maximal doses of sulfonylureas.

Contraindication for metformin
1. Malabsorption or GI disturbances/GI intolerance
2. Low BMI, less than 21 kg/m^2, marked weight loss
3. Organ failure:
   - Creatinine: >1.4 mg/dL, eGFR<30
   - Liver failure: Acute/chronic
   - Cardiac failure, hypotension/sepsis
4. Active vitamin B12 deficiency
5. Metabolic acidosis

Insulin secretagogues
Agents that affect the ATP-sensitive K$^+$ channel

Sulfonylureas
They specifically bind to a receptor that closes an ATP-sensitive potassium channel of the pancreatic β cell, thus depolarizing the cell membrane. This results in an influx of extracellular calcium through voltage gated calcium channels, which causes insulin granules to move toward the cell surface, facilitating exocytosis. Thus, sulfonylureas have an insulinotropic effect on pancreatic β cells.

They can reduce fasting sugars 40–70% mg/dL and HbA1c by 1–2%, immediate action.

- **First generation:** Tolbutamide, chlorpropamide.
- **Second generation:** Glibenclamide (glyburide), glipizide, gliclazide, glimepiride.
- **Third generation:** Glimiperide

Contraindications to sulfonylureas: Hypersensitivity, renal insufficiency is a relative contraindication (Glipizide and gliclazide are preferred, glibenclamide is avoided), hepatic insufficiency, Type 1 DM, diabetic ketoacidosis.

Nonsulfonylureas-Meglitinides
- **Repaglinide and nateglinide** are not sulfonylureas but interact with the ATP-sensitive potassium channel. Owing to their short half-life, these are given with each meal or immediately before to reduce meal related glucose excursions.
- **Advantages of megltinides:** Flexibility in mealtime dosing—Ramzan drug, no significant increase in bodyweight, can be utilized in mild to moderate renal failure and lesser hypoglycemia.

Agents that Enhance GLP-1 Receptor Signaling—Incretin-based Therapy
- **Glucagon-like peptide-1 analogs**
  - The injectable GLP-1 analogs such as liraglutide, exenatide, lixisenatide, dulaglutide and albiglutide imitate the effects of endogenous GLP-1, thereby stimulating pancreatic insulin secretion in a glucose dependent fashion, suppressing pancreatic glucagon output, slowing gastric emptying, and decreasing appetite.
  - Their main advantage is weight loss, which can be significant in some of the patients.
  - Limiting side effects of these agents are nausea and vomiting, particularly early in the course of treatment.
  - Chances of pancreatitis and pancreatic and thyroid cancers are a matter of concern
- **Dipeptidyl peptidase 4 (DPP-4) inhibitors, Gliptins**
  - An alternative approach to the use of GLP-1 analogs is to inhibit dipeptidyl peptidase 4 to conserve endogenous GLP-1. DPP-4 enhances the incretin effect.
  - The enzyme dipeptidyl peptidase 4 (DPP-4) rapidly inactivates GLP1. Inhibition of this enzyme thus potentiates the effect of endogenous GLP1 secretion.
  - *Drugs available:* **Linagliptin (5 mg OD), saxagliptin (5 mg OD), alogliptin, sitagliptin (100 mg OD) and**

vildagliptin (50 mg OD/BD) and teneligliptin (20-40 mg) and evogliptin (5 mg OD)
- *Side effects:* Adverse effects (AEs) such as constipation, nasopharyngitis, urinary tract infection, myalgia, arthralgia, headache, and dizziness are the commonly reported AEs with the use of these agents. Worsening of heart failure rare risk for pancreatitis has been reported.
- **Teneligliptin** is a newer, more potent DPP-4 inhibitor which is safe in renal failure.

α-Glucosidase Inhibitors

Drugs in this group: Acarbose, miglitol and voglibose.
Mechanism of action: α-glucosidase is an enzyme present on the brush border of the small intestine. It is needed for the breakdown of oligosaccharides (carbohydrates) into simple sugars (before carbohydrates can be absorbed) in the intestinal lumen.
- **Major side effects:** These drugs are poorly tolerated and may produce diarrhea, flatulence, and abdominal distension. They are due to increased delivery of unabsorbed oligosaccharides to the large intestine where it undergoes fermentation.
- **Advantages:** They are not as potent as other oral hypoglycemic drugs in lowering the HbA1c but they are unique because it reduces the postprandial glucose rise even in patients with type 1 DM. They do not produce hypoglycemia.

Thiazolidinediones

Drugs in this group: Thiazolidinediones (more conveniently known as the "glitazones") includes **pioglitazone**, rosiglitazone and troglitazone. Troglitazone and rosiglitazone are withdrawn due to increased incidence of liver failure and increased cardiovascular risk, respectively in patients using it.

Mechanism of action: Thiazolidinediones reduce insulin resistance by binding to **peroxisome proliferator-activated receptor gamma (PPAR-γ)**.
- **Side effects:** Include
  - Weight gain of 2-3 kg (due to fluid retention as well as increase in adiposity), fluid retention and heart failure
  - Mild anemia and osteoporosis (increased propensity to bone fractures), bladder carcinoma

Sodium-glucose co-transporter 2 (SGLT2) inhibitors
- Dapagliflozin (5-10 mg/day), remogliflozin (100 mg BD), empagliflozin (25 mg/day), ertugliflozin canagliflozin (100-300 mg/day).
- Sodium-dependent glucose cotransporters (SGLT) are found in the intestinal mucosa of the small intestine and the proximal tubules of the nephrons.
- They provide insulin-independent glucose-lowering by blocking glucose reabsorption in the proximal renal tubule. The capacity of tubular cells to reabsorb glucose is reduced by SGLT2 inhibitors leading to increased urinary glucose excretion and consequently, correction of the hyperglycemia
- The adverse effects of SGLT2 inhibitors may include fatigue, hypoglycemia, increased urine output, increased hematocrit, and **mycotic genital or urinary tract infections.**
- Other side effects include hypotension, acute kidney injury, bone fracture and auto-amputations.
- Bring about a reduction in HbA1c 0.7-1%.
- Dose reduction is needed in renal insufficiency.

Insulin Treatment

Insulin is necessary for all patients with type 1 DM and many patients with type 2 DM.

General Indications for Insulin Therapy
See **Table 14.24**.

Table 14.24: Indications for insulin therapy.

• Type 1 DM • Diabetic ketoacidosis (DKA) • Hyperosmolar hyperglycemic state	Diabetes under following conditions: • Pregnancy (preferably prior to pregnancy) • Acute severe illness needing hospitalization • Perioperative/intensive care unit setting • Patients with acute coronary syndrome (MI) • Patients on high dose corticosteroids • Inability to tolerate or contraindication to oral antiglycemic agents • Newly diagnosed type 2 diabetes with significantly elevated blood glucose levels (patients with severe symptoms or DKA) • Patient no longer achieving therapeutic goals on combination antiglycemic therapy

Insulin Preparations

Properties of various insulin preparations
The commonly used insulin preparations and their duration of action are presented in **Table 14.25**.

Insulin Analogs/Newer Insulins (Table 14.26 and Fig. 14.13)

Insulin analogs are prepared by modifying human insulin and have replaced soluble and isophane insulins, especially type 1 diabetes mellitus. Insulin analogs have more flexibility and convenience. In contrast to soluble insulin (which should be injected 30 minutes before eating), rapid-acting insulin analogs can be given immediately before, during, or even after meals. Long-acting insulin analogs (better than isophane insulin) maintain "basal" insulin levels for up to 24 hours, and may be given once daily.

Patients on regular insulin regimens may develop repeated episodes of hypoglycemia between meals (during some part of the day) and particularly at night. Insulin analogs are useful in such patients. The various preparations include:

Insulin Lispro

- It is first human insulin analog produced by recombinant DNA technology utilizing a nonpathogenic strain of *E. coli*.
- Glucose-lowering activity: More rapid onset of action (<15 minutes), early peak (60-90 minutes) and a shorter duration of glucose-lowering activity (<5 hours).
- **Disadvantages:** Because of its short duration of action

Table 14.25: Duration of action (in hours) of various insulin preparations.

Class	Type	Onset of effect (hours)	Peak effect (hours)	Effective duration of action (hours)
Rapid acting	Insulin analogs: Lispro, aspart, glulisine	<0.25	0.5–1.5	2–4
Short-acting	Regular (crystalline, soluble, plain)	0.5–1	2–3	3–6
	Semilente	0.5–1	2–6	10–12
Intermediate	Isophane (NPH)	2–4	4–10	10–16
	Lente (excess zinc ions)#	1–3	6–12	18–24
Long-acting	Protamine zinc (PZI)	2–4	14–24	36
	Ultralente	2–4	18–24	36
	Insulin analogs: Glargine, detemir	1–4	None	18–24

#Lente (intermediate acting) insulin is mixtures of semilente and ultralente in the ratio of 30:70, respectively.

Table 14.26: Insulin analogs.

Short-acting	Long-acting
Lispro	Glargine
Aspart	Detemir
Glulisine	Degludec

Insulin Aspart and Insulin Glulisine

They are also short-acting insulin analogs similar to lispro.

Insulin Glargine

- It is a human "peakless" bioengineered insulin analog that has a long duration of action and has an acidic pH.
- **Glucose-lowering activity:** After a lag time of 4–6 hours, the flat peakless effect last for 24 hours.
- **Mechanism of action:** After injection into the subcutaneous tissue, **acidic form of insulin becomes neutral and forms microprecipitate.** They **release small amounts** of insulin **very slowly.** It results in a relatively constant concentration for 24 hours without a pronounced peak.
- **Advantages:** It is given **once daily** as subcutaneous injection generally at bedtime. **Hypoglycemia does not develop.**
- **Disadvantages:** As insulin glargine is in acid form, it may cause **increased pain at the injection site.** Its acid nature also **limits its ability to mix with other insulins.**

Insulin Detemir

- It is long acting, basal soluble human insulin analog and has a neutral pH.

Advantages

- Because of its neutral pH, it causes **least pain** at the site of injection.
- It binds to albumin via its fatty acid chain which allows this analog to remain liquid and soluble following injection. It has prolonged mode of action due to its attachment to fatty acid.
- Neither renal nor hepatic impairment exert influence over its pharmacological effects.
- No gain of weight.
  - It is effective when administered once or twice daily and combined with the basal soluble analog insulin and/ or with oral hypoglycemic drugs or pre-meal short acing insulin regimen. Insulin detemir and the rapid-acting analog insulin aspart or lispro, it closely mimic near normal insulin profiles and improves glycemic control than more conventional insulin therapy.

Insulin Degludec

- It is a long-acting (>40 hours) human insulin analog.
- **It forms** soluble multi-hexamers at the site of subcutaneous injection and releases monomers slowly to give an ultra-long peakless phmacokinetic (PK) profile. It reduces

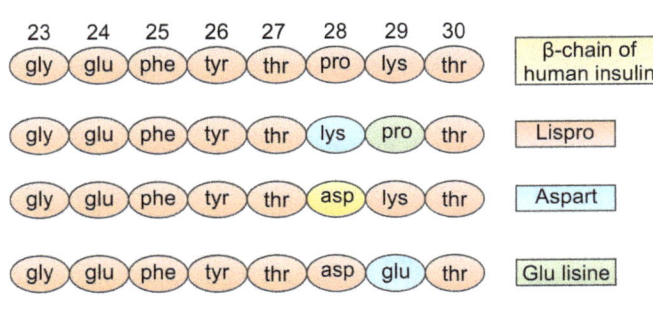

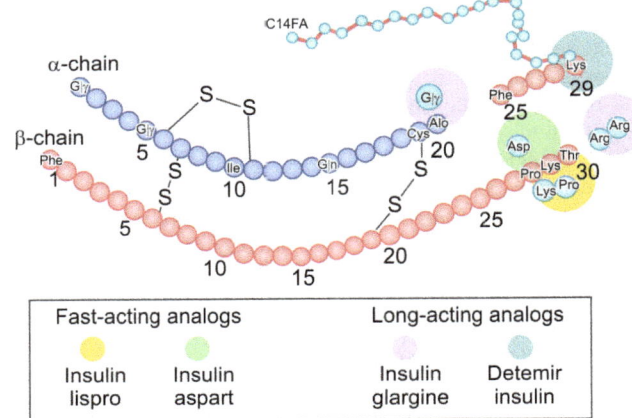

Fig. 14.13: Amino acid structure of insulin and insulin analogs.

variability of concentration in the plasma with once daily regimen.

Advantages of degludec
- **Peakless insulin**
- Excellent improvement in HbA1c, superior fasting plasma glucose (FPG) reduction
- Less hypoglycemia. Reduction of up to 36% in nocturnal hypoglycemia
- Flexibility: Dosing flexibility: **Administration any time on any day.**
- Schematic representation of duration of action of insulin profiles in diabetes mellitus is depicted in **Figure 14.14**
- Merits and demerits of newer insulin/insulin analogs (**Table 14.27**).

Complications of Insulin Therapy
- **Hypoglycemia during insulin treatment:** It is the most common complication of insulin therapy and causes anxiety for both patients and relatives. It occurs due to imbalance between injected insulin and a patient's normal diet, activity, and basal insulin requirement. The risk of hypoglycemia is more before meals, during the night, and during exercise. Irregular eating habits, unusual exertion and alcohol excess may precipitate hypoglycemic episodes.
- **At the injection site**
  - **A shallow injection** causes intradermal (rather than subcutaneous) delivery of insulin resulting in **painful, red lesions** or even scarring. Abscess at injection site is extremely rare.
  - **Local allergic reactions:** May occur at the injection site early in therapy. These include local itching, erythematous and indurated lesions, and discrete subcutaneous nodules. They usually resolve spontaneously.
  - Fatty lumps, called as lipohypertrophy, may develop due to overuse of a single injection site due to lipogenic effects of the injected insulin. It may occur with any type of insulin.
  - **Insulin resistance and anti-insulin antibodies:** Most common cause of mild insulin resistance is obesity. Insulin resistance may be associated with antibodies directed against the insulin receptor.
- **Weight gain:** Many patients may gain weight on insulin treatment, especially if the insulin dose is increased inappropriately. This may be prevented by diet restriction, exercise, and addition of metformin.
- Generalized allergic (urticaria and anaphylactic) reactions are very rare.

Algorithm of therapy for type 2 diabetes mellitus is depicted in **Flowchart 14.4**.

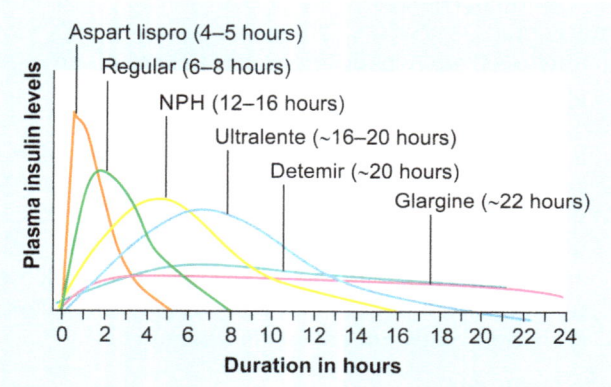

Fig. 14.14: Insulin therapy in diabetes mellitus. Schematic representation of duration of action of insulin profiles.

Table 14.27: Merits and demerits of newer insulin/insulin analogs.

Merits	Demerits
• Better mimicking of physiological insulin secretion • Better control of glucose levels in the fasting, inter-digestive and post prandial period • Lesser risk of hypoglycemia (especially nocturnal) • No need to be injected half an hour before meals • More predictable action profile independent of dose/site of injection/exercise • Greater flexibility with short acting analogs • Compliance is improved with long acting analogs as once a day insulin	• No significant different in adverse effects when compared to standard insulins • Worsening retinopathy with Lispro (homologous to IGF-1) • Carcinogenicity: Concerns over glargine carcinogenicity • High cost

Glycosylated Hemoglobin and Fructosamine

Glycosylated Hemoglobin (HbA1c)
- HbA1c is a minor component of adult hemoglobin (HbA) and its important subgroup is glycosylated hemoglobin (HbA1c). HbA1c has an irreversibly attached glucose and is known as glycosylated hemoglobin.
- **Normal level:** Glycosylated hemoglobin is expressed as a percentage of the normal hemoglobin (standardized range 4–6.1%). In general, the goal of diabetic treatment is to obtain a value below 7%. It should be as close to normal (<6%) as possible without significant hypoglycemia.
- **Significance:** The percentage of glycosylated hemoglobin can be measured and its value provides an excellent assessment of overall state of **glycemic control during the preceding 3 months.**
- Although the glycosylated hemoglobin level provides a rapid assessment of glycemic control, blood glucose level should also be tested to know the control.

Glycosylated Plasma Proteins ("Fructosamine")
- It may also be measured as an index of diabetic control. It measures glycation of all serum proteins and the major component being **glycosylated albumin.** Since albumin accounts for most of the protein in blood, the measurement of fructosamine, for practical purposes, measures glycated albumin. As albumin has a turnover of about 2 weeks, fructosamine reflects **glycemia over the preceding 2–3 weeks** (shorter period).

Chapter 14: Endocrinology 501

Flowchart 14.4: Stepwise approach for the management of type 2 diabetes.

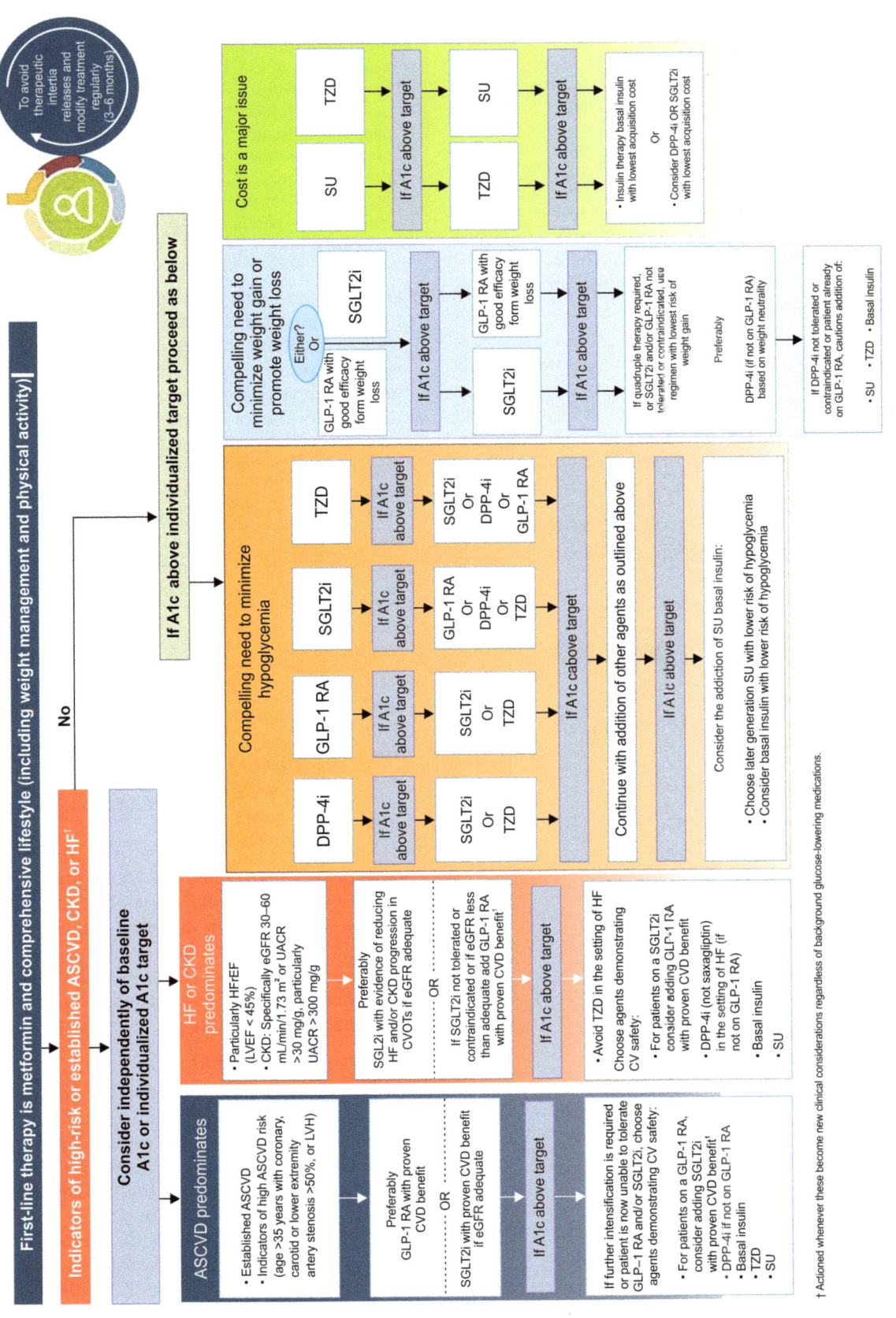

- It is **useful in diabetic patients with anemia or hemoglobinopathy and in pregnancy** (when hemoglobin turnover is changeable).

Complications of Diabetes

Classification of complications of diabetes is presented in **Box 14.12**.

Diabetic Ketoacidosis

Diabetic ketoacidosis (DKA), a medical emergency is a state of metabolic decompensation, which occurs due to a severe deficiency of insulin. More **common and marked in type 1 diabetes** and is rare but may also occur in type 2 diabetes. It is usually seen in previously undiagnosed diabetes mellitus. Precipitating factors are listed in **Box 14.13**.

Mechanism/pathogenesis (Fig. 14.15): Cardinal biochemical features of DKA: **(1) hyperglycemia, (2) hyperketonemia (and ketonuria), and (3) metabolic acidosis.** DKA develops due to the combined effects (1) relative or absolute **insulin deficiency** and (2) counter-regulatory **glucagon excess.** Other hormones such as catecholamines (e.g., epinephrine), cortisol, and growth hormone are also produced in excess.

Consequences of Insulin Deficiency and Glucagon Excess

- **Severe hyperglycemia:** The blood glucose levels of 500–700 mg/dL.

> **Box 14.12:** Complications of diabetes.
>
> **Acute Metabolic Complications**
> - Diabetic ketoacidosis (DKA)
> - Hyperosmolar hyperglycemic state (hyperosmolar non-ketotic diabetic coma)
> - Lactic acidosis
> - Hypoglycemia
>
> **Chronic (Long-term) Complications**
> A. **Vascular Complications**
> 1. **Microvascular**
>   - Ophthalmic
>   - Diabetic retinopathy (non-proliferative and proliferative)
>   - Cataract
>   - Glaucoma
>   - Peripheral neuropathy
>   - Sensory
>   - Motor
>   - Sensory motor
>   - Autonomic neuropathy
>   - Renal
>   - Nephropathy: Microalbuminuria, macroalbuminuria
>   - Chronic kidney disease
>   - Foot disease
> 2. **Macrovascular**
>   - Coronary artery disease
>   - Peripheral vascular disease
>   - Cerebrovascular disease
>
> B. **Nonvascular Complications**
> - Gastroparesis
> - Infections
> - Skin changes (dermatological complications)
> - Hearing loss.

> **Box 14.13:** Precipitating factors.
>
> Precipitating factors of diabetic ketoacidosis (DKA) in a known patient with DM.
> - Infections (pneumonia, urinary tract infections, sepsis, gastroenteritis)
> - Acute pancreatitis
> - Alcohol Intoxication
> - Inadequate insulin
> - Infarction (cerebral, coronary, mesenteric, peripheral)
> - Severe stress (e.g., physical, emotional)
> - Hyperthyroidism, pheochromocytoma
> - Drugs (e.g., thiazides, corticosteroids, cocaine)
> - Pregnancy.

- **Diuresis and dehydration:** Hyperglycemia causes a hyperosmolar state, which induces an **osmotic diuresis** leading to volume depletion **and dehydration** (characteristic features of ketoacidosis). There is loss of electrolyte, particularly of sodium and potassium.
- **Ketonemia** and **ketonuria:** When the **rate of production of ketone bodies exceeds the rate of utilization** by peripheral tissues, it results in **ketonemia** and **ketonuria.**
- **Metabolic acidosis:** Acetoacetic acid and β-hydroxybutyric acid are strong acids and are responsible for the acidotic state. If the excretion of ketone bodies in the urinary is compromised by dehydration, it results in **systemic metabolic ketoacidosis (high-anion gap).**

Clinical Features of DKA

- DKA may present as the initial symptom complex that leads to a diagnosis of type 1 DM for the first time, but more commonly, it develops in patient with already diagnosed diabetes mellitus.
- Clinical features of diabetic ketoacidosis are those of uncontrolled diabetes with acidosis. Patients typically present with **polyuria, polydipsia,** and other symptoms of progressive hyperglycemia.
- **Other clinical features** include **nausea, vomiting, weakness, weight loss,** lethargy, anorexia, leg cramps, blurred vision, and shortness of breath. Vomiting is an ominous symptom because it precludes oral replacement of fluid losses; severe volume depletion may follow quickly.
- **Abdominal pain** is classically periumbilical and sometimes may be so severe that may be confused with a surgical acute abdomen (such as acute pancreatitis or ruptured viscus).

Physical Findings in DKA

- Findings secondary to **dehydration and acidosis:** These include **dry skin** and mucous membranes, **reduced jugular venous pressure, tachycardia, hypotension** (postural or supine), cold extremities/peripheral cyanosis, depressed mental function, and **Kussmaul (deep, rapid hyperventilation) respirations.**
- **Fruity** (sickly-sweet) **smell** of ketones on the patient's **breath** allows an instant diagnosis.
- **Hypothermia:** Body temperature is either normal or low in uncomplicated DKA. Presence of fever suggests infection.
- Mental apathy, confusion, psychomotor retardation, hyporeflexia, and hypotonia may be observed.

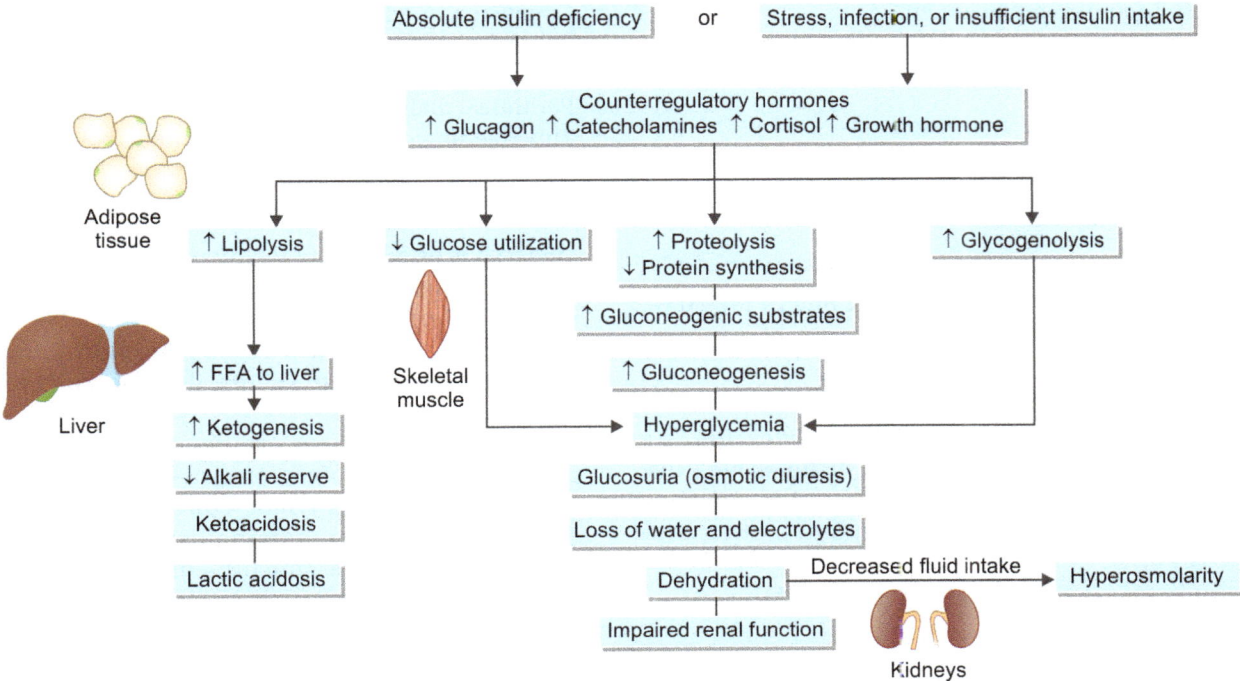

Fig. 14.15: Pathogenesis of diabetic ketoacidosis.

- Abdominal tenderness.
- **Symptoms and signs of cerebral edema:** Headache, altered sensorium, seizures, bowel/bladder incontinence, papilledema, bradycardia, hypertension, and respiratory arrest.

Complications: Acute gastric dilatation/erosive gastritis, cerebral edema, hyperkalemia/hypokalemia, hypoglycemia, infections, myocardial infarction, mucormycosis, and ARDS.

Investigations
- **Urine examination:** Shows glucose and ketones.
- **Plasma levels** of following is to be estimated:
  - **Glucose** levels are raised (hyperglycemia) often markedly.
  - **Ketone bodies** are raised.
- **Serum electrolytes:**
  - **Potassium** levels are normal or raised in the initial stages despite a total body deficit of potassium. This is because, metabolic acidosis shifts potassium from intracellular compartment to extracellular compartment. The levels drop once the treatment is started.
  - **Sodium** levels are usually low, particularly if the patient has repeated vomiting and continued to drink water (pseudohyponatremia).
  - **Bicarbonate** levels are low. Value <12 mmol/L indicates severe acidosis.
  - **Phosphorus** level may be high initially despite a total body deficit of phosphorus.
- **Blood:**
  - Leukocytosis invariably occurs in DKA; this represents a stress response and may not necessarily indicate infection.
  - *ABG:* Reveals high-anion gap metabolic acidosis.
  - Blood urea nitrogen (BUN) is usually raised due to prerenal failure produced from volume depletion.
- Infection screen: Full blood count, blood and urine culture, C-reactive protein, chest X-ray.
- Serum amylase may be elevated.
- **ECG:** To rule out myocardial infarction.

Management
Start with ABCs, bilateral IVs (often require multiple medications), monitor, ECG.
- Search for the underlying etiology/inciting event (infection).

IV fluids
- Patients are often loss of more than 6 L. Start with 10–20 cc/kg in fluid depleted patients.
- May need to repeat fluid boluses for hydration → consider providing 200 mL/h of IV fluid
- NS is the typical fluid of choice

Insulin:
- Insulin infusion at 0.1–0.14 units/kg IV per hour is recommended → continue the insulin drip rate the same until serum bicarbonate and anion gap are improving.
  - If serum glucose is dropping (or once it drops to <250–300 mg/dL), begin dextrose 5% 50–200 mL/hour.

Hyponatremia—corrects with hyperglycemia treatment. If hyponatremic after correction, use NS for fluid repletion.

Potassium
- If K >5.2 mEq/L, no replacement is necessary, and insulin can be started.
- If K is 3.3–5.2 mEq/L, provide PO K (20 mEq) and peripheral IV at 10 mEq/hour while starting insulin.
- If K <3.3 mEq/L, hold insulin until >3.3. Start PO and IV potassium.

Magnesium is often low due to hypokalemia. If the patient is hypokalemia and hypomagnesemia, provide 1–2 g $MgSO_4$ IV.

Phosphorus <1 requires replacement.

Bicarbonate: Correct bicarbonate for patients with pH <6.9.

Supportive care
- Intubation, mechanical ventilation
- Antibiotics
- Renal replacement
- Treatment of complications

Complications of DKA

Mortality is less that 10%. Death occurs due to infection, thrombosis, cerebral edema, and shock.

Hyperglycemic Hyperosmolar State (HHS)

- It is **metabolic emergency,** which usually occurs as a complication of **uncontrolled type 2 diabetes mellitus.** Patients usually present in **middle or later life** (presently it is increasingly seen in younger adults), often with previously undiagnosed diabetes.
- This syndrome has a high mortality rate (>50%).

Characteristics

Characteristics of hyperglycemic hyperosmolar state: It is a syndrome characterized by:
- **Severe hyperglycemia** [>30 mmol/L (600 mg/dL)]
- **Hyperosmolality** (serum osmolality >320 mOsm/kg)
- Extreme **dehydration in the absence of significant hyperketonemia** (<3 mmol/L) **or ketoacidosis** (pH >7.3, bicarbonate >15 mmol/L) **(Fig. 14.16)**.

Precipitating factors for HHS:
- Infections
- Physical and emotional stress
- Inadequate fluid intake
- Cerebrovascular accidents
- Myocardial infarction
- Concurrent medication, e.g., thiazide diuretics, steroids, immunosuppressive agents, phenytoin and osmotic agents like mannitol
- Peritoneal dialysis and hemodialysis
- Tube feeding of high-protein formulas/consumption of glucose-rich fluids/parenteral nutrition

Clinical Features

- **Onset:** It is usually more **insidious** in onset compared to DKA. It presents with a several-week history of polyuria, weight loss, and diminished oral intake.
- **Dehydration:** Characteristic **clinical features** on presentation are **due to volume depletion and extreme dehydration.**
- **Central nervous system manifestations:** These include alteration in the level of consciousness ranging from mental confusion, stupor or coma, **convulsions** (sometimes Jacksonian in type), hemiballism/hemichorea and transient hemiplegia. Impairment of consciousness is directly related to the degree of hyperosmolality.
- Milder GI symptoms
- Infections, particularly pneumonia or pyelonephritis and gram-negative sepsis are very common.
- Hyperosmolar state may predispose to stroke or myocardial infarction.
- Bleeding and acute pancreatitis may accompany HHS.

Physical examination: Shows severe dehydration, hyperosmolality, hypotension, tachycardia and altered mental status.

Laboratory Findings

- **Plasma glucose:** Markedly raised and usually **around 1,000 mg/dL** (range 600–2,400 mg/dL)
- **Serum osmolarity:** Usually extremely high.
- **Prerenal azotemia** with raised BUN and creatinine.

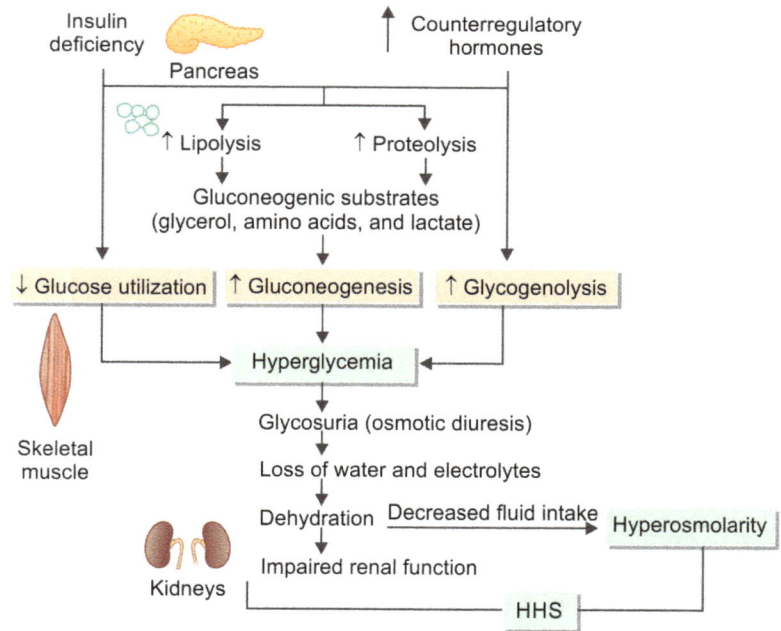

Fig. 14.16: Pathogenesis of hyperglycemic hyperosmolar state (HHS).

- **Plasma bicarbonate:** A mild metabolic acidosis with **marginal decrease** in plasma bicarbonate (about 20 mmol/L) is seen. Marked decrease in plasma bicarbonate (<10 mmol/L) indicates lactic acidosis.

Management

- **Fluid replacement:** The average fluid deficit is much higher than DKA and is about **10 L.** It should be corrected intravenously. Initially 2–3 L isotonic (0.9%) saline should be administered over 1–2 hours. Subsequently, half-strength (0.45%) saline should be given. Once the plasma glucose reaches 300 mg/dL, use 5% dextrose-saline solution. CVP should be monitored in patients with cardiac disease.
- **Insulin:** Regular insulin should be administered as low-dose intravenous infusion as in DKA. The goal is to achieve the plasma glucose around 200 mg/dL.
- **Potassium supplementation** is needed early (as in DKA).
- **Lactic acidosis:** Treat with intravenous sodium bicarbonate.
- **Infections:** With suitable antibiotics.
- **Anticoagulants:** To prevent thrombosis.

Hypoglycemia

Whipple's triad: It is the most convincing documentation of hypoglycemia.
- **Symptoms** consistent with **hypoglycemia**
- **Low plasma concentration** of blood glucose ≥70 mg/dL (3.9 mmol/L) measured with a precise method (not a glucose monitor)
- **Relief of symptoms after** the **plasma glucose level is raised.**
  The ADA recommends a plasma glucose threshold of 54 mg/dL for the diagnosis of clinically significant hypoglycemia.

Causes of hypoglycemia in adults:
- Drugs: Insulin or insulin secretagogues, alcohol and others
- Critical illness: Hepatic, renal or cardiac failure, sepsis, malaria, inanition
- Hormone deficiency: Cortisol, glucagon and epinephrine (in insulin-deficient diabetes)
- Non-islet cell tumor
- Endogenous hyperinsulinism: Insulinoma, functional beta-cell disorders (nesidioblastosis), noninsulinoma pancereatogenous hypoglycemia, postgastric bypass hypoglycemia, insulin autoimmune hypoglycemia, antibody to insulin, antibody to insulin receptor, insulin secretgogue
- Accidental, surreptitious, or malicious hypoglycemia

Significance: Hypoglycemia is a dangerous complication, and more serious than hyperglycemia. Prolonged hypoglycemia may cause permanent damage to the brain.

Pathogenesis
Clinical features
- **Blood glucose level and symptom development:** Symptoms due to hypoglycemia usually occur with plasma glucose at:
  - Level of 60 mg/dL in nondiabetic individuals
  - Higher levels (80 mg/dL) in poorly controlled diabetic patients
  - Lower levels in well-controlled diabetic patients.
- **Symptoms** fall into two main groups:
  1. *Related to acute activation of the autonomic nervous system (neurogenic symptoms):* These are produced by excessive secretion of adrenaline and symptoms include sweating, tremor, tachycardia, anxiety, and hunger. Adrenergic symptoms predominate, when hypoglycemia is of rapid onset (e.g., insulin reactions).
  2. *Those secondary to glucose deprivation of the brain (neuroglycopenia):* It causes dizziness, headache, clouding of vision, blunted mental acuity, and loss of fine motor skill, confusion, abnormal behavior, convulsions, and loss of consciousness. Central nervous system symptoms predominate, when hypoglycemia is of gradual onset. Patients with longstanding diabetes may not develop warning adrenergic symptoms **(hypoglycemic unawareness)** due to severe neuropathy and are at a greater risk of central nervous dysfunction.

Management

- **Oral carbohydrate:** If hypoglycemia is detected early, it may be corrected by ingestion of carbohydrate (preferably in an easily absorbable form).
- **Intravenous dextrose:** It is given in serious hypoglycemia, when there is impaired mental functions, and prolonged hypoglycemia is anticipated (e.g., with depot-insulin and oral sulfonylureas like chlorpropamide). 100 mL of 25% dextrose is administered. Oral carbohydrate should be given as soon as the patient is able to eat.
- **Glucagon:** Glucagon in the dose of 0.5–1 mg subcutaneously or intramuscularly may be given when there is severe hypoglycemia. It may be repeated if necessary after 10 minutes. Glucagon stimulates hepatic glycogenolysis. But it may not be effective in severe and prolonged hypoglycemia due to depot-insulins. It should not be used for the treatment of hypoglycemia due to oral hypoglycemic drugs.
- **Octreotide:** It is useful for patients who develop recurrent hypoglycemia following dextrose infusion.
- **Other measures** are aimed at preventing recurrence of hypoglycemia. These include adjusting the dose of oral hypoglycemic drugs, changing the timing of insulin injections, adjustments in diet and physical activity/exercise, etc.

CHRONIC COMPLICATIONS OF DIABETES

Pathogenesis of chronic complications of diabetes is multifactorial and includes: (1) hyperglycemia (glucotoxicity) is the main mediator, (2) insulin resistance, and (3) obesity.

Hyperglycemia
Effects of Hyperglycemia
See **Figure 14.17.**

Chapter 14: Endocrinology

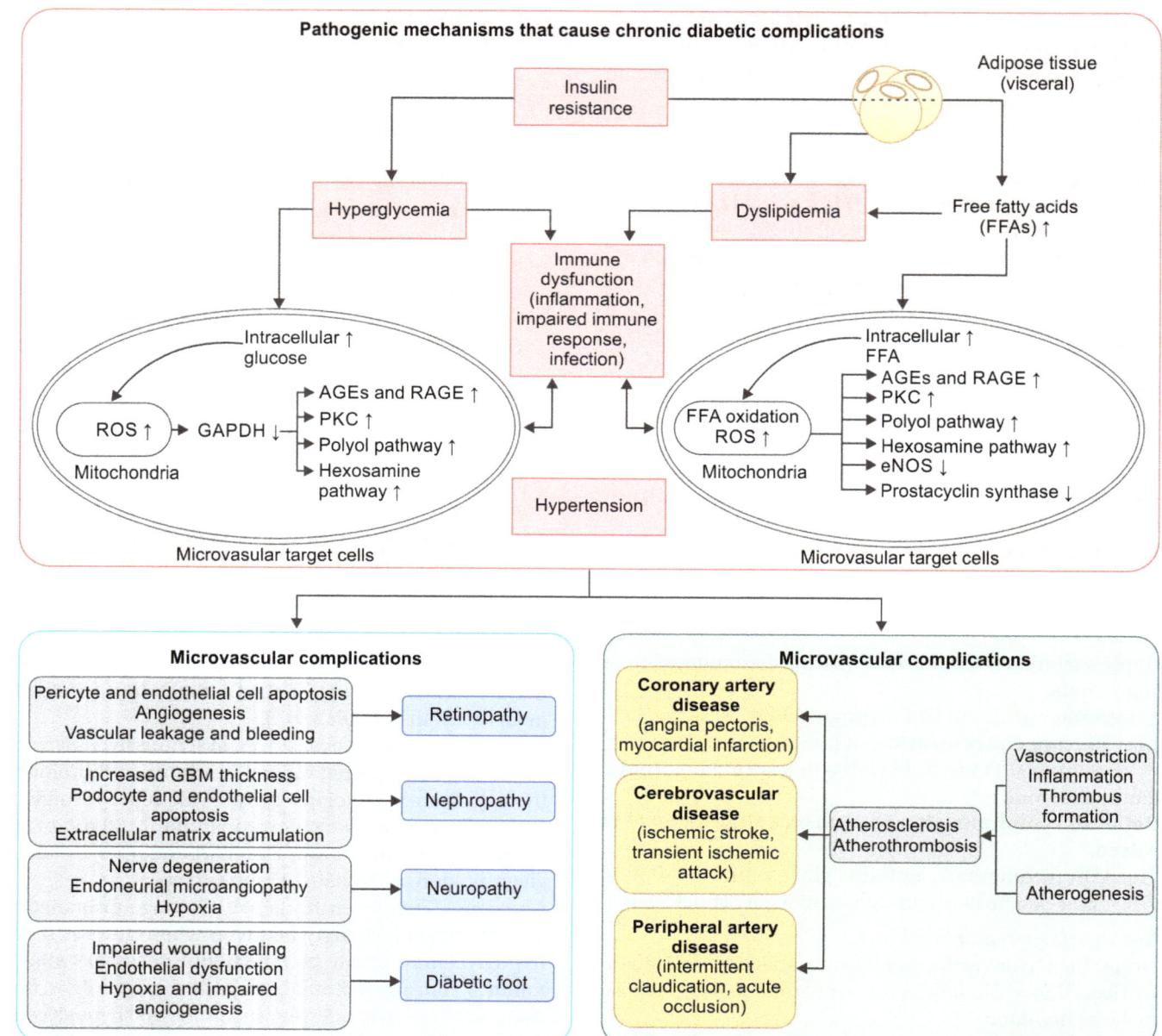

Fig. 14.17: Pathogenesis of chronic complications of DM due to hyperglycemia.

Cardiovascular Complications of Diabetes

The lesions of large- and medium-sized muscular arteries are the **most common causes of mortality** in long-standing diabetes. These include:

Atherosclerosis: Diabetes is one of the major modifiable risk factor for atherosclerosis and other cardiovascular morbidities. The main cardiovascular complications of diabetes are accelerated atherosclerosis. The **atherosclerosis is more severe and occurs at earlier age.** Diabetics have **increased levels of** plasminogen activator inhibitor (**PAI-1**), which **inhibits fibrinolysis and favors development of atherosclerotic plaques. Renal arteries** also develop **severe atherosclerosis.** The atherosclerotic lesions can manifest in a variety of ways:

- **Myocardial infarction:** It is due to atherosclerosis of the coronary arteries and is the **most common cause of death in diabetics.** Diabetics have greater risk of coronary artery disease and cardiovascular complications than nondiabetics. Risk for cardiovascular disease is more even in pre-diabetics.
- **Gangrene of the lower/upper extremities:** Patient may also present with intermittent claudication. Gangrene may results from advanced vascular disease and is more common in diabetics.
- **Renal vascular insufficiency.**
- **Cerebrovascular accidents** (stroke).

Diabetic Nephropathy

Diabetic nephropathy is the term used for **collective lesions that often occur together in the diabetic kidney.** About **30–40% of all diabetics** develops nephropathy and is **leading cause of chronic kidney disease (CKD) and end-stage renal** disease (ESRD). It is a leading cause of death and disability in diabetes and is more common in type 1 DM than type 2 DM.

Pathogenesis: Diabetic glomerulosclerosis represents a part of the generalized diabetic microangiopathy.

Clinical features: The natural history of diabetic nephropathy follows a fairly predictable sequence of events.

- **Glomerular hyperperfusion** and **renal hypertrophy** develops in the first years after the onset of DM. It is associated with an **increase of the glomerular filtration rate** (GFR). It shows nephromegaly (enlargement of kidneys).
- During the first 5 years of DM, **thickening of the glomerular basement membrane,** glomerular hypertrophy, and expansion of mesangial volume occur as the GFR returns to normal.
- **Microalbuminuria:** After 5–10 years, many patients start excreting **small amounts of albumin in the urine.** It is the **earliest manifestation** of diabetic nephropathy in which the urine has low amounts of albumin (>20 mg/day, but <300 mg/day). Microalbuminuria defined as the **persistent elevation of the urinary albumin excretion of 20–300 mg/L** (or 20–200 μg/min) in an early morning urine sample. It is also a well-established marker for increased cardiovascular morbidity and mortality in either type 1 or type 2 diabetics. Normal individual excrete albumin <20 mg/day. It indicates early and possibly reversible glomerular damage. Type 2 diabetes is more likely to have microalbuminuria (or overt nephropathy) at diagnosis. This is because of the long duration of abnormal glucose metabolism in type 2 DM. Hence, patients with type 2 DM should be screened at the time of diagnosis for the presence of microalbuminuria.
- **Nephropathy with macroalbuminuria:** Without specific interventions, diabetics will develop **overt nephropathy with macroalbuminuria** (>300 mg of urinary albumin per day), usually associated with hypertension. From this stage, the renal disease is irreversible. There is a steady decline in glomerular filtration rate at a rate of about 1 mL/minute/month. The stage of macroalbuminuria may progress to nephrotic syndrome.
- **End-stage renal disease:** The overt nephropathy may progress to ESRD. Patient develops azotemia, renal failure, and uremia.

Management

- **Prevention:** Control of glycemia can reverse microalbuminuria in some patients. Stop smoking and control dyslipidemia.
- **Management of diabetic nephropathy**
  - *Glycemic control:* Insulin is the antidiabetic of choice, regular and rapid acting are preferred, biguanides are contraindicated, if eGFR <30. SGLT2 inhibitors can be used till eGFR >45. Sulfonylureas, Glitazones, and Acarbose are avoided.
  - *Blood pressure control:* Recommended BP <140/90 mmHg.
  - ACE inhibitors and ARBs are first line for BP control
  - *Dietary modification*: Protein restriction, as it reduces hyperfiltration and intraglomerular pressure. Up to 0.8 g/day is recommended by the ADA. Sodium restriction to <2,300 mg/day is also mandated.
  - *Miscellaneous:* Treat UTI aggressively. Lipid lowering by HMG CoA reductase inhibitors.

Ophthalmologic Complications of Diabetes Mellitus

Diabetes can produce different lesions in the eye. These include:

- **Diabetic retinopathy** (damage to the retina and iris) can lead to blindness.
- **Cataract** is denaturation of the protein and other components of the lens of the eye and leads to opacity of lens. Cataract develops early in diabetics than in the general population. Sustained very poor control of diabetes and ketosis can cause an acute cataract (snowflake cataract). Fluctuations in blood glucose level can cause refractive variability due to osmotic changes within the lens (the absorption of water into the lens can produce temporary hypermetropia). This clinically presents as fluctuating difficulty in reading and it resolves with control of the diabetes.
- **External ocular palsies:** The 6th and the 3rd cranial nerves **(Tolosa-Hunt syndrome)** are the most commonly affected. These nerve palsies usually recover spontaneously within 3–6 months.
- Glaucoma.

Diabetic Neuropathy

Classification of Diabetic Neuropathy

See **Box 14.14**.

Management

- **Strict glycemic control, foot care**
- **Mononeuropathies are usually self-limiting** and do not require any specific therapy. Explanation and reassurance about remission within months may be necessary.
- **Neuritic pain** of diabetic neuropathy may be treated with nonsteroidal anti-inflammatory drugs (opiates-tramadol,

---

Box 14.14: Classification of diabetic neuropathy.

Diffuse neuropathy: Distal symmetrical neuropathy (DSPN)
- Small fiber
- Large fiber
- Mixed (most common)
  - **Mononeuropathy (mononeuritis multiplex)**
    - Isolated cranial/ peripheral nerve
    - Mononeuritis multiplex
  - **Radiculopathy or polyradiculopathy**
    - Radiculoplexus neuropathy
    - Thoracic radiculopathy
  - **Nondiabetic neuropathies common in diabetes**
    - Pressure palsies
    - CIDP
    - Treatment-induced painful small fiber neuropathy
  - **Autonomic neuropathy**

oxycodone), tricyclic antidepressants (amitriptyline, imipramine), duloxetine, venlafaxine mexiletine, valproate and anticonvulsants (e.g., phenytoin, carbamazepine, gabapentin, or pregabalin). Duloxetine is an antidepressant, potent dual reuptake inhibitor of serotonin and noradrenaline is useful in refractory cases.

- **Transepidermal nerve stimulation (TENS):** Beneficial in some patients.
- **Topical capsaicin containing creams:** May be occasionally beneficial.
- **Orthostatic/postural hypotension:** Responds to sleeping with the head of the bed raised, avoiding sudden upright position, full-length elastic support stockings and increased salt intake. Rarely, fludrocortisone, α-adrenoceptor agonist (midodrine) are needed.

Dermatological Complications of Diabetes Mellitus

- **Skin infections:** Due to immune dysfunction, e.g., carbuncles and furuncles and intertrigo
- Balanoposthitis
- **Vaginal candidiasis/balanitis:** Due to immune dysfunction
- **Diabetic ulcers:** Due to peripheral neuropathy and ischemia
- **Xanthomatoses:** Due to hyperlipoproteinemia
- Necrobiosis lipoidica diabeticorum (NLD)
- Diabetic dermopathy (shin spots)
- Tight waxy skin the dorsum of the hands with joint contractures in type 1 DM—digital sclerosis
- Acanthosis nigricans
- **Acrocordans/skin tags:** Marker of insulin resistance
- Granuloma annulare
- **Diabetic blisters:** Bullosis diabeticorum

Musculoskeletal Complications in Diabetes

- **Diabetic muscle infarction:** Painful muscle swelling, usually in thigh
- Neuropathic arthropathy (Charcot joint)
- Carpal tunnel syndrome
- Dupuytren's contracture
- Flexor tenosynovitis
- Adhesive capsulitis (frozen shoulder)
- Diabetic cherioarthropathy—"prayer sign", "table top test"
- Diabetic sclerodactyly

Gestational Diabetes Mellitus

Gestational diabetes mellitus (GDM) is defined as **glucose intolerance (diabetes) that develops or is first recognized during pregnancy.** Typically it is asymptomatic and usually remits after delivery. However, there is an increased risk of type 2 diabetes in later life and maintaining a low bodyweight and keeping physically active can reduce this risk (**Box 14.15**).

Oral Glucose Tolerance Test

Diagnosis is based on an OGTT performed at 24–28 weeks of gestation in women with moderate to high risk.

Criteria for Diagnosis of GDM

See **Table 14.28**.

Box 14.15: Importance of diagnosis of gestational diabetes mellitus.

Fetal risk with GDM
- Fetal macrosomia
- Intrauterine fetal death
- Respiratory distress
- Hypoglycemic fetuses
- Polyhydramnios
- Hypocalcemia
- Increased incidence of shoulder dystocia
- Fetal hyperbilirubinemia
- Transient tachypnea of the newborn

Risk for off springs of women with GDM: Increased risk of obesity and diabetes

Risk for women with GDM: Increased risk of obesity and diabetes in future.
- Increased incidence of preeclampsia
- Cesarean section

Table 14.28: Criteria for diagnosis of gestational diabetes mellitus.

Time (hour)	Upper limit of normal values (mg/dL)	
	Whole blood (O'Sullivan)	Plasma (Carpenter and Coustan)
0 (fasting)	85	95
1	160	180
2	140	155
3	125	140

(Two or more of these values must be abnormal).

Management

- **Aim:** To normalize the maternal blood glucose and reduce excessive growth of fetus.
- **Insulin:** Initiate insulin therapy when target glucose levels exceed despite nutritional therapy. Insulin does not cross the placenta.
- **Dietary modification:** Reduce the consumption of quick-acting refined carbohydrate. Treatment for other patients with diet in the first instance, although most may require insulin at some stages during pregnancy.
- Many oral hypoglycemic drugs cross the placenta and should be avoided because of the potential risk to the fetus. However, *metformin and/or glyburide/glibenclamide* are considered safe to use in pregnancy.

METABOLIC SYNDROME

Metabolic syndrome (previously known as syndrome X or insulin resistance syndrome) refers to the clustering of cardiovascular risk factors and includes abdominal obesity, hyperglycemia, dyslipidemia (high TGs, low HDL), and elevated blood pressure. The pathophysiological hallmark is insulin resistance.

Clinical diagnosis: National Cholesterol Education Program's Adult Treatment Panel III (ATP III)
- Waist circumference of more than 102 cm in men and more than 88 cm in women;
- Triglyceride levels of at least 150 mg per dL;

- High-density lipoprotein cholesterol levels of less than 40 mg per dL in men and less than 50 mg per dL in women;
- Blood pressure of at least 130/85 mm Hg; and
- Fasting glucose levels of at least 110 mg per dL

Associated Risks
- Cardiovascular diseases
- Type 2 diabetes mellitus
- Polycystic ovary syndrome
- Sleep-disorders breathing
- Chronic kidney disease
- Nonalcoholic fatty liver disease

Treatment
- Components of therapy include:
  - Exercise
  - Hypocaloric diet
  - Weight reduction
  - Diet high in fibers
- Control of diabetes, hypertension, and lipid abnormalities by various drugs.
- In the absence of diabetes, hypoglycemic drugs (e.g., metformin, acarbose) are not recommended to control insulin resistance.

OBJECTIVE-BASED SELF-EVALUATION

LONG QUESTIONS

1. Classify diabetes mellitus. Enumerate the ADA criteria for diagnosis of diabetes. List the classes of antidiabetic agents with examples.
2. List the complications of diabetes mellitus. Discuss the pathophysiology, clinical features, and management of diabetic ketoacidosis.
3. List the acute complications of diabetes mellitus. Discuss the pathophysiology, clinical features, and management of hyperglycemic hyperosmolar state.
4. List the chronic complications of diabetes mellitus. Discuss the pathophysiology, clinical features, and management of diabetic nephropathy.
5. Discuss the etiology, clinical features, and management of Addison's disease.
6. Discuss the etiology, clinical features, and management of Cushing syndrome.
7. Discuss the etiology, clinical features, and management of acromegaly.
8. Discuss the etiology, clinical features, and management of Graves' disease.
9. Discuss the etiology, clinical features, and management of hypothyroidism.
10. Discuss the etiology, clinical features, and management of diabetes insipidus.

SHORT ANSWER QUESTIONS

1. Hypopituitarism
2. Sheehan's syndrome
3. Thyroid function tests
4. Subclinical hypothyroidism
5. Antithyroid drugs
6. Eye signs in Graves' disease
7. Myxedema coma
8. Hashimotos thyroiditis
9. Adverse effects of glucocorticoids
10. Common indication and contraindications of steroids
11. Pheochromocytoma
12. Gestational diabetes
13. Metabolic syndrome
14. Maturity onset diabetes of the young
15. Latent autoimmune diabetes in adults
16. Medical nutrition therapy for diabetes
17. Insulin analogs/newer insulins
18. Glycosylated hemoglobin
19. Hypoglycemia
20. Classification of diabetic neuropathy
21. Dermatological Complications of diabetes mellitus
22. Cardiovascular complications of diabetes
23. Incretin-based therapy
24. Acute adrenal crisis
25. Sick euthyroid syndrome
26. Thyroid storm
27. Hyperprolactinemia
28. Conns syndrome

MULTIPLE CHOICE QUESTIONS

1. All of the following hormones are produced by the anterior pituitary pituitary, *except*:
   a. Adrenocorticotrophic hormone
   b. Growth hormone
   c. Oxytocin
   d. Prolactin
2. Which of the following is the most common sign of Cushing's syndrome?
   a. Amenorrhea
   b. Hirsutism
   c. Obesity
   d. Purple skin striae
3. A 40-year-old woman presents to your clinic complaining of difficulty swallowing, sore throat, and tender swelling in her neck. She has also noted fevers intermittently over the past week. On physical examination, she is noted to have a small goiter that is painful to the touch. Her erythrocyte sedimentation rate (ESR) of 53 mm/h, and a thyroid-stimulating hormone (TSH) of 21 µIU/mL. What is the most likely diagnosis?
   a. Autoimmune hypothyroidism
   b. Graves' disease
   c. Ludwig's angina
   d. Subacute thyroiditis

4. Infarction of pituitary gland following postpartum hemorrhage is called:
   a. Sheehan's syndrome
   b. Kallmann syndrome
   c. Nelson's syndrome
   d. Wolfram syndrome
5. Thyrotoxicosis without hyperthyroidism is seen in:
   a. Graves' disease
   b. Toxic multinodular goitre
   c. Subacute thyroiditis
   d. Toxic adenoma
6. Endocrine cause of clubbing includes all, *except*:
   a. Cushing's syndrome
   b. Acromegaly
   c. Graves disease
   d. Hyperparathyroidism
7. Delayed relaxation of tendon reflexes is characteristically seen in:
   a. Addison's disease
   b. Hypothyroidism
   c. Hypoparathyroidism
   d. Diabetes mellitus
8. Mutations in hepatocyte nuclear factors or in glucokinase results in which type diabetes:
   a. Type 1 diabetes
   b. Type 2 diabetes
   c. Maturity-onset diabetes of the young
   d. Latent autoimmune diabetes in adults
9. All of the following are long-acting insulin analogs, *except*:
   a. Insulin Aspart
   b. Insulin Glargine
   c. Insulin Detemir
   d. Insulin Degludec
10. Best antihypertensive agent in a diabetic patient to reduce microalbuminuria is:
    a. Amlodipine
    b. Atenolol
    c. Furosemide
    d. Telmisartan

=== ANSWERS ===

1. c   2. c   3. d   4. a   5. c
6. a   7. b   8. c   9. a   10. d

Infectious Diseases

CHAPTER OUTLINE

- Measles (Rubeola)
- Rubella (German Measles)
- Mumps
- Infectious Mononucleosis
- Chickenpox (Varicella)
- Shingles (Herpes Zoster)
- Arboviral Diseases
- Dengue Fever
- COVID-19
- Diphtheria
- Plague
- Botulism
- Pertussis
- Typhoid
- Food Poisoning
- Dysentery
- Amebiasis
- Cholera
- Leptospirosis
- Rickettsial Diseases
- Candidiasis
- Mucormycosis
- Malaria
- Kala-azar or Visceral Leishmaniasis
- Sepsis
- HIV/AIDS
- Sexually Transmitted Infections
- Syphilis
- Pyrexia of Unknown Origin (PUO)

VIRAL INFECTIONS

MEASLES (RUBEOLA)

- Measles virus, the cause of measles is an RNA virus of the genus Morbillivirus in the family Paramyxoviridae.
- Measles is highly contagious; approximately 90% of susceptible household contacts acquire the disease.
- Maximal dissemination of virus occurs by droplet spray during the prodromal period (catarrhal stage).

Clinical Features

Measles has three clinical stages:

1. Incubation Stage

- This stage lasts for about 6–21 days to the first prodromal symptoms and another 2–4 days to the appearance of the rash.
- **Period of infectivity** is from *4 days before and 2 days after* the onset of rash. Patients with compromised immunity can shed virus for the entire duration of illness.

2. Prodromal Stage with an Enanthem (Koplik Spots) and Mild Symptoms

- Usually lasts for 3–5 days and is characterized by low-grade to moderate **fever, dry cough, coryza,** and **conjunctivitis**.
- **Koplik spots (Fig. 15.1A):** Pathognomonic sign of measles are grayish white dots, usually as small as grains of sand, that have slight, reddish areolae; occasionally they are hemorrhagic.
- Usually tends to occur opposite the lower molars but can spread irregularly over the rest of the buccal mucosa.
- Rarely, they are found within the midportion of the lower lip, on the palate, described as "grains of salt on a red background" and on the lacrimal caruncle.
- They appear usually within 12–18 hours and disappear rapidly.
- Koplik's spots begin to slough when the exanthem appears.
- The conjunctival inflammation and photophobia may suggest measles before Koplik spots appear. In particular, a transverse line of conjunctival inflammation, sharply demarcated along the eyelid margin, may be of diagnostic assistance in the prodromal stage.

3. Final Stage with a Maculopapular Rash (Exanthem) (Fig. 15.1B) Accompanied by High Fever

- Usually starts as faint macules on the upper lateral parts of the neck, behind the ears along the hairline, posterior parts of the cheek.
- Individual lesions become increasingly maculopapular as the rash spreads rapidly over the entire face, neck, upper arms, and upper part of the chest within approximately first 24 hours.
- During the succeeding 24 hours, the rash spreads over the back, abdomen, entire arm, and thighs.
- As it finally reaches the feet on the 2nd–3rd day, it begins to fade on the face. Associated with lymphadenopathy, conjunctivitis, and pharyngitis.
- In hemorrhagic measles (**black measles**), bleeding may occur from the mouth, nose, or bowel.

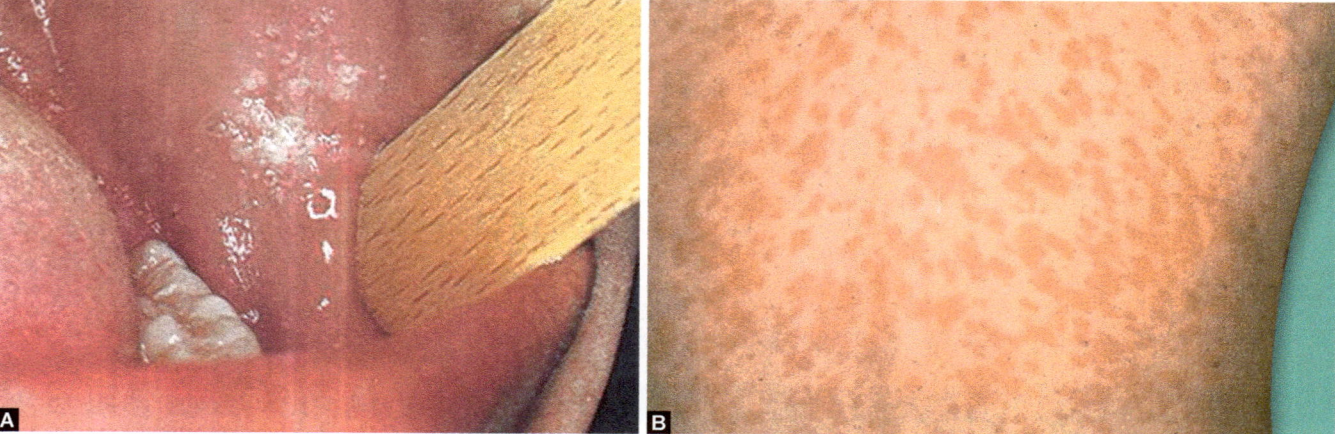

Figs. 15.1A and B: (A) Koplik spots—pathognomonic of measles, which appears as grayish white dots on the buccal mucosa; (B) Maculopapular rashes in measles.

- Complete absence of rash (modified measles) is rare, except:
  - In patients who have received immunoglobulin (Ig) during the incubation period.
  - In some patients with HIV infection.
  - Occasionally in infants younger than 9 months of age who have appreciable levels of maternal antibody.

Diagnosis

- Diagnosis is usually apparent from the characteristic clinical picture; laboratory confirmation is rarely needed.
- Testing for measles IgM antibodies is recommended in some situations. Measles IgM is detectable for 1 month alter illness, but sensitivity of IgM assays may be limited in the first 72 hours of the rash illness.

Complication (Box 15.1)

They are more common in older children and adults.

Treatment

There is **no specific antiviral therapy** and it is entirely supportive.
- **Antipyretics** (acetaminophen or ibuprofen) for fever
- **Bed rest**
- **Maintenance of an adequate fluid intake**
- **Vitamin A supplementation:** Recommended by the American Academy of Pediatrics for Children:
  - From 6 months to 2 years of age who are hospitalized for measles and its complications.
  - Older than 6 months of age with measles and immunodeficiency.
  - Recommended regimen as a single dose of:
    - 100,000 IU orally for children 6 months to 1 year
    - 200,000 IU for children 1 year and above
    - Children with ophthalmologic evidence of vitamin A deficiency should be given additional doses the next day and 4 week later.
- **Treatment of secondary bacterial infections:** Prompt identification and treatment of secondary bacterial infections (with appropriate antibiotics).
- **Measles encephalitis:** Aerosolized and IV ribavirin may be useful.

Box 15.1: Complications of measles.

Due to virus replication
- Acute laryngotracheobronchitis (croup) in young children
- Giant-cell pneumonitis in immunocompromised children

Due to secondary bacterial infections
Common:
- Otitis media
- Bronchitis
- Bronchopneumonia
- Gastroenteritis

Others:
- Noma/cancrum oris
- Gangrenous stomatitis
- Diarrhea due to undernutrition

Less common:
- Transient hepatitis
- Myocarditis
- Conjunctivitis
- Keratitis
- Corneal ulcers

Postinfectious: Rare CNS complications
- **Early:** Postmeasles encephalomyelitis
- **Late:** Measles inclusion body encephalitis (MIBE) and subacute sclerosing panencephalitis (SSPE)

Others:
- Guillain-Barré syndrome
- Hemiplegia
- Cerebral thrombophlebitis
- Retrobulbar neuritis
- Exacerbate underlying *Mycobacterium tuberculosis*
- Measles pneumonia in HIV-infected patients is often fatal

Prevention

- **Passive immunization** with intramuscular injection of human normal immune globulin (0.25 mL/kg; maximum: 15 mL) is effective for prevention and attenuation of measles within 6 days of exposure.
- **Active immunization:** It is achieved by giving subcutaneous injection live-attenuated measles virus. All children aged 12–15 months should be given measles vaccination. It can be given simultaneously in combination with rubella and

mumps vaccines (MMR vaccine). Further MMR dose is given at the age of 4 years. This vaccination offer protection for at least 15 years.

RUBELLA (GERMAN MEASLES)

Rubella is infection caused by a **Rubella virus,** which is an enveloped RNA virus and member of the Togaviridae family. The name is derived from the Latin, meaning *little red.*

- **Mode of spread via respiratory droplet infection:** Maximum infectivity from up to 10 days before the onset to 2 weeks after the onset of the rash.
- After an incubation period of 14–21 days, the primary symptom of rubella virus infection is the appearance of a rash (exanthema) on the face, which spreads to the trunk and limbs and usually fades after 3 days.
- The skin manifestations are called "**blueberry muffin lesions**".

Clinical Features

Clinical features depends on age of the patient and divided into acquired and congenital rubella. Symptoms are mild or absent in children under 5 years.

Acquired Rubella

- **Prodromal or catarrhal phase:** Characterized by malaise, fever, headache, and mild conjunctivitis. Lymphadenopathy (particularly suboccipital, postauricular, and posterior cervical lymph nodes) may be observed during the second week after exposure. **Forchheimer** spots (small petechial lesions on the soft palate) are suggestive but not diagnostic. Splenomegaly may be found.
- **Eruptive or exanthematous phase:** Occurs within 7 days of the initial symptoms. Characterized by **pinkish red, macular rashes** first appear behind the ears and on the forehead and then spread downward to the trunk and limbs. These rashes usually last for 2–3 days. May be associated with polyarthritis and generalized lymphadenopathy, which may persist for 2 weeks.
- **Complications** are rare. These include secondary bacterial infection of lung, arthralgia (common in females), hemorrhagic manifestations due to thrombocytopenia and postinfectious encephalitis.

Congenital Rubella Syndrome

It is the most serious consequence of rubella virus infection of mother during first trimester pregnancy.

- **Classical triad of congenital rubella syndrome:**
  - Cataract
  - Cardiac abnormalities
  - Deafness
- **Others:**
  - *Congenital heart diseases:* Patent ductus arteriosus, ventricular septal defect, pulmonary stenosis
  - *Eye diseases:* Corneal clouding, cataracts, chorioretinitis, microphthalmia, blindness
  - *CNS:* Mental retardation, microcephaly
  - *Deafness*
  - *Others:* Hepatosplenomegaly, myocarditis, interstitial pneumonia, and metaphyseal bone lesions.

- **Mode of spread:** From the transplacental transmission of the virus from an infected mother to the fetus.
- **First trimester infections** lead to abnormalities in 85% of cases and greater damage to organs.
- **Second trimester infections** lead to defects in 16%. More than 20 weeks of pregnancy fetal defects are uncommon.

Expanded Rubella Syndrome

This additionally includes the following manifestations:
- Hepatosplenomegaly
- Thrombocytopenic purpura
- Intrauterine growth retardation
- Myocarditis
- Interstitial pneumonia
- Humoral and cellular immunodeficiency.

Diagnosis

Diagnosis is clinically made. However, laboratory diagnosis is needed especially in pregnancy.
- Detection of rubella specific IgM by ELISA in serum, confirmed by demonstration of IgG seroconversion (or a rising titer of IgG) in a serum taken 14 days later.
- Detection of viral genome in throat swabs (or oral fluid), urine and the products of conception (in the case of intrauterine infection).

Treatment

- No specific therapy is available.
- Symptom-based treatment is given for various manifestations, such as fever and arthralgia.

Prevention

- **Passive immunization:** Human immunoglobulin can reduce the symptoms but does not prevent the teratogenic effects.
- **Active immunization:** Active immunization is by giving live-attenuated rubella vaccine.
- **Indications:** Should be given to all children at the age of 15 months along with MMR vaccine. A second dose is given to young females between the age of 11 and 13 years and all seronegative females of child-bearing age.

MUMPS

- Mumps is an acute systemic viral infection caused by paramyxovirus (RNA virus) and is characterized by swelling of the parotid glands.
- **Mode of spread:** The virus is transmitted by the respiratory route (1) by droplet infection, (2) by direct contact, or (3) through saliva and fomites. Humans are the only natural hosts of the mumps virus. The peak infectivity is 2–3 days before the onset of the parotitis and for 3 days afterward.
- **Incubation period** is about 15–20 days (average 18 days).

Clinical Features

Primarily affects school-aged children and young adults (peaks at 5–9 years of age) and is uncommon before 2 years of age.
- **Prodromal symptoms:** Nonspecific and includes malaise, low-grade fever, myalgia, anorexia, headache, and tenderness at the angle of the jaw.

- **Parotid gland enlargement:** Prodromal symptoms are followed by severe pain over the parotid glands due to parotitis. Parotitis produces either unilateral or bilateral parotid swelling (75% of cases). It is accompanied by obliteration of the space between the earlobe and the angle of the mandible. The chief complaints at this stage are difficulty in eating, swallowing, and talking. Submandibular gland involvement is less frequent.

Complications of Mumps

For complications of mumps *see* **Box 15.2**.

Diagnosis

On the basis of the clinical features in atypical cases, diagnosis is confirmed by following investigations:
- **Serological test:** Demonstration of a mumps-specific IgM response in a blood or oral fluid during infection is diagnostic.
- **Demonstration virus:** Culture of virus or identification by genome [polymerase chain reaction (PCR)] or antigen detection assays, from saliva, throat swab, urine, and CSF.

Treatment

- Mumps is generally a benign, self-resolving illness.
- Treatment is symptom-based and supportive. Adequate nutrition and mouth care. Analgesics to relieve pain.

Prevention

MMR vaccine: To be given at the age of 15 months.

INFECTIOUS MONONUCLEOSIS (GLANDULAR FEVER)

Etiology

Caused by Epstein–Barr virus (EBV). It is a herpes virus that infects and replicates in B lymphocytes in the submucosal lymphoid tissue of nasopharynx and oropharynx.

Age: Peak incidence in 14–16 years for females and 16–18 years for males. Subclinical infection is very common.

Mode of transmission is largely through saliva (e.g., kissing hence the nickname kissing disease).

Incubation period: 7–10 days.

Clinical Features

Usually presents with nonspecific prodromal symptoms followed by the classical triad of (1) fever, (2) severe pharyngitis, and tonsillitis, and (3) lymphadenopathy (particularly posterior cervical lymph node enlargement but sometimes generalized) and hepatosplenomegaly.

Other features: Petechial rashes on palate and maculopapular skin rash, the latter develops in 90% of patients who have received ampicillin or amoxicillin (inappropriately) for the sore throat.

Investigations

- **Peripheral blood smear:** In >90% of, two-thirds are lymphocytes, 20–40% atypical lymphocytes. The atypical lymphocytes are large with larger eccentric and folded nuclei with a lower nuclear-to-cytoplasm ratio.
- **Liver function tests:** Raised liver enzymes
- **Serological tests:**
  - *Demonstration of heterophile antibodies:* The following tests will be useful for demonstration of heterophile antibodies.
    - Paul-Bunnell test is characteristically positive: Sheep red blood cells agglutinate in the presence of heterophile antibodies.
    - Monospot test is a sensitive slide test: Horse red cells agglutinate on exposure to heterophile antibodies.
  - *Demonstration specific antibodies against EBV antigens:* These are demonstrated by ELISA.
    - Antibody against viral capsid antigens (anti-VCA): These antibodies are initially of IgM type and later of IgG type (which persists for life).
    - Antibodies to Epstein–Barr nuclear antigen (EBNA): This can be demonstrated by polymerase chain reaction (PCR).

Complications of EBV Infection (Box 15.3)

- Chronic fatigue syndrome
- **Hematological complications:**
  - Hemolytic anemia and thrombocytopenia
  - Aplastic anemia, thrombotic thrombocytopenic purpura of hemolytic-uremic syndrome, and disseminated intravascular coagulation (DIC)
- Glomerulonephritis, interstitial nephritis, hepatitis, myocarditis, and pericarditis
- Splenic rupture
- **Cardiac:** Myocarditis and pericarditis
- **Hepatic:** Reyes syndrome
- **Skin:** Ampicillin associated rash (Jarisch–Herxheimer reaction) and oral hairy leukoplakia
- Neurologic complications, e.g., meningitis, encephalitis, transverse myelitis, and Guillain–Barré (GB) syndrome
- Airway obstruction due to marked enlargement tonsils/severe pharyngeal edema
- **Oncogenesis:** Nasopharyngeal carcinoma, Burkitt's lymphoma, Hodgkin disease

Treatment

- Infectious mononucleosis is usually a self-limiting disease and majority requires no specific treatment and recovery rapidly.
- Symptomatic treatment includes rest, acetaminophen, etc.

Box 15.2: Complications of mumps.

- Epididymo-orchitis (30%) in adults can lead to infertility
- Oophoritis
- Mumps pancreatitis
- Mumps meningitis (5–10%), encephalitis. CSF reveals a lymphocytic pleocytosis
- Mumps myocarditis
- Others: Mastitis, hepatitis, polyarthritis, transient hearing loss, labyrinthitis, and electrocardiographic abnormalities
- Abortion (if infection occurs in the first trimester of pregnancy)
- Thrombocytopenic purpura

Box 15.3: Complications of EBV infection.

* Chronic fatigue syndrome.
* Hematological complications:
  * Hemolytic anemia and thrombocytopenia.
  * Aplastic anemia, thrombotic thrombocytopenic purpura of hemolytic-uremic syndrome, disseminated intravascular coagulation (DIC).
* Glomerulonephritis, interstitial nephritis, hepatitis, myocarditis, pericarditis.
* Splenic rupture.
* Cardiac: Myocarditis, pericarditis.
* Hepatic: Reyes syndrome.
* Skin: Ampicillin associated rash (Jarisch-Herxheimer reaction), oral hairy leukoplakia.
* Neurologic complications, e.g., meningitis, encephalitis, transverse myelitis, and Guillain-Barré (GB) syndrome.
* Airway obstruction due to marked enlargement tonsils/severe pharyngeal edema.
* EBV-associated oncogenesis:
  * Benign EBV-associated proliferations
    - Oral hairy leukoplakia, primarily in adults with AIDS
    - Lymphoid interstitial pneumonitis, in children with AIDS
  * Malignant EBV-associated proliferations
    - Nasopharyngeal carcinoma
    - Burkitt lymphoma
    - Hodgkin disease
    - Lymphoproliferative disorders
    - Leiomyosarcoma in immunodeficient including AIDS

- Corticosteroids are indicated when there are neurological complications (e.g., meningitis, encephalitis, severe hemolysis, marked thrombocytopenia, and marked tonsillar enlargement causing respiratory obstruction.

HERPESVIRUSES INFECTING HUMANS

Herpes viruses are double-stranded DNA viruses. The various diseases caused by them are listed in **Table 15.1**.

CHICKENPOX (VARICELLA)

- Chickenpox is caused by ubiquitous and extremely contagious primary infection with varicella-zoster virus (also called as human herpesvirus 3). It is usually a benign illness of childhood (5–9 years of age).
- Varicella zoster virus (VZV) is a dermotropic and neurotropic virus and is a member of the family Herpesviridae.
- It causes two distinct clinical entities: varicella (chickenpox) and herpes zoster (shingles). Primary infection is chickenpox and usually occurs in childhood. The virus remains latent; which reactivate later in life giving rise to herpes zoster.

Mode of Transmission

- By droplet infection from the upper respiratory tract.
- Direct contact with discharge from ruptured lesions on the skin.

Table 15.1: Disease caused by various herpesviruses in human beings.

Virus	Diseases
Herpes simplex	
• Type 1	Herpes labialis (herpes febrilis/cold sore—**Fig. 15.2A**), kerato conjunctivitis, dendritic corneal ulcer, pulp space infections (whitlows), encephalitis with temporal lobe involvement, genital herpes (40%), pneumonitis, tracheobronchitis, ulcerative stomatitis, esophagitis
• Type 2	Genital herpes (60%), neonatal infections
Cytomegalovirus	Congenital infections (intrauterine growth retardation), perinatal infections, infections in the immunocompromised patients (pneumonitis, retinitis)
Epstein-Barr virus (EBV)	Infectious mononucleosis, Burkitt's lymphoma, nasopharyngeal carcinoma, hairy leukoplakia in AIDS patients
Varicella-zoster virus	Chickenpox, herpes-zoster (shingles)
Human herpesvirus 6	Exanthem subitum (sixth disease), Roseola subitum-slapped cheek appearance **(Fig. 15.2B)**
Human herpesvirus 7	Exanthem subitum (sixth disease)
Human herpesvirus 8	Kaposi's sarcoma, multicentric Castleman's disease

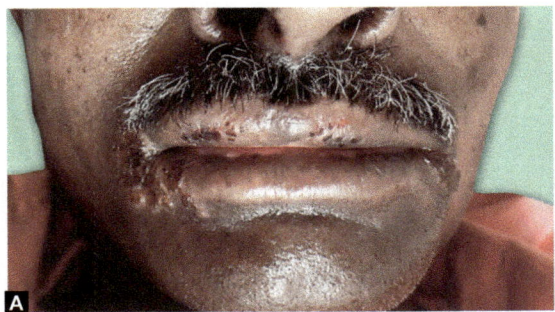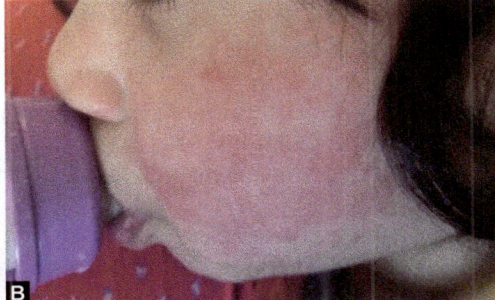

Figs. 15.2A and B: (A) Herpes labialis/febrilis caused by herpes simplex type 1 virus; (B) Roseola subitum-slapped cheek appearance in humanherpes virus 6 infection.

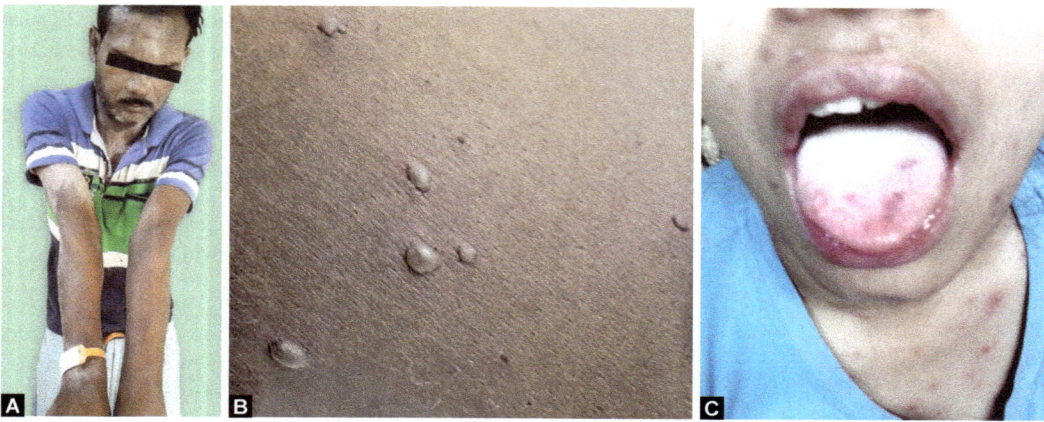

Figs. 15.3A to C: Lesions in chickenpox: (A) Involvement of face and body; (B) Vesicles; (C) Chickenpox exanthema (widespread) and enanthem (rash/small spots on the mucous membranes).

- Humans are the only reservoirs of VZV. Chickenpox is contagious till pustules disappear.
- **Incubation period** is about 10–21 days.

Clinical Features

- **Distribution of skin lesions:** Chickenpox presents with characteristic rash on the 2nd day of illness that first appears on the trunk followed by the face **(Fig. 15.3A)**, and finally on the limbs. Maximum lesions are found on the trunk and minimum on the periphery of the limbs (centripetal distribution).
- **Appearance of skin lesions**
- Rash appear first as **small pink macules** and **progress to papules, vesicles (Fig. 15.3B) and pustules within 24 hours**. Finally, these lesions dry up and form scabs.
- New lesions develop in crops every 2–4 days and each crop is associated with fever. Thus, lesions at all stages of development are seen in any area at the same time.
- Infectivity lasts for up to 4 days before the lesions appear till the last vesicles crust over.
- In immunocompromised patients the skin lesions are hemorrhagic and are numerous. Dissemination to other organs is quite common.
- Enanthem is rash/small spots on the mucous membranes **(Fig. 15.3C)** may also be seen.

Complications of Chickenpox

For complications of chickenpox see **Table 15.2**.

Diagnosis

- Mainly clinical, by recognition of the skin rash.
- If needed, it may be confirmed by:
  - Detection of antigen (direct immunofluorescence) or DNA (PCR) of fluid aspirated from vesicles.
- Serology is used to identify seronegative individuals at risk of infection
- Isolation of virus by culture of vesicular fluid.
- **Tzanck smear:** Prepared by scraping of the base of the vesicular lesion. It shows multinucleated giant cells and epithelial cells with eosinophilic intranuclear inclusion bodies. Its sensitivity is low (60%).

Table 15.2: Complications of chickenpox.

• Secondary bacterial infection of skin lesions	• Myocarditis
• CNS (rare)	• Acute glomerulonephritis
▪ Cerebellar ataxia	• Corneal lesions
▪ Encephalitis	• Arthritis, osteomyelitis
▪ Aseptic meningitis	• Bleeding diatheses
▪ Transverse myelitis	• Hepatitis
▪ Guillain-Barré syndrome	• Reye's syndrome with aspirin use
• Varicella pneumonia (interstitial)	• Perinatal varicella
	• Congenital varicella (extremely uncommon)

Management

- No treatment is needed in majority of patients.
- Medical management of immunologically normal patient is by prevention of avoidable complications. These include good hygiene (daily bathing), meticulous skin care (to avoid secondary bacterial infection).
- Avoid aspirin use in children to prevent Reye's syndrome.
- Symptomatic treatment for itching/pruritus includes antihistamines and local calamine lotion.
- Secondary bacterial infection is managed with local antiseptic or systemic antibiotics (e.g., cloxacillin).

Antiviral Therapy

- Not required for uncomplicated primary VZV infection in children.
- **Drugs used:** Antiviral drugs that are used include acyclovir (15 mg/kg by mouth five times daily), valacyclovir (1 g three times daily), or famcyclovir (250 mg three times daily) and famcyclovir (500 mg TID) for 5–7 days.
- **Indications:** Though in healthy children, antiviral drugs may reduce the duration of disease when administered within 24 hours of symptoms. However, they are usually not recommended but are indicated in the following cases:
  - For uncomplicated chickenpox when the patient presents within 24–48 hours of onset of vesicles.
- All patients with complications.
- Immunocompromised patients and pregnant women, regardless of duration of vesicles. More severe disease in

immunocompromised patients requires initial parenteral therapy. Immunocompromised patients may shed virus for a prolonged period and may require prolonged treatment.

Prevention

Three methods for the prevention of VZV infections are:
1. **Live-attenuated vaccine:** It is given to prevent chickenpox in immunocompetent children and adults who are at a high risk of infection. It is contraindicated in pregnant or immunocompromised patients.
2. **Passive prophylaxis using zoster immune globulin (ZIG) or varicella-zoster immune globulin (VZIG):**
   - It may be given to individuals who are susceptible, those patients having high risk of severe disease or complication of chickenpox (e.g., immunocompromised, steroid treated or pregnant women with history of significant exposure). It should be given within 96 hours of exposure.
   - It is given prophylactically to newborn infants, infant whose mother develops chickenpox within 5 days before or within 48 hours after delivery.

SHINGLES (HERPES ZOSTER)

Initial infection with VZV produces chickenpox. After this initial infection, VZV persists in latent form in the dorsal root ganglion of sensory nerves or cranial nerve ganglia. Shingles arises from the reactivation of latent virus later in life.

Clinical Features

- **Age:** It may occur at any age but most common in the elderly.
- **Skin lesions:** The onset of the skin rash is usually preceded (3–4 days before discrete vesicles occur in the skin) by severe pain **(burning discomfort)** in the affected dermatome. Though **rash is similar to chickenpox**, classically they are unilateral and restricted to a sensory nerve (i.e., dermatomal) distribution **(Fig. 15.4A)**. This is associated with a brief dissemination of virus causing viremia and can produce distant satellite "chickenpox" lesions. Virus is from freshly formed vesicles may also cause chickenpox in susceptible contacts. Chickenpox may be contracted from a patient suffering from shingles but not vice versa. Occasionally, paresthesia may develop without rash ("zoster sine herpete").
- **Dermatome involved:** Most commonly involves **thoracic dermatomes or ophthalmic division of the trigeminal nerve** (vesicles may develop on the cornea and can produce corneal ulceration leading to blindness). Bowel and bladder dysfunction may develop with sacral nerve root involvement. Occasionally it may cause cranial nerve palsy, myelitis or encephalitis.

Complications of Shingles (Herpes Zoster)

- **Herpes zoster ophthalmicus**, leading to loss of vision
- **Ramsay Hunt syndrome (Fig. 15.4B):** It develops due to geniculate ganglion involvement and characterized by involvement of cranial nerves (V and VII). A triad of (1) ipsilateral facial paralysis/palsy (ipsilateral loss of taste and buccal ulceration), (2) ear pain, and (3) vesicles/rashes in the external auditory canal and auricle is seen. It may be mistaken for Bell's palsy.
- **Postherpetic neuralgia is seen in** 10–15% of people with shingles. It results in troublesome persistent pain for 1–6 months or longer, following healing of the skin rash. It is more common in elderly patients.
- **Granulomatous cerebral angiitis** is a cerebrovascular complication. It leads to a stroke-like syndrome in patients with shingles, especially in an ophthalmic distribution.

Management

- **Early therapy with acyclovir or related agents** (refer treatment of chickenpox) reduce both early- and late-onset pain, especially in patients above 65 years.
- **Postherpetic neuralgia: Analgesics** along with **amitriptyline** 25–100 mg daily or gabapentin (start with 300 mg daily and slowly increasing to 300 mg twice daily or more). **Capsaicin cream** (0.075%) may be of some help.

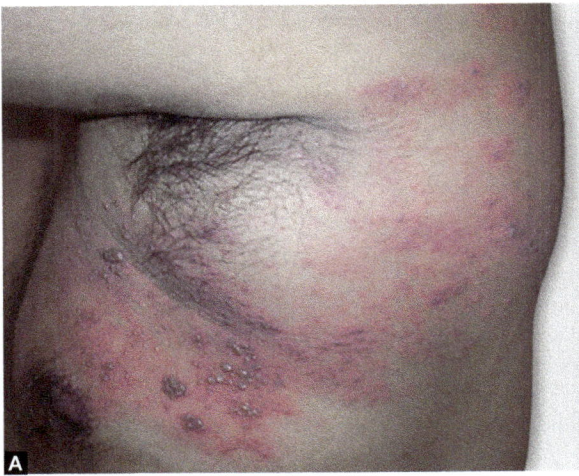 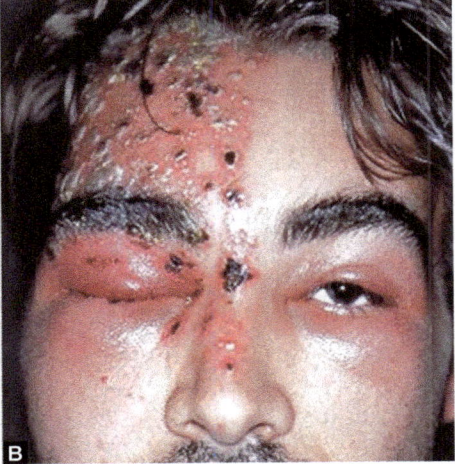

Figs. 15.4A and B: (A) Herpes zoster-dermatomal involvement; (B) Ramsay Hunt syndrome.

Table 15.3: Disease caused by arbovirus.

Family	Common diseases	Family	Common diseases
Arenaviridae	• Lymphocytic choriomeningitis • Lassa fever • Arena viruses	Flaviviridae	**Mosquito-borne:** • Japanese encephalitis • West Nile encephalitis • St. Louis encephalitis • Yellow fever • Dengue fever **Tick borne:** • Kyasanur Forest disease (KFD) • **Direct contact:** Ebola disease
Bunyaviridae	• California encephalitis • Rift Valley fever • Sandfly fever • Crimean-Congo hemorrhagic fever • Hanta virus—hemorrhagic fever with renal/cardiopulmonary syndrome	Togaviridae	• Chikungunya disease • Sindbis disease • Eastern equine encephalitis • Western equine encephalitis • Venezuelan encephalitis

Table 15.4: Diseases caused by arbovirus and their manifestation.

	Flu-like syndrome	Encephalitis	Hepatitis	Hemorrhage	Shock
Dengue	+	−	+	+	+
Yellow fever	+	−	+	+	+
St. Louis encephalitis	+	+	−	−	−
West Nile encephalitis	+	+	−	−	−
Venezuelan encephalitis	+	+	−	−	−
Western equine encephalitis	+	+	−	−	−
Eastern equine encephalitis	+	+	−	−	−
Japanese encephalitis	+	+	−	−	−

(+ = Present; − = Absent)

ARBOVIRAL DISEASES

For arboviral diseases *see* **Tables 15.3 and 15.4**.

DENGUE FEVER

☐ It is caused by four distinct subgroups of dengue viruses, types 1, 2, 3, and 4 (DEN 1-4).
☐ Dengue infection of humans occurs from bites of *Aedes aegypti* mosquitoes.
☐ WHO classifies dengue viral infections into nonsevere dengue (with and without warning signs) and severe dengue **(Table 15.5 and Flowchart 15.1)**.

Clinical Features

After the incubation period of 5–8 days, the illness begins abruptly and is followed by the three phases: (1) Febrile phases, (2) critical phase, (3) recovery phase.

Febrile Phase

☐ Presents with high-grade fever that usually lasts 2–7 days.
☐ May have flushing of face, body ache, myalgia, arthralgia, severe backache (**'break–bone' fever**), retro-orbital pain and headache.
☐ Sore throat and conjunctival redness in some patients.

Table 15.5: Classification of dengue viral infections.

Non-severe dengue without warning signs	Non-severe dengue with warning signs	Severe dengue

Propable dengue
• Travel to endemic area
• Fever with two of the following criteria:
  ▪ Nausea and vomiting
  ▪ Rashes
  ▪ Body pain
  ▪ Positive Tourniquet test
  ▪ Leucopenia
  ▪ Absence of warning signs
  ▪ Laboratory–confirmed dengue
	Presence of warning signs
	• Abdominal pain of tenderness
	• Persistent vomiting
	• Clinical fluid accumulation
	• Mucosal bleed
	• Lethargy and restlessness
	• Liver enlargement 2 cm
	• **Laboratory:** Increase in hematocrit concurrent with rapid decrease in platelet count
		• Severe plasma leakage leading to:
		  ▪ Dengue shock syndrome (DSS)
		  ▪ Fluid accumulation with respiratory distress
		• Severe bleeding
		As evaluated by clinician:
		• Severe organ involvement
		  ▪ Liver: AST or ALT ≥1,000
		  ▪ CNS: Impaired consciousness
		  ▪ Heart and other organs

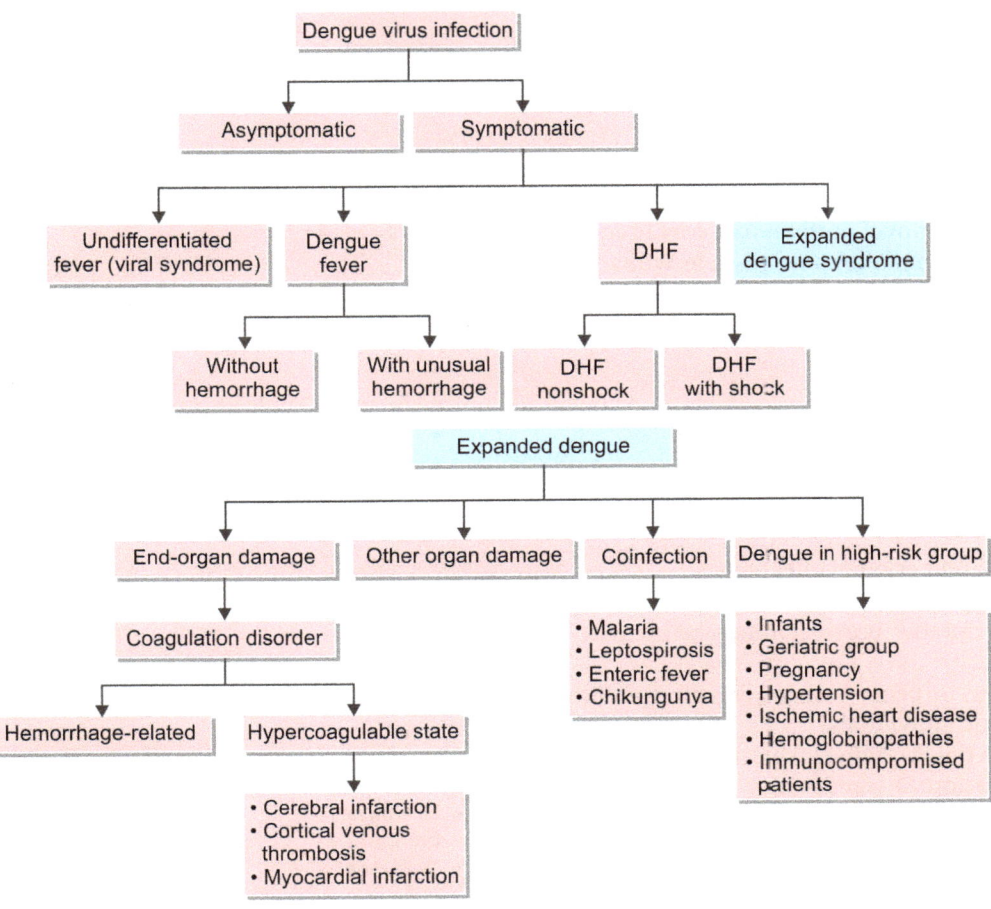

Flowchart 15.1: Dengue virus infection.

- Anorexia, nausea, and vomiting.
- Tenderness upon pressure on eyeball.
- A positive tourniquet test may be present.

Critical Phase
- Plasma leakage may happen which usually lasts 24–48 hours.
- Fall in WBC and platelet counts may precede plasma leakage
- May develop pleural effusion and ascites
- Shock and organ failure occurs when a critical volume of plasma is lost through leakage. It is often preceded by warning signs.

Recovery Phase
- If the patient survives the 24–48 hours critical phase, a gradual reabsorption of extravascular fluid takes place in the following 48–72 hours.
- Rash of 'isles of white in the sea of red'.
- Some patients may experience pruritus, particularly on hands and feet.
- Bradycardia.

Severe Dengue
- Evidence of plasma leakage
- High or progressively rising hematocrit
- Pleural effusions or ascites
- Circulatory compromise or shock significant bleeding
- Altered level of consciousness (lethargy of restlessness, coma, convulsions)
- Severe gastrointestinal involvement (persistent vomiting, increasing or intense abdominal pain, jaundice)
- Severe organ impairment (acute liver failure, acute renal failure, encephalopathy or encephalitis, cardiomyopathy).

Diagnosis
- Leucopenia, thrombocytopenia, and elevated live enzymes.
- Virus isolation from blood (within first 5 days).
- Serum NS1 antigen is highly specific and is positive early in the course of illness.
- Molecular methods like RT-PCR or nucleic acid sequence base amplification (NASBA) to detect viral RNA.
- Rising viral antibody titers IgG and IgM (start after 5 days of onset).
- In patients with severe dengue, chest radiograph to look for pleural effusion, and ultrasound abdomen for ascites and gallbladder wall thickening.

Overview of Management
- Managing patients in early febrile phase of dengue—**antipyretics like paracetamol**
- Recognizing early stage of plasma leakage or critical phase and initiating fluid therapy—IV fluids normal saline
- Patients with warning signs need to be referred to a tertiary care hospital

- Early diagnosis management of complications like shock, bleeding, and organ impairment.
- During the early febrile phase, it is often not possible to predict clinically whether a patient with dengue will progress to severe disease. Therefore, daily monitoring of patients is crucial.

COVID-19

At the end of 2019, a novel coronavirus was identified as the cause of a cluster of pneumonia cases in Wuhan, China. The WHO designated the disease COVID-19 and the virus is designated severe acute respiratory syndrome coronavirus 2 (SARS-CoV-2).

Transmission

- Person-to-person:
  - Mainly via respiratory droplets
  - Direct contact with mucous membrane (eyes/nose/mouth)
- Viral shedding and period of infectivity
  - It can be transmitted prior to the onset of symptoms and throughout the course of illness, particularly early in the course.
  - Transmission can occur during incubation period (from asymptomatic individuals)
  - Duration of viral shedding is variable.
- Risk of transmission: Depends on :
  - Type and duration of exposure
  - Use of preventive measures
  - Amount of virus in respiratory secretions
  - Environmental contamination—it is a potential source, especially in hospitals. Period of infectivity is ~6 days
- Risk of reinfection: Some antibodies are protective; not definitely established yet.

Pathogenesis

For pathogenesis of severe acute respiratory syndrome *see* **Figure 15.5**.

Binding of Spike protein to ACE-2 Receptors
↓
Uncoating
↓
Replication of viral genomic RNA by RNA-dependent-RNA-polymerase
↓
Translation of viral proteins
↓
Viral assembly into vesicles in the Golgi apparatus
↓
Exocytosis

Clinical Features

- **Incubation period:** <14 days
- Majority are asymptomatic
- **Spectrum of disease:**
  - *Mild:* no/mild pneumonia

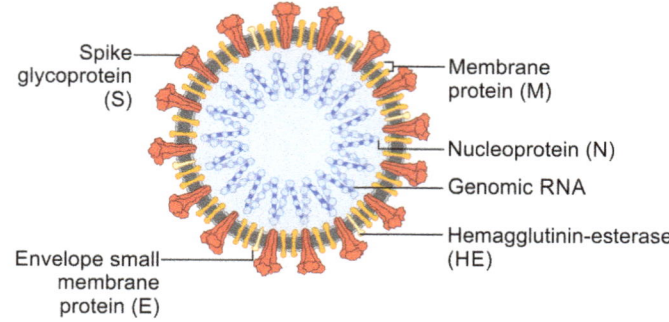

Fig. 15.5: Pathogenesis of severe acute respiratory syndrome coronavirus 2 (SARS-CoV-2)

- *Severe:* >50% lung involvement. Dyspnea, hypoxia seen.
- *Critical:* Respiratory failure, Shock, MODS
- Death
- Most common manifestation—Pneumonia—fever, cough, dyspnea, bilateral lung infiltrates on imaging.

Other features:	Hypoxia
❖ Conjunctivitis	❖ Fever
❖ Fatigue	❖ Dry/wet cough
❖ Confusion	❖ Dyspnea (new or worsening)
❖ Chest pain	❖ Anosmia or other smell abnormalities
❖ Nausea/vomiting	
❖ Diarrhea	❖ Ageusia or other taste abnormalities
❖ Chills/rigor	
❖ Headache	❖ Sore throat
❖ Rhinorrhea	❖ Myalgia
❖ Tachypnea	

Complications

- ARDS
- Cardiac arrhythmias
- Acute cardiac injury
- Shock
- Guillain-Barré syndrome
- DVT and pulmonary embolism
- Acute stroke
- Children – Kawasaki disease, Toxic shock syndrome
- Cytokine release syndrome
- Secondary infection.

Risk Factors for Severe Illness

Clinically:	Comorbidities:
❖ Hypoxia—SpO$_2$ <94%	❖ Age >50 years
❖ HR >100 bpm	❖ DM
❖ RR >30 cpm	❖ HTN
❖ SBP <90 mm Hg	❖ Lung disease (COPD, BA, Post-TB sequelae)
❖ Altered mental status	❖ CKD
	❖ CLD
	❖ HIV
	❖ Malignancy (Hematologic, Solid organ tumors)
	❖ Immunosuppression
	❖ Obesity

Laboratory Diagnosis
- Lymphopenia with N/L >3.5
- CRP >100
- Ferritin >300
- LDH >245
- D-dimer >1,000 ng/mL
- High AST/ALT
- High PT/INR
- High Trop-T
- AKI
- Increased CPK.

Imaging
- **Chest X-ray:** Normal in early/mild
- **CT chest:**
  - *Ground glass opacities (GGO):* 83% cases
  - GGO with mixed consolidation
  - Pleural thickening
  - Interlobular septal thickening
  - Air bronchograms.
- **Less common findings:**
  - Bronchiectasis
  - Pleural effusions
  - Pericardial effusion
  - Lymphadenopathy
  - Crazy pavement pattern (GGO with superimposed septal thickening).

Chest CT Severity Score
20 lung regions evaluated on chest CT using a system attributing scores of 0, 1, and 2, if parenchymal opacification involved 0%, less than 50%, or equal or more than 50% of each region. The CT-SS is defined as the sum of the individual scored in the 20 lung segment regions, which may range from 0 to 40 points **(Fig. 15.6)**.

Diagnosis
- Clinical suspicion:
  - New-onset fever/cough/dyspnea
  - History of contact with a COVID positive case/suspect within last 14 days
  - History of travel within last 14 days
  - History of work in health care settings
  - History of comorbidities/ risk for severe illness
- RT-PCR:
  - Preferred diagnostic test for COVID-19.
  - Specimens: Nasopharyngeal swab/Nasal swab from both anterior nares/nasal or nasopharyngeal wash or aspirate/oropharyngeal swab.
  - RT-PCR positive for SARS-CoV-2 indicated COVID-19 disease present.
  - Detectable SARS-CoV in upper respiratory tract specimens may persist for weeks after symptom onset.
  - Prolonged viral detection does not indicate ongoing infectiousness.
  - Lower respiratory tract specimens (expectorated sputum, tracheal aspirate, and BAL fluid) for RT-PCR may be reserved for hospitalized patients. Induced sputum is not recommended for testing.
- **Serology:** Detect SARS-CoV-2 antigens nucleocapsid or Spike protein. Uncertain sensitivity and specificity.
- **Imaging:** CXR/CT thorax – Bilateral peripheral and lower zone involvement.
- ECG
- Blood tests.

Basic Investigations
- CBC
- ESR, CRP
- LFT
- RFT
- RBS

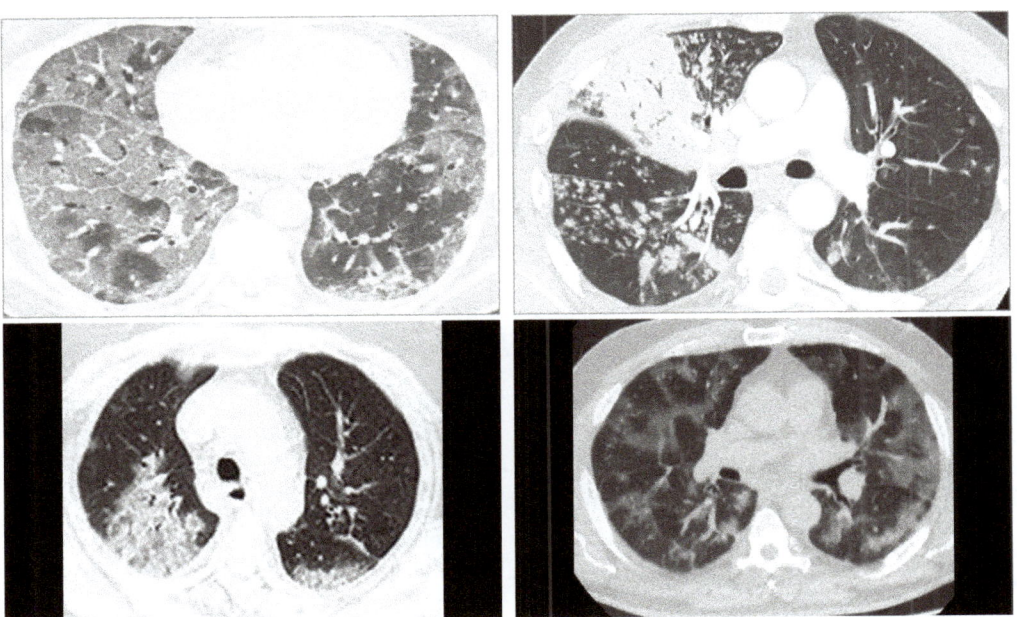

Fig. 15.6: CT findings in COVID pneumonia.

> **Box 15.4: Treatment for COVID-19.**
>
> - **General:**
>   - No dietary restriction.
>   - Good hydration
>   - RBS <180
>   - Continue ACE/ARBs, if present
>   - Avoid NSAIDs other than PCR
>   - Avoid nebulization (aerosolization of the virus)
>   - *Oxygen supplementation:* Hudson's/Venturi/HFNC/NIV/Mechanical ventilation.
> - **Category A (ICMR):** Asymptomatic/Mild symptoms:
>   - Tablet Oseltamivir 75 mg 1-0-1 x 5 days
>   - Tablet Azithromycin 500 mg 0-1-0 x 5 days
>   - Tablet HCQ 400 mg stat → 100 mg 1-0-1 x 4 days
>   - Tablet Zinc 50 mg 0-1-0 x 7 days
>   - Tablet Vit C 500 mg 1-1-1 x 7 days
>   - Injection Enoxaparin 40 mg s/c OD x 7 days (if D-dimer increased or CXR/CT suggestive of GGO)
> - **Category B (ICMR):** Symptomatic with mild-moderate pneumonia with no signs of severe disease, RR 15–30 cpm, SpO_2 90–94% at room air:
>   - Cat A treatment PLUS
>   - IV Antibiotics, if indicated
>   - Tablet N-acetyl-cysteine 600 mg 1-1-1, if cough +
>   - Injection Dexamethasone 6 mg 1-0-0 x 10 days or till discharge, whichever is shorter.
>   - Continuous SpO_2 monitoring
>   - Oxygen via nasal prongs or Hudson's mask.
> - **Category C (ICMR):** Symptomatic with severe pneumonia, RR >30 CPM, SpO_2 <90% at room air or 90–94% with O_2, ARDS, Septic shock.
>   - Category A and B treatment PLUS
>   - *If septic shock:* Injection Sepsivac 0.3 mL I/D OD
>   - NIV/MV
>   - Inotropes, if required
>   - Novel therapy as per clinical discretion: Discussed later

> **Box 15.5: Drugs approved for the treatment of COVID-19.**
>
> **Remdesivir:**
> - Acts against RNA-dependent RNA polymerase of SARS-CoV-2.
> - Indicated in those on supplemental oxygen/mechanical ventilation/ECMO.
> - Contraindicated in deranged LFT, GFR <30 mL/min
> - Should not be used concurrently with HCQ
> - Pregnancy is NOT a contraindication.
>
> **IL-6 pathway inhibitors:** Tocilizumab, Sarilumab, siltuximab.
> - Observational data revealed decreased risks of intubation and/or death
> - Associated with an increased risk of secondary infections
>
> **Hydroxychloroquine (HCQ)/chloroquine**
> - It was recommended initially, but FDA revoked emergency use authorization in June 2020, due to increased arrhythmias
> - Contraindications for HCQ:
>   - QTc >500
>   - Porphyria
>   - Myasthenia gravis
>   - Retinal pathology
>   - Epilepsy
>   - Hypokalemia <3
>   - Pregnancy is NOT a contraindication.
>
> **Convalescent plasma:** High neutralizing antibody titers is hypothesized to have clinical benefit when given early in the course of disease, however recent studies have not shown significant benefit
>
> **Lopinavir/Ritonavir:** Though recommended initially, clinical trials have failed to demonstrate efficacy
>
> **Favipiravir:**
> - An RNA polymerase inhibitor
> - Used in mild disease
>
> **Ivermectin:** In vitro activity against SARS-CoV-2, various clinical trials of ivermectin are underway.
>
> **Bamlanivimab:**
> - Recombinant neutralizing human IgG1-kappa monoclonal antibody directed against the spike (S) surface protein of SARS-CoV-2, derived from antigen specific B-cells of a convalescent COVID-19 patient.
> - Binds to the receptor binding domain (RBD) of the S protein at a position overlapping the ACE-2 binding site.
> - Emergency Use Authorization (EUA) on 9th November 2020 for mild/moderate COVID-19 disease
>
> **Casirivimab and Imdevimab:**
> - Casirivimab IgG1 kappa and Imdevimab IgG1 lambda, recombinant human IgG1 monoclonal antibodies that bind simultaneously to the receptor binding domain of SARS CoV-2's spike protein, and thereby preventing the entry of virus into the host cells.
> - EUA by FDA on November 21st 2020. Approved for treatment of mild-to-moderate COVID-19 in adults
>
> **Baricitinib:** Janus kinase inhibitor used as a treatment for adults with moderate to severe Rheumatoid arthritis.
>
> **Foralumab:** Anti CD3 monoclonal antibody, which induces T regulatory cells, resulting in IL-10 mediated anti inflammatory effect.
>
> **AZD7442:** It is a combination of two long-acting antibodies (LAABs) derived from convalescent patients after SARS-CoV-2 infection. The LAABs were optimized with half-life extension and reduced Fc receptor binding.
>
> Other agents that have been proposed for COVID-19 therapy include the HCV antivirals sofosbuvir plus daclatasvir, the selective serotonin receptor blocker fluvoxamine, famotidine, colchicine, vitamin D, and zinc

Others
- D-dimer
- Ferritin
- LDH
- PT/INR
- Trop-T
- Procalcitonin
- ABG

Treatment (Box 15.4)

- **Influenza–like Illness (ILI):** Fever (>38°C) + cough with onset <10 days not requiring admission.
- **Severe acute respiratory infection (SARI):** Fever (>38°C) with cough with onset <10 days requiring admission.

Drugs Approved for the Treatment of COVID-19

For drugs approved for the treatment of Covid-19 *see* **Box 15.5.**

BACTERIAL INFECTIONS

DIPHTHERIA

- Diphtheria is caused by *Corynebacterium diphtheriae*
- The disease is transmitted by droplet infection from active cases or carriers
- The incubation period is about 1 week.

Clinical Features

- Its manifestations may be local (due to the membrane) or systemic (due to exotoxin).
- Insidious in onset with a sore throat and fever being the usual manifestation. The fever is moderate but there is usually marked tachycardia.

Respiratory Diphtheria

- **Pharyngeal diphtheria:** It is characterized by marked tonsillar and pharyngeal inflammation and the presence of a pseudomembrane. There may be regional often tender lymphadenopathy (cervical lymph nodes), and along with marked edema of submandibular areas produces the so-called **"bull-neck"** appearance (swelling of the neck). Pharyngeal diphtheria is associated with the greatest toxicity.
- **Laryngeal diphtheria:** It is usually represents extension of the membrane from the pharynx. Extension and sloughing of membranes may produce fatal airway obstruction. It usually presents with a husky voice, a brassy cough and later dyspnea and cyanosis due to respiratory obstruction.
- **Nasal diphtheria:** It is restricted to the nasal mucosa and is characterized by the presence of a unilateral, serosanguineous (frequently blood-stained) nasal discharge.

Cutaneous Diphtheria

It is uncommon but occurs in individuals with poor personal hygiene and with burns. It produces round, deep, "punched-out" skin ulcers with undermined edges and is covered by a gray-yellow or gray-brown adherent membrane. The ulcers occur more commonly on the lower and upper extremities, head and trunk. Constitutional symptoms are not common.

Complications

- **Airway (laryngeal) obstruction:** It may occur with advanced diphtheria. Airway obstruction may be either due to the sloughed pseudomembrane or extension of the pseudomembrane to the larynx or into the tracheobronchial tree (bronchopulmonary diphtheria). It is mainly observed in children because of their small airways.
- **Cardiac complications:** These include **myocarditis** with arrhythmias, cardiac failure, and ECG changes. They often develop weeks after initial episode of diphtheria. These are usually reversible.
- **Neurological complications** occur in 75% of cases.
  - **Palatal palsy** may develop after 10 days.
  - **Polyneuropathy** with weakness and paresthesia may develop 3–5 weeks after the onset of diphtheria.
  - **Paralysis of accommodation** may manifest as difficulty in reading small print.
  - Encephalitis can occur rarely.
- **Other complications** include pneumonia, renal failure, encephalitis, cerebral infarction, and pulmonary embolism.

Diagnosis

- The diagnosis is based on the demonstration of the characteristic diphtheritic membrane
- Demonstration of the organism by Albert staining
- Culture of the organism on Loeffler's medium.

Management

- Isolation and strict bed rest.
- Antidiphtheritic toxin should be given as early in the course of diphtheria as possible. 20,000–40,000 units for pharyngeal/laryngeal disease of <48 hours duration, 40,000–60,000 units for nasopharyngeal disease, and 80,000–120,000 units for >3 days of illness or diffuse neck swelling
- Benzylpenicillin (1,200 mg four times daily IV) or amoxicillin (500 mg three times daily) is given for 2 weeks. Patients allergic to penicillin are given erythromycin (500 mg four times daily for 14 days).
- Tracheostomy may become necessary for respiratory distress.
- **Contact prophylaxis:** Single dose of penicillin G benzathine (600,000 units intramuscularly—IM) or oral erythromycin (500 mg four times daily for 7–10 days).
- Vaccines include diphtheria, pertussis, tetanus (DPT) and diphtheria tetanus (DT).

PLAGUE

- Plague, known as "black death", is caused by *Yersinia pestis*, a gram-negative, nonmotile bacillus.
- Three types of plague: Bubonic, septicemic, and pneumonic.
- The most common route of infection in humans is after bite of a plague-infected rat flea.

Clinical Features

Bubonic Plague

- Presents in a week after exposure
- Presents with fever with chills, weakness, nausea and vomiting
- May have swollen painful lymph nodes in the groin or axilla. These are called the buboes that are rarely fluctuant or suppurative.
- Complications include secondary septicemia, pneumonia, and meningitis.
- The mortality rate for untreated bubonic plague is 60%.

Septicemic Plague

- Septicemic plague may occur as a complication of untreated bubonic plague or pneumonic plague (secondary septicemic plague) and can develop in the absence of obvious signs of primary disease (primary septicemic plague).

- Septicemic plague presents with high fever, chills and malaise, but without any lymph node enlargement. Patients may develop septic shock and DIC with vasculitis.
- Gangrene of the tip of the nose or digits, due to small artery thrombosis may appear in advanced stages of the disease (Black death).
- Left untreated, the mortality approaches 100%.

Pneumonic Plague

- Pneumonic plague may occur by primary respiratory infection, or as a complication of the bubonic and septicemic forms of the disease (secondary pneumonia).
- Presents within 1–6 days of exposure.
- It begins abruptly with intense headache, weakness, pyrexia, vomiting, abdominal pain and diarrhea. Chest pain, cough, dyspnea and hemoptysis develop thereafter.
- Complications are respiratory failure, septic shock, etc., and mortality is high.

Diagnosis

- Smears from blood, sputum, bubo aspirate, and cerebrospinal fluid may be stained with Gram, Giemsa, or Wayson's stains to demonstrate bipolar staining coccobacilli (safety pin appearance).
- Cultures of various tissue fluids.
- Serological tests for antibodies.

Treatment

- With prompt use of antibiotics fatality rate decreases below 5% for bubonic plague and below 10% for septicemic and pneumonic plague.
- Effective medications include Streptomycin, Gentamicin, and Ciprofloxacin. Total duration of treatment is 10 days.

BOTULISM

It is caused by **Clostridium botulinum.**

Classification

- Food-borne botulism occurs due to ingestion of preformed toxin in contaminated food. It is the most common form of botulism.
- Wound botulism develops from toxin produced by infection of a wound.
- Infantile botulism results from ingestion of spores, which on germination in the gut, produce toxin.

Clinical Features

- Incubation period varies from 2 hours to 8 days.
- Initial presentation includes gastrointestinal symptoms followed rapidly by involvement of cranial nerves, causing diplopia, dysphagia, and dysarthria.
- This is followed by progressive, descending motor paralysis, and then, diaphragmatic paralysis and death.
- Wound botulism is similar except that GI upset does not occur.
- Infant botulism is characterized by onset of constipation, followed by weakness in sucking, crying, or swallowing. This is followed by progressive bulbar and extremity muscle weakness.

Diagnosis

- Diagnosis of botulism is based on clinical features.
- Conditions often confused with botulism include GB syndrome, myasthenia gravis, tick paralysis, diphtheria.

Treatment

It includes supportive care with assisted ventilation prevention of secondary infection and administration of antitoxin (not available in India).

PERTUSSIS (WHOOPING COUGH)

- Caused by *Bordetella pertussis*
- Spread is by droplet infection.
- Incubation period: 1–2 weeks.

Clinical Features

- The first stage (catarrhal phase) is characterized by upper respiratory catarrh with conjunctivitis and dry cough.
- Followed by severe bouts of cough lasting for weeks.
- Characteristic whoop and may have cyanosis. Pertussis is most contagious in the catarrhal and early paroxysmal stages.

Complications

- Bronchopneumonia
- Bronchiectasis
- Encephalitis
- Convulsions
- Conjunctival hemorrhage
- Prolapsed rectum.

Diagnosis

- Peripheral blood lymphocytosis may be seen in well-established cases.
- The diagnosis can be confirmed by the isolation of *B. pertussis*.
- PCR to detect *B. pertussis*
- Direct fluorescent antibody test.

Management

- Erythromycin for 7–14 days is the recommended treatment. Azithromycin and clarithromycin are equally effective and have lesser side effects than erythromycin.
- A cough suppressant like methadone can reduce the severity of coughing paroxysms.

TYPHOID (ENTERIC FEVER)

Enteric fever is the general term, which includes **both typhoid and paratyphoid** fever. It is an acute systemic illness characterized by fever, headache, and abdominal discomfort.

Causative Agent

- Enteric fevers are caused by **Salmonella typhi** and **Salmonella paratyphi.** Salmonella are gram-negative,

flagellate, motile, nonsporulating, facultative anaerobic bacilli (rods). Boiling or chlorination of water and pasteurization of milk destroy the bacilli.
- Typhoid fever (enteric) is an **acute systemic disease** caused by infection with *Salmonella typhi* (also known as Salmonella enterica serovar Typhi). Paratyphoid fever is a clinically similar but milder disease caused by *Salmonella paratyphi* (Salmonella enterica serovar Paratyphi A, B or C).

Source of Infection

Humans are the only natural reservoir and include:
- **Patient suffering from disease:** Infected urine, feces, or other secretions from patients.
- **Chronic carriers of typhoid fever:** S. typhi or S. paratyphi **colonizes in the gallbladder, urinary bladder**, or biliary tree.

Mode of Transmission

- From **person-to-person contact**.
- **Ingestion** of **contaminated food** (especially dairy products) and shellfish or **contaminated** food, milk or **water**. Chronic carriers, often food handlers transmit the disease.
- **Direct spread:** Rare by **finger-to-mouth contact** with feces (fecal-oral route), urine, or other secretions is rare.

Incubation period: Usually 10–14 days and for paratyphoid it is shorter.

Pathogenesis

- The typhoid bacilli *(Salmonella)* are **ingested through contaminated food or water are** able to **survive in gastric acid of the stomach and** reach mucosa of small intestine.
- In the small intestine, they penetrate the **ileal mucosa**, reach the submucosa, and are **phagocytosed by the macrophages in the Peyer's patches.**
- They are **carried to** the **mesenteric lymph node** via lymphatics **and** enter the **bloodstream via** the **thoracic duct causing** bacteremia.
- They colonize reticuloendothelial tissues **(liver, gallbladder, spleen, bone marrow),** and multiply further and re-enter bloodstream causing **massive bacteremia** (occurs toward the end of incubation period) and disease clinically manifests.
- In the intestine, the bacilli are localized to the **Peyer's patches and lymphoid follicles** of the terminal ileum. They cause inflammation, plateau-like elevations of Peyer's patches and necrosis, which results in characteristic **oval typhoid ulcers.**

Clinical Features

- Onset is gradual and nonspecific. Patients usually present with fever, anorexia, headache, abdominal pain, bloating, nausea, and vomiting.
- **Fever:** The temperature rises in a step-ladder fashion **(step-ladder fever)** to 40–41°C for 4 or 5 days in some cases. The hallmark of typhoid fever is continuous, persistent fever, often lasting 4–8 weeks in untreated patients.
- Early intestinal manifestations include constipation (especially in adults) or mild diarrhea (in children).

Physical Findings

- In the early stages abdominal tenderness, hepatosplenomegaly, lymphadenopathy and a scanty maculopapular rash ("rose spots") are found.
- **Rose spots or rose-red spots:** These are small 2–4 mm, pale-red maculopapular lesions on the skin that fade/blanch on pressure appear on the chest and abdomen, which occur during first week and usually last only 2–3 days. They result from bacterial embolism and *Salmonella* can be cultured from the biopsy of these lesions.
- **Mild hepatosplenomegaly:** Spleen is soft and palpable (around the 7–10th day) may be accompanied by tender hepatomegaly.
- **Relative bradycardia:** The pulse is often slower than would be expected from the height of the fever.
- **Intestinal manifestations:** By the end of 1st week, constipation is succeeded by diarrhea and abdominal distension, with tenderness in the right iliac fossa. The stools are loose and greenish in color and characteristically described as "pea-soup". Intestinal complications often develop in the 3rd or 4th week of illness.
  - *If untreated by the end of 2nd week:* Patient may be profoundly ill.
  - *By 3rd week:* Toxemia increases and patient may develop coma and die.
  - The 4th week of the illness is characterized by gradual improvement.

Complications of Typhoid

For complications of typhoid see **Box 15.6**.

Laboratory Diagnosis

For laboratory diagnosis see **Box 15.7**.

Treatment

- **General management:** These include bed rest, isolation, and maintenance of nutrition and fluid intake.

Box 15.6: Complications of typhoid.

- **General complications:** Toxemia, dehydration, peripheral circulatory failure, DIC.
- **Intestinal complications:** The most common intestinal complication is ileus. **Perforation** of typhoid ulcer and **hemorrhage from the ulcer** may occur at the end of the second week or during the third week of the illness.
- **Extraintestinal complications:**
  - *Neurological:* Delirium **(muttering delirium),** psychosis, **seizures,** coma vigil, catatonia, meningitis, encephalopathy, GB syndrome peripheral neuritis and deafness.
  - *Miscellaneous:* **Myocarditis,** endocarditis, pericarditis, pneumonia, **cholecystitis,** pyelonephritis, glomerulonephritis, osteomyelitis, arthritis, periostitis, hepatitis, thrombophlebitis. Patients with **sickle cell disease are susceptible to** *Salmonella* **osteomyelitis.**
- **Carrier state:** Persistence of bacilli in the **gallbladder or urinary tract** may result in passage of bacilli in the feces or urine and causes a "carrier state" which is the source of infection to others. After clinical recovery, about 5–10% will continue to excrete *S. typhi* for several months and they are termed convalescent carriers.

> **Box 15.7: Laboratory diagnosis of typhoid fever.**
>
> ❖ **Total leukocyte count:** It shows **leukopenia with relative lymphocytosis. Eosinophils are usually absent.**
> ❖ **Isolation of Bacilli:**
>   □ *Blood culture:* This is the "Gold Standard" investigation for diagnosis of typhoid. The maximum positivity of blood culture is in **first week** of fever in 90% of patients and remains positive in second week till the fever subsides. Blood culture rapidly becomes negative on treatment with antibiotics. During early phase, bone marrow culture aspirate is more sensitive than blood culture, even after a brief prior antibiotic treatment.
>   □ *Stool cultures:* It is almost as valuable as blood culture and become positive in the **third week.**
>   □ *Urine culture:* It reveals the organism in approximately 25% of patients by **third week.**
> ❖ **Widal test/reaction:** Classic Widal test **measures** agglutinating **antibodies against** *O, H* and **Vi antigens** of *S. typhi* and H antigens of *S. paratyphi* A and B, but **lacks sensitivity and specificity.** Widal test (immunological reactions) becomes positive from **end of the first week till fourth week.** There are many false-positive (anamnestic reaction) and occasional false-negative Widal reactions. Vi antigen is alone detected in the carrier state. The mean sensitivity, specificity, NPV and PPV of Widal test remains below 80%. Therefore, Widal test should not be used as a diagnostic tool to rule out typhoid fever unless supported by invasive clinical pictures and other confirmatory tests.
> ❖ **Other serologic tests:** They are available for the rapid diagnosis of typhoid fever with a higher sensitivity.
> ❖ **Molecular methods:** PCR detects flagellin, somatic gene and Vi gene.

Table 15.6: Various antibiotic regimens in typhoid fever.

Drug	Dosage and duration of treatment
Ceftriaxone	75 mg/kg/day for 7–14 days
Chloramphenicol	3–4 g/day till the fever subsides, followed by 2 g/day, for a total duration of 14 days.
Amoxicillin	4–6 g/day in four divided doses for 14 days
Cotrimoxazole	Trimethoprim 640 mg + sulfamethoxazole 3,200 mg in two divided doses daily for 14 days
Ciprofloxacin	500–750 mg twice daily for 14 days
Ofloxacin	400–800 mg/day for 14 days
Cefotaxime	50–75 mg/kg/day for 7–14 days
Cefixime	20 mg/kg/day for 10–14 days
Azithromycin	1 g once a day for 7 days
Aztreonam	50–100 mg/kg/day for 14 days

- **Antibiotic therapy:** Several antibiotics are effective in enteric fever and various drug regimens are presented in **Table 15.6.** It must be guided by culture and sensitivity report.
- **Multidrug resistant strains:** Certain strains of *S. typhi* (especially in India) are resistant to chloramphenicol, amoxicillin, and cotrimoxazole are called as multidrug-resistant strains. These should be treated with ciprofloxacin.
- **NARST (Nalidixic acid resistant *Salmonella typhi*):** Sometimes, strains that are sensitive to ciprofloxacin in vitro may not respond to ciprofloxacin. They are usually resistant to nalidixic acid when tested in vitro. These patients need treatment for longer duration with ciprofloxacin or with ceftriaxone.
- **Corticosteroids:** It is indicated in patients with severe toxemia, central nervous system manifestations and DIC. Intravenous dexamethasone is given in the dose of 3 mg/kg as a loading dose, followed by 1 mg/kg every 6 hourly for 24 hours.

Treatment of Complications

Intestinal perforation and hemorrhage occur in the 3rd or 4th week of illness are managed accordingly.

Carrier state in typhoid:

- **Asymptomatic carrier state:** About 3–5% of patients develop long-term asymptomatic carrier state. Many carriers does not give history of typhoid fever and are probably had an undiagnosed mild infection.
- **Chronic carriers:** These carriers are usually older than 50 years and females with gallstones. *S. typhi* resides in the gallbladder, urinary bladder and even within the gallstones. They are intermittently excreted into the stool, thereby contaminating water or food. Vi antigen is positive in carriers.
- Chronic carriers should be given ciprofloxacin/ampicillin for 4 weeks. Cholecystectomy may be needed in some patients.

Prevention

- **Improved sanitation and living conditions:** It is most important method to prevent typhoid fever. These measures include good hygiene, clean water, proper sewage disposal and proper water treatment. Travelers are advised to avoid drinking untreated water, ice in drinks, and eating ice creams.
- **Vaccination:** Three available typhoid vaccines are:
  - *Inactivated injectable:* two in number
    - Heat-killed, phenol-extracted, whole-cell vaccine—because of several adverse reactions, this is not used at present.
    - Vi-polysaccharide-parenteral administration in individuals >2 years; single dose.
  - *Oral live-attenuated vaccines:* Ty21a, a live, attenuated vaccine containing the *S. typhi* strain Ty21a is oral administered in individuals >6 years; one capsule every other day for three doses.

FOOD POISONING

- Food poisoning is an **illness contracted by eating contaminated food.**
- In most cases, food that causes food poisoning is contaminated by bacteria, such as *Salmonella* or *Escherichia coli* (*E. coli*), or a virus, such as the norovirus. Some toxins can cause food poisoning within a short time. Vomiting is the main symptom of food poisoning

Causes of Food Poisoning

For causes of food poisoning *see* **Box 15.8.**

> **Box 15.8:** Causes of food poisoning.
>
> **Infective (bacteria or their toxins)**
> - Due to toxin
>   - Preformed toxins, e.g., *Staphylococcus aureus*, *Bacillus cereus*
>   - Enterotoxins released in the intestine, e.g., *Vibrio cholerae*, *E. coli*, *Clostridium perfringens*, *Clostridium difficile*
> - Due to intestinal mucosal damage
>   - Invasion of mucosa, e.g., reovirus
>   - Invasion and destruction of mucosa, e.g., *Shigella*, *Yersinia enterocolitica*, *Salmonella*, *Entamoeba histolytica*, *Bacillus anthracis*.
>
> **Noninfective**
> - Allergic type, e.g., shellfish.
> - Nonallergic type, e.g., scombrotoxin (fish), fungi (*Amanita phalloides*).
> - Chemicals, e.g., detergents, pesticides.

Various organism causing food poisoning and their symptoms are summarized in **Table 15.7.**

DYSENTERY

Dysentery is defined as an acute inflammation of the large intestine (colitis) characterized by diarrhea with blood and mucus in the stools. Two causes are bacillary and amebic infections.

Bacillary Dysentery (Shigellosis)

- Bacillary dysentery is an acute **necrotizing infection** of the **distal small bowel and colon** caused mostly by one of **Shigella** species. *Shigella* species that cause colitis are classified into four major subgroups namely: *dysenteriae* (most virulent), *flexneri*, *boydii* and *sonnei*. Bacillary dysentery is one of the **most common causes of bloody diarrhea**. Other organisms causing bacillary dysentery include *E. coli* O157:H7, *Salmonella*, *Campylobacter*, etc.
- *Shigella* **produces toxin** (endotoxin as well as an exotoxin) that has cytotoxic, neurotoxic, and enterotoxic effects. When inflammation is severe, ileus, toxic megacolon, gross hemorrhage, and perforation may develop.
- **Source of infection: Humans** are the only natural reservoir.
- **Mode of transmission:** By **ingestion** through fecal-oral route or via fecally contaminated water and food. It can be acquired by oral contact with any contaminated surface (e.g., clothing, towels, and unwashed hands after defecation or skin surfaces) or flies.
- **Incubation period:** It ranges from **1 to 3 days.**

Clinical Features

- **Severity of infection:** Disease severity varies from mild to severe. *S. sonnei* produces mild infection, *S. flexneri* infection is usually more severe, and *S. dysenteriae* may produce fulminating infection resulting in death within 48 hours.

Table 15.7: Various organism causing food poisoning and their symptoms.

Organism	Incubation	Symptoms	Foods
Campylobacter jejuni	2–5 days	Diarrhea, vomiting, headache, fever, muscle pain	Poultry, dairy products, water
Salmonella enteritidis	12–36 hours	Abdominal cramps, headache, fever, nausea, diarrhea	Poultry, meat, eggs and egg products, sliced melons
Escherichia coli	3–4 days	Diarrhea, vomiting, mild fever	Undercooked ground beef, unpasteurized cider
Listeria monocytogenes	3–70 days	Flu-like, meningitis, encephalitis, spontaneous abortion	Unpasteurized milk, ice cream, ready-to-eat, lunch meats
Clostridium perfringens	10–12 hours	Abdominal pain, nausea, diarrhea fever, headache, vomiting usually absent	Stews, gravies, beans
Clostridium botulinum (intoxication)	4 hours to 8 days	Vomiting; constipation; diplopia, dysphagia, dysarthria, paralysis, death	Baked potatoes, fish, garlic/oil mixtures, low-acid canned foods
Staphylococcus aureus (intoxication)	1–7 hours	Nausea, retching, abdominal cramps, diarrhea	Ready-to-eat, reheated foods, dairy products, protein foods
Bacillus cereus (intoxication)	30 minutes to 6 hours (emetic) or 6 to 15 hours (diarrheal)	Nausea, vomiting, watery diarrhea	Rice products, starchy foods, casseroles, puddings, soups
Hepatitis A	10–50 days	Sudden fever, vomiting, jaundice	Water (ice), shellfish, ready-to-eat, fruit juices, vegetables
Norwalk virus	10–50 hours	Nausea, diarrhea, headache, mild fever	Water, shellfish, raw vegetables and fruits
Rotavirus	1–3 days	Vomiting, diarrhea, mild fever	Ready-to-eat, water and ice
Giardia lamblia	3–25 days	Fatigue, nausea, weight loss, abdominal cramps	Water, ice, raw vegetables
Cryptosporidium parvum	1–12 days	Severe diarrhea, may have no symptoms	Water, raw foods, unpasteurized cider, ready-to-eat

Table 15.8: Complications of bacillary dysentery.

Intestinal	Extraintestinal
• Rectal prolapse • Toxic megacolon • Colonic perforation	• Bacteremia • Meningismus, seizures • Transient peripheral neuropathy • Reiter syndrome • Hemolytic-uremic syndrome (HUS) • Thrombotic thrombocytopenic purpura

- Symptoms start 24–48 hours after ingestion and usually presents as frequent small quantity of stools containing blood, mucus and purulent exudate with little fecal material (dysentery). This is accompanied by fever, colicky abdominal pain and tenesmus. Severe cases may show signs of systemic toxicity, dehydration and electrolyte disturbances.
- Physical examination may show tenderness over the colon in the left iliac fossa and hyperactive bowel sounds.

Complications
The complications are described in **Table 15.8**.

Diagnosis
- **Stool culture** is required for confirmation of *Shigella* infection.
- **Sigmoidoscopy** shows red and swollen mucosa covered by mucus on the surface. The submucus veins are obscured.
- Enzyme immunoassay used for detecting Shiga toxins in stools.
- PCR for *Shigella* DNA in stools.

Management
- Fluid and **electrolyte** deficits should be corrected by oral rehydration therapy or, if diarrhea is severe, by intravenous replacement of water and electrolyte loss.
- **Antibiotic therapy:** Infections caused by *S. dysenteriae* and *S. flexneri* should be given ciprofloxacin (500 mg twice daily for 3 days). Second-line agents include azithromycin and ceftriaxone.
- **Antidiarrheal medication** should be avoided. Codeine or loperamide may be given to control diarrhea in adults without dysentery.

AMEBIASIS

Etiology
- Amebiasis is an **infection caused by protozoan *Entamoeba histolytica***
- *E. histolytica* has three distinct stages:
  1. **Trophozoite stage:** Amebic trophozoites are seen in the stools of patients with acute symptoms.
  2. **Precyst stage:** In the colon, the trophozoite develops into a cyst through an intermediate form termed the precyst.
  3. **Cyst stage: Amebic cysts are the infecting stage** and are found only in stools. They are spherical and have thick chitin walls, and usually four nuclei.

- **Source of infection:** Humans are the only known reservoir for *E. histolytica*. It is reproduced in the colon of infected individual and passes in the feces.
- **Mode of infection:** It is **acquired by fecal-oral route** through ingestion of materials contaminated with human feces containing *E. histolytica*. Pathogenesis of amebiasis is depicted in **Figure 15.7**.
- **Incubation period:** About 2–6 weeks.

Amebic Colitis
Amebic colitis can present in two forms: Amebic dysentery and nondysenteric amebic colitis.

Amebic Dysentery
Pathogenesis:
- The amebic cysts are passed in the stool of infected individuals and the **cysts can contaminate water, food, or fingers.**
- These cysts are tetra-nucleated and can remain viable for weeks to months. However, these are destroyed in temperature below 5°C or above 40°C.
- Amebic dysentery results from ingestion (fecal-oral transmission) of *E. histolytica* cysts. **Amebic cysts colonize the epithelial surface of the terminal ileum and** undergo further nuclear division, and release trophozoites. The trophozoites are carried to the large intestine and may colonize any part of the large intestine, but **most frequently in the cecum and ascending colon causing amebic colitis.** They produce the characteristic "flask-shaped" amebic ulcers with a narrow neck and broad base. These patients pass both cysts and trophozoites in the stool.
- Most often, the amebic infection remains subclinical. However, antibody response usually occurs even without local invasion. These asymptomatic patients should be treated to prevent transmission of infection to others and development of amebic colitis at a later period.
- **Ameboma** is a common complication of amebic dysentery. It is a localized granuloma, which presents as a palpable mass in the rectum or causes a filling defect in the colon on radiography.
- **Trophozoite may penetrate blood vessels and reach the liver through** portal vein. In the liver they multiply and produce amebic liver **abscesses** in about 40% of patients with amebic dysentery. The liquid contents of this abscess have a characteristic pinkish color, which may later change to chocolate-brown (like anchovy sauce).
- They can also travel to lungs and brain.

Clinical features of intestinal amebiasis (amebic dysentery):
- It may produce **dysentery of varying severity.** It presents with intermittent diarrhea consisting of **foul smelling** (offensive), **loose, watery stools** that may contain **mucus and blood.** Sometimes diarrhea alternate with constipation.
- **Other symptoms include abdominal pain**/cramp (especially right lower quadrant which may simulate acute appendicitis), flatulence, and weight loss. Sometimes it is accompanied by systemic symptoms such as headache, fever, nausea, and anorexia. Less commonly, it may present

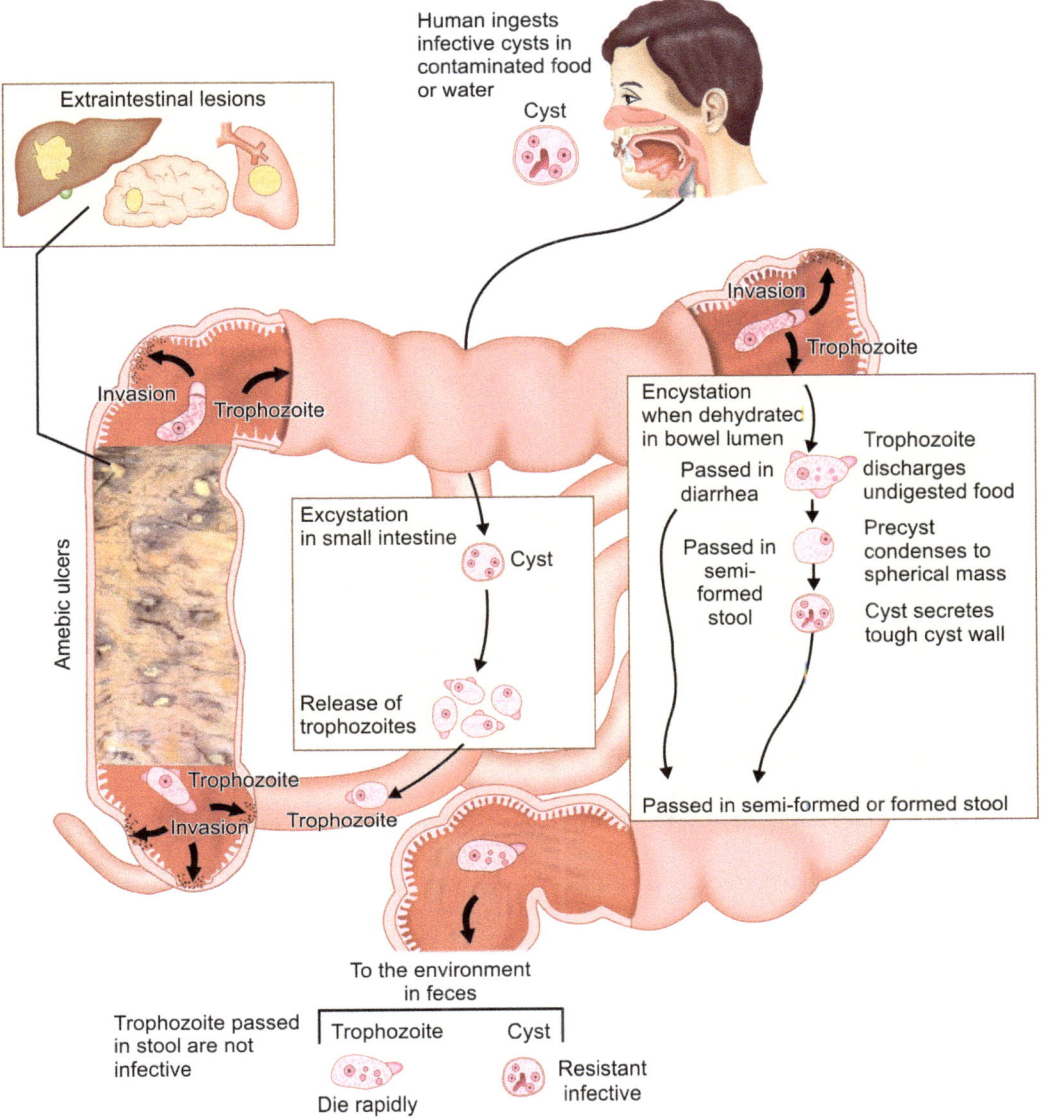

Fig. 15.7: Pathogenesis of amebiasis.

as acute amebic dysentery, resembling bacillary dysentery or acute ulcerative colitis.
- **Physical examination:** There may be tenderness over the cecum (*amebic typhlitis*), ascending colon and over the left iliac fossa **(amebic point or Manson-Barr point)** and tender hepatomegaly.

Complications
For complications of amebiasis *see* **Table 15.9**.

Diagnosis
- **Microscopic examination of stool:** Presence of motile trophozoites containing red blood cells (hematophagous trophozoites) in fresh sample of stool will confirm the diagnosis. If a fresh stool sample cannot be examined immediately, it should be preserved with a fixative such as polyvinyl alcohol or kept cool (4°C). Presence of amebic cysts alone does not imply disease.
- **Sigmoidoscopy** and barium enema may show the characteristic "flask-shaped" ulcers with normal surrounding mucosa. The aspirated material or scrapings from the ulcer or biopsy of the ulcer may show the trophozoites. Colonic exudate obtained by sigmoidoscopy may microscopically show trophozoites.
- **Serologic tests:** Indirect hemagglutination test, ELISA, or counter immunoelectrophoresis can detect antibodies in the blood. They are more useful in extraintestinal amebiasis.

Table 15.9: Complications of amebiasis.

Intestinal complications	Extraintestinal complications
• Massive hemorrhage	• Amebic liver abscess
• Ameboma	• Pleuropulmonary amebiasis
• Perforation and peritonitis	• Hepaticobronchial fistula
• Toxic megacolon in fulminant cases	• Amebic pericarditis
• Postdysenteric colitis	• Cutaneous amebiasis
• Rectovaginal fistula	
• Chronic infection with stricture formation	

Table 15.10: Treatment for amebiasis.

Condition	Drug	Adult dosing
Asymptomatic	Paromomycin (OR)	25 to 35 mg/kg/day PO in three divided doses × 7 days
	Iodoquinol (OR)	650 mg PO TID × 20 days
	Diloxanide furoate (Luminal agent only)	500 mg PO TID × 10 days
Intestinal disease* (mild to moderate)	Metronidazole (OR)	500 to 750 mg PO TID × 7–10 days
	Tinidazole (followed by luminal agent as above)	2 g PO daily × 3 days
Liver abscess or severe intestinal disease	Metronidazole (OR)	750 mg PO or IV TID × 10 days
	Tinidazole (followed by luminal agent as above)	2 g PO daily × 5 days

*Nitazoxanide 500 mg PO BID × 3 days may be considered as an alternative to nitroimidazoles for mild to moderate amebiasis, followed by a luminal agent.

- Amebic fluorescent antibody test is positive in about 90% of patients with liver abscess and in 60–70% with active colitis.
- Detection of E. histolytica antigen or DNA in a stool sample.

Treatment of Amebiasis
See **Table 15.10**.

Differences between Amebic Dysentery and Bacillary Dysentery
For differences between amebic dysentery and bacillary dysentery see **Table 15.11**.

CHOLERA
- Cholera is an acute illness that results from colonization of the small intestine by *Vibrio cholerae*.
- The disease is characterized by its epidemic occurrence and explosive, severe diarrhea with rapid depletion of extracellular fluid and electrolytes.
- The major pathogenic strain has a somatic antigen (O1). It is called serogroup O1

Clinical Features
- The incubation period is about 12–48 hours.
- Explosive onset of watery diarrhea without pain or colic follows vomiting (vomiting may be absent). The characteristic "rice-water" stool consists of clear fluid with flecks of mucus. Several liters of isotonic fluid may be lost within hours, leading rapidly to profound shock.
- In extreme cases, there may be signs of severe dehydration. The skin is cold, clammy, and wrinkled (washer women's skin) with loss of skin turgor. The blood pressure drops, and the pulse becomes rapid and thready.
- Occasionally, a very severe form of the disease occurs in which the loss of fluid into the dilated bowel kills the patient

Table 15.11: Differences between amebic dysentery and bacillary dysentery.

Features	Amebic dysentery	Bacillary dysentery
Macroscopic		
Number of motions	6–8 motions/day	Over 10 motions/day
Amount of stool	Relatively copious	Relatively small
Odor	Offensive	No odor
Nature	Blood and mucus mixed with feces	Blood and mucus, no feces
Color	Dark red	Bright red
Reaction	Acidic	Alkaline
Consistency	Not adherent to the container	Adherent to the container
Microscopic		
RBC	In clumps	Discrete or in rouleaux
Pus cells	Few	Numerous
Macrophages, Ghost cells	Very few	Numerous
Eosinophils, Pyknotic bodies	Present	Scarce
Causative agent	Trophozoites of E. histolytica	Motile bacteria
Charcot-Leyden crystals	Present	Absent

before typical gastrointestinal symptoms appear. This is known as "cholera sicca".

Diagnosis
- "Hanging drop" preparation of the stool demonstrates the characteristic motile organisms.
- Culture of the stool or a rectal swab can isolate and identify the organism.

Treatment
- Vigorous intravenous fluid and electrolyte therapy should be continued till the patient is hemodynamically stable and vomiting subsides.
- Oral rehydration also attempted along with IV fluids, if tolerated.
- Tetracycline, Cotrimoxazole, and Ciprofloxacin.

LEPTOSPIROSIS
Etiology
- It is caused by *Leptospira interrogans*, which is pathogenic. The organism is a tightly coiled spirochete with one axial filament.
- Human infection can occur either by direct contact with urine or tissue of an infected animal or indirectly through contaminated water, soil or vegetation. Transmission may occur through cuts, mucous membranes (nasopharynx, conjunctiva, and vagina), and possibly unabraded skin.

Clinical Features

- High-grade fever with chills and rigors
- Headache
- Myalgia
- Conjunctival suffusion
- Nausea, vomiting, and abdominal pain
- Cough and pharyngitis
- Lymphadenopathy
- Hepatosplenomegaly
- Meningitis
- Skin rashes.

Weil's Syndrome

- Weil's syndrome is not a specific subgroup of leptospirosis; it is simply severe leptospirosis.
- It can develop as the second phase of a biphasic illness or as a progressive illness.
- The overall picture in Weil's syndrome is striking, and is characterized by intense jaundice, mental status changes, hemorrhage, purpura or petechiae, and renal failure.
- Hemorrhagic manifestations are common.

Investigations

- Anemia
- Neutrophilia
- Thrombocytopenia
- Raised erythrocyte sedimentation rate (ESR).
- Deranged renal function—Urea and creatinine
- Deranged liver function
- Prolongation of prothrombin time
- Urine examination shows microscopic hematuria, pyuria, and proteinuria.
- Levels of creatinine phosphokinase (CPK) are elevated in 50% of cases
- Chest radiograph may show patchy bronchopneumonia and a small pleural effusion.
- CSF may be abnormal in up to 90% of cases.
- Serum IgM antibodies in the second phase of illness.

Treatment

- A variety of antimicrobial agents have been found to be effective in vitro, but the recommended drugs are given below:
  - Intravenous penicillin, ampicillin, ceftriaxone, or doxycycline
- Renal failure and jaundice require meticulous attention of fluid and electrolyte therapy. Renal failure may require dialysis.
- Anemia and thrombocytopenia may require blood transfusion.

RICKETTSIAL DISEASES

- Rickettsiae are obligate intracellular gram-negative parasites.
- Most are zoonoses spread to humans by arthropods (except Q fever) **(Table 15.12)**.

Treatment

- Tetracycline is the drug of choice Or Doxycycline 100 mg BID PO × 7-15 days.
- Chloramphenicol 500 mg qid PO × 7-15 days/IV Chloramphenicol 150 mg/kg per day for 5 days.
- **Coxiella endocarditis:** Combination therapy–Tetracycline + Co-trimoxazole/ Tetracycline + Rifampicin.

Table 15.12: Examples of rickettsial diseases and their features.

Diseases	Rickettsial agent	Insect vector	Mammalian reservoir	Clinical features
Typhus Group				
Epidemic typhus	R. prowazekii	Louse	Human	Fever/chills, myalgia, headache, rash (No eschar) all over body except palm, sole and face
Murine typhus (Endemic typhus)	R. typhi	Flea	Rodents	Fever, myalgia, headache, rash (No eschar), trunk, extremities, milder form of illness
Scrub typhus	R. tsutsugamushi	Mite	Rodents	Fever, headache, **rash with eschar** cigarette burn sign, lymphadenopathy
Spotted Fever Group				
Indian tick typhus	R. conorii	Tick	Rodent, Dog	Fever, headache, **rash with eschar**, first appear on wrist and ankle
Rocky mountain spotted fever	R. rickettsii	Tick	Rodents, Dogs	Fever, headache, rash (No eschar)—first appear on wrist and ankle, palms and soles involved, systemic complications—respiratory, cardiovascular, central nervous, renal and hepatic system
Rickettsial pox	R. akari	Mite	Mice	Mild illness, fever, headache, vesicular rash with eschar, lymphadenopathy, resemblance to chickenpox
Others				
Q fever	C. burnetii	Nil	Cattle, sheep, goats	Fever, headache, fatigue, pneumonia, endocarditis, no rash
Trench fever	Rochalimaea/ Bartonella quintana	Louse	Human	Fever, splenomegaly, bone pains, maculopapular rash.

FUNGAL INFECTIONS

CANDIDIASIS (MONILIASIS)
- Infection of skin or mucous membranes (e.g., oral cavity and vagina) is called moniliasis.
- *Candida albicans* is the most common cause of candidiasis.
- It causes the following conditions of medical importance:
  - Oral thrush: Conditions that favor oral *Candida* infection include use of broad-spectrum antibiotics, xerostomia, immune dysfunction (e.g., diabetes, immunosuppressive therapy, HIV infection, etc.) or the presence of removable prostheses. Furthermore, about one in four patients with lichen planus will have superimposed candidiasis.
  - Vaginal candidiasis occurs more commonly in diabetics.
  - Cutaneous candidiasis presenting as intertriginous infection and paronychia.

Treatment
- Topical application of antifungal agents like nystatin, clotrimazole, or miconazole.
- Swallowing nystatin suspension or sucking on clotrimazole troches for esophageal candidiasis.
- Systemic antifungal agent ketoconazole or itraconazole for 2 weeks.
- Severe systemic infections may require intravenous fluconazole, or Amphotericin B.
- Echinocandins are newer class of antifungals that include caspofungin, micafungin, and anidulafungin. These agents have limited toxicity, are safe in presence of renal or hepatic impairment, have minimal drug interactions, and importantly, have broad-spectrum activity against most *Candida spp.*

MUCORMYCOSIS
- It represents a group of **life-threatening infections** caused by fungi of the order Mucorales.
- *Rhizopus oryzae* (in the family Mucoraceae) is by far the most common cause of infection.

Risk Factors
- **Impaired immune system:** Mucormycosis typically **cause infection primarily in patients with diabetes or defects in phagocytic function** (e.g., associated with prolonged neutropenia or glucocorticoid treatment), solid organ or hematopoietic stem cell transplantation (HSCT), or malignancy.
- **Elevated levels of free iron:** Supports fungal growth in serum and tissues. Hence patients with raised levels of free iron also have increased risk. In iron-overloaded patients with end-stage renal failure, treatment with deferoxamine (iron chelator for the human host) predisposes to the development of rapidly fatal disseminated mucormycosis. Deferoxamine serves as a fungal siderophore, directly delivering iron to the mucorales.

Clinical Categories
Mucormycosis can be divided into at least six clinical categories based on clinical presentation and the involvement of a particular anatomic site. These are: (1) rhinocerebral (most common in diabetics), (2) pulmonary (in patients undergoing hematopoietic stem cell transplant), (3) cutaneous, (4) gastrointestinal, (5) disseminated, and (6) miscellaneous.

Rhinocerebral mucormycosis (Fig. 15.8):
- The **initial symptoms** of rhinocerebral mucormycosis are **nonspecific** and include **eye or facial pain** and **facial numbness** followed by the onset of **conjunctival suffusion, blurring of vision**, and soft tissue swelling.
- If untreated, infection usually spreads from the ethmoid sinus to the orbit, resulting in compromise of extraocular muscle function and **proptosis**, typically with **chemosis**. Onset of signs and symptoms in the contralateral eye, with resulting bilateral proptosis, chemosis, vision loss, and ophthalmoplegia, is ominous and suggests the development of cavernous sinus thrombosis.
- Upon visual inspection, infected tissue may appear to be normal during the earliest stages of fungal spread and then progresses through an erythematous phase, with or without edema, before the onset of a violaceous appearance and finally the development of a black necrotic eschar.

Definitive Diagnosis
- Diagnosis requires a positive culture from a sterile site (e.g., a needle aspirate, a tissue biopsy specimen, or pleural fluid). A probable diagnosis of mucormycosis can be done by culture from a nonsterile site (e.g., sputum or bronchoalveolar lavage).
- Biopsy with histopathologic evidence of invasive mucormycosis is the most sensitive and specific modality for definitive diagnosis. Biopsy reveals characteristic wide (6–30 m), thick-walled, ribbon-like, aseptate hyphal elements that branch at right angles.

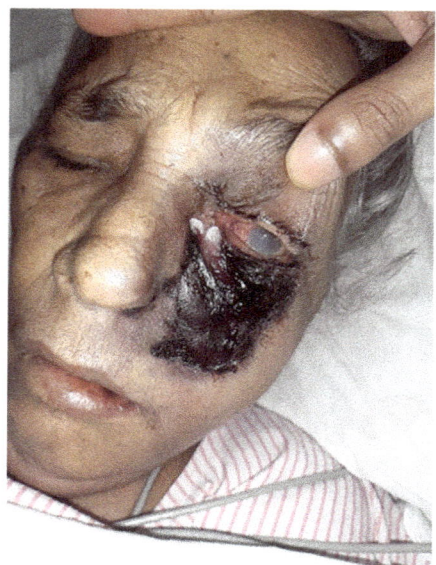

Fig. 15.8: Rhinocerebral mucormycosis.

Treatment: Surgical Debridement Plus

- **Amphotericin B deoxycholate:** 1 mg/kg per day.
- **Liposomal AmB (LAmB):** 5–10 mg/kg per day. However, dose escalation of LAmB to 10 mg/kg per day for CNS mucormycosis may be considered in light of the limited penetration of polyenes into the brain.
- **Amphotericin B lipid complex (ABLC):** 5–7.5 mg/kg.
- Echinocandin-lipid polyene combinations in primarily diabetic patients with rhino-orbital-cerebral mucormycosis.

PROTOZOAL INFECTIONS

MALARIA

- Malaria is a protozoan disease caused by *Plasmodium*. Human malaria is usually caused by one of four species of the genus *Plasmodium* namely (1) *P. falciparum*, (2) *P. vivax*, (3) *P. ovale* and (4) *P. malariae*. Occasionally a species of malaria usually found in primates namely *P. knowlesi* (simian parasite) can affect man.
- *P. falciparum* causes the most severe form of malaria than the other *Plasmodium* species. *P. vivax* is the most common cause of malaria in India.
- **Mode of transmission:** By the bite of female anopheles mosquitoes. Malaria can also be transmitted through contaminated blood transfusions.

Life Cycle of the Malarial Parasite (Fig. 15.9) and Pathogenesis

The life cycle of *Plasmodium* species is simple because it involves only humans and mosquitoes. However, the development of the parasite is complex, because it passes through several morphologically distinct forms. Malarial parasites pass its life cycle in two different hosts namely: (1) human (intermediate host) and (2) female anopheles mosquito (definitive host).

Human Cycle

- Human cycle (infection) starts with the introduction of infectious sporozoite by the bite of infected female anopheles mosquito. The sporozoite is found in the salivary glands of mosquitoes. During mosquito bite, the mosquito takes a blood meal and sporozoites are released into the human's blood. The different stages of human cycle are:
  - *Pre-erythrocytic (Primary exo-erythrocytic) stage:*
    - Sporozites cannot directly enter erythrocyte to start its erythrocyte stage, but undergoes development inside liver cells. The infection of the liver and development of sporozites into merozoites is referred to as the pre-erythrocytic (exo-erythrocytic) stage. Within minutes of entry of sporozites into the human blood (those which are not destroyed by the immune response),

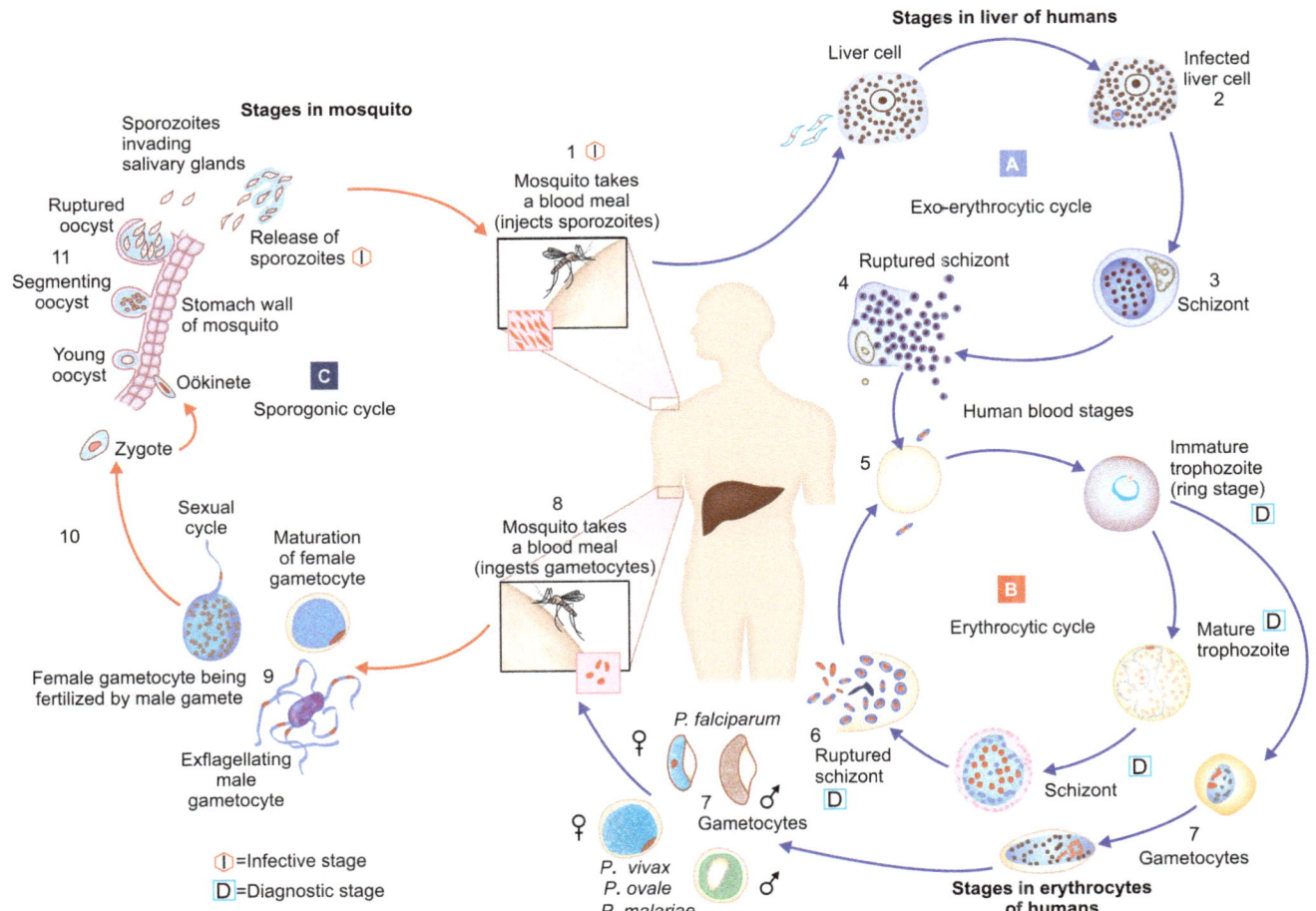

Fig. 15.9: Life cycle of malarial parasites (refer text for description).

they are carried via the bloodstream and are rapidly (within 30 minute) taken up by the liver. They enter liver cells and these malaria parasites multiply by asexual reproduction (intrahepatic schizogony), releasing about 30,000 merozoites (asexual, haploid forms) when each infected liver cells ruptures. This stage is asymptomatic and during this phase, the parasites are not found in the peripheral blood. The infected hepatocytes rupture and release merozoites into the bloodstream.
- During *P. falciparum* infection, rupture of swollen liver cells usually occurs within 8-12 weeks. *P. falciparum* and *P. malariae* have no persistent exoerythrocytic phase but a new outbreak of fever may result from multiplication of parasites in red cells, which have not been eliminated by treatment and immune processes.
- In contrast, *P. vivax* and *P. ovale* releases merozoites into the bloodstream weeks to months after initial infection.
- *Hypnozoite (latent) stage:*
  - The pre-erythrocytic phase disappears completely in *P. falciparum*, whereas a few parasites persist in the liver cells as dormant forms in *P. vivax* and *P. ovale*. The resting phase of parasite (latent phase) is called as hypnozoite. These hypnozoites are capable of developing into merozoites months or years later, causing relapsing malarial infection. Thus, the first attack of clinical malaria may develop long after the individual has left the endemic area.
- *Erythrocytic stage:*
  - Once merozoites are released from the liver into the bloodstream, they rapidly invade erythrocyte by penetration of the membrane. Within the red cells (erythrocytic stage) asexual division occurs.
  - Asexual forms: In the red cells parasite develop through the stages of asexual forms changing from merozoite to trophozoite, to schizont and finally appearing as 8-24 new merozoites. These asexual forms of parasite can be demonstrated in the thick blood smears.
- *Ring form:* It is the first stage of the parasite in the red cell and is characterized by the presence of a single chromatin mass (ring form).
- *Trophozoite:* During this, the parasite assumes an irregular or ameboid shape.
- *Schizont:* It is the next stage the parasite has consumed two-thirds of the RBC's hemoglobin and has grown to occupy most of the cell. It shows multiple chromatin masses, each of which develops into a merozoite. Rupture of the schizont releases merozoites into the blood. This causes fever and the periodicity of fever depends on the species of parasite.
□ **Merozoites:** Rupture of the red cell containing merozoites releases the merozoites into the bloodstream. These merozoites are capable of invading additional new erythrocyte and repeating the cycle. The characteristic clinical features of malaria such as paroxysmal fever, chills, and rigors develop during the release of these merozoites into the blood.
□ Each cycle of the above process is called erythrocytic schizogony. The periodicity of such cycle takes about 48 hours in *P. falciparum, P. vivax* and *P. ovale* and about 72 hours in *P. malariae. P. vivax* and *P. ovale* mainly attack reticulocytes and young erythrocytes, whereas *P. malariae* tends to attack old erythrocytes; *P. falciparum* will parasitize any stage of erythrocyte.
□ **Sexual forms:** Most malaria parasites within the red cells develop into daughter merozoites. A few merozoites within erythrocytes develop not into trophozoites but undergo a different pathway of development into sexual forms called gametocytes (male and female gametocytes). These gametocytes are not released from the red cells until taken up by a feeding mosquito to complete the life cycle. These gametocytes are ingested by the mosquito during a blood meal when mosquito bites the infected human.

Mosquito Cycle

□ A female anopheles mosquito during its blood meal from an infected patient ingests both sexual and asexual forms of parasite, but it is only the mature sexual forms (gametocytes) capable of development.
□ The male and female gametocytes of malarial parasite fuse inside the mid-gut (stomach) of the mosquito to form a zygote.
□ The zygote matures to form an ookinete, which penetrates the gut wall and form an oocyst.
□ The oocyst matures and forms numerous sporozoites. These sporozoites have special predilection toward the salivary glands and reach maximum concentration in the salivary ducts of mosquito. The mosquito at this stage is capable of transmitting malarial infection.
□ During the blood meal these sporozoites are inoculated into the new human host, thus completing the life cycle of *Plasmodium*.

Clinical Features

Vivax, Ovale, and Malariae Malaria

□ **Incubation period:**
- *P. vivax:* 2 weeks
- *P. ovale:* 2 weeks
- *P. malariae:* 4-5 weeks.

□ **Fever with chills and rigors:** In vivax and ovale malaria infections, the characteristic tertian interval (48 hours interval between spikes or fever on alternate days) may be seen. In *P. malariae* infections, the quartan interval (72 hours interval between spikes or fever every 3rd day) may be seen.
□ Headache and body pain
□ Jaundice
□ *Vivax* and *ovale* malarias have a persistent hepatic cycle (Hypnozoites) that may give rise to relapses.
□ Occasionally, vivax malaria can produce complications similar to those of falciparum malaria.

Falciparum Malaria (Malignant Tertian or Subtertian Malaria)

- **The incubation period:** 1–2 weeks
- Prodromal symptoms like malaise, headache, myalgia, anorexia, and mild fever may last for several days before the onset of the classical "malarial paroxysms"
- In a classical malarial paroxysm suddenly the patient feels inexplicably cold and apprehensive. Mild shivering follows, which quickly turns into violent shaking with teeth rattling. There is intense peripheral vasoconstriction and goose flesh. The rapid increase in temperature may trigger febrile convulsions. The rigor lasts up to 1 hour. This is followed by a hot flush with throbbing headache, palpitations, tachypnea, prostration, postural syncope, and vomiting. The temperature reaches its peak. Finally, a drenching sweat breaks off and the fever defervesce over the next few hours. The exhausted patient sleeps off. The whole paroxysm lasts about 8–12 hours.
- Neurological complications of falciparum malaria can manifest as acute headache, irritability, agitation, seizures, psychosis, and impaired consciousness.

Severe Manifestations and Complications of Falciparum Malaria

Criteria for severe and complicated malaria are described in **Table 15.13**.

Table 15.13: Criteria for severe and complicated malaria.

Severe malaria is defined as one or more of the above occurring in the absence of an identified alternative cause and in the presence of *P. falciparum* or *P. knowlesi* parasitemia.

Manifestation	Features
World Health Organization criteria from 1990	
1. Cerebral malaria	Unarousable coma not attributable to any other cause, with a Glasgow Coma Scale score ≤9; Coma should persist for at least 30 minutes after a generalized convulsion
2. Severe anemia	Hematocrit <15% or hemoglobin ≤5 g/dL the presence of parasite count >10,000/µL
3. Renal failure	Urine output <400 mL/24 hours in adults (<12 mL/kg/24 hours in children) and a serum creatinine >265 µmol/L (>3.0 mg/dL) despite adequate volume repletion
4. Metabolic (lactic) acidosis	Metabolic acidosis is defined by an arterial blood pH of <7.35 with a plasma bicarbonate concentration of <22 mmol/L; hyperlactatemia is defined as a plasma lactate concentration of 2–5 mmol/L and lactic acidosis is characterized by a pH <7.25, and a plasma lactate >5 mmol/L.
5. Pulmonary edema or acute respiratory distress syndrome (ARDS)	Breathlessness, bilateral crackles, and other features of pulmonary edema. The acute lung injury score is calculated on the basis of radiographic densities, severity of hypoxemia, and positive end-expiratory pressure
6. Hypoglycemia	Whole blood glucose concentration of less than 2.2 mmol/L (less than 40 mg/dL)
7. Hypotension and shock (algid malaria)	Systolic blood pressure <50 mm Hg in children 1–5 years or <70 mm Hg in patients ≥5 years; cold and clammy skin or a core-skin temperature difference >10°C
8. Abnormal bleeding and/or disseminated intravascular coagulation	Spontaneous bleeding from the gums, nose, gastrointestinal tract, retinal hemorrhages and/or laboratory evidence of disseminated intravascular coagulation
9. Repeated generalized convulsions	≥3 generalized seizures within 24 hours
10. Hemoglobinuria	Macroscopic black, brown or red urine; not associated with effects of oxidant drugs or enzyme defects (like G6PD deficiency)
Added World Health Organization criteria from 2000	
11. Impaired consciousness	Various levels of impairment may indicate severe infection although not falling into the definition of cerebral malaria. These patients are generally arousable.
12. Prostration	Extreme weakness, needs support
13. Hyperparasitemia	5% parasitized erythrocytes or >250,000 parasites/µL (in nonimmune individuals)
14. Hyperpyrexia	Core body temperature above 40°C
15. Jaundice (Hyperbilirubinemia)	Plasma or serum bilirubin >50 mcmol/L (3 mg/dL)
Other (Not included in WHO)	
16. Severe thrombocytopenia	Platelet counts less than 10,000/ mm^3
17. Fluid and electrolyte disturbances	Dehydration, postural hypotension, clinical evidence of hypovolemia
18. Vomiting of oral drugs	Patients with persistent vomiting may have to be admitted for parenteral therapy
19. Complicating or associated infections	Aspiration bronchopneumonia, septicemia, urinary tract infection, etc.
20. Malarial retinopathy	In children dying with cerebral malaria, malarial retinopathy was found to be a better indicator of malarial coma. Similar retinopathy in an adult has also been reported

Investigations

Microscopy
- **Blood smears:** Diagnosis of malaria rests on the demonstration of asexual forms of the parasites in peripheral blood smears. Both thin and thick smears should be examined **(Fig. 15.10)**.
- **Quantitative buffy coat analysis (QBC):** In this test, the centrifuged buffy coat is stained with a flurochrome (e.g., acridine orange) that "lights up" malarial parasites when viewed under UV light.

Other Laboratory Findings
Rapid diagnostic tests: Detection of *P. falciparum*-specific histidine-rich protein-2 (HRP-2) and lactate dehydrogenase antigens in finger prick blood samples..
- **Blood:**
  - Normochromic normocytic anemia, thrombocytopenia.
  - Total leukocyte count is low to normal, but neutrophil leukocytosis may be observed in severe infections.
- **Acute-phase protein:** ESR, plasma viscosity, and levels of C-reactive protein are high.
- **Coagulation study:** In severe infections, prothrombin time, and partial thromboplastin time may be prolonged and antithrombin III levels are decreased.
- **Other findings in severe malaria:** In complicated malaria there may be metabolic acidosis and:
  - Low-plasma concentrations of glucose, sodium, bicarbonate, calcium, magnesium, and albumin.
  - Elevated levels of lactate, BUN, creatinine, muscle, and liver enzymes, bilirubin, and gamma globulin.
- *Neuroimaging in cerebral malaria* may show brain swelling, cortical infarcts, and hyperintense areas in white matter.

Management

Management of Uncomplicated Malaria
P. vivax malaria:
- Chloroquine is the drug of choice. It is given at a dose of 600 mg base (four tablets) stat, followed by 600 mg base (four tablets) on second day, followed by 300 mg base (two tablets) on third day.
- Primaquine is given at a dose of 15 mg daily for 14 days. It destroys the hypnozoite phase in the liver.

P. falciparum malaria:
- Chloroquine resistance in falciparum malaria is common and therefore, WHO recommends combination therapy for *P. falciparum* malaria.
- Artemisinin derivatives produce faster relief. This is known as **artemisinin-based combination therapy or ACT**. These combinations can then be taken for shorter durations than artemisinin alone.
- These combinations include
  - Artemether + Lumefantrine
  - Artesunate + Mefloquine
  - Dihydroatemisinin + Piperaquine
  - Artesunate + Sulfadoxine-Pyrimethamine.
- The ACT used in the national programme in India is artesunate + sulfadoxine –Pyrimethamine. It is given as:
  - 200 mg Artesunate along with Sulfadoxine 1,500 mg and Pyrimethamine 75 mg on day 1.
  - 200 mg Artesunate on days 2 and 3.
- ACTs can be given in second and third trimester of pregnancy. Recommended treatment in first trimester of pregnancy is quinine.
- To prevent spread of disease the patient should receive Primaquine in a single dose of 45 mg.

KALA-AZAR OR VISCERAL LEISHMANIASIS

Etiology
- Kala-azar (visceral leishmaniasis) is a generalized visceral infection by the organism *Leishmania donovani*. It affects the monocytes and macrophages of liver, spleen, bone marrow, and lymph nodes.
- The flagellated forms (promastigotes) of the organism develop within the female sandflies (*Phlebotomus argentipes*), which convey the disease to humans **(Fig. 15.11)**.

Clinical Features
- Some patients present with a low-grade fever, whereas others present with a high-grade, intermittent fever showing a double rise of temperature in 24 hours (camel-hump fever)
- Generalized pigmentation, particularly over face is common (kala-azar means black fever).
- Anemia, generalized lymphadenopathy
- Massive splenomegaly and hepatomegaly.

Investigations
- Anemia, granulocytopenia, and thrombocytopenia.
- Low-serum albumin and high-serum globulin, especially IgG.
- Mild elevation in bilirubin, AST/ALT, and alkaline phosphatase.
- Demonstration of amastigotes (LD bodies) in stained smears of aspirates of bone marrow, liver, spleen, lymph nodes or buffy coat of peripheral blood. Bone marrow is positive in 50–70% cases while splenic aspirate is positive in 70–90% cases.

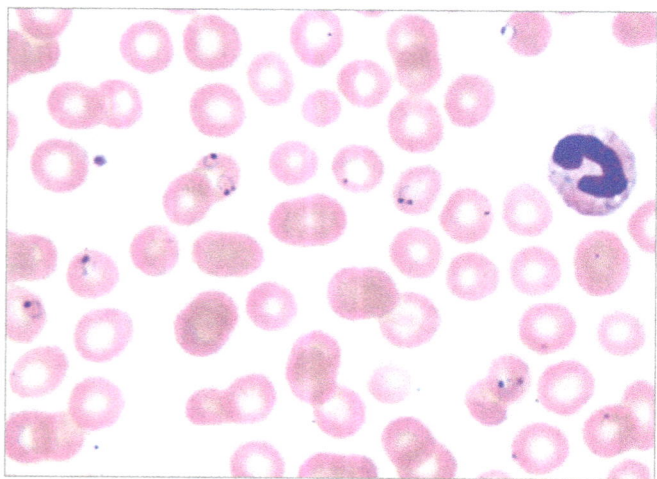

Fig. 15.10: Blood smears of malarial parasites.

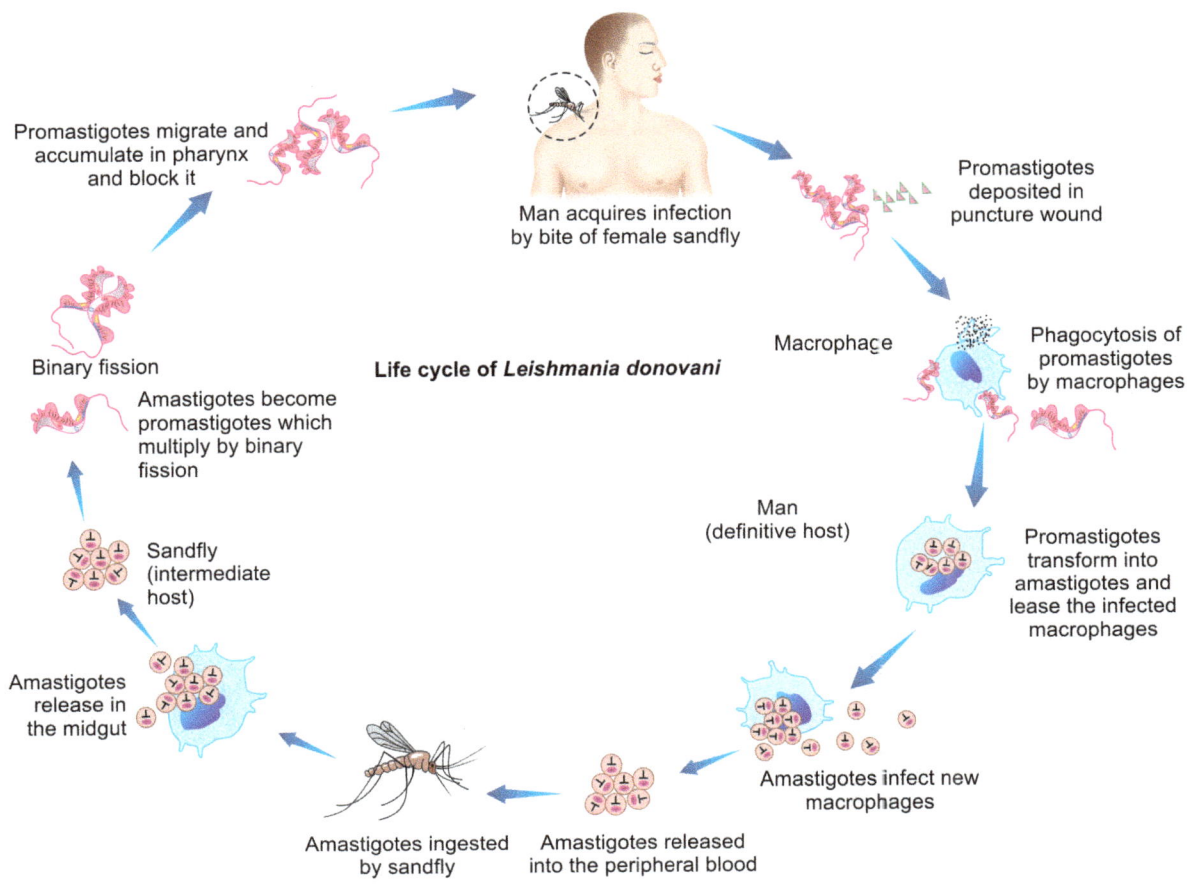

Fig. 15.11: Life cycle of *Leishmania donovani*.

- Culture of the aspiration in the Novy-MacNeal-Nicolle (NNN) medium for the organism.

Treatment
- Pentavalent antimonials
- Pentamidine
- Amphotericin B
- Miltefosine.

SEPSIS

Systemic Inflammatory Response Syndrome (SIRS)
- SIRS is the body's response to a clinical insult (e.g., infection, inflammation, stress, trauma, burns)
- Must have at least two of the following:
  - Temperature >38.5°C or <36°C
  - Heart rate >90 beats/min
  - Respiratory rate >20 breaths/min or $PaCO_2$ <32 mm Hg
  - WBC >12,000 cells/mm³, <4,000 cells/mm³, or >10% immature (band) forms.

Sepsis
Systemic inflammatory response syndrome plus suspected or confirmed infection (documented via cultures or visualized via physical exam/imaging). Latest definition of sepsis—*Sepsis is defined as life-threatening organ dysfunction caused by the dysregulated host response to infection.* (Sepsis = suspected infection PLUS q SOFA = 2) q SOFA- 3 criteria: Hypotension-systolic BP <100 mm Hg, altered mental status-GCS <13, respiratory rate >22 **(Table 15.14)**.

Table 15.14: Difference between severe sepsis and septic shock.

Severe sepsis	Septic shock

All three must be met within 6 hours:
1. Documentation of a **suspected source** of infection
2. Two or more manifestations of **SIRS** criteria:
  a. Temperature >38.3°C/101°F or <36°C/96.8°F
  b. Heart rate >90
  c. Respiratory rate >20
  d. WBC >12 or <4 or >10% bands
3. **Organ dysfunction,** evidenced by any one of the following:
  a. SBP <90 or MAP <65, or a SBP decrease of more than 40 pts
  b. Cr >2.0 or urine output <0.5 cc/kg/hour for 2 hours
  c. Bilirubin >2 mg/dL (32.4 mol/L)
  d. Platelet count <100
  e. INR >1.5 or PTT >60
  f. Lactate >2 mmol/L
4. Or if a provider documents severe sepsis, r/o sepsis, possible sepsis, or septic shock
	1. There must be documentation of septic shock present and
	2. **Tissue hypoperfusion** persisting in the hour after crystalloid fluid administration, evidenced by:
	  a. SBP <90
	  b. MAP <65
	  c. Decrease in SBP by >40 points from the patient's baseline
	  d. Lactate ≥4
	3. Or if the criteria are not met, but there is provider documentation of septic shock or suspected septic shock

Etiology

- Bacteria: Gram positive or gram negative
- Fungi
- Protozoa or rickettsiae.

Risk Factors for Sepsis

For risk factors for sepsis see **Table 15.15**.

Management of Sepsis (Table 15.16)

- Initial resuscitation – IV fluid Normal saline @30 mL/kg
- Send blood cultures
- Identify organ dysfunctions
- Control the source of sepsis
- Initiate broad spectrum antibiotics
- Vasopressors and inotropes to combat hypotension
- **Steroids:** If shock is not responding to initial fluid resuscitation
- Management of organ dysfunction (Ventilator support, Dialysis).

Table 15.15: Risk factors for sepsis.

Risk factors for sepsis	
Genetic polymorphism • Cytokine response • Coagulation • Mannose-binding protein	Intrinsic Factors • Age • Nutrition • Comorbidities • Vaccination
Procedures • Urinary catheters • IV cannula • Wound dressings	Community Factors • Contacts • Disease outbreaks • Specific exposure
Surgeries	Hospital Factors • Duration of stay • ICU stay • Local strain sensitivity patterns

Table 15.16: Early goal directed therapy (EGDT) for sepsis.

6-hour severe sepsis/septic shock bundle	24-hour severe sepsis and septic shock bundle

• **Early detection:** Obtain serum lactate level.
• **Early blood culture/antibiotics:** Within 3 hours of presentation.
• **Hypotension (SBP <90, MAP <65) or lactate >4 mmol/** Initial fluid bolus 20–40 mL of crystalloid (or colloid equivalent) per kg of body weight.
• **Vasopressors:**
  ▪ Hypotension not responding to fluid
  ▪ Titrate to MAP >65 mm Hg.
• **Septic shock or lactate >4 mmol/L:**
  ▪ CVP and ScvO$_2$ measured.
  ▪ CVP maintained >8 mm Hg.
  ▪ MAP maintain >65 mm Hg.
• **PRBCs (packed RBCs) if hematocrit <30%.**
• **Inotropes**
	• **Glucose control:** Maintained on average <150 mg/dL
	• **Drotrecogin alfa (activated):** Administered in accordance with clinical situation
	• **Steroids:** For septic shock requiring continued use of vasopressors for equal to or greater than 6 hours
	• **Lung protective strategy:** Maintain plateau pressures <30 cm H$_2$O for mechanically ventilated patients
	• **DVT prophylaxis**
	• **Early enteral nutrition**
	• **Stress ulcer prophylaxis**

HUMAN IMMUNODEFICIENCY VIRUS (HIV)/ ACQUIRED IMMUNODEFICIENCY SYNDROME (AIDS)

Characteristic Features

- The human immunodeficiency virus (HIV) causes Acquired immunodeficiency syndrome (AIDS)
- Former names of the virus include: Human T-cell lymphotropic virus (HTLV-III), lymphadenopathy associated virus (LAV), AIDS-associated retrovirus (ARV).
- Discovered independently by Dr Luc Montagnier, Dr Anthony Gallo, and Dr Jay Levy in 1983–84.
- It is an RNA virus belonging to the *Lentivirus* genus of the Retroviridae family
- HIV occurs in two genetically different but related main forms—HIV-1 and HIV-2 (**Fig. 15.12**).
- AIDS is defined as:
  - Clinical diagnosis of any stage 4 condition with confirmed HIV infection; OR
  - Immunological diagnosis with confirmed HIV infection and CD4+ <350/µL regardless of presence of symptoms.

Routes of Transmission of HIV

Routes of transmission of HIV have been described in **Table 15.17**.

Pathogenesis of HIV infection have been described in **Figure 15.13**.

Clinical Manifestations of HIV/AIDS

Acute Seroconversion

- An acute viral illness develops about 6 weeks after exposure.
- It presents with high fever, skin rash, headache, muscle pain, joint pain, and lymphadenopathy.
- This illness is self-limiting and lasts for 2–3 weeks.
- Usually, the person is in the "window period" and hence seronegative but during the recovery phase HIV antibody test often turns positive.
- Diagnosis can be diagnosed by nucleic acid amplification tests that detect viral genetic material from patient specimens p24 antigen.

Asymptomatic Carrier Stage

- The individual is asymptomatic but is potentially infectious for others.
- This stage may last for 5–10 years.
- Laboratory abnormalities may include anemia, leukopenia, lymphopenia, reduce CD4+ counts

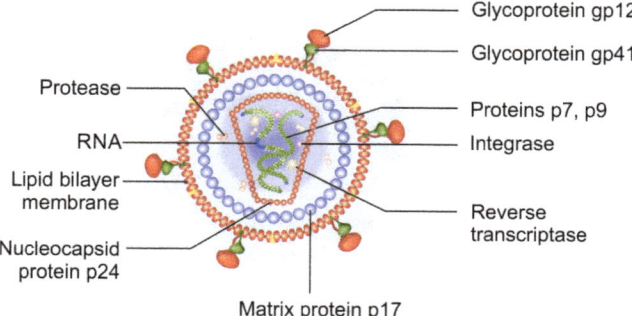

Fig. 15.12: Diagrammatic representation of structure of the human immune deficiency virus (HIV)-1 virion.

Table 15.17: Exposure route and percentage of transmission of HIV.

Exposure route	HIV transmission
Blood transfusion	90–95%
Perinatal	20–40%
Sexual intercourse:	
• Vaginal	0.05–0.1%
• Anal	0.065–0.82%
• Oral	0.005–0.01%
Injecting drugs use	0.63–2.14%
Needle stick exposure	0.13%
Mucous membrane splash to eye, oronasal	0.09%

Persistent Generalized Lymphadenopathy (PGL)

☐ Lymph node enlargement at two or more extra-inguinal sites that are noncontiguous that persist for more than 3 months in the absence of any other illness. The lymph nodes are more than 1 cm in size.
☐ Biopsy reveals nonspecific lymphoid hyperplasia.

HIV Constitutional Disease and AIDS-related Complex (ARC)

☐ ARC is diagnosed in a patient who has at least two of the following for more than 3 months.
 • Fever more than 38°C
 • Weight loss of more than 10% of body weight

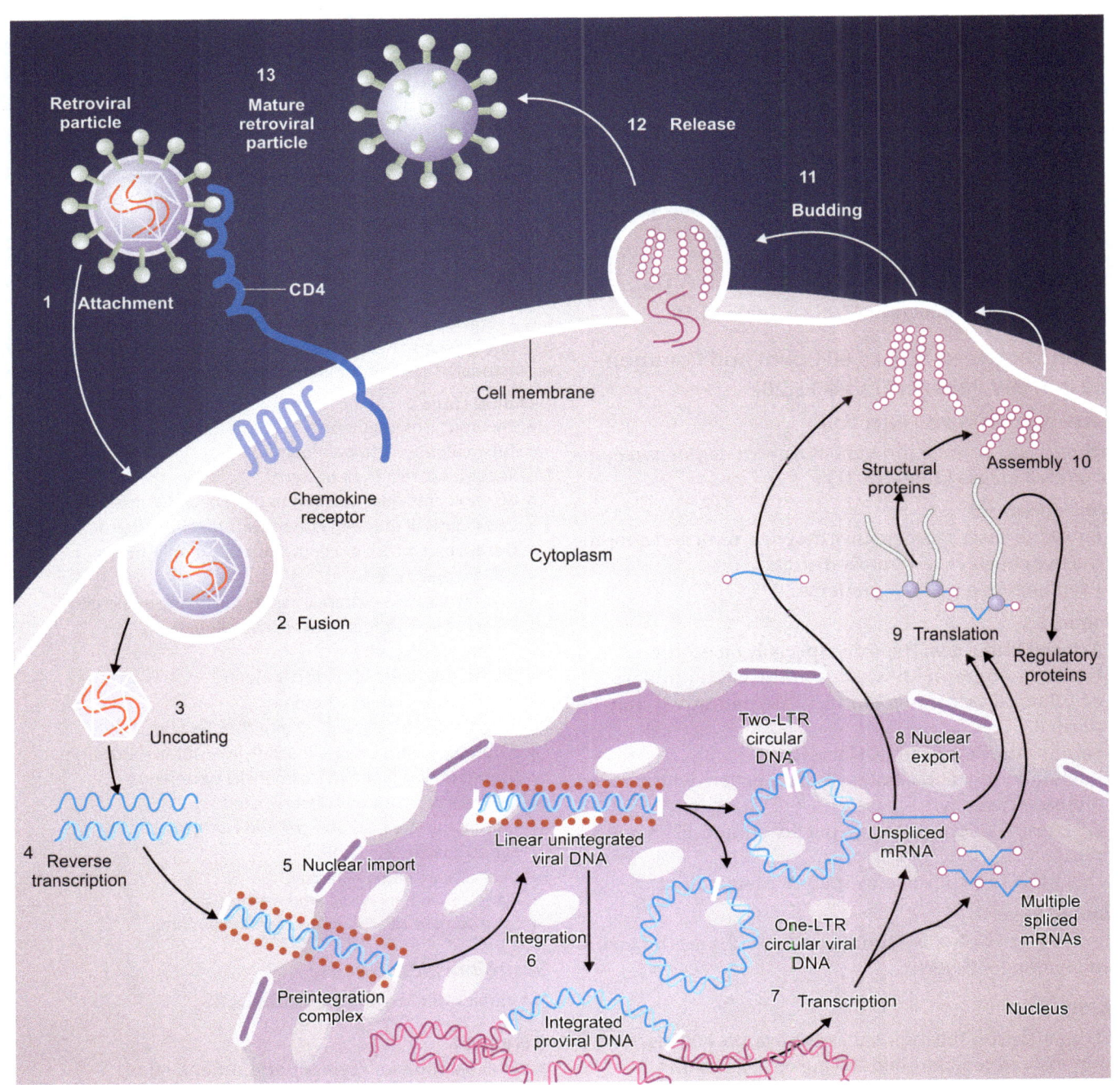

Fig. 15.13: Pathogenesis of HIV/AIDS.

- PGL
- Diarrhea
- Fatigue and night sweats
- Lymphopenia, leukopenia, and thrombocytopenia
- Reduced helper cells.
- Cutaneous energy.

❏ The condition of ARC with minor opportunistic infections like oral candidiasis is known as constitutional disease.

Full-blown AIDS

Within a few months of showing features of ARC, the CD4+ count drops 500/m³ and the patient develops a number of life-threatening infections and cancers.

HIV Clinical Staging and Classification

❏ Two clinical staging systems, namely the WHO and the Centers for Disease Control (CDC), are in use and are listed below **(Box 15.9 and Table 15.18)**.
❏ Note that the WHO clinical stage is used in low- and middle-income countries while the CDC clinical categories are used in high-income countries
❏ Clinical features of full-blown AIDS can be categorized into certain well-defined patterns (described further).

Oppurtunistic Infections and Cancers in AIDS

For infection and cancers in AIDS see **Table 15.19**.

Relation between CD4+ Cell Count and Common Illness in HIV Patients (Table 15.20)

Pneumocystis jiroveci Infection

Pneumocystis jiroveci (previously known as *Pneumocystis carinii*) is a fungus **(Table 15.21)**.

Clinical features:
❏ Subacute onset of progressive dyspnea, fever and nonproductive cough → respiratory distress
❏ Examination reveals crepitations.

Diagnosis:
❏ **Arterial blood gas:** Hypoxia especially on exertion
❏ Chest radiograph shows a ground-glass appearance or bilateral infiltrates but in some patients it may be normal.
❏ Serum shows elevated LDH levels.
❏ Pulmonary functions show restrictive pattern with reduced diffusion capacity.
❏ CT chest/Gallium-67 shows patchy ground-glass appearance.
❏ Diagnosis is established by sputum examination.

Management:
The drug of choice is trimethoprim/sulfamethoxazole combination for 21 days.

Prophylaxis
❏ Trimethoprim 160 mg + sulfamethoxazole 800 mg/day.
❏ Aerosolized pentamidine 300 mg once a month OR
❏ Dapsone 50 mg bid.

Box 15.9: WHO clinical staging classification of HIV infection.

Primary HIV Infection
❖ Asymptomatic
❖ Acute retroviral syndrome

Clinical Stage I
❖ Asymptomatic
❖ Persistent generalized lymphadenopathy

Clinical Stage 2
❖ Unexplained moderate weight loss (<10% of body weight)
❖ Recurrent upper respiratory tract infections (sinusitis, tonsillitis, otitis media, pharyngitis)
❖ Herpes zoster
❖ Angular cheilitis
❖ Recurrent oral ulceration
❖ Papular pruritic eruptions
❖ Seborrheic dermatitis
❖ Fungal nail infections

Clinical Stage 3
❖ Unexplained severe weight loss (>10% of body weight)
❖ Unexplained chronic diarrhea for longer than one month
❖ Unexplained persistent fever (above 37.5°C for >1 month)
❖ Persistent oral candidiasis
❖ Oral hairy leukoplakia
❖ Pulmonary tuberculosis
❖ Severe bacterial infections (e.g., Bacteremia, meningitis, pneumonia, empyema, bone, or joint infection)
❖ Acute necrotizing ulcerative stomatitis, gingivitis or periodontitis
❖ Unexplained anemia (<8 g/dL), neutropenia (<500/μL) or HIV associated immune thrombocytopenia (<50,000/μL) for >1 month

Clinical stage 4
❖ Pneumocystis pneumonia
❖ Tuberculosis—extrapulmonary
❖ Pneumonia, recurrent bacterial
❖ Disseminated non tuberculous mycobacterial infection
❖ Candidiasis of esophagus, trachea, bronchi, or lungs
❖ Disseminated coccidioidomycosis or histoplasmosis
❖ CNS Toxoplasmosis
❖ Cryptococcosis—extrapulmonary (including meningitis)
❖ Progressive multifocal leukoencephalopathy
❖ HIV encephalopathy
❖ Cryptosporidiosis, chronic (>1 month)
❖ Isosporiasis, chronic (>1 month)
❖ Chronic Herpes simplex (>1 month) infection
❖ Cytomegalovirus disease (outside liver, spleen and nodes)
❖ Recurrent non-typhoidal Salmonella bacteremia
❖ Leishmaniasis, atypical disseminated
❖ Lymphoma (cerebral or B-cell non-Hodgkin's)
❖ Kaposi's sarcoma
❖ Cervical carcinoma—invasive
❖ Symptomatic HIV-associated nephropathy
❖ Symptomatic HIV-associated cardiomyopathy

Gastrointestinal Disease

For causes of diarrhea see **Table 15.22**.

Treatment:
❏ Nitazoxanide for cryptosporidium infection.
❏ TMP-SMX for isosporiasis.

Table 15.18: CDC clinical staging classification of HIV infection.

Category A	Category B	Category C
• Asymptomatic • Primary HIV infection • Persistent generalized lymphadenopathy	• **Constitutional symptoms:** fever (38.5°C) or diarrhea for >1 month • Oropharyngeal Candidiasis • Oral hairy leukoplakia • **Herpes zoster:** Involving two separate episodes or more than one dermatome • Persistent vulvovaginal Candidiasis • Pelvic inflammatory disease, especially tubo-ovarian abscess • Cervical dysplasia (moderate or severe)/cervical carcinoma in situ • Bacillary angiomatosis • Listeriosis • Idiopathic thrombocytopenic purpura • Peripheral neuropathy	Same as WHO stage 4, with the following modifications: • Pulmonary tuberculosis included • Recurrent Salmonella septicemia
Note: Based on the absolute CD4+ counts, the stages may be further classified as follows:		
CD4+ count >500: **A1** CD4+ count >200–499: **A2** CD4+ count <200: **A3**	CD4+ count >500: **B1** CD4+ count >200–499: **B2** CD4+ count <200: **B3**	CD4+ count >500: **C1** CD4+ count >200–499: **C2** CD4+ count <200: **C3**

Table 15.19: Infection and cancers in AIDS.

Infections	Cancers
• *Pneumocystis jiroveci* • *Candida* • *Cryptococcus* • *Toxoplasma* • Typical/atypical mycobacteria • Amebiasis	• Kaposi's sarcoma • B-cell lymphoma of brain • Others

Table 15.20: Relation between CD4+ cell count and common illness in HIV patients.

CD4+ count	Illnesses
200–350/µL	• Herpes simplex • Tuberculosis • Oral and vaginal thrush • Herpes zoster
100–200/µL	• *Pneumocystis jiroveci* pneumonia • *Candida* esophagitis
50–100/µL	• Cryptococcal meningitis • AIDS dementia • Toxoplasma encephalitis
<50/µL	• Progressive multifocal leukoencephalopathy • *Mycobacterium avium* complex • Cytomegalovirus infection

Table 15.21: Treatment of *Pneumocystis jiroveci* infection.

Mild cases	Moderate to severe cases (PaO$_2$<70 mm Hg)
• Trimethoprim + sulfamethoxazole • Trimethoprim + dapsone OR • Pentamidine IV OR • Atovaquone	• Trimethoprim + sulfamethoxazole OR • Pentamidine OR • Clindamycin + primaquine • In all cases, add prednisolone

Table 15.22: Causes of diarrhea in HIV.

Infections	HIV related
• *Salmonella* • *Shigella* • *Campylobacter* • *Escherichia coli* • *Cryptosporidium* • *Giardia* • *Isospora* • *Microsporidium* • *Entamoeba histolytica* • CMV • *Mycobacterium avium complex*	• HIV invading gut epithelium **GI malignancies** • Lymphoma • Kaposi's sarcoma

Oral Manifestations of HIV/AIDS
See **Box 15.10**.

Neurological Disease

AIDS Dementia Complex (ADC)
It precedes the white matter of lateral and posterior columns of the spinal cord resulting in spastic paraparesis and sensory ataxia. The onset is subacute.

Viral Infections

- Progressive multifocal leucoencephalopathy (PML) is caused by the polyoma virus [JC virus (JCV)] and is characterized by focal neurological abnormalities including blindness, aphasia, hemiparesis, and ataxia that progress to altered sensorium and death within 6 months.
- MRI → white matter lesions in areas of the brain corresponding to clinical deficits.
- Confirmation is by PCR to identify JCV DNA in CSF.
- Treatment is mainly by starting ART.

> **Box 15.10:** Oral manifestations of HIV/AIDS.
> - Xerostomia
> - Candidiasis
> - Oral hairy leukoplakia
> - Periodontal diseases such as linear gingival erythema and necrotizing ulcerative periodontitis
> - Kaposi's sarcoma
> - Bacillary angiomatosis
> - Human papilloma virus-associated warts
> - Ulcerative conditions including herpes simplex virus lesions, recurrent aphthous ulcers, and neutropenic ulcers.
> - Hairy tongue
> - HIV—salivary gland disease, and pigmentation disorders
> - Rarely—lymphoma, tuberculosis, MAC infection

Fungal Infections

- Cryptococcal meningitis may present with headache and fever.
- Cryptococcal antigen and culture are usually positive, both in serum and CSF.
- India ink staining on CSF may show the organisms.
- Treatment is by administering amphotericin B and flucytosine for 2 weeks followed by fluconazole for 8–10 weeks.

Protozoan Infections

- Toxoplasma encephalitis presents with headache, confusion, seizures, ataxia and focal deficits.
- A contrast CT scan → single or multiple contrast enhancing lesions often with surrounding hypodensity due to edema.
- Patients are seropositive for antitoxoplasma IgG antibodies.
- Treatment is by a combination of pyrimethamine + sulfadiazine + leukovorin for at least 6 weeks.
- Prophylaxis indicated in toxoplasma-seropositive patients with a CD4+ count <100 cells/µL. One double-strength tablet of TMP-SMX daily is the preferred regimen.
- If patients cannot tolerate TMP-SMX, alternative is dapsone + pyrimethamine + Leukovorin.

Mycobacterium Avium Complex (MAC)

- Usually occurs if CD4+ <50/µL
- Often presents with disseminated multiorgan infection (hepatomegaly, splenomegaly, and lymphadenopathy) along with fever, night sweats, weight loss, fatigue, diarrhea, and abdominal pain.
- Anemia and raised alkaline phosphatase are common.
- Blood, bone marrow or lymph node aspirate may grow the organisms
- Chemoprophylaxis: Azithromycin or clarithromycin
- Treatment includes use of clarithromycin + ethambutol + rifabutin.

Laboratory Diagnosis of HIV Infection

Antibodies against the virus are detectable within 3–12 weeks after infection. Most commonly, enzyme-linked immunosorbent assay (ELISA) is employed for screening while confirmation is done by Western blot test (**Flowchart 15.2**).

- Other findings include lymphopenia, leukopenia, thrombocytopenia, and decrease in T4–helper cells (CD4+ counts).

Flowchart 15.2: Testing algorithm used to determine the HIV infection.

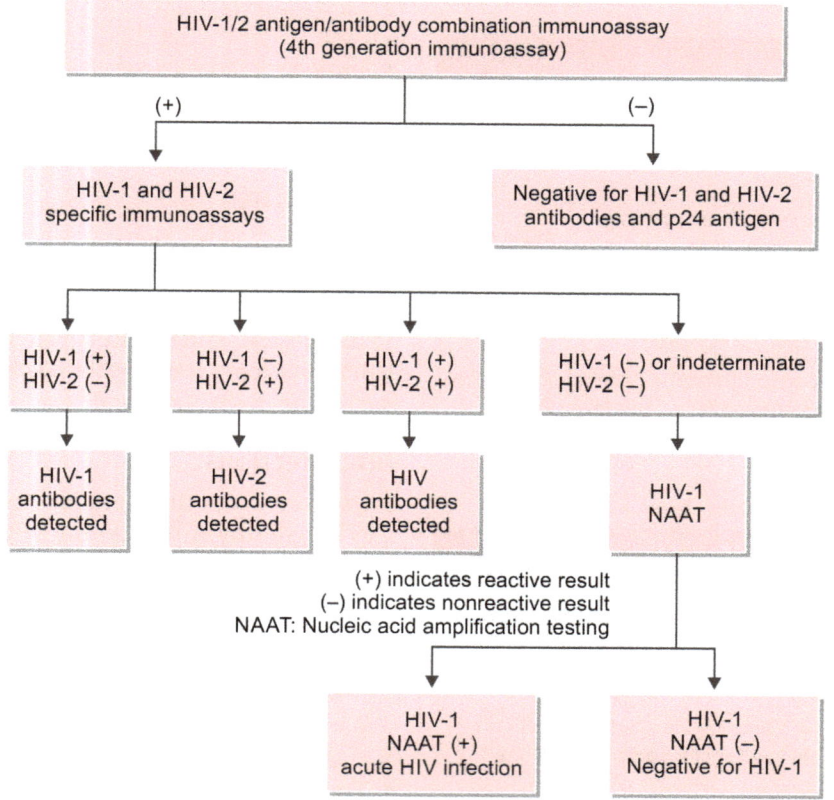

- Other tests include
  - Antigen detection (p24 assays) and
  - Polymerase chain reaction (PCR) for measuring the amount of viral particles (HIV RNA) in the blood (viral load).

Management of a Patient with HIV Infection

General Measures

- These include balanced diet, quitting smoking and intake of alcohol, adequate rest and practice of safer sex so as to avoid infection of partner and also to avoid infection with other organism that may hasten the progress of the disease.
- An important aspect of treatment is counseling and proper education of the patient.
- **Treatment of common opportunistic infections in AIDS (Table 15.23)**

Antiretroviral Drugs

For antiretrovial drugs see **Box 15.11**.

Indications for Antiretroviral Therapy

For indications for antiretroviral therapy see **Table 15.24**.

Table 15.23: Treatment of common opportunistic infections in AIDS.

Opportunistic infection	First line treatment	Alternate treatment
Pneumocystis jiroveci	See text	See text
Toxoplasma	Pyrimehamine +sulfadiazine	Pyrimethamine +clindamycin
Cryptococcus	Amphotericin +Flucytosine	Amphotericin
Isospora belli	Co-trimoxazole	–
Candida (mucosal)	Clotrimazole OR fluconazole	Ketoconazole
Candida (systemic)	Amphotericin	–
Cytomegalovirus	Ganciclovir	Foscarnet 60 mg/kg TID
H. simplex (oral)	Acyclovir	–
H. simplex (encephalitis)	Acyclovir	Vidarabine
Herpes Zoster (local)	Acyclovir	–
Herpes zoster (disseminated)	Acyclovir	Vidarabine

Antiretroviral Regimens

Most commonly used regimens include a PI with two NRTIs, or one NNRTI with two NRTIs or three NRTIs.

Box 15.11: Antiretroviral drugs.

Nucleoside reverse transcriptase inhibitors (NRTIs):
- Zidovudine
- Didanosine
- Zalcitabine
- Stavudine
- Lamivudine
- Abacavir
- Emtricitabine

Non-nucleoside reverse transcriptase inhibitors (NNRTIs):
- Nevirapine
- Delavirdine
- Efavirenz

Nucleotide reverse transcriptase inhibitor (nRTI): Tenofovir disoproxil fumarate

Fusion inhibitors: Enfuvirtide

Protease inhibitors (PIs)
- Indinavir
- Ritonavir
- Saquinavir
- Nelfinavir
- Amprenavir
- Lopinavir/ritonavir
- Atazanavir
- Fosamprenavir
- Tipranavir
- Darunavir

Integrase inhibitors: Raltegravir

CCR5 inhibitors: Maraviroc

Entry inhibitor (Post attachment): Ibalizumab

Others:
- Amprenavir
- Fosamprenavir
- Nelfinavir
- Saquinavir
- Tipranavir/ritonavir

Cobicistat:
- CYP3A4 inhibitor without antiretroviral activity
- Used as a boosting agent.
- Increases plasma drug concentrations, half-life and maximum plasma concentrations, thus improving the potency of the antiviral agent.
- This allows lower and less frequent dosing of the parent drug, thus reducing the burden of pills.

Table 15.24: Indications for antiretroviral therapy.

Clinical category	CD4+cell count	Plasma HIV RNA	Recommendations
Symptomatic HIV disease (stage 3 and 4)	Any value	Any value	Start HAART
Asymptomatic	<200/mm³	Any value	Start HAART
Asymptomatic	200–350/mm³	Any value	Start HAART
Asymptomatic	350/mm³	100,000	Some experts recommend Starting HAART
Asymptomatic	350/mm³	<100,000	Defer HAART

Box 15.12: Combination of drugs.

Preferred regimens
INSTI + 2 NRTIs preferred:
1. Bictegravir-emtricitabine-tenofovir alafenamide
2. Dolutegravir + tenofovir alafenamide-emtricitabine
3. Dolutegravir-abacavir-lamivudine

Note: Tenofovir alafenamide-emtricitabine is the preferred NRTI combination

Alternative regimens
INSTI-based regimens:
- Elvitegravir/cobicistat-emtricitabine-tenofovir alafenamide
- Raltegravir plus tenofovir alafenamide-emtricitabine

PI-based regimens:
- Atazanavir (boosted with ritonavir or cobicistat) plus tenofovir alafenamide-emtricitabine
- Darunavir (boosted with ritonavir or cobicistat) plus tenofovir alafenamide-emtricitabine

NNRTI-based regimens:
- Doravirine plus tenofovir alafenamide-emtricitabine
- Efavirenz plus tenofovir alafenamide-emtricitabine
- Efavirenz-emtricitabine-tenofovir disoproxil fumarate

When tenofovir (TAF or TDF) and abacavir cannot be used:
- Darunavir (boosted with ritonavir or cobicistat) plus dolutegravir
- Darunavir (boosted with ritonavir or cobicistat) plus lamivudine
- Dolutegravir-lamivudine

Recommended Combination of Drugs
See **Box 15.12**.

Immune Reconstitution Inflammatory Syndrome

- The constellation of clinical symptoms, signs or investigational parameters resulting from such inflammatory response is called immune reconstitution inflammatory syndrome (IRIS).
- Treatment includes continuation of primary therapy against the offending pathogen and continuation of effective HAART and judicious use of anti-inflammatory agents.
- In severe cases, a short course of steroids may be indicated.

Post-exposure Prophylaxis (PEP) Regimens

- 3-drug regimen recommended-2 NRTIs plus a third drug [preferably an integrase strand transfer inhibitor (INSTI), or a ritonavir-boosted protease inhibitor (PI)].
- Preferred regimen (CDC 2016):
  - Tenofovir 300 mg plus Emtricitabine 200 mg PO OD PLUS
  - Dolutegravir 50 mg orally once daily or Raltegravir 400 mg orally twice daily
  - PEP should be initiated promptly, preferably within 1–2 hours postexposure and is continued for 4 weeks.

SEXUALLY TRANSMITTED INFECTIONS

Sexually transmitted disease (STD) are a group of communicable diseases that are transmitted predominantly by sexual contact and caused by a wide range of bacterial, viral, protozoal, and fungal agents and ectoparasites (**Table 15.25**).

Table 15.25: Sexually transmitted infections.

Bacterial agents	Viral agents
• Neisseria gonorrhea • Chlamydia trachomatis • Haemophilus ducreyi • Mycoplasma hominis • Ureaplasma urealyticum • Calymmatobacterium granulomatis • Shigella spp. • Group B Streptococcus • Bacterial vaginitis associated organisms	• Human (alpha) herpesvirus • Human (beta) herpesvirus • Hepatitis B virus • Human papillomavirus • Molluscum contagiosum virus. • Human immunodeficiency virus
Protozoal agents	**Fungal agents**
• Entamoeba histolytica • Giardia lamblia • Trichomonas vaginalis	Candida albicans **Ectoparasites** Phthirus pubis Sarcoptes scabiei

Gonorrhea

Gonorrhea is a sexually transmitted infection (STI) due to the gram-negative diplococcus, *Neisseria gonorrheae*.

- **Mode of transmission:** Genital-genital, genital-anorectal, oro-genital or oro-anal contact or from mother-to-child transmission during delivery.
- **Incubation period:** usually 2–10 days following exposure.
- **Clinical features:**
  - *Gonococcal infections in men:* Acute urethritis
  - *Gonococcal infections in women:* Gonococcal cervicitis and vaginitis. It may be asymptomatic in up to 80% of women.
  - *Anorectal and pharyngeal gonorrhea:* are usually asymptomatic.
  - Ocular gonorrhea.
  - *Disseminated gonococcal infection (DGI):* Arthritis of one or more joints (asymmetric and migratory), pustular skin lesions, fever, and tenosynovitis. Gonococcal endocarditis or meningitis may rarely occur.
  - Acute perihepatits (Fitz-Hugh-Curtis syndrome) is a rare complication of PID, and is thought to occur through direct extension of *N. gonorrheae* from fallopian tube to liver capsule and peritoneum along the paracolic gutters. Patients present with sharp, pleuritic right upper quadrant pain.
- **Diagnosis**
  - **Gram's staining and culture** of urethral exudates, genital, rectal, pharyngeal or ocular secretions show gram-negative intracellular monococci and diplococci.
  - **Sterile pyuria:** Urine may show polymorphonuclear leucocytes with a negative urine culture report.
- **Complications:**
  - *In females:* It causes pelvic inflammatory disease PID (pelvic inflammatory disease). Local complications such as endometritis, salpingitis, tubo-ovarian abscess, bartholinitis, peritonitis, and perihepatitis.
  - *In male patients:* Periurethritis, epididymitis epididymo-orchitis, and prostatitis.
  - *Newborns:* Ophthalmia neonatorum in newborns.
- **Treatment (Box 15.13)**

Box 15.13: Treatment of gonorrhea.

- One of the following regimens is recommended at present:
  - Cefixime 400 mg orally (single dose)
  - Ceftriaxone 250 mg intramuscularly (single dose)
  - Spectinomycin 2 g intramuscularly (single dose)
- If quinolone and azithromycin resistance is not a problem:
  - Ciprofloxacin 500 mg orally (single dose)
  - Ofloxacin 400 mg orally (single dose)
  - Levofloxacin 250 mg orally (single dose)
  - Azithromycin 2 g orally (single dose)
- For epididymo-orchitis doxycycline 100 mg twice daily for 14 days along with one dose of ceftriaxone or ciprofloxacin.

Nongonococcal Urethritis

For nongonococcal urethritis see **Table 15.26**.

Treatment
- Doxycycline 100 mg twice daily for 7 days OR
- Azithromycin 1G orally.

Alternatives
- Erythromycin base 500 mg four times for 7 days OR
- Ofloxacin 300 mg twice daily for 7 days OR
- Levofloxacin 500 mg once daily for 7 days
- All sex partners in last 60 days should be evaluated and treated
- Sexual abstinence till completion of treatment.
- Points with NGU reviewed 2–3 weeks after treatment to confirm resolution of symptoms and treatment of sexual contacts.
- Should be checked for other STIs including syphilis and HIV, results of tests checked during review.

Table 15.26: Causes of nongonococcal urethritis.

Chlamydia trachomatis (15–40%)	Mycoplasma genitalium (15–25%)
Others (20–50%) • Trichomonas vaginalis • Ureaplasma urealiticum • Herpes simplex virus (in absence of skin lesions) • Adenovirus • Hemophilus	Miscellaneous In association with urinary tract infection, bacterial prostatitis, urethral stricture, phimosis, secondary to instrumentation of the urethra, congenital abnormalities, chemical irritation, tumors

SYPHILIS

- Syphilis (lues) is a **chronic,** systemic infection **caused by spirochete *Treponema pallidum*** is usually **sexually transmitted.** Spirochetes are gram-negative, slender corkscrew-shaped bacteria **(Fig. 15.14).**
- **Mode of transmission:**
  - **Sexual contact:** It is the usual mode of spread.
  - **Transplacental transmission:** From mother with active disease to the fetus (during pregnancy) → congenital syphilis.
  - **Blood transfusion**
  - **Direct contact:** With the open lesion is rare mode of transmission.
- **Classification:** Classification of syphilis is shown in Table 15.27.

Acquired Syphilis

Primary syphilis

Primary chancre (Fig. 15.15): It is the classical lesion of primary syphilis.
- **Location:** The primary chance develop at the site of inoculation.
  - *In males:* **Penis or scrotum** in males (in heterosexual) and in homosexual males, it may occur in the anal canal, rectum, or within the mouth
  - *In females:* **Cervix, vulva,** and **vaginal** wall.
- Primary chance is single, firm, **nontender (painless)**, slightly raised, **red papule** (chance) up to several centimeters in diameter. It rapidly becomes eroded to create a clean-based shallow ulcer. Because of the induration surrounding the ulcer, it is designated as **hard chancre**.

Regional Lymphadenitis

Secondary Syphilis

Mucocutaneous lesions: These are painless, superficial lesions, and contain spirochetes and are infectious.
- **Skin rashes (75%):** They begin as **discrete red-brown macules (Fig. 15.16A)**
- **Condylomata lata (10%):** In moist, warm, intertriginous areas of the skin, such as the **anogenital region (perineum, vulva, and scrotum)**, inner thighs, and axillae **(Fig. 15.16B)**.
- **Mucosal lesions (30%):** Usually occurs in the mucous membranes of **oral cavity** (**lip, oral** mucosa, tongue, palate, and pharynx) or vulva, vagina, or glans penis

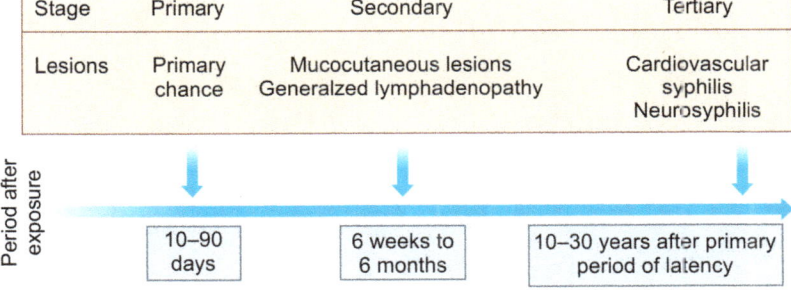

Fig. 15.14: Course of syphilis (if untreated).

Table 15.27: Classification of syphilis.

Acquired syphilis	Congenital syphilis
A. Primary syphilis B. Secondary syphilis C. Latent syphilis D. Late syphilis (tertiary) • Late latent • Benign tertiary • Quaternary syphilis (cardiovascular and neurosyphilis)	• Intrauterine death and perinatal death. • Early (infantile) • Late (tardive)

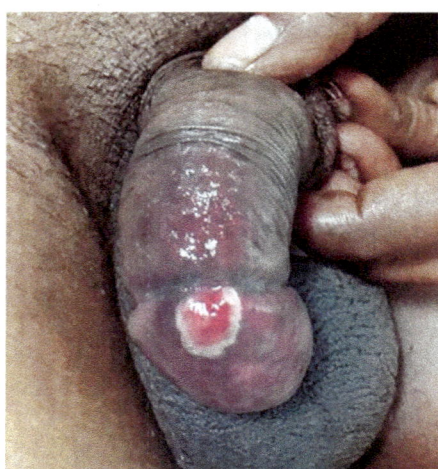

Fig. 15.15: Primary chancre.

as **silvery-gray superficial** mucosal **erosions**. They are surrounded by a red serpiginous periphery and are usually painless. Rarely, they may coalesce to produce characteristic "snail track" ulcers in the mouth.
❒ **Generalized painless lymphadenopathy:** Generalized, firm nontender lymphadenopathy occurs in about 50% of patients. They involve especially **epitrochlear nodes**
❒ **Less common manifestations** include meningitis, cranial nerve palsies, anterior or posterior uveitis, hepatitis, gastritis, glomerulonephritis (proteinuria, nephrotic syndrome or hemorrhagic glomerulonephritis), or arthritis and periostitis.

Latent syphilis:
❒ **Early latency (within 1 year of infection):** During this period syphilis may be transmitted sexually.
❒ **Late latency (begins at 1 year of infection):** During this, the patient is no longer sexually infectious. Pregnant women with latent syphilis may infect the fetus in utero.

Late (Tertiary) Syphilis

Late latent syphilis:
❒ This phase may persist for many years or for life.
❒ No symptoms or signs of syphilis.
❒ More than 60% of patients suffer little or no ill health even without treatment.

Benign tertiary (gummatous) syphilis:
❒ It is called benign because of its response to therapy rather than its clinical manifestations.
❒ It may develop after 3–10 years after initial infection.
❒ **Structures involved:** Skin (frequently at sites of trauma as nodules or ulcers), mucous membranes (mouth, pharynx, larynx, or nasal septum appear as punched-out ulcers), bone (e.g., skull, tibia, fibula, and clavicle) muscle, or viscera (e.g., liver- hepar lobatum, spleen).

Quaternary syphilis:
❒ **Cardiovascular syphilis**
  • May present many years after initial infection.
  • Most **frequently involves the aorta** (the ascending aorta aortic valve and/or the coronary ostia, the aortic arch) and known as syphilitic aortitis.
  • Clinical features include angina, features of aortic incompetence, and aortic aneurysm.
❒ **Neurosyphilis:** It may take years to develop. It may be asymptomatic or symptomatic.
  • *Asymptomatic neurosyphilis:* It is detected by CSF examination, which shows pleocytosis (increased numbers of inflammatory cells), elevated protein levels, or decreased glucose. Antibodies can also be detected in the CSF, which is the most specific test for neurosyphilis.
  • *Symptomatic disease:* Takes one of several forms
    ▪ Chronic meningovascular disease: Chronic meningitis → involves base of the brain, cerebral convexities and spinal leptomeninges.

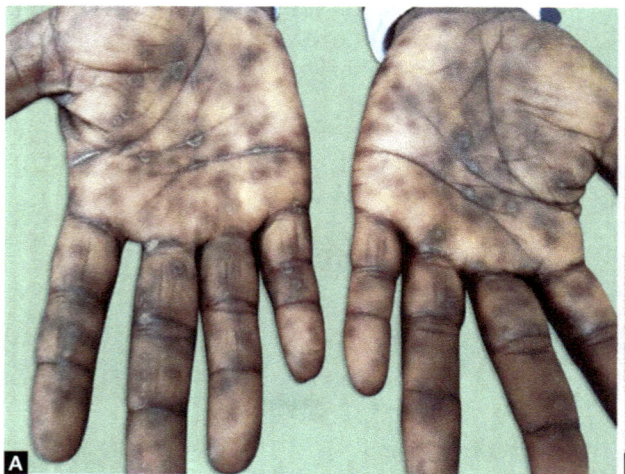 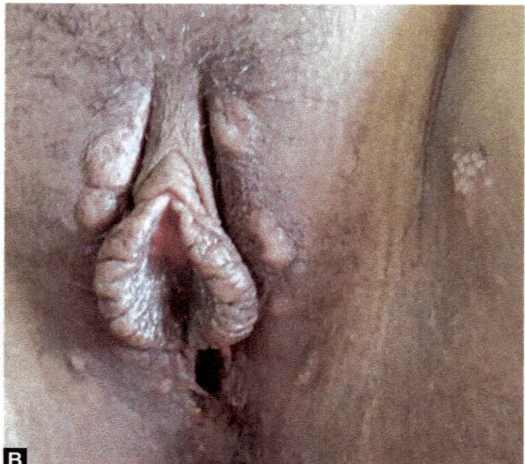

Figs. 15.16A and B: (A) Symmetrical skin rashes of secondary syphilis on palm; (B) Condyloma lata.

- Tabes dorsalis: It is characterized by **demyelination of posterior column, dorsal root, and dorsal root ganglia**.
- General paresis of insane: Shows generalized brain parenchymal disease with dementia; hence called as general paresis of insane.

Congenital Syphilis

- **Intrauterine death and perinatal death.**
- **Early (infantile) congenital syphilis**: It manifests within the **first 2 years of life** and often manifested by **nasal discharge (rhinitis)** and congestion **(snuffles)**. They resemble features of secondary syphilis.
- A **desquamating or bullous eruption/rash** can lead to epidermal sloughing of the skin, mainly in the hands, feet, around the mouth and anus. Also may show condyloma lata.
- **Skeletal abnormalities**: Syphilitic osteochondritis (inflammation of bone and cartilage is more distinctive in the nose → produces characteristic **saddle nose deformity**), syphilitic periostitis (involves the tibia and leads to anterior bowing, or **saber shin**).
- Others organs involved include **liver** (diffuse fibrosis) and **lungs (airless-pneumonia alba)**.

Late (tardive) congenital syphilis:
- Manifests **2 years after birth**, and about 50% of untreated children with neonatal syphilis will develop late manifestations and take the form of "stigmata" relating to early damage to developing structures, particularly teeth and long bones **(Table 15.25)**.

> **Box 15.14:** Stigmata of congenital syphilis.
> - Hutchinson's incisors (anterior-posterior thickening with notch on narrowed cutting edge)
> - Mulberry molars (imperfectly formed cusps/deficient dental enamel)
> - High-arched palate
> - Maxillary hypoplasia
> - Saddle nose
> - Rhagades (radiating scars around mouth, nose and anus following rash)
> - Salt and pepper scars on retina (from choroiditis)
> - Corneal scars (from interstitial keratitis)
> - Sabre tibia (from periostitis)
> - Bossing of frontal and parietal bones (healed periosteal nodes)

- **Distinctive manifestation is Hutchinson's triad is:** (1) **interstitial keratitis, Hutchinson's teeth** (small widely spaced screwdrivers or peg-shaped upper central incisors, with notches in the enamel), and (2) **eighth-nerve deafness**. Stigmata of congenital syphilis are listed in **Box 15.14**.

Laboratory Diagnosis

Demonstration of Treponema pallidum.
- Dark-field microcopy:
- Direct fluorescent antibody T.pallidum (DFA-TP) test
- Serological tests **(Table 15.28)**

Management

Management of syphilis is described in **Table 15.29**.

Table 15.28: Sensitivity of serological tests in untreated syphilis.

Test	Stage of disease (percent positive [range])			
	Primary	Secondary	Latent	Tertiary
VDRL	78 (74–87)	100	95 (88–100)	71 (37–94)
RPR	86 (77–99)	100	98 (95–100)	73
FTA-ABS*	84 (70–100)	100	100	96
Treponemal agglutination*	76 (69–90)	100	97 (97–100)	94
EIA	93	100	100	

*FTA-ABS and TP-PA are generally considered equally sensitive in the primary stage of disease.

Table 15.29: Management of syphilis.

Stage	Drug	Regimen
Primary	Procaine penicillin	6,00,000 units IM once daily for 12 days
	Oxytetracycline	500 mg orally four times daily for 15 days
	Doxycycline	100 mg orally two times daily for 15 days
	Benzathine penicillin	2.4 mega (million) units IM single dose (1.2 million units in each buttock)
Secondary	Procaine penicillin	6,00,000 units IM once daily for 15 days
	Benzathine penicillin	2.4 million units IM single dose
Early latent	Benzathine penicillin	2.4 million units IM single dose
Late latent/tertiary	Benzathine penicillin	2.4 million units IM weekly for 3 weeks
Cardiovascular	Benzathine penicillin	4 million units IM weekly for 3 weeks
Neurosyphilis	Crystalline penicillin	18–24 million units/day for 10–14 days
	Procaine penicillin PLUS Probenecid	2.4 million units/day IM for 10–14 days FLUS 500 mg QID for 10–14 days

PYREXIA OF UNKNOWN ORIGIN (PUO)

Fever of minimum 3 weeks' duration with daily temperatures raising more than 101°F and the cause of which is not diagnosed even after investigating in hospital for 1 week.

Types
- Classic PUO
- Nosocomial PUO
- Neutropenic PUO
- HIV-associated PUO.

Common Causes of Prolonged Fever
Common causes of prolonged fever are listed in **Table 15.30**.

Investigations
Investigations for PUO are listed in **Table 15.31**.

Treatment
- Treatment of underlying cause detected after investigations
- Empirical broad-spectrum antibiotics
- Empirical antitubercular treatment.

Table 15.30: Common causes of prolonged fever.

Infections:	Neoplasms:	Connective tissue disorders:
• Tuberculosis • Malaria • Typhoid • Infective endocarditis • Urinary tract infections • Perinephric abscesses • Liver abscess • Abdominal abscesses • Pelvic inflammatory diseases • HIV infection	• Lymphomas • Leukemia • Gastrointestinal malignancies • Metastatic tumors of liver • Hypernephroma • Atrial myxomas	• Systemic lupus erythematosus • Rheumatoid arthritis • Temporal arteritis • Polyarteritis nodosa (PAN)
Miscellaneous: • Drug fever (sulfonamides, aminoglycosides, penicillin) • Multiple pulmonary thromboembolism • Hemolytic anemia • Thyroiditis • Granulomatous hepatitis • Cyclic neutropenia.	**Psychogenic fevers:** • Habitual hyperthermia • Factitious fever • Fabricated fever	**Periodic fevers:** Familial Mediterranean fever (polyserositis).

Table 15.31: Investigations for PUO.

Laboratory tests:	Serological tests:	Radiographic examination:
• Complete blood picture • ESR • Peripheral smear examination • Urine routine and microscopy • Blood and urine culture • Renal and liver function tests • Mantoux test	• ASO titer • Rheumatoid factor • Antinuclear antibodies • Viral antibody titers • Brucella agglutination test	• Chest radiography • Barium GI series • Echocardiography • Ultrasonography of abdomen and pelvis • CT scan of abdomen and thorax • PET scans.
Biopsy: • Bone marrow biopsy • Liver biopsy • Lymph node biopsy	**Diagnostic surgical procedures:** • Peritoneoscopy • Laparoscopy • Bronchoscopy • Exploratory laparotomy	

OBJECTIVE-BASED SELF-EVALUATION

SHORT ANSWER QUESTIONS

1. Discuss the modes of transmission and clinical staging of HIV infection.
2. Discuss enteric fever under the headings: (a) Causative agent, (b) Clinical features, (c) Complications, (d) Diagnosis, and (e) Management.
3. Discuss the clinical features, complications, and management of infectious mononucleosis.
4. Discuss the etiology, clinical features, complications, and treatment of malaria.
5. Discuss syphilis under headings: (a) Causative agent, (b) Clinical features, (c) Diagnosis, and (d) Management.
6. Discuss the clinical features, complications, and management of dengue fever.
7. Discuss the clinical features, complications, and management of leptospirosis.
8. Discuss the clinical features, complications, and management of COVID-19.

9. Discuss the clinical features, complications, and management of infectious mononucleosis.
10. Discuss the clinical features, complications, and management of diphtheria.

SHORT ANSWER QUESTIONS

1. Post-exposure prophylaxis for HIV after needlestick injury
2. List four common opportunistic infections in HIV/AIDS
3. WHO staging of HIV
4. Enumerate antiretroviral drugs
5. List the differences between bacillary and amoebic dysentery
6. Oral manifestations of HIV/AIDS
7. Complications of mumps/measles/rubella
8. Congenital rubella syndrome
9. Define PUO. List the types
10. Clinical features/stigmata of congenital syphilis
11. Complications of gonorrhea
12. Define sepsis and SIRS
13. List the complications of malaria
14. List the common causes of food poisoning
15. Complications of chickenpox
16. Ramsay-Hunt syndrome
17. Mucormycosis

MULTIPLE CHOICE QUESTIONS

1. A week after his return to the USA from India a 45-year-old man he develops fevers and a blood test confirms the presence of falciparum malaria. What is the most appropriate treatment:
   a. Quinidine
   b. Chloroquine
   c. Artesunate
   d. Praziquantel

2. A young executive developed abdominal pain, diarrhea and fevers 1 week prior to his return. On examination, he has a fever of 38.5°C relative bradycardia and diffuse abdominal pain. Stool microscopy shows pus cells and red blood cells, culture is awaited. What is the most likely organism?
   a. *Plasmodium falciparum*
   b. Norwalk virus
   c. Rotavirus
   d. *Salmonella* species

3. A 16-year-old student with fever and sore throat has gray plaques on his tonsils, cervical lymphadenopathy, and splenomegaly. What is the most likely diagnosis?
   a. *Streptococcus* infection
   b. *Borrelia vincenti* infection
   c. Diphtheria
   d. Infectious mononucleosis

4. A 14-year-old student presents with 1-day history of rash, which has followed a 3-day history of cold-like symptoms and conjunctivitis. The rash began as a maculopapular eruption in the postauricular region but has rapidly spread to his face and upper body. On examination, white papules are visible inside his mouth. What diagnosis fits best with this clinical picture?
   a. Scarlet fever
   b. German measles
   c. Measles
   d. Adenovirus infection

5. A 19-year-old woman has just returned from a holiday is severely dehydrated and gives a history of passing voluminous watery stools that look like rice water, mixed with mucus and blood. Blood testing reveals a raised hemoglobin, markedly raised urea and raised creatinine. What diagnosis fits best with this clinic picture?
   a. Cholera
   b. Typhoid fever
   c. *Salmonella*
   d. Amoebic dysentery

6. A sewage worker presents with a high temperature and myalgia, especially in his legs. After a short improvement, he develops jaundice 6 days later. On examination, his temperature is 39°C, he is jaundiced and has hepatosplenomegaly. Leukocytes 17×10^9/L, bilirubin 325 mmol/L, AST 70 U/L, ALT 45 U/L, creatinine 248 mmol/L, HbsAg-negative. What is the most likely diagnosis?
   a. Hepatitis A
   b. Infectious mononucleosis
   c. Leptospirosis
   d. Budd–Chiari syndrome

7. An 20-year-old man who has not received childhood vaccine presents with meningism, orchitis and unilateral parotitis. What is the most likely diagnosis?
   a. Epstein–Barr virus infection
   b. HIV
   c. Rubella
   d. Mumps

8. A 44-year-old man returns from a trip to the jungles of northern Thailand with high-grade fever, bodyache, severe myalgia and a rash which on limbs and has now spread to involve the trunk. Malaria films are negative. What diagnosis fits best with this clinical picture?
   a. Dengue fever   b. Malaria
   c. Hepatitis A   d. Influenza

9. HIV patients with a CD4 count <200/mm³ should receive appropriate prophylaxis against *Pneumocystis jiroveci* (formerly called *Pneumocystis carinii*) pneumonia. What is the most appropriate medication?
   a. Ampicillin   b. Erythromycin
   c. Co-trimoxazole   d. Corticosteriods

10. A HIV positive patient but in the stable phase of the disease is best monitored with which biomarker?
    a. C-reactive protein
    b. CD4 lymphocyte count
    c. Erythrocyte sedimentation rate
    d. Polymerase chain reaction

11. A patient with HIV presents with a sudden onset of confusion. CMV encephalitis is suspected. What treatment should be commenced?
    a. Ganciclovir
    b. Aciclovir
    c. Ceftriaxone
    d. Dexamethasone

12. Which of the following is not an AIDS defining illness?
    a. Aspergillosis
    b. Cytomegalovirus retinitis
    c. Candidiasis
    d. *Mycobacterium tuberculosis*

13. A internee has a needlestick injury after taking blood from a patient known to be HIV positive. What is the most appropriate immediate management after hand washing for 10 minutes?
    a. Continue handwashing for a further 20 minutes
    b. Antiretroviral therapy
    c. Test for hepatitis B and C
    d. Broad-spectrum antibiotics

14. A 23-year-old man who lives with his male partner consults you for an opinion. He has suffered anal discharge and pruritis for the past 3 days. There are also some symptoms of dysuria. A urethral smear reveals intracellular diplococci. What is the most likely infective agent to fit with this clinical picture?
    a. *Neisseria gonorrhoeae*
    b. *Chlamydia trachomatis*
    c. *Treponema pallidum*
    d. Herpes simplex type 2

15. A 22-year-old male has recently had unprotected sex and has notices the development of a firm lesion on his penis. He states it begin as a small bump which then ulcerated and the became a firm lesion. It is not painful. He has associated inguinal lymphadenopathy which is not painful. You suspect syphilis. Which test if positive will confirm primary syphilis?
    a. Widal
    b. Paul-Bunnell
    c. VDRL
    d. Monospot

ANSWERS

1. c   2. d   3. d   4. c   5. a
6. c   7. d   8. a   9. c   10. b
11. a   12. a   13. b   14. a   15. c

CHAPTER 16: Emergencies in Medicine

CHAPTER OUTLINE

- List of Common Emergencies in Medical Practice
- **Hypersensitive Reactions**
  - Urticaria (Hives)
- Angioedema
- Systemic Anaphylaxis

LIST OF COMMON EMERGENCIES IN MEDICAL PRACTICE

Emergencies in Cardiology (Acute Coronary Syndrome, Acute Heart Failure, Infective Endocarditis, Arrythmias) BLS/ACLS	Chapter 9
Emergencies in Pulmonology (Acute Severe Asthma, Pulmonary Embolism, Acute Exacerbation of COPD)	Chapter 8
Emergencies in Endocrinology (Diabetic Ketoacidosis, Hyperosmolar Non-ketotic State, Hypoglycemia, Hyperthyroid Crisis, Myxedema Coma, Acute Adrenal Insufficiency)	Chapter 14
Emergencies in Nephrology (Pyelonephritis, Obstructive Uropathy, Acute Renal Failure, Hyponatremia, Hyperkalemia)	Chapter 10
Emergencies in Gastroenterology/Hepatology (Gastrointestinal Bleed, Fulminant Hepatic Failure, Acute Pancreatitis)	Chapters 6 and 7
Hematology/Oncological Emergencies (Disseminated Intravascular Coagulation, Thrombocytopenia, Blood Transfusion Reaction)	Chapter 12
Neurological Emergencies (Stroke, Subarachnoid Hemorrhage, Meningitis Encephalitis, Status Epilepticus)	Chapter 11
Allergy, Anaphylaxis	Discussed in this chapter

HYPERSENSITIVITY REACTIONS

The characteristic features of hypersensitivity reactions are given in **Table 16.1**.

URTICARIA ("HIVES")

- Urticaria (also known as hives) is produced due to localized edema of dermis secondary to a temporary increase in capillary permeability. The term angioedema is used if edema involves subcutaneous or submucosal layers.

Types: Acute urticaria is the presence of urticaria for less than 6 weeks and chronic if it persists for more than 6 weeks.

- Urticaria may be brought out by either immunologic or nonimmunologic mechanisms. Urticaria is triggered by a wide variety of antigens or by physical stimuli, including cold, pressure, and sunlight. They produce local degranulation of mast cells by various mechanisms such as: (1) Type I hypersensitivity, (2) spontaneous mast cell degranulation (chronic urticarial), (3) chemical mast cell degranulation, and (4) autoimmunity (chronic urticaria).

Clinical Manifestations

- Urticaria is common and can be seen in persons of all ages.
- The common triggers are cold, heat, sweating, exercise, pressure, vibration, and sunlight. **Dermographism**, literally "skin writing," is the most common form of physical urticaria.
- Urticarial eruptions may involve any area of the body from the scalp to the soles of the feet.
- Urticarial lesions represent local area of edema involving only the superficial portions of the dermis. On certain body sites (e.g., the lips, hands), the edema spreads deeper into subcutaneous tissue and is referred to as angioedema.
- They are well-circumscribed wheals, pink-to-light red in color, with erythematous raised serpiginous borders blanched center. Size of the lesions vary from one millimeter to several centimeters.
- Almost always pruritic and individual wheals come and go within 24 hours and those lesions lasting up to 6 weeks are called as acute urticaria. If the urticaria recurs over a period of 6 weeks or more it is known as chronic urticaria.
- When individual lesions last more than 36–48 hours and leave postinflammatory hyperpigmentation or palpable purpura, it is called as urticarial vasculitis.
- Urticaria may be associated with headache, dizziness, nausea, vomiting, abdominal pain, diarrhea, and arthralgias.

Table 16.1: Characteristic features of hypersensitivity reactions.

Type	I (immediate)	II (cytotoxic)	III (immune complex)	IV (delayed)
Antigens	Pollens, molds, mites, food drugs and parasites	Cell surface or tissue bound	Exogenous (viruses, bacteria, fungi, parasites) autoantigens	Cell/tissue bound
Mediators	IgE and mast cells	IgG, IgM, and complement	IgG, IgM, IgA, and complement	Cytotoxic T-cells, activated macrophage
Time taken for reaction to develop	5–10 minutes	6–36 hours	4–12 hours	48–72 hours
Pathological feature	Edema, vasodilatation, mast cell degranulation, eosinophils	Antibody-mediated damage to target cells	Acute inflammatory reaction (neutrophils), vasculitis	• Perivascular inflammation, mononuclear cells, fibrin • Granulomas: Caseation and necrosis in TB
Prototype disorder/diseases produced	• Asthma (extrinsic) • Anaphylaxis (systemic and localized) • Urticaria, eczema • Angioedema • Allergic rhinitis • Food allergies	• Autoimmune hemolytic anemia, transfusion reactions, hemolytic disease of newborn • Good pasture's syndrome Pernicious anemia • Myasthenia gravis	Autoimmune diseases (e.g., SLE, glomerulonephritis rheumatoid arthritis) Serum sickness, Arthus reaction	• Tuberculosis • Contact dermatitis • Leprosy • Transplant rejection
Diagnostic tests	• Skin-prick tests • Specific IgE in serum	• Coombs' test • Indirect immunofluorescence	Immune complexes, complement levels	Skin test—erythema induration (e.g., tuberculin test)
Treatment	• Antigen avoidance • Antihistamines, corticosteroids (usually topical) • Leukotriene receptor antagonists • Sodium cromoglicate • Epinephrine (adrenaline) for life-threatening anaphylaxis	• Exchange transfusion • Plasmapheresis • Immunosuppressives/cytotoxic drugs	• Corticosteroids • Immunosuppressives/cytotoxic drugs • Plasmapheresis • Anti-TNF antibody, anti-B-cell antibody, anti-CTLA-4 antibody	• Immunosuppressives • Corticosteroids, removal of antigen

(Ig: immunoglobulin; TB: tuberculosis; TNF: tumor necrosis factor)

Management

Management of urticaria depends on its severity and the duration.
- **Mild urticaria limited to the skin:** Antihistamines (diphenhydramine) or the newer nonsedating agents (terfenadine, cetirizine, and loratadine).
- **Severe urticaria:** Short-term corticosteroids (up to 1 mg/kg).
- **Chronic urticaria:** Find the cause and remove the causative antigen. Antihistamines, omalizumab and cyclosporine, for 8–16 weeks may be beneficial.

Allergy

- Allergy is defined as a hypersensitivity reaction induced by exposure to an otherwise harmless exogenous substance (known as an allergen), generally environmental.
- In an allergic reaction, initial exposure to allergen triggers the production of specific IgE antibodies by activated B-cells. These IgE antibodies bind to the surface of mast cells via high-affinity IgE receptors.
- The first dose of allergen (priming dose) which sensitizes the immunologic system (B lymphocyte). On re-exposure, the allergen (shocking dose) binds to membrane-bound IgE which activates the mast cells, releasing vasoactive mediators (the early phase response) and causing a type I hypersensitivity reaction and the symptoms of allergy. This may be followed by late phase reaction and is mediated by basophils, eosinophils, and macrophages.
- Examples: Asthma, anaphylaxis, rhinitis, urticaria, angioedema, eczema, and food hypersensitivity.

ANGIOEDEMA

Angioedema is defined as a well-demarcated localized edema involving the deeper layers of the skin, including the subcutaneous tissue and submucosal tissues.

Etiology

It is an IgE-mediated reaction that causes direct release of histamine from the mast cells. It follows a variety of allergens. It may develop due to insect sting, drug reaction, food allergy, and exposure to other biological products. Rarely, angiotensin-converting enzyme (ACE) inhibitors may produce angioedema due to increased levels of bradykinin. Most of the cases are idiopathic.

C1-esterase Inhibitor Deficiency

C1-esterase (C1INH) inhibitor is a complement protein that inhibits spontaneous activation of classical complement pathway. C1-esterase inhibitor also regulates kinin cascade, activation of which increases local bradykinin levels and produces local pain and swelling. Both C1-esterase inhibitor and C1 levels are low. C1INH deficiency produces bradykinin. Deficiency of C1INH may be hereditary or acquired disorder.

- **Hereditary angioedema:** It is an autosomal dominant disorder, which is caused due to C1 esterase inhibitor (C1INH) deficiency. Angioedema develops either spontaneously or following infection or injury (e.g., dental injury). Onset is usually in early childhood. The attacks become worse at puberty and usually its frequency and severity decreases after the age of 50 years and may even disappear totally. Diagnosis confirmed by low levels of C1INH (in 85% cases) or dysfunctional C1INH (in 15% cases).
- **Mutations in chromosome 11; autosomal dominant inheritance:**
    - *Type I C1ID:* In 85% patients, there is no detectable protein.
    - *Type II C1ID:* In 15% patients, dysfunctional proteins are detected.
- **Acquired C1INH deficiency:** It presents in a manner similar to the hereditary angioedema but the onset occurs in the fifth and sixth decades of life. It is due to appearance of an autoantibody. It may occur with B-cell lymphoma, multiple myeloma, Waldenstrom's macroglobulinemia, and chronic lymphocytic leukemia.

Clinical Features

- Angioedema may occur at any age but is most common in young adults.
- It presents with well-defined, nonpitting swelling, usually nonpruritic. It may be associated with urticaria lesions.
- Angioedema up to 6 weeks is called acute and if it lasts beyond 6 weeks is called chronic.
- It may involve any area of the body but often affects periorbital, lips **(Fig. 16.1)** and genital areas.
- Angioedema of the upper respiratory tract may cause laryngeal obstruction which may be life threatening.
- Involvement of gastrointestinal system may produce abdominal colic, with or without nausea and vomiting.

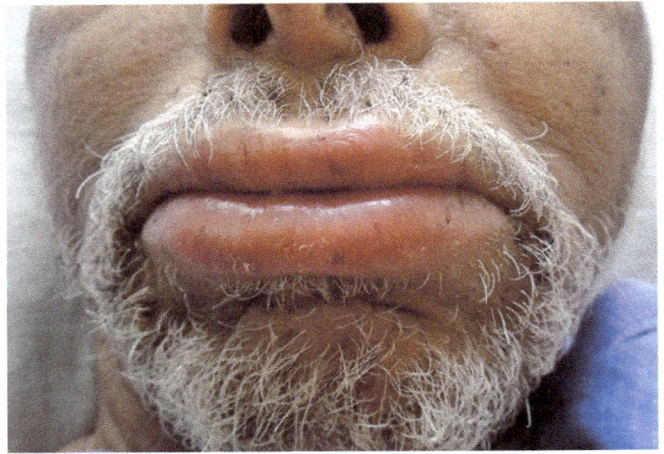

Fig. 16.1: Angioedema.

- Angioedema does not produce residual discoloration unless there is extravasation of RBCs.

Treatment

- Identification of the etiologic factor(s) and remove the offending agent if possible.
- Antihistamines to control the lesions, e.g., diphenhydramine cetirizine, desloratadine.
- Observe for any evidence of airway obstruction and if present manage in a fashion similar to those with anaphylaxis.
- Acute attack should be controlled with epinephrine.
- Chronic angioedema not responding to maximal dosages of antihistamines, glucocorticosteroids, and other immunomodulating agents (e.g., methotrexate, cyclosporine) may be considered.
- During severe attacks of hereditary angioedema due to C1INH deficiency, fresh frozen plasma is lifesaving as it provides C1-esterase inhibitor. Danazol is useful to prevent episodes of hereditary angioedema.
- Newer therapy for hereditary angioedema: Purified C1 inhibitor concentrate, recombinant C1INH—**Conestat alfa,** bradykinin receptor antagonist—**Icatibant** and kallikrein inhibitor—**Ecallantide.**

SYSTEMIC ANAPHYLAXIS

Definition: Systemic anaphylaxis is a life-threatening form of immediate (appears within minutes after systemic exposure to specific antigen) type 1 hypersensitivity reaction mediated by IgE. It is a systemic response that develops when mast cells (possibly basophils) are provoked to secrete mediators with potent vasoactive and smooth muscle contractile activities.

Causes

It occurs in sensitized individuals and requires prior sensitization occurs to inciting antigen, either alone or in combination with a hapten. It usually occurs when allergen is administered parenterally and it is less likely after oral ingestion, inhalation, or cutaneous or ocular topical contact. The causes of systemic anaphylactic reactions are listed in **Box 16.1**.

Anaphylaxis may be triggered by extremely small doses of antigen, e.g., the minute dose of antigen is used in skin testing for various forms of allergies.

Mechanism **Initial exposure to antigen:** The sensitizing antigen (allergen) from its site of entry is presented to T-cells which differentiate into T_H2 cells. IL-l3 secreted by T_H2 cells **enhances IgE production by B-cells. IgE gets attached to mast cells and basophils.**

- **During subsequent exposure to antigen,** the antigen (allergen) binds to the IgE antibodies previously bound to the mast cells and produces IgE-induced degranulation of mast cells and basophils. It results in the liberation of a number of mediators. Mediators released by mast cells include preformed mediators (stored in secretory granules) and secondary mediators (newly synthesized products) **(Fig. 16.2)**.

> **Box 16.1: Causes of systemic anaphylactic reactions.**
>
> **Anaphylaxis: IgE-Mediated Mast Cell Degranulation**
> 1. **Proteins:**
>   - Foreign proteins (e.g., antisera),
>   - Foods (peanuts, fish and shellfish, egg, milk, soya products)
>   - Food additives (aspartame, monosodium glutamate)
> 2. **Drugs:**
>   - Antibiotics (penicillins, cephalosporins, tetracyclines, trimethoprim-sulfamethoxazole, cancomycin, nitrofurantoin)
>   - Chemotherapeutic agents
>   - Hormones (e.g., insulin, vasopressin, parathormone)
>   - Enzymes (chymotrypsin, penicillinase, streptokinase).
>   - Intravenous anesthetic agents (suxamethonium, propofol)
>   - Latex
> 3. **Biological agents:**
>   - Blood
>   - Tetanus, rabies, and diphtheria antitoxins
>   - Anti-thymocyte globulin
>   - Vaccines
> 4. **Insect bites and stings:**
>   - Honey bee (bee venom)
>   - Wasps (wasp venom)

Anaphylactoid reactions (pseudoallergic reactions/non-IgE mediated):
- They are indistinguishable from anaphylactic reactions.
- Most non-IgE-dependent foreign agents do not require antigen processing (sensitization) and can elicit a mast cell activation response on first antigenic exposure itself. However, they may be associated with IgG and IgM antibodies and not IgE. These antibodies activate the complement system through classical pathway and produce activated complement components and may cause direct release of preformed mediators from mast cells and basophils.
- Anaphylactoid reactions are short lived because these involve only degranulation of mast cells and not cytokine synthesis.
- Causes of anaphylactoid reactions are given in **Box 16.2**.

Clinical Features (Tables 16.2 and 16.3)

The anaphylactic response appears within minutes after systemic exposure to specific antigen.

Diagnostic Criteria for Anaphylaxis

> Anaphylaxis is likely when **one of the following three** criteria occurs:
> - Acute skin and/or mucosal symptoms (e.g., hives, pruritus, flushing, lip/tongue/uvula swelling) and one of the following:
>   - Respiratory symptoms (e.g., wheezing, stridor, shortness of breath, hypoxia)
>   - Hypotension or associated end-organ dysfunction (e.g., hypotonia, syncope, incontinence)
> - Exposure to probable allergen for the patient and two or more of the following:
>   - Skin/mucosal tissue involvement
>   - Respiratory symptoms
>   - Hypotension or end-organ dysfunction
>   - Persistent gastrointestinal symptoms (e.g., emesis, abdominal pain)
> - Decreased blood pressure after exposure to known allergen for the patient:
>   - Adults: Systolic blood pressure < 90 mm Hg or >30% decrease in systolic blood pressure
>   - Infants and children: Hypotension for age or >30% decrease in systolic blood pressure

Treatment

Anaphylaxis is an acute medical emergency and its early recognition is mandatory, since death occurs within minutes to hours after the first symptoms.

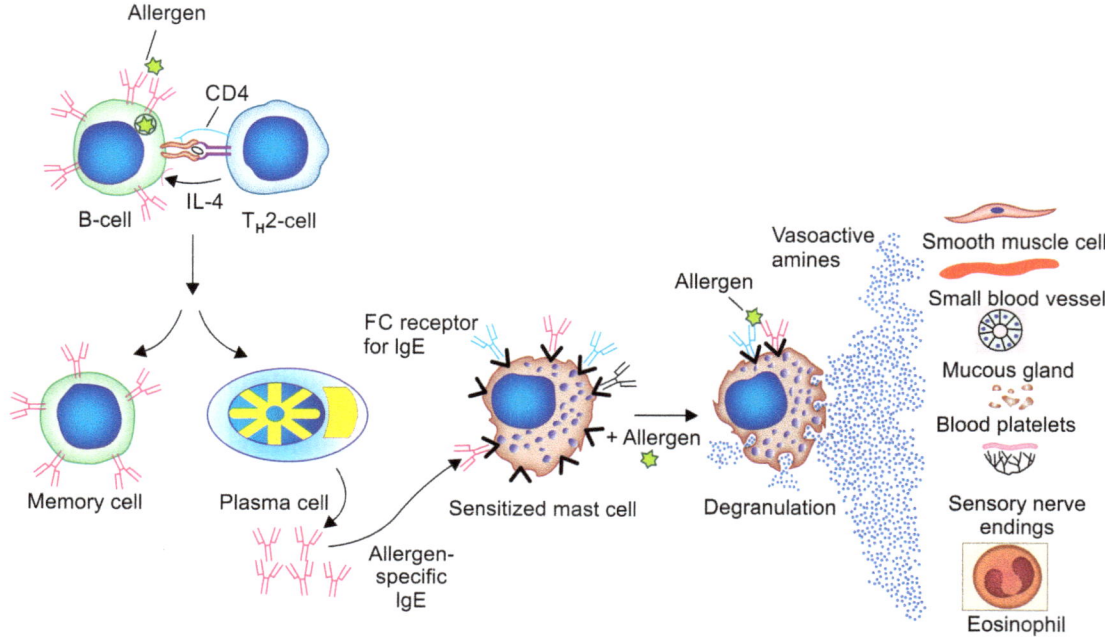

Fig. 16.2: Mechanism of systemic anaphylaxis.

> **Box 16.2:** Anaphylactoid reactions (pseudoallergic reactions/non-IgE mediated).
>
> *Anaphylactoid: Non-IgE-mediated mast cell degranulation*
> 1. **Drugs:**
>   - Aspirin and nonsteroidal anti-inflammatory drugs (NSAIDs)
>   - Vancomycin
>   - Narcotics (e.g., codeine, morphine, opiates)
>   - Radiocontrast media/dye
> 2. **Physical:**
>   - Exercise
>   - Exposure to cold
> 3. **Autoimmune**
> 4. **Narcotics/vancomycin**
> 5. **Idiopathic**

Table 16.2: Clinical features of systemic anaphylaxis.

Cutaneous	Respiratory
• Itching (pruritus) • Hives (urticaria) • Skin erythema with or without angioedema • Flushing • Insect stings	• Intense bronchospasm resulting in respiratory distress • Dyspnea and wheeze • Laryngeal edema resulting in hoarseness and laryngeal obstruction • Pulmonary edema
Gastrointestinal	**Cardiovascular**
• Nausea • Vomiting • Abdominal cramps • Diarrhea	• Tachycardia • Hypotension • Arrhythmias • Shock and collapse
Central nervous system	
• Confusion • Feeling of impending doom • Apprehension • Metallic taste • Altered levels of consciousness	**Biphasic anaphylaxis** is recurrence of symptoms that develops following the apparent resolution of the initial anaphylactic episode with no additional exposure to the causative agent

Table 16.3: Clinical features of systemic anaphylaxis depending on severity.

Severity	Features
Mild	Cutaneous features only: pruritus, erythema, urticaria, or mild angioedema
Moderate	The above plus more severe angioedema and/or vomiting, abdominal pain and/or mild dyspnea or tightening of throat
Severe	The above plus respiratory difficulty (laryngeal edema or asthma) and/or hypotension

- **Prevent further contact with allergen,** e.g., removal of bee sting.
- **Ensure airway patency:** Fatal outcomes in anaphylaxis are mainly due to either airway constriction or hypotension.
- **Oxygen alone via a nasal catheter or with nebulized salbutamol/albuterol,** oxygen 4–6 L/min.
  - If progressive hypoxia develops, either endotracheal intubation or tracheostomy with intermittent positive ventilation is mandatory for oxygen delivery.
- **Administer adrenaline (epinephrine) intramuscularly** into the thigh and is the most critical drug to administer. Earlier administration during the course of an anaphylactic event is better.
  - **Adult:** 0.3–0.5 mg (0.3–0.5 mL of a 1:1,000 solution) IM in the lateral thigh, repeated at 10–15-minute intervals if necessary.
  - **Child:** 1:1,000 dilution at 0.01 mg/kg or 0.1–0.3 mL administered IM in the lateral thigh, repeated at 10–15-minute intervals if necessary.
  - 0.5 mL of 1:1,000 solution sublingually in cases of major airway compromise or hypotension.
  - 3–5 mL of 1:10,000 solution via central line
  - 3–5 mL of 1:10,000 solution diluted with 10 mL of normal saline via endotracheal tube.
  - For protracted symptoms that require multiple doses of epinephrine, an IV epinephrine drip may be useful; the infusion is titrated to maintain adequate BP.

Administer antihistamines: They may prevent the progression of urticaria and pruritus, but does not reverse hypotension or tissue edema by directly opposing effects of mast cell activation, e.g., chlorphenamine 10 mg IM or slow IV injection, diphenhydramine, 50–100 mg IM or IV.
- **Administer corticosteroids:** Hydrocortisone 200 mg IV stat (not effective for the acute event as takes 4 hours to act; but alleviate recurrence of bronchospasm, urticaria, and hypotension).
- **Glucagon** could reverse refractory bronchospasm and hypotension in patients who are taking β-adrenergic antagonists. Recommended dosage is 1–5 mg intravenously bolus slowly over 5 minutes followed by an infusion at 5–15 µg/min titrated to clinical response.
- **Provide supportive treatments:**
  - *Bronchodilators:* They relieve bronchospasm, e.g., nebulized $β_2$-agonists/salbutamol and aminophylline, 0.25–0.5 g IV.
  - *Hypotension:* Immediately assume the Trendelenburg position (prevent progression to anaphylactic shock). Shock is treated with intravenous fluids (if needed with dopamine) to restore or maintain blood pressure. **Extracorporeal membrane oxygenation (ECMO)** has been tried.

Chapter 16: Emergencies in Medicine

OBJECTIVE-BASED SELF-EVALUATION

SHORT ANSWER QUESTIONS

1. List types of hypersensitivity reaction with examples.
2. How will you manage acute anaphylactic shock?
3. Discuss the clinical features of angioedema.

MULTIPLE CHOICE QUESTIONS

1. A 45-year-old man with no past medical history attends the emergency department with an episode of acute onset breathlessness and chest pain. He has recently returned from a business trip had been complaining of a painful, swollen left leg. Which is an appropriate next step?
   a. Intra-arterial thrombolysis
   b. Intravenous thrombolysis followed by CPR for 90 minutes
   c. Intravenous thrombolysis followed by CPR for 30 minutes
   d. Transthoracic echocardiography to image the right ventricle

2. A 73-year-old man is brought to the emergency department in cardiac arrest. He was found by his career unconscious on the floor. ECG reveals polymorphic ventricular tachycardia. Which is the next most appropriate management option?
   a. Increase dose of adrenaline
   b. Increase shock energy
   c. Lidocaine IV
   d. Magnesium sulfate IV

3. A 55-year-old man with a history of depression overdoses of his antihypertensive medication (beta-blocker). His blood pressure is recorded as 96/60 mm Hg and his pulse is 45. A 12 lead ECG reveals a heart block. From the options below, which is the first step in this patient's management?
   a. Activated charcoal
   b. Atropine
   c. Observation
   d. Temporal transvenous cardiac pacing

4. A 76-year-old man with history of left ventricular dysfunction secondary to ischemic heart disease had developed sudden onset rapid, irregular palpitations, and felt breathless so he called the emergency services. He has a heart rate of around 156 and the blood pressure is 60 systolic. The 12 lead ECG showed atrial fibrillation. From this list, which is the treatment of choice for this patient?
   a. Atenolol intravenously
   b. Amiodarone intravenously
   c. Digoxin intravenously
   d. Direct current cardioversion (DCCV)

5. A 26-year-old gentleman is admitted to the emergency department after a motor vehicle accident. You are asked to review the patient. He is fully oriented to time, place and person. On questioning, the patient cannot provide any information about the accident; the last he remembers was getting into the car in order to attend a meeting. What course of management would you advise?
   a. Admit the patient for observation and consciousness charting
   b. CT scan head
   c. Discharge home with advice to return if any deterioration
   d. MRI head

6. A 18-year-old female presents acutely unwell. Six weeks previously she had been diagnosed with hypothyroidism by her general practitioner. On examination she appears unwell and mildly dehydrated. She has a temperature of 37.5°C and has a BMI of 21.3 kg/m². Her blood pressure is 72/44 mm Hg, with a pulse of 100 beats per minute. In the meantime what is the most appropriate immediate management of this patient?
   a. Intravenous cefotaxime
   b. Intravenous glucose
   c. Intravenous fluids and hydrocortisone
   d. Intravenous thyroxine (T4)

7. A 70-year-old lady had a GI bleed 10 months ago related to NSAID use for osteoarthritis. At that time an endoscopy showed a duodenal ulcer which was treated. She now represents with an acute hematemesis. Her Hb on admission is 5.6 g/dL. OGD is performed, showing a single bleeding vessel on the posterior wall of the duodenum. Injection sclerotherapy is attempted but fails to stop the bleeding. What is the next step in her management?
   a. Glypressin
   b. IV omeprazole
   c. Octreotide
   d. Urgent referral to on-call surgeons

8. A school girl is brought to the emergency department by her parents. She took a number of paracetamol tablets, but did not intend to kill herself. Which of the following is the best indicator of the degree of hepatocellular damage?
   a. Aspartate transaminase level
   b. Bilirubin level
   c. INR
   d. Paracetamol level
   e. Quantity of paracetamol ingested

9. A patient presents with acute hereditary angioedema. On examination there is evidence of stridor. How do you manage this patient?
   a. Adrenaline   b. Itacibant
   c. Chlorphenamine   d. Hydrocortisone

10. What immunoglobulin if present in low levels can be associated with anaphylaxis?
    a. IgG   b. IgE
    c. IgM   d. IgD

ANSWERS

| 1. b | 2. d | 3. b | 4. d | 5. b |
| 6. c | 7. d | 8. c | 9. b | 10. b |

Viva Voce: Instruments, Procedures, and X-rays

CHAPTER 17

CHAPTER OUTLINE

Instruments and Procedures
- Gastric Lavage Tube
- Laryngoscope
- Metal Tracheostomy Tube
- Endotracheal Tube
- Ambu Bag
- Ryles Tube—Nasogastric Tube
- Suction Catheter
- Foley Catheter
- Insulin Syringe
- Tuberculin Syringe
- Trucut Biopsy Gun
- Lumbar Puncture Needle
- Intravenous Drip Set
- Intravenous Cannula
- Oxygen Mask
- Inhaler Devices
- Urinometer
- Westergren Tube

Discussion of Common X-rays

The viva voce session consists of discussion on drugs, instruments, procedures, X-rays, and general viva.

INSTRUMENTS AND PROCEDURES

GASTRIC LAVAGE TUBE (FIG. 17.1)

Description
It is used for gastrointestinal decontamination to empty the stomach of toxic substances by the sequential administration and aspiration of small volumes of fluid via an orogastric tube. Other names are Ewald's tube/Boas tube.

Indications
For decontamination after oral consumption of poison.

Contraindications
- Corrosive ingestions or esophageal disease
- Hydrocarbon or petroleum distillate ingestion
- Convulsion
- Cardiac dysrhythmias
- The poison ingestion is not toxic at any dose.
- The poison ingestion is adsorbed by charcoal and adsorption is not exceed by quantity ingestion.
- Presentation many hours (>3 hours) after poisoning
- A highly efficient antidote, such as NAC is available

Technique
Box 17.1 describes the technique of performing orogastric lavage.

Box 17.1: Technique of performing orogastric lavage.

Select the correct tube size
- Adults and adolescents: 36–40 French
- Children: 22–28 French

Procedure
1. If there is potential airway compromise, endotracheal intubation should precede
2. The patient should be kept in the left lateral decubitus position. Because the pylorus points upward in this orientation, this positioning theoretically helps prevent the xenobiotic from passing through the pylorus during the procedure.
3. Before insertion, the proper length of tubing to be passed should be measured and marked on the tube. The length should allow the most proximal tube opening to be passed beyond the lower esophageal sphincter.
4. After the tube is inserted, it is essential to confirm that the distal end of the tube is in the stomach.
5. Any material present in the stomach should be withdrawn and immediate instillation of activated charcoal should be considered for large ingestions of xenobiotics that are known to be adsorbed by activated charcoal.
6. In adults, 250-mL aliquots of a room temperature saline lavage solution is instilled via a funnel or lavage syringe. In children, aliquots should be 10–15 mL/kg to a maximum of 250 mL.
7. Orogastric lavage should continue for at least several liters in an adult and for at least 0.5–1.0 L in a child or until no particulate matter returns and the effluent lavage solution is clear.
8. After orogastric lavage, the same tube should be used to instill activated charcoal if indicated.

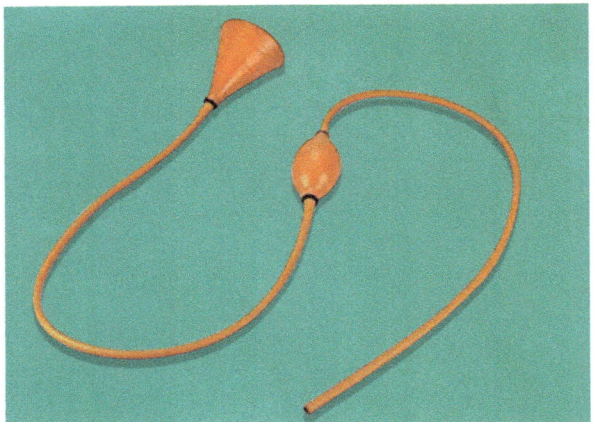

Fig. 17.1: Gastric lavage tube.

Complications

- Aspiration of gastric contents (3% of patients)
- Esophageal rupture (rare)
- Laryngospasm
- Bradycardia

LARYNGOSCOPE (FIG. 17.2)

Description

Laryngoscopes are usually left-handed tools designed to facilitate visualization of the larynx. A laryngoscope consists of a handle, a blade, and a light source (Fig. 17.3). The most commonly used blades include the curved Macintosh and the straight Miller blades.

Indications

- Patients requiring emergent intubation include those who experience acute respiratory failure, an altered mental status that needs airway protection, and inadequate oxygenation and ventilation.
- Nonemergent intubation occurs in the perioperative setting as patients may require general anesthesia.

Contraindications

- Patients who have supraglottic or glottic pathology.
- A relative contraindication to laryngoscopy includes patients with anatomy that does not allow successful laryngoscopy use, injuries to the area, or physiologic status that is not conducive to the procedure.

METAL TRACHEOSTOMY TUBE (FIG. 17.4)

Description

It consists of three parts—outer cannula with flange (neck plate), inner cannula, and an obturator.

Indications

- Upper airway obstruction (e.g., stridor)
- Prolonged intubation
- Facilitation of ventilation support
- For management of pulmonary secretions

ENDOTRACHEAL TUBE (FIG. 17.5)

Description

It is a tube constructed of polyvinylchloride (PVC) that is placed between the vocal cords through the trachea to provide

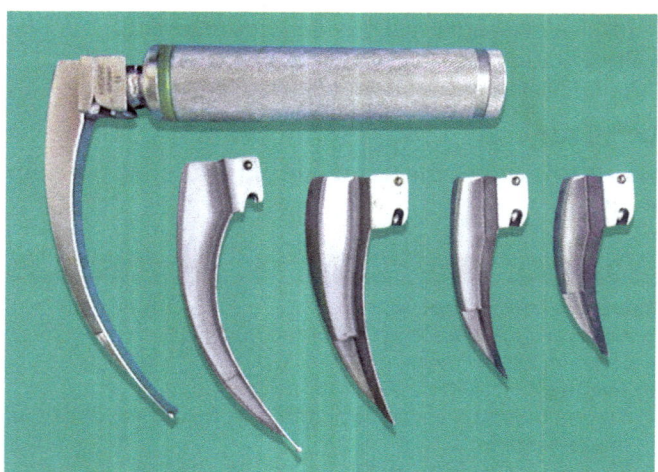

Fig. 17.2: Laryngoscopes.

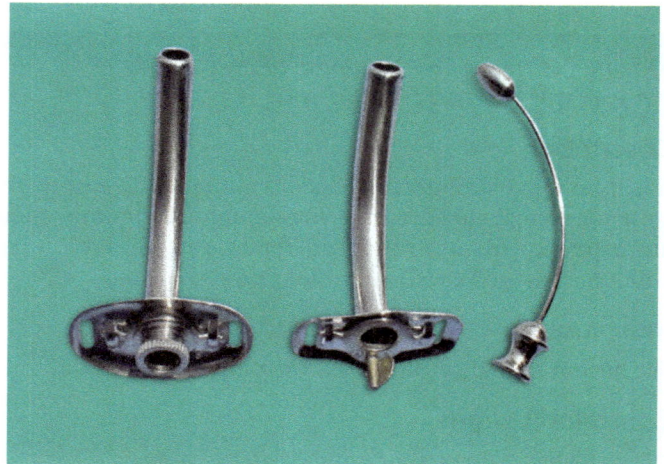

Fig. 17.4: Metal tracheostomy tube.

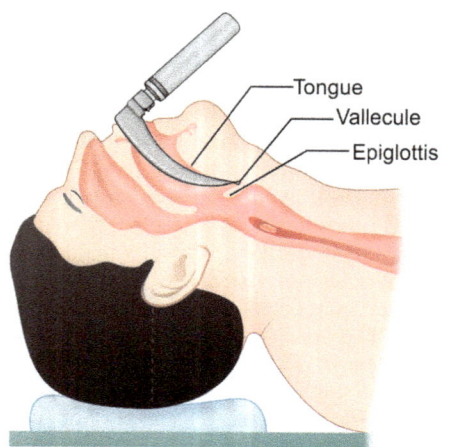

Fig. 17.3: Laryngoscopy.

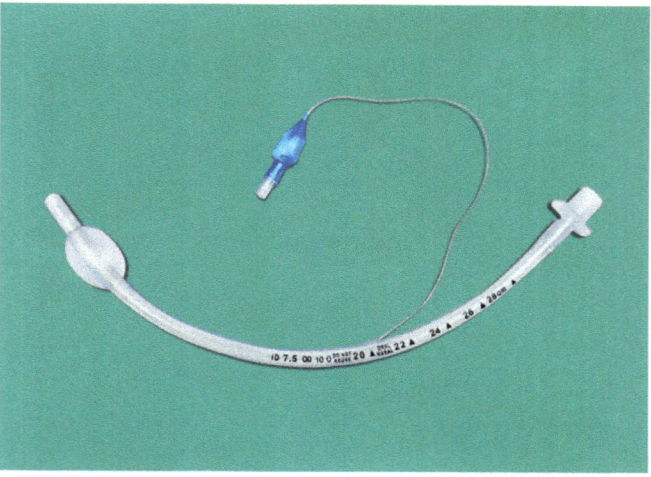

Fig. 17.5: Endotracheal tube.

oxygen and inhaled gases to the lungs. It also serves to protect the lungs from contamination, such as gastric contents and blood parts of endotracheal (ET) tube.

The Tube
The endotracheal tube has a length and diameter. The endotracheal tubes (ETTs) size refers to its internal diameter in millimeters (mm). PVC is not radiopaque, and thus a radiopaque linear material is included throughout the length of the tube to make it easier to visualize the placement on X-ray. Ideally, the distal tip of the ETT is 4 cm (± 2 cm) above the carina on chest X-ray in adults.

The Cuff
A cuff is an inflatable balloon at the distal end of the ETT. The inflated cuff produces a seal against the tracheal wall; this prevents gastric contents from entering the trachea and facilitates the execution of positive pressure ventilation. The cuff inflates by attaching an appropriate size syringe (10–20 mL for adult ETT) to the pilot balloon.

The Bevel
To facilitate placement through the vocal cords and to provide improved visualization ahead of the tip, the ETT has an angle or slant known as a bevel.

The Murphy's Eye
Endotracheal tubes have a built-in safety mechanism at the distal tip known as Murphy's eye, which is another opening in the tube positioned in the distal lateral wall.

The Connector
Endotracheal tube connectors attach the ETT to the mechanical ventilator tubing or an Ambu bag.

Indications
- Acute respiratory failure, inadequate oxygenation, or ventilation
- Airway protection in a patient with depressed mental status
- In the perioperative setting, endotracheal tubes may be placed in many clinical circumstances, including patients receiving general anesthesia, surgery involving
- Less frequently to manage increased intracranial pressure or to manage copious secretions or bleeding from the airway

Contraindications
- Severe airway trauma or obstruction that does not allow safe placement of the tube
- Severe cervical spine injury, which requires complete immobilization
- Those patients with Mallampati III/IV classification suggesting potentially difficult airway management.

AMBU BAG (FIG. 17.6)
Description
A *bag valve mask (BVM), Ambu bag* or generically as a *manual resuscitator* or "self-inflating bag" is a hand-held device

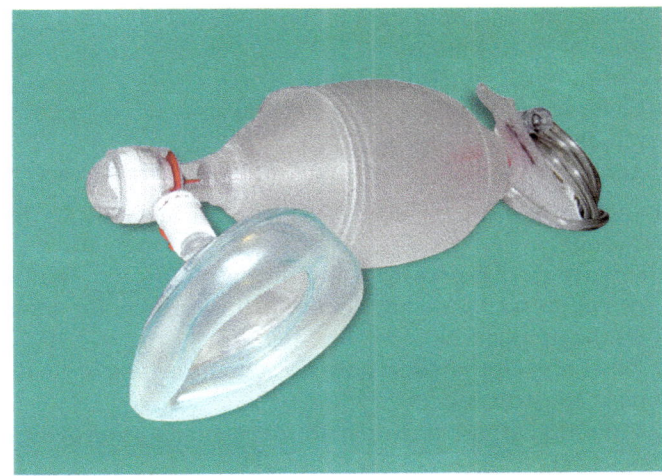

Fig. 17.6: Ambu bag.

commonly used to provide positive pressure ventilation to patients who are not breathing or not breathing adequately.

The BVM consists of a flexible air chamber (the "bag", roughly a foot in length), attached to a face mask via a shutter valve.

Ambu is the acronym for "artificial manual breathing unit".

Complications
- Air to inflate the stomach (called gastric insufflation)
- Lung injury from overstretching (called volutrauma)
- Lung injury from overpressurization (called barotrauma)

RYLES TUBE—NASOGASTRIC TUBE (FIG. 17.7)
Description
It is a flexible tube made of rubber or plastic, and it has bidirectional potential. It can be used either to feed or remove the contents of the stomach, including air, to decompress the stomach, or to remove small solid objects and fluid, such as poison, from the stomach.

Indications
Diagnostic indications for nasogastric (NG) intubation include the following:

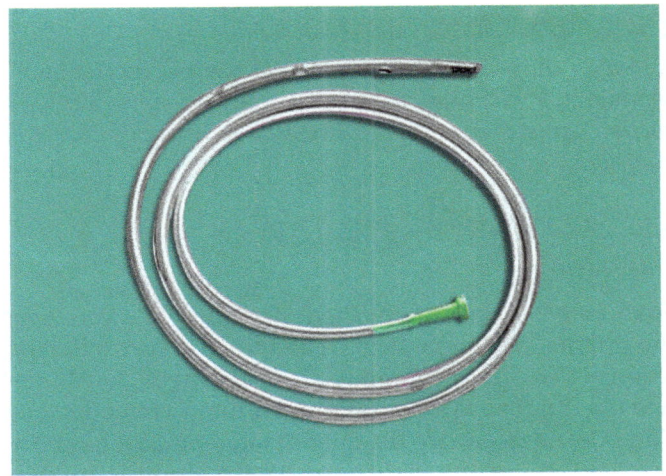

Fig. 17.7: Nasogastric tube.

- Evaluation of upper gastrointestinal (GI) bleeding (i.e., presence and volume)
- Aspiration of gastric fluid content
- Identification of the esophagus and stomach on a chest radiograph
- Administration of radiographic contrast to the GI tract

Therapeutic indications for NG intubation include the following:
- Gastric decompression, including maintenance of a decompressed state after endotracheal intubation, often via the oropharynx
- Relief of symptoms and bowel rest in the setting of small-bowel obstruction
- Aspiration of gastric content from recent ingestion of toxic material
- Administration of medication
- Feeding
- Bowel irrigation

Contraindications

Absolute contraindications for NG intubation include the following:
- Severe midface trauma
- Recent nasal surgery

Relative contraindications for NG intubation include the following:
- Coagulation abnormality
- Esophageal varices
- Recent banding of esophageal varices
- Alkaline ingestion (the tube may be kept, if the injury is not severe)

Verification of Position of Ryles Tube

- Verify proper placement of the NG tube by auscultating a rush of air over the stomach using the 60 mL Toomey syringe or by aspirating gastric content.
- Obtaining a chest radiograph
- Colorimetric capnography is another valid method for verifying NG tube positioning in mechanically ventilated patients.

SUCTION CATHETER (FIG. 17.8)

A *suction catheter* is a medical device used to extract bodily secretions, such as mucus or saliva from the upper airway. A *suction catheter* connects to a *suction machine* or *collection canister*.

FOLEY CATHETER (FIG. 17.9)

Description

Foley catheter (named for Frederic Foley, who produced the original design in 1929): The tube has two separated channels, or *lumens*, running down its length. One lumen opens at both ends and drains urine into a collection bag. The other has a valve on the outside end and connects to a balloon at the inside tip. The balloon is inflated

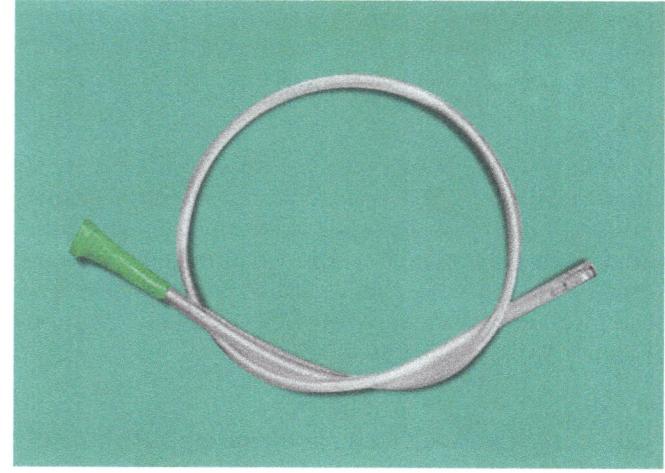

Fig. 17.8: Suction catheter.

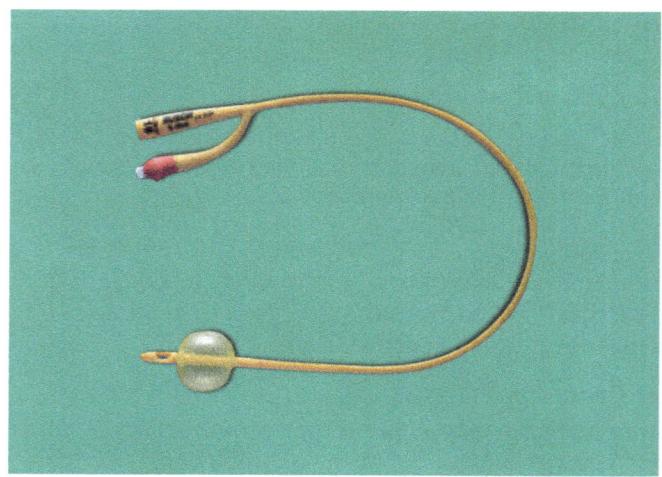

Fig. 17.9: Foley catheter.

with sterile water when it lies inside the bladder to stop it from slipping out. Saline should not be used to inflate the bulb, as it can crystallize within. Air must not be used to inflate, as it will float over the urine. Coatings include polytetrafluoroethylene, hydrogel, or a silicon elastomer—the different properties of these surface coatings determine whether the catheter is suitable for 28-day or 3-month indwelling duration.

Indications

- Acute retention of urine
- Chronic retention of urine with overflow
- In cases of neurogenic bladder
- In surgery involving bladder and prostrate
- In all perineal operations
- Intravesical chemotherapy
- To carry out urethrography
- To monitor urine output

Contraindications

Urethral trauma is the only absolute contraindication to placement of a urinary catheter.

SAHLI'S HEMOGLOBINOMETER (FIGS. 10A AND B)

It is used to estimate hemoglobin.
Method used is—acid hematin method.

NEUBAUER CHAMBER/HEMOCYTOMETER (FIG. 17.11)

Description
The Neubauer chamber is a thick crystal slide with the size of a glass slide (30 × 70 mm and 4-mm thickness). In a simple counting chamber, the central area is where the cell counts are performed.

Use: It is used to count red blood cell (RBC)/white blood cell (WBC).

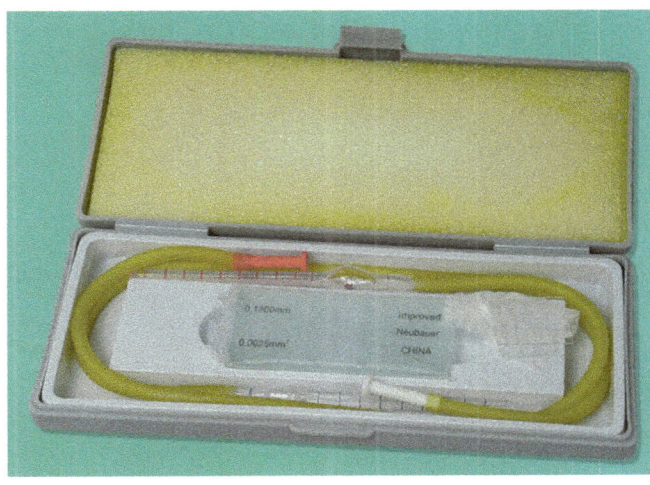

Fig. 17.11: Neubauer chamber/hemocytometer.

INSULIN SYRINGE (FIG. 17.12)

Description
Syringes for insulin users are designed for standard U-100 insulin. The dilution of insulin is such that 1 mL of insulin fluid has 100 standard "units" of insulin. Even 40 IU syringes are available.

Use: It is used for subcutaneous insulin administration.

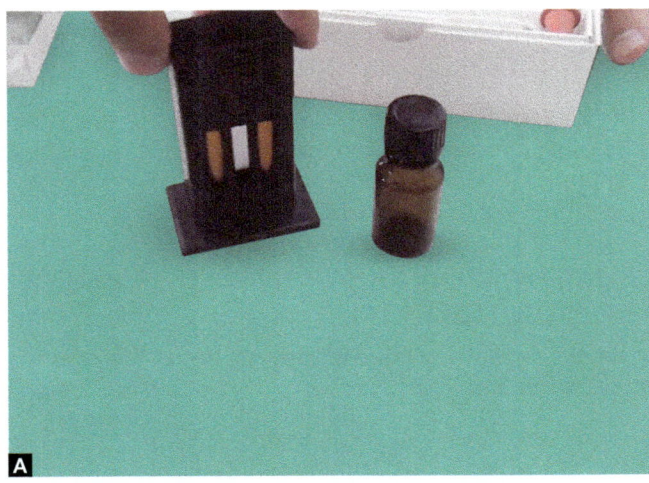

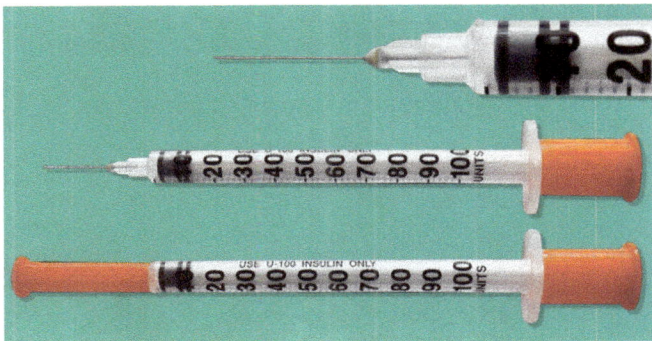

Fig. 17.12: Insulin syringe.

TUBERCULIN SYRINGE (FIG. 17.13)

Tuberculin syringes are small *syringes* with fine *needles* that hold up to one half to one cubic centimeter of fluid, used to administer medication (antigen) under the skin and perform a tuberculosis test called purified protein derivative (PPD)/Mantoux test.

Insulin 40 versus Insulin 100 versus Tuberculin Syringe

U-40 insulin *syringes* markings on the barrel are up to 40 *units*, while in U-100 markings are up to 100 *units*. While in case of 1 mL *tuberculin syringes* the markings are in up to 1 mL.

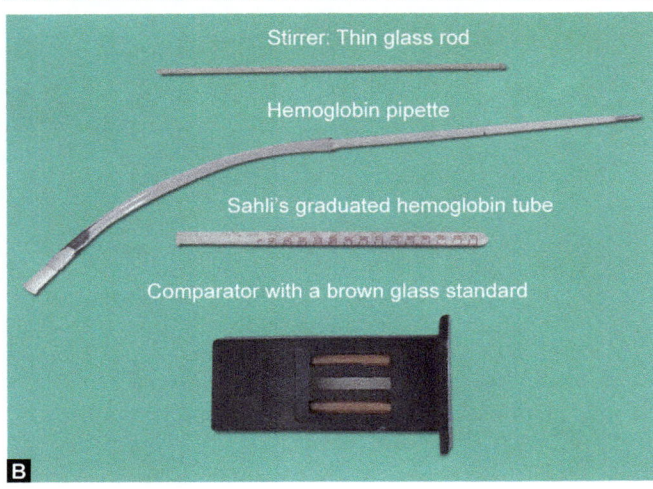

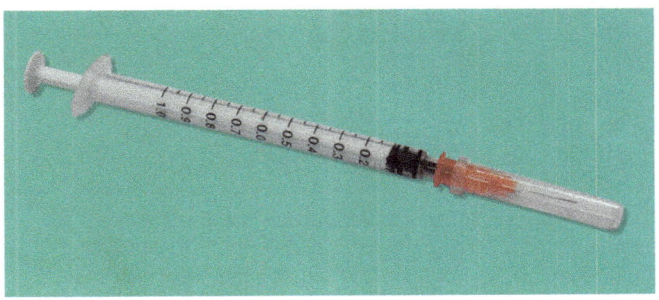

Fig. 17.13: Tuberculin syringe.

Figs. 10A and B: Sahli's hemoglobinometer.

VIM SILVERMAN LIVER BIOPSY NEEDLE (FIG. 17.14)

Description

It has *three parts*:
- Cannula
- Stylet/trocar
- Prong/fork/bifid needle—longer than needle and it protrudes out of the needle. It has a very sharp cutting edge and has longitudinal grove. This retains the tissue when the needle and cannula are withdrawn.

Indications for Liver Biopsy
- In evaluation of jaundice
- Liver cirrhosis
- **Storage disorders:** Glycogen storage disease, hemochromatosis, and Wilson's disease
- Granulomatous lesions, such as tuberculosis and sarcoidosis
- **Infections:** Viral hepatitis and parasitic (amebic liver abscess).
- To diagnose benign and malignant neoplasms

Contraindications of Liver Biopsy
- Bleeding diathesis
- Hemangiomas
- Hydatid cyst
- Severe ascites

Complications of Liver Biopsy
- Hemorrhage
- Infection
- Adjacent structures can be injured (gallbladder, colon, and blood vessels)
- Rarely, there can be precipitation of hepatic coma.

TRUCUT BIOPSY GUN (FIG. 17.15)

Description

A needle with a gap near its tip is passed into the lesion. A surrounding sheath with a cutting tip is passed down the needle. The sheath cuts a specimen corresponding to the gap in the needle. The needle and sheath, with the specimen, are then removed from the patient.

Use: It is used for tissue biopsy—liver/kidney

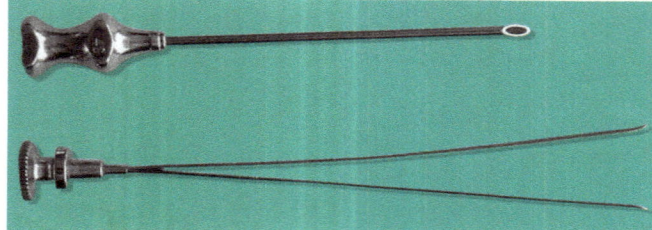

Fig. 17.14: Vim Silverman liver biopsy needle.

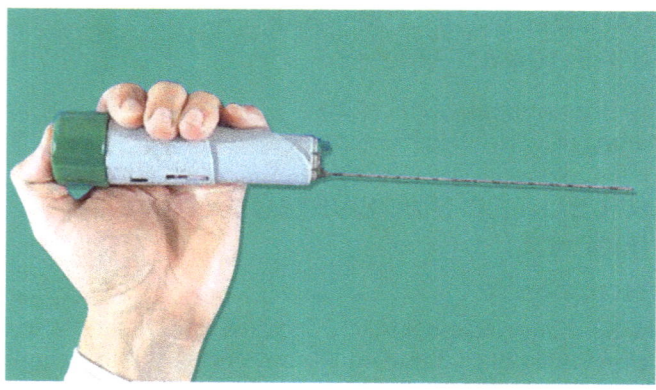

Fig. 17.15: Trucut biopsy gun.

BONE MARROW ASPIRATION NEEDLE (KLIMA NEEDLE) (FIG. 17.16)

Indications

Indications are the diagnosis and management of acute leukemia, staging for lymphoma, evaluation of pancytopenia, thrombocytopenia, investigation of anemia, fever (pyrexia of unknown origin), lymphadenopathy, and hepatosplenomegaly.

Contraindications
- Bleeding disorders and coagulopathy
- Local skin infection/osteomyelitis

Sites
- Posterior superior iliac spine and anterior superior iliac spine
- Sternum and tibial tuberosity

BONE MARROW BIOPSY NEEDLE (JAMSHIDI NEEDLE) (FIG. 17.17)
- Biopsy done when bone marrow tap is dry
- Also for infiltrative disorders

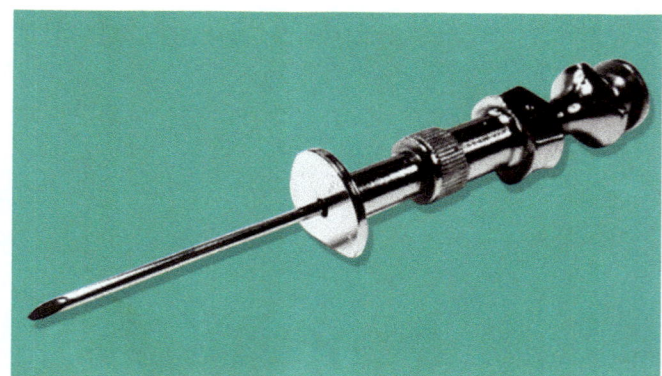

Fig. 17.16: Bone marrow aspiration needle (Klima needle).

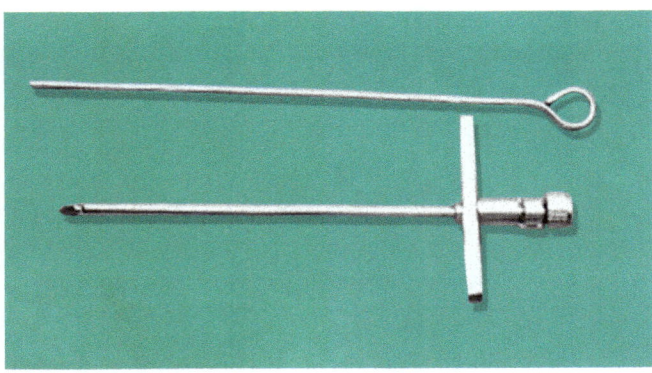

Fig. 17.17: Bone marrow biopsy needle (Jamshidi needle).

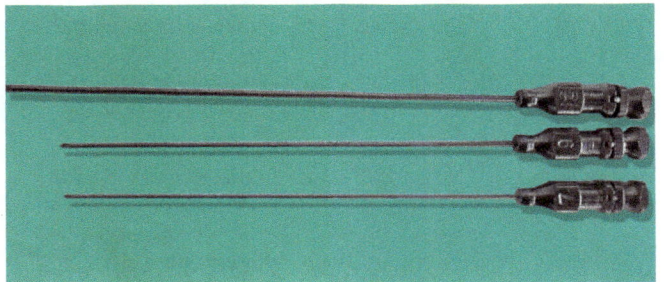

Fig. 17.18: Lumbar puncture needle.

LUMBAR PUNCTURE NEEDLE (FIG. 17.18)

Description

Lumbar puncture (LP) is the technique done to obtain cerebrospinal fluid (CSF) sample and also provides an indirect measure of intracranial pressure (ICP), usually between L3 and L4 (3rd *lumbar space*) through the dura and into the spinal canal.

Indications for Lumbar Puncture

Diagnostic Indications

- Meningitis
- Encephalitis
- Subarachnoid hemorrhage
- Primary or metastatic malignancy (e.g., acute leukemias and lymphoma)
- *Demyelinating diseases*: Multiple sclerosis
- Subacute sclerosing panencephalitis (SSPE)
- Guillain–Barré syndrome
- Injecting the radiopaque dye for myelography

Therapeutic Indications

- Spinal anesthesia and epidural analgesia
- Intrathecal injection of chemotherapeutic drugs for CNS prophylaxis/relapse of acute lymphoblastic leukemia (ALL), and lymphomas
- Therapeutic CSF drainage in cases of normal pressure hydrocephalus

Contraindications for Lumbar Puncture

- Raised intracranial pressure and coagulopathy
- Local infective lesion
- Bony deformities at site of puncture

Complications of Lumbar Puncture

- *Postspinal headache*
- Herniation of cerebellum through the foramen magnum due to raised intracranial pressure
- Introduction of infection by the LP needle through the infected skin or subcutaneous tissue

INTRAVENOUS DRIP SET (FIG. 17.19)

It is used for administering intravenous fluids, drugs, and blood products.

Intravenous fluids are administered through thin, flexible plastic tubing called an *infusion set* or *primary infusion tubing/administration set* (Perry et al., 2014). The infusion tubing/administration set connects to the bag of IV solution. Primary IV tubing is either a macro-drip solution administration set that delivers 10, 15, or 20 gtt/mL, or a micro-drip set that delivers 60 drops/mL. Macro-drip sets are used for routine primary infusions. Micro-drip IV tubing is used mostly in pediatric or neonatal care, when small amounts of fluids are to be administered over a long period of time (Perry et al., 2014). The drop factor can be located on the packaging of the IV tubing.

Primary IV tubing is used to infuse continuous or intermittent fluids or medication. It consists of the following parts (**Fig. 17.20**):

- **Backcheck valve:** It prevents fluid or medication from traveling up the IV.
- **Access ports:** These are used to infuse secondary medications and give IV push medications.
- **Roller clamp:** It is used to regulate the speed of, or to stop or start, a gravity infusion.
- **Secondary IV tubing:** It is shorter in length than primary tubing, with no access ports or backcheck valve; when connected to a primary line via an access port, it is used to infuse intermittent medications or fluids. A *secondary tubing administration set* is used for secondary IV medication.

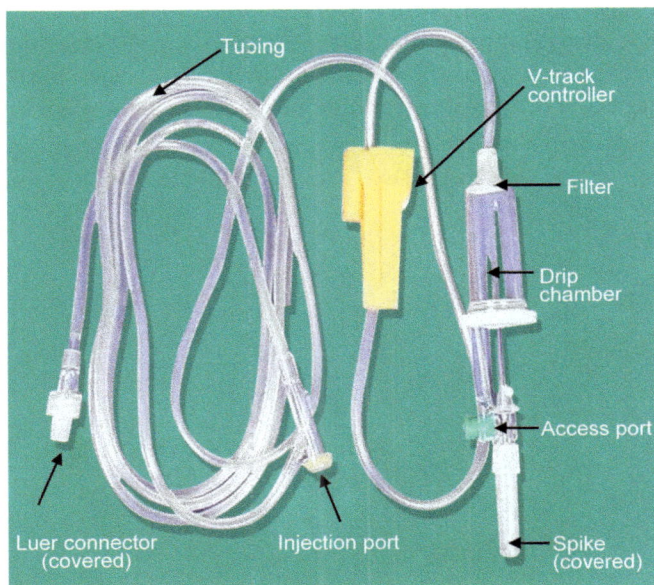

Fig. 17.19: Intravenous (IV) drip set.

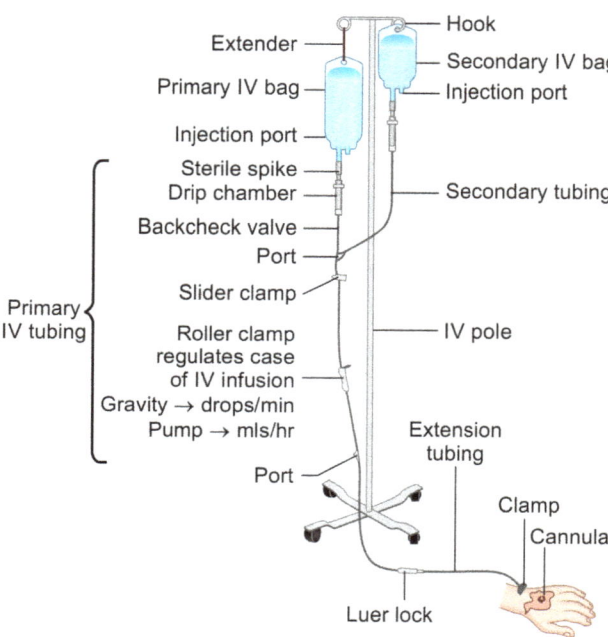

Fig. 17.20: Primary intravenous (IV) tubing.

Flow Rate Calculation

When calculating the flow rate of IV solutions, remember that the number of drops required to deliver 1 mL varies with the type of administration set. Administration sets are of two types:
1. Macro-drip set (delivers 10–20 drops/mL)
2. Micro-drip set (60 drops/mL)

Flow rate = Volume of infusion in mL × Drip factor (in drops/mL)/Time of infusion in minutes

INTRAVENOUS CANNULA

It is used for administering intravenous fluids, drugs, and blood products (**Table 17.1**).

OXYGEN MASK (FIG. 17.21)

It is used for administering oxygen.

An *oxygen mask* provides a method to transfer breathing oxygen gas from a storage tank to the lungs. Oxygen masks may cover only the nose and mouth (oral nasal mask) or the entire face (full-face mask). They may be made of plastic, silicone, or rubber.

Table 17.1: Color coding of intravenous cannula.

Size	Color	Length	Flow rate (mL/min)	Uses
14 G	Orange	45	250–300	• Used for adolescent and adult major surgery and trauma • Infusion of large amount of fluids or colloids
16 G	Gray	45	150–240	• Adolescent and adult major surgery and trauma • Infusion of large amount of fluids or colloids
18 G	Green	45	100–120	• Adolescent and adult major surgery and trauma • Infusion of large amount of fluids or colloids
20 G	Pink	32	55–80	• Older children, adolescent and adult • Ideal for IV infusion and blood infusion • Medication administration • Emergency management
22 G	Blue	25	22–50	• Older children, adolescent and elderly adult • IV infusion with moderate flow rates • Medication administration
24 G	Yellow	19	23	• Infant toddler, older children • Major surgery and trauma among children • Can administer fluids and medication
26 G	Voilet	19	10–15	• Neonate, infant and elderly adults • Suitable for infusion but infusion rate is low

INHALER DEVICES

Inhaler devices can be meter dose inhaler, dry powder inhalers, or nebulizers (**Figs. 17.22 to 17.25; Tables 17.2 to 17.4**).

Inhalant Drugs

- Broncodilators—salbutamol, formeterol, ipratropium, and tiotropium
- **Corticosteroids:** Beclomethasone, budesonide, and fluticasone
- **Mucolytic agents:** Acetylcysteine
- **Antimicrobials:** Ribaviran and tobramycin
- **Immune modulators:** Cyclosporine and interferon-α
- Anesthetics—opioids

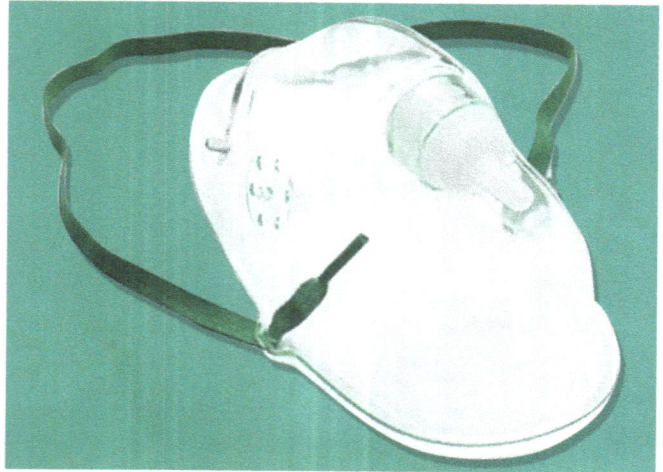

Fig. 17.21: Oxygen mask.

A *spacer* is a device used to increase the ease of administering aerosolized medication from a metered-dose inhaler (MDI). It adds space in the form of a tube or "chamber" between the

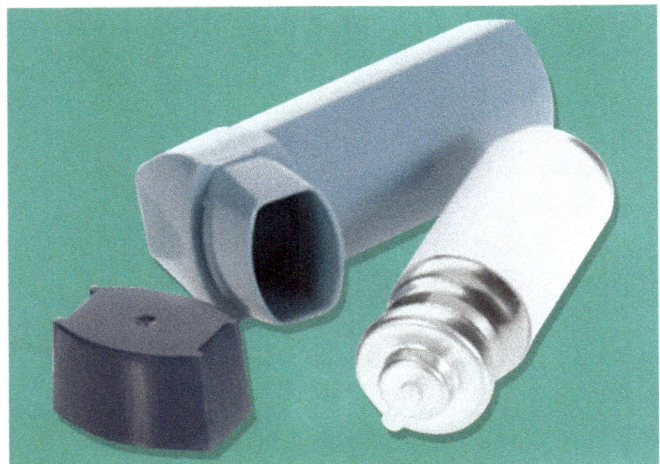

Fig. 17.22: Metered dose inhaler.

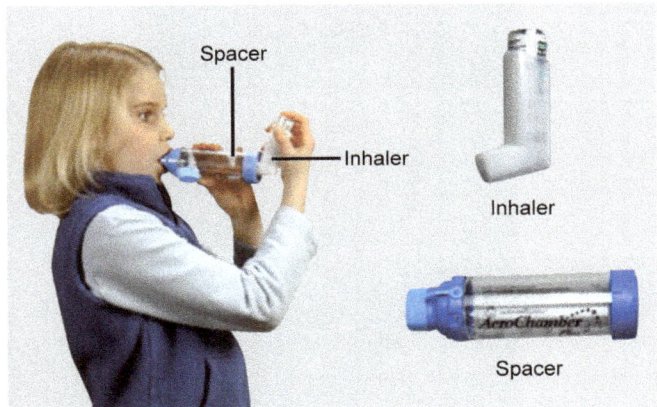

Fig. 17.23: Spacer.

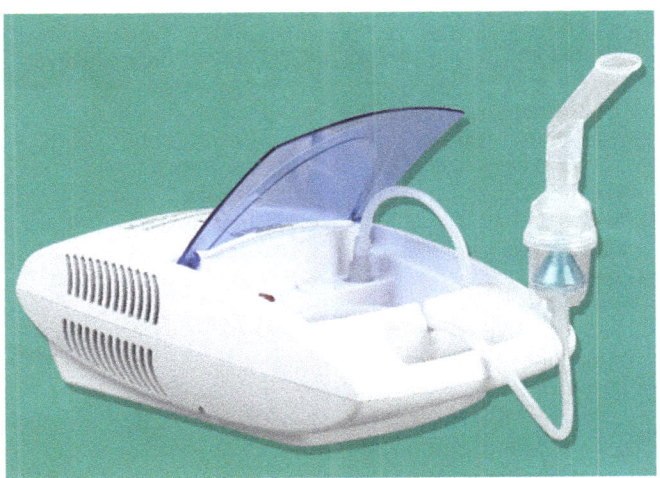

Fig. 17.25: Nebulizers.

Table 17.2: Metered dose inhaler.

Advantages	Disadvantages
• Rapid application • Handling • Multidose	• Hand–breathe coordination • Ineffective use in poor ventilated patients • Oropharyngeal deposition and local side effects

Table 17.3: Dry powder inhalers.

Advantages	Disadvantages
• Less patient coordination required • Spacer not necessary • Compact portable • No propellant • Usually higher lung deposition than a pMDI	• Work poorly, if inhalation is not forceful enough • Many patients cannot use them correctly • Most types are moisture sensitive • Need to reload capsule each time

(pMDI: pressurized metered-dose inhalers)

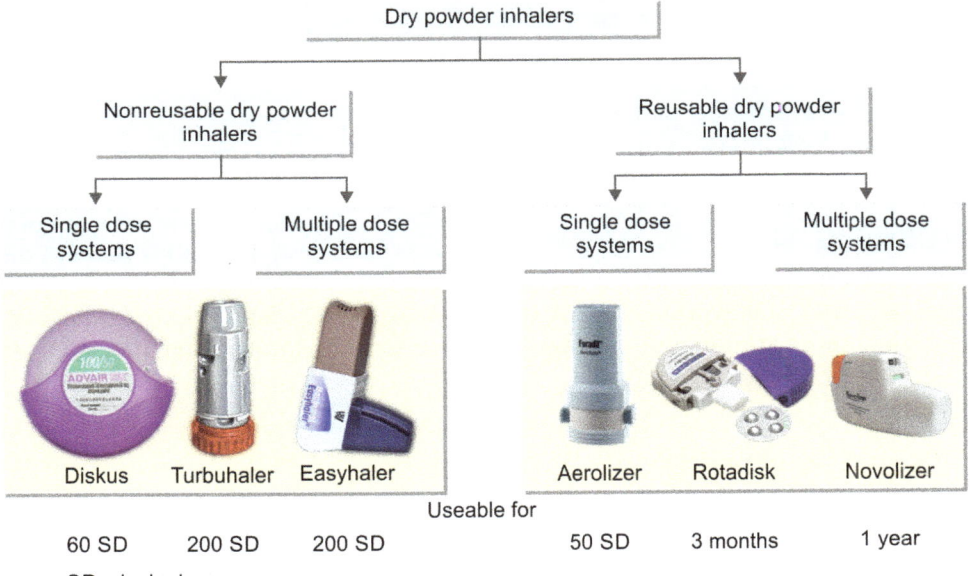

Fig. 17.24: Dry powder inhalers.

Table 17.4: Nebulizers.

Advantages	Disadvantages
• Provide therapy for patients who cannot use other inhalation modalities (e.g., MDI and DPI) • Allow administration of large doses of medicine • Patient coordination not required • Effective with tidal breathing • Dose modification possible • Can be used with supplemental oxygen	• Decreased portability • Longer set-up and administration time • Higher cost • Electrical power source required • Contamination possible

mouth and canister of medication. Most spacers have a one-way valve that allows the person to inhale the medication while inhaling and exhaling normally; these are often referred to as *valved holding chambers* (VHC).

URINOMETER (FIG. 17.26)

Urinometer is an instrument used to measure the specific gravity of urine.

There are three parts of urinometer. They are as illustrated in **Figure 17.26**:
1. **The float:** It is the air-containing part.
2. **Weight:** The lower end of urinometer
3. **Stem:** It has calibrations with numbers marked to measure the specific gravity.

Normal values of specific gravity are 1.003–1.030. It signifies the relative mass density. Specific gravity of urine is a measure of concentrating ability of kidneys and is determined to get information about its tubular function.
- **Increased specific gravity in urine:** Diabetes mellitus, nephritic syndrome, fever, and dehydration
- **Decreased specific gravity in urine:** Diabetes insipidus, chronic renal failure (low and fixed at 1.010) due to loss of concentrating ability of tubules, and compulsive water drinking.
- **Isosthenuria:** This is condition where there is fixed specific gravity. The specific gravity of the urine remains at 1.010 regardless of the volume of water consumption by the person. It occurs specifically in chronic renal disease.

WESTERGREN TUBE (FIG. 17.27)

The Westergren method requires collecting 2 mL of venous blood into a tube containing 0.5 mL of sodium citrate. It should be stored no longer than 2 hours at room temperature or

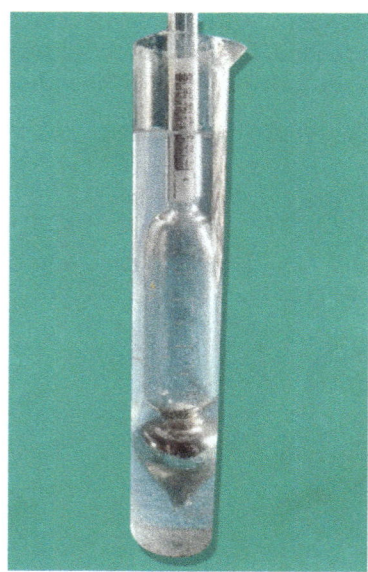

Fig. 17.26: Urinometer.

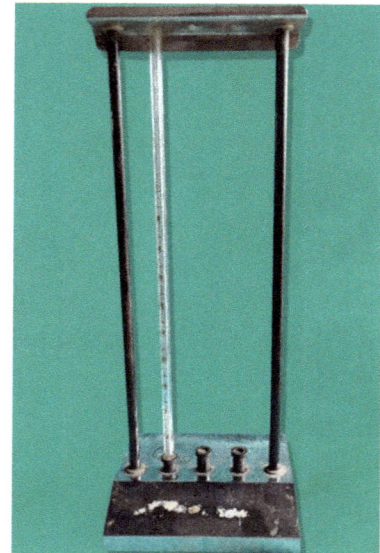

Fig. 17.27: Westergren tube.

6 hours at 4°C. The blood is drawn into a Westergren–Katz tube to the 200 mm mark. The tube is placed in a rack in a strictly vertical position for 1 hour at room temperature, at which time the distance from the lowest point of the surface meniscus to the upper limit of the red cell sediment is measured. The distance of fall of erythrocytes, expressed as millimeters in 1 hour, is the erythrocyte sedimentation rate (ESR).

DISCUSSION OF COMMON X-RAYS

Figures 17.28 to 17.49 discuss about common X-ray.

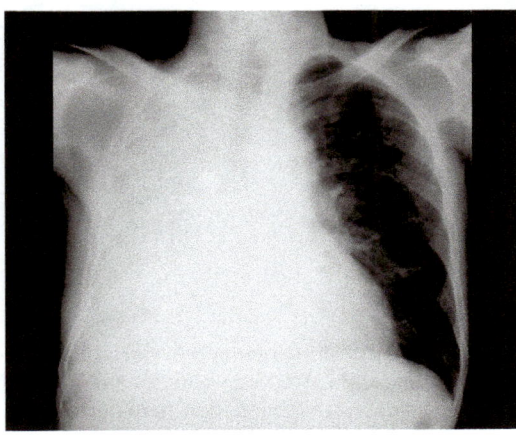

Fig. 17.28: Chest X-ray posteroanterior (PA) view showing homogenous opacity on the right hemithorax with trachea shifted to same side suggestive of right-sided collapse/pneumonectomy.

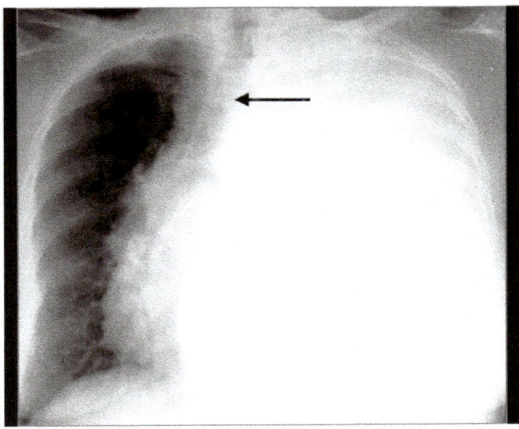

Fig. 17.29: Chest X-ray posteroanterior (PA) view showing homogenous opacity on the left hemithorax with trachea shifted to opposite side suggestive of left-sided massive pleural effusion.

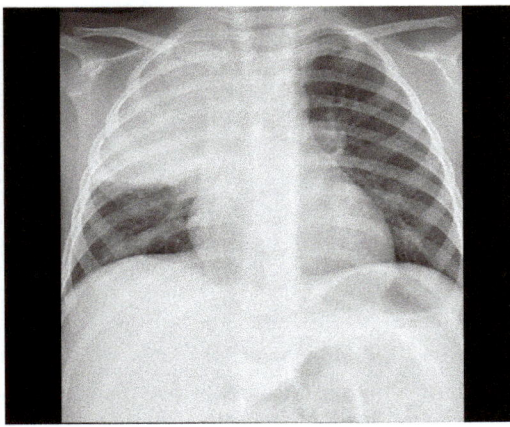

Fig. 17.30: Chest X-ray posteroanterior (PA) view showing—trachea central, cardiophrenic and costophrenic angles are normal, homogenous opacity in right upper zone with air bronchogram suggestive of right upper lobe pneumonia.

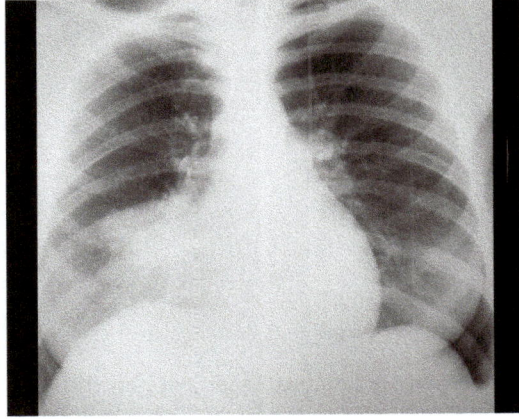

Fig. 17.31: Chest X-ray posteroanterior (PA) view showing—trachea central, cardiophrenic and costophrenic angles are normal, homogenous opacity in right mid and lower zone with air bronchogram, right heart border is not clear (Silhouette sign) suggestive of right middle lobe pneumonia.

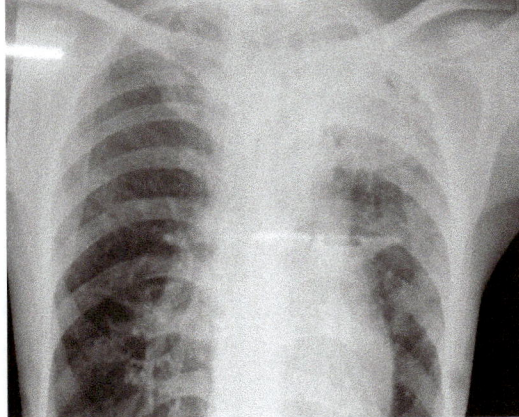

Fig. 17.32: Chest X-ray posteroanterior (PA) view showing—trachea central, cardiophrenic and costophrenic angles are normal, nonhomogenous opacity in left upper zone with cavity with air crescent sign suggestive of aspergilloma—crescent sign of Monad.

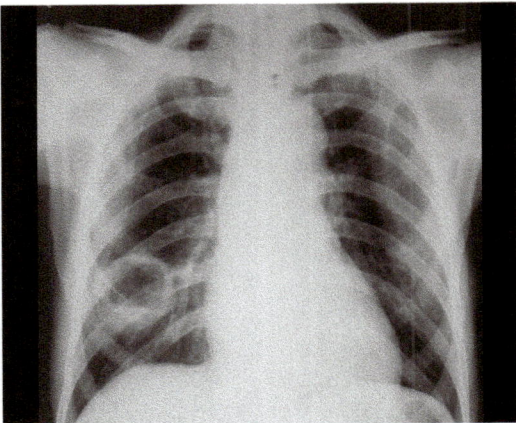

Fig. 17.33: Chest X-ray posteroanterior (PA) view showing—trachea central, cardiophrenic and costophrenic angles are normal, and thick walled cavity with air fluid level suggestive of lung abscess.

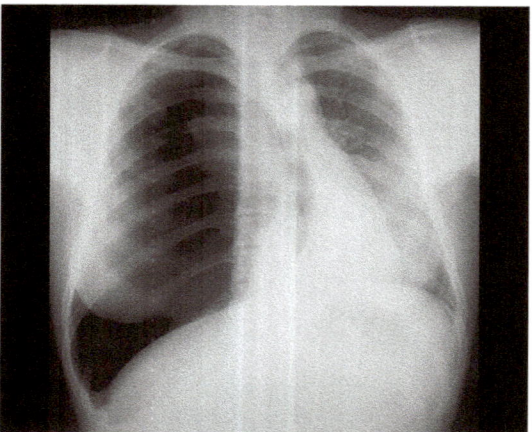

Fig. 17.34: Chest X-ray posteroanterior (PA) view showing— trachea and mediastinum deviated to left, cardiophrenic and costophrenic angles are normal, homogenous hyperlucency in right hemithorax suggestive of right-sided pneumothorax.

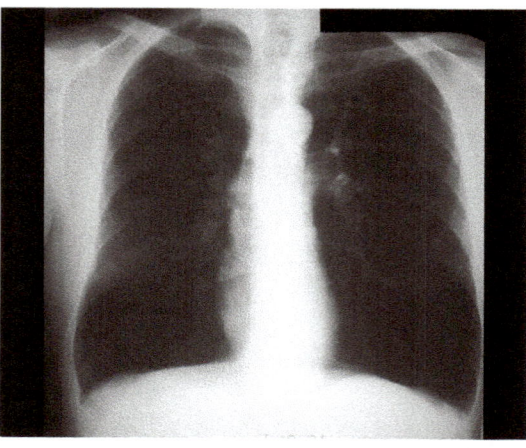

Fig. 17.35: Chest X-ray posteroanterior (PA) view showing—trachea central, cardiophrenic and costophrenic angles are normal, bilateral hyperlucent lung fields with hyperinflation, flattened diaphragm and tubular heart suggestive of bilateral emphysema.

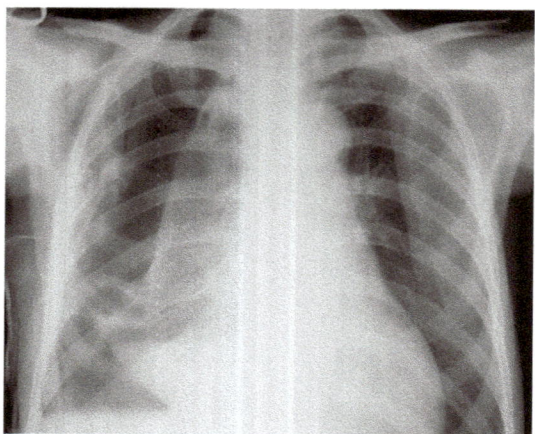

Fig. 17.36: Chest X-ray posteroanterior (PA) view showing tracheal shift to left, hyperlucency in right hemithorax with collapse lung margin (visceral pleural line) with obliteration of costophrenic angle with multiple air fluid levels suggestive of hydropneumothorax.

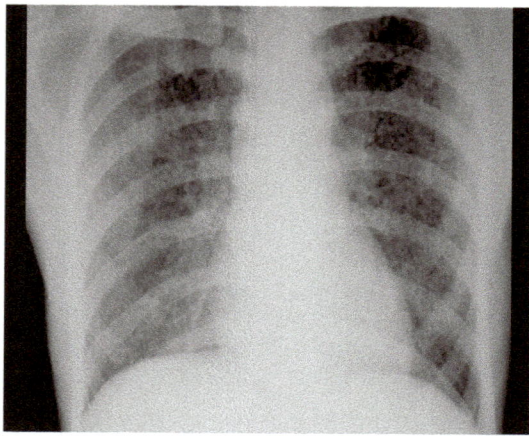

Fig. 17.37: Chest X-ray posteroanterior (PA) view showing small millet sized (1–3 mm) shadows in bilateral lung fields suggestive of miliary mottling.

Differential diagnosis (D/D) for miliary mottling:
- Miliary tuberculosis
- Tropical pulmonary eosinophilia
- Sarcoidosis
- Pneumocystis

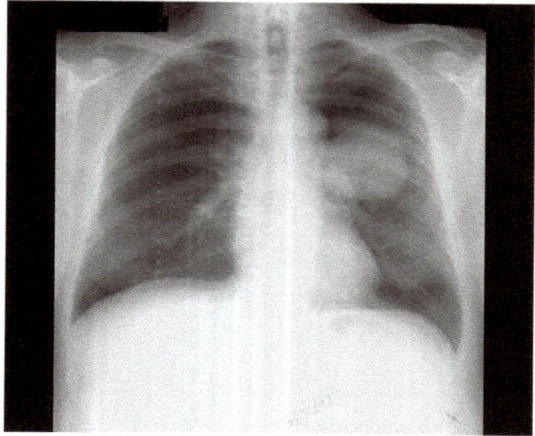

Fig. 17.38: Chest X-ray posteroanterior (PA) view showing rounded homogenous lesion in the right mid-zone—solitary pulmonary nodule.

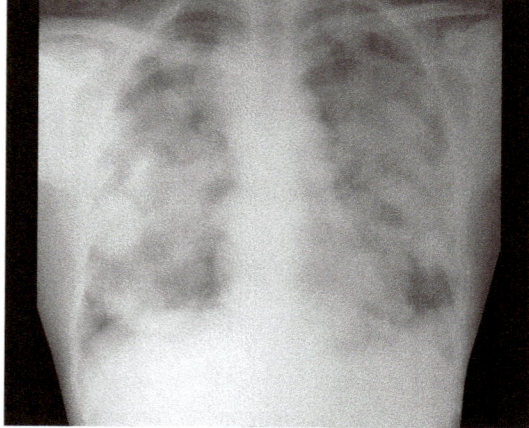

Fig. 17.39: Chest X-ray posteroanterior (PA) view showing multiple rounded nodular opacities in bilateral lung fields—Cannon ball metastasis: Primary—breast, thyroid, bowel, testes, kidney and choriocarcinoma.

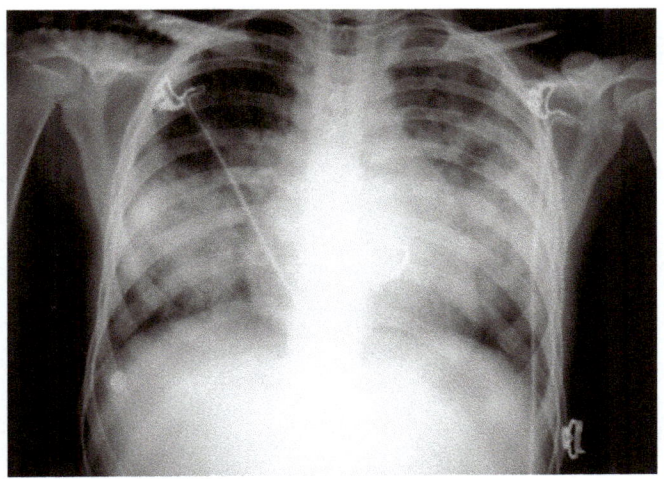

Fig. 17.40: Chest X-ray posteroanterior (PA) view showing cardiomegaly with bilateral nonhomogenous opacity in mid and lower zones (bat wing appearance) suggestive of pulmonary edema. Also patient has metallic mitral valve prosthesis.

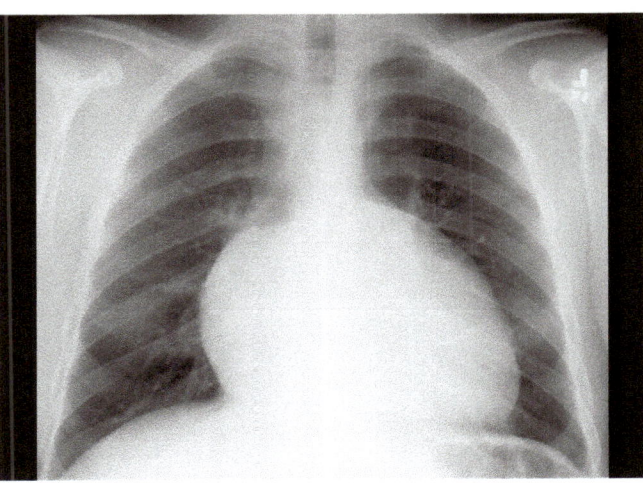

Fig. 17.41: Chest X-ray posteroanterior (PA) view showing gross cardiomegaly with stenciled heart borders, lungs clear, suggestive of pericardial effusion.

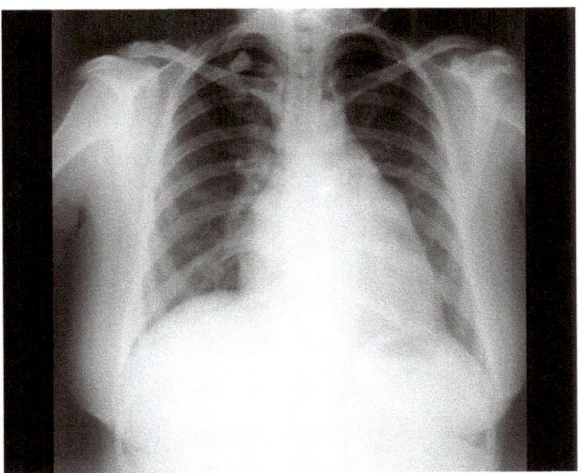

Fig. 17.42: Chest X-ray posteroanterior (PA) view showing cardiomegaly with features of mitral valve disease—splaying of carina, double atrial shadow, straightening of left heart border, enlarged left atrial appendage, and prominent pulmonary artery.

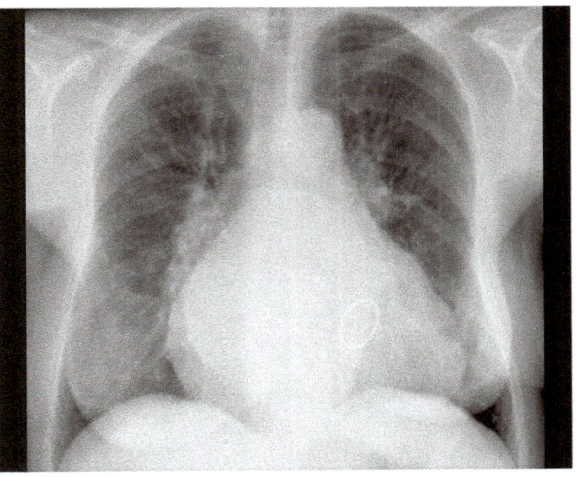

Fig. 17.43: Chest X-ray posteroanterior (PA) view showing cardiomegaly with features of mitral valve disease—splaying of carina, double atrial shadow, straightening of left heart border, mitral valve metallic prosthesis, enlarged left atrial appendage, prominent pulmonary artery, and prominent upper lobe veins (Stag Antler sign).

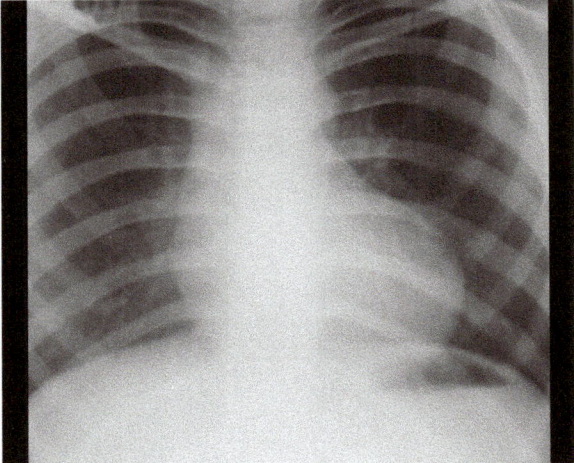

Fig. 17.44: Chest X-ray posteroanterior (PA) view showing pulmonary oligemia with upturned apex (right ventricle) suggestive of tetrology of Fallot (Cour-en-Sabot).

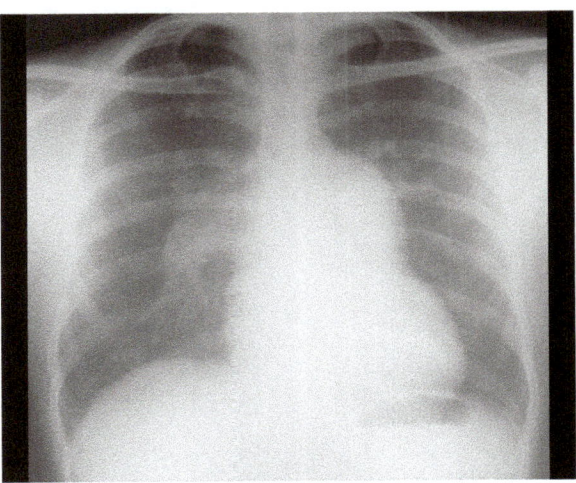

Fig. 17.45: Chest X-ray posteroanterior (PA) view showing mild cardiomegaly, prominent pulmonary artery, pulmonary plethora, prominent right atrium—suggestive of atrial septal defect—Jug Handle appearance.

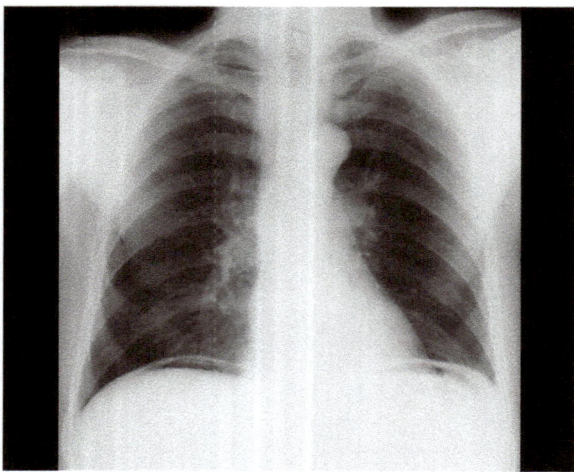

Fig. 17.46: Chest X-ray posteroanterior (PA) view showing free air under bilateral hemidiaphragm—pneumoperitoneum.

Causes:
- Hollow viscus perforation
- Post laparotomy/laparoscopy
- Subphrenic abscess
- Tubal insufflation (Rubins test)

Minimum amount of air needed to produce this—1 cc

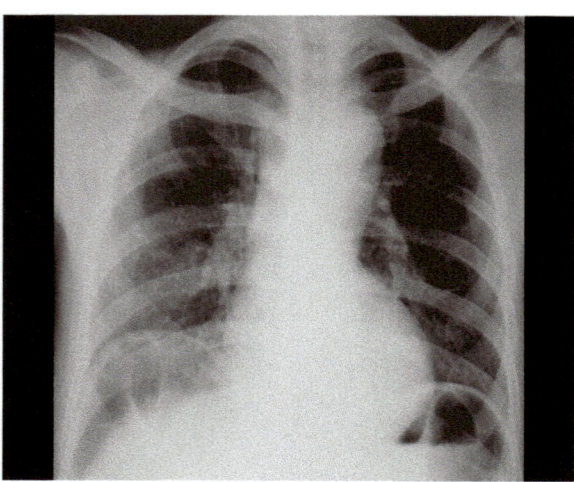

Fig. 17.47: Chest X-ray posteroanterior (PA) view showing interposition of transverse colon between liver and right hemidiaphragm—Chilaiditi syndrome.

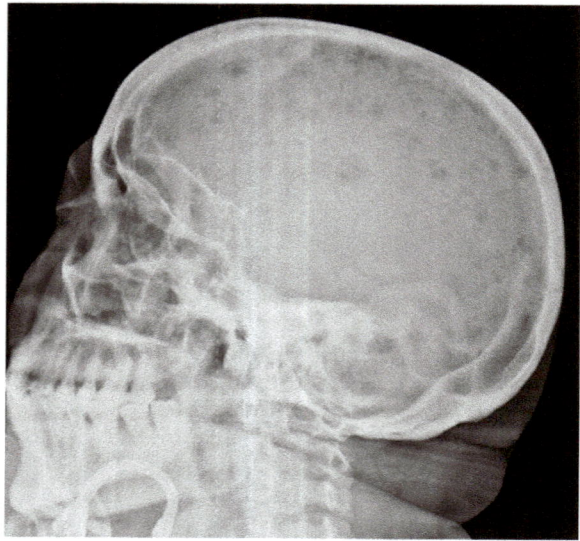

Fig. 17.48: Lateral X-ray of skull showing multiple punched out lesions.

Differential diagnosis (D/D): Myeloma, metastasis, and rarely Langerhans cell histiocytosis

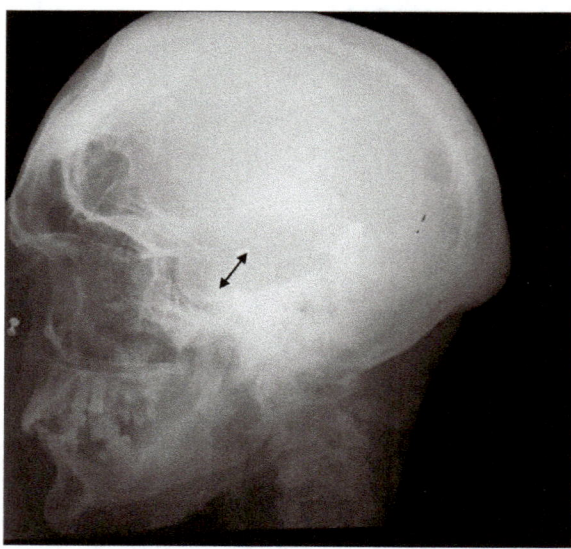

Fig. 17.49: Lateral skull X-ray showing prognathism, thickened skull vault, prominent air sinuses, enlarged sella turcica—suggestive of acromegaly.

18 CHAPTER

Normal Laboratory Values

CHAPTER OUTLINE

- Laboratory Values of Clinical Importance
- Commonly Used Formulas in Medicine

LABORATORY VALUES OF CLINICAL IMPORTANCE

The laboratory reference values in this appendix are divided into different section namely—(1) hematology and coagulation (**Table 18.1**), (2) clinical chemistry of blood (**Table 18.2**), (3) lipid profile (**Table 18.3**), (4) urea and electrolytes (**Table 18.4**), (5) thyroid function tests (**Table 18.5**), (6) urine (**Table 18.6**), and (7) cerebrospinal fluid (**Table 18.7**), and short list of routinely used formulas in medicine (**Table 18.8**).

1. *Hematology and coagulation* (**Table 18.1**)
2. *Clinical chemistry of blood* (**Table 18.2**)
3. *Lipid profile* (**Table 18.3**)
4. *Renal function tests* (**Table 18.4**)
5. *Thyroid function tests* (**Table 18.5**)
6. *Urine* (**Table 18.6**)
7. *Cerebrospinal fluid* (**Table 18.7**)
8. *Short list of routinely used formulas in medicine* (**Table 18.8**)

Table 18.1: Hematology and coagulation.

Component (specimen)	Reference value	
	Conventional	SI units
RBCs and hemoglobin:		
RBC count:		
• Males	4.5–5.5 × 10^{12}/L (mean 5.0 × 10^{12}/L)	
• Females	3.8–4.8 × 10^{12}/L (mean 4.3 × 10^{12}/L)	
RBC diameter	6.7–7.7 μm (mean 7.2 μm)	
RBC indices (absolute values)		
• Mean corpuscular volume (MCV)	82–100 fL	
• Mean corpuscular hemoglobin (MCH)	27–32 pg	
• Mean corpuscular hemoglobin concentration (MCHC)	31–35 g/dL	
• Red cell distribution width (RDW)	11.5–14.0%	
RBC lifespan	120 days	
Erythrocyte sedimentation rate (ESR) (whole blood)		
• Westergren, 1st hour:		
▪ Males	0–15 mm 1st hour	
▪ Females	0–20 mm 1st hour	
▪ Children	0–10 mm 1st hour	
• Wintrobe, 1st hour:		
▪ Males	0–9 mm 1st hour	
▪ Females	0–20 mm 1st hour	
Ferritin (serum):		
• Males	20–300 ng/mL	20–300 μg/L
• Females	15–200 ng/mL	15–200 μg/L
Folate (serum)	3–20 μg/L	3–20 ng/mL

Contd...

Contd...

Component (specimen)	Reference value	
	Conventional	SI units
Hematocrit (PCV):		
• Males	38–47%	
• Females	36–46%	
• Infants (cord blood)	45–70%	
Haptoglobin (serum)	40–240 mg/dL	0.4–2.4 g/L
Hemoglobin (Hb):		
• Adult hemoglobin (HbA)	95–98%	
• Males	13.0–17.0 g/dL	
• Females	12.0–15.0 g/dL	
• Hemoglobin A_2 (HbA$_2$)	1.5–3.5%	
• Hemoglobin, fetal (HbF) in adults	<0–2%	
• HbF, children under 6 months	<5%	
Iron, total (serum):	50–150 µg/dL	7–25 µmol/L
• Total iron binding capacity (TIBC)	310–340 µg/dL	45–73 µmol/L
• Iron saturation	20–45%	0.20–0.45
Osmotic fragility:		
• Slight hemolysis	At 0.45–0.39 g/dL NaCl	
• Complete hemolysis	At 0.33–0.36 g/dL NaCl	
• Mean corpuscular fragility	0.4–0.45 g/dL NaCl	
Reticulocytes:		
• Adults	0.5–2.5%	
• Infants	2–6%	
• Newborn (cord blood)	1–7%	
Transferrin saturation:		
• Male	25–56%	
• Female	14–51%	
Vitamin B_{12} (serum):		
• Body stores	10–12 mg	
• Daily requirement	2–3 µg	
• Serum level	280–1,000 pg/mL	
Autohemolysis test (whole blood)	0.4–4.50%	0.004–0.045
Autohemolysis test with glucose (whole blood)	0.3–0.7%	0.003–0.007
Leukocytes:		
Differential leukocyte count (DLC):		
• P (polymorphs or neutrophils)	40–70% (2,000–7,500/µL)	
• L (lymphocytes)	20–40% (1,500–4,000/µL)	
• M (monocytes)	2–10% (200–800/µL)	
• E (eosinophils)	1–6% (40–450/µL)	
• B (basophils)	<1% (10–100/µL)	
Total leukocyte count (TLC):		
• Adults	4,000–11,000/µL	
• Infants (full term, at birth)	10,000–25,000/µL	
• Infants (1 year)	6,000–16,000/µL	
Platelets and coagulation:		
Bleeding time (BT):		
• Ivy's method	2–7 min	
• Template method	2–9 min	
Clot retraction time (clotted blood):		
• Qualitative	Visible in 60 min (complete in <24 hours)	
• Quantitative	48–64% (55%)	
Clotting time (CT):		
• Lee and White method	4–11 minutes	
D-dimer (plasma)	220–740 ng/mL	

Contd...

Contd...

Component (specimen)	Reference value	
	Conventional	SI units
Fibrinogen (plasma)	200–400 mg/dL	
Fibrin split (or degradation) products (FSP or FDP)	<10 µg/mL	<10 mg/L
Partial thromboplastin time with kaolin (PTTK) or activated partial thromboplastin time (APTT/aAPTT)	30–40 seconds	
Platelet count	150,000–450,000/µL	
Prothrombin time (PT) (Quick's one stage method)	11–16 seconds	
Thrombin time (TT)	15–19 seconds (control ± 2 seconds)	

(RBC: red blood cell)

Table 18.2: Clinical chemistry of blood.

Component	Specimen	Reference value	
		Conventional	SI units
Alpha fetoprotein (AFP), adults	Serum	0–8.5 ng/mL	0–8.5 µg/L
Aminotransferases (transaminases) • Aspartate (AST and SGOT) • Alanine (ALT and SGPT)	 Serum Serum	 12–38 U/L 7–41 U/L	 0.20–0.65 µkat/L 0.12–0.70 µkat/L
Amylase	Serum	20–96 U/L	0.34–1.6 µkat/L
Bilirubin: • Total • Direct (conjugated) • Indirect (unconjugated)	Serum	 0.3–1.3 mg/dL 0.1–0.4 mg/dL 0.2–0.9 mg/dL	 5.1–22 µmol/L 1.7–6.8 µmol/L 3.4–15.2 µmol/L
CA-125	Serum	0–35 U/mL	0–35 Ku/L
Calcium—ionized	Whole blood	4.5–5.3 mg/dL	1.12–1.32 mmol/L
Calcium—total	Serum	8.7–10.2 mg/dL	2.2–2.6 mmol/L
Chloride	Serum	102–109 mEq/L	102–109 mmol/L
C-reactive proteins	Serum	0.2–3.0 mg/L	0.2–3.0 mg/L
Creatine kinase (CK), total: • Males • Females	Serum	 51–294 U/L 39–238 U/L	 0.87–5.0 µkat/L 0.66–4.0 µkat/L
Creatine kinase MB (CKMB)	Serum	0–5.5 ng/mL	0–5.5 µg/L
Gamma glutamyl transpeptidase (transferase) (γ-GT)	Serum	9–58 IU/L	0.15–1.00 µmol/L
Glucose (fasting): • Normal • Impaired fasting glucose (IFG) • Diabetes mellitus	Plasma	 70–100 mg/dL 101–125 mg/dL >126 mg/dL	 <5.6 mmol/L 5.6–6.9 mmol/L >7.0 mmol/L
Glucose (2-hour postprandial): • Normal • Impaired glucose tolerance (IGT) • Diabetes mellitus	Plasma	 <140 mg/dL 140–200 mg/dL >200 mg/dL	 <7.8 mmol/L 7.8–11.1 mmol/L >11.1 mmol/L
Glycated hemoglobin (HbA$_{1c}$)	Whole blood	4.0–6.0%	20–42 mmol/mol Hb
Lactate dehydrogenase (LDH)	Serum	115–221 U/L	2.0–3.8 µkat/L
Muramidase	Serum	5–20 µg/mL	
5-nucleotidase	Serum	0–11 U/L	0.02–0.19 µkat/L
Phosphatases: • Acid phosphatase • Alkaline phosphatase	Serum	 0–5.5 U/L 33–96 U/L	 0.90 µkat/L 0.56–1.63 µkat/L
Prostate-specific antigen (PSA)	Serum	0–4.0 ng/mL	0–4.0 µg/L

Contd...

Contd...

Component	Specimen	Reference value	
		Conventional	SI units
Proteins—total: • Albumin • Globulins • Albumin/globulin ratio	Serum	6.7–8.6 g/dL 3.5–5.5 g/dL 2.0–3.5 g/dL 1.5–3:1	67–86 g/L 35–55 g/L 20–35 g/L
Rheumatoid factor	Serum	<15 IU/mL	<15 kU/L
Troponins—cardiac (cTn): • Troponin I (cTnI) • Troponin T (cTnT)	Serum Serum	0–0.08 ng/mL 0–0.01 ng/mL	0–0.8 µg/L 0–0.1 µg/L
Urea nitrogen (BUN)	Blood	7–20 mg/dL	2.5–7.1 mmol/L
Uric acid: • Males • Females	Serum	3.1–7.0 mg/dL 2.5–5.6 mg/dL	0.18–0.41 µmol/L 0.15–0.33 µmol/L

(AST: aspartate aminotransferase; SGOT: serum glutamic oxaloacetic transaminase; ALT: alanine aminotransferase; SGPT: serum glutamic pyruvic transaminase)

Table 18.3: Lipid profile.

Component	Reference value	
	Conventional	SI units
Total serum cholesterol:		
Desirable for adults	<200 mg/dL	<5.17 mmol/L
Borderline high	200–239 mg/dL	5.17–6.18 mmol/L
High undesirable	>240 mg/dL	>6.21 mmol/L
LDL cholesterol:		
Desirable range	100–130 mg/dL	<3.34 mmol/L
Borderline high	130–159 mg/dL	3.36–4.11 mmol/L
High	160–189 mg/dL	4.11–4.20 mmol/L
Very high	>190 mg/dL	>4.21 mmol/L
HDL cholesterol:		
Low	<40 mg/dL	<1.03 mmol/L
High, protective range	>60 mg/dL	>1.55 mmol/L
Triglycerides	<160 mg/dL	<2.26 mmol/L

(HDL: high-density lipoprotein; LDL: low-density lipoprotein)

Table 18.4: Renal function tests.

Analyte	Reference value	
	Conventional	SI units
Sodium	136–146 mEq/L	136–146 mmol/L
Potassium	3.5–5.0 mEq/L	3.5–5.0 mmol/L
Chloride	95–107 mEq/L	95–107 mmol/L
Urea	20–40 mg/dL	3.3–6.6 mmol/L
Creatinine	0.6–1.2 mg/dL	53–106 µmol/L

Table 18.5: Thyroid function tests.

Thyroid function tests	Specimen	Reference value	
		Conventional	SI units
Radioactive iodine uptake (RAIU) 24 hours		5–30%	
Thyroxine (T4) total	Serum	5.4–11.7 µg/dL	70–151 nmol/L
Triiodothyronine (T3) total	Serum	77–135 ng/dL	1.2–2.1 nmol/L
Thyroid-stimulating hormone (TSH)	Serum	0.4–4.25 µU/mL	0.4–4.25 mU/L

Table 18.6: Normal urine values.

Component	Reference value
Volume—24 hours	600–1,800 mL (variable)
pH	5.0–9.0
Specific gravity—quantitative (random)	1.002–1.028 (average 1.018)
Protein—24 hours urine	<150 mg/day
Protein—qualitative (random)	Negative
Glucose—quantitative—24 hours urine	50–300 mg/day
Glucose—qualitative (random)	Negative
Urobilinogen—24 hours urine	1.0–3.5 mg/day
Microalbuminuria (24 hours)	0–30 mg/24 hours (0–0.03 g/day) (0–30 µg/mg creatinine) (0–0.03 g/g creatinine)

Table 18.7: Normal values of cerebrospinal fluid (CSF).

Component	Reference value — Conventional	Reference value — SI units
CSF volume	120–150 mL	
Appearance	Clear and colorless	
CSF pressure	60–150 mm water	
pH	7.31–7.34	
Total proteins	20–40 mg/dL	0.14–0.45 g/L
Glucose	40–80 mg/dL	2.3–4.5 mmol/L
Chlorides	720–750 mg/dL	
Cells: • Polymorphs • Lymphocytes	Usually absent 0–5/µL	

COMMONLY USED FORMULAS IN MEDICINE (TABLE 18.8)

Table 18.8: Commonly used formulas in medicine.

Electrolyte disorders	
Plasma osmolality	2 Na⁺ (mEq/L) + Serum glucose (mg/dL)/18 + BUN (mg/dL)/2.8
Corrected sodium	Increase Na⁺ by 1.6 mEq/L for each 100 mg% (when serum glucose >100 mg%)
Total body sodium deficit	(Desired sodium – measured sodium) × Body weight × [0.6 (men) or 0.5 (women)]
Potassium deficit	1 mmol/L decrease → approximately 200–400 mmol loss of total body K⁺
Urine–plasma electrolyte ratio (in chronic hyponatremia)	Urinary (sodium + potassium)/plasma sodium: • >1 (fluid restriction up to less than 500 mL/day) • =1 (500–700 mL/day) • <1 (fluid restriction up to 1 L)
Water deficit (in hypernatremia)	Water deficit = (Plasma sodium – 140) × TBW/140
TTKG (trans-tubular potassium gradient) in hypokalemia	Urinary potassium × plasma osmolality/serum potassium × urinary osmolality >4 indicates renal loss of potassium
Corrected calcium	0.8 × (4 – serum albumin) + serum calcium
Acid–base disorders	
Anion gap (serum)	(Sodium + potassium) – (bicarbonate + chloride) • 8–16 mEq/L (old methods) • 5–11 mEq/L (new techniques)
Urine anion gap	Urine sodium + potassium – chloride –25 to –50 (normal range)

Contd...

Contd...

Delta ratio	(Serum anion gap − 12)/(24 − serum bicarbonate) • <0.4 hyperchloremic normal anion gap acidosis • <1 high AG and normal AG acidosis • >2 high AG acidosis and a concurrent metabolic alkalosis
Respiratory acidosis	*Acute*: 10 increase in pCO_2 → 1 increase in bicarbonate *Chronic*: 10 increase in pCO_2 → 4 increase in bicarbonate
Respiratory alkalosis	*Acute*: 10 decrease in pCO_2 → 2 decrease in bicarbonate *Chronic*: 10 decrease in pCO_2 → 5 decrease in bicarbonate
Metabolic acidosis	pCO_2 = 1.5 (bicarbonate) + 8 ± 2
Metabolic alkalosis	10 increase in bicarbonate → pCO_2 increases by 6
Nephrology	
Renal failure index	Urine Na/(Urine Cr/PCr)
Cockcroft–Gault GFR	(140 − Age) × (Body weight in kg) × (0.85 if female)/(72 × Cr)
Fractional excretion of sodium (FENa)	(Serum Cr × Urine Na)/(Serum Na × Urine Cr)%
Hematology	
Corrected reticulocyte count	Reticulocyte % × (Hb/15)
Reticulocyte production index	= Corrected reticulocyte count/maturation time • At a hemoglobin of 15, the maturation time = 1 day • At a hemoglobin of 12, the maturation time = 1.5 days • At a hemoglobin of 8, the maturation time = 2 days • At a hemoglobin of 5, the maturation time = 2.5 days
Mentzer index	(MCV, in fL) divided by (RBC, in millions per μL) Less than 13, thalassemia is said to be more likely
Parenteral iron in iron deficiency anemia	[2.3 × body weight (kg) × Hb deficit (g/dL)] + 1,000 mg (to replenish stores)
Respiratory system	
A–a gradient	PAO_2 − PaO_2 [PAO_2 = (FiO_2 × 713) − $PaCO_2$/0.8; PaO_2 is obtained from the ABG]
Cardiology	
Corrected QT	QT/√RR (Bazett's formula)
MAP	Systolic BP + (2 × diastolic BP)/3
Miscellaneous	
BMI	W/H^2 (W = weight in kg and H = Height in meters)

(AG: anion gap; BMI: body mass index; BUN: blood urea nitrogen; GFR: glomerular filtration rate; MAP: mean arterial pressure; MCV: mean corpuscular volume; pCO_2: partial pressure of carbon dioxide)

Index

Page numbers followed by '*b*' refer to box, '*f*' refer to figure, '*fc*' refer to flowchart and '*t*' refer to table.

A

Abciximab 276
Abdomen 65*f*
    four quadrants of 64*f*
    lower 58
    percussion of 67
    quadrants of 64
    regions of 65
    shape of 64
Abdominal pain 49, 166, 301, 528
    causes of 58*t*
    recurrent episodes of 161
Abdominal swelling 51
    causes of 52*t*
Abortions 436
Abscess 305
    diagnostic aspiration of 202
    formation 305
    metastatic 238
    myocardial 306
    ring 306
Absolute basophil count 419
Absolute insulin deficiency 502
Absorption
    atelectasis 239
    storage 386
    transport 386
Acanthosis nigricans 455
Acebutolol 284
Acetaminophen 512
Achalasia predisposes 159
Acid
    base balance 343
    fast bacilli 225, 252
    neutralizing 162
    regurgitation 157
Acidosis 349, 502
Acquired immunodeficiency syndrome 538, 540, 541*t*
    oral manifestations of 542*b*
    pathogenesis of 539*f*
Acral paresthesia 451
Actinomyces israelii 249
Activated partial thromboplastin time 404, 409
Acute aortic
    dissection 287
    regurgitation 300
Acute cardiogenic pulmonary edema 314
Acute coronary syndrome 271, 272, 273*fc*, 273*t*, 277, 287
    clinical features of 274
    complications of 274
    management of 277*fc*
    signs of 274*t*
Acute diarrhea 54*t*, 151, 152
    causes of 54, 91, 91*t*
    management of 153*fc*
Acute hepatitis 57, 179*f*
    causes for 181, 181*t*
Acute kidney injury 340, 349*t*
    causes of 341*f*, 342*t*
    classification of 340, 340*t*, 342*t*
    clinical features of 342*t*
    complications of 343, 344*b*
    network classification 340, 341*f*

Acute lymphoblastic leukemia 412, 563
    clinical features of 414*t*
Acute lymphocytic leukemia 409, 412, 413*t*
    treatment of 412*fc*
Acute mitral regurgitation 296
    causes of 296
Acute myeloid leukemia 412, 413*t*, 418
    treatment of 413*fc*
Acute myocardial infarction 275*f*, 275*t*, 277*b*, 316, 527
    management of 276
    signs of 274*t*
    symptoms of 274*t*
Acute pyelonephritis 351
    pathogenesis of 350*f*
Acute respiratory distress syndrome 94, 186, 257, 258, 258*t*, 259, 259*fc*, 260, 260*f*
    pathophysiology of 258
Acute respiratory failure 258
    causes of 258*b*
Acute respiratory syndrome coronavirus 520
Acute rheumatic carditis, clinical features of 290
Acute rheumatic fever 288
    diagnosis of 291
    management of 292
Acute systemic disease 525
Acute tubular necrosis 334, 342
Acute viral hepatitis 176
    complications of 180*t*
Acyclovir 343
Adams-Stokes attacks 318
Adaptive immune system 442
Addison's disease 35, 144, 450, 483, 484, 484*f*
    cardinal features of 484
    clinical features of 484
Adefovir dipivoxil 184
Adenocarcinoma 155
Adenomas, adrenal 482
Adenosine deaminase 235
Adenosylcobalamin 386
Adenovirus 350
Adipokines 455
Adipose tissue 455
Adrenal crisis 485
Adrenal disorders 281
Adrenal gland 479, 479*t*
    disorders 479
Adrenal vein catheterization 483
Adrenalectomy, bilateral 482, 484
Adrenaline 213, 323, 328
Adrenocortical insufficiency 483
    causes of 483
    clinical features of 484*t*
Adrenoleukodystrophy 483
Adrenomyeloneuropathy 483
Adventitious sounds 85, 109, 109*fc*
    discontinuous 109
Adverse drug reactions 323
Aerobic exercise 330, 495
Agnosia 355
Agranulocytosis 472
Air
    bronchograms 521
    space pneumonia 249
Airflow
    limitation, chronic 215
    narrowing 206

    obstruction 217
    reversal of 238
Airway 322, 327
    disease 240
        chronic obstructive 215
        small 215
    hyperreactivity 206, 215
    hyperresponsiveness 206
    obstruction 17, 523
    patency, advanced techniques for 323
    remodeling 207
    responsiveness 209
    smooth muscle 211, 213
Alabaster skin 461
Alanine
    aminotransferase 170, 171, 179, 574
    transaminase 31
Alar chest 97
Albumin 334
    glycosylated 500
    gradient, serum-ascites 197, 198*t*
    levels 435
Albuminuria 344*f*
Alcohol 161, 189, 258
    chronic 320, 437
    consumption 495
    intake 280
    metabolism 436
Alcoholism
    chronic 62
    sign of 60
Aldosterone antagonist 199, 278, 312
Aldosteronism, primary 281
Alemtuzumab 263
Alfacacidol 451
Aliskiren 285
Alkaline phosphatase 31, 171, 179, 424
Allergens 211
Allergic bronchopulmonary aspergillosis 260, 261*t*
Allergic reactions 277, 500
Allergic status, measurement of 210
Allogeneic bone marrow transplantation 416
Allogeneic transplantation 413
Allopurinol 200
All-trans-retinoic acid 413, 435
Almotriptan 359
Alogliptin 497
Alpha 1-antitrypsin, deficiency of 220
Alpha-fetoprotein 173, 201, 573
Alpha-ketoglutarate, decarboxylation of 436
Alpha-tocopherol transfer protein 445
Alport syndrome 340
Alteplase 277
Alveolo-capillary junction 89
Amanita phalloides 200
Amastigotes, demonstration of 536
Ambu bag 559, 559*f*
Ambulatory blood pressure monitoring 281
Ambulatory peritoneal dialysis 346
Amebiasis 528
    complications of 529*t*
    pathogenesis of 529*f*
    treatment of 530, 530*t*
Amebic abscess 202
Amebic colitis 528

Amebic complement fixation test 202
Amebic dysentery 528, 530, 530t
Amebic liver abscess 202
Amebic typhlitis 529
Ameboma 528
Amenorrhea 464
Amikacin 233
Amiloride 285, 467
Amino acid
    decarboxylation of 439
    structure 499f
Aminoglycosides 232
Aminophylline 213
Aminosalicylate agents 167
Aminotransferases 170, 573
Amiodarone 187, 316, 323
Amitriptyline 359, 508, 517
Amlodipine 270, 284, 488
Amoxicillin 164, 199, 200, 308, 343, 351
    plus aminoglycosides 352
Amoxiclav 253
Amphetamines 161
Amphotericin B 537
    deoxycholate 533
    lipid complex 533
Ampicillin 308, 351
    intravenous 352
Amygdala 367
Amylin 457
Amyloidosis 320, 348
    generalized 238
Amylophagia 384
Anaerobic bacterial infection 241
Anagrelide 420
Anaphylactoid reactions 554, 555b
Anaphylaxis, diagnostic criteria for 554
Anchovy sauce 202
Ancillary tests 379
Ancylostoma 261
Androgens 400
Anemia 28, 29, 61, 204, 269, 345, 380, 400
    acquired hemolytic 391t
    acute hemolytic 397
    causes of 346b
    classification of 381t
    dimorphic 421
    etiology of 382t
    hypochromic microcytic 398, 399t
    investigation of 562
    macrocytic 421
    normochromic 398t, 438
    normocytic 398t
        normochromic 415, 398
    severe 395
    signs of 381f, 382t
    stimulates erythropoietin 395
    supportive therapy for 398
    symptoms of 381f
    treatment of 421
Anesthesia induction 486
Aneurysm formation 267
Angina 118, 267t, 283, 294, 298
    abdominal 118
    atypical 268
    decubitus 118
    episodic 118
    functional classification of 119
    pectoris 267, 300
        management of 269
    precipitate factors for 267
    severity of 268
    types of 118
Angioedema 263, 552, 553f
    chronic 553
    hereditary 553

Angiography, coronary 269
Angiotensin receptor
    antagonists 312
    blocker 285, 286
Angiotensin-converting enzyme 552
    inhibitors 277, 285, 286, 312, 315
Anistreplase 277
Ankle jerk reflexes 437
Ann Arbor classification 424t
Anorexia 144, 221
    causes of 144b
    nervosa 437
Antacids 157
Anthropometry 43, 454
Anti anginal drug 271t
    second-line 232, 270
    treatment 269
Anti-apoptotic gene 418
Anti-B lymphocyte therapy 340
Antibiotic 219
    intravenous 352
    prophylaxis 185
    regimen 308, 526t
    therapy 199, 238, 255, 257, 351, 526, 528
        duration of 241
        parenteral 241
Antibody 304
    bound platelets 402
    complexes 336
Anticholinergic 218
    agents 146
    drug 218
Anticoagulants 276, 505
Anticoagulation
    chronic 325
    indications for 295
    therapy 312
Antidepressants 316
Antidiabetic drugs, oral 493
Antidiarrheal agents 154
Antidiuretic hormone, exogenous 467
Antiepileptic drug 367, 367t, 368t
    therapy 367
Antifungal agents 261
Antigen 304
    defection 374
    description of 516
    prostate-specific 573
    types of 206
Antiglomerular basement membrane antibody 336
Antihemophilic globulin 405
Antihistamines 555
Antihistaminic agents 145
Antihypertensive agents 287t, 454
Antihypertensive drug 284f, 284t
    therapy 283
Anti-inflammatory drugs 507
Anti-inflammatory therapy 238
Anti-insulin antibodies 500
Antilymphocyte globulin 400
Antimicrosomal antibody 468
Antimotility drugs 154
Antimucolytic agents 218
Antimuscarinic drug 218
Antioxidant 220, 435
Antiparkinsonian drugs 146
Antiphospholipid antibody syndrome 328
Antiplatelet antibody 403
Antiplatelet therapy 270, 276, 362
    intravenous 276
Antipsychotics 146
Antipyretics 512, 519
Antiretroviral drugs 543, 543b
Antiretroviral therapy, indications for 543, 543t
Antistreptolysin O antibodies 291

Antistreptozyme test 291
Antithrombin therapy 276
Antithrombotic factors, deficiency of 328
Antithyroglobulin 478
    antibody 468
Antithyroid
    drugs 472
    peroxidase 478
        antibody 468
Antitrypsin 220
Antituberculous drugs 231
    classification of 231, 232t
    effects of 232, 232t
Antiviral therapy 516
Anuria 333
    causes of 334, 334b
Aorta 319, 546
    abdominal 14, 66f
    aneurysm of 283
    coarctation of 320
Aortic area 299
    auscultation of 139, 139f
Aortic dissection 118, 283
Aortic pulsations 126
Aortic regurgitation 125-127, 130, 132, 135, 137-140, 142, 290, 299, 301t
    acute 299
    causes of 300b
    chronic 300
    murmur of 138
    symptoms 299
Aortic stenosis 123, 126, 127, 132, 137, 138, 142, 268, 298, 309
    classification of 298, 298b
    etiology of 298, 298b
    severe 269
    supravalvular 298
    symptomatic triad of 298
Aortic valve replacement 299
Apex
    abnormalities of 125
    beat 294, 296, 299, 300
    displacement of 125
    pulse deficit, demonstration of 10f
Aphasia 305, 355
Apical impulse 96, 99, 124, 125
Apical pansystolic murmur 297
Aplastic anemia 29, 400, 514
    causes of 400, 400t
    severe 400
Aplastic crisis 394
Apnea 378
    test 378
        procedure of 378
Apoptotic tumor cells, plenty of 427
Appendicitis 58
Apraxia 355
Arbovirus 518t
Arrhythmia 269, 290, 450
    types of 315
Arterial blood gas 217, 222, 540
    analysis 210, 260
Arterial disease 493
Arterial oxygen saturation 252, 419
Arterial pulse, assessment of 9
Arteritis, coronary 267
Artery disease, peripheral 271
Arthritis 292
Arthropod-borne viruses 372
Asbestosis 257
Ascaris lumbricoides 261
Aschoff body 290
Ascites 59, 76, 189, 196
    assessment for 77

causes of 76, 77, 198t
etiology of 76t
examination of 78, 78t
pathogenesis of 197t
praecox 76
severe 562
signs of 78, 79f
treatment of 192
Ascitic fluid
infection, classification of 197
nature of 197
Ascorbic acid 433
Ashrafian sign 301
Askanazy cells 478
Aspartate aminotransferase 31, 171, 179, 183, 275, 574
Aspergilloma 230, 238, 261
Aspergillosis, bronchopulmonary 260
Aspergillus 303
fumigatus 230, 261
Aspiration 241, 246, 259
abscess 241
pneumonia 249
Aspirin 160, 187, 276, 278, 292
Asthma 207t, 223, 224t, 261, 263
acute 214fc
allergic 213
bronchial 206, 211t, 224, 239
cardiac 211t
characteristics of 206
classification of 206, 206b
control, assessment of 210t
COPD overlap syndrome 224
drug-induced 215
early-onset 207t
episodic 209
global initiative for 206, 209
late-onset 207t
management of 213f
occupational 215
pathogenesis of 207, 208f
phenotype 213
risk of 207, 208f
severe 209, 212, 213t
severity of 214t
Ataxia 354
telangiectasia 410
Atelectasis 239
classification 239
nonobstructive 239
obstructive 239
passive 239
relaxation 239
Atenolol 284
Atheroembolism 267
Atherosclerosis 266, 283, 455, 506
advanced 267
pathogenesis of 266
risk of 339
Atorvastatin 363
Atrial arrhythmias 311
Atrial fibrillation 142, 283, 294, 295, 296, 299, 316
classification 316
complexes 10
complications 316
electrocardiogram of 316f
etiology of 316, 316t
signs 316
symptoms 316
Atrial flutter 317
electrocardiogram of 317f
Atrial septal defect 21, 126, 131, 132, 134, 135, 142, 320
Atrioventricular blocks 318
complete 318
first-degree 318
second-degree 318
third-degree 318
Atrophic autoimmune thyroiditis 474, 478
Atrophic hypothyroidism 484
Atropine 323
Attack
acute 358
severe 359
Aura
duration of 358
language 358
motor 358
sensory 358
types of 358
visual 358
Auscultation, sequence of 131
Ausculto percussion method 70, 70f
Austin-Flint murmur 138, 300
Autoantibody 469
adrenal 485
screening 348
Autohemolysis test 572
Autoimmune
adrenal insufficiency 483
cytopenias 417
disease 445, 484, 489
disorders 471, 475
hemolytic anemia 399
classification of 400b
polyglandular syndrome, type 2 478
Autoimmunity 551
Autologous stem cell transplantation 422
Autonomic failure 19, 324
Autonomic nervous system 347, 505
Autosplenectomy 393
Axillary lymph nodes 40
Azathioprine 182, 438
Azilsartan 285
Azithromycin 219, 253
Azotemia 333, 336
lymphocytosis 486

B

Bacillary dysentery 527, 530, 530t
complications of 528t
Bacillus Calmette-Guerin 231
Backcheck valve 563
Backwash ileitis 166
Baclofen 374
Bacteremia 251, 303
Bacteria 240
eradication of 238
Bacterial endocarditis prophylaxis 308
Bacterial peritonitis, spontaneous 58, 199
Bacteriuria, asymptomatic 350, 351
Bacteroides 202
fragilis 371
Bag-of-worms appearance 291
Balanitis 508
Bald tongue 29f
Ball valve thrombus 294
Balloon
dilatation 299
tamponade 193
Barbiturates, long-term of 437
Bariatric surgical techniques 457
Barium swallow 190
Barlow's disease 441
Barlow's syndrome 297
Barotrauma 559
Barrel-shaped chest 97, 97f
Barrett's esophagus 155, 156, 158
Bartonella 305, 307

Basal ganglia 451
Basic thyroid evaluation 467f
Basilar migraine 356
Bat's wing 259
B-cell lymphoma 553
Becker's sign 301
Bell's palsy 375, 375f
medical treatment of 376
sequelae of 376
Bell's phenomenon 375f
Benazepril 285
Bendopnea 90
Benzathine penicillin G 292
Benzodiazepines 474
Berger's disease 340
Beriberi
acute fulminant cardiovascular 436
dry 436
infantile 436
wet 436
Bernheim effect 299
Berry's node 40
Beta-adrenoceptor blocker therapy 312
Beta-blockers
cardioselective 270
nonselective 194
Beta-cell
destruction, mechanisms of 490
hyperplasia 491
Betahistine 457
Beta-thalassemia
pathogenesis of 396f
syndromes 396t
Betaxolol 284
Bicarbonate 504
secretion 159
Bicuspid aortic valve disease 299
Biguanides 496
Bilirubin
conjugated 31
metabolism 171f
unconjugated 31
Binet staging 417t
Biopsy, cardiac 311
Biotin 433
Biotinidase 440
deficiency 440
Birmingham paradox 12
Bisoprolol 284
Bisphosphonate 161
intravenous 450
Bite cells 398f
Bitot's spot 435, 435f
Black fever 536
Black measles 511
Black nails 35
Bladder 351
neck obstruction 352
Blast crisis phase 414
Blastocystis hominis 240
Bleeding
colonic 52
diathesis 562
disorders 562
probable site of 335t
time 402, 441, 572
Blood
ammonia
estimation 189
levels 194
chronic 146
clinical chemistry of 571, 573t
concentrations 440
cultures 305
examination 243

glucose level 494, 505
pressure 17, 18, 115, 141, 283, 294, 296
　control 281, 507
　cuff, placement of 18f
　diastolic 17, 280
　examination of 17
　high 280t
　maintenance of 362
　optimize 327
　systolic 17, 280
smears 536
tests 210, 311
transfusion 400, 428, 545
　complications of 429, 429t
urea 408
　nitrogen 149, 503, 576
vessels 283
　erosion of 228
viscosity 419
Blue nails 35
Blue sclera 29f
Blueberry muffin lesions 513
Blunt chest trauma 259
Body
　hair 60
　iron stores, elevation of 203
　mass index 45, 46, 50, 83, 115, 217, 432, 576
　sodium deficit, total 575
Boerhaave's syndrome 144
Bone
　density 444
　disease, pathogenesis of 345
　formation 397f
　marrow 29, 395
　　aspiration needle 562, 562f, 563f
　　biopsy 235, 562
　　failure 411
　　involvement 426
　　study 415
　　transplantation 397, 412, 430, 430t
　matrix proteins 443
　mineral density 444
　mineralization of 442
　pain 440
　resorption, markers of 448
　sclerosis of 452
　softening disease 442
Bordetella pertussis 524
Botulism 524
Bow legs 443f
Bowel disease 36
Bowel sounds 66
　auscultation of 66f
Bozzolo sign 301
Brachial pulse, palpation of 14, 14f
Bradbury-Eggleston syndrome 19
Bradyarrhythmia 315
Bradycardia 10, 24, 525, 558
Bradycardic drug 270
Bradykinin receptor antagonist 553
Bradypnea 16
Brain
　abscess 238
　biopsy 374
　death 378
　　diagnosis of 378
　edema, diffuse 377
　involvement 204
　lesions, bilateral structural 62
　natriuretic peptide 311
Brainstem reflexes 378
Brazilian purpuric fever 26
Break-bone fever 518
Breath sounds 84, 108, 243
　bronchovesicular 108

diminished intensity of 109t
intensity, grading of 107
normal physiology of 107
vesicular 108
Breathing 322, 323, 327
　abnormal patterns of 16
　advanced 323
　patterns, types of 16f
　sleep-disorders 509
Breathlessness 91b, 91t, 216, 228, 251
　acute severe 91
　description of 91
Brittle finger nails 384
Broadbent's sign 133
Brock's syndrome 226, 236
Bromocriptine 281, 464
Bronchial breathing 243
　types of 108
Bronchial disease 262
Bronchial inflammation 206
Bronchial thermoplasty 212
Bronchial tumors 239
Bronchiectasis 215, 236, 237f, 239, 250, 262, 524
　causes of 236b
　complications of 238
　diffuse 236
　dry 237, 239
　focal 236
　postobstructive 236
　proximal 236, 260
　sicca 237, 239
　types of 236f
Bronchoalveolar lavage 252
Bronchodilator 212, 218, 555
　therapy 212
Broncholith 226, 230
Bronchopneumonia 249, 250, 252, 256, 524
　acute 256
　chest X-ray of 256f
Bronchorrhea 87
Bronchoscopy 237
Bronchospasm 215, 450
Brown bowel syndrome 445
Brown-Vialetto-Van Laere syndrome 437
Bruce protocol, modified 268
Brugada syndrome 318
Brugia malayi 263
Bruits 66
Bubonic plague 523
Budd-Chiari syndrome 22, 57, 63, 198, 200, 419
　acute 200
　causes of 200t
　chronic 200
　clinical features 200
　fulminant 200
Buffalo hump 480f
Buffy coat analysis, quantitative 536
Bullous eruption 547
Bumetanide 285
Bupropion 457
Burdwan fever 26
Burkitt lymphoma 426, 428f
　categories of 427t
Burning feet syndrome 439
Burr cells 348

C

Cabergoline 464, 482
Cabot-Locke murmur 139
Cachexia 47
Calcitonin 450
Calcium 442
　carbonate 451
　channel

　　antagonists 270, 284
　　blockers 146, 270, 271, 364, 488
　citrate 451
　deposition of 442
　distribution of 446
　gluconate 451
　homeostasis 445, 446
　　hormonal regulators of 447t
　levels, regulation of 446
　metabolism 447f
　phosphorus balance 343
　plasma levels of 442
　sensitizer 313
　urinary excretion of 444
Campylobacter 154, 527
Canadian Cardiovascular Society 119
Cancer 217
　colorectal 58
Candesartan 285
Candida 303, 304, 307
　albicans 532
　infection 492
Candidiasis 532
Cannon ball metastasis 568f
Capillary fragility test 401
Capreomycin 233
Captopril 285
　test, oral 483
Caput medusa 80
Carbamazepine 146, 200, 368, 374, 438, 466
Carbapenem 352
Carbenoxolone 281
Carbimazole 472, 474
Carbohydrate 436, 439, 495, 498
　metabolism 170
　oral 505
Carbon dioxide 217
Carbon monoxide transfer test 209
Carbon tetrachloride 200
Carboxymaltose 385
Carcinoid syndrome 201, 302, 438
Carcinoma 437
　adrenal 482
　bronchogenic 262
　colon 463
　　risk of 167
　hepatocellular 201, 201t, 456
　intramucosal 158
Cardiac apex, types of 125f
Cardiac arrest 318, 321, 323
　causes of 318, 318t, 321, 321b
　diagnosis of 321
　identification of 322
　management 318
Cardiac arrhythmias 119, 120, 315, 324, 520
　classification of 315t
Cardiac disease 128f
　structural 120, 324
Cardiac disorders 147
Cardiac failure, congestive 35, 36f, 245, 292
Cardiac injury
　acute 520
　biochemical markers of 274
Cardiac limb syndrome 123
Cardiac pain, ischemic 117
Cardiac resynchronization therapy 312
Cardiac tamponade 22, 118
Cardiac troponins 275
Cardiogenic pulmonary edema 259, 260, 313, 314
Cardiomyopathy 318, 455
　classification of 318, 319f
　etiology 318
　primary 320
　secondary 320
Cardiopulmonary disease 120, 324

Cardiorenal syndrome 311
Cardiorespiratory disease 328
Cardiovascular disease 262, 335, 339, 348, 509
Cardiovascular disorders 217
Cardiovascular system 3, 85, 91, 114, 116, 117, 122, 127, 380, 422
    examination 114
Carditis 290, 292
    evidence of 291
    manifestations of 290
Carey-Coombs murmur 138, 290
Carnitine, formation of 440
Carotenemia 436
Carotid arteries 299
Carotid pulse
    palpation of 13
    right 14f
Carotid shudder 299
Carpal tunnel syndrome 475, 508
Carpopedal spasm 450, 451
Carrier protein 405
Carvallo's sign 138
Carvedilol 284
Casal's necklace 438, 438f
Castell's sign 73f
Castell's method 73
Castleman disease 37
Cat scratch disease 42
Catacrotic pulse 11
Catheter aspiration 248
Cavernous bronchial breathing 229
Cefadroxil 308
Cefotaxime 199, 219
Ceftazidime 199
Ceftriaxone 219, 253
Cefuroxime 352
Celiac disease 58, 471
Cell growth, control of 435
Central cyanosis 32, 61
    demonstration of 32f
Central nervous system 3, 274, 347, 412, 413, 422, 437
    causes 145
    complications 282
    manifestations 504
    symptoms 473
Cephalexin 308
Cephalosporin 351, 352
    oral 351
    third-generation 199, 219
Cerebellar artery, posterior inferior 363
Cerebellum 437
Cerebral edema 185, 186, 283
    signs of 503
    symptoms of 503
Cerebral function 360
Cerebral hemispheres
    functions of 355
    lobes of 355f
Cerebral infarction 361
Cerebral malaria 536
Cerebrospinal fluid 411, 563, 571
    normal values of 575t
Cerebrovascular accident 282, 350, 360, 504, 506
Cerebrovascular disease 360
Cerebrum 389
Ceruloplasmin 172
Cervical lymph node 37
    examination of 37
    posterior 513, 514
    superficial 37
Cervical venous hum 28, 28f
Chancre, primary 545, 546f
Charcot's triad 176
CHARGE syndrome 123
Cheilitis 438

Chelation therapy 203
Chemical
    mast cell degranulation 551
    pleurodesis 248
Chemotherapy 161, 201, 414
    alternative 413
    antituberculous 232, 236
    short-course 232
Chest 221
    asymmetry of 96, 98t
    compressions 322
    deformity 96, 97t, 123
    dynamics, measurement of 102
    examination of 96, 96t
    expansion, examination of 103f
    lower posterior 101, 102f
    movement
        causes of 102
        measurement of 102t
    pain 82, 92, 114, 117, 228, 251, 268, 268t, 294
        causes of 117, 117f, 118
        differential diagnosis of 117
        episodes of 159
        respiratory causes of 92
    physiotherapy 218
    radiograph 475
    syndrome, acute 393-395
Chickenpox 515
    complications of 516, 516t
    lesions in 516f
Chilaiditi syndrome 570f
Child-Pugh classification, modified 189t
Child-Turcotte-Pugh score 189t
Chipmunk facies 30f, 397f
Chlamydia 305
    pneumonia 253
Chloroquine 397
Chlorpropamide 466
Chlorthalidone 285
Cholangiopancreatography 173
    endoscopic retrograde 173
Cholecalciferol 441
Cholelithiasis 395
Cholera sicca 530
Cholestasis 171, 200
Cholestyramine 472
Chondroectodermal dysplasia 123
Chorea 290, 291
    causes of 293
    onset of 291
    treatment of 292
Christmas disease 405
Chromogranin A 487
Chronic asthma 207, 209
    management of 212t
    stepwise management of 212
Chronic bronchitis 215, 217, 218t, 222f, 223, 223t, 239, 247
    types of 215
Chronic diarrhea 54t, 151
    causes of 54t, 91, 91t, 152, 153t
Chronic hepatitis 179f, 181, 182
    B 182, 183fc
        infection 182
        viruses 201
    C 184
        viruses 201
    causes of 181t
    D 185
Chronic immune disorders 400
Chronic kidney disease 29, 333, 344, 346f, 349b, 349t, 506, 509
    causes of 344, 345t, 348
    classification 344f

    clinical features of 345t
    treatment of 449
Chronic liver disease 29, 219, 309
    peripheral signs of 59
Chronic mitral regurgitation 296
    causes of 296
Chronic obstructive pulmonary disease 31, 94, 99, 123, 125, 215, 215b, 217b, 219f, 223, 224, 224t, 250, 258, 271, 325
    complications of 217
    pathogenesis of 216fc
Chronic renal failure 346, 444
    management of 348
Chronic respiratory failure 258
    causes of 258b
Churg-Strauss syndrome 263
Chvostek's sign 450, 451
Chylothorax 242, 245
Chymase inhibitors 287
Ciliary dysfunction syndrome 236, 238
Cinacalcet 449
Ciprofloxacin 199, 233, 352, 526
Circulation 323
Circulatory failure 325
    causes 325
    classification 325
Cirrhosis 51, 181, 184, 188, 197
    absence of 197
    alcoholic 188, 201
    biliary 189
    cause of 59f
    classification of 188f
    complications of 188, 189t
    drug-induced 189
    end stage of 188
    etiology of 62, 63t
    morphological classification of 189t
    signs of 63t
    treatment of 203
Citrus fruits 441
Clarithromycin 253, 308
Clevidipine 288
Clindamycin 308
Clofibrate 466
Clonazepam 368
Clonidine patch 286
Clopidogrel 270, 276, 278
Closed-angle glaucoma 269
Clostridioides 57
Clostridium
    botulinum 524
    difficile infection 153
Clotting disorders 403
Clotting time 441, 572
Cloxacillin 516
Clubbing
    atypical presentation of 34
    cyanosis 61
    grades of 33
Cluster headache 359, 360b
    clinical features 359
    diagnostic criteria for 359
    management of 360
Coagulation 446, 571
    abnormality 560
    disorders 401t
    studies 411, 536
Coagulopathy 563
Cobalamine 433
Cobb's syndrome 297
Cobbler's chest 97
Cobblestone 168
Cocaine 161
Coccidioides immitis 240
Coenzyme 387, 436, 439

Coin test 111
　demonstration of 111f
Cold
　pressure testing 268
　shock 325
Cole-Cecil murmur 139, 300
Colitis, infectious 58
Collagen, formation of 440
Collapse, treatment of 240
Collar rash 438
Colonic disorders 151
Coma 341, 377, 378
　assessment of 378
　classification of 377, 378t
　confusion 377
　consciousness 377
　drowsiness 377
　lethargic 377
　obtundation 377
　stupor 377
Common bile duct 174
Common femoral artery, palpation of 14
Community-acquired pneumonia 250, 250b, 251t, 252t
　antibiotic treatment for 253t
　complications of 251
　types of 251
Complete blood count 306, 421, 435
Compression atelectasis 239
Concomitant drug therapy 476
Condylomata lata 545, 546f
Conestat alfa 553
Confirmatory aldosterone suppression test 483
Congenital heart diseases 316, 320, 324, 513
　classification of 320t
Conjunctiva 30, 175f
Conn's syndrome 482
Connective tissue disorders 63
Consciousness, loss of 120, 465
Constipation 55, 58, 145
　causes of 146, 146b
　etiology of 55, 55t
　functional 146, 146b
　primary causes of 146
　secondary causes of 146
Continuous murmurs 135
　classification of 136
　differential diagnosis of 136
Convulsions 305, 524
Cooley's anemia 395
Coombs' test 392, 426
Copper metabolism, normal 203
Cor pulmonale 222, 238, 324
　causes of 325b
　chronic 325
　clinical features 324
　etiology 324
　features of 94
　signs 325
　symptoms 325
Cornea, calcification of 448
Corneal xerosis 435
Coronary artery
　atherosclerosis 267f
　bypass graft 128, 269, 271, 272, 278, 279, 315
　disease 267, 278, 279, 282, 283, 294, 296, 298, 310, 311, 463
　severe 268
Coronary sinus septal defect 320
Corrigan's sign 13, 301
Cortical bone, subperiosteal resorption of 448
Corticospinal tracts 389
Corticosteroids 212, 213, 218, 219, 260, 281, 292, 399, 407, 526, 555, 564
　oral 218

　therapy, side effects of 486
　trial of 210
Corticotropin-releasing hormone test 485
Corynebacterium diphtheriae 523
Cotrimoxazole 351
Cotswold's modification 424t
Cough 86, 216, 221, 223, 251, 263
　chronic 228
　classification of 86t
　production 86
　　mechanism of 86
　reflex 86fc, 254
　severe persistent productive 236
　types of 86, 87t
Courvoisier's law 75, 176
COVID pneumonia 521f
COVID-19 520
　treatment of 522, 522b
Coxiella 305
　burnetii 249, 307
　endocarditis 531
Coxsackie B 490
Cranial nerve 374
　diseases of 374
　palsy 370
C-reactive protein 252
Creatine kinase 475
Creatinine phosphokinase 531
Crepitation, mechanism of 109
Cretinism 474
Crigler-Najjar syndrome 176
Crocodile tears 376
Crohn's disease 34, 58, 161, 167, 167f, 168, 168f, 400
　clinical features of 168
Cruveilhier Baumgarten murmur 66, 67f
Cryoglobulinemia, mixed 181
Crypt abscesses 168
Cryptic miliary tuberculosis 234, 235
Cryptosporidium infection 540
Crystalluria 343
Cubilin 386
Curling ulcers 161
Cushing's disease 35, 479, 482
Cushing's syndrome 43, 281, 283, 454, 479, 480f, 481, 481b, 481fc
　causes of 479, 479t
　clinical features of 480f, 480t
　exogenous 482
　features of 481
Cushing's triad 185
Cushing's ulcers 161
Cyanosis 31, 93, 223
　atypical presentation of 32
　cardiac 32
　etiology of 31
　mixed 31
　peripheral 31, 32
　true 31
Cyclophosphamide 428
Cycloserine 232, 233
Cyclosporine 233, 281
Cyst 239, 528
Cystic fibrosis 241, 250, 254
Cystitis 58, 351
Cytomegalovirus 350, 401, 423, 490
Cytotoxins 160

D

Dahl sign 221
D-dimer test 409
de Carvallo's sign 295, 302
de Lange'ssyndrome 123
de Musset's sign 301
de Quervain's thyroiditis 477

Death, cause of 344
Deep cervical lymph nodes 37
Deep tendon reflex 29
Deep vein thrombosis 36, 121, 217, 309, 328, 362
　clinical features of 329
　risk factors of 328
　treatment of 329
Dehydration 502
　severity of 154t
Dehydroascorbic acid 440
Dehydrogenase deficiency 437
Delphian node 40
Dementia 373, 438
Dendritic cells 207
Dengue virus infection 519fc
　classification of 518t
Dennison sign 301
Denosumab 450
Dental
　caries 145, 452
　procedures 308
Deoxythymidine monophosphate 387
Depression 286, 347, 438
Dermatitis 438, 440
　atopic 206
　exfoliative 436
Dermatome 517
Dermatopathy 469
Dermographism 551
Dermopathy 468
　diabetic 508
　infiltrative 471
Desensitization 212
Desmopressin 466
Destroy activated suppressor cells 400
Device therapy 312
Dexamethasone 371
　suppression test 481, 483
Dextrocardia 237f
Diabetes insipidus 465
　causes of 465, 465b
　central 465, 466
　types of 465
Diabetes mellitus 181, 268, 334, 335, 489, 495, 500f
　cardiovascular complications of 506
　chronic complications of 505
　classical triad of 492
　classification of 489b
　clinical features of 492
　complications of 502, 502b, 508
　diagnosis of 494, 494f
　etiopathogenesis of 489
　gestational 508, 508b, 508t
　juvenile 489
　management of 494
　ophthalmologic complications of 507
　risk factors of 494
　treatment of 203
　type 1 484, 492
　　pathogenesis of 489, 490f
　　treatment of 496t
　type 2 491, 492, 509
　　pathogenesis of 490, 491f
　　pathophysiology of 492f
　　treatment of 496t
　types 3C 493
Diabetic ketoacidosis 16, 493, 502
　complications of 504
　pathogenesis of 503f
Diabetic nephropathy 506
　management of 507
Diabetic neuropathy 324, 507
　classification of 507, 507b
Dialysis
　dementia 347
　disequilibrium 347

Diamond-Blackfan syndrome 401
Diaphragm 137
Diaphragmatic movements 102
    examination of 102f
Diarrhea 53, 54t, 151, 154, 154t, 167, 438
    causes of 152t, 541t
    inflammatory 53, 54, 151-153
    large-volume 151
    secretory 151, 152
    small-volume 151
    types of 53
    watery 54, 151, 153
Diastolic murmurs 135
    configuration of 137f
Diazepam 258
Diazoxide 288
Dicrotic pulse 11
Didanosine 187
DiGeorge syndrome 123, 450
Digital index 34
Digital rectal examination 350
Digoxin 312, 474
Dihydropyridine 270, 286
    calcium antagonists 270, 271
Dihydrotachysterol 451
Dihydroxyphenylalanine 487
Diltiazem 270, 284
Dimercaptosuccinic acid 351
Dipeptidyl peptidase inhibitor 501
Diphtheria 523
Dipstick tests 350
Direct Coombs' test 417
Direct mucosal injury 160
Direct renin inhibitor 285, 287
Directly observed treatment, short course 233
Dirofilaria 261
Disseminated intravascular coagulation 408, 409t, 411, 413, 514
    pathogenesis of 408f
Distal small
    bowel 527
    intestine 440
Diuresis 502
Diuretic therapy 311
Diverticulitis 58
Diverticulosis 58
Dobutamine 328
Dock's murmur 139
Domiciliary oxygen therapy, long-term 218
Domperidone 358
Dopamine 328
    agonists 464
    antagonists 145
    receptor agonists 464
Dorsal root ganglia 547
Dorsalis pedis artery 15
Dorsalis pedis artery, palpation of 15, 15f
Dosulepin 359
Dotatate pet scan 462
Down's syndrome 122, 410
Doxazosin 285
Doxorubicin 428
Doxycycline 248, 253
Drowsiness 341
Drug
    classes 330t
    prophylaxis 359, 359b
    sensitivity testing 230
    therapy 211, 218, , 218t, 311, 456
        secondary prevention 278
Drummond sign 301
Dry powder inhalers 565f
Dubin-Johnson syndrome 176
Dullness
    lower border of 69f
    upper border of 69f

Duloxetine 508
Dumdum fever 26
Duodenal gastric reflux 161
Duodenal ulcer 162t, 164
Duodenum 159, 383
    diseases of 159
Dupuytren's contracture 60, 61f, 508
    causes of 61
Duroziez's sign 301
Dwarfism 488
Dysarthrias 355
Dysentery 154, 154t, 527, 528
Dyslipidemia 455, 508
Dyspepsia 55, 147
    causes of 55, 55b, 147b
    criteria for 55
    functional 57, 147, 148t
    symptoms of 147t
Dysphagia 55, 154, 155fc, 157, 159
    causes of 155
    high-grade 158
    low-grade 158
Dyspnea 82, 88, 90, 114, 120, 217, 221, 223, 263, 293, 296, 341
    acute 91, 258, 311
    chronic 91
    exertional 300
    mechanism of 89
    severity 217
Dysrhythmias, cardiac 557

E

Ecchymosis 441
Eclampsia 281
Ectopic thyroid tissue, description of 468
Eculizumab 399
Eczema 206
Edema 35, 36, 93, 120, 336
    acute pulmonary 287
    cardiogenic 259
    examination of 35
    generalized 238, 338
    treatment of 339
Ehlers-Danlos syndrome 300
Ehrlich's aldehyde test 173
Eisenmenger's syndrome 313, 320, 321
Electric digital thermometer 23
Electrolyte
    balance 349, 412
    disorder 349
    imbalances 152
Eletriptan 359
Elevated serum aminotransferases, causes of 170
Ellis-Van creveld syndrome 43, 123
Emboli, formation of 304
Emergency response system, activation of 322
Emesis, mechanism of initiation of 53
Emphysema 215, 217, 219, 222f, 223, 223t, 247
    features of 217
    obstructive 226
    pathogenesis of 221f
    types of 220, 220f
Empirical therapy 370
Empyema 238, 242
    aspiration of 246
    clinical features of 245b
    thoracis 245
        management of 246
Enalapril 278, 285
Enalaprilat 288
Encephalitis 373, 524
Encephalopathy 186, 437
    chronic hepatic 194
    hypertensive 282, 287

Endocarditis 290
    acute 303, 303t
    noninfective 308
    postoperative 303
    subacute 303t, 304, 306
Endocardium 290, 308
Endocrine 59, 281, 345
    abnormality 347, 372
    diseases 144
    disorders 147
Endocrinology 460
Endocrinopathy 153
Endopeptidase inhibitor 313
Endoscopic hemostasis therapy 150
Endoscopic variceal band ligation 194
Endoscopy 162
Endothelin receptor antagonist 313
Endotracheal tube 558, 558f, 559
Entamoeba histolytica 202
Entecavir 184
Enterobacteriaceae 249, 251
Enterococcal endocarditis 307
Enterococcus faecalis 202
Enteroviruses 372
Enzymes 160, 171, 275, 275f
Eosinophilia 210, 348, 486
    asthmatic pulmonary 260
Eosinophils 207, 348
Eosinophiluria 341
Epicardial coronary artery 279
Epigastric pain 57, 57t, 157
    syndrome 148
Epigastric pulsations 127
    causes of 127
    demonstration of 127f
Epigastrium 161
Epilepsy 364
    pyridoxine-dependent 439
    syndromes 365
Epinephrine 213, 555
Epiphyseal growth plate 443, 444
Epiphyses 443f
Episodes, hemorrhagic 341
Epistaxis 341
Epithelial defensive factors 156
Epitrochlear lymphadenopathy, causes of 42
Epitrochlear nodes 546
Eplerenone 278, 285
Eprosartan 285
Epsilon-aminocaproic acid 409
Epstein-Barr
    nuclear antigen 514
    virus 422, 427, 514
Eptifibatide 276
Erb's maneuver 139f
Erb's neoaortic area 116
Erectile dysfunction 493
Erenumab 359
Ergocalciferol 441
Ertapenem 253
Erythema marginatum 290
Erythrocyte 440
    sedimentation rate 179, 252, 275, 394, 408, 424, 478, 531, 566, 571
    thiamine transketolase activity 437
    transaminase activity 439
    transketolase 437
Erythrocytosis 201, 418
Erythroid hyperplasia, marked 395
Erythromycin 292
Erythropoiesis, ineffective 395
Erythropoietin 281, 419
Escherichia coli 154, 407, 526
Esmolol 288
Esomeprazole 163

Esophageal disease 557
Esophageal dysphagia, causes of 56t, 155t
Esophageal procedures 308
Esophageal varices 192f, 560
    banding of 193f, 560
Esophagitis 155
    infectious 56, 156
Esophagus 159
    achalasia of 158
    diseases of 154
    gastroesophageal junction of 159
    perforated 118
    squamous carcinoma of 159
Estimate estimated glomerular filtration rate 333t
Ethacrynic acid 285, 449
Ethambutol 232, 233
Ethionamide 232, 233, 438
Etoposide 428
Euthyroidism 467
Exacerbation
    acute 219
    antibiotic for 238
    treatment of severe 212
Exercise tolerance test 268
Exertional angina pectoris 268
Exhaled nitric oxide, fraction of 210
Exophthalmos 468, 470f
Extensive colitis 166
External Waldeyer's ring 37, 40
Extracorporeal membrane oxygenation 555
Extremity degenerative joint disease 455
Eye
    involvement, features of 204
    signs 469, 470b
Ezetimibe 330

F

Fabry's disease 298
Facial
    edema 36
    hair 62f
    muscles, ipsilateral contraction of 451
    nerve 374
        anatomy 375f
        palsy, causes of 374, 374t
    pallor 475
    weakness 373
Falciparum malaria 535
    complications of 535
False hemoptysis 87, 88, 88t, 261, 262t
Famcyclovir 516
Fanconi anemia 410
Fat
    metabolism, abnormal 491, 492
    restriction of 495
Fatigue 296
    syndrome, chronic 514
Fatty acid oxidation 491
Fatty diarrhea 54, 151, 153
Fatty liver 187, 200
    alcoholic 187
    causes of 187b
Fatty streaks 266
Felbamate 368
Felodipine 270
Femoral pulse, examination of 14f
Fenoldopam 288
Fentanyl 146
Ferritin 380
Fetal hemoglobin 380
Fetor hepaticus 62
Fever 24, 83, 121, 251, 336
    acute 24
    aseptic 25
    biphasic 26

    chronic 24
    clinical pattern of 25f
    enteric 524
    glandular 26, 514
    goal 26
    grading of 24
    intermittent 24
    low-grade 228, 263
    malta 26
    patterns of 24
    rat bite 26
    relapsing 24, 26
    remittent 24
    sandfly 26
    subacute 24
    types of 24
Fiber 495
    supplementation 146
Fibric acid analogs 330
Fibrin degradation 409
Fibrinolytics, fibrin specific 277
Fibrosis, degree of 181
Filariasis 36f
Fine-needle aspiration cytology 468, 478
First-line antituberculous drugs 231, 232
Fish-mouth valves 290
Fistula
    arteriovenous 136
    bronchopleural 245
Fits 341
Fitz-Hugh-Curtis syndrome 57
Flagella 160
Flail chest 97
Flat chest 97
Flatulent dyspepsia 147
Flexor tenosynovitis 508
Fludrocortisone 486
Fluent aphasias 355
Fluid
    balance 343
    intravenous 253
    replacement 505
    retention 349
    thrill 77
        demonstration of 78f
Flunarizine 359
Fluocinolone acetonide 471
Fluorescent in situ hybridization 410
Fluorine 452
Fluoroquinolone 219
Folate deficiency 390
Foley catheter 560, 560f
Folic acid 387, 433, 439
    metabolism 387
    role of 387, 387f
    supplementation 395
Follicle-stimulating hormone 461
Food poisoning, causes of 527b
Forchheimer spots 513
Formiminoglutamic acid 387, 387f
Fosinopril 285
Fothergill's disease 374
Fouchet's test 173
Fragmentation syndromes 174
Free tetrahydrothyronine 473, 476
Free triiodothyronine 473
Fremanezumab 359
French paradox 12
Fresh frozen plasma 185, 409, 429
Frey' syndrome 376
Friction fremitus 104
Friedlander's pneumonia 256
Friedreich's sign 22
Friedrich's ataxia 320
Frohlich's syndrome 43

Frovatriptan 359, 359]
Fructosamine 500
Fulminant hepatic failure
    causes of 185t
    complications of 185t
Fungal
    infections 532, 542
    toxin 201
Funnel chest 97
Furosemide 146, 285, 311, 449

G

Gabapentin 368, 374
Gaertner's method 22
Gait
    antalgic 444
    ataxia 437
Galcanezumab 359
Galinstan 23
Gallavardin phenomenon 299
Gallbladder, examination of 75
Gamma glutamyl transpeptidase 573
Gangrene 506
Gastric
    crisis 373
    disorders 437
    electrical stimulation 145
    emptying 157
    hyperacidity 161
    insufflation 559
    juice, aspiration of 236
    lavage tube 557, 557f
    outflow obstruction 164
    ulcer 162t
        benign 162f
        chronic nonhealing 164
Gastritis, chronic 437
Gastroenterology 144
Gastroesophageal junction 156, 159
Gastroesophageal reflux disease 57, 155, 156f, 456
    complications of 157, 157t
    diagnostic tests for 157b
    treatment of 157b
Gastrointestinal bleeding 51, 52, 148, 346
    types of 52t
Gastrointestinal disease 63, 540
Gastrointestinal disorders 147, 456
Gastrointestinal system 553
Gastrointestinal tract 49, 51, 55, 59, 140, 147, 241, 303, 438
    examination 49
    procedure 308
Gastroparesis 57
Gatifloxacin 253
Gemifloxacin 219, 253
Gene therapy 395
Genitourinary tract 242, 303
Geographic tongue 63
Geophagia 384
Gerhardt's sign 301
German measles 513
Ghon complex 226
    fate of 226
Ghon lesion 225
Giant platelets 420
Giardia lamblia 147
Gibson's murmur 139, 320
Gilbert's syndrome 170, 176
Glasgow coma scale 378t
Gliptins 497
Glitazones 498
Glomerular diseases 335, 336
    causes of 335b
    diabetic 334
    primary 337

Glomerular dysfunction 306
Glomerular filtration rate 333, 507, 576
Glomeruli 336
Glomerulonephritis 335, 337t, 348, 514
    crescentic 337
    focal segmental 305, 307
    hemorrhagic 546
    primary 335
    rapidly progressive 337
Glomerulosclerosis
    diabetic 348
    focal 337, 340
    segmental 337, 340
Glossitis 438
Glucagon 502, 555
Glucocorticoids 145, 187, 479
    administration of 483
    adverse effects of 487t
    responsive hyperplasia 483
Gluconeogenesis 439
Glucose
    6-phosphate dehydrogenase 174, 382, 392
        deficiency 397
    intolerance, mild 487
    levels, normal 494
    tolerance, normal 490
Glucotoxicity 505
Glutamyl transpeptidase 172
Glutaric acidemia 437
Glycemic control 507
Glyceryl trinitrate 270
Glycogen storage disease 562
Glycosaminoglycans, accumulation of 469
Glycoside, cardiac 312
Glycosuria 335
Glycosylated plasma proteins 500
Goblet cells 158
Goiter 468
Gonorrhea 544
    anorectal 544
    pharyngeal 544
    treatment of 545b
Gout 286
Graham-Steel murmur 139, 295
Gram's staining 197, 544
Granular casts 341
Granulocyte colony-stimulating factor 419
Granulocytopenia 536
Granuloma annulare 508
Granulomatous cerebral angiitis 517
Grave's thyrotoxicosis 36
Graves' disease 36, 468, 469, 473
    hyperthyroidism of 471
    investigation of 471
    treatment of 471
Graves' orbitopathy 469
Great artery, transposition of 34, 132
Ground glass opacities 521
Growth
    deceleration 43
    hormone 461
Guanabenz 286
Guanfacine 286
Guillain-Barré syndrome 19, 514, 520, 563
Gum swelling 441
Gustatory lacrimation 376
Gustatory sweating 376
Gynecomastia 60, 60f, 61f
    causes of 60b

H

Hackett's grading system 71f
Haemophilus influenzae 217, 249, 251, 393, 395
Hair, loss of 60
Hairy cell leukemia 413, 414

Ham's test 392
Hamman's mediastinal crunch 111
Haptoglobin 383
Hard chancre 545
Harrison's sulcus 221, 443
Hartnup's disease 438
Harvey's sign 79, 79f, 300
Hashimoto's thyroiditis 474, 478, 484
    pathogenesis of 474
    treatment of 478
Haverhill fever 26
Headache 355, 356, 363, 436
    classification of 355, 356t
    cluster 359, 360b
    postspinal 563
    primary 355, 356, 360t
    red flags of 358t
    secondary 355, 356
    types 356f
Hearing, sensorineural loss of 340
Heart
    block, complete 20
    border
        description of 128
        right 128, 129f, 222, 302
    burn 157, 161
    disease 303
        acquired 116
        chronic rheumatic 288
        congenital 122
        coronary 476
        cyanotic 34
        ischemic 266, 267f, 271, 272ff, 294, 315, 316
        peripartum 320
        structural 119
    disorders 198
    failure 283, 298, 306, 309, 310, 450
        acute 309
        advanced 311
        biventricular 309
        cause of 310t, 311
        chronic 309
        clinical manifestations of 310
        compensated 309
        congestive 21, 290, 317, 320, 436
        diastolic 309
        high-output 309
        left-sided 309
        low-output 309
        management of 311, 313
        right side 309, 325
        severe 278, 311
        signs of 310t
        symptoms of 121, 296, 301, 310t
        systolic 309, 314f
        treatment of 312, 325
        types of 309
    lung transplantation 325
    rate 327
    sounds 131, 133f, 142
        diastolic 132
        frequency of 130
        soft first 296, 296f
    topographical areas of 123, 131
    transplantation 313
Heat stroke 26
Heimlich maneuver 322
Heinz body 398
    preparation 392
Helicobacter pylori 160
    diagnostic tests for 163t
    infection 148, 164t
Hemagglutination 202
Hemangiomas 562
Hematemesis 52, 88, 89t, 148, 149, 149t, 261, 262t

Hematochezia 52
Hematological disorders 262
Hematological tests 189
Hematopoiesis, extramedullary 420
Hematopoietic stem cell transplantation,
        types of 430
Hematuria 283, 305, 335, 336, 340
    microscopic 335
    progressive 340
    recurrent macroscopic 340
Heme
    iron 384
    synthesis 439
Hemianopia, bitemporal 463
Hemicraniectomy 362
    decompressive 362
Hemiparesis 370
Hemiplegia 305, 361
Hemithorax circumference 103f
Hemochromatosis 562
    hereditary 202
Hemocytometer 561f
Hemoglobin 217
    A 380, 397
    concentration 380
    electrophoresis 392, 394
    fetal 572
    glycated 573
    glycosylated 500
    maintenance of 397
    normal 380
    structure 380
Hemoglobinopathy 392
    types of 392t
Hemolysis 204
    cause of 392
    evidences of 394
    extravascular 391f
    intravascular 391f
    location of 390
Hemolytic anemia 29, 170, 175f, 390, 445
    chronic nonspherocytic 397
    classification of 390
    clinical features of 390, 392t
    diagnosis of 390
    evidence of 399
    treatment of 392
Hemolytic crises 394, 395
Hemolytic uremic syndrome 405, 407, 514
    pathogenesis of 407f
Hemophilia 429
    A 403
    B 405
Hemoptysis 87, 88, 89t, 149, 149t, 228, 230, 236,
        238, 261, 262t, 293
    causes of 87, 88t, 230, 261, 262t
    clinical clues of 87
    diagnosis of 88t
    treatment of 238
    true 87, 88, 88t, 261, 262t
Hemorrhage 277, 267, 408, 440
    adrenal 483
    conjunctival 524
    gastrointestinal 149f, 341
    intracerebral 361
    intracranial 361
    petechial 437
    postpartum 461
    subperiosteal 441
Hemorrhagic disorder, severe 405
Hemosiderin 380, 383
Hemosiderosis 396
    cardiac 396
Hemothorax 242
Henoch-Schonlein purpura 335

Heparin, unfractionated 276, 277
Hepatic elastography 173
Hepatic encephalopathy 185, 193, 194t, 195
  acute 194
  treatment of 196t
  types of 193, 195t
Hepatic failure
  hyperacute 185
  severe 185
  subacute 185
  subfulminant 185
Hepatitis 200
  A 176, 177, 180
    virus 176, 177, 180, 185
  alcoholic 187
  autoimmune 181, 189
  B 177, 180, 348
    antigen 183
    core antigen 177
    phases of 182t
    plus 185
    surface antigen 180
    virus 177, 179f, 180, 180t, 182, 183, 429
  C 177, 178, 180, 348
    virus 177, 180, 181t, 184, 184t, 185
  D 178, 180
    virus 177, 180, 429
  delta 177, 178, 180
  drug-associated chronic 181
  E 177, 178, 180
    antigen 183
    virus 177, 180
  failure, fulminant 185
  fulminant 179
  types of 177
Hepatobiliary disorders 170
Hepatocellular dysfunction 185
Hepatojugular reflux 22
Hepatorenal syndrome 195, 196
  types of 196t
Hepatosplenomegaly 513, 525, 531
Hepatotropic viruses 177t
Hepcidin 203, 384
  significance of 384
Hernia, hiatus 156, 158, 158f
Herpes simplex virus 372
Herpes zoster 517, 517f
  ophthalmicus 517
Hess test 401, 402, 405, 441
Hiccups 145
High altitude pulmonary edema 314
High-density lipoprotein 330, 455, 492, 574
High-frequency sounds 127, 128
Hill's sign 301
Hip circumference 46
Histamine 209
Histidine, metabolism of 387f
Histoplasma capsulatum 240
Hodgkin's cells 422
Hodgkin's disease 337
Hodgkin's lymphoma 422, 426t, 425t, 426, 427t, 439
  classification of 422, 423f, 423t
  Rye's classification of 423t
  treatment of 424t
Holocarboxylase synthetase, deficiency of 440
Hooking maneuver 72
Hoover's sign 221
Hormone
  adrenocorticotropic 461
  anterior pituitary 460
  antidiuretic 334, 465
  deficiency 505
Horn cells, anterior 354
Horse-shoe dullness 76, 76f, 77, 79f

Human immunodeficiency virus 24, 538, 401,
    538f, 541t, 548
  infection 231
    classification of 541t
    clinical staging classification of 540b
    laboratory diagnosis of 542
  oral manifestations of 542b
  pathogenesis of 539f
Hungry-bone syndrome 450
Huntington's disease 293
Hurler's syndrome 43
Hürthle cells 478
Hutchinson's teeth 547
Hydatid cyst 562
Hydralazine 286, 288
  nitrate 312
Hydrocarbon 557
Hydrochlorothiazide 285, 451
Hydrocortisone 486
  sodium succinate 213
Hydroflumethiazide 285
Hydrogels 457
Hydrophilic glycosaminoglycans, accumulation
    of 471
Hydropneumothorax 249
Hydrothorax 242
Hydroxyapatite 446
Hydroxycarbamide 394, 420
Hydroxydaunorubicin 428
Hydroxytryptamine 166
Hydroxyurea 263, 420
Hyperaldosteronism 482
  primary 482
  secondary 482, 483
Hyperapnea 16
Hyperbilirubinemia 188
  congenital nonhemolytic 176
  fluctuating 170
  types of 171t
  unconjugated 175
Hypercalcemia 201, 281, 448, 449, 486
  acute 449
  causes of 449, 450t
  psychological stress 161
Hypercalciuria 448
Hyperchloremic acidosis, mild 448
Hypercholesterolemia 475
Hyperestrogenism
  causes of 60
  effects of 60
Hyperglycemia 60, 363, 490, 502, 504, 505, 506f
Hyperglycemic hyperosmolar state 504
  characteristics of 504
  pathogenesis of 504f
Hyperinflation, features of 217
Hyperinsulinism, endogenous 505
Hyperkalemia 286, 311, 337, 341, 344, 349, 486
Hyperkeratosis 435
  follicular 435
Hyperleukocytosis, treatment of 412
Hyperlipidemia 329, 330, 338
  causes of 330, 330f, 339
  classification 330
  management 330
Hypermagnesemia 344
Hypermetabolic state 420, 468
  symptoms of 415
Hypernatremia 323, 343, 465
Hyperoxia test 32
Hyperparathyroidism 446
  causes of 446, 447t
  classification of 446, 447t
  clinical features of 446
  manifestations of 448
  primary 448
  treatment of 349

Hyperperfusion, glomerular 507
Hyperphosphatemia 341, 344, 349
  treatment of 349
Hyperplasia 207, 215, 216
  congenital adrenal 484
Hyperprolactinemia 464
  causes of 464, 464b
Hyperpyrexia 25, 26
Hypersecretory syndromes 162
Hypersensitivity reactions 551, 552t
Hypersomnia 194
Hypertension 36, 126, 132, 268, 280, 281, 282t,
    316, 336, 483
  causes of 280, 281b
  classification of 280, 280f, 280t
  complications of 282, 487
  control of 363
  essential 281, 335
  etiology 280
  high-renin 281
  mild-to-moderate 336
  paradoxical 18
  primary 280
Hypertensive retinopathy 282, 282f
  grading of 282b
Hyperthermia 26, 363, 473
  malignant 26
Hyperthyroid crisis 473
  causes of 473
  treatment of 473
Hyperthyroidism 269, 467, 468, 469, 471
  amiodarone-induced 469
  apathetic 469
  causes of 468b
  diagnosis in 473fc
  iodine-induced 469
  primary 449
Hypertonic saline 238
Hypertriglyceridemia 281, 475
Hypertrophic cardiomyopathy 125, 127, 132, 320
Hypertrophic obstructive cardiomyopathy 123,
    125, 135, 137, 138
Hypertrophy 207, 216
Hyperuricemia 341, 344
Hyperventilation 268
  hysterical 451
Hypervitaminosis
  D 445
  treatment of 445
Hypoalbuminemia 197, 338, 453
Hypocalcemia 341, 344, 349
  treatment of 349
Hypocapnia 329
Hypocomplementemia 336
Hypofibrinogenemia 429
Hypoglycemia 186, 201, 486, 500, 505
Hypoglycemic drugs, oral 496
Hypogonadism 464
Hypokalemia 311, 483
Hypomagnesemia 311
Hyponatremia 286, 311, 343, 363, 462, 476, 486, 503
Hypoparathyroidism 450
  causes of 450
  functional 450
  idiopathic 450
  infantile 450
  surgical 450
Hypophosphatemia 448
Hypopituitarism 460, 484
  causes of 461b
  symptoms of 462
Hypoproteinemia 198
Hyposplenism 394
Hypotension 18, 186, 277, 363, 450, 462, 555
  cause of 18, 18f

Index

consequent systemic 461
orthostatic 19, 120, 324
postural 19, 508
Hypothalamic disease 467
Hypothalamic disorder 372
Hypothermia 26, 328, 476, 502
causes of 26
Hypothesis 454
Hypothyroidism 454, 462, 467, 472, 474, 476fc
central 474
clinical features of 475t
etiology of 474b
features of 478
period of 478
primary 464, 474
secondary 467, 474
signs of 477
symptoms of 477
treatment of 475
Hypovolemia 328, 349, 363
Hypoxemia 329
Hypoxia 9

I

Ibuprofen 146, 215, 512
Icterus 29, 93
conjunctival 170
demonstration of 30f
Idiopathic hypereosinophilic syndrome 263
Ifosfamide 428
Iliac bruit 67f
Imipramine 508
Immature lymphoid cells 425
Immotile cilia syndrome 254
Immune
complex deposits 336
disorders, acquired 425
function 435, 440
hypersensitivity 261
modulators 564
reconstitution inflammatory syndrome 544
thrombocytopenic purpura 402, 402f, 403, 403t, 471
treatment of 403b
tolerance induction 404
Immunity, cell-mediated 435
Immunization
active 178, 512, 513
passive 512, 513
Immunoglobulin 552
A 342
intravenous 400
M 180
Immunophenotype 422
Immunoradiometric assay 481
Immunosuppressive
agents 182, 254
therapy 400
Immunotherapy 212
Impaired bilirubin conjugation 174
Impaired glucose
intolerance, phase of 490
tolerance 489
Impaired respiratory muscle function 89
Implantable cardioverter defibrillator 312
Indapamide 285
Indinavir 200, 343
Indirect challenge tests 209
Indomethacin 215
Indoor air pollution 250
Induction chemotherapy 413
Infarction
adrenal 483
crisis 393
persistent aura without 358

Infections 144, 186
bacterial 523
chronic 147, 400
control of 454
evidence of 304
prevention of 218
severity of 527
source of 227, 528
spread of 228
treatment of 218, 412
Infectious diseases 153, 511
Infective endocarditis 296, 302, 308b, 400
consequences of 302
diagnosis of 306, 306b
prophylaxis 308b
signs of 122, 122f, 305f
Inferior sinus venosus 320
Inflammatory
bowel disease 58, 153, 166
disorder 266
reaction 291
Influenza 522
Inhaled nitric oxide 395
Inherited metabolic liver disease 189
Inhibits prostaglandin synthesis 445
Injection sclerotherapy 193
Insane, general paralysis of 373
Inspiratory intercostal retraction 97
Insulin 561
absolute deficiency of 489
analogs 498, 499t, 500t
aspart 499
deficiency 489
consequences of 502
glulisine 499
preparations 498, 499t
profiles 500f
requirement 492
resistance 281, 489, 500
consequences of 455, 491
phases of 492
syringe 561, 561f
therapy 493, 500f
complications of 500
indications for 498, 498t
Insulin-induced hypoglycemia test 485
Insulinoma Stein-Leventhal syndrome 454
Intercellular cement substances, formation of 440
Intercostals catheter 248
Interferon gamma release assays 230
Interlobar fissure
major 95f
minor 95f
Interlobular septal thickening 521
International League against Epilepsy 364t
Interosseous membrane, calcification of 452f
Intestinal bleeding, small 52
Intestine 226
diseases of 164
Intra-aortic balloon pumping 315
Intracellular fluid 446
Intracorpuscular defects 174
Intracranial bleed 287
Intracranial pressure 16, 186, 372, 376, 436, 563
Intrauterine death 547
Intrauterine growth retardation 513
Intravascular hemolysis 398
diagnosis of 392t
Intravenous cannula 564
color coding of 564t
Intravenous drip set 563, 563f
Intravenous isotonic saline 451
Intravenous sorafenib 201
Intubation, indications for 214
Invasive fibrous thyroiditis 479

Invasive pulmonary aspergillosis 261
Ionized calcium, importance of 446
Ionositol 433
Iopanoic acid 472
Irbesartan 285
Iron 439
absorption 383
balance
negative 384
regulation of 384
binding capacity, total 203, 385, 572
deficiency
advanced 384
anemia 28, 35, 384, 384f, 385t
stages of 384
distribution of 380, 383t
excretion 383
functions of 384
isomaltoside 385
metabolism 380, 383f
overload 394, 397
therapy, oral 384
transport of 383
Irregular rhythm, causes of 10
Irritable bowel syndrome 58, 164
management of 166fc
Ischemia 296
acute mesenteric 58
chronic mesenteric 58
symptoms of 278
Ischemic neurological deficit, reversible 361
Ischemic stroke 361
hemorrhagic conversion of 361
treatment of 362
Isolated organ tuberculosis 228
Isolated systolic hypertension, causes of 281
Isoniazid 200, 232, 233
therapy, prolonged 438
Isoproterenol 328
Isosorbide
dinitrate 270
mononitrate 270
Isosthenuria 566
Isotonic exercise 294
Isotretinoin 435
Isradipine 284
Ivabradine 271, 312

J

Jaccoud's arthritis 290
Jack-in-box sign 291
Jacksonian march 364
Jamshidi needle 562, 563f
Janeway lesions 305
Jarisch-Herxheimer reaction 514
Jaundice 30, 31, 51, 59, 174, 189
acholuric 175
cholestatic 174, 175
classification of 174t
deep 175f
hemolytic 174
hepatocellular 174, 175
mild 175, 175f
neonatal 397
types of 30, 175t
Jaw
enlargement of 463f
thrust method 322
Jejunum, proximal 383
Jod-Basedow phenomenon 469
Jones criteria 291
modified 291
Jug handle appearance 569f
Jugular vein 296
internal 19
right 19f

Jugular venous pressure 11f, 9f, 21f, 22f, 23, 115, 294, 299, 302, 310
Jugular venous pulse 19, 115, 294
    causes of 20
    examination of 19
Jugular venous system 19
Jugulodigastric lymph nodes 38f
Jugulo-omohyoid lymph nodes 39f

K

Kala-azar 536
Kanamycin 233
Kawasaki disease 37, 520
Kearns-Sayre syndrome 484
Keith-Wagener-Barker classification 282b
Keratitis 376
   interstitial 547
Keratomalacia 435
Ketoacidosis 58
Ketoconazole 482
Ketogenic diet 367
Ketonemia 502
Ketones, smell of 502
Ketonuria 502
Ketosis 490
Key-Hodgkin murmur 139
Kidney 76t, 348, 351, 442
   disease 449
   enlargement, causes of 75, 75t
   examination of 75
   functions of 333, 340
   injury molecule 343
Kikuchi-Fujimoto disease 37
Kimura disease 37
Kinesia paradox 12
Klebsiella pneumonia 240, 249, 251, 256
Klima needle 562, 562f
Klinefelter syndrome 44
Knuckle pigmentation 29f
Koch's disease 225
Koilonychia 29f, 35
Koplik's spots 511, 512f
Korotkoff's sound 12, 17
   types of 17
Korsakoff's psychosis 437
Kronig's isthmus 106, 106f
Kussmaul's sign 22
Kwashiorkor 36, 453, 453f
Kyasanur forest disease 26

L

La Ortner's syndrome 294
Labetalol 284, 288
Labyrinthine disorders 145
Lacrimal gland enlargement 61
Lactate dehydrogenase 31, 198, 242-244, 275, 392, 398
Lactoferrin 383
Lactose intolerance 58
Lacunar syndrome 362
Lady Windermere syndrome 236
Laennec's cirrhosis 189
Lamivudine 184
Lamotrigine 368, 374
Lancisi's sign 302
Landolfi's sign 301
Langerhans cell histiocytosis 570
Lanreotide 464
Lansoprazole 163
Laryngeal diphtheria 523
Laryngeal obstruction 523
Laryngoscope 558, 558f
Laryngospasm 450, 558
Lasmiditan 359

Latent autoimmune diabetes 490, 493
Latent syphilis, late 546
Latent tuberculosis 231
Laxatives 146
   types of 146t
Left bundle branch block 131, 132, 277
Left heart
   border 128, 129f, 295f
   failure, clinical features of 313
Left ventricular
   failure 16, 127, 140, 283, 310
   hypertrophy 123
   infarction 328
   third heart sound 297
Leg
   flapping tremors in 62f
   ulcers, chronic 395
Legionella 252, 305
   pneumophila 249, 251, 256
Legionnaire's disease 24
Leishmania donovani, life cycle of 537f
Lennox-Gastaut syndrome 365
Leptospira interrogans 530
Leptospirosis 530
Lesions, periventricular 437
Lethargy 296
Leucoencephalopathy, multifocal 541
Leukemia 303, 409, 426
   classification of 409t
   eosinophilic 263
   etiology of 410
Leukemia, acute 410, 411
   myelogenous 414t
   promyelocytic 413, 435
Leukemia, chronic 414
   lymphatic 337
   lymphocytic 37, 410t, 416, 417, 417t, 553
   myelocytic 410t
   myeloid 37, 410, 414, 416f, 416t
Leukocyte 244, 440
   alkaline phosphatase 415, 419
   count 572
   esterase test 350
   poor plasma 412
   vitamin C 441
Leukonychia 61f
Leukopenia 254
Leukostasis 411
Leveen shunt 199
Levetiracetam 368
Levine's sign 268
Levofloxacin 219, 233, 253
Levosimendan 313
Levothyroxine 478
   sodium 475
Libman-Sacks endocarditis 309
Lichen planus 181
Light's criteria 243
Ligneous thyroiditis 479
Limb, ischemic 294
Linagliptin 497
Lincoln sign 301
Linea nigra 64
Lip breathing, pursed 17, 100f
Lipid
   abnormalities 339
   management 269
   metabolism
      abnormalities 347
      regulation of 435
   pneumonia 250
   profile 571, 574t
Lipid-rich necrotic core 266
Lipiduria 338, 339
Lipoid pneumonia 250

Lipoprotein, low-density 266, 329, 330, 455, 492, 494, 574
Liposuction 457
Liraglutide 457
Lisinopril 285
Listeria monocytogenes 370, 371
Lithium 472, 474
   nephrotoxicity, reversible 467
Live-attenuated vaccine 517
   oral 526
Liver 76t
   anomalous lobe of 70f
   biochemistry 170, 306
   biosynthetic function of 172
   cell failure, chronic 50
   cirrhosis of 59, 59f
   dullness 129f
   examination 68
   failure, acute 186t
   function test 149, 170, 171, 188, 252, 411, 514
   functions of 170, 170b
   involvement 204
   palm 60
   palpation of 68f, 69f
   shrunken 189
   span 68, 69, 69f, 69t
   transplantation 182, 199, 202
Liver abscess 57
   bacterial 202
   pyogenic 202
Liver biopsy 176, 183, 190, 203, 204, 235
   complications of 562
   contraindications of 562
Liver disease 36, 144
   alcoholic 187, 187t
   cholestatic 445
   chronic parenchymal 181
   end-stage 183, 507
Lobar pneumonia 249, 252, 254
Local injection therapy 201
Locomotor brachii 301
Loeffler's fibroblastic endocarditis 263
Loeffler's syndrome 261
Loin pain 305
Loop diuretics 199, 311
Looser's zones 444
Loperamide 146
Losartan 285
Loud first heart sound 294
Low-cardiac output, symptoms of 121
Löwenstein-Jensen slopes 230
Lower abdominal pain 58
   causes of 58t
Lower gastrointestinal bleeding 51, 52, 149t, 151
   causes of 52t, 53t, 151f
   management of 152fc
Lower motor neuron 354
   disease, signs of 354, 355t
   facial palsy 376, 376t
Lower urinary tract 335
   infections 350
   origin 335
Ludwig's angina 118
Lugol's iodine 474
Lumbar puncture 563
   contraindications for 563
   indications for 563
   needle 563, 563f
Lung
   cancer 217
   capacity, total 456
   diseases of 325
   function tests 209
   infiltrates, bilateral 520
   injury, acute 258

lobes 95f
lower margin of 96f
lymphatic drainage of 93
parenchymal disease of 262
persists 247
primary tuberculosis of 225
resonance 105
secondary tuberculosis of 227f
topographical percussion of 106
tuberculosis of 229t
vascular diseases of 88, 262
volumes, measurement of 217
Lung abscess 238, 240, 251, 567f
    causes of 240b
    classification 240
    complications of 241
    etiology 240
    large 241
Lung disease 242, 257t, 324
    chronic obstructive 215
    interstitial 34
    occupational 257
    suppurative 236
Luteinizing hormone 461
Lymph node 37, 39, 40f, 42f, 417
    axillary group of 40
    enlarged 239
    epitrochlear group of 42
    group of 37, 38f
    inguinal 42
    mediastinal 42
    mesenteric 42
    occipital 39f
    postauricular 39f
    posterior triangle 39f
    right axillary 40
    submandibular 38f
    submental group of 38f
    supraclavicular 39, 39f
Lymphadenopathy 36, 416, 531
Lymphatic drainage 94f
Lymphatic obstruction 197
Lymphatic spread 226, 228
Lymphocyte 207
Lymphocytic infiltration 478
Lymphoid
    follicles 525
    neoplasm 425
        classification of 426t
Lymphoma 303, 422
    follicular 425

M

Macrocytic anemia 386
Macrolide antibiotics 238
Macronodular cirrhosis 189
Macular rashes 513
Magnesium lubeluzole 363
Malabsorption
    causes of 165fc
    classification of 165fc
    signs of 165f
    symptoms of 165f
    syndrome 54, 153, 164, 450
Malabsorptive procedures 457
Malaise 336, 533
Malaria
    complicated 535t
    severe 536
Malarial parasites
    blood smears of 536f
    life cycle of 533, 533f
Malarial paroxysms 535
Maldigestion 54, 153
Mallory-Weiss syndrome 144

Malnutrition, types of 453f
Mammary artery, internal 271
Mammillary bodies 437
Manson-Barr point 529
Mantoux test 231, 231f, 561
Marantic endocarditis 309
Marasmic kwashiorkor 453
Marasmus 309, 452, 453f
Marcus-Gunn jaw-winking phenomenon 376
Marfan's syndrome 44, 123, 300
Masked hypertension 281
Mass movement 376
Massive ascites 76, 78
Massive bacteremia 525
Massive hemoptysis 87, 261
    causes of 87, 88t, 262t
Massive proteinuria 338
Massive splenomegaly 414, 415
Mast cell 207
    degranulation, spontaneous 551
Maturity onset diabetes of young 493
    types of 493t
Maxillary sinuses 463f
May's sign 22
Mayan's sign 301
Measles 511
    complications of 512b
    encephalitis 512
Medical adrenalectomy 482
Medical nutrition therapy 494
Mefenamic acid 215
Megaloblastic anemia 28, 387, 388t
Meglitinides 497
    advantages of 497
Meigs' syndrome 198
Melatonin 359
Melena 52, 148
Memantine 359
Membranous
    glomerulonephritis 340
    nephropathy 337
Memory disturbances 437
Menaquinone 446
Meningeal syphilis 373
Meningitis 238, 369, 371t
    acute bacterial 369
    aseptic 372
    bacterial 370
    classic signs of 370
    classification of 369, 370t
    features of 372
Meningococcal septicemia 486
Meningovascular disease, chronic 546
Meningovascular syphilis 373
Menke's disease 172
Menstrual cycles 24
Mentzer index 576
Mepolizumab 263
Meropenem 352
Merozoites 534
Mesial temporal lobe epilepsy syndrome 366
Metabolic
    abnormalities 120, 347
    acidosis 576
    alkalosis 576
    bone disease 345
    diseases 335
    disorders 146, 147, 349
    syndrome 46, 281, 508
Metal tracheostomy tube 558, 558f
Metaphyseal bone lesions 513
Metaplasia, intestinal 158
Metastasis, differential diagnosis of 570
Metastatic malignancy 483
Metered dose inhaler 565, 565f, 565t

Metformin 457, 496
Methacholine bronchial provocation test 209
Methemoglobinemia 399
    causes of 399t
    treatment of 399t
Methicillin-resistant *Staphylococcus aureus* 250, 255
Methimazole 472, 474
Methotrexate 187, 200, 428
Methyclothiazide 285
Methylcobalamin 386
Methyldopa 286
Methylmalonyl coenzyme A metabolism 387f
Methysergide 359
    treatment 293
Metoclopramide 358, 486
Metolazone 285
Metoprolol 284
Metyrapone 482
    test 485
Meyers-Kouwenaar syndrome 263
Microalbuminuria 334, 335, 507
Microangiopathic hemolytic anemia 406, 429
Microcytic anemia 439
Microcytic hypochromic
    anemia, differential diagnosis for 385t
    red blood cell 386f
Microhematuria 196
Micronodular cirrhosis 189
Micronutrient deficiencies 452, 453
    signs of 432, 432t
    symptoms of 432, 432t
Microthrombi, formation of 406
Microvascular angina 118
Microvascular thrombi 408
Middle lobe pneumonia, right 255f
Middle lobe syndrome 226, 236
Middleton's maneuver 72, 72f
Midface trauma, severe 560
Migraine 356, 358t
    attack 358
    aura 357
    catamenial 356
    chronic 359
    classical 356, 357
    classification 356
    clinical features 357
    complications of 358
    diagnostic criteria 358
    familial hemiplegic 356
    hemiplegic 356
    management 358
    pathogenesis 356
    treatment of 359fc
    vestibular 356
Migrainosus infarction 358
Migrating polyarthritis 290
Miliary pulmonary
    disease 228
    infiltrates 263
Miliary recruits 249
Miliary tuberculosis
    classical 234
    nonreactive 234
Milkmaid's grip 291
Miller-Moses test 465
Mill-Wheel murmur 139
Milrinone 327
Miltefosine 537
Mineral supplements 454
Minocycline 248
Minoxidil 286
Mitotane 482
Mitral facies 294
Mitral regurgitation 125, 127, 130, 131, 134, 135, 137, 138, 142, 295, 296

causes of 296b
complications of 297b
murmur of 297
uncomplicated 296
Mitral stenosis 127, 130, 131, 137, 138, 139f, 142, 269, 293, 295f, 301, 309
    auscultation for 139
    causes of 293t
    complications of 295, 295t
    congenital 293
    murmur of 138, 294
    severity of 295
Mitral valve
    apparatus 296
        calcification of 293
    disease 569f
    prolapse 123, 297
    replacement 296
Mitral valvotomy 296
Mitral valvular disease 316
Moexipril 285
Mollaret's meningitis 372
Monckeberg's sclerosis 18
Monkey fever 26
Monoclonal gammopathies 181
Mononucleosis, infectious 231, 514
Monospot test 514
Mood disorders 445
Moon facies 480f
Moraxella catarrhalis 217, 249, 251
Morning cough 216
Morphine 146
    sulfate 315
Morquio's syndrome 43
Mosquito cycle 534
Motilin receptor agonists 145
Motility disorders 56
Moxifloxacin 219, 253
M-protein 289
Mucociliary
    apparatus 254
    clearance 238
Mucocutaneous candidiasis syndrome 450
Mucocutaneous lesions 545
Mucolytic agents 564
Mucopolysaccharides, accumulation of 475
Mucopurulent relapse 216, 217
Mucopurulent sputum 254
Mucosal lesions 168, 545
Mucosal ulcerations 168
Mucus
    hypersecretion of 216
    instools 146, 146t
    passage of 167
    plugs 239
    secretion, surface 159
Muddy conjunctiva 30
Muehrcke's nails 61
Mueller's maneuver 138
Muller's sign 301
Multidrug-resistance
    protein 176
    strains 526
Multifactorial disease 490
Multinodular goiter 472
Multiorgan dysfunction syndrome 408
Multiple acyl-coenzyme A 437
Multiple endocrine neoplasia syndromes 448t
Multiple lentigines syndrome 43
Multiple myeloma, clinical features of 422t
Multisystem inflammatory disease 288
Mumps 513
    complications of 514, 514b
Mural endocardium 302
Murmur 116, 127, 134, 138, 142, 290, 297, 304

change of 304
early diastolic 135, 137, 290, 300
early systolic 137
ejection systolic 268
grading of 136
late diastolic 135
late systolic 298
maximum intensity of 138
mid-diastolic 135, 294, 302
mid-systolic 299f
pansystolic 137, 296, 320
presystolic accentuation of 295
radiation of 137f
right-sided 137
timing of 135f
Murphy's eye 559
Murphy's sign 75
Muscarinic antagonists 218
Muscarinic receptor agonist 145
Muscle
    dysfunction 347
    infarction, diabetic 508
    spindles 89
    twitching 450
Muscular dysfunction 451
Muscular dystrophy 275, 320
Musculoskeletal
    disorders 217
    system 303
Myalgias 263
Myasthenia gravis 471
Mycobacteria 224
    characteristics of 225
    classification 224
Mycobacterium
    abscessus 224
    africanum 225
    atypical 224b
    avium 224
    bovis 225
    chelonae 224
    gordonae 224
    kansasii 225
    leprae 224
    marinum 225
    microti 225
    szulgai 224
    tuberculosis 224, 225, 230, 231
    ulcerans 225
Mycophenolate mofetil 479
Mycoplasma 252, 253
    pneumonia 249, 256
Mycotic genital tract infections 498
Myelodysplastic
    neoplasm 418
    syndromes 410, 418, 421
Myelofibrosis, primary 420
Myeloid neoplasms, classification of 418
Myeloma, differential diagnosis of 579
Myeloproliferative diseases 417
Myeloproliferative neoplasm 414, 418, 418t
Myocardial function, impaired 274
Myocardial hibernation 312
Myocardial infarction 274, 283, 296, 309, 504, 506
Myocardial perfusion scanning 269
Myocardial stunning 312
Myocarditis 290, 513, 523
Myocardium 290
    dysfunctional 310
Myoclonic epilepsy, juvenile 365
Myoclonic jerks 373
Myoglobin 275
Myopathic disorders 146
Myxedema 36f, 281, 471f
    clinical picture of 474

coma 476
    management of 477t
facies 475
management of 477
primary 474

N

Nadolol 284
Nails
    red 35
    white 35, 61f
Naltrexone 457
Naproxen 215
Naratriptan 359
Narcotic overdose 259
Nasal diphtheria 523
Nasal discharge 547
Nasogastric tube 559, 559f
Nasopharynx 530
Nausea 49, 52, 336
    causes of 53t, 144, 144t
Nebivolol 284
Nebulizers 565f, 566t
Neck
    circumference 46
    pain, anterior 478
Necrobiosis lipoidica diabeticorum 508
Neisseria
    gonorrheae 544
    meningitides 370
Nelson's syndrome 482
Neoplasia 153
Neoplasms 240
Nephritic syndrome, acute 336b
Nephritis 340
    hereditary 340
    interstitial 514
Nephrocalcinosis 448, 449
Nephrogenic diabetes insipidus 466
Nephrolithiasis 58
Nephrotic syndrome 198, 337, 337b, 338f, 339, 423, 546
    causes of 337, 337b
Nephrotoxic drugs 349
Nerves, peripheral 389
Nervous dyspepsia 147
Nervous system
    function 444
    peripheral 347
    structure of 354f
Neubauer chamber 561f
Neurocardiogenic syncope 120, 324
Neurogenic pulmonary edema 314
Neurogenic shock 325
    management of 328
Neurogenic theory 357
Neuroglycopenia 505
Neurokinin-1 145
Neuroleptic malignant syndrome 25, 26
Neurologic
    disorders 146
    medications 454
    syncope 120
Neurological disease 541
Neurology 354
Neuromuscular irritability 450, 451
Neuropathic pain 27
Neuropathy 201
    distribution of 437
Neuroprotection 363
Neurosyphilis 372, 546
    asymptomatic 372, 546
    symptomatic 372
Neurotransmitter synthesis 439
Neurovascular disease 356

Neurovascular syncope 120
Nevus araneus 59
New-onset angina 279
Niacin 433, 438
Nicardipine 270, 284, 288, 488
Nicorandil 271
Nicotinamide 439
    treatment 438
Nicotinic acid 330
Niemann-Pick disease 37
Nifedipine 270, 284
Night blindness 435
Night sweats 24, 228
Nimodipine 363
Nisoldipine 285
Nitazoxanide 540
Nitrofurantoin 351
Nitroglycerin 288
Nixon's method 73, 74f
Nocturnal angina 118
Noisy breathing 92
Nonalcoholic
    fatty liver disease 187, 189, 509
    steatohepatitis 187, 201, 456
    steatosis 187
Nonbacterial thrombotic endocarditis 309
Noncardiac pain 117
Noncardiogenic pulmonary edema 313, 314
Noncaseating granulomas 168
Nondihydropyridine calcium antagonists 270
Nonendocrine 471
Nonfluent aphasias 355
Nonfunctioning pituitary tumors 460
Nongastric diseases 160
Nongonococcal urethritis 545
    causes of 545t
Non-heme iron 384, 440
Non-Hodgkin lymphoma 181, 426, 427t
    development of 425t
    grading of 425t
    management of 427t
Nonmegaloblastic macrocytic anemia, causes of 390t
Nonnarcotic drugs 259
Nonorganic dyspepsia 147
Nonpharmaceutical agents 215
Nonpitting pedal edema 471f
Nonshockable rhythms 323
Non-ST elevation myocardial infarction 273, 278
Nonsteroidal anti-inflammatory drug 36, 57, 121, 149, 156, 160, 162, 186, 211, 281, 342, 358
Non-ST-segment elevation
    acute coronary syndrome 278
    myocardial infarction 273
Nonsulfonylureas 497
Nonthyroid diseases 467
Nontuberculous empyema 246
Nonulcer dyspepsia 147
Noonan's syndrome 43, 123
Noradrenaline 328
Norfloxacin 199
Nosocomial pneumonia 250
Nuclear cardiology 310
Nucleic acid amplification
    technology 235
    tests 230
Nutrition 432
    anthropometry 432
    disorders 217
    status 454t

O

Obesity 480f
    causes of 454, 455t
    complications of 454
    endocrine manifestations of 455, 455t
    etiology of 454
    hypoventilation syndrome 93
    mechanical complications of 455
    metabolic complications of 454
    risk factors of 454, 455t
    treatment of 456, 456t, 457f
Obliterative fibrous pleuritis 228
Obstipation 55
Obstructive jaundice 174, 175
    causes of 175f
Obstructive sleep apnea 281, 456
Occasionally cranial nerve palsies 370
Occult mitral stenosis 310
Octreotide 464
Ocular palsies 373
Oculomotor dysfunction 437
Oddi dysfunction 147
Odynophagia 55, 155, 157
    causes of 55, 155, 156b
Ofloxacin 199, 233
Oligomenorrhea 464
Oliguria 333, 336
    causes of 333, 333t
    temporary 336
Oliver's sign 99, 128
    demonstration of 101f, 129f
Olmesartan 285
Omega-3 fatty acid 330
Omeprazole 163
Oolycythemia 418b
Ophthalmic division 517
Ophthalmopathy 469
Ophthalmoplegia 437
Ophthalmoplegic migraine 356
Opiates 258, 507
    intravenous 276
Opioids 486
Oppurtunistic infections 540
Oral cavity 303, 308
Oral cavity examination 63, 93
    buccal mucosa 63
    gums 63
    lips 63
    palate 63
    pharynx 63
    teeth 63
    tongue 63
Oral contraceptives 281
Oral glucose tolerance test 462, 508
Oral mucosa 32f
    pigmentation of 63
Oral rehydration 454
    solution 454
Oral ulcers, causes of 63, 63t
Orbitopathy 468
Organic tricuspid regurgitation 302
Oropharyngeal dysphagia, causes of 55t, 155t
Oropharyngeal tuberculosis 225
Oroya fever 26
Orthopnea 89, 90, 90t, 294, 296
Osler nodes 305, 307
Osler sign 18
Osmotic
    diarrhea 151, 152, 153
    fragility 392, 395
Osteitis fibrosa cystica 346, 448
Osteoarthritis 455
Osteoarthropathy, hypertrophic 201
Osteoid matrix 440
    mineralization of 442
Osteomalacia 346, 442-444
    causes of 444t
Osteomyelitis 228, 238
Osteopenia 444f
Osteoporosis 201, 346, 442
Osteosclerosis 346
Osteosclerotic myeloma 422
Oval typhoid ulcers 525
Ovarian tumor 198
Oxcarbazepine 368, 374
Oxidants 220
Oxygen 219, 253
    concentrations of 212
    content, optimize 327
    exchange, failure of 257
    mask 564
    therapy 218
Oxymetholone 400
Oxyphil cells 478

P

P gene 177
Pacemaker leads 302
Packed cell volume 418
Packed red cells 428
Paget's disease 10
Pain 374
    abdomen 55
    acute severe 395
    behaviors 27
    biliary 147
    crampy abdominal 167
    description of 56
    diffuse abdominal 58
    duration of 374
    episodic 161
    types of 27
Painful crisis, acute 395
Palatal palsy 523
Palliative therapy 411
Pallor 28
    grading of 28
    over conjunctiva 28f
Palm
    hyperpigmentation of 30f
    pigmentation of 484f
Palmar click 301
Palmar erythema 60
Palpable heart sounds 126
Palpable splenomegaly 71f
Palpation 51, 67, 99
    breast bud 61f
    method of 99
Palpitation 114, 119
    causes of 119
    types of 119
Pamidronate 450
Pancarditis 290
Pancolitis 166
Pancreatic beta-cell destruction 489
Pancreatic exocrine insufficiency 445
Pancreatic neoplasms 147
Pancreaticobiliary disorders 55, 147
Pancreatitis 186
    chronic 147
Pancytopenia 398, 399t, 414
Pandigital clubbing 237
Pantoprazole 163
Pantothenic acid 433, 439
Papillary muscles 296
Papilledema 283, 450
Paraaminosalicylic acid 232, 233
Para-aortic lymphadenopathy 42
Paracetamol 200, 519
Paradox 12
Paradoxical split 132
Paraesophageal hernia, mixed 158
Paralysis 354
Parasternal heave, examination of 126f

Parasternal pulsation, left 125
Parathormone 442
Parathyroid
    hormone 444
    surgery 449
Parenteral iron therapy 384
Parenteral nutrition 440
Parenteral therapy 517
Parenteral thiamine 437
Paresis, localized 364
Paresthesia 450
Parietal cell antibody 388
Parkinson's disease 19, 26, 324
Parotid gland enlargement 514
Paroxysmal hypertension 18, 486, 487
Paroxysmal nocturnal
    dyspnea 89, 89f, 90, 90t, 294
    hemoglobinuria 398, 430
Pasireotide 464, 482
Patent ductus arteriosus 34, 123, 125-128, 131, 135, 139, 142
Paul-Bunnell test 514
Peakless insulin 500
Pectus carinatum 97f
Pectus excavatum 97f, 441
Pedal edema 35f, 49, 114, 120
    nonpitting type of 36f
    pitting type of 36f
Pellagra 438
Pelvic inflammatory disease 544
Penicillin
    G benzathine 293
    resistant 371
    sensitive 370, 371
    V 292, 293
Pentamidine 537
Pentavalent antimonials 537
Pentose phosphate pathway 437
Pentoxifylline 471
Peptic strictures 156
Peptic ulcer 448
    complications of 162b
    disease 159, 160
    pathogenesis of 159
Percutaneous coronary intervention 269, 271, 272, 277-277
Pericardial effusion 569f
Pericardial knock 133
Pericardial rub 134
Pericardial tamponade 328
Pericarditis 22, 118, 290
    constrictive 22, 22f, 269
    suppurative 306
Pericardium 290
Perifollicular hemorrhages 441
Perihepatitis 57
Perinatal death 547
Perindopril 285
Perineum 545
Perioral paresthesia 451
Periorbital edema 336
Periorbital puffiness 475
Peripheral blood
    film 395, 398
    smear 388f, 395f, 397f, 398f, 408, 411, 417, 514
Peristalsis
    direction of 65t
    visible 65
Peritoneum, inflammation of 197
Peritonitis, dialysis-related 58
Pernicious anemia 387, 390f, 471, 484
Persistent ductus arteriosus 320
Pertussis 524
Petechiae 441
Petroleum distillate ingestion 557

Petrosal venous sinus catheterization 482
Peutz-Jeghers syndrome 35
Peyer's patches 525
Pharyngeal diphtheria 523
Pharyngitis 336
Pharynx 336
Phenobarbitone 438
Phenothiazines 145, 316
Phenoxybenzamine 488
Phenoxymethylpenicillin 292
Phentermine 457
Phentolamine 288
Phenyl
    alkylamines 270
    butazone 200, 215
Phenytoin 146, 200, 368, 374, 438
Pheochromocytoma 281, 438, 486, 487t
Philadelphia chromosome 410, 414, 415, 415f
Phobias 347
Phosphorus 504
    plasma levels of 442
Phosphorylated derivatives 439
Phrynoderma 435
Phthinoid chest 97
Phylloquinone 432, 445
Pickwickian syndrome 93, 456
Pigeon breast deformity 443
Pigeon chest 97, 444
Pindolol 284
Pioglitazone 498
Piperacillin-tazobactam 351, 352
Pistol shot femorals 301
Pitting edema, grading of 35, 35f
Pituitary disease 467
Pituitary function 463
Pituitary gigantism 462
Pituitary gland, infarction of 461
Pituitary hormones 460, 461t
Pituitary tumor 460, 462
Plague 523
Plasma 441
    aldosterone concentration 483
    cardiac biomarkers 274
    cell 168
        dyscrasias 421
    concentration, low 505
    cortisol levels 481
    fibrinogen 409
    glucose, fasting 500
    insulin 492
    level, normal 172
    noradrenaline 487
    potassium levels 482
    protease enzyme 406
    proteins 172
    renin activity, suppressed 483
    vitamin C level 441
Plasmapheresis 474
Plasminogen activator inhibitor 455
Plasmodium
    cycle of 534
    falciparum 398
Platelet
    count, low 149
    defects, qualitative 402
    disorders 401, 401t
    function disorders, classification of 402t
    inhibition 362
    transfusion
        contraindications of 429t
        indications of 429t
Platynychia 384
Platypnea 90
Pleura 247
    lymphatic drainage of 93
    parts of 94f

Pleural biopsy 236, 243
Pleural diseases 257
Pleural effusion 228, 242
    causes of 242, 242t
    classification of 242t
    diagnosis of 245, 245fc
Pleural fluid 242t, 245
    analysis 235
    aspiration of 236
    glucose concentration 244
    parameters 244t
        interpretation of 243
    tumor markers 243
Pleural rub 110, 110t
Pleuritic chest pain 92
Pleuritic pain 237
    mild analgesics for 253
Pleurodesis, types of 249
Plummer nails 35
Plummer's disease 469
Plummer-Vinson syndrome 384
Pluripotent hematopoietic stem cell 414
Pneumococcal conjugate vaccine 255
Pneumococcal pneumonia 251, 254
    risk factors for 254
Pneumococcal polysaccharide vaccine 255
Pneumococcal sepsis 254
Pneumocystis jiroveci 240, 249, 540
    infection, treatment of 541t
Pneumonia 217, 238, 249, 250, 362
    atypical 256
    chronic eosinophilic 263
    classification of 249, 249b
    empiric regimens for 253t
    healthcare-associated 250
    hospital-acquired 250
    idiopathic acute eosinophilic 262
    interstitial 249, 513
    necrotizing 249
    noninfective 250
    nonresolving 254
    primary 249t
    suppurative 249
    ventilator associated 250
Pneumonic plague 524
Pneumonitis
    chemical 250
    radiation 250
Pneumothorax 118, 217, 246, 247, 253
    classification of 246fc
    right sided 247f
    traumatic 247
    treatment of 248
POEMS syndrome 422
Polyangiitis 335
    microscopic 335
Polycystic kidney diseases 348
Polycystic ovary syndrome 445, 455, 509
Polycythemia 200, 201, 418
    classification of 418
    primary 418
    secondary 217, 418, 420t
    vera 418-420, 420t
        complications of 419t
Polydipsia 465, 483
    primary 334, 466
Polygenic disorder 455
Polyglandular autoimmune syndrome 484, 485
Polymerase chain reaction 163, 252, 514, 543
Polymyositis 201, 275
Polyneuropathy 493, 523
Polyoma virus 350
Polyuria 334, 465, 483
    causes of 334, 334b
Polyvinylchloride 558

Index

Pontain's murmur 28, 139
Pontiac fever 26
Popliteal artery 14
    palpation of 14, 15f
Popliteal lymphadenopathy 42
Porphyria 201
    cutanea tarda 181
Portal hypertension 189, 190, 190f, 197
    classification of 190
    clinical features of 191t
    combination of 197
    complications of 191b
    obstruction of 191fc
    treatment of 192t
Portal vein thrombosis 57
Portal venous pressure, measurement of 190
Portosystemic encephalopathy 194t
Posterior circulation syndrome 362
Postherpetic neuralgia 517
Postprandial distress syndrome 148
Postprandial plasma glucose 462
Postrenal proteinuria 334
Post-streptococcal glomerulonephritis 336
Post-tuberculous bronchiectasis 230
Potassium
    balance 343
    channel activators 270
    deficit 575
    iodide, saturated solution of 472
    perchlorate 472
    supplementation 505
Pott's disease 228
Pott's spine 80
Prader's orchidometer 61f
Pramlintide 457
Prasugrel 270, 276
Prazosin 285
Preauricular lymph nodes 38f
Prednisolone 182, 292, 339, 428, 450
Prednisone 478
Preeclampsia 281
Pregabalin 374
Prerenal azotemia 504
Presyncope 120, 298, 324
Presystolic murmur 135, 294
Pretibial fever 26
Pretibial myxedema 36, 468, 471
Primaquine 397
Primidone 368
Prinzmetal angina 118, 279
Procainamide 316
Procaine penicillin 292
Proctitis 166
Proctosigmoiditis 166
Prodromal viral symptoms 478
Prolactinoma 464
Prominent pulmonary artery 569f
Pronator sign 291
Prophylactic antibiotics 192
Prophylactic anticonvulsants 364
Prophylaxis 178, 193, 184t, 199, 308
    passive 517
    regimens, post-exposure 544
Propranolol 284, 359, 471
Proprotein convertase subtilisin 330
Propyl thiouracil 472, 474
Prosopalgia 374
Prostacycline analog 287
Prostaglandin analogs 163
Prostate, enlarged 352
Prostatitis 351
Prostheticvalve endocarditis 303
Protease-antiprotease imbalance 220
Protein 244
    acute phase 435
    energy malnutrition 452
    losing pneumopathy 238
    loss
        consequences of 338t
        nature of 338
        proportion of 338
        retinol-binding 432
Proteinuria 196, 283, 334, 336, 343, 546
    classification of 334t
    glomerular 334
    orthostatic 334, 508
    overflow 334
    transient 334
    types of 334, 334t
Proteolysis 220
Proteus vulgaris 202
Proton pump inhibitors 157, 163, 164
Protozoal infections 533, 542
Protozoan *Entamoeba histolytica* 528
Provitamin A carotenoids 434
Proximal muscle, weakness of 444
Pruritus 341
Pseudoallergic reactions 554, 555b
Pseudo-Cushing's syndrome 479
Pseudocyanosis 31
Pseudohypertension 18
Pseudomonas aeruginosa 240, 249, 251, 371
Pseudoparalysis 441
Pseudo-Pelger-Hüet cells 421
Pseudosyncope, causes of 120
Pseudotumor cerebri 436
Psychiatric
    illness 147
        medications 454
        problems 347
        syncope 120
Psychoses 347
Psychosomatic disorders 119
Puddle sign 78, 79f
Pulmonary artery 123
    hypertension 134
Pulmonary bullae 222
Pulmonary capillary wedge pressure 313f
Pulmonary circulation, diseases of 325
Pulmonary cyanosis 32
Pulmonary disease 226, 456
Pulmonary edema 283, 297, 313
    causes of 313, 314t
    classification of 313
Pulmonary embolectomy 325
Pulmonary embolism 20, 118, 217, 328, 329, 362, 520
Pulmonary eosinophilia, simple 261
Pulmonary eosinophilic syndromes 261
Pulmonary fibrosis, progressive 257
Pulmonary function tests 217, 222, 238
Pulmonary hypertension 20, 222, 223, 295, 296, 320, 325
    primary 325
    symptoms of 121
    treatment of 219
Pulmonary infarction 240, 262
    clinical features of 329
Pulmonary nodule 568f
Pulmonary oligemia 569f
Pulmonary pulsations 126
Pulmonary regurgitation 137, 138
    murmur of 295
Pulmonary rehabilitation 218
Pulmonary stenosis 20, 123, 126, 132, 137, 138, 321
Pulmonary thromboembolism, recurrent 325
Pulmonary tuberculosis 224, 229, 230, 262, 235
    complications of 228t
    primary 226
    progressive 226, 227
    sequel of 230
    symptoms of 228
Pulmonary valvular
    ejection 134
    stenosis 309
Pulmonary venous pressure 309
Pulsatile liver 140
    palpation of 140f
Pulsatile swelling 99
Pulsation, systolic 140
Pulse 9, 10, 115, 141, 300
    character of 11
    deficit 10
    Doppler sonography 200
    grading of 10
    peripheral 13, 13f, 300
    pressure, normal 10
    rate 9
    wave, component of 11, 11f
    waveforms 12f
Pulsus
    alternans 11, 12, 13f
    anacroticus 11
    bigeminus 11
    bisferiens 11, 13, 301
    dicroticus 11
    paradoxus 12, 13f
    parvus et tardus 11
Pupils 185
Pyelonephritis 58
Pyrazinamide 232, 233, 438
Pyrexia of unknown origin 548, 562
Pyridoxamine 439
Pyridoxine 433, 439
Pyruvate, decarboxylation of 436

Q

Q fever 26, 249
Quaternary syphilis 546
Quinapril 285
Quincke's edema 36
Quincke's sign 301
Quinidine 200, 316
Quinine 397
Quinolone 232, 352
Q-wave infarctions 272

R

Rabeprazole 163
Rachitic
    chest 97
    rosary 443
Radial artery 271
    palpation of 9, 9f
Radioactive iodine ortechnetium, uptake of 467
Radioiodine 472
    ablation 472
Ramipril 285
Ramsay Hunt syndrome 517, 517f
Ranke complex 226
Ranolazine 270, 271
Rash 263
    complete absence of 512
Rasmussen's aneurysm 230
Reads syndrome 297
Recent nasal surgery 560
Rectal bleeding 167
Rectal temperature 23
Recti
    diastasis of 65
    divarication of 65, 65f
Red blood cell 174, 381, 385, 561, 573
    disorders of 380
    transfusion 428t

Red cell 348
   casts 336, 348
   concentrates 428
   destruction 346
   nucleated 397f
   transfusion 385
Red current-jelly sputum 256
Reed-Sternberg cells 422
Reflux
   abdominojugular 22f
   tests for 157
Refractory angina 118
Refractory ascites, treatment of 199
Refractory epilepsy, treatment of 367
Regional lymphadenitis 225, 545
Regular aerobic exercises 283
Rehydration, adequate 449
Reid index 216
Reitan's number connection test 194
Renal abnormalities 406
Renal artery bruit 66f
Renal biopsy 337, 339, 348
Renal calculi, recurrent 448
Renal complications 283, 306
Renal disease 144, 147
   active 348
Renal dysfunction 283
Renal excretion 440
Renal failure 186, 305, 311
   acute 287, 340, 344t
   index 576
   progressive 283
Renal function tests 411, 571, 574t
   progressive loss of 337
Renal hypertrophy 507
Renal ischemia 334
Renal osteodystrophy 345
Renal parenchymal disease 281
Renal pelvis 335
Renal prostaglandin synthesis 466
Renal replacement 504
Renal system 333
Renal tubular epithelial cells 341
Renal vascular insufficiency 506
Renin hypertension, normal 281
Renin-angiotensin-aldosterone system 197
Renovascular disease 286
Resectional surgery 241
Reserpine 286
Resistant hypertension 287
   treatments for 287
Resistant rickets 442
Respiration 16
   muscles of 16
   paradoxical 12
   types of 16, 16f
Respiratory acidosis 576
Respiratory alkalosis 189, 329, 576
Respiratory control, diseases of 325
Respiratory depressant drugs 258
Respiratory diphtheria 523
Respiratory disease 93, 100, 101t
Respiratory disorders 147
Respiratory distress 393
Respiratory failure 94t, 186, 217, 222, 238, 257, 258, 258t
   features of 94, 257
   perioperative 257
Respiratory infection 218
   severe acute 522
Respiratory movements 96, 101f
   examination of 101, 101f
Respiratory procedure 308
Respiratory rate 16, 93, 115
Respiratory stimulants 219

Respiratory symptoms 228, 245, 262
Respiratory syndrome coronavirus, pathogenesis of severe acute 520f
Respiratory system 3, 82, 85, 86, 91, 93, 206, 237, 247, 445
   abnormal signs in 97
   complaints 82
   examination of 82, 94
   signs of 99t
Respiratory tract 241, 303, 308
   lower 95, 99, 104, 241
Respiratory tree, components of 220
Resuscitation, cardiopulmonary 322, 322t
Reticulocyte 395
   production index 576
Retinal lesions 263
Retinal migraine 356
Retinol 432
Retinopathy 493
   diabetic 507
Retrosternal burning 161
Retrovirus 538
Reye's syndrome 186
Rheumatic aortic stenosis 298
Rheumatic carditis 291
Rheumatic chorea, management of 293
Rheumatic endocarditis 290
Rheumatic fever 293
   categories of 293t
   pathogenesis of 289f
   prevention of 293t
   signs of 122
Rheumatic heart disease 289f, 316
Rheumatic mitral stenosis 293
Rheumatoid arthritis 147, 257, 400, 471
   juvenile 37
Rhinitis 547
   allergic 206
Rhinocerebral mucormycosis 532, 532f
Rhino-orbital-cerebral mucormycosis 533
Rhizopus oryzae 532
Rhonchi 109t
   classification of 109, 109t
Rhythm 10, 323
Rib crowding 104
   examination of 104f
Riboflavin 433, 437
   pure deficiency of 438
Richter syndrome 416
Rickets 442, 443f
   features of 443f
   treatment of 443
Rickettsial diseases 531, 531t
Riedel's thyroiditis 479
Riedels lobe 70
Rifampicin 232, 233
Rifampin 233
Rifle criteria 340
Right bundle branch block 131, 132
Right ventricular
   failure 296, 310
   infarction 328
Riley-Day syndrome 19, 281
Ritonavir 200
Rituximab 400, 407, 472
   intravenous 479
Rizatriptan 359
Roger's murmur 139
Roller clamp 563
Rosai-Dorfman syndrome 37
Rose spots 525
Rosenbach's sign 301
Rose-red spots 525
Rosuvastatin 363
Roth spots 305

Rotor syndrome 176
Roux-en-Y gastric bypass 457
Rubella 490, 511, 513
   acquired 513
   virus 513
Rubella syndrome 123
   congenital 513
Rugger jersey 346
   appearance 347f
Rye's classification 422, 423t
Ryle's tube 362, 559
   position of 560
Rytand's murmur 139

S

Saddle nose deformity 547
Sahli's hemoglobinometer 561, 561f
Salicylic acid 433
Salivary cortisol, late-night 481
Salmonella 154, 393, 526, 527
   paratyphi 524, 525
   typhi 524, 525
Salt loading test, oral 483
Salt-and-pepper appearance 449
Saxagliptin 497
Scalene lymph nodes 40f
Scars 64, 98, 128
   visible 99
Schamroth's sign 34f
   demonstration of 33f
Schilling test, stages of 389f
Schistocytes, presence of 408
Schmidt syndrome 485
Sclera, unexposed 30
Sclerodactyly, diabetic 508
Scleroderma 247
Sclerosing thyroiditis 479
Sclerosis, multiple 374
Sclerotherapy 193
   complications of 193
Scoliosis 239
   acquired 96
   causes of 96, 99t
   congenital 96
Scorbutic rosary 97, 441
Scrotum 545
Scurvy
   infantile 441
   types of 440
Seborrheic dermatitis 438, 439
Second heart sound 132, 296f
   component of 300
Seizures 364, 366, 366t, 443
   absence 365
   antileptic drugs in 367t
   atonic 365
   causes of 366, 366b
   classification of 364, 364t
   complex partial 365
   febrile 366
   focal 364
   generalized 364
   myoclonic 365
   unclassified 364
   unknown onset 364
Sensitive slide test 514
Sensory 451
Sentinel headaches 363
Sepsis 339, 537, 538t
   management of 538
   risk factors for 538, 538t
   severe 537t
   syndrome 325
Septic
   embolism 307, 240

infarcts 305
shock 328, 537t
Septicemia 238, 258
Septicemic plague 523
Sequestration crisis 393, 394
Seroconversion, acute 538
Serological test 255, 291, 305, 514, 529, 547
Serotonin 145
syndrome 25
Serum
alkaline phosphatase 201, 443
ascites albumin gradient 197
aspartate transferase 475
biochemistry 348
ceruloplasmin levels 204
cholesterol 339
copper 204
cortisol 476
creatine phosphokinase 476
electrolytes 503
enzymes 170
globulins 172
immunoglobulins 238
ionized calcium 451
lactate dehydrogenase 475
osmolarity 504
periostin 210
phosphate 443
proteins 188
retinol level 435
thyroid stimulating hormone 467, 475
thyroxine, total 467
triiodothyronine, total 467
urate 348, 411
uric acid 419
vitamin B12 419
Serum albumin 172, 339
concentration 197
Serum bilirubin 170
levels 30
Serum calcium 443, 479
concentrations, correction of 448
Serum ferritin 203
levels reflect 383
Serum glutamic
oxaloacetic transaminase 574
pyruvic transaminase 574
Serum iron 203, 385
profile 203, 385t
Seven s's of innocent murmurs 138
Sexually transmitted infections 544, 544t
Sheehan's syndrome 461
treatment of 462
Shelley sign 301
Sherman sign 301
Shigella 154
produces toxin 527
Shigellosis 527
Shingles 517
Shock 258, 325
anaphylactic 327
cardiogenic 278, 327, 328, 328b
causes of 326t
extra-cardiac obstructive 328
hypovolemic 328
management of 327
stages of 325, 326t
types of 325, 326, 326fc, 327t
Shockable rhythms 323
Shone's complex 298
Short stature, cause of 43, 488t
Shoshin beriberi 436
Shoulder 322
drooping 98f
examination of drooping of 96

Shunt 199, 320
fraction 257
Sibutramine 281, 457
Sick euthyroid syndrome 477
Sick sinus syndrome 9
Sickle cell
anemia 390, 392t, 393f
crisis 395
disease 352
Sickle solubility test 394
Sickling test 394
Sick-sinus syndrome 317
Sideroblastic anemias 398
types of 399t
Sideropenic dysphagia 384
Sigmoidoscopy 528, 529
Sildenafil 269
Silicosis 225, 257
Sinus 98
venosus defects 320
X-rays 237
Sitagliptin 497
Situs inversus 237f
Sjogren's disease 37
Sjogren's syndrome 156
Skeletal abnormalities 547
Skeletal fluorosis 452
Skeletal health 472
Skeletal manifestations 448
Skin 93, 226, 303, 345
fold measurements 432
fold thickness 44, 432
lesions 290
appearance of 516
distribution of 516
over abdomen 64
prick tests 210
rashes 545
tags 508
xerosis of 435f
Skinfold
callipers, types of 45f
triceps 45, 45f
Skoda's sign 125
Skull, plain films of 463
Slit-lamp examination 204
Small bowel disorders 151
Small duct obstruction 174
Snuffles 547
Sodium
balance 343
bicarbonate 323
ferric gluconate 385
fractional excretion of 343, 576
intake 280
iopodate 474
nitroprusside 288
valproate 374
Soft tissue calcification 449
Solitary toxic adenoma 473
Somatic pain 27
Somatostatin receptor ligands 464
Somatotrope pituitary adenoma 462
Sore throat, previous history of 289
Sotos syndrome 44
Sound production 109
mechanism of 108t
Speech therapy 363
Spherocytes 395
Spherocytosis, hereditary 395, 395f
Sphingolipid biosynthesis 439
Spider angiomas 59
Spider nevi 59
demonstration of 60f
Spider telangiectasia 59

Spinal cord 389
Spine 347f
deformity of 98, 98f
examination of 96
Spino-acromion distance 103f
examination of 102
Spinocerebellar syndrome 445
Spinoscapular distance, examination of 102, 103f
Spirochete treponema pallidum 545
Spirometry 209
Spironolactone 285
Spleen 75, 75t, 76t
examination of 70
palpation 72f
percussion sign 73
surface marking of 71f
Splenectomy 395, 397, 407
Splenic enlargement 71
Splenic irradiation 421
Splenomegaly, treatment of 421
Spontaneous pneumothorax 246
secondary 247, 248
types of 247, 248f
Sputum 87, 216, 228, 236, 255, 256
culture of 230
microscopic examination of 229
tests 210
Stable angina 118, 268, 273t
management of 272fc
pectoris 268
Stable plaques 267
Staphylococcal pneumonia 255
Staphylococcus
aureus 202, 240, 249-252, 255, 304
epidermidis 303
pneumoniae 253
Starry sky appearance 428f
Starry sky pattern 428
Statin 271, 276, 363
therapy 278
Status anginosus 118
Status asthmaticus 209
Status epilepticus 368
etiology of 369
management of 369, 369t
Status migrainosus 358
Steatosis 187
ST-elevation myocardial infarction 272, 273
Stem cell therapy 430
clinical application of 430t
Stem cell transplantation 395, 400, 416
Stenosis 279
Stents, types of 271
Step-ladder fever 525
Stercobilinogen 175
Sterile pyuria 544
Sternoclavicular pulsations 127
Sternocleidomastoid muscle 16
Steroid 327, 372
contraindications of 486t
hormone 454
modulation 439
indications of 486t
therapy 486
types of 485t
Sticky sputum 87
Still's murmur 139
Stokes-Adams-Morgagni attacks 318
Stomach 159
diseases of 159
Stomatitis 438
Stone 352
Stony dullness 242
Stool
antigen test 163
microscopic examination of 529

Streptococcal
　antibody tests 291
　antigens 336, 348
　infection 291
　　primary 336
　super antigens 289
Streptococcus
　agalactiae 371
　milleri 202
　pneumoniae 217, 240, 249-251, 371
　pyogenes 240, 249
　viridans 304
Streptokinase 246, 277
Streptomycin 232, 233
Stress 281
　echocardiography 269, 310
　emotional 119
　testing 269
　ulcers 161
Strict glycemic control 507
Stridor 110
String sign 168
Stroke 283, 360
　acute 520
　　ischemic 362
　classification of 361fc
　complete 360
　hemorrhagic 361
　progressing 360
　risk factors for 361, 361t
　types of 361
Strongyloides stercoralis 147
Subarachnoid hemorrhage 282, 287, 363, 370
　clinical features of 363
　risk factors for 363t
Subclinical hyperthyroidism 471, 474, 477
　cardiac effects of 477
　causes of 477, 478b
　effects of 477
Subclinical hypothyroidism, causes of 477b
Subcutaneous emphysema, description of 104
Subcutaneous fat 47
Subcutaneous nodules 290
Subcutaneous tissue 454, 475
Subepithelial collagen, deposition of 207
Subhyaloid hemorrhage 363
Sublingual glyceryl trinitrate 268
Sublingual immunotherapy 212
Submucosal glands 207
Subtertian malaria 535
Subvalvular aortic stenosis 298
Succussion splash 67, 111
Sucralfate 163
Sucrose lysis 392
Suction catheter 560, 560f
Sudden cardiac death 318
　causes 318, 318t
Sudden infant death syndrome 224
Sulfadiazine 293, 343
Sulfamethoxazole 351, 397
Sulfisoxazole 293
Sulfonamides 200, 397
Sulfonylureas 497
Sumatriptan 359
Supraclavicular fossa 80
Supraventricular tachycardia, paroxysmal 317, 317f
Sweat electrolytes 238
Syncope 114, 120, 294, 324, 366, 366t
　causes of 324, 324b
　exertional 298
Syndrome of inappropriate secretion of antidiuretic hormone 373
Syndromic lymphadenopathy 37
Synkinesis 376

Synthetic cannabinoids 145
Syphilis 545, 547t
　acquired 545
　benign tertiary 546
　cardiovascular 546
　classification of 546t
　congenital 547, 547b
　course of 545f
　late 546
　management of 547, 547t
　primary 545
　secondary 545, 546f
Syphilitic osteochondritis 547
Syphilitic periostitis 547
Systemic anaphylactic reactions, causes of 554b
Systemic anaphylaxis 553
　clinical features of 555t
　mechanism of 554f
Systemic corticosteroids 211
Systemic diseases 335, 337
Systemic hypertension 294
Systemic immunological diseases 335
Systemic inflammatory response syndrome 537
Systemic lupus erythematosus 29, 37, 259, 267, 296, 400
Systemic mastocytosis 161
Systemic metabolic ketoacidosis 502
Systemic miliary tuberculosis 228
Systemic thromboembolism 294
Systolic click-murmur syndrome 297
Systolic collapse 22
Systolic dysfunction 309
Systolic murmurs 135, 136, 295
　configuration of 136f

T

Tabes dorsalis 373, 547
Tachyarrhythmia 315
Tachycardia 10, 251, 258, 290, 436
Tachycardiac palpitations 119
Tachypnea 16, 242, 258
Tactile fremitus 104
Tadalafil 269
Takayasu's disease 15
Tall stature 44, 489
　causes of 44, 489, 489t
Tamoxifen 187, 479
T-cell lymphotropic virus 410
Telbivudine 184
Telithromycin 253
Telmisartan 285
Temporal artery skin thermometer 23
Temporal lobe seizures 365
Tenderness 104
Tendon xanthoma 268
Tenecteplase 277
Teneligliptin 498
Tenesmus 55, 167
Tenofovir 184
Tense ascites 76, 78
Tension pneumothorax 247
Tensiontype headache 360
Terazosin 285
Terbutaline 213
Terlipressin 192
Tesofensine 457
Testicular atrophy 60
Testosterone enanthate 461
Tetany, causes of 451, 451t
Tetracycline 187, 200, 248
Tetrahydrofolate 387, 387f
　formation of 386
Tetralogy of Fallot 126, 315, 321, 321f, 569f
Thalamus, degeneration of 437

Thalassemia 390, 395, 397f
Thalassemic facies 396
Thermometers 23
Thiacetazone 232
Thiamine 432, 436
　deficiency 436, 437
　causes of 436, 436t
Thiazide diuretics 466
Thionamides 472
Thoracic dermatomes 517
Thorax, diseases of 325
Throat swab culture 291
Thrombectomy, endovascular mechanical 362
Thrombocytopenia 401, 401t, 407, 411, 536, 562
　autoimmune 399
　purpura 513
　severe 406
Thrombocytosis 403
　causes of 403t
Thromboembolic disease 361
Thromboembolism 296, 311
Thrombolysis 277
　indications for 277b
Thrombolytic agent 277, 277t
Thrombolytic therapy 277, 278b, 329
　complications of 277
Thrombosis 267, 399, 405
Thrombotic occlusion 266
Thrombotic thrombocytopenia purpura 405, 406, 514
　pathogenesis of 406f
Thunderclap 363
Thyroglobulin 467
Thyroid 475
　antibodies 478, 479
　auto antibody tests 468
　cartilage 46
　disease 467
　disorders 467
　function test 467, 476, 478, 479, 571, 574t
　gland, ultrasound of 468, 478
　hormone
　　deficiency of 474
　　synthesis 472
　lymphoma 478
　orbitopathy 469
　overactivity 468
　peroxidase antibodies 476
　radionuclide 478
　stimulating hormone 461, 473, 476, 574
　stimulating immunoglobulins 468
　storm 473
Thyroidectomy
　preparation for 472
　subtotal 472, 473
Thyroiditis 477
　autoimmune 181
　chronic autoimmune 474
　creeping 478
　goitrous autoimmune 474, 478
　subacute 477
Thyrotoxic crisis 473
Thyrotoxicosis 273, 281, 316, 468
　clinical features of 470t
　complication of 473
　eye signs of 470b
　factitia 469
　primary 467
　symptoms of 478
Thyrotropin 467
Thyrotropin-releasing hormone 462
　stimulation test 467
Tiagabine 368
Tic douloureux 374
Ticagrelor 270, 276

Tidal percussion 106, 106f
Timolol 284
Tirofiban 276
Tissue damage 274
Tobramycin 352
Tocopherol 445
Todd's paralysis 364
Tolosa-Hunt syndrome 507
Tongue
    color of 63
    dry 63
Tonsil 226
    white patch of 63
Topiramate 368
Torcetrapib 330
Torsade de Pointes 316, 316f
Torsemide 285
Touraine-Solente-Gole syndrome 34
Tourniquet test 401, 402, 405
Toxic
    gas, inhalation of 236, 259
    industrial inhalants 215
    inhalation 258
    megacolon, signs of 167
    multinodular goiter 469, 473
    reaction 320
    shock syndrome 520
    solitary adenoma 469
Toxicity
    chronic 436
    types of 436
Trachea 96, 99, 568f
Tracheal breath sounds 108
Tracheal tug 128
    sign 99
Tracingtrachea 100f
Trail's sign 96, 98f
Tramadol 507
Trandolapril 285
Transaminases 170, 411
Transcription-polymerase chain reaction 415
Transepidermal nerve stimulation 508
Transesophageal echocardiography 295, 297, 306
Transferrin 383
Transient ischemic attack 361, 282, 394
Transient neurologic symptoms 406
Transmural inflammation 168
Transplacental transmission 545
Transthoracic echocardiography 306
Trans-tubular potassium gradient 575
Traube's sign 301
Traube's space 73, 73f, 242
    obliteration of 73
    percussion of 73, 107, 107f
Trauma, severe 259
Treitz ligament 80
Tremor 373
Trephine biopsy 426
Treponema pallidum 372
Trepopnea 90
Tretinoin 435
Triamcinolone acetate 471
Triamterene 285
Tricarboxylic acid 437
Tricuspid area, auscultation of 139
Tricuspid opening snap 302
Tricuspid regurgitation 131, 137, 138, 140, 142, 302
    auscultation of 139f
    causes of 302
    functional 296, 302
Tricuspid stenosis 130, 131, 134, 138, 140, 301
    causes of 302b
Trigeminal nerve 374
Trigeminal neuralgia 374
    causes of 374

Trigger islet cell destruction 490
Triglycerides 432
Trimetazidine 270, 351
Triptans 359
Triradiate pelvis 444
Trophozoite stage 528
Tropical pulmonary eosinophilia 263
Trousseau's sign 408, 450
Trucut biopsy gun 562, 562f
Tube drainage 246
Tubercular meningitis 371
    complications of 372
Tuberculin 230
    skin test 230
    syringe 561, 561f
    test 235
Tuberculosis 37, 217, 225, 227, 234f, 234t, 247, 552
    active 231t
    chest X-ray of 229f
    endobronchial 230, 236
    extrapulmonary 233
    infection, high-risk of 231t
    intestinal 225
    postprimary 227
    primary 225
    reinfection of 229t
    secondary 227
    treatment regimen for 233t
Tuberculous
    empyema 228, 246
    foci 232, 232t
    meningitis 370
    pleural effusion 235
Tubing administration set, secondary 563
Tubular heart 222f
Tubulointerstitial proteinuria 334
Tumor 239, 352
    adrenal 482
    endobronchial 236
    necrosis factor 167, 552
Turner syndrome 43, 123
Twin beating pulse 11
Tympanic temperature 23
Typhoid 524
    complications of 525, 525b
    fever 26f, 526t
Typical chest pain 268
Tyrosine kinase inhibitors, second-generation 416
Tzanck smear 516

U

Ulcer
    aphthous 63, 168
    diabetic 508
    dyspepsia 147
    multiple 159
    recurrent 164
Ulcerative colitis 58, 166
    treatment of 167fc
Ulnar paradox 12
Ultrasound, endoscopic 162, 173
Umbilicus 80t
Umblical hernia 66f
Unstable angina 118, 272, 274, 278, 279
    management of 272
Upper gastrointestinal bleeding 51, 52, 148, 149t
    causes of 52t, 149t
Upper gastrointestinal endoscopy 190
Upper lobe 227
    pneumonia, right 255f
    right 241
Upper motor neuron 354
    disease, signs of 354, 355t
    facial palsy 376, 376t

Upper respiratory tract 157, 241
    examination 84
    infections 350
    system, examination of 94
Urea
    breath test 163
    nitrogen 574
Urease test, rapid 163
Uremia 340
Uremic toxins 345
Ureters 351
Urethra 335
Uric acid levels, measurement of 426
Urinary bladder 335
Urinary copper 204
Urinary incontinence 456
Urinary N-methylnicotinamide 439
Urinary obstruction, chronic 352
Urinary potassium loss 483
Urinary retention, acute 58
Urinary tract
    causes of 335f
    obstruction 349
Urinary tract infection 349, 350, 498
    classification of 350
    clinical spectrum of 350t
    complicated 351t
    signs of 350t
    symptoms of 350t
    uncomplicated 351t
Urine 306
    acute retention of 560
    analysis 341
    biochemistry 348
    cola-colored 336
    culture 348
    examination 238, 339, 350
    levels 439
    microscopy 348
    red 336
    tests 173
    turns dark yellow 175
    urobilinogen 173
    values, normal 575t
    volume 333
Urinometer 566, 566f
Urogenital system 3
Urokinase 277
Urticaria 551

V

Vagal activation 274
Vaginal candidiasis 508
Vagus nerve stimulation 367
Valacyclovir 516
Valley fever 26
Valproate 368, 508
Valproic acid 200
Valsartan 285
Valve
    damage 305
    holding chambers 566
    leaflets 296
Valvular aortic stenosis 298
Valvular disease 269
Valvular dysfunction 306
Valvular endocarditis 290
Valvular heart disease 293
Valvuloplasty 299
Vancomycin 308
Vanillylmandelic acid 282
Vardenafil 269
Variant angina 118, 268
Variceal banding 193

Variceal bleeding 151, 191
  acute 192
  prevention of 193, 194t
  recurrent 194
Varicella 515
Varicella-zoster
  immune globulin 517
  virus 256, 515
Varicose veins 455
Vasculitis 240, 335, 349
Vasoconstrictor therapy 192
Vasodepressor syncope 120, 324
Vasodilatation 436
Vasopressin 193, 323, 327
  antagonists 313
  stimulation test 482
Vasovagal syncope 120, 324
  classical 120, 324
Veins, direction of flow of 80f
Venesection 203
Venlafaxine mexiletine 508
Venous
  obstruction 197
  paradox 12
  stasis 455
  thrombosis 200
Ventilation
  mechanical 214
  noninvasive 214
Ventilatory defect severity, obstructive 217
Ventilatory support, mechanical 219
Ventricular septal defect 21, 123, 125-127, 131, 135, 138, 142, 320
Ventricular tachyarrhythmia 322
Ventricular tachycardia 315, 315f
  causes of 315t
  clinical features of 316t
Verapamil 146, 270, 285
Vertebra, collapse of 444
Vertigo 355
  occasional attacks of 356
Very low-density lipoprotein 455
Vessel wall, condition of 13
Vibrio cholerae 530
Vigabatrin 368
Vim Silverman liver biopsy needle 562f
Vincent's angina 118
Vincristine 263, 428
Viral encephalitis 373
Viral gastroenteritis 58
Viral hepatitis 175f, 179t
  B 179
  chronic 181
  clinical feature of 179
  etiology of 177t
  serological markers for 180t
Viral infections 511
Viral meningitis 372
Virchow node 39
Visceral
  crisis 373
  leishmaniasis 536
  pain 27
Visible mass 65
Vision
  blurring of 532
  loss of 305
  normal 434
Visual field 464
  defects 356
  examination 463
Vital examination 93
Vital signs 9
Vitals examination 9, 115

blood pressure 17
pulse 9
respiration 16
Vitamin
  A 434
    functions of 434
    micronutrient deficiencies of 452
    prophylactic 436
    supplementation 512
    toxicity 436
  A deficiency 435, 435f
    causes of 435t
  B complex 436
  B_1 432
  B_{10} 433
  B_{11} 433
  B_{12} 419, 433
    absorption, mechanism of 386f
    deficiency 354, 388
    metabolism 386
    role of 386, 387f
  B_2 433, 437
  B_3 433, 438
    deficiency 438
  B_4 433
  B_5 433, 439
  B_6 433, 439
  B_7 433
  B_8 433
  B_9 433
  C 432, 433, 440, 441
    deficiency, causes of 440
  D 432, 441
    activation of 345
    adequate consumption of 443
    analogs, synthetic 449
    dependent rickets 442
    hereditary 442
    nutritional deficiency of 443
    physiology of 442f
    receptor 442
    role of 444, 444t
    supplementation 339
  D deficiency 174
    causes of 442
  D_2 441
  D_3 441
  E 445
  K 172, 432, 445, 446
    antagonists 446
    deficiency 405
    dependent factors 446
  K_2 446
  supplements 454
  water-soluble 432, 436, 440
Vocal fremitus 84, 103
  demonstration of 104f
Voice, hoarseness of 92, 294
Volutrauma 559
Vomiting 49, 52, 144
  causes of 53t, 144, 144t
  chronic 144
von Willebrand disease 405, 429
von Willebrand factor 403
  functions of 405f
  gene 405
Voriconazole 261
Vulnerable plaque 267
Vulva 545

W

Waist circumference 46
Waist-hip ratio 46
  examination of 46f

Waldenstrom's macroglobulinemia 553
Waldeyer's ring 423
Warfarin 278
Warning signs 476
Water
  deprivation test 465, 466f
  retention 345
Water-borne infection 178
Waterhouse-Friderichsen syndrome 370, 408, 485, 486
Watson's water hammer pulse 301
Weakness 221, 354
Wegener's granulomatosis 95, 257, 337
Weight gain, causes of 454, 455t
Weight loss 147, 221
  causes of 147, 147b
  severe 222
  types of 147
Weil's syndrome 531
Weingarten syndrome 263
Wells scoring system 329
Wernicke's
  aphasia 355
  disease 26, 437
  encephalopathy 437
Westergren tube 566, 566f
Westergren-Katz tube 566
Wheeze 82, 109t
  classification of 109, 109t
Whipple's triad 505
Whispering pectoriloquy 110
White blood cell 153
White cells 348
White coat hypertension 18, 281
Whooping cough 524
Wide pulse pressure, signs of 301t
Wilkins score 295
William's syndrome 123, 298
Wilson's disease 63, 171, 172, 203, 293, 562
Wimberger ring sign 441, 441f
Winter bronchitis 294
Winter cough 216
Winterbottom sign 40
Wolff-Chaikoff effect 469
Wolff-Parkinson-White syndrome 317
Wuchereria bancrofti 263

X

Xanthelasma 268
Xanthomatoses 508
Xanthurenic acid excretion 439
Xerophthalmia 435
Xerosis 435

Y

Yersenia
  enterocolitica 469
  pestis 523

Z

Zidovudine 187, 200
Ziehl-Neelsen stain 225
Zieves syndrome 62
Zinc acetate 204
Zoledronic acid 450
Zollinger-Ellison syndrome 159
Zolmitriptan 359
Zonisamide 368
Zoonotic disease 178
Zoster immune globulin 517
Zoster sine herpete 517

EU GSPR Authorised Reprsentative
Logos Europe, 9 rue Nicolas Poussin
1700, La Rochelle, France
Phone: +33 (0) 6 67 93 73 78
E-mail: contact@logoseurope.eu